ATLAS OF
PEDIATRIC PHYSICAL
DIAGNOSIS
SECOND EDITION

ATLAS OF
PEDIATRIC PHYSICAL
DIAGNOSIS
SECOND EDITION

Edited by

Basil J. Zitelli, M.D.
Associate Professor of Pediatrics
University of Pittsburgh
School of Medicine
University Pediatric Diagnostic Referral Service
Children's Hospital of Pittsburgh

Holly W. Davis, M.D.
Associate Professor of Pediatrics
University of Pittsburgh
School of Medicine
Medical Director
Emergency Department
Children's Hospital of Pittsburgh

Foreword by
Frank A. Oski, M.D.
Given Professor of Pediatrics
The Johns Hopkins University
School of Medicine
Baltimore

Ⅿ WOLFE

Library of Congress Cataloging-in-Publication Data
Atlas of pediatric physical diagnosis / edited by Basis J. Zitelli,
    Holly W. Davis; foreword by Frank A. Oski. - 2nd ed.
        p.cm.
    Includes bibliographical references and index.
    ISBN 0-397-44618-7
    1. Children-Diseases-Diagnosis. 2. Physical diagnosis.
1. Zitelli, Basil J. (Basil John), 1946- . II. Davis, Holly W., 1945-
[DNLM: 1. Diagnosis-in infancy & childhood-atlases. 2. Physical Examination-in infancy and
childhood-atlases. WS17 A881]
RJ50.A86 1991
618.92'00754-dc20
DNLM/DLC   91-19571
for Library of Congress   CIP

British Library Cataloging-in-Publication Data
Atlas of pediatric physical diagnosis. - 2nd edn.
    1. Zitelli, Basil J. II. Davis, Holly W.
    618.9200754

ISBN 0-397-44618-7

Editor:	Dimitry Popow
Art Director:	Jill Feltham
Designer:	Jeffrey S. Brown
Illustrators:	Wendy Jackelow
	Alan Landau (1st ed)
	Laura Pardi (1st ed)

10 9 8 7 6 5 4 3

Printed in Singapore by Imago Productions (FE) PTE Ltd.

Reprinted in Singapore 1992, 1993

© Copyright 1992 Gower Medical Publishing. Reprinted in 1993 by Wolfe Publishing, an
imprint of Mosby-Year Book Europe Limited.

ISBN: 0-397-44618-7

For full details of all Mosby-Year Book Europe Limited titles, please write to
Mosby-Year Book Europe Limited, Lynton House, 7-12 Tavistock Square,
London WC1H 9LB, England.

FOREWORD

Sir William Osler once wrote, "There is no more difficult art to acquire than the art of observation." Doctors Basil Zitelli and Holly Davis have done a great deal of observing and recording to assist you in acquiring the skills necessary to become a better than average clinician.

The more you see, the more you will know. Although there is no true substitute for experience, the superb collection of photographs and drawings in the *Atlas of Pediatric Physical Diagnosis* is the next best thing to being there.

Spending the time with more than 1,400 figures will result in your heightened capacity to make a prompt and correct diagnosis. Look, read, and enjoy, secure in your knowledge that you are learning some valuable pediatric lessons.

Frank A. Oski, M.D.
Given Professor of Pediatrics
The Johns Hopkins University
School of Medicine

To our parents, who were our first teachers

Hannah L. Zitelli and Patsy A. Zitelli
Ruth Holmes Davis and William S. Davis

To my wife Suzanne and my children
Matthew, Daniel, Benjamin, and Anne Zitelli
and to
Betty Due Reilly Sullivan, Sue Evans Hughes,
and
Mary Newton McKendry Van Horn Thompson

To those exceptional teachers we have had, whose dedication,
enthusiasm and creativity helped make the acquisition, application
and sharing of knowledge more fun than hard work, and who
inspired us not only to perform to the best of our ability, but also to
become teachers as well as physicians

John Altrocchi, Ph.D., Morton Bogdanoff, M.D.,
Arthur Ferguson, Ph.D., Henry Furrie, Paul C. Gaffney, M.D.,
Arthur Glaeser, Robert Kudra, Hans Lowenbach, M.D.,
Lois A. Pounds, M.D., Francis G. Reilly, M.D.,
Elizabeth Robenheimer,Elizabeth Seipel, Estelle Tankard, Doris
Turner, Catherine M. Wilfert, M.D.,
William H. Zinkham, M.D., J.R. Zuberbuhler, M.D.

To our residents and students, whose eagerness to learn and to put
their knowledge to use keeps us learning actively and makes teaching
so rewarding

PREFACE
TO THE SECOND EDITION

For many disorders, visual recognition is a major factor in making the correct diagnosis. Thus, the experienced clinician who has seen the spectra of different disorders has a distinct advantage.

This book was developed for students, residents, nurses, and practitioners who care for children to aid them in the diagnosis of pediatric disorders by way of rapid visual examination or review of simple laboratory tests. Our goal is to broaden the visual experience of the clinician.

The enthusiastic response to the first edition led us to believe that a second edition was not only possible but necessary. Every chapter has been reviewed, revised, and updated. New information and diagnostic techniques have been included. Additional contributors have provided greater depth and dimension to the *Atlas*, and created new chapters in pediatric urology and pulmonary disorders. Our book is by no means encyclopedic, but rather presents an overview of problems that lend themselves to visual diagnosis. The accompanying text deliberately emphasizes pertinent historical factors, visual findings, techniques of examination, and diagnostic methods rather than therapy. We have attempted to select disorders that are common and/or important, and where relevant, to describe the spectrum of clinical findings. It is our hope that this *Atlas* will continue to serve as a useful and practical reference for anyone who cares for children.

Basil J. Zitelli, M.D.
Holly W. Davis, M.D.

ACKNOWLEDGEMENTS

The *Atlas* is the product of the unstinting efforts of many dedicated people. The authors devoted much time, effort, and expertise, and gathered photographs largely from their patient populations and clinical material at Children's Hospital of Pittsburgh. Most of these were taken and produced by our Medical Media Department. Douglas Sellers, Norman Rabinovitz, Norman Snyder, Russell Weleski, Laura Dugan, William Winstein, Jr., and Kathleen Muffie, aided by Eric Jablonowski and Suzanne Mikesell, deserve credit for being at our beck and call.

Cynthia Vogt, coordinator of the Neuroradiology teaching file; Bernadette Marshalek and Sandra Williams, coordinators of the Radiology teaching files; along with Georgette Babbit, Theresa Buffo, Jeanette Ference, Tracy Fisher, Bruce Gyms, Jodie Henrickson, Linda Jacobs, William Thomas, and Christine Tuttle of the Radiology file room deserve high praise for scouring their files to find the numerous radiographs, CT, MRI, and bone scans we needed.

Nancy Dunn and Dolores Blumstein of the Blaxter Medical Library at Children's Hospital of Pittsburgh were most helpful in locating and double-checking the many references we used.

We thank the staff at Gower Medical Publishing who have logged countless hours in the process of design, layout, and production of the final product.

Darlene Chiponis and Joy Harris in proofreading the first edition.

Special acknowledgment is due to David Kazimer for his tireless work on nearly half of the new manuscripts for the second edition and for his care and talent in helping design many of the new tables, to Helen Shorner for her comparable work on the first edition, and to Susan Gelnett who made major secretarial contributions to both editions. Further, we must acknowledge the assistance provided by all the other secretaries who prepared manuscripts for individual authors.

We would also like to express our gratitude to numerous colleagues around the country who generously shared clinical photographs and radiographs with us, and to the many patients and families who graciously allowed us to include their pictures.

Finally, we would like to thank the many thousands of people who have found the first edition of the *Atlas* so useful for their praise, support, and suggestions. We hope their thoughts and our labors have resulted in an improved text that will be of help to all who care for children.

CONTENTS

CONTRIBUTORS   xi

1 GENETICS: COMMON CHROMOSOMAL DISORDERS
Mark W. Steele
General Principles	1.1
Abnormalities of Autosomes	1.7
Abnormalities of Sex Chromosomes	1.11
Molecular Cytogenetic Syndromes	1.13
Other Imprinting Syndromes	1.16
Chromosomal-Like Syndromes	1.18
Prenatal Diagnosis	1.22

2 NEONATOLOGY
Michael J. Balsan, Ian R. Holzman
General Physical Examination Techniques	2.1
The Placenta	2.7
Birth Trauma	2.9
Congenital Anomalies	2.12
Primitive Reflexes	2.15
Respiratory Distress	2.15
Newborn Stools	2.18

3 DEVELOPMENTAL-BEHAVIORAL PEDIATRICS
Heidi Feldman, Roberta E. Bauer
Gross Motor Development	3.1
Fine Motor Development	3.7
Cognitive Development	3.10
Language Development	3.13
Social Development	3.16
Variations in Developmental Patterns	3.18
Cerebral Palsy	3.19
Mental Retardation	3.22
Specific Language and Reading Disorders	3.24
Visual Impairment	3.28

4 PEDIATRIC ALLERGY AND IMMUNOLOGY
David P. Skoner, Andrew H. Urbach, Philip Fireman
Immunological Hypersensitivity Disorders	4.1
Immunological Deficiency Disorders	4.19
Abnormal Function of the Immune System: Suspicion and Evaluation	4.20
Phagocytic Disorders	4.30
Complement System Disorders	4.31
Mucosal Barrier Disorders	4.32
Diagnostic Techniques	4.32

5 PEDIATRIC CARDIOLOGY
F. Jay Fricker, Sang C. Park, Cora C. Lenox
Physical Diagnosis of Congenital Heart Disease	5.1
Cyanosis and Clubbing	5.1
Syndrome-Associated Physical Findings	5.3
Signs of Bacterial Endocarditis	5.7
Laboratory Aids in the Diagnosis of Congenital Heart Disease	5.7

6 CHILD ABUSE AND NEGLECT
Holly W. Davis, Mary Carrasco
Epidemiology	6.1
Physical Abuse	6.2
Sexual Abuse	6.18
Examination Techniques	6.19
Physical Findings	6.22
Specimen Collection	6.24
Passive Abuse or Neglect	6.27
Emotional Abuse	6.28

7 PEDIATRIC RHEUMATOLOGY
Andrew H. Urbach
Juvenile Rheumatoid Arthritis	7.1
Dermatomyositis	7.5
Systemic Vasculitis	7.7
Scleroderma	7.13
Systemic Lupus Erythematosus	7.16

8 PEDIATRIC DERMATOLOGY
Bernard A. Cohen, Holly W. Davis, Susan B. Mallory, John A. Zitelli
Papulosquamous Disorders	8.3

Vesiculopustular Disorders	8.17
The Reactive Erythemas	8.19
Bites, Stings and Infestations	8.23
Acne	8.27
Tumors and Infiltrations	8.28
Neonatal Dermatology	8.32
Hemangiomas	8.35
Nevi and Melanomas	8.38
Disorders of Pigmentation	8.41
Disorders of Hair and Nails	8.43
Complications of Topical Skin Therapy	8.47

9 PEDIATRIC ENDOCRINOLOGY
David Finegold

The Anterior Pituitary Gland	9.1
Normal Growth	9.3
Specific Hormonal Imbalances	9.6
Sexual Maturation	9.14
Insulin-Dependent Diseases	9.20

10 PEDIATRIC NUTRITION AND GASTROENTEROLOGY
J. Carlton Gartner Jr.

Nutrition	10.1
Anthropometric Measurements and Laboratory Tests	10.3
Gastroenterology	10.8
Vomiting	10.9
Diarrhea	10.11
Chronic Liver Disease	10.14

11 PEDIATRIC HEMATOLOGY AND ONCOLOGY
J. Malatack, Julie Blatt, Lila Penchansky

Hematology	11.1
Anemias Due to Decreased Red Cell Production	11.3
The Hemolytic Anemias	11.10
Bleeding Disorders	11.22
Oncology	11.26
Cancer in Children	11.26
Laboratory Aids to Diagnosis	11.34

12 PEDIATRIC INFECTIOUS DISEASE
Holly W. Davis, Raymond B. Karasic

Infectious Exanthems	12.1
Mumps (Epidemic Parotitis)	12.16
Bacterial Skin and Soft-Tissue Infections	12.18
Infectious Lymphadenitis	12.26
Bacterial Bone and Joint Infections	12.35
Congenital and Perinatal Infections	12.43

13 NEPHROLOGY
Demetrius Ellis

Glomerular Disorders	13.1
Hematuria	13.3
Vesicoureteral Reflux	13.7
Developmental/Hereditary Disorders	13.9
Renovascular Hypertension	13.18
Chronic Renal Failure	13.19

14 PEDIATRIC UROLOGIC DISORDERS
Mark F. Bellinger

Prenatal Urinary Tract Dilation	14.1
Cryptorchidism in the Neonate	14.2
Hydronephrosis	14.3
Cutaneous Urinary Diversion	14.5
Exstrophic Anomalies	14.6
Anomalies of the Male Genitalia	14.9
Lesions of the Female Genitalia	14.15
Ambiguous Genitalia	14.17

15 PEDIATRIC NEUROLOGY
Henry B. Wessel

Neurocutaneous Syndromes	15.1
Central Nervous System Malformations	15.7
Increased Intracranial Pressure	15.13
Facial Weakness	15.17
Neuromuscular Disorders	15.18
The Hypotonic Infant	15.22

16 PEDIATRIC PULMONARY DISORDERS
Blake E. Noyes, David M. Orenstein

Cough	16.1
Stridor	16.9

Wheezing	16.11
Cystic Fibrosis	16.12
Apnea and Sudden Infant Death Syndrome	16.15
Diagnostic Techniques	16.16

17 PEDIATRIC SURGERY

Don K. Nakayama

Respiratory Distress	17.1
Vomiting	17.7
Gastrointestinal Bleeding	17.14
Abdominal Pain	17.18
Abdominal Masses	17.20
Head and Neck	17.25
Chest Wall	17.29
Abdominal Wall	17.30
Anus	17.35

18 PEDIATRIC AND ADOLESCENT GYNECOLOGY

Pamela Murray, Holly W. Davis, Melissa Hamp

Normal Female Genitalia	18.1
Gynecologic Evaluation	18.3
Genital Tract Obstruction	18.9
Genital Trauma	18.11
Nontraumatic Vulvovaginal Disorders	18.13
Pregnancy	18.30

19 PEDIATRIC OPHTHALMOLOGY

Kenneth P. Cheng, Albert W. Biglan, David A. Hiles

Anatomy of the Visual System	19.1
Evaluation of Vision	19.3
Refractive Errors	19.4
Strabismus	19.6
Amblyopia	19.13
Diseases of the Eyes and Surrounding Structures	19.14
Retina	19.28
Ocular Trauma	19.37

20 ORAL DISORDERS

M.M. Nazif, Holly Davis, D.H. McKibben, Mary Ann Ready

Normal Oral Structure	20.1
Normal Mixed Dentition	20.3
Natal and Neonatal Abnormalities	20.5
Developmental Abnormalities	20.6
Discoloration	20.10
Caries	20.12
Infections	20.12
Trauma	20.16

21 ORTHOPEDICS

Timothy Ward, Holly W. Davis, Edward N. Hanley Jr.

Development of the Skeletal System	21.1
Musculoskeletal Trauma	21.3
Disorders of the Spine	21.24
Disorders of the Upper Extremity	21.30
Disorders of the Lower Extremity	21.33
Generalized Musculoskeletal Disorders	21.46

22 PEDIATRIC OTOLARYNGOLOGY

Timothy P. McBride, Holly W. Davis, James S. Reilly

Ear Disorders	22.1
Nasal Disorders	22.14
Disorders of the Paranasal Sinuses	22.22
Oropharyngeal Disorders	22.30
Upper Airway Obstruction	22.37

CONTRIBUTORS

Michael Balsan, M.D.
Assistant Professor of Pediatrics, Obstetrics and Gynecology
University of Pittsburgh, School of Medicine
Magee-Women's Hospital
Children's Hospital of Pittsburgh

Roberta E. Bauer, M.D.
Director, Division of Developmental Pediatrics
Akron Children's Hospital Medical Center
Assistant Professor of Pediatrics
Northeastern Ohio University College of Medicine
Akron, Ohio

Mark F. Bellinger, M.D.
Associate Professor of Surgery/Division of Urology
University of Pittsburgh, School of Medicine
Chief, Pediatric Urology
Children's Hospital of Pittsburgh

Albert Biglan, M.D.
Adjunct Associate Professor of Ophthalmology
University of Pittsburgh, School of Medicine

Julie Blatt, M.D.
Associate Professor of Pediatrics
University of Pittsburgh, School of Medicine
Division of Pediatric Hematology, Oncology
Children's Hospital of Pittsburgh

Mary M. Carrasco, M.D.
Assistant Professor of Pediatrics
University of Pittsburgh, School of Medicine
Director, Family Intervention Center
Children's Hospital of Pittsburgh

Kenneth Cheng, M.D.
Clinical Instructor of Ophthalmology
University of Pittsburgh, School of Medicine

Bernard A. Cohen, M.D.
Assistant Professor of Dermatology and Pediatrics
Director, Pediatric Dermatology
Children's Hospital of Pittsburgh

Holly W. Davis, M.D.
Associate Professor of Pediatrics
University of Pittsburgh, School of Medicine
Medical Director, Emergency Department
Children's Hospital of Pittsburgh

Demetrius Ellis, M.D.
Professor of Pediatrics
University of Pittsburgh, School of Medicine
Director, Pediatric Nephrology
Children's Hospital of Pittsburgh

Heidi M. Feldman, M.D., Ph.D.
Associate Professor of Pediatrics
University of Pittsburgh, School of Medicine
Division of Child Development
Children's Hospital of Pittsburgh

David N. Finegold, M.D.
Associate Professor of Pediatrics
University of Pittsburgh, School of Medicine
Division of Pediatric Endocrinology
Children's Hospital of Pittsburgh

Philip Fireman, M.D.
Professor of Pediatrics
University of Pittsburgh, School of Medicine
Director, Allergy, Immunology, and
  Rheumatology
Children's Hospital of Pittsburgh

Frederick J. Fricker, M.D.
Associate Professor of Pediatrics
University of Pittsburgh, School of Medicine
Division of Pediatric Cardiology
Children's Hospital of Pittsburgh

J. Carlton Gartner, Jr., M.D.
Professor of Pediatrics
University of Pittsburgh, School of Medicine
Director, University Pediatric Diagnostic
  Referral Service
Children's Hospital of Pittsburgh

Melissa Hamp, M.D.
Assistant Professor of Pediatrics
Michigan State University, College of Human
  Medicine
Director of Adolescent Medicine

Director of Combined Internal Medicine–Pediatric
Residency Program
Hurley Medical Center
Flint, Michigan

Edward N. Hanley, Jr., M.D.
Chairman, Department of Orthopedic Surgery
Carolinas Medical Center
Charlotte, North Carolina

David A. Hiles, M.D.
Clinical Professor of Ophthalmology
Chief, Division of Pediatric Ophthalmology
Department of Ophthalmology
University of Pittsburgh, School of Medicine
Director, Pediatric Ophthalmology
Children's Hospital of Pittsburgh

Ian R. Holzman, M.D.
Professor of Pediatrics
Chief, Division of Newborn Medicine
Mount Sinai Medical Center
New York, New York

Raymond B. Karasic, M.D.
Associate Professor of Pediatrics
University of Pittsburgh, School of Medicine
Divisions of Pediatric Emergency Medicine and
Pediatric Infectious Diseases
Children's Hospital of Pittsburgh

Cora C. Lenox, M.D.
Professor Emeritus of Pediatrics
University of Pittsburgh, School of Medicine
Division of Pediatric Cardiology
Emeritus Staff
Children's Hospital of Pittsburgh

J. Jeffrey Malatack, M.D.
Associate Professor of Pediatrics
University of Pittsburgh, School of Medicine
University Pediatric Diagnostic Referral Service
Children's Hospital of Pittsburgh

Timothy P. McBride, M.D.
Assistant Professor of Otolaryngology
Georgetown University School of Medicine

Director of Pediatric Otolaryngology
Georgetown University Medical Center

David H. McKibben, D.M.D.
Clinical Assistant Professor of Pediatric
  Dentistry
University of Pittsburgh, School of Medicine
Assistant Director, Dental Services
Children's Hospital of Pittsburgh

Susan B. Mallory, M.D.
Associate Professor of Internal
  Medicine (Dermatology) and
  Dermatology in Pediatrics
Washington University School of Medicine
Director, Pediatric Dermatology
St. Louis Children's Hospital

Pamela J. Murray, M.D., M.H.P.
Assistant Professor of Pediatrics
University of Pittsburgh, School of Medicine
Director, Adolescent Medicine
Children's Hospital of Pittsburgh

Don K. Nakayama, M.D.
Associate Professor of Pediatric Surgery
University of Pittsburgh, School of Medicine
Director, Benedum Pediatric Trauma Program
Children's Hospital of Pittsburgh

Mamoun M. Nazif, D.D.S., M.D.S.
Professor of Pediatric Dentistry
University of Pittsburgh, School of Medicine
Director, Dental Services
Children's Hospital of Pittsburgh

Blake E. Noyes, M.D.
Research Instructor in Pediatrics
University of Pittsburgh, School of Medicine
Co-Director of Cystic Fibrosis Center
Children's Hospital of Pittsburgh

David M. Orenstein, M.D.
Associate Professor of Pediatrics
University of Pittsburgh, School of Medicine
Associate Professor of Instruction and Learning
(Exercise Physiology)

University of Pittsburgh, School of Education
Director, Cystic Fibrosis Center
Director, Pediatric Pulmonology
Children's Hospital of Pittsburgh

Sang C. Park, M.D.
Professor of Pediatrics
University of Pittsburgh, School of Medicine
Division of Pediatric Cardiology
Children's Hospital of Pittsburgh

Lila Penchansky, M.D.
Associate Professor of Pathology
University of Pittsburgh, School of Medicine

Mary Ann Ready, D.M.D.
Public Health Pediatric Dentist
U.S. Public Health Service
Indian Hospital
Crowe Agency, Montana

James S. Reilly, M.D.
Professor, Department of Surgery
Division of Otorhinolaryngology
University of Alabama at Birmingham
Otorhinolaryngologist in Chief
Children's Hospital of Alabama

David P. Skoner, M.D.
Associate Professor of Pediatrics
University of Pittsburgh, School of Medicine
Division of Allergy, Immunology and
Rheumatology
Children's Hospital of Pittsburgh

Mark W. Steele, M.D.
Associate Professor of Pediatrics and Human
  Genetics
University of Pittsburgh, Schools of
  Medicine and Public Health
Clinical Geneticist
Children's Hospital of Pittsburgh

Andrew H. Urbach, M.D.
Associate Professor of Pediatrics
University of Pittsburgh, School of Medicine
University Pediatric Diagnostic Referral Service
Children's Hospital of Pittsburgh

W. Timothy Ward, M.D.
Assistant Professor of Orthopedic Surgery
University of Pittsburgh, School of Medicine
Division of Pediatric Orthopedic Surgery
Associate Director Benedum Pediatric Trauma
Program
Children's Hospital of Pittsburgh

Henry B. Wessel, M.D.
Associate Professor of Pediatrics and Neurology
University of Pittsburgh, School of Medicine
Division of Child Neurology
Director EMG Lab and MDA Clinic
Children's Hospital of Pittsburgh

John A. Zitelli, M.D.
Pittsburgh, Pennsylvania

GENETICS: COMMON CHROMOSOMAL DISORDERS

Mark W. Steele, M.D.

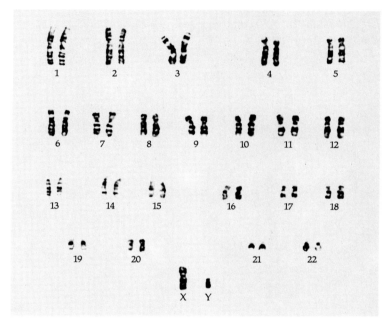

FIG. 1.1 Photomicrographs show that this is a G-banded male kary-otype (a female would have two X chromosomes and no Y chromosome). The horizontal banding produced by the Giemsa staining technique allows for precise identification of homologous chromosomes.

GENERAL PRINCIPLES

The Nature of Chromosomes

The human hereditary factors are located in the genes (the genome): 10 percent (about 100,000) structural genes that code for proteins (such as enzymes), and the other 90 percent whose functions are not clear. The genes are composed of deoxyribonucleic acid (DNA) and are stored in intranuclear cell organelles called chromosomes. Each chromosome contains one linear DNA molecule folded over onto itself several times, as well as ribonucleic acid (RNA) and proteins. Since all genes exist in pairs, all chromosomes must likewise exist in pairs. The members of each pair of genes are called alleles; and of each pair of chromosomes, homologues. The conventional depiction of the constitution of homologues in the nucleus is called the cell's karyotype (Fig. 1.1). If, at any gene locus, the alleles are identical, that gene locus is said to be homozygous. If the alleles are not identical, the gene locus is heterozygous.

Except for gametes, normal human cells contain 23 pairs of chromosomes, 46 in all. One of these pairs is concerned, in part, with inducing the primary sex of the embryonic gonads. These sex chromosomes are called the X and Y chromosomes, and they are not genetically homologous except in a few areas. Females have two X chromosomes while males have an X and a Y chromosome. The remaining 22 pairs are called autosomes and determine non-sex-related (somatic) characteristics.

During most of a cell's life cycle, chromosomes are diffusely spread throughout the nucleus and cannot be morphologically identified. Only when the cell divides does chromosome morphology become apparent (Fig. 1.2). The in vitro life cycle and the cellular division, or mitosis, of a somatic cell are illustrated

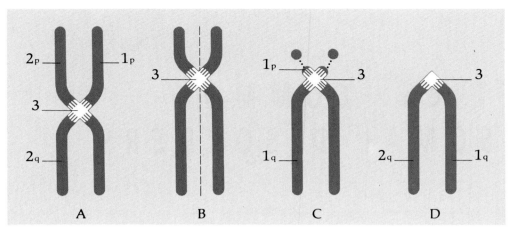

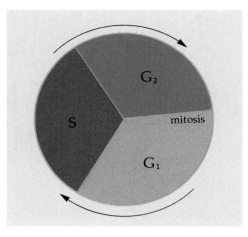

FIG. 1.2 Morphology of a chromosome during metaphase. **A,** metacentric chromosome with centromere (3) in middle. **B,** submetacentric chromosome with centromere off center. **C,** acrocentric chromosome with centromere near one end. **D,** telocentric chromosome (not found in humans) with centromere at one end. The DNA of the chromosome has replicated to form two chromatids: 1p and 1q represent one complete chromatid, 2p and 2q the other complete chromatid. The chromosome will then divide longitudinally, as shown in **B.**

FIG. 1.3 The in vitro life cycle of a somatic cell. The interphase lasts 21 hours and can be divided into three stages: G_1 (7 hours)—cell performs its tasks; S (7 hours)—DNA replicates; G_2 (7 hours)—cell prepares to divide (mitosis).

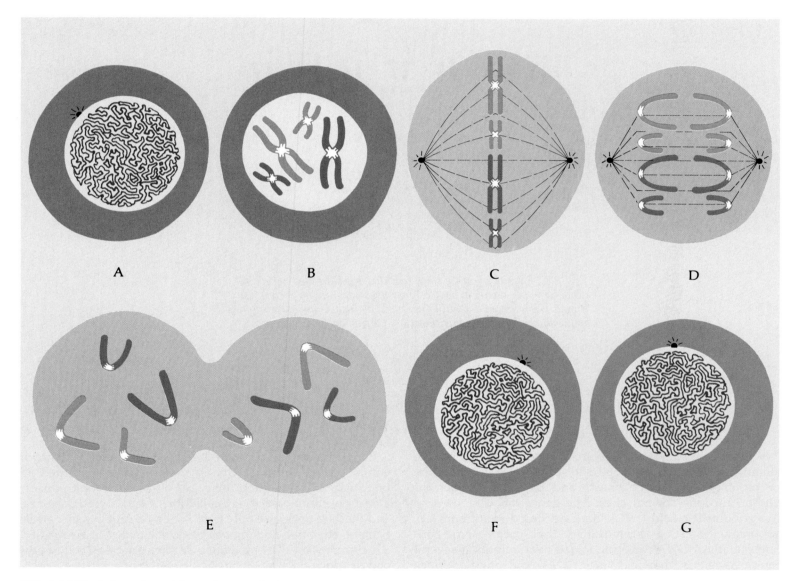

FIG. 1.4 Mitosis lasts about 1 hour, during which time the cell divides. **A,** interphase cell at end of G_2. **B,** prophase—replicated DNA condenses and is visible. **C,** metaphase—46 duplicated chromosomes align randomly on spindle and can be photographed for karyotyping. **D,** anaphase—chromosomes divide longitudinally, and half of each one moves to the opposite poles of the cell. **E,** telophase—cell wall divides. **F,** and **G,** interphase at G_1—two daughter cells each with 46 chromosomes.

GENETICS: COMMON CHROMOSOMAL DISORDERS

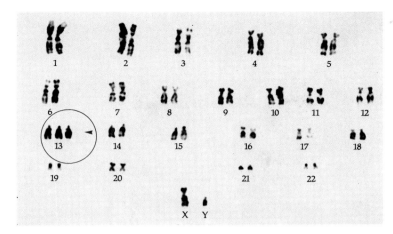

FIG. 1.5 Karyotype of a patient with trisomy 13 demonstrates aneuploidy. Note the extra chromosome 13, causing the cell to have 47 instead of 46 chromosomes.

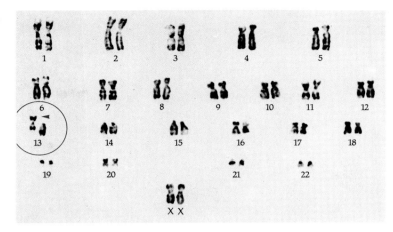

FIG. 1.6 Pericentric inversion (arrow) of chromosome 13.

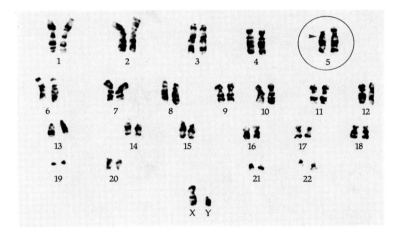
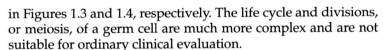

FIG. 1.7 Deletion (arrow) of the p arm of chromosome 5 (cri du chat syndrome).

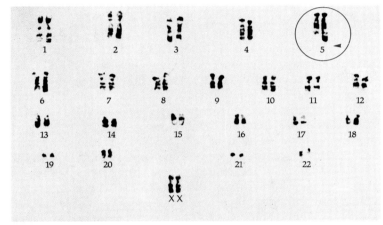

FIG. 1.8 Unbalanced translocation. The additional DNA was translocated onto the q arm of chromosome 5. The abnormality was inherited from a normal carrier father (Fig. 1.9) with a balanced reciprocal translocation between the q arms of chromosome 3 and chromosome 5. The patient died of multiple birth defects, and in essence had a partial trisomy of the distal portion of the q arm of chromosome 3.

in Figures 1.3 and 1.4, respectively. The life cycle and divisions, or meiosis, of a germ cell are much more complex and are not suitable for ordinary clinical evaluation.

Any somatic cell that can divide in tissue culture can be used for chromosomal (cytogenetic) analyses. The most convenient tissue source is peripheral blood from which lymphocytes can be stimulated to divide during 2 or 3 days' incubation in tissue culture media. After death, lung tissue is best to culture for chromosomal analyses, although the process requires a 4- to 6-week incubation period. When a treatment decision requires urgency, preliminary chromosomal evaluation can be made within 4 to 24 hours using uncultured bone marrow aspirate.

An abnormality in chromosome number less than an even multiple of 23 (the haploid number) is called aneuploidy (Fig. 1.5). Usually, aneuploidy is 45 or 47 chromosomes; rarely, multiples of the X or Y chromosome will result in individuals with 48 or 49 chromosomes. If aneuploidy occurs in a gamete as a result of a chromosomal division error (nondisjunction or anaphase lag) during meiosis, all cells will be affected in the fertilized embryo. Subsequently, the parents' recurrent risk for another chromosomally abnormal offspring is increased to

approximately 1 to 2 percent. The reason for this increased risk is obscure, but such couples should seek prenatal diagnostic counseling. About half of such abnormal offspring will have a chromosomal abnormality different from that of the proband.

If the one-celled embryo (zygote) is chromosomally normal and aneuploidy occurs after fertilization in an embryonic somatic cell because of a division error during mitosis, only one or two lines of embryonic cells will be affected. The remaining embryonic cells will be chromosomally normal. This mixed chromosomal state is called mosaicism, and cannot have been inherited since it occurred after conception. However, with a mosaic child, the parents' recurrent risk may still be increased over that of the general population (to 1 to 2 percent as above) since the zygote may have been aneuploid to start with. In the latter case, the chromosomally normal cell line resulted from a division error during somatic cell mitosis.

Chromosomes can be normal in number (diploid), but still be abnormal in structure. Inversions (Fig. 1.6), deletions (Fig. 1.7), and translocations (Fig. 1.8) are examples of structural chromosomal abnormalities. These abnormalities can arise as new (sporadic) mutations in the egg or sperm from which the embryo was formed, in which case the parents' recurrent risk

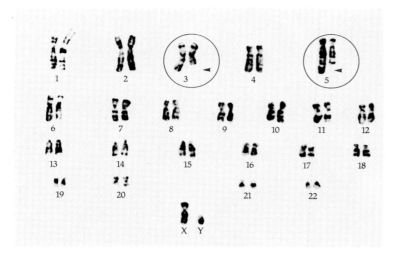

FIG. 1.9 A "balanced" reciprocal translocation of chromosomes 3 and 5 in a normal male (the father of the defective newborn in Fig. 1.8).

for another chromosomally abnormal offspring is again 1 to 2 percent. However, the abnormality may also be inherited from a phenotypically normal carrier parent (Fig. 1.9).

About 1 in 350 normal individuals carries a balanced, structurally abnormal set of chromosomes. "Balanced" here means that the structural abnormality does not appear on cytogenetic analysis to have resulted in any net loss or gain of genetic material. If the balanced chromosomal abnormality runs in the family (i.e., is inherited from a parent), the carrier is usually phenotypically normal. However, if the carrier state resulted from a new mutation, there is a sixfold increased risk that the carrier will have some degree of mental retardation (albeit, most such carriers are still phenotypically normal).

Incidence of Chromosomal Abnormalities

At least 25 percent and perhaps as many as 40 percent of all pregnancies terminate in spontaneous abortion. Most such abortions are so early in gestation that pregnancy is not recognized. The earlier the abortion, the more probable that the fetus had a chromosomal abnormality. Of first trimester abortuses, 62 percent are chromosomally abnormal, compared to 5 percent of later abortuses. On the average, 50 percent of all spontaneous abortuses are chromosomally abnormal, with triploidy (69 chromosomes), trisomy 16, and 45XO being by far the most common findings (Fig. 1.10). While the former two are not found among liveborns, 45XO is relatively common and results in Turner syndrome. Nevertheless, 98 percent of embryos with Turner syndrome abort. Since most chromosomally abnormal embryos abort spontaneously, it is not surprising that the incidence of chromosomal abnormalities among liveborns in general is only about 6 in 1,000, or that it is about 50 in 1,000 among stillborns and other perinatal deaths.

When to Suspect a Chromosomal Abnormality

Chromosomal abnormalities, either in number or structure, are likely to have a detrimental effect on the phenotype. Aneuploidy of an autosome either is lethal or interferes significantly with physical and mental development. However, aneuploidy

INCIDENCE OF CHROMOSOMAL ABNORMALITIES*	
Among Spontaneous Abortuses	**%**
1st trimester	62
After 1st trimester	5
Type of Abnormality	
Trisomy 16	8
Other trisomies	18
Triploidy	8
45XO	9
Miscellaneous	7
Overall incidence	50
Among Liveborns	**per 1000**
Abnormality of autosomes	4.0
Trisomies	1.4
Balanced rearrangements	2.0
Unbalanced rearrangements	0.6
Abnormality of sex chromosomes	2.2
In males (XXY, XYY, mosaics)	3.0
In females	1.4
45XO	0.1
XXX, mosaics	1.3
Overall incidence	6.2

*About one-quarter of all conceptuses are chromosomally abnormal. About 50 in 1000 stillborns have a chromosomal abnormality.

FIG. 1.10

of an X or Y chromosome may have little effect on the phenotype. Aneuploidy is not an entirely random event, and familial clustering is well known.

Carriers of an inherited, reciprocal translocation are usually genetically balanced and are subsequently normal. Carriers of a *de novo* reciprocal translocation, however, may not be entirely genetically balanced since the incidence of mental retardation in such individuals is about six times greater than that in the general population. In either case, conceptions are likely to be genetically unbalanced, and may abort spontaneously or be born with major congenital anomalies. A history of unexplained infertility, multiple spontaneous abortions (three or more), and particularly the prior birth of a defective baby to the couple or to a close relative should make one suspect that one of the parents carries a balanced chromosomal translocation. A chromosome study on the couple is thus indicated, and if translocation is found, they should seek prenatal diagnostic counseling.

A normal person who carries a balanced reciprocal translocation can produce six chromosomal types of gamete. On fertilization, these would result in either a normal conceptus, a carrier conceptus like the normal carrier person, two types of immediately lethal conceptus due to gross chromosomal imbalances (that is, too much and/or too little DNA), and two types of abnormal conceptus due to lesser chromosomal imbalances. Whether or not the latter two will abort spontaneously or come to term as defective liveborns cannot be predicted in advance solely on theoretical grounds. Therefore, genetic coun-

GENETICS: COMMON CHROMOSOMAL DISORDERS

EXAMPLES OF CONGENITAL ANOMALIES*

Category	Minor	Major
Craniofacial	Bony occipital spur Flat occiput Slight micrognathia (3)	Choanal atresia Severe scaphocephaly Cleft lip and/or palate (1.5)
Eye	Inner epicanthal folds (4) Short palpebral fissures	Coloboma of iris Cataract
Auricle	Sinus Skin tags (2)	Severely malformed Rudimentary
Skin	Raised hemangioma Cafe au lait spots	Multiple hemangiomas Posterior webbed neck
Hand	Simian crease (20) Duplication of thumbnail Rudimentary polydactyly Clinodactyly of the fifth digit (10)	Polydactyly Absence of thumbs Complete cutaneous syndactyly Absence of all metacarpals
Foot	Partial syndactyly of second and third toes (2) Recessed fifth toes	Absence of nails Equinovarus
Other skeletal regions	Shieldlike chest Cubitus valgus	Short thoracic cage Absence of radius
Miscellaneous	Diatasis recti (>3 cm) Ectopic femoral testes	Neural tube defects Severe hypospadias

*Except as noted in parentheses, the incidence of each is 1 in 1000 liveborns.

FIG. 1.11

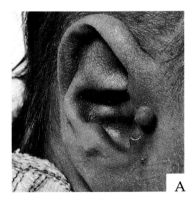
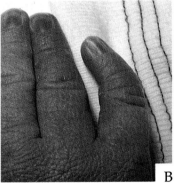
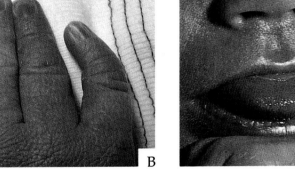
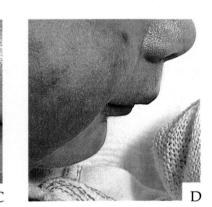

A B C D

FIG. 1.12 Clinical photographs show several minor anomalies seen at birth. **A,** preauricular skin tag. **B,** clinodactyly of the fifth finger. **C,** macroglossia. **D,** micrognathia. (Courtesy of Dr. Christine L. Williams, New York Medical College)

seling in such situations simply must depend on knowledge of what has happened before in similar situations.

Past experience suggests the following: if a carrier has already produced a chromosomally defective liveborn, one knows that such defective fetuses can come to term. Consequently, that carrier's recurrent risk for another defective liveborn is about 20 percent. However, if a carrier has only produced spontaneous abortions, it is less likely that such defective fetuses can come to term. Consequently, that person's risk for producing a chromosomally defective liveborn is only about 4 percent. Finally, if a couple of whom one spouse is a carrier has not yet experienced any pregnancies, their risk for a chromosomally defective liveborn is estimated to be about 10 percent. The sex of the carrier parent does not affect these risks.

Physical anomalies at birth are categorized as minor or major types (Figs. 1.11, 1.12, and 1.13). Minor anomalies, such as epicanthal folds (in Caucasians), simian creases, and raised hemangiomas, are of little physiologic significance, and each one occurs in less than 4 percent of the population. In contrast, major anomalies, such as coloboma of the iris (see Chapter 19), polydactyly, and multiple hemangiomas, have a greater adverse effect on the individual.

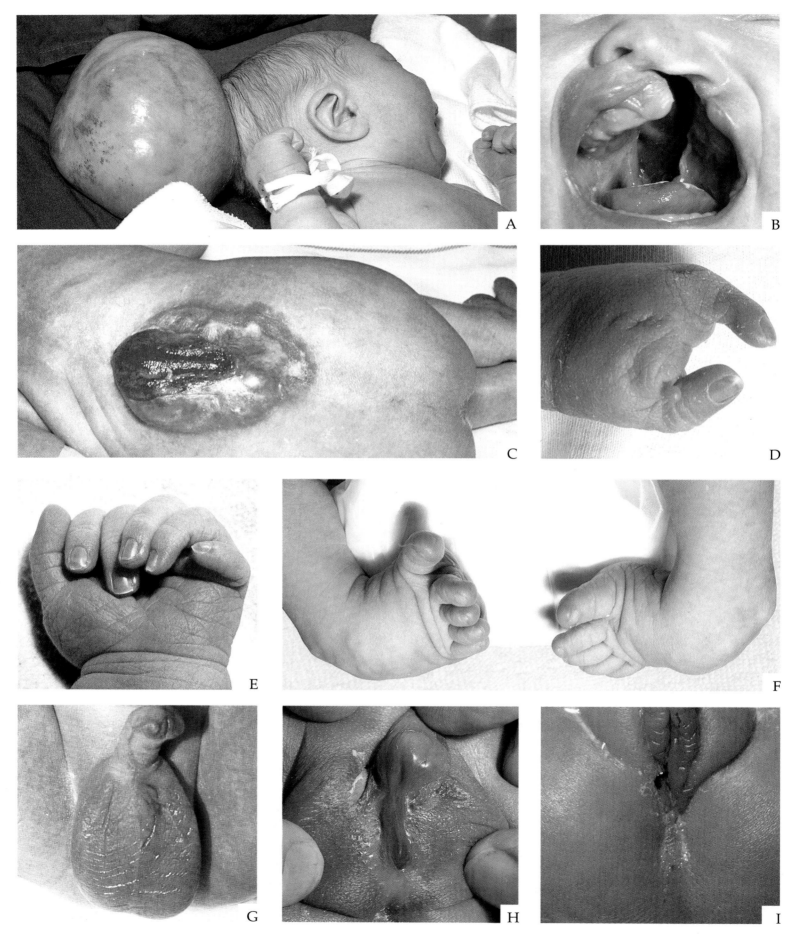

FIG. 1.13 Clinical photographs show several major anomalies seen at birth. **A,** encephalocele. **B,** cleft lip and palate. **C,** meningomyelocele. **D,** lobster-claw hand. **E,** polydactyly (postaxial). **F,** bilateral clubfoot. **G,** hypospadias. **H,** fused labia with enlarged clitoris. **I,** imperforate anus. (Courtesy of Dr. Christine L. Williams, New York Medical College)

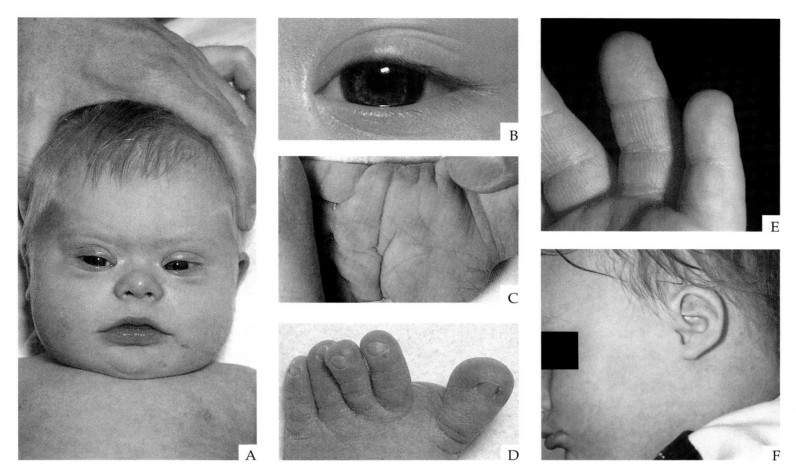

FIG. 1.14 Clinical photographs show several minor anomalies associated with Down syndrome. **A,** typical facies (note epicanthal folds). **B,** Brushfield spots. **C,** simian crease. **D,** wide space between first and second toes. **E,** short fifth finger. **F,** small ears.

Among 7,000 newborn infants surveyed, 45 percent had one or more minor anomalies; 9 percent had three or more. Many of these minor anomalies represent the effects of multifactorial inheritance, i.e., they are simply familial. About 1.5 percent of newborns have at least one major anomaly, and this incidence is severalfold greater among prematures. Infants with a single major anomaly (e.g., congenital heart disease, polydactyly, cleft lip) do not present an increased incidence of minor anomalies and usually represent multifactorial or simple mendelian inheritance. In contrast, infants with two or more major anomalies usually show an increased incidence of minor anomalies and often represent a specific syndrome of congenital anomalies. Most such syndromes, particularly when there are two or more primary defects in morphogenesis, represent the effects of simple mendelian inheritance; a few represent the effect of environmental teratogens on the fetus in utero (e.g., rubella, maternal alcohol ingestion, antiepileptic medication). About 10 percent of these syndromes represent the effect of unique or known chromosomal abnormalities, with translocations illustrating the former and aneuploidies such as trisomy 21 (Down syndrome) or 45XO (Turner syndrome) characteristic of the latter.

ABNORMALITIES OF AUTOSOMES
Down Syndrome

The worldwide incidence of Down syndrome among liveborns is 1 in 700, with 45 percent of affected individuals being born to women over 35 years of age. In the United States, the incidence is somewhat lower: about 1 in 1,100 liveborns and only 20 percent born to women over age 35. This difference represents the effect of elective infertility among older U.S. women, and, to a lesser extent, the impact of prenatal diagnosis leading to selective abortion of Down syndrome fetuses. The incidence of Down syndrome among conceptuses is three times greater than among liveborns, but about two-thirds of Down syndrome fetuses spontaneously abort.

There is no single physical stigma of Down syndrome; rather, the clinical diagnosis rests on a gestalt of many minor and a few major anomalies. Although any one of the minor anomalies may be found in a normal person, it is the constellation of several anomalies in one individual that characterizes Down syndrome (Fig. 1.14). These minor anomalies include brachycephaly, inner epicanthal folds, upward slanting eyes, Brushfield spots, small ears, a small upturned nose with sad-

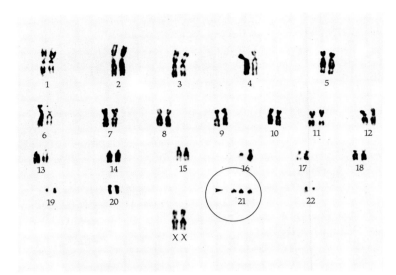

FIG. 1.15 Karyotype of a Down syndrome patient indicates trisomy 21.

FIG. 1.16

RISK OF DOWN SYNDROME IN LIVEBORNS (BY MATERNAL AGE)	
Age (years)	Risk Factor
<25	1 in 1600
25–29	1 in 1100
30–34	1 in 700
35–39	1 in 250
40–42	1 in 80
>42	1 in 40

Note: Risk for any chromosomal abnormality in liveborns: maternal age <35 years—1 in 400; 35 to 40 years—1 in 100; >40 years—1 in 50.

dle bridge, a small mouth with protruding tongue which fissures with age, a short neck with redundant skin-folds, simian crease(s), clinodactyly of the fifth finger(s) with single digital crease due to hypoplasia of the middle phalanx, and a wide space between first and second toes. The number of such anomalies varies in any particular case.

Other features of Down syndrome are infection-prone dry skin; relatively short stature; rapid aging with premature graying of hair; hypotonia during infancy; wide, flat iliac wings; and a narrow acetabular angle on radiographs. Adult males have reduced libido and are usually impotent (or perhaps sterile). Adult females may have normal libido and are fertile; about one-third of their liveborns may have Down syndrome, the rest should be normal. In both sexes, puberty is delayed.

Several major anomalies are commonly associated with Down syndrome. Congenital heart disease is found in 45 percent of cases, particularly atrioventricular communis and ventricular septal defects. About 7 percent have a gastrointestinal anomaly, most often duodenal atresia. There is also an increased incidence of thyroid disorders (particularly of the autoimmune type) in Down syndrome individuals, their mothers, and their close relatives. Individuals with Down syndrome should have their thyroid function checked annually by blood T_4 and TSH_6 testing. Acute and neonatal leukemia occur 15 times more frequently than in the general population. In newborn infants, much of this is represented by transient leukemoid reactions (with complete remission likely) rather than true leukemia. Quantitative abnormalities are found in many enzyme systems. However, the most consistent major anomaly is mental retardation.

With rare exceptions, Down syndrome individuals are mentally retarded. The degree of retardation varies, with intelligence quotients (IQs) ranging from 20 to 80, and is significantly related to the environment in which the Down syndrome child is raised. A warm, accepting, stimulating home upbringing with early special education maximizes the child's intellectual potential. With such an upbringing, over 95 percent are highly trainable to educable retardates who, as adults, should be capable of a semi-independent existence within the parents' home or in a sheltered workshop. This is facilitated by the fact that their social quotients (SQs) are relatively higher than their IQs. Additionally, mosaic Down syndrome individuals tend to be somewhat brighter than their nonmosaic counterparts, given a comparably positive rearing. There may even be a slight positive correlation between parental IQ and that of their Down syndrome child, but whether this reflects genetic or environmental influences is not known. With rare exceptions, institutionalization is contraindicated, since it has been found to have an extremely negative effect on the patients' mental development.

The apparent decline in both IQ and SQ with age in Down syndrome individuals may be largely an artifact of testing, particularly in children younger than 12 years. Most Down syndrome children should be tested between the ages of 6 and 8 years for the best estimate of their intellectual potential. Given proper rearing, most Down syndrome children will have an IQ between 45 and 55, though rare cases are known with IQ scores between 60 and 85. Autopsy analyses of brains from Down syndrome persons revealed the neuropathologic changes of Alzheimer's disease in 1.6 percent of 20- to 38-year-old individuals and in 100 percent of those older than 40 years. In the 42- to 69-year-old group, the Alzheimer pathologic findings were considered severe in 60 percent of the cases. Nevertheless, only about 25 percent of older individuals with Down syndrome exhibit clinical manifestations of Alzheimer's disease. The reason for the clinical–pathologic discordance is not known. The life span of Down syndrome individuals is less than that of the general population.

The etiology of Down syndrome is trisomy 21 (Fig. 1.15). In 94 percent of cases, this is a consequence of meiotic nondisjunction. The extra chromosome 21 is maternally derived in 95 percent of instances, paternally derived in 5 percent. Aneuploidy in offspring increases with maternal but not paternal age. Consequently, a couple's risk of having a liveborn child with Down syndrome is directly correlated with maternal age (Fig. 1.16). However, once a couple has had a trisomy 21 child, their recurrent risk for a child with some chromosomal abnormality (Down syndrome in half of the cases) is 1 to 2 percent at any maternal age.

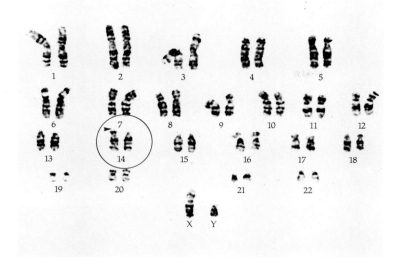

FIG. 1.17 *Karyotype of a Down syndrome patient shows 14/21 centric fusion translocation.*

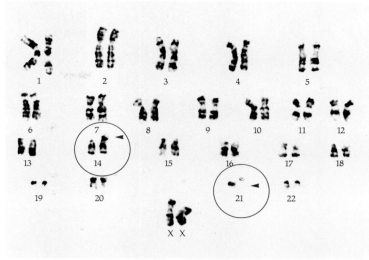

FIG. 1.18 *Karyotype of a normal female 14/21 centric fusion translocation carrier (the mother of the Down syndrome patient in Fig. 1.17).*

About 2 percent of Down syndrome cases are chromosomal mosaics with a mixture of normal and trisomy 21 cells. Although mosaicism represents a chromosomal division error occurring after conception, recurrent risk for the couple is still 1 to 2 percent, since 80 percent of mosaics represent trisomy 21 zygotes.

About 4 percent of Down syndrome cases represent a centric fusion translocation between the long arm of a chromosome 21 and those of either a 14, 15, 13 (Fig. 1.17) or a 21, 22 acrocentric chromosome. Of these, about one third are inherited from a clinically normal, balanced carrier (Fig. 1.18); the remainder are sporadic. Chromosome studies should therefore be performed on the parents and siblings of a translocation Down syndrome individual. If a parent carries a 21/21 translocation, all liveborns will have Down syndrome; for the remaining 21/centric fusion translocations, the empiric recurrent risk for a Down syndrome liveborn is 2 percent if the father is the carrier and 10 percent if the mother is the carrier. In United States, Canada, and other highly industrialized Western nations, 20 percent of Down syndrome individuals die by age 5 years (most from congenital heart disease), 55 percent by age 60 years and 86 percent by age 68 years. The improved longevity in Down syndrome means that a significant proportion of affected individuals will survive both their parents. Consequently, contingency care plans for the Down syndrome child should be made early.

Trisomy 13 and 18

Trisomy 13 and 18 are relatively rare chromosomal abnormalities, the incidence being about 1 in 8,000 liveborns for trisomy 18 and 1 in 20,000 for trisomy 13. About 95 percent of trisomy 18 fetuses abort early, while trisomy 13 fetuses rarely abort spontaneously. The major physical features of each abnormality are listed in Figure 1.19, and illustrated in Figures 1.20 and 1.21. There is often much overlap in physical findings between the two syndromes, making it occasionally difficult to distinguish one from the other solely on the basis of clinical evaluation. Both syndromes result in severe mental retardation and usually lead to death within 1 year. Therefore, heroic attempts at medi-

PHYSICAL ABNORMALITIES IN TRISOMY 13 AND 18 SYNDROMES*

Abnormality	Trisomy 13	Trisomy 18
Severe developmental retardation	††††	††††
>90% dead within 1st year	††††	††††
Cryptorchidism in males	††††	††††
Low-set, malformed ears	††††	††††
Multiple major congenital anomalies	††††	††††
Prominent occiput	†	††††
Cleft lip and/or palate	†††	†
Micrognathia	††	†††
Microphthalmos	†††	††
Coloboma of iris	†††	†
Short sternum	†	†††
Rocker-bottom feet	††	†††
Congenital heart disease	††	††††
Scalp defects (of skin)	†††	†
Flexion deformities of fingers	††	††††
Polydactyly	†††	†
Hypoplasia of nails	††	†††
Hypertonia in infancy	†	†††
Apneic spells in infancy	†††	†
Midline brain defects	†††	†
Persistence of Hgb F	††††	†
Horseshoe kidney	†	†††

Relative frequency: ††††, usual; † rare.

FIG. 1.19

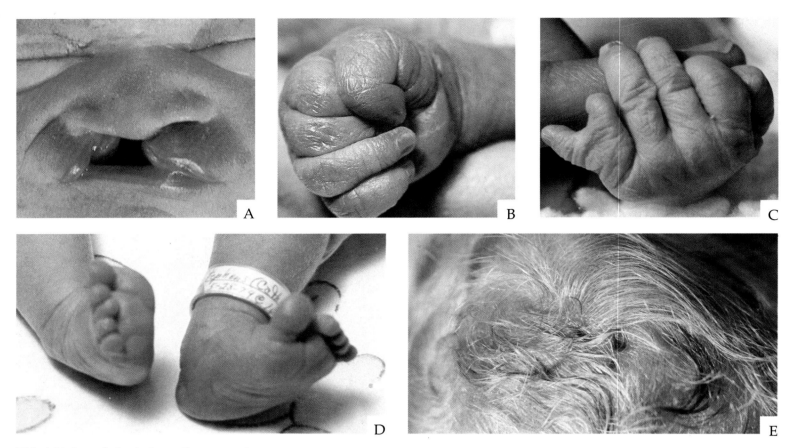

FIG. 1.20 *Several physical manifestations of trisomy 13.* ***A,*** *facies showing midline defect.* ***B,*** *clenched hand with overlapping fingers.* ***C,*** *preaxial polydactyly.* ***D,*** *equinovarus deformity.* ***E,*** *typical punched-out posterior scalp lesions. (****A,*** *courtesy of Dr. T. Kelly, University of Virginia Medical Center, Charlottesville.* ***B–E,*** *courtesy of Dr. Kenneth Garver, West Penn Hospital, Pittsburgh)*

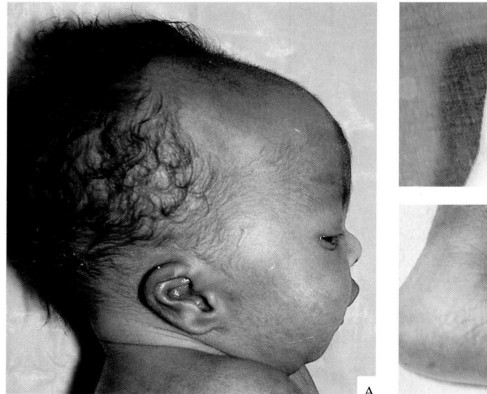

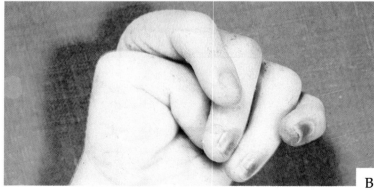

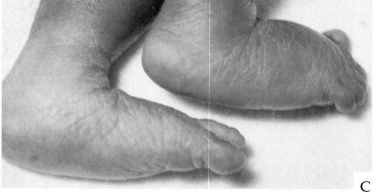

FIG. 1.21 *Several physical manifestations of trisomy 18.* ***A,*** *typical profile reveals prominent occiput and low-set, posteriorly rotated malformed auricles.* ***B,*** *clenched hand showing typical pattern of overlapping fingers.* ***C,*** *rocker-bottom feet. (****A,*** *courtesy of Dr. Kenneth Garver, West Penn Hospital, Pittsburgh)*

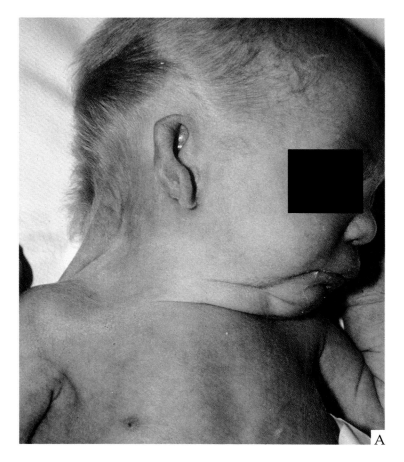

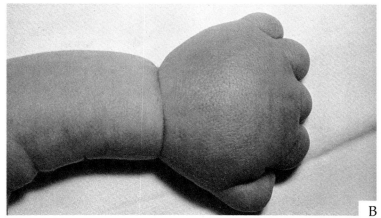

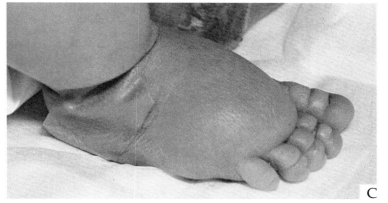

FIG. 1.22 Clinical photographs show several physical manifestations associated with Turner syndrome. **A,** web neck, widespread nipples, abnormal ears, and micrognathia. **B,** and **C,** lymphedema of hands and feet.

cal intervention should not be encouraged. With improved general health care, rare cases of survival for 10 to 30 years have been reported (although with significant developmental delay). Chromosomal mosaicism may allow a somewhat better prognosis, particularly for trisomy 18. A relatively normal albeit mildly retarded 20-year-old female with diploid/trisomy 18 chromosomal mosaicism has been reported.

As in Down syndrome, meiotic nondisjunction is the mechanism for the chromosome error in most cases of trisomy 13 and 18, with risk increasing with maternal age. Occasionally, cases result from centric fusion translocations (spontaneous or inherited) or postconception mosaicism. The recurrence risk for another chromosomally abnormal liveborn is 1 to 2 percent at any maternal age (but higher when resulting from an inherited translocation); prenatal diagnosis of fetal chromosomal abnormalities is recommended with subsequent pregnancies.

About 20 percent of liveborns with the physical features of trisomy 13 are chromosomally normal, probably resulting from single-gene-dominant mutations, or, less often, recessive inheritance. Less common are chromosomally normal liveborns with the physical features of trisomy 18. Such instances may constitute variants of Smith-Lemli-Opitz syndrome (autosomal-recessive trait) or may be the result of maternal ingestion of methotrexate early in pregnancy. The occasional infant who has survived methotrexate embryopathy has had normal intelligence. However, the prognosis for these other chromosomally normal mimics of trisomy 13 or 18 is little better than that for the other two. Unfortunately, the negative prognosis is often resisted by parents, physicians, and other health care providers, resulting in fruitless medical-surgical interventions

with subsequent frustration and bitterness by all involved. Early frank discussions of the realities may be painful, but in the long run may be better for all concerned.

ABNORMALITIES OF SEX CHROMOSOMES
Turner Syndrome

This is one of the three most common chromosomal abnormalities found in early spontaneous abortions; in fact, only 2 percent of affected fetuses are ever born. The phenotype is female. Primary amenorrhea, sterility, sparse pubic-axillary hair, underdeveloped breasts, and short stature (4.5 to 5 feet) are the usual manifestations. These women have an infantile uterus, and their ovaries are only strands of fibrous connective tissue. Other physical features may include webbing of the neck, cubitus valgus, a low hairline, shield chest, and coarctation of the aorta (in 20 percent of cases) (Fig. 1.22). Newborns often have lymphedema of the feet and/or hands which can reappear briefly during adolescence. Mental development is usually normal. However, average full-scale IQ is somewhat lower than that of the general population, the deficit reflecting a decrease in performance rather than verbal IQ. Schooling and behavioral problems seem to be the same as in age-matched controls. Difficulties with spatial orientation, such as map reading, may be a problem. The classic physical findings of Turner syndrome may be absent or so minimal in the newborn period that the diagnosis is missed. The first indication may be unexplained short stature in later childhood and/or failure of

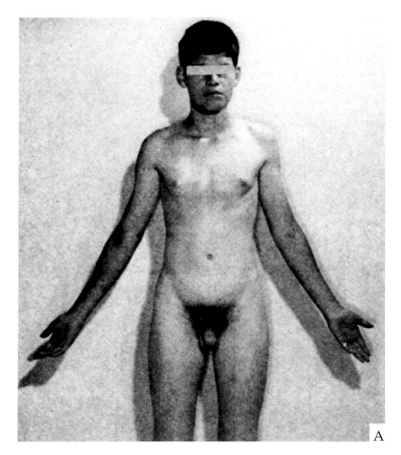

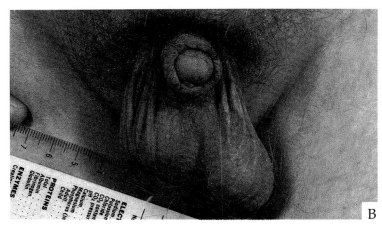

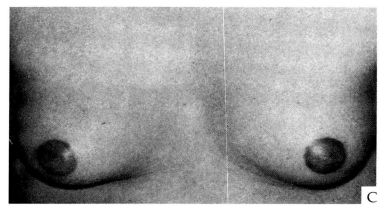

FIG. 1.23 Clinical photographs show several physical manifestations of Klinefelter syndrome. **A,** eunuchoid body habitus, relatively narrow shoulders, increased carrying angle of arms, female distribution of pubic hair, normal penis, small scrotum due to small size of testes. **B,** small testes and penis. **C,** gynecomastia. (**B,** courtesy of Dr. Peter Lee, University of Pittsburgh School of Medicine **C,** reproduced by permission from Gardner LI (ed): Endocrine and Genetic Diseases of Childhood, ed. 2. Philadelphia, WB Saunders, 1975)

the secondary sex characteristics to develop by late adolescence. Thus, a chromosome study is indicated as part of the diagnostic workup of adolescent girls with either or both of these complaints.

The chromosome error in 60 percent of individuals with Turner syndrome is 45XO. Most often, the missing sex chromosome is paternally derived, so the risk of Turner syndrome does not increase with parental age. Another 15 percent of individuals with Turner syndrome are mosaics (XO/XX, XO/XX/XXX, or XO/XY). The physical stigma may be less marked in mosaics, some of whom may be fertile. If an XY cell line is present, the intraabdominal gonads should be removed since they are prone to malignant change. The remaining cases of Turner syndrome have 46 chromosomes, including one normal plus one structurally abnormal X. The latter may have a short (p) arm deletion or may be an isochrome duplication of the long (q) arm of the X chromosome; usually it is paternally derived.

While loss of the short arm of an X chromosome results in full-blown Turner syndrome, deletion of the long arm usually produces only streak (fibrous) gonads with consequent sterility, amenorrhea, and infantile secondary sex characteristics. A buccal smear for sex chromatin is a poor diagnostic test for Turner syndrome since mosaics, partial deletions, and isochromes can be sex chromatin-positive. If the diagnosis is clinically suspected, a G-banded chromosome study should be ordered. Should the affected child be 45XO or a mosaic, the parental recurrent risk for a chromosomally abnormal liveborn

is 1 to 2 percent, but may be higher if a parent carries a structurally abnormal X chromosome.

Prenatal diagnosis of chromosomally abnormal fetuses should be discussed with the parents, and the *relatively* good prognosis for Turner syndrome liveborns should not be overlooked. Girls with Turner syndrome should receive appropriate hormone therapy during adolescence to develop their secondary sex characteristics and stimulate menses. Although hormonal efforts to promote growth have not yet been very successful, newer therapeutic approaches hold promise for the future.

A chromosomally normal phenotypic mimic of Turner syndrome is Noonan syndrome (see Chapter 5, Cardiology). This autosomal-dominant trait occurs in 1 of 1,000 liveborns and affects both sexes. Microcephaly, pulmonary stenosis, and normal stature are more common than in Turner syndrome; unfortunately, about half of affected individuals are mildly to moderately mentally retarded. Noonan females menstruate and are fertile, but males are usually sterile. Most cases represent fresh mutations, and the empiric recurrent risk without a family history is 10 percent.

Klinefelter Syndrome

About 20 percent of aspermic adult males have Klinefelter syndrome, as do 1 in 250 males over 6 feet tall. The physical stigmata usually are not obvious until puberty, at which time the normal onset of spermatogenesis is blocked by the pres-

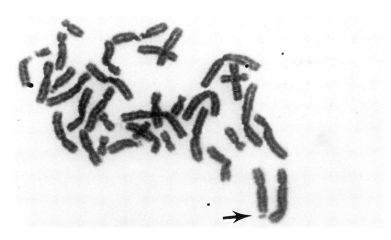

FIG. 1.24 *Fragile X chromosome marker in lymphocyte culture. Partial metaphase plate shows the chromosome break at Xq27* arrow *characteristic of fragile X syndrome (solid Giemsa stain).*

ence of two X chromosomes. Consequently, the germ cells die, the seminiferous tubules become hyalinized and scarred, and the testes become small. Testosterone levels are below the normal adult male level, though the level varies from case to case (the average is about half normal). This then leads to a wide range of virilization in these cases. At one extreme is the eunuchoid male with a small penis and gynecomastia (Fig. 1.23); at the opposite extreme is the virile mesomorph with a normal penis. Scoliosis may develop during adolescence. Libido may be reduced in adult males, virtually all of whom are sterile. Libido may be improved by testosterone therapy, but whether this reflects a pharmacologic or a psychologic effect is not clear. Homosexuality is not more common with Klinefelter syndrome than in the general population. The average full-scale IQ of men with Klinefelter syndrome is 98, which is about the same as the general population. There is a mild decrease in verbal (but not performance) IQ which might account for the increased incidence of school difficulties. However, behavioral problems are no more common than in the population at large.

Testosterone treatment should begin at about 11 or 12 years of age if in vivo levels do not result in virilization. Such treatment will also prevent gynecomastia, which occurs in 40 percent of cases. Once gynecomastia occurs, it can only be corrected by surgery.

The karyotype in Klinefelter syndrome is XXY in 80 percent of cases and mosaic (XY/XXY) in the other 20 percent. Rarely, the latter may be fertile. About 60 percent of cases reflect a chromosome error in oogenesis, 40 percent an error in spermatogenesis. Risk of having an affected child increases with maternal age. Males with more than two X chromosomes (XXXY, XXXXY) are usually mentally retarded and are more likely to have skeletal and other major congenital anomalies such as cleft palate, congenital heart disease (particularly PDA), and microcephaly. The parents' recurrent risk for another chromosomally abnormal liveborn is 1 to 2 percent; prenatal diagnosis with subsequent pregnancies should be discussed.

XXX and XYY Syndromes

Triple X females have no characteristic physical stigmata. However, intelligence is reduced, and about one fourth are mildly retarded. Educational, but not behavioral problems, are more common than in age-matched controls. The parental risk for an XXX daughter increases with maternal age. XXX females are fertile, and the offspring are usually chromosomally normal. About 1 in 1,000 liveborn females are triple X.

About 1 in 350 males over 6 feet tall are XYY. Such males have no pathognomonic physical stigmata, and average IQ is normal. The prevalence of XYY males in a prison population is manyfold greater than their proportion in the general population. This had led to the erroneous conclusion that XYY males must be overly aggressive and antisocial, presumably due to the extra Y chromosome. In fact, XYY males are typically neither. Educational and behavioral problems in XYY young boys are the same as in age-matched controls. Their disproportion in prisons—usually for nonaggressive crimes—is for reasons that remain unclear. Since XYY males reflect a chromosomal error in their father's spermatogenesis, the recurrent risk does not increase with parental age. XYY males are fertile, and the offspring are usually chromosomally normal. Because parents of XXX females and XYY males have the usual 1 to 2 percent recurrent risk for chromosomally abnormal liveborns, prenatal diagnosis should be discussed. It also would be advisable for XXX females and XYY males to consider prenatal diagnosis with their own pregnancies.

Sex and Gender

Sex is determined by chromosomes, but gender is a psychosocial definition. It is the latter which should be the prime consideration to the medical practitioner. When sex and gender are not compatible, anatomic, physiologic, and psychosocial considerations should determine the final gender assignment of the individual. Finally, although XO, XXY, XYY, and XXX fetuses can be detected in utero by amniocentesis and in newborns by routine chromosome screening, the relatively benign clinical course of these conditions should be an important factor in deciding to pursue such genetic diagnostic approaches.

MOLECULAR CYTOGENETIC SYNDROMES

Advances in molecular genetics during the last 5 years have provided new insights into the genetic pathogenesis of several syndromes often associated with specific cytogenetic abnormalities.

Fragile X Syndrome

It has been long recognized that there is a significant excess (about 25 percent) of males in moderately to severely mentally retarded populations. Much of this inordinate male representation is the result of defective recessive X-linked genes. These may represent new mutations or inheritances from normal heterozygous (carrier) mothers. About 1 in 150 individuals, usually male, has some form of X-linked mental retardation—including one fifth with fragile X syndrome.

In 1969, Herbert Lubs noted the in vitro cytogenetic marker now called "fragile X" in short-term lymphocyte cultures. However, its clinical significance was not realized until a 1977 report by G.R. Sutherland in Australia. Under tissue culture conditions which starve the cell of its ability to synthesize thymidilic acid, one sees a chromosome break at Xq27, the distal part of the long arm of the X chromosome (Fig. 1.24), in cells of individuals clinically affected with fragile X syndrome.

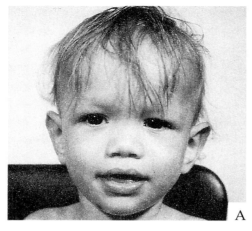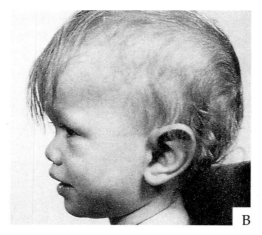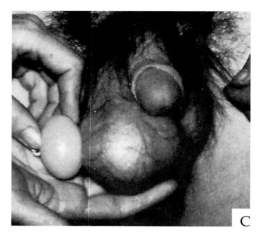

FIG. 1.25 Physical findings in fragile X syndrome. **A** and **B**, note the long, wide, and protruding ears, elongated face and flattened nasal bridge. **C**, macroorchidism in adult male with fragile X syndrome due to interstitial testicular edema. (**A** and **B**, reproduced by permission from Simko A, Hornstein L, Soukup S, Bagamery N: Fragile X syn- drome: recognition in young children. Pediatrics 1989;83(4):547– 552. **C**, reproduced by permission from Hagerman RJ: Fragile X syn- drome, in Lockhart JD (ed): Current Problems in Pediatrics. Chicago, Year Book Medical Publishers, 1987, vol. XVII, no II, 632)

By pedigree analysis, about 1 in 1,100 males has the fragile X gene but only 80 percent (1;1,400) show clinical manifestations. About 1 in 750 females has the fragile X gene but only 30 per- cent (1/2,500) are clinically affected (i.e., the fragile X gene is 80 percent penetrant in males, 30 percent penetrant in females). Females with the fragile X gene usually are heterozy- gotes and, when clinically normal, are called "carrier females." Having only one X chromosome, males with the fragile X gene are of course hemizygous and, when clinically normal, are called "transmitting males."

Males with fragile X syndrome are moderately to severely mentally retarded; about two thirds have an IQ between 20 and 49 (range <20 to 69). The IQ may decline with age. The majority have speech delay, short attention span, hyperactivity, persistence of mouthing objects, and poor motor coordination. While autism is no more frequent than in other mentally retarded children, disciplinary problems, temper tantrums, poor eye contact, avoidance of socialization, and rocking are common. Physical stigmata may include long or wide or pro- truding ears, long face, prominent jaw, flattened nasal bridge, and high arched palate (Fig. 1.25A,B). Some have "velvety" skin, hyperextensible joints, and mitral valve prolapse. Relative macrocephaly is more likely tnan microcephaly. Macro- orchidism is found in 80 percent of adult and 20 percent of pre- pubescent males as a consequence of interstitial testicular edema (Fig. 1.25C), although affected males may still be fertile.

Females with fragile X syndrome are somewhat less retard- ed than males; about 60 percent fall in the 35 to 69 IQ range and 20 percent are of low normal or normal intelligence. However, even among the latter, learning disabilities, mood disorders such as unipolar and bipolar disease, schizoid per- sonality, and significant disturbances in affect, socialization, and communication are common. The physical features often seen in males with fragile X syndrome are less likely to be found in females.

In most clinically affected patients, the fragile X chromo- some marker can be detected in peripheral blood lymphocytes cultured in special medium, as described previously. Detection is somewhat less feasible using tissue cultures of skin fibro- blast or of fetal aminocytes. The range of expression in cul- tured lymphocytes is 1 to 50 percent positive cells (average 25 percent in affected males, 15 percent in affected females). Occasionally, a normal person will express the fragile X chro- mosome marker in no more than 1 in 200 cells. This is of no known significance. Males and females who carry the fragile X gene (by pedigree analysis) but are clinically normal are unlikely to express the fragile X chromosome marker in vitro. Since this test requires special media, the clinician must speci- fy the fragile X test when sending a blood sample to the genet- ics laboratory for analysis.

The genetics of fragile X syndrome are complex. A transmit- ting male who has the fragile X gene (FXG) but is phenotypi- cally normal will transmit the FXG to all his daughters, but they also will be normal. However, his daughters' children may be affected by fragile X syndrome. An explanation pro- posed by Charles D. Laird in 1987 stated that the FXG lies in or near Xq27 and can exist in one of two abnormal states. The ini- tial state (mutation) is benign, that is, it has no clinical effects and is found in the normal transmitting male and his daugh- ters. However, after passing through meiosis in the daughters, the benign FXG can be converted to the malignant FXG. Sons receiving the malignant FXG from their mothers are affected with fragile X syndrome, as are some of their daughters. Only the malignant form of the FXG can be detected in vitro by the fragile X chromosome test.

Laird invoked the new concept of genetic imprinting as the underlying mechanism. Genetic imprinting simply means that as the genome passes through meiosis in males and females, it is normal for parts of it to be functionally altered. Conse- quently, by the time of conception, the maternally and pater- nally derived haploid genomes are doing different things so that one set of each must be present for normal human embryogenesis. The actual biochemical processes involved in such physiologic genetic imprinting are as yet unknown.

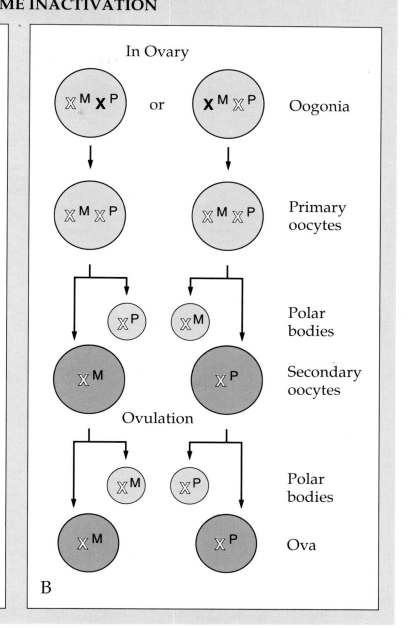

FIG. 1.26 Functional behavior of the X chromosome in XX females. **A,** somatic and premeiotic germ cells. Implantation occurs 5 days after conception, at which time in each female cell either X^M or X^P is randomly genetically inactivated and remains so in each of the cell's descendents. Because the process is random, by determining the proportion of cells with an inactive X^M or inactive X^P in each of a large population of women, a Gaussian population distribution of women is generated. That is, most women in the population will have an approximate 50/50 mix of cells, in which each cell expresses either X^M or X^P. However, some women will have by chance more cells with an inactive X^M and vice versa. **B,** meiotic germ cells. When a female germ cell enters into the first prophase of meiosis, X-inactivation is abolished; both X chromosomes become genetically active through fertilization and continue so until embryonic uterine implantation. Then, as in **A,** above, random X inactivation in XX females occurs all over again.

However, as with fragile X syndrome, genetic imprinting can have pathologic consequences. Although women have two X chromosomes, only one is genetically active in each cell. Whether the active X chromosome in each cell is maternally or paternally derived is simply random (Fig. 1.26A). However, in germ cells, at some point during meiosis, both X chromosomes become active (Fig. 1.26B). If the clinically benign FXG is on the previously inactive X chromosome in a germ cell, the Xq27 area on that X chromosome is permanently deactivated during meiosis, that is, it is *pathologically imprinted*. The imprinted Xq27 area represents the malignant state of the FXG. A male inheriting this imprinted X, having only one X chromosome, can make no Xq27 gene products and therefore has fragile X syndrome. If the benign FXG is on the previously active X chromosome in a germ cell, nothing changes during meiosis, so a male who inherits this X chromosome gets only the

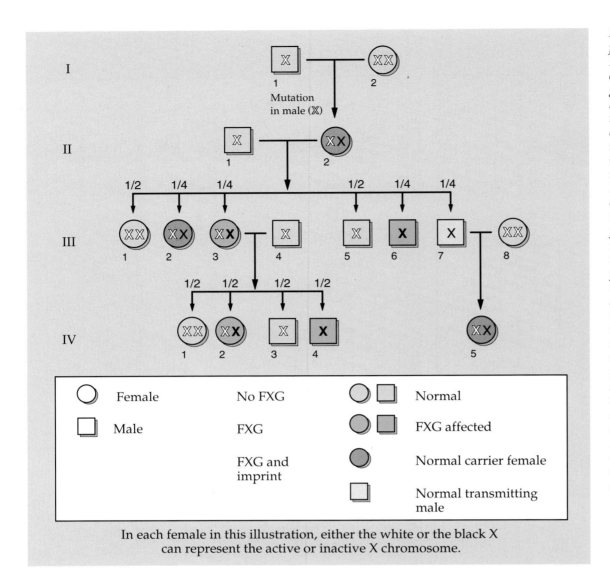

In each female in this illustration, either the white or the black X can represent the active or inactive X chromosome.

FIG. 1.27 Inheritance pattern of fragile X gene (Laird hypothesis). Because each XX female cell has only one X chromosome that is genetically active, the cell will be harmed only if the malignant (i.e., imprinted) FXG is on its active X chromosome (since that cell could make no Xq27 gene products). Consequently, females with the malignant FXG will have fragile X syndrome only if, by chance, over 50 percent of their cells meet this criterion. Otherwise, these females will be normal and indistinguishable clinically or by fragile X chromosome testing from females with the benign FXG (e.g., III2 vs III3). This becomes an issue in genetic counseling, when the normal sibs of a person with fragile X syndrome wish to know their risk of having a child with fragile X syndrome. In the present figure, III1,2,5,7, IV1,3, and even III3 and IV2 could represent such normal siblings. Fortunately, molecular genetic analysis (using DNA probes for RFLPs closely linked to the FXG) of multiple family members can sort out who is who in many— although not all—cases.

benign FXG and is normal. To a lesser extent, females inheriting the malignant FXG sometimes may be clinically affected with fragile X syndrome (Fig. 1.27).

If a normal woman (whose own father is normal) has a child affected with fragile X syndrome, each of her subsequent sons has a 35 percent risk of being affected with the syndrome, and each subsequent daughter has a 15 percent risk. If a woman has fragile X syndrome, each of her sons has a 50 percent risk of being affected with it, and each daughter a 25 percent risk. A male affected with fragile X syndrome will have normal sons because they will get his Y chromosome; however, he will transmit the malignant FXG to each daughter, although each will have only a 50 percent risk of being affected with fragile X syndrome.

Prenatal diagnosis of fragile X syndrome in the fetus is possible by assaying cultured amniocytes or cultured chorionic villous samples for the in vitro fragile X chromosome marker (see section on Prenatal Diagnosis). However, as this approach is not completely reliable, it should be supplemented by molecular genetic restriction fragment length polymorphism (RFLP) analysis of the family. Together, the two techniques allow reliable prenatal diagnosis of fragile X syndrome in the fetus in most family pedigrees. The family molecular genetic analysis should be done prior to initiating a pregnancy to be certain it can be informative.

OTHER IMPRINTING SYNDROMES
Prader-Willi and Angelman Syndromes

Two other syndromes associated with chromosomal abnormalities and imprinting are Prader-Willi and Angelman syndromes (Fig. 1.28 and 1.29). Newborns affected with Prader-Willi syndrome (PWS) usually are markedly hypotonic. Decreased fetal movement in utero and a breech fetal position are often noted. While birth is usually at term, birth weights tend to be below 3,000 g. In neonates, poor sucking and swallowing reflexes predispose to choking episodes that can cause respiratory problems. The cry may be weak. Although Moro and deep tendon reflexes often are decreased, the neurologic evaluation is otherwise unremarkable. Motor development is delayed and most patients are mildly to moderately mentally retarded (IQ range 35 to 85), with particular delay in speech. Hypotonia abates over the next 2 to 3 years, but patients develop uncontrollable appetite which rapidly produces marked obesity. The distribution of excess fat is particularly thick over the lower trunk, buttocks, and proximal limbs (Fig. 1.28A). Although the facies are not particularly dysmorphic, they are similar in most PWS patients. The eyes often are described as "almond shaped," and strabismus is common. The bifrontal diameter is narrow and the face is "fat" (particularly around the cheeks and chin), the mouth is "fishlike" in shape, and the ears may be slightly dys-

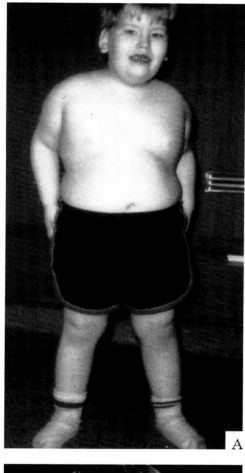

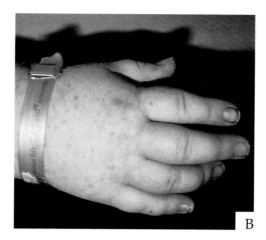

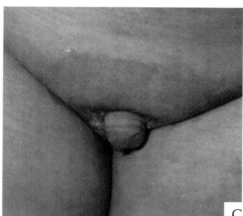

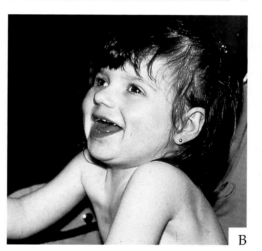

FIG. 1.28 Prader-Willi syndrome. **A,** this patient demonstrates the marked obesity characteristic of PWS. Excess fat is distributed over the trunk, buttocks, and proximal extremities. **B** and **C,** small hands (and feet) and hypoplastic penis and scrotum are other typical features. (**A,** courtesy of Dr. Jeanne M. Hanchett, The Rehabilitation Institute of Pittsburgh. **B** and **C,** courtesy of Dr. Holly W. Davis, Children's Hospital of Pittsburgh)

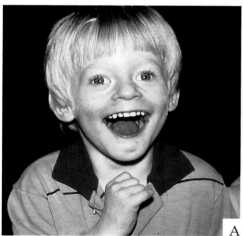

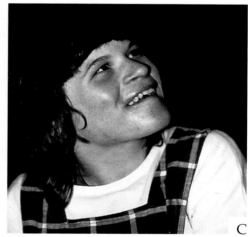

FIG. 1.29 Angelman syndrome. **A–C,** three patients with typical facies. Note the maxillary hypoplasia, large mouth—often with protruding tongue—and the prognathism. (Courtesy of Drs. C.A. Williams and J. Hendrickson, University of Florida, Gainesville)

plastic. Hypopigmentation is common, the patient usually has blond to light brown hair, blue eyes, and sun-sensitive fair skin. Picking of skin sores can become a problem. Hands and feet are noticeably small from birth, and the stature of the older child and adult is short (Fig. 1.28B). The penis and testes remain small, and the scrotum is atrophic in males with PWS (Fig. 1.28C), although the penis can be enlarged by testosterone therapy. If the testes are cryptorchid, surgical correction should be attempted. Menarche in females is delayed to absent and menses, when present, are sparse and irregular. The gonadotrophic hormone levels are reduced in both sexes. No patient with PWS has been known to reproduce.

Of particular concern in older children with PWS are the problems of emotional lability and extreme temper tantrums. These, and the overeating can often be partly ameliorated by intensive inpatient behavioral modification programs followed by longitudinal parental support and followup in the home. Interestingly, despite having a normal basal metabolic rate, weight reduction requires significantly more severe caloric restriction in these patients than in normal persons. Diabetes mellitus can develop in the older child, and its incidence is correlated with the severity of obesity. Although it tends to be insulin-resistant, the condition does respond well to treatment with oral hypoglycemic agents. Life expectancy is

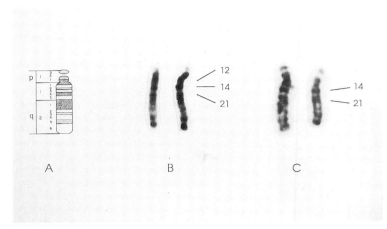

FIG. 1.30 High resolution banding in Prader-Willi syndrome. The diagram of a high resolution analysis of chromosome 15 is shown on the left. In pair "B" both chromosomes are normal, while in pair "C" the band q12 is deleted from the paternally derived chromosome 15 (rightmost) in a patient with PWS. Note that in higher resolution chromosome preparations, banding patterns become more and more subdivided. This allows detection of increasingly smaller structural abnormalities. However, as the number of bands increases, cytogenic analysis becomes progressively more difficult. To avoid error, the clinician should provide sufficient medical information to help the laboratory personnel decide specifically where to look for very small structural abnormalities in the parent's karyotype. Blanket requests for high resolution chromosome studies should be avoided.

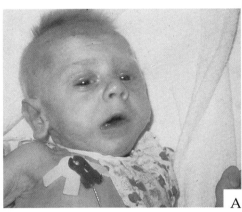
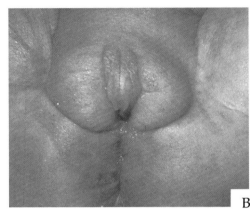

FIG. 1.31 Smith-Lemli-Opitz syndrome. **A,** note the anteverted nostrils, low-set ears, small chin, and clenched hand. **B,** hypospadias, cryptorchidism, or ambiguous genitalia as shown here also may be seen. (Courtesy of Dr. W. Tunnessen, Johns Hopkins Medical Center, Baltimore)

shortened by cardiorespiratory complications related to the extreme obesity (Pickwickian syndrome).

Angeleman syndrome (AS) was described about 10 years after PWS was first recognized in 1956. Except for the tendency to hypopigmentation, the clinical phenotypes of AS and PWS are quite different. Patients with AS are severely mentally retarded. Speech is impaired to absent, and inappropriate paroxysms of laughter are common. Physical features include microbrachycephaly, maxillary hypoplasia, large mouth with protruding and "flickering" tongue, prognathism, and short stature (in adults) (Fig. 1.29A–C). The gait is ataxic, with a tip-toe walk and jerky arm movements resembling those of a marionette, hence its designation as the "happy puppet syndrome." Akinetic or major motor seizures are common. While survival to adulthood is possible, none has been known to reproduce.

Although most cases of PWS and AS are sporadic, occasional instances of affected sibs are known. About 60 percent of patients with PWS and AS have a detectable chromosomal abnormality. On high resolution chromosome analysis, the Giemsa band q12 is deleted from the long arm of a chromosome 15 (15q12-) (Fig. 1.30). By both microscopic and molecular genetic analyses, the chromosomal abnormality appears to be the same in patients with PWS and AS, but with one difference. In PWS, the abnormal chromosome 15q12- is always derived from the patient's father, while in AS it is derived from the patient's mother. Because the parental chromosome studies usually are normal, the abnormal 15q12- in PWS and AS represents a new germ cell mutation in the PWS patient's father or the AS patient's mother. Given the low (about 1 to 2 percent) risk of recurrence for subsequent sibs of a given patient, it appears most likely that such familial cases represent parental germ cell mosaicism for the new mutation.

About 40 percent of patients with PWS and AS have microscopically normal chromosomes. However, some of these have DNA abnormalities in the 15q12 area on molecular genetic analysis, although again, the parental derivation of the DNA abnormality is on the paternally derived chromosome in PWS and maternally derived chromosome in AS. The remaining patients with PWS and AS appear to have completely normal #15 chromosomes by present means of analyses. However, some of these patients with PWS, and perhaps all, have been shown to have parental disomy for their #15 chromosomes. That is, both #15 chromosomes present are maternally derived so that, in effect, no paternal 15q12 area is present. Presumably, future research might show that in AS with normal #15 chromosomes, both are paternally derived so that, in effect, no maternal 15q12 area would be present.

All this means that normal genes in the 15q12 area are somehow imprinted during parental germ cell meiosis. Consequently, normal genes in the 15q12 area are functionally different after paternal and maternal meiosis. Normal human development requires one representation of normal paternal 15q12 genes and one of normal maternal 15q12 genes to be present in the embryo. If normal paternal 15q12 genes are missing (by whatever mechanism) the result is PWS, indicating that a double dose of normal maternal 15q12 genes cannot compensate for the lack of any normal paternal 15q12 genes. Likewise, lack of any normal maternal 15q12 genes results in AS.

CHROMOSOMAL-LIKE SYNDROMES

As already mentioned, some syndromes without a detectable chromosomal abnormality have clinical features that can suggest a chromosomal disorder, and these enter into the differen-

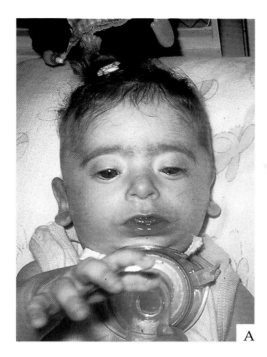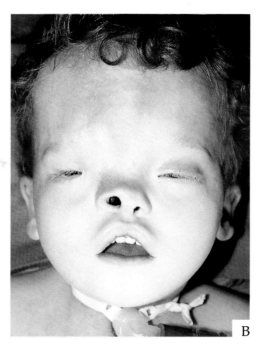

FIG. 1.32 CHARGE association. **A,** note small left eye with ptosis; low-set, posteriorly rotated, anomalous auricles; small chin. Choanal atresia necessitated tracheotomy. **B,** another infant with CHARGE association reveals broad forehead, widespread eyes with narrow palpebral fissures, hypoplastic right nares, low-set ears, and Cupid's bow mouth. (**A,** courtesy of Dr. W. Tunnessen, Johns Hopkins Medical Center, Baltimore. **B,** courtesy of Dr. Timothy McBride, Georgetown University Medical Center)

tial diagnosis of the latter. Some of the more common of the syndromes in this class include the Smith-Lemli-Opitz, CHARGE, VATER, Cornelia de Lange, Noonan, and fetal alcohol syndromes.

Smith-Lemli-Opitz Syndrome

This is an autosomal recessive, simple, mendelian genetic disorder, although it shares many physical features in common with trisomy 18. Affected infants tend to be small for gestational age, and often are born via breech presentation after a pregnancy noted for decreased fetal movements. Patients have microcephaly with prominent occiput and narrow frontal area. Facial stigmata include eyelid ptosis, epicanthal folds, strabismus, low-set or posteriorly rotated ears, broad nasal tip with upturned nares, and micrognathia (Fig. 1.31A). Simian crease of the palm and syndactyly of the second and third toes are characteristic; in males, hypospadias with cryptorchidism or even ambiguous genitalia are other usual findings (Fig. 1.31B). Clenched hands, digital abnormalities, cataracts, cleft palate or bifid uvula also are seen in some cases. Radiographs may reveal stippled epiphyses. Structural abnormalities of the CNS (at times associated with seizures), heart, GI tract, and/or kidneys are common. Initial hypotonia progresses to hypertonia with irritable behavior, shrill screaming, and feeding problems. Affected infants fail to thrive. Eighty percent die by age 18 months, most in the first year. Only a few have survived longer than 4 years, and these were moderately to severely mentally retarded.

Being an autosomal recessive disorder, the recurrent risk for a couple with an affected child is 25 percent for each subsequent conception. This risk can be reduced by artificial insemination of the mother using a healthy, unrelated sperm donor. Prenatal diagnosis also may be attempted using high resolution ultrasound of the fetus to look for intrauterine growth retardation and major organ structural abnormalities.

CHARGE Association

CHARGE is an acronym for a nonrandom association of features including *c*oloboma of the retina or, less commonly the iris; *h*eart abnormalities; *a*tresia of the choanae; *r*etarded growth and mental development; *g*enital hypoplasia in males, and *e*ar anomalies that can include deafness. The minimal diagnostic criteria should include abnormalities in four of the six categories—of which at least one must be coloboma or choanal atresia (Fig. 1.32). Cleft lip and/or palate and renal abnormalities sometimes are found, as is the DiGeorge sequence. The latter includes congenital heart disease (particularly abnormalities of the aortic arch, right subclavian artery, or ventricular septal defect); agenesis or hypoplasia of the thymus with decreased T-cell production and impaired cell-mediated immunity; partial or, less often, complete absence of the parathyroid glands manifested by hypocalcemia and neonatal tetany; and often a facies characterized by wide-spaced, slightly downslanting eyes, anteverted nares, a short philtrum, and small abnormal ears). Infants with CHARGE association often die early as consequence of their congenital anomalies, but many survive to adulthood. Although there is developmental delay, the IQ range is broad (range<30 to 80). Older males often have a micropenis that responds to testosterone therapy, while older females usually have amenorrhea and poor development of secondary sex characteristics.

In the neonate, CHARGE association must be differentiated from chromosomal disorders such as trisomy 13 or 18, as well as from the more benign nonchromosomal VATER association. Although chromosome studies should be normal in CHARGE association, when the DiGeorge sequence is present a small interstitial deletion of chromosome 22 at q11 may be found on occasion, with high resolution cytogenetic techniques.

The etiology of CHARGE association is unknown, but most likely it is heterogeneous. Although most cases are sporadic, instances of affected sibs and an affected parent and offspring

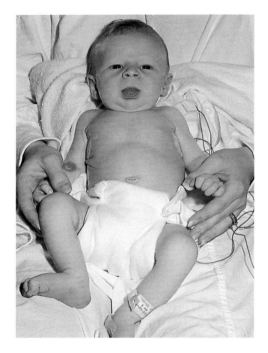

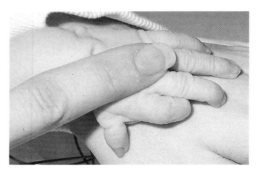

FIG. 1.33 Although this child with VATER association has a relatively normal facial appearance, radial dysplasia and an abnormal thumb are present.

have been reported. The risk of recurrence for a couple with one affected child is about 4 percent; however, if there are two affected sibs, this rises to approximately 25 percent for each subsequent conception. If an affected parent has an affected child, the risk of recurrence is most likely 50 percent. Prenatal diagnosis may be attempted with high resolution ultrasound to detect major structural abnormalities in the fetus.

VATER Association

VATER is another acronym for a nonrandom association of *v*ertebral and *a*nal anomalies, *t*racheoesophageal fistula with *e*sophageal atresia, and *r*adial and/or *r*enal abnormalities. Most affected newborns have anomalies in all five categories. The acronym can be expanded to VACTERL to include congenital heart disease (particularly ventricular septal defect, which again is found in a majority of cases) and, less often, other *l*imb defects (Fig. 1.33). Vertebral anomalies include hemivertebrae and sacral abnormalities. Limb deformities consist of radial aplasia or hypoplasia, abnormal thumbs, polydactyly, and syndactyly. Renal abnormalities include unilateral agenesis and, less commonly, ectopic or horseshoe kidney. The etiology of VATER association is unknown. Virtually all cases are sporadic, and no chromosomal abnormalities have been detected. The prognosis for growth and development in infants who survive infancy is good. Most have normal intelligence and eventually achieve normal stature. Consequently, to make optimal management decisions, it is important to distinguish VATER syndrome from more dire chromosomal abnormalities (such as trisomy 18) or nonchromosomal abnormalities such as CHARGE association.

For the purpose of genetic counseling, VATER association also must be differentiated from Towne syndrome, an autosomal dominant, simple, mendelian genetic disorder which shares some features. However, in Towne syndrome there often is a positive family history involving at least two generations, and ear abnormalities including microtia, as well as preauricular and facial skin tags, while vertebral anomalies and tracheoesophageal fistula are unusual. The prognosis for

growth and development in Towne syndrome patients is good as well. However, the risk for recurrence of Towne syndrome with a positive family history could be 50 percent, while for VATER syndrome the risk should be less than 2 percent. Prenatal diagnosis for both conditions would depend on detecting structural anomalies in the fetus by high resolution ultrasound.

De Lange or Cornelia de Lange Syndrome

De Lange or Cornelia de Lange syndrome is characterized by intrauterine growth retardation and persistent failure to thrive, severe to moderate mental retardation, and microcephaly with flat occiput and low hairline. Facial features include long, curly eyelashes, bushy eyebrows which by 16 months meet at the midline (synophrys), small nose with anteverted nostrils, long philtrum, downturned mouth with thin lips (the upper lip may have a midline break, the lower a corresponding notch), and small chin (Fig. 1.34A). Micromelia (small hands and feet) is another characteristic finding (Fig. 1.34B). Hirsutism, cutis marmorata, proximally placed thumbs (Fig. 1.34B), flexion contractures of the elbows, aplasia or hypoplasia of limbs, and in males hypospadias with cryptorchidism are common, as are significant abnormalities of various other major organs. Affected adults are short, with average IQ <35(range 4 to 85). Menses may be normal in older females, who often have a bicornuate uterus.

The incidence of de Lange syndrome is estimated at 1 in 100,000 liveborns. The etiology is unknown but probably is heterogeneous. Although most cases are sporadic, affected sibs are found in 2 to 5 percent of families with normal parents. A small minority of patients with features similar to those of de Lange syndrome have a duplication involving the lower half (q21→qter) of a chromosome 3. In effect, these patients have a partial 3q trisomy. This chromosomal abnormality may be a new spontaneous mutation, but more often is inherited from a normal parent carrying a balanced chromosomal rearrangement. Various other nonspecific chromosomal abnormalities

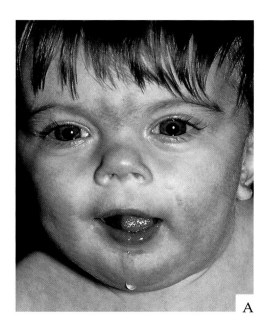

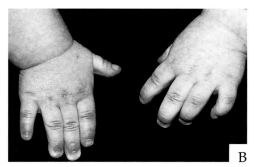

FIG. 1.34 Cornelia de Lange's syndrome. **A,** note heavy eyebrows with developing synophrys, long eyelashes, small upturned nose, long philtrum, small mouth with thin lips. **B,** small hands, hypoplastic proximally placed thumb, small fifth finger with mild clinodactyly. (Courtesy of Dr. A.H. Urbach, Children's Hospital of Pittsburgh)

A

B

occasionally have been found in individuals with features typical of de Lange syndrome. When there is a chromosome abnormality, the recurrent risks and prenatal diagnosis are as previously discussed in this chapter. Nevertheless, most patients with de Lange syndrome reveal normal chromosomes even when high resolution techniques are used. It is possible that these cases represent the effect of a new spontaneous dominant gene mutation. In this scenario, instances of affected sibs could suggest gonadal mosaicism for the dominant mutation in one of the normal parents. A more likely etiology for most cases of de Lange syndrome is a submicroscopic chromosome duplication/deletion, possibly in 3q21→qter (that is, a "contiguous gene syndrome"). The latter implies the duplication/deletion of several unrelated but physically contiguous genes resulting in a syndrome of congenital anomalies. In any event, if a normal couple has a child with de Lange syndrome and the results of chromosome studies for every member are normal by high resolution cytogenetic techniques, the recurrent risk is 2 to 5 percent. After the birth of a second affected sib the subsequent risk of recurrence approaches 25 percent. Prenatal diagnosis depends on finding intrauterine growth retardation and/or major structural abnormalities in the fetus by high resolution ultrasound.

Finally, there have been several case reports of women mildly affected with de Lange syndrome whose offspring were both affected and normal. However, in several of these reports the diagnosis has been questioned. In any event, the recurrent risk in such parent-child cases could be as high as 50 percent for each conception.

Noonan Syndrome

Noonan syndrome is most likely an autosomal dominant, simple, mendelian genetic disorder affecting both males and females that shares many clinical features with Turner syndrome. Consequently, when females are affected, Turner syndrome enters the differential diagnosis.

Some clinical features can help distinguish Noonan from Turner syndrome in affected females, although a chromosome study is mandatory to confirm the diagnosis. Females with Turner syndrome are of normal intelligence and invariably have short stature. Approximately 20 percent have congenital heart disease, usually coarctation of the aorta, and most are sterile with primary amenorrhea. In contrast, up to 50 percent of females with Noonan syndrome can have normal stature and 25 percent are mildly mentally retarded. Although 45 percent have congenital heart disease, the most common form is pulmonary valvular stenosis. They also have normal menses and are fertile. Conversely, most males affected with Noonan syndrome have cryptorchidism and are sterile. The facies are characterized by a broad forehead and hypertelorism with an antimongoloid slant that includes epicanthi and ptosis (particularly unilateral). Coarse, curly hair is more characteristic of Noonan than Turner syndrome, although both have low hairlines (see Cardiology Chapter). Among the several features the two syndromes share, lymphedema of the hands and feet in the neonatal period and pterygium colli (webbed neck) seen later in infancy are highly diagnostic (see Fig. 1.22).

Noonan syndrome is seen in about 1 in 1,000 liveborns. Most cases are sporadic, but some are inherited from an affected mother, in which case the risk of recurrence is 50 percent for each subsequent conception. If there is no family history, and careful evaluation of the parents reveals no evidence of Noonan syndrome, the risk of recurrence after the birth of one affected child is approximately 10 percent. Prenatal diagnosis of an affected fetus depends largely on finding characteristic structural abnormalities via high resolution ultrasound.

Fetal Alcohol Syndrome

The effect of exposure to significant levels of serum alcohol during gestation results in a constellation of clinical features that can resemble trisomy 18, Smith-Lemli-Opitz syndrome, or Noonan syndrome. Although the teratogenic effects were first

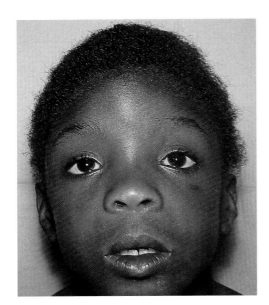

FIG. 1.35 Fetal alcohol syndrome. Note the poorly formed philtrum; slightly narrow and widespread eyes, with inner epicanthal folds and mild ptosis; hirsute forehead; short nose; and relatively thin upper lip.

noted in 1968 in France, these were not widely known until 5 years later through the reports of K.L. Jones working with the late D.W. Smith in the United States. Hallmarks of the syndrome are short palpebral fissures, smooth philtrum and a thin, smooth upper lip. Other features include mild microcephaly, short nose, and hypoplasia of the nails and distal digits (particularly the fifth toes). Occasionally, affected infants have eyelid ptosis, epicanthal folds, strabismus, small raised hemangiomata, cervical vertebral abnormalities, congenital heart disease, renal anomalies, and hypoplasia of the labia in females (Fig. 1.35).

Newborns with fetal alcohol syndrome tend to be small for gestational age, and have poor catch-up growth. They are hypotonic, irritable, and tremulous. Most older children tend to be thin, hyperactive, and over 80 percent have some delay in mental development—particularly fine motor function. Their IQs range from 50 to 80. Affected infants with the characteristic dysmorphology are said to have fetal alcohol syndrome, while those without the dysmorphology but with the development problems are said to have fetal alcohol effects.

The breakdown products of ethanol (particularly acetaldehyde) ingested by the mother during the pregnancy are the source of fetal alcohol syndrome/effects. Maternal Antabuse® treatment during pregnancy is contraindicated, because it also raises serum acetaldehyde levels. Although there may be no absolutely safe level of maternal alcohol consumption *throughout* pregnancy (particularly in the first trimester), the risk of teratogenesis clearly increases dramatically with increasing degrees of maternal ethanol consumption. Major evidence of fetal alcohol syndrome/effects is observed in 30 to 50 percent of offspring of mothers who are chronic severe alcoholics (over 7 drinks/day), whereas more subtle effects result from 4 to 6 drinks/day. Prematurity and/or low birth weight for gestational age can result from 2 to 3 drinks/day. It is estimated that some fetal alcohol effects can be seen in 1 of 300 to 1,000 liveborns, depending on population drinking norms. The risk to the fetus of occasional maternal alcoholic binges is not clear, but such drinking is best avoided. It is also unclear why some babies are affected and others are not,

despite equivalent degrees of maternal alcoholism. This fact may reflect some polygenic maternal and/or fetal difference in ethanol/acetaldehyde metabolism. Prenatal diagnosis may be attempted with high resolution ultrasound aimed at detecting intrauterine growth retardation and major structural abnormalities. Also, maternal serum α-fetoprotein may be reduced at 16 weeks' gestation if the fetus has fetal alcohol syndrome.

PRENATAL DIAGNOSIS

The standard technique for prenatal diagnosis of fetal chromosome abnormalities is by transabdominal amniocentesis at 16 weeks' gestation. This is often performed in the obstetrician's office under local anesthesia. Results are usually available in 23 days or less (minimum 10 days) and should be over 99 percent reliable. Early prenatal diagnosis of fetal chromosomal abnormalities is possible at 9 to 12 weeks' gestation by trans-cervical (less commonly transabdominal) chorionic villus sampling (CVS), with results available in 13 days or less. However, CVS is presently limited to a few highly experienced practioners in tertiary care medical centers. While diagnostic accuracy should be over 98 percent, in 10 percent of instances technical problems or other ambiguities necessitate an amniocentesis at 16 weeks. Both CVS and amniocentesis must be carried out in conjunction with sonography to determine fetal number and viability, gestational age, and placental location. The procedure-related fetal loss (death) rate for amniocentesis is about 1 percent and for CVS about 1.5 to 2 percent. Consequently, when couples are counseled on the need for prenatal diagnosis of fetal chromosomal abnormalities, one must strive to ensure that they understand their relative risk of having an abnormal liveborn as compared with their risk of losing the pregnancy as a result of the procedure.

Prenatal diagnosis of fetal chromosomal abnormalities is an option that should be considered and discussed when a pregnant woman is 35 years of age or older, when a couple has had a previous child with a chromosomal abnormality, or when a parent is known to carry a chromosomal rearrangement. Another indication, still considered experimental, is the finding of a low maternal serum α-fetoprotein level at 16 weeks' gestation, as this has been associated with increased risk for Down syndrome, trisomy 18, and trisomy 13. Unfortunately, maternal serum α-fetoprotein tests may not be reliable unless performed in very experienced, high-volume laboratories. This screening method has a relatively low specificity even under the best of circumstances, thereby leading to excessive confirmatory amniocenteses on women with normal fetuses.

Because of the potential for loss of a normal fetus associated with invasive procedures such as amniocentesis and CVS, intensive research is underway to attempt cytogenetic analyses of fetal cells that may be present in maternal blood by 9 weeks' gestation. Using molecular Y chromosome probes, the preliminary results indicate that these cells could allow a very reliable fetal sex determination. Such fetal cells are usually nucleated RBCs. They do not divide, negating the usual metaphase cytogenetic type of analysis. However, they can be analyzed cyteogentically in interphase using molecular cytogenetic DNA probes. It is hoped that this noninvasive technique for prenatal fetal cytogenetic analysis will be available within a few years.

An increasingly useful technique for monitoring fetal development in utero is ultrasound scanning (sonography). This

GENETICS: COMMON CHROMOSOMAL DISORDERS

technique can allow detailed visualization of the fetus by passing high-frequency sound waves through the mother's abdomen and uterus. There is yet no evidence that this causes structural, physiologic, or genetic damage to the mother or fetus.

Level I ultrasound is now used routinely by most obstetricians as an office procedure to monitor pregnancies. Usually this is done between 12 and 20 weeks' gestation, but it can be carried out at any gestational age. Level I ultrasound allows the clinician to confirm gestational age by measuring fetal crown-rump and femoral length, and biparietal diameter. Serial measurements of the latter compared with abdominal diameter often can detect microcephaly. Fetal viability, cardiac activity, number, position, and growth, as well as placental location, amniotic fluid volume, and pelvic adequacy can be evaluated by the clinician using Level I ultrasound. Often, initial suspicions of major fetal structural defects, such as anencephaly and spina bifida cystica, can arise indicating the need for further higher resolution (levels II and III) ultrasound evaluation and/or other prenatal diagnostic procedures.

High resolution sonography allows much more detailed evaluation of fetal morphology. Although the equipment used is more sophisticated than that in Level I ultrasound, the main difference resides in the expertise of the sonographer. High resolution ultrasound of the fetus is performed in tertiary care medical centers by radiologists, cardiologists, and perinatologists specially trained and highly experienced in this technique. Some examples of major fetal structural abnormalities that can be diagnosed by high resolution ultrasound prior to 26 weeks' gestation include craniospinal defects such as anencephaly, spina bifida cystica, hydrocephalus, microcephaly, encephalocele, and cysts, all of which can be detected in 95 percent of instances with over 99 percent reliability; GI anomalies such as omphalocele, gastroschisis, diaphragmatic hernia, and duodenal atresia (90 percent detection rate); GU anomalies such as obstructive uropathy, renal agenesis, and infantile polycystic kidneys (95 percent detection rate); skeletal dysplasia such as osteogenesis imperfecta, abnormal limbs, and achondroplasia (95 percent detection rate). Detection of fetal cardiac anomalies is best left to specialists in fetal echcardiography (80 to 95 percent detection rate over 99 percent reliability). Detection of fetal structural anomalies such as duodenal atresia may be the first indication of a fetal chromosomal abnormality such as Down syndrome. If possible, this should be confirmed by prenatal chromosome studies on the fetus. Finally, in those rare instances when fetal biopsy or fetal blood sampling may be diagnostically indicated in the second or third trimester, the procedure is guided by ultrasound.

BIBLIOGRAPHY

Buyse ML (ed): *Birth Defects Encyclopedia*. New York, Alan R. Liss, 1990.

Childs B (ed): *Molecular Genetics in Medicine*. New York, Elsevier, 1987.

Epstein CJ: Down syndrome, in Scriver CR, Beaudet AL, Sly WS, Valle D (eds): *The Metabolic Basis of Inherited Disease*, ed 6. New York, McGraw-Hill, 1989, 291–326.

Gelehrter TD, Collins FS: *Principles of Medical Genetics*. Baltimore, Williams & Wilkins, 1990.

Goodman RM, Gorlin RJ: *The Malformed Infant and Child*. New York, Oxford University Press, 1983.

Hagerman RJ: Fragile X syndrome, in Lockhart JD (ed): *Current Problems in Pediatrics*. Chicago, Year Book, 1987, vol XVII(11).

Jones KL: *Smith's Recognizable Patterns of Human Malformation*, ed 4. Philadelphia, WB Saunders, 1988.

Knoll JHM, Nicholls RD, Magenis RE, et al: Angelman and Prader-Willi syndromes share a common chromosome 15 deletion but differ in parental origin of the deletion. *Am J Med Genet* 1989;32:285–290.

Laird CD: Proposed mechanism of inheritance and expression of the human fragile X syndrome of mental retardation. *Genetics* 1987;117:587–599.

Ledbetter DH, Cavenee WK: Molecular cytogenetics, in Scriver CR, Beaudet AL, Sly WS, Valle D (eds): *The Metabolic Basis of Inherited Disease*, ed 6. New York, McGaw-Hill, 1989, 343–371.

McKusick VA: *Mendelian Inheritance in Man*, ed 9. Baltimore, Johns Hopkins University Press, 1990.

Milunsky A: *Genetic Disorders and the Fetus*, ed 2. New York, Plenum, 1986.

Nussbaum RL, Ledbetter DH: Fragile X syndrome, in Scriver CR, Beaudet AL, Sly WS, Valle D (eds): *The Metabolic Basis of Inherited Disease*, ed 6. New York, McGraw-Hill, 1989, 327–341.

Ratcliffe SG, Paul N (eds): *Prospective Studies on Children with Sex Chromosome Aneuploidy*. March of Dimes Original Article Series 22(2). New York, Alan R. Liss, 1986.

Steele MW, Golden WL: Syndromes of congenital anomalies, in Kelley VC (ed): *Practice of Pediatrics*. Philadelphia, JB Lippincott, 1984.

Thompson JS, Thompson MW: *Genetics in Medicine*, ed 4. Philadelphia, WB Saunders, 1986.

Weaver DD: *Catalog of Prenatally Diagnosed Conditions*. Baltimore, Johns Hopkins University Press, 1989.

Yu W-D, Wenger SL, Steele MW: X chromosome imprinting in fragile X syndrome. *Hum Genet* 1990;85:590–594.

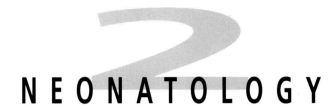

NEONATOLOGY

Michael J. Balsan, M.D. ◆ Ian R. Holzman, M.D.

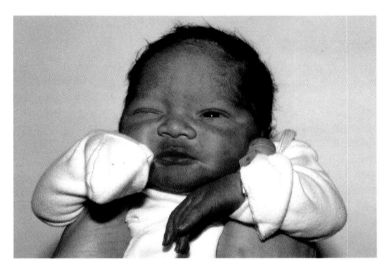

FIG. 2.1 Examination techniques. Holding an infant under the arms and gently rocking him calms the infant and reflexively induces eye opening.

GENERAL PHYSICAL EXAMINATION TECHNIQUES

The purposes of the routine newborn examination are to assess the infant's gestational age, to document normal growth and development for a given gestational age, to uncover any signs of birth-related trauma or congenital anomalies, and lastly, to determine the overall health and condition of the infant. Examination of the newborn requires specialized techniques, given the lack of cooperation on the part of the patient, the infant's small size, and developmental immaturity. If possible, the newborn should be examined in the presence of one or both parents, to reassure them about normal variations and to discuss any abnormal findings. The baby should remain at least partially clothed through as much of the examination as possible, although a complete and thorough examination is imperative. The examiner's hands should be warm, to minimize the chance that the infant will become uncomfortable due to heat loss.

As much observation as is feasible must be accomplished before disturbing a quiet infant. By visual inspection one can readily assess skin and facies; general tonus and symmetry of movement; respiratory rate, retractions, and color; and abdominal contour. Auscultation of the heart and lungs should be done before more stressful portions of the examination, which are likely to make the infant fussy. Allowing the baby to suck on a pacifier or gloved finger can be helpful in quieting him. The latter also allows for an assessment of sucking strength as well as of integrity of the palate. Lifting the infant under the arms (Fig. 2.1) and gently rocking him (such that the head swings toward and away from the examiner) is usually calming. This maneuver also induces a reflexive opening of the eyes, which facilitates the ophthalmologic examination. Sucking also induces eye opening and can be useful. Such maneuvers may be necessary to convince the examiner that the patient does not have a congenital cataract or an intraorbital mass (see Pediatric Ophthalmology, Chapter 19) requiring prompt intervention.

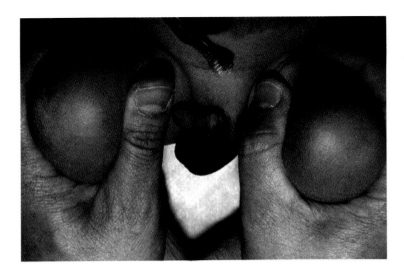

FIG. 2.2 Ortolani's maneuver. The proper hand positioning for this maneuver is demonstrated. Abducting the femur produces a palpable "clunk" in the infant with congenital hip dislocation.

When examining the abdomen it is often helpful to gently flex the hip on the side being examined, since this relaxes the abdominal muscles. Most structures in the abdomen are smaller (pyloric olive), softer (liver), more superficial (spleen tip), or deeper (kidneys) than expected. The use of any part of the hand other than the fingertips is to be discouraged, since maximal sensitivity is essential.

Careful evaluation of the hip joints is a crucial part of every newborn examination because identification and early treatment of congenital dislocation can prevent later disability. While asymmetry of buttocks and skin creases or of femoral length can be clues to dislocation, the performance of at least one of a number of active motion tests is essential. Ortolani's maneuver involves placing the third or fourth finger over the greater trochanter, and the thumb on the medial aspect of the thighs (Fig. 2.2). The thighs are adducted and then abducted with the fingers pushing toward the midline and the thumbs away. A definite "clunk" can be felt and often heard if the femoral head has been dislocated and "clunks" back into the acetabulum. Often, higher pitched clicks and snaps can be heard and felt which do not represent anything more than tendons passing over bone or cartilage.

Assessment of Gestational Age

One of the unique considerations in the examination of the newborn is the assessment of the infant's gestational age. Accurate determination should be the first part of any newborn examination since this provides the context for the remainder of the evaluation. No differential diagnosis of newborn disease can be made without knowing whether the infant is premature or full-term, and whether the infant is small, large, or appropriate 'for gestational age. While an accurate menstrual and pregnancy history usually provides firm evidence of gestational age, there are many cases in which data such as the date of the last menses or the date of the onset of fetal movement are either unavailable or unreliable.

A number of different investigators (see Bibliography) have developed examination criteria, both morphologic and neurologic, for the assessment of gestational age. While these criteria are generally useful because of the ordered patterns

of fetal development, no single feature or even small group of features can be relied upon to develop at the same rate in all infants. In fact, assessment of paired structures, such as ears, may reveal slightly different degrees of maturation from one side to the other. Thus, all of the available methods involve *numerous* physical and neurologic items, and at best have a 2-week range of error.

While morphologic criteria tend to be uninfluenced by events occurring around the time of delivery, neurologic findings may be unreliable in the presence of a number of conditions, including depression secondary to medication, asphyxia, seizures, metabolic diseases, infections, and severe respiratory distress. Even morphologic criteria may be inaccurate if the infant is born with severe edema, growth retardation, or suffers effects from maternal drug use. Such factors must be considered in estimating gestational age.

With the above caveats clearly in mind, Figure 2.3 illustrates one of a number of published data tables used in the estimation of the gestational age of newborns. In this version, there are six morphologic and six neurologic criteria which, in aggregate, yield an estimate of gestational age based on an examination performed at 12 to 24 hours of life. Individual findings are scored on a scale from 0 to 5, and the total score is compared with the chart shown on the right of Figure 2.3.

PHYSICAL MATURITY

Among the most striking differences among infants of various gestational ages is the quality of the skin. As intrauterine development proceeds, the chemical nature of skin changes. There is a gradual decrease in water content and a thickening of the keratin layer. The most premature infants (24 to 28 weeks) exhibit nearly translucent, paper-thin skin (Fig. 2.4) which is easily abraded. A diffuse red hue and a prominent venous pattern are characteristic. At term, the skin no longer appears thin, and the general color is a pale pink. Some superficial peeling and cracking around the ankles and wrists may be visible. Post-term infants (42 to 44 weeks) often have more diffuse peeling and cracking of the skin as the outermost layers are sloughed (Fig. 2.5).

The general quality of scalp hair changes during development from rather fine, thin hair (24 to 28 weeks) to coarser and thicker hair at term. There are, of course, racial differ-

Physical Maturity

	0	1	2	3	4	5
Skin	Gelatinous, red, trans-parent	Smooth, pink, visible veins	Superficial peeling &/or rash, few veins	Cracking, pale area, rare veins	Parchment, deep cracking, no vessels	Leathery, cracked, wrinkled
Lanugo	None	Abundant	Thinning	Bald areas	Mostly bald	
Plantar creases	No crease	Faint red marks	Anterior transverse crease only	Creases anterior two thirds	Creases cover entire sole	
Breast	Barely perceptible	Flat areola, no bud	Stippled areola, 1-2 mm bud	Raised areola, 3-4 mm bud	Full areola, 5-10 mm bud	
Ear	Pinna flat, stays folded	Slightly curved pinna, soft, slow recoil	Well-curved pinna, soft but ready recoil	Formed & firm with instant recoil	Thick cartilage, ear stiff	
Genitals: male	Scrotum empty, no rugae		Testes descending, few rugae	Testes down, good rugae	Testes pendulous, deep rugae	
Genitals: female	Prominent clitoris & labia minora		Majora & minora equally prominent	Majora large, minora small	Clitoris & minora completely covered	

Maturity Rating

Score	Wks.
5	26
10	28
15	30
20	32
25	34
30	36
35	38
40	40
45	42
50	44

Neuromuscular Maturity

FIG. 2.3 Gestational age assessment. The six morphologic and six neurologic criteria, in aggregate, yield an estimation of gestational age. (Reproduced with permission from Ballard J, Novak KK, Driver M, et al: A simplified score of assessment of fetal maturation of newly born infants. J Pediatr 1979; 95:769.

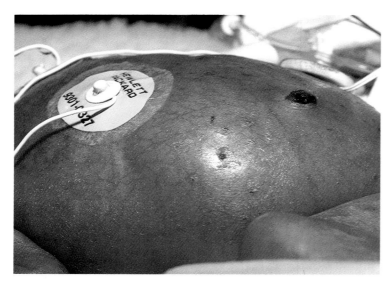

FIG. 2.4 Premature skin. This premature infant demonstrates translucent, paper-thin skin with a prominent venous pattern.

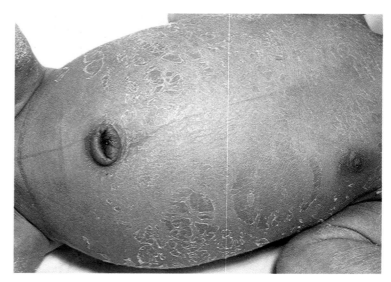

FIG. 2.5 Postterm skin. Peeling and cracking of the skin are characteristic of the infant delivered after 42 weeks' gestation.

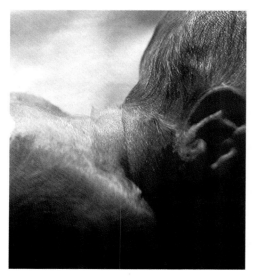

FIG. 2.6 Lanugo. This fine body hair resembling "peach fuzz" is present on infants of 24 to 32 weeks' gestation.

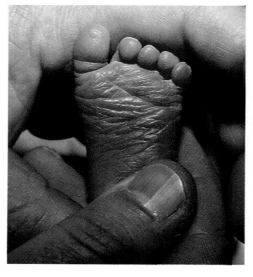

FIG. 2.7 Sole creases. Transverse sole creases cover approximately one-half the sole in this infant, indicating a gestational age of approximately 34 weeks.

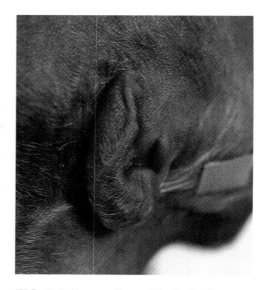

FIG. 2.8 Ear cartilage. The lack of cartilage and easy foldability (lack of recoil) is evident in the ear of this premature infant at 26 weeks.

ences in hair quality which can make this change difficult to assess. A second type of hair, known as lanugo, appears and disappears during development. Lanugo is very fine body hair which resembles "peach fuzz." It is absent prior to the 20th to 22nd weeks, becomes diffuse until 30 to 32 weeks, and then begins to thin. Assessment of presence and extent of lanugo hair is best accomplished by observing the back tangentially (Fig. 2.6).

Transverse creases begin to appear on the anterior portion of the soles of the feet at approximately 32 weeks (Fig. 2.7). By 36 weeks of gestation, the anterior two-thirds of the sole is covered with creases. To adequately assess this feature, it is necessary to stretch the skin over the sole gently so as to distinguish wrinkling from true creases. Infants with congenital neurologic dysfunction involving the lower extremities may lack normal creases, as might infants born with severe

pedal edema. It is sometimes possible to learn something about gestational age long after birth by reviewing the sole prints made for identification in many hospitals.

Breast tissue, which is responsive to maternal hormonal influences, shows a progressive development as gestational age advances. Infants of gestational ages less than 28 weeks have barely perceptible breast tissue (see Fig. 2.4). With advancing age, these tissues show progressive development (see Fig. 2.5), and occasionally, a term infant is noted to have active glandular secretions termed "witch's milk."

Cartilaginous development proceeds in an orderly manner during gestation, and can be assessed by examination of the external ear. While the normal incurving of the upper pinnae begins at 33 to 34 weeks and is complete at term, it is more reliable to assess the extent of cartilage in the pinnae by feeling its edge and folding the ear (Fig. 2.8). Until approximately

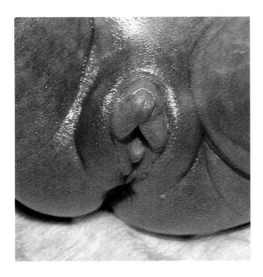

FIG. 2.9 Premature female genitalia. Prominence of the labia minora in a premature female infant at 28 weeks.

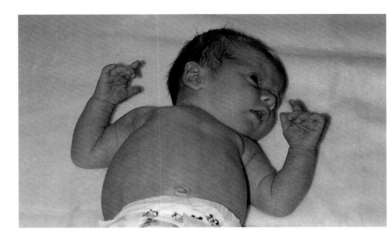

FIG. 2.10 General posture. The typical, marked flexor posture of the term infant.

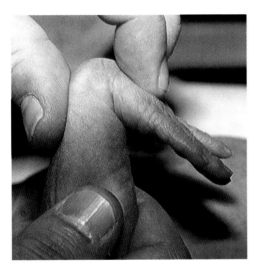

FIG. 2.11 Square-window test. The position for assessing the square window is shown. The 45° angle seen between palm and forearm is consistent with a gestational age of 30 to 32 weeks.

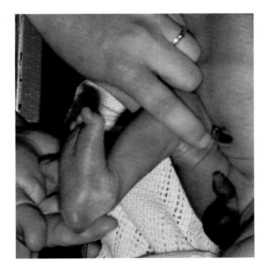

FIG. 2.12 Knee flexion. The position for assessing knee flexion is shown. Note the decreased knee flexibility of this term infant.

32 weeks, there is only minimal recoil of a folded ear, but by term, there is instant recoil.

The appearance of the genitalia can be used to assess gestational age. In the male, the testes descend into the scrotum during the last month of gestation, but they are often palpable in the inguinal canal by 28 to 30 weeks. The appearance of rugae on the scrotum parallels testicular migration. Absence of testicular descent will alter the appearance of the scrotum at term. Clearly, congenital cryptorchidism complicates this evaluation. In the female, the labia majora tend to be overshadowed by the clitoris and labia minora until 34 to 36 weeks (Fig. 2.9). In cases of fetal malnutrition, lack of subcutaneous fat which should normally be present in the latter part of gestation can interfere with assessment of the female genitalia.

NEUROMUSCULAR MATURITY

There are numerous neurologic tests and observations which can be used in attempting to assess gestational age. Most examiners use those that seem to best cover the various facets of neurologic function, including range of motion, tone, reflexes, and posture. None are particularly reliable in the face of illness, and the entire neurologic examination is best done between 12 and 24 hours after birth to allow recovery from the stress of delivery.

The resting supine posture of infants changes with advancing gestational age. The mature infant exhibits a marked flexor posture of the extremities in comparison to the extensor posture of the premature infant (Fig. 2.10).

Tests for flexion angles assess a combination of muscle tone, ligament and tendon laxity, and flexion-extension development. The inexperienced examiner usually assumes that the most premature infant will be the most flexible, but observation of flexion angles demonstrates that this is false. The square-window test of the wrist (Fig. 2.11) is performed by gently flexing the hand upon the wrist and assessing the resultant angle. Infants less than approximately 32 weeks can be flexed only to 45° to 90°, while term infants undergo full flexion. Sometime between birth and adulthood this flexion ability is lost. Examination of the flexion of the knees reveals a different pattern of development, with decreasing flexibility as gestational age increases (Fig. 2.12). It is essential to emphasize gentleness in these evaluations, since any result can be achieved if the examiner applies undue force.

Active tone and reflex responsiveness may be assessed by examining arm recoil. In this maneuver, the supine infant's forearms are fully flexed for 5 seconds, extended by pulling on the hands, and then released. As gestational age increases, the flexion response of the infant is more pronounced.

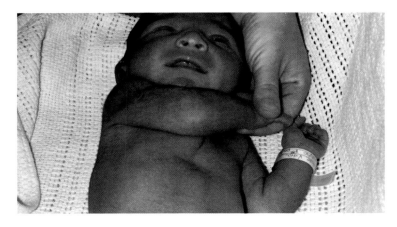

FIG. 2.13 *Scarf sign. The elbow cannot be drawn, with gentle traction on the upper extremity, across this term infant's chest. This is in contrast to the marked flexibility of a preterm infant.*

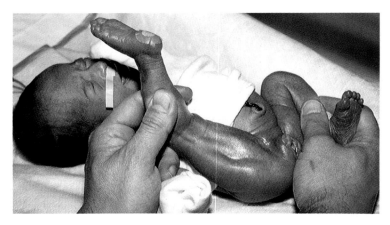

FIG. 2.14 *Heel-to-ear maneuver. The position for assessing the heel-to-ear maneuver is demonstrated. The degree of extension seen is consistent with a 28- to 30-week infant.*

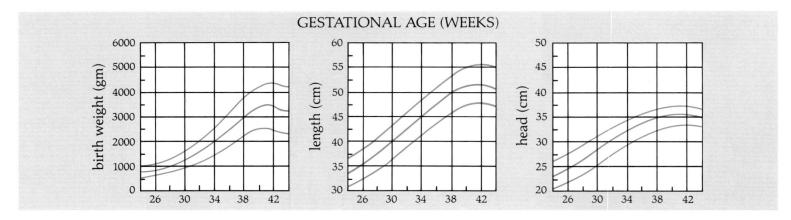

FIG. 2.15 *The mean (± 2 standard deviations) weight, length, and head circumference for infants born at various gestational ages. Infants above or below the curves are considered too large or too small for gestational age. (Reproduced with permission from Usher R, McLean F: Intrauterine growth of liveborn Caucasian infant at sea level. J Pediatr 1969; 74:901.)*

Resting tone of the upper extremities can be assessed by eliciting the scarf sign. Gentle traction of the upper extremities across the chest in a rostral direction ("placing a scarf on the infant") while examining the position of the elbow will reveal a decreasing displacement of the elbow as gestational age increases (Fig. 2.13).

In a similar manner, resting tone of the lower extremities can be assessed by the heel-to-ear maneuver. With the infant on its back, a foot is moved as near to the ipsilateral ear as possible without exerting undue force. The pelvis must be kept flat during the evaluation. The most premature infants can easily touch their heel to their ear (Fig. 2.14). This becomes somewhat more difficult after 30 weeks, and impossible by approximately the 34th week of gestational age.

Abnormalities of Growth

One of the important advances in neonatal medicine has been the realization that the size of an infant at birth does not necessarily reflect gestational age (Fig. 2.15). The parameter most commonly affected is weight, especially in infants who are small for gestational age. A number of terms have been applied to small infants, including "small for gestational age (SGA)," "intrauterine growth retardation (IUGR)," and "fetal malnutrition (FM)." The last is probably most descriptive of those infants whose weight is inappropriately low in relation to length and head circumference. These infants, who appear long and thin, often have an obvious loss of subcutaneous tissue which is best seen over the buttocks and within the folds of the neck.

The relationship between weight, length, and head circumference can be useful in understanding the etiology of the small size. Conditions that affect growth during the third trimester of pregnancy, such as preeclampsia, tend to interfere with the normal acquisition of fatty tissue while sparing brain growth (and thus head circumference) and linear growth. These infants have an asymmetrical form of growth retardation. In more severe cases, the onset of protein catabolism will affect muscle mass. By comparing length or head circumference percentiles to the weight percentile at any given gestational age, one can detect growth retardation even if the actual weight still falls within two standard deviations of normal. Often infants who are postmature (>42 weeks) have some decrease in weight compared to length or head circumference. Problems beginning earlier than the third trimester tend to produce more generalized growth retardation (Fig. 2.16). In the more premature infants, such global decreases in growth often complicate assessment of gestational age since the tools are rather limited in infants born at 24 to 28 weeks' gestation. Two of the most important causes of generalized growth retardation are chromosomal syndromes and congenital infections. A thorough investigation of such

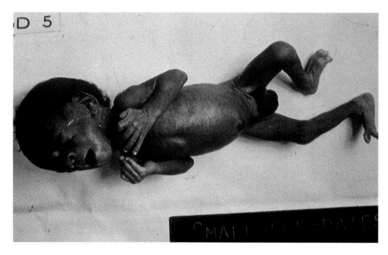

FIG. 2.16 Intrauterine growth retardation. This term baby weighed only 1.7 kg. The head appears disproportionately large for the thin, wasted body. This resulted from placental insufficiency late in pregnancy. Hypoglycemia may be a complication. (Courtesy of TALC, Institute of Child Health)

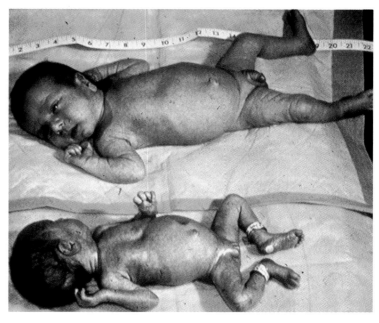

FIG. 2.17 Discordant twins. This is a pair of markedly discordant dizygotic twins. Disturbed placentation accounted for the marked reduction in size of the smaller twin.

FIG. 2.18 Large-for-gestational age infant. This infant of a diabetic mother weighed 5.0 kg at birth, and exhibits the typical rounded facies.

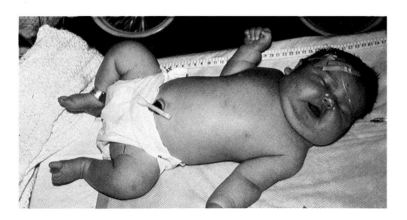

problems should be undertaken in any unexplained instance of generalized growth retardation.

Multiple gestation pregnancies often produce infants who are both premature and symmetrically small. Size discordancy (>10 percent difference in weight) between identical twins is fairly common, as their placentas can share vascular connections, resulting in overperfusion of one twin and underperfusion of the other. This leads to a marked difference in size, with the growth of underperfused twin being symmetrically retarded. Discordancy may also occur in dizygotic twins (Fig. 2.17) if one of the pair has inadequate placentation. Rarely, one of a pair of twins may be afflicted with a chromosomal abnormality or a congenital infection, while the other is normal.

Infants who are too large for gestational age (LGA) are often the products of pregnancies in diabetic or prediabetic mothers. The effect is usually noted during the third trimester, with infants at term weighing greater than 8 pounds. Weight is the most affected parameter but length and head circumference are often increased as well. Infants of diabetic mothers often are identifiable by their macrosomia, round facies (Fig. 2.18), and sometimes by plethora and hirsutism (especially of the pinnae). They may also demonstrate visceromegaly, with enlargement particularly of the liver and heart.

While infants greater than 8 pounds are more likely to be from diabetic pregnancies, a significant number of large term infants are the products of normal pregnancies. Nevertheless, all LGA infants should be routinely screened for hypoglycemia, and their mothers investigated for the possibility of undiagnosed diabetes mellitus. Two fairly unusual syndromes can also serve as the cause for excessive newborn size: (1) cerebral gigantism, or Soto syndrome, in which infants have macrosomia, macrocephaly, large hands and feet, and ultimately poor coordination and variable mental deficiency; and (2) Beckwith-Wiedemann syndrome, whose prominent features include macrosomia, macroglossia, omphalocele, linear ear fissures, and neonatal hypoglycemia (see Endocrinology, Chapter 9).

THE PLACENTA

Careful examination of the placenta can prove to be a valuable aid in the diagnosis and treatment of the newborn infant. It is most unfortunate that it has been relegated to an "afterbirth" and is often immediately discarded without knowing the condition of the offspring. After trimming the membranes and cord, the normal ratio of fetal to placental weight is approximately 4–7 to 1. The configuration, color,

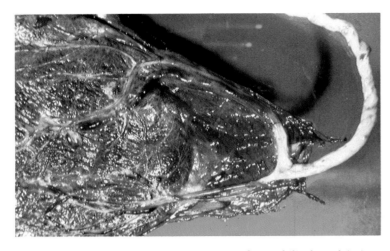

FIG. 2.19 Velamentous cord insertion. The umbilical cord is inserted into the amniotic membranes rather than into the placental disc. This leaves the umbilical vessels relatively unprotected and predisposes them to rupture.

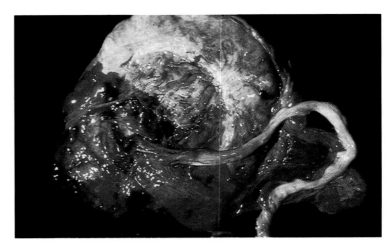

FIG. 2.20 Circumvallate placenta. There is extension of villous tissue beyond the chorionic surface, with a well-defined hyalinized fold at the edge of the chorionic plate.

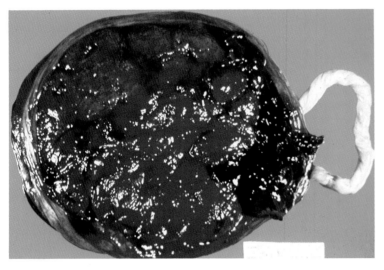

FIG. 2.21 Abruptio placenta. Examination of this placenta reveals a small abruption site, with an adherent blood clot along the margin.

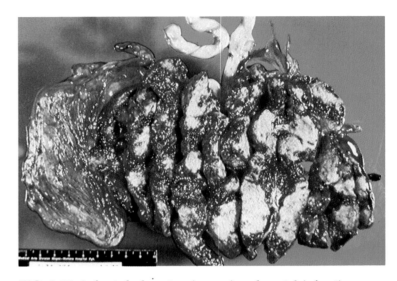

FIG. 2.22 Infarcted placenta. A massive placental infarction comprising the majority of the villous surface is shown. Such an extensive infarction compromises fetal nutrition and oxygenation.

condition of the membranes, insertion of the cord, and condition of both the fetal and maternal surfaces are all relevant.

The insertion of the umbilical cord into the placenta, which can be central, eccentric, marginal, or velamentous, can be important in understanding unexplained asphyxia or blood loss. In a velamentous insertion (Fig. 2.19), the cord is inserted into the membranes rather than into the disc, leaving the umbilical vessels unprotected for a variable distance. These vessels are more prone to rupture, with resultant fetal hemorrhage (vasa previa).

At times, placentation itself is abnormal. In a circumvallate placenta (Fig. 2.20), the villous tissue projects beyond the chorionic surface, with a hyalinized fold at the edge of the chorionic plate. This type of placentation has been reported to be a cause of antepartum bleeding, premature labor, and increased perinatal mortality.

Premature placental separation (abruptio placenta) can lead to an accumulation of blood behind the placenta (Fig. 2.21). Although the bleeding is usually of maternal origin,

fetal blood loss may also occur. Large abruptions may lead to poor growth, fetal asphyxia, or even death. It is important to distinguish a true abruption, where an adherent clot compresses the maternal surface, from the nonadherent collection of blood which forms upon normal placental separation.

Placental infarctions (Fig. 2.22) are among the more common, easily diagnosed abnormalities. They tend to occur along the margin of the placenta, and can vary in color from red to yellowish-white. When small, they are usually of little significance. However, large (>30 percent of placental volume) central infarcts can be clinically significant by reducing the placental surface available for fetal oxygenation and nutrition. Infarcts are most common in pregnancies complicated by hypertension.

Chorioamnionitis (Fig 2.23), inflammation of the fetal membranes, is an immediate clue to potential neonatal infection. Upon gross examination, the membranes lack their normal sheen and translucency, appearing gray or yellow. Inflammation, confirmable by microscopic examination, can

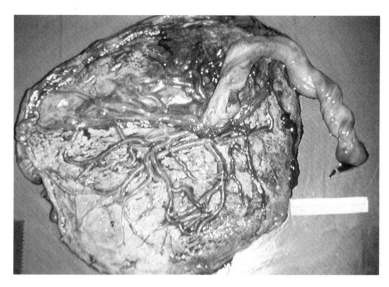

FIG. 2.23 *Chorioamnionitis. This is a placental specimen from a pregnancy with documented amniotic fluid infection. The surface of the membranes is opaque and shows yellowish discoloration.*

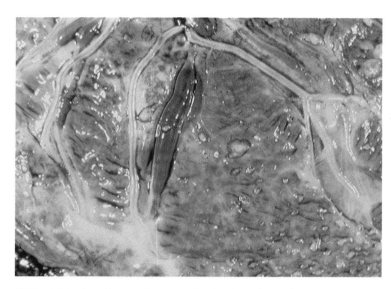

FIG. 2.24 *Amnion nodosum. The fetal surface of this placenta from a pregnancy with oligohydramnios demonstrates multiple nodules consistent with amnion nodosum. This finding suggests a strong possibility of renal agenesis or dysgenesis.*

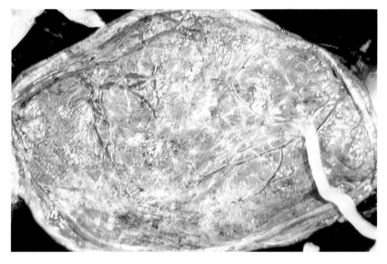

FIG. 2.25 *Monochorionic, monoamniotic placenta. Examination of this placenta from monozygotic twins reveals no dividing membranes, thus assuring monozygosity.*

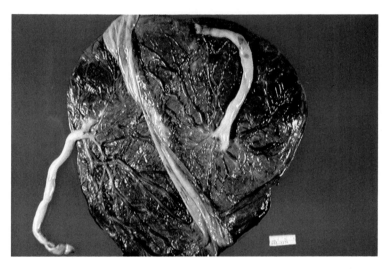

FIG. 2.26 *Dichorionic, diamniotic placenta. The presence of two amniotic sacs and separate chorions in this twin placenta precludes determination of zygosity.*

also be found in the fetal vessels of the chorionic plate and the umbilical cord.

In pregnancies in which the quantity of amniotic fluid is decreased (oligohydramnios), examination of the amnion may also reveal shiny, gray, flat nodules known as amnion nodosum (Fig. 2.24). The presence of these nodules can be an immediate clue to the diagnosis of renal dysfunction or agenesis in the newborn. Since such infants may also have hypoplastic lungs and dysmorphic features (such as occurs in Potter syndrome) this early clue to the diagnosis can be most helpful to the physician and family.

In multiple gestation deliveries, a careful placental evaluation is crucial. The major distinction to be made is whether there is a single chorion or outer layer of the fetal membranes. When twins are present in a single amniotic cavity, and thus a single chorion (Fig. 2.25), monozygosity is as-sured. For all practical purposes, a single chorion which bridges two amniotic sacs is also evidence for monozygotic twins. In this instance, it is essential to carefully examine the membranes at the site of connection of the two amniotic sacs. When two chorions and two amnions (or a total of four membranes at their interface) are present (Fig. 2.26), twins may be either monozygotic or dizygotic. Approximately 36 percent of monozygotic twins are dichorionic.

BIRTH TRAUMA

In the vast majority of cases, a newborn infant is left relatively unscathed by the birth process. However, there are times when both transient and permanent stigmata of birth trauma are evident. Prompt identification of such injuries is not only important for good management, it can also prevent

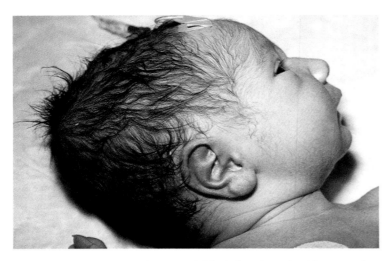

FIG. 2.27 Caput succedaneum. This infant has significant scalp edema as a result of compression during transit through the birth canal. The edema crosses suture lines.

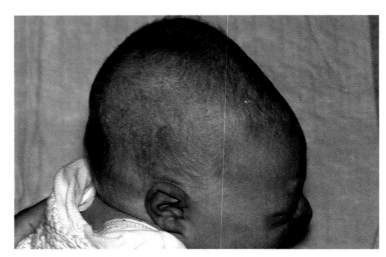

FIG. 2.28 Cephalohematoma. In this infant with bilateral cephalohematomas, the midline sagittal suture remained palpable, confirming the subperiosteal location of the hematomas.

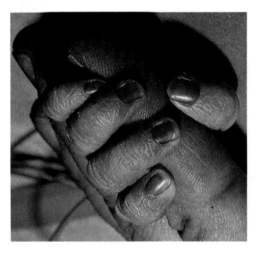

FIG. 2.29 Meconium staining. The marked discoloration of this infant's fingernails resulted from longstanding meconium staining of the amniotic fluid prior to delivery.

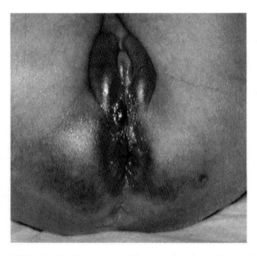

FIG. 2.30 Bruising. This severe bruising of the perineum was the result of a difficult breech labor and delivery.

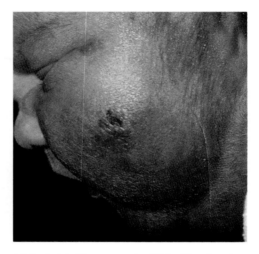

FIG. 2.31 Fat necrosis. This discolored nodular lesion on the cheek is characteristic of subcutaneous necrosis of fat secondary to forceps trauma.

inappropriate speculation, diagnostic tests, and treatment. This section will review some of the more common birth-related physical signs and appropriate therapy.

Caput Succedaneum

Normal transit of the fetal head through the birth canal induces both molding of the skull and scalp edema, especially if labor is prolonged. The edema, which can be massive, is known as a caput succedaneum (Fig. 2.27). Much of this edema is present at birth and tends to overlie both the occipital bones and portions of the parietal bones, bilaterally. In some cases, bruising of the scalp may also be present (especially if a vacuum extractor was employed). The presence of a caput requires no therapy, and spontaneous resolution within a few days is the rule. At times, it can be difficult to distinguish a caput from a rare but serious subgaleal (subaponeurotic) hematoma, which is a collection of blood within scalp tissues extending under the epicranial aponeurosis. Such infants, however, will show signs of progressive hypovolemia. While the exact source and location of bleeding may be unclear initially, awareness of the possibility of massive

blood loss extending under a large portion of the scalp, and prompt replacement can be lifesaving.

Cephalohematoma

Often, confusion arises between the diagnosis of a caput and that of a cephalohematoma. The latter is a localized collection of blood beneath the periosteum of one of the calvarial bones. It is distinguished from a caput by the fact that its borders are limited by suture lines, usually those surrounding the parietal bones. However, diagnosis can be difficult in the immediate newborn period when there may be overlying scalp edema. Cephalohematoma can be bilateral (Fig. 2.28), but it is more often unilateral. On palpation, the border feels elevated and the center depressed. Most patients have an uncomplicated course of slow resolution over 1 or more months, with possible calcification. Occasionally complications are seen, the most common being jaundice, resulting from breakdown and resorption of a large hematoma. Secondary anemia should also be considered when the hematoma is large. Underlying hairline skull fractures occur with some regularity, but are rarely of clinical significance. The exception is the uncommon

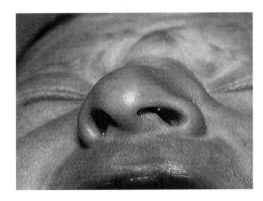

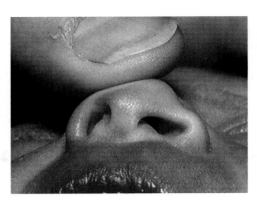

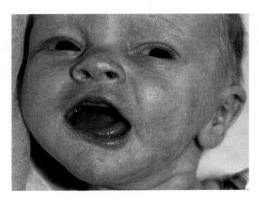

FIG. 2.32 Nasal deformity. This infant incurred dislocation of the triangular cartilage of the nasal septum during delivery. Inspection of the nose reveals deviation of the septum to the right and asymmetry of the nares (left). When the septum is manually moved toward the midline, the asymmetry persists, confirming the dislocation (right).

FIG. 2.33 Facial nerve palsy. This infant incurred injury to the right facial nerve, resulting in loss of the nasolabial fold on the affected side, and asymmetrical movement of the mouth. The side of the mouth which appears to droop is the normal side.

development of a leptomeningeal cyst. Radiologic investigation for an underlying depressed fracture is indicated in those infants whose histories suggest significant trauma, and those having depressed levels of consciousness and/or neurologic abnormalities on examination. Another potentially serious, though rare, complication is infection. This is more likely to occur when the integrity of the overlying skin is broken. Needle aspiration of a cephalohematoma is contraindicated because of the risk of introducing microorganisms.

Meconium Staining

Meconium is noted in the amniotic fluid in as many as 10 percent of deliveries. The meconium may have been recently expelled or may have been present in the amniotic fluid for hours or days. Since the timing of the passage of meconium may have significance for the diagnosis of asphyxia, it is useful to examine infants for the presence of meconium staining. Apparently, it takes at least 4 to 6 hours of contact before staining of the umbilicus, skin, and nails occurs (Fig. 2.29). Often, the meconium-stained infant is postmature and has diffuse peeling of the skin as well as a shriveled, stained umbilical cord.

Bruises and Petechiae

Superficial bruising can occur whenever delivery is difficult. This is relatively common with breech presentations (Fig. 2.30), and can include swelling and discoloration of the labia and of the scrotum (to be distinguished from an incarcerated inguinal hernia). When bruises are extensive, significant secondary jaundice may develop as the extravasated blood is broken down and resorbed. In those infants in whom a nuchal cord is found at delivery, the presence of diffuse petechiae around the head and neck is a common occurrence and does not warrant further investigation. The appearance of new bruises or petechiae after delivery should alert the physician and nurse to the possibility of a bleeding disorder.

Fat Necrosis

Many infants delivered with the aid of forceps show forceps marks after delivery, which tend to fade over 24 to 48 hours.

Occasionally, a well-circumscribed, firm nodule with purplish discoloration may appear at the site of a forceps mark. This is felt to represent fat necrosis (Fig. 2.31), and resolves spontaneously over weeks to months. The phenomenon may occur at other sites of trauma as well.

Nasal Deformities

Abnormalities of the nose are commonly seen after delivery, the majority consisting of transient flattening or twisting of the nose induced during transit through the birth canal. Less than 1 percent of nasal deformities are due to actual dislocations of the triangular cartilage of the nasal septum. These can be differentiated from positional deformities by manually moving the septum to the midline and observing the resultant shape of the nares. In a true dislocation, marked asymmetry of the nares persists (Fig. 2.32). Returning the septum to its proper position can be accomplished in the nursery with the guidance of an otolaryngologist. Failure to recognize and treat dislocation may lead to permanent deformity.

Peripheral Nerve Damage

Injury to the peripheral nervous system, especially the facial and brachial nerves, is one of the more common serious occurrences related to birth. Unilateral facial nerve palsy is the most common peripheral nerve injury, with an incidence as high as 1.4 per 1,000 live births. Injury can be the result of direct trauma from forceps or of compression of the nerve against the sacral promontory while the head is in the birth canal. With pronounced nerve injury, there is decreased facial movement and forehead wrinkling on the side of the palsy, eyelid elevation, and flattening of the nasolabial folds and corner of the mouth (Fig. 2.33). Crying accentuates the findings, with the most obvious sign being asymmetrical movement of the mouth. The side which appears to droop when crying is the normal side. The differential diagnosis includes Möbius syndrome (usually bilateral) and absence of the depressor anguli oris muscle, which may be associated with cardiac anomalies. The latter condition is distinguishable from facial nerve palsy by the absence of any involvement of the forehead, eyelid, or nasolabial area. The prognosis for facial nerve palsies is excellent, and recovery usually

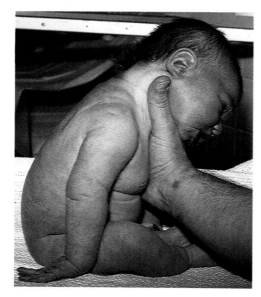

FIG. 2.34 Brachial plexus injury. Traction injury to C5, C6, and C7 (Erb) spinal cord segments produces this palsy. The infant shown demonstrates the characteristic posture of the limply adducted and internally rotated arm.

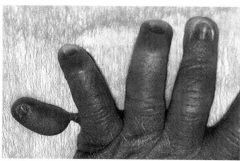

FIG. 2.35 Supernumerary digit. This is the common position for a sixth digit. The thin pedicle distinguishes this anomaly from true polydactyly.

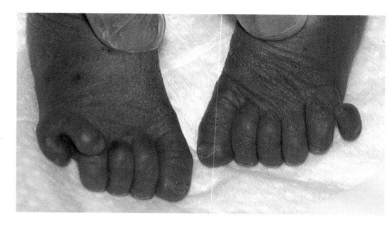

FIG. 2.36 Polydactyly. True bilateral polydactyly of the fifth toe is seen in this infant.

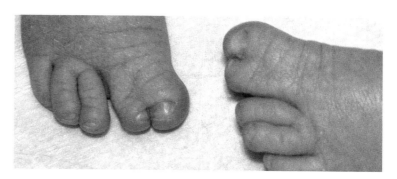

FIG. 2.37 Syndactyly. This child demonstrates bilateral fusion of the soft tissue between the first and second toes.

occurs within the first month. In the meantime, prevention of corneal drying is essential. Surgery is reserved for cases in which clear-cut severing of the facial nerve has occurred.

The incidence of brachial plexus trauma with current obstetric management is approximately 0.7 per 1,000 live births. The mechanism of injury in most instances is traction on the plexus during delivery. Although lesions have classically been divided into those affecting upper spinal segments (Erb palsy) and those affecting lower segments (Klumpke palsy), the distinction may not be clear-cut in some cases. Injury to the C5 and C6 fibers is most often identified by the child's arm hanging limply adducted and internally rotated at the shoulder, and extended and pronated at the elbow (Fig. 2.34). Appropriate deep-tendon reflexes are absent. It may be difficult to confirm sensory deficit, and autonomic fibers are often intact. Diagnosis is made clinically, but electromyography may be indicated to assess severity of injury and to determine prognosis in patients not showing improvement after 6 to 8 weeks. Treatment should be deferred for at least 7 to 10 days; then, specific physical therapy and splinting should be undertaken. Most infants with brachial plexus palsies demonstrate complete recovery in the first few months of life. The earlier recovery begins, the better the long-term prognosis.

CONGENITAL ANOMALIES

There are innumerable congenital anomalies, many of a minor nature, which can be noted at birth. While any single minor malformation may be of little medical consequence, the identification of three or more in a single infant may be a clue to more serious errors of morphogenesis. A careful family history, including examination of the parents and siblings, can often place these malformations in proper perspective.

Digits

The majority of minor external anomalies involve the hands, feet, and head. One of the more common abnormalities of digitation, especially in black infants, is the presence of a supernumerary digit (Fig. 2.35). These are most often located lateral to the fifth digit, either on the hand or foot. They are distinguishable from true polydactyly because of the small pedicle which attaches them to the fifth digit. The supernumerary digit may have a fingernail, but often lacks bones. While usually of no consequence, they have, on occasion, been associated with major CNS malformations. Removal may be accomplished by applying a ligature around the pedicle (assuming it is thin and lacks palpable bony tissue) as close as possible to the surface of the fifth digit, and allowing for the digit to fall off naturally. This usually takes approximately 1 week. Care should be taken to observe for infection. True polydactyly (duplication of digits) may also be seen (Fig. 2.36). It is most common on the feet, but can also occur on the hands. There may be a family history of this anomaly, or it may occur in association with other, more serious patterns of malformation. While removal is not required, it may be

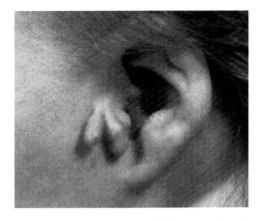

FIG. 2.38 Ear tags. Multiple preauricular skin tags were seen as an isolated finding in this patient.

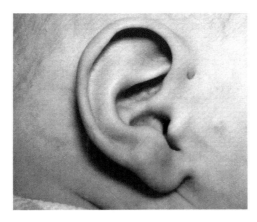

FIG. 2.39 Aural fistula. A pronounced congenital ear pit is seen anterior to the tragus. Its only significance is that it may become infected.

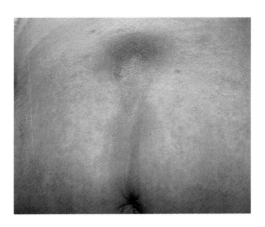

FIG. 2.40 Pilonidal sinus. This midline sinus overlying the sacrum did not extend to the spinal cord.

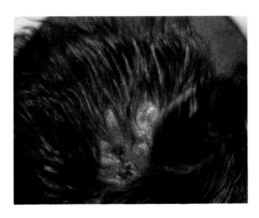

FIG. 2.41 Localized ectodermal dysplasia. An extensive punched-out area lacking all normal dermal elements is seen in the midline of the scalp of this child with trisomy 13.

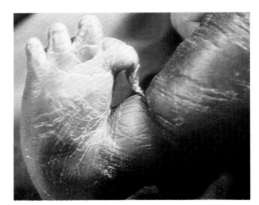

FIG. 2.42 Amniotic bands. A lower extremity amniotic band caused amputation of the toes and constriction around the lower leg.

indicated cosmetically. Syndactyly, fusion of the soft tissues between digits, is relatively common (Fig. 2.37). Once again, a family history can be helpful.

External Ear

Careful morphologic examination of the external ear may reveal a number of minor anomalies. One of the more common is the presence of preauricular skin tags located anterior to the tragus (Fig. 2.38). They may be unilateral or bilateral, and represent remnants of the first branchial arch. Although often of little consequence, they may be seen in more serious malformations of branchial arch development involving multiple structures of the head and neck. Surgical removal may be indicated for cosmetic purposes.

A second, often overlooked malformation is the presence of ear pits or congenital aural fistulas located anterior to the tragus (Fig. 2.39). These may be familial, occur twice as often in females, and are more common in blacks. They are of little consequence beyond the fact that they may become infected.

Midline Defects

While major malformations of the spinal column such as myelomeningocele are readily identifiable (see Pediatric Neurology, Chapter 15), diagnostic differentiation between two other midline defects—pilonidal sinuses and congenital dermal sinuses of the lumbar and sacral spine—can be difficult. A pilonidal sinus tends to be located over the sacrum (Fig. 2.40). The surface opening is usually larger than that of a dermal sinus, but the tract rarely extends into the spinal canal. Therefore, while infection can occur, CNS extension is unlikely. A congenital dermal sinus is usually located over the lower lumbar region, with a sinus tract that can extend farther down the spinal column. The external orifice may be a small dimple or an easily visible opening surrounded by hair. Recognition is important, as there may be an underlying spinal dysraphism, and infection of the tract can extend to the CNS. Both types of sinuses may coexist in the same infant. If diagnostic differentiation is difficult, radiographic and neurosurgical evaluations may be indicated.

Another form of midline defect may occur over the posterior parietal scalp and consists of a localized area of ectodermal dysplasia (Fig. 2.41). This lesion appears "punched out" and lacks all normal dermal elements. It may be associated with chromosomal anomalies, especially trisomy 13, but may be present in otherwise normal infants. Similar lesions, often located on the extremities, are to be distinguished from those on the scalp, since they often represent a dermatologic defect known as cutis aplasia.

Amniotic Bands

A number of serious structural deformations can result from early in utero amniotic rupture and subsequent bandline compression or amputation. The band-induced abnormalities generally affect the limbs, digits, and craniofacial structures (Fig. 2.42). This phenomenon is usually sporadic.

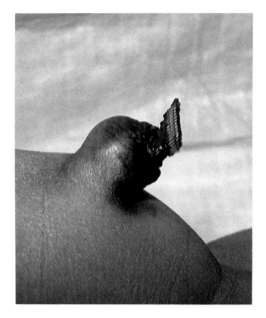

FIG. 2.43 Umbilical hernia. This prominent umbilical hernia was noted at birth in an otherwise normal black infant.

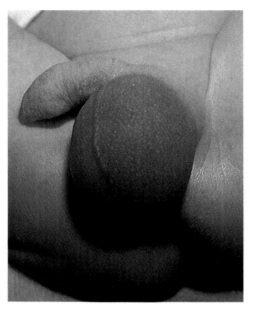

FIG. 2.44 Scrotal swelling. This infant demonstrates a unilateral hydrocele which was noted at birth. Transillumination was consistent with the diagnosis.

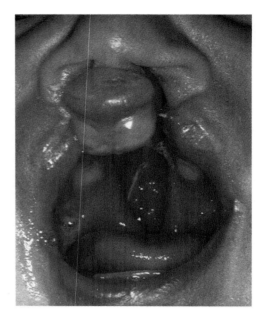

FIG. 2.45 Cleft lip. A prominent bilateral cleft lip coupled with a complete cleft palate is seen in an infant with trisomy 13. The cleft extends from the soft to the hard palate, exposing the nasal cavity.

Umbilical Hernia

An umbilical hernia is a common finding, especially in black infants (Fig. 2.43). The incidence of this defect of the central fascia beneath the umbilicus is also higher in premature infants and those with congenital thyroid deficiency. It is important to distinguish between this relatively benign fascial defect and the more serious defects of those somites which form the peritoneal, muscular, and ectodermal layers of the abdominal wall underlying the umbilicus, resulting in an omphalocele. In the latter condition, a portion of the intestine is located outside of the abdominal wall (see Pediatric Surgery, Chapter 17). When large, the distinction is obvious, but in its mildest form it will resemble a fixed hernia of the umbilicus. A true umbilical hernia requires no therapy, since the majority resolve spontaneously in the first few years of life. Those that remain after the age of 3 years can be surgically repaired. Attempts to reduce the hernia with tape or coins are ineffective. Incarceration is rare.

Scrotal Swelling

Swelling of the scrotum in the neonate is a relatively common finding, especially in breech deliveries. While the differential diagnosis includes hematomas, infections, testicular torsion, and tumors, the great majority of cases are attributable to hydroceles or fluid accumulation in the tunica vaginalis. Palpation reveals an extremely smooth, firm, egg-shaped mass which brightly transilluminates (Fig. 2.44). When the hydrocele is noncommunicating, one can often get above the mass with a palpatory thumb and finger and feel a normal spermatic cord. The testicle may be difficult to palpate, but is usually visible upon transillumination. It should be noted that with inguinal hernias, the prolapsed intestine may transilluminate as well, but usually presents visible septa under high-intensity light. Furthermore, on palpation there is significant thickening of the spermatic cord. While a hydrocele may persist for months, the majority resolve spontaneously. There is a high association with inguinal hernias, especially in those hydroceles which persist. In such cases, the spermatic cord is often noticeably thickened. Given the association with hernias, the possibility of bowel incarceration should be kept in mind. Surgical repair is indicated when a hydrocele persists for more than 6 months, or when it is associated with findings suggestive of an inguinal hernia. See Chapter 17 for a more detailed discussion of inguinal hernias.

Oral Clefts

Cleft lip and/or palate are among the most common facial anomalies (Fig. 2.45). These defects represent failure of lip fusion (at 35 days) and, in some cases, subsequent failure of closure of the palatal shelves (at 8 to 9 weeks). While many cases occur spontaneously, others appear to be inherited, and in a minority of instances the defect is one manifestation of a chromosomal disorder. Adequate assessment necessitates careful examination of all the structures of the head and neck and their relationship to each other. For example, cleft palate may be coupled with mandibular hypoplasia (Pierre Robin anomaly), resulting in significant respiratory obstruction. Because of associated eustachian tube dysfunction, otitis media is an almost invariable complication of cleft palate. Specialized feeding techniques are often necessary for these infants. Even in the absence of an overt cleft, palpation and visualization of the palate and uvula should be routine, since clefts of the soft palate (associated with a bifid uvula and a midline notch at the posterior border of the hard palate) can lead to later speech problems.

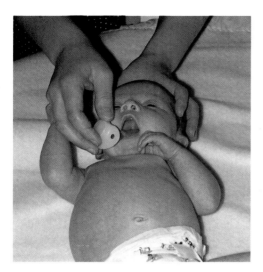

FIG. 2.46 Rooting reflex. The infant opens his mouth and turns his head towards the pacifier stimulating his cheek.

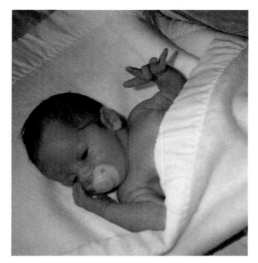

FIG. 2.47 Sucking reflex. Vigorous sucking movements are initiated when an object is placed in the infant's mouth.

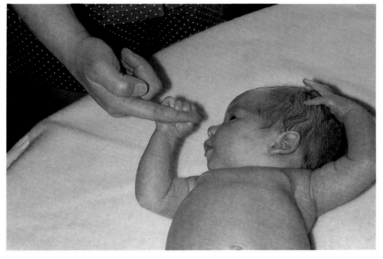

FIG. 2.48 Grasp reflex (palm). Transverse stimulation of the mid-palm leads to a grasp by the infant.

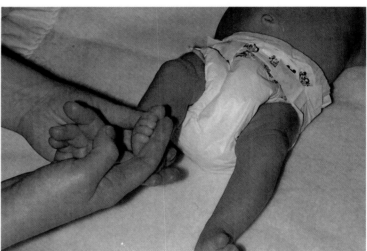

FIG. 2.49 Grasp reflex (sole). Transverse stimulation of the mid-sole triggers a grasp by the infant.

PRIMITIVE REFLEXES

Normal newborns exhibit a large number of easily elicited primitive reflexes which are often altered or absent in the infant with neurologic impairment. These reflexes may be transiently depressed in the infant who has experienced difficulty in achieving the transition between intra- and extrauterine existence. The persistent absence or asymmetry of one or more of these reflexes may be a clue to the potential presence of neuromuscular abnormalities requiring further investigation (see Developmental Pediatrics, Chapter 3).

The rooting reflex may be elicited by lightly stimulating the infant's cheek and observing his reflexive attempts to bring the stimulating object to his mouth (Fig. 2.46). The sucking reflex is activated by placing an object in the infant's mouth and observing the sucking movements (Fig. 2.47). The grasp reflex is illustrated in Figures 2.48 and 2.49, where transverse stimulation of the mid-palm or mid-sole leads to flexion of the digits or toes around the examiner's fingers.

The Moro reflex (Fig. 2.50) evaluates both vestibular maturation and the relationship between flexor and extensor tone. Elicitation of the reflex involves a short (10 cm), sudden drop of the head when the infant is supine. The full response in-

volves extension of the arms, "fanning" of the fingers, then upper extremity flexion followed by a cry. An incomplete but identifiable reflex becomes apparent at approximately 32 weeks of gestation, and by 38 weeks, it is essentially complete. The more immature infants demonstrate extension of the arms and fingers, but no true flexion or sustained cry. Marked asymmetry of response may be associated with focal neurologic impairment.

These, and a host of other less commonly utilized reflexes are termed "primitive" because they are present at or shortly after birth, and normally disappear after the first few months of life. Just as their absence may indicate neurologic impairment at birth, their abnormal persistence may also be cause for concern.

RESPIRATORY DISTRESS

The differential diagnosis and the subsequent management of the infant with respiratory distress are the most frequent challenges encountered by the practitioner of newborn medicine. Problems posed by prematurity, the failure of the necessary transition to extrauterine existence, infectious complications, metabolic derangements, and various congenital and

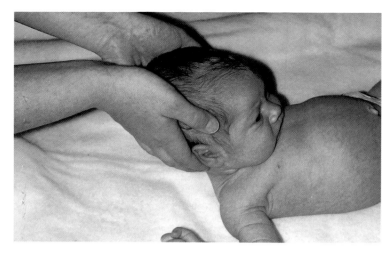

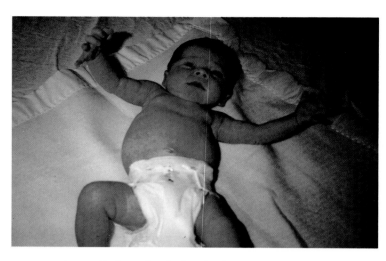

FIG. 2.50 *The Moro reflex. To elicit the reflex, the head is supported and allowed to drop to the level of the bed (***left***). The initial extension* *response to vestibular stimulation is shown at the* ***right***. *The complete response includes secondary flexion and cry.*

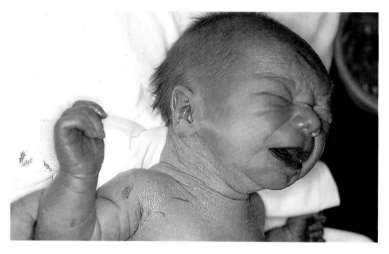

FIG. 2.51 *Cyanosis. This critically ill infant exhibits cyanosis and poor skin perfusion.*

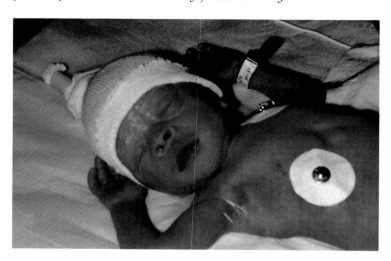

FIG. 2.52 *Flaring. Reflexive widening of the nares may be seen in infants with respiratory distress.*

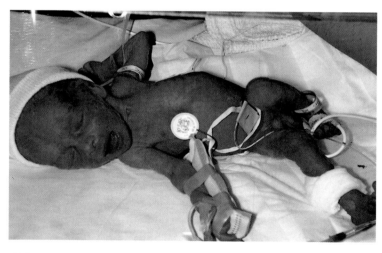

FIG. 2.53 *Retractions. The inward collapse of the lower anterior chest wall can be seen in this premature infant with respiratory distress syndrome.*

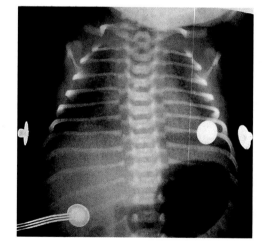

FIG. 2.54 *Respiratory distress syndrome. Note the "ground glass" appearance and the presence of air bronchograms.*

acquired abnormalities of the cardiopulmonary system may all lead to a similar presentation in the newborn period.

Infants with respiratory distress may present with tachypnea and/or cyanosis (Fig. 2.51), and varying degrees of a triad of signs termed grunting, flaring, and retractions ("GFR"). Grunting is a characterstic involuntary guttural expiratory sound made by infants as they exhale against a closed glottis in an attempt to maintain their expiratory lung volume. Flar-

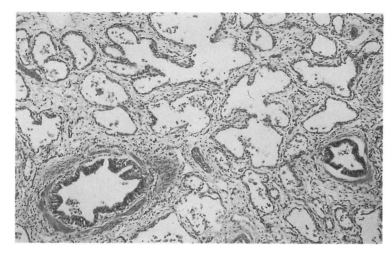

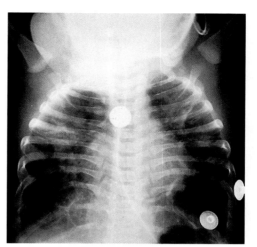

FIG. 2.56 Broncho-pulmonary dyspla-sia. Note the alternating areas of hyperinflation and atelectasis.

FIG. 2.55 Bronchopulmonary dysplasia. Histologic features include inflammation and fibrosis.

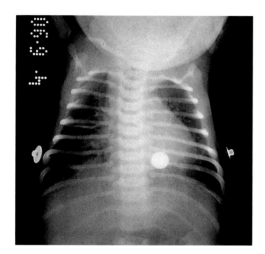

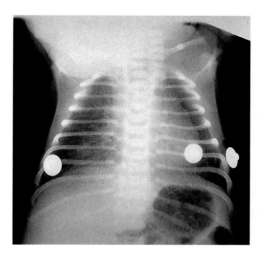

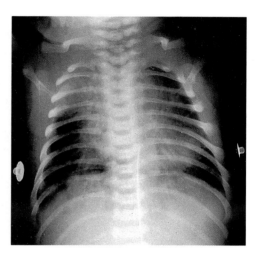

FIG. 2.57 Transient tachypnea of the newborn. Radiograph reveals a number of streaky perihilar densities, and a visible fluid density in the right major fissure.

FIG. 2.58 Congenital pneumonia. Cultures from the lungs of this infant were positive for Group B Streptococcus. Note the similarity to previous radiographs.

FIG. 2.59 Meconium aspiration. The radiograph reveals irregularly distributed areas of hyperaeration and consolidation.

ing refers to the reflexive opening of the nares during inspiration in such infants (Fig. 2.52). Retractions are the result of increased respiratory effort with high negative intrathoracic pressures leading to an inward collapse of the relatively compliant chest wall of the newborn during inspiration (Fig. 2.53).

Classic respiratory distress syndrome (RDS) is caused by a combination of lung immaturity secondary to preterm delivery, and surfactant deficiency. The radiographic findings in such infants consist of a "ground glass" appearance (small airway and alveolar atelectasis) and "air bronchograms" (an outline of the large airways superimposed upon the relatively airless lung parenchyma) (Fig. 2.54). Infants with RDS usually need supplemental oxygen therapy and often require mechanical ventilatory assistance.

Most infants with RDS recover without sequelae. However, a small proportion develop a chronic lung condition known as bronchopulmonary dysplasia. Histologically, this condition is characterized by varying degrees of inflammation and fibrosis (Fig. 2.55). The chest x-rays of such infants exhibit areas of hyperinflation alternating with atelectasis (Fig. 2.56).

The most common cause of respiratory distress in the newborn period among term infants is transient tachypnea of the newborn (TTN). Thought to be related to the delayed removal of fetal alveolar fluid, this condition is more common in infants born by cesarean section. Radiographic findings may include streaky perihilar shadows caused by dilated lymphatics and/or visible fluid densities within the intralobar fissures (Fig. 2.57). As its name implies, TTN resolves over time, usually with minimal supportive care.

Unfortunately for the clinician, the early clinical and radiographic findings in infants with potentially life-threatening congenital pneumonias may mimic those seen in RDS or TTN (Fig. 2.58). This diagnostic uncertainty leads to early treatment of many of these infants with antibiotics until bacterial cultures, serial chest radiographs, and clinical improvements reassure the practitioner that the discontinuation of such antibiotics is warranted.

Meconium aspiration, discussed in the section of newborn stools, may also manifest with respiratory distress. The radiographic findings consist of irregularly distributed areas of hyperaeration and consolidation throughout the lung parenchyma (Fig. 2.59).

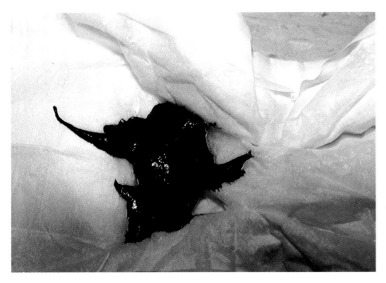

FIG. 2.60 Meconium. A typical, sticky, greenish-black meconium stool is shown. This consists of accumulated intestinal cells, bile, and proteinaceous material formed during intestinal development.

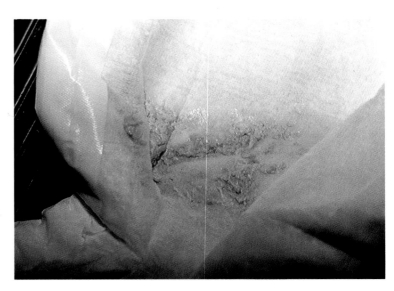

FIG. 2.61 Transitional stool. At 2 to 3 days following delivery, stools become greenish-brown and may contain some milk curds.

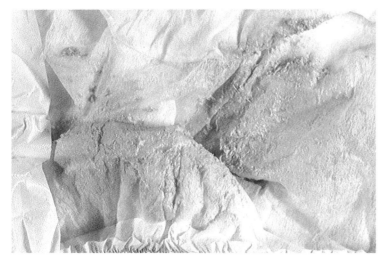

FIG. 2.62 Breast-milk stool. The stools of breast-fed infants are yellow, soft, mild smelling, and typically have the consistency of pea soup.

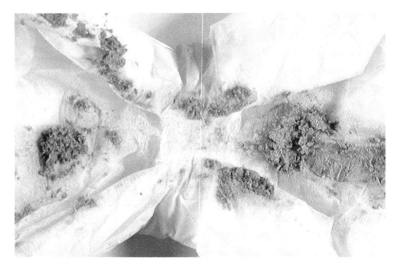

FIG. 2.63 Formula stool. Infants fed commercial formulas typically have darker, firmer stools than do breast-fed infants.

Congenital heart disease (Chapter 5), and various anomalies of the thoracic cavity or the lung itself (Chapter 16) also commonly manifest with signs of respiratory distress in the newborn, and should be included in the differential diagnosis when evaluating such infants.

NEWBORN STOOLS

An infant's first few bowel movements consist of accumulated intestinal cells, bile, and proteinaceous material formed during intestinal development. The material, termed meconium (Fig. 2.60), is a sticky greenish-black product mirroring the shape of the fetal intestine. When passed prior to delivery into the amniotic fluid, it can, if aspirated into the lung, cause a potentially life-threatening disorder known as meconium aspiration syndrome. Such early passage is generally precipitated by fetal distress or asphyxia. Failure to pass meconium in the first 2 days of life may indicate intestinal obstruction due to stenosis, atresia, or Hirschsprung disease. The possibility of cystic fibrosis with a meconium ileus should also be considered. In premature infants, failure to pass meconium may reflect meconium plug syndrome (small left colon syndrome), which appears to be a disorder of maturation of intestinal motility. In most cases, a Gastrografin® enema leads to prompt passage of meconium without recurrence.

By the third day of life, stools change in character, and become what are known as transitional stools (Fig 2.61). They are greenish-brown to yellowish-brown in color, less sticky than meconium, and may contain some milk curds. In some infants who are fed generous quantities of milk during the first few days, the stool may have an increased liquid component which contains undigested sugar. This diarrheal stool will resolve with moderation in the quantity of feeding, since it is caused by the osmotic effect of undigested lactose.

After the third to fourth day, the quality and frequency of stool are often functions of the type of milk given. Breast-fed infants have stools which are yellow to golden in color, mild smelling, and pasty in consistency, resembling pea soup (Fig. 2.62). Although it is commonly held that the mother's diet directly affects the frequency and consistency of a breast-fed infant's stool, there is little scientific information on this subject. Infants fed cow's milk–based formula have pale yellow to light brown stools which are firm and somewhat more offensive in odor (Fig. 2.63).

There is a wide range of normal stool frequency in neonates. Many infants have a stool after each feeding for the first several weeks, due to an active gastrocolic reflex. Other normal infants may have one stool every few days. In general, infants fed cow's milk formula have stools less frequently than those taking breast milk.

A careful history, with emphasis on an infant's stool pattern, feeding history, and any parental attempts (laxatives, rectal manipulation) to induce bowel movements can be extremely important. Normal weight gain in the face of true diarrhea is unusual. Difficulty in passing stools (straining, crying, decreased frequency) may reflect local irritation from anal fissure formation, rather than true constipation. The use of a topical lubricant and stool softeners can often overcome constipation. Failure of such measures suggests the possibility of significant pathology (see Chapter 17 for further discussion).

BIBLIOGRAPHY

Avery GB (ed): *Neonatology—Pathophysiology and Management of the Newborn*, ed 3. Philadelphia, JB Lippincott, 1987.

Ballard JL, Novak KK, Driver M: A simplified score for assessment of fetal maturation of newly-born infants. *J Pediatr* 1979;95:769–774.

Dubowitz LV, Dubowitz C, Goldberger C: Clinical assessment of gestational age in the newborn infant. *J Pediatr* 1970;77:1–10.

Fox H: Pathology of the Placenta, in *Major Problems in Pathology*, Philadelphia, WB Saunders, vol. 7, 1978.

Jones KL: *Smith's Recognizable Patterns of Human Malformation*, ed 4. Philadelphia, WB Saunders, 1988.

Painter MJ, Bergman I: Obstetrical trauma to the neonatal central and peripheral nervous system. *Semin Perinatol* 1982;VI(1):89–104.

Scanlon JW, Nelson T, Grylack LJ, Smith YF: *A System of Newborn Physical Examination*. Baltimore, University Park Press, 1979.

DEVELOPMENTAL–BEHAVIORAL PEDIATRICS

Heidi Feldman, M.D. Ph.D. ◆ Roberta E. Bauer, M.D.

Developmental-behavioral pediatrics is the study of the acquisition of functional skills during childhood, and of variations in sequence or timing that indicate developmental disorders and disabilities. Traditionally, developmental pediatrics concerns itself with cognitive and motor competence and with constitutionally based physical and mental disabilities that limit adaptive functioning. In contrast, behavioral pediatrics emphasizes behavioral and emotional characteristics, and the interaction of family and social variables on these characteristics. We prefer a union of the terms. Developmental-behavioral pediatrics thus emphasizes that cognitive and motor skills interact with social and emotional characteristics in both normal and disordered development.

The goal of this chapter is to familiarize the reader with developmental-behavioral issues faced in routine pediatric practice. The first half discusses the fundamental principles of development and applies them to each major domain of functioning. Within each domain is a discussion of developmental milestones, methods of assessment, signs of developmental variation, and approaches to children who show developmental delay or deviant patterns. The second half describes several developmental disorders including definitions, diagnostic criteria, the role of physical examination in evaluation, and relevant physical findings.

Principles of Normal Development

For ease of description and investigation, development is commonly discussed in terms of domains of function: gross motor skills refer to the use of the large muscles of the body; fine motor skills, to the use of small muscles of the hands; cognition, to the use of higher mental processes, including thinking, memory, and learning; language, to the comprehension and production of meaningful symbolic communication; and social/emotional functioning, to emotional reactions to events and interactions with others. In fact, these domains are interdependent. Cognitive abilities in infancy cannot readily be distinguished from sensorimotor functioning. Similarly, mature social functioning depends on competent language abilities. Perceptual abilities interact with fine motor skills as well as with cognitive abilities. Within each domain, developmental change is generally orderly and predictable.

Developmental Assessment

A central component of health maintenance is developmental surveillance. In surveillance, the physician uses all clinical tools, history, physical examination, screening tests and other assessment techniques to determine a child's developmental status. Observations of the child's level in each developmental domain can often be accomplished in the course of a complete physical examination. This promotes a longitudinal view of the child, and allows parental concerns to be addressed. A formal developmental screening or assessment can be arranged if there are severe or persistent concerns.

Standardized screening methods, such as the Denver Developmental Screening Test, also play an important role in evaluation. Physicians typically use screening tests at selected health maintenance visits, most often at the 9-month visit and again at either the 24-month or the 36-month visit. These tests allow physicians to distinguish normal development from delays and deviations in unselected populations. However, they are inappropriate instruments for populations at risk, who require comprehensive assessment. Screening instruments are better measures of severe developmental delays than of mild delays; some children with minor developmental problems may be missed. Others, however, who are developing normally may fail a screening test because of shyness, unfamiliarity with the examiner or the materials, or other factors unrelated to developmental competence. When parents have concerns about their child's developmental standing, the screening test can be used to confirm but not to describe the nature of the problem. If parental concerns persist despite negative findings, a full evaluation is in order. To ensure that the child's performance is representative of his or her ability, screening tests should be performed when the child is physically well, familiar with the setting and examiner, and under minimal stress.

GROSS MOTOR DEVELOPMENT
Early Reflex Patterns

At birth, a neonate's movements consist of alternating flexions and extensions that usually are symmetric, and vary in strength with the infant's state of wakefulness. Though they appear to be purposeless, these involuntary reflexes indicate

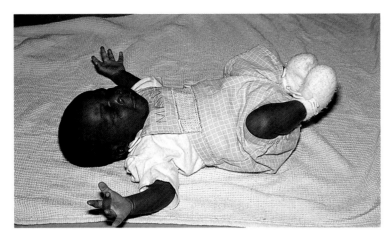

FIG. 3.1 First phase of the Moro response. Symmetric abduction and extension of the extremities follow a loud noise or an abrupt change in the infant's head position.

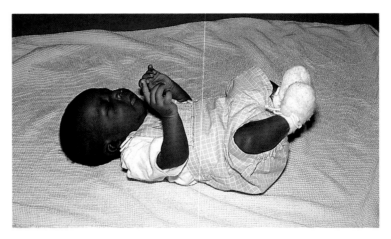

FIG. 3.2 Second phase of the Moro response. Symmetric adduction and flexion of the extremities, accompanied by crying.

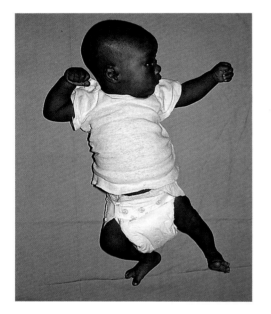

FIG. 3.3 Asymmetric tonic neck reflex (ATNR). Flexion of the arm and leg on the occipital side and extension on the chin side create the "fencer position."

FIG. 3.4

PRIMITIVE REFLEXES AND PROTECTIVE EQUILIBRIUM RESPONSES

Reflex	Appearance	Disappearance
Moro	Birth	4 months
Hand grasp	Birth	3 months
Crossed adductor	Birth	7 months
Toe grasp	Birth	8–15 months
ATNR	2 weeks	6 months
Head righting	4–6 months	Persists voluntarily
Protective equilibrium	4–6 months	Persists voluntarily
Parachute	8–9 months	Persists voluntarily

Different sources may vary on the precise timing of the appearance and disappearance of these primitive and equilibrium responses.

that the patterns of movement requiring the integrated activity of multiple muscle groups are present even at birth.

Perhaps the best known of these patterns is the Moro response. This reflex can occur spontaneously following a loud noise, but typically, it is elicited during the course of physical examination by an abrupt change in the infant's head position. The first phase of the response consists of symmetric abduction and extension of the arms with extension of the trunk (Fig. 3.1). The second phase is marked by adduction of the upper extremities, as in an embrace, and frequently is accompanied by crying (Fig. 3.2). The Moro reflex gradually disappears by 4 months of age, secondary to the development of cortical functioning. In children up to 4 months of age, the Moro response can be used to evaluate the integrity of the central nervous system, and to detect peripheral problems such as congenital musculoskeletal abnormalities or neural plexus injuries.

Another early reflex pattern is called the asymmetric tonic neck reflex (ATNR) (Fig. 3.3). A newborn's limb motions are strongly influenced by head position. If the head is directed to one side, either by passive turning or by inducing the infant to follow an object to that side, extensor muscle tone increases on that side, as well as in the flexor muscles on the opposite side. This response is not often seen immediately after birth, when the child has high flexor tone throughout the body, but it usually appears by 2 to 4 weeks of age. The ATNR allows the child to sight along the arm to the hand, and is considered one of the first steps in the coordination of vision and reaching. This reflex disappears by 6 months of age, secondary to the development of cortical functioning.

With the emergence of voluntary control from higher cortical centers, muscular flexion and extension become balanced. Primitive reflexes are replaced by reactions that allow children

DEVELOPMENTAL–BEHAVIORAL PEDIATRICS

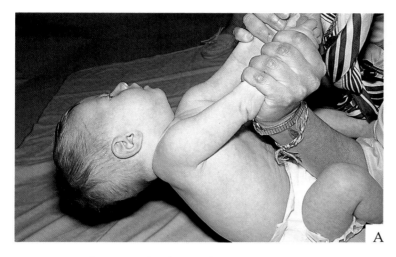
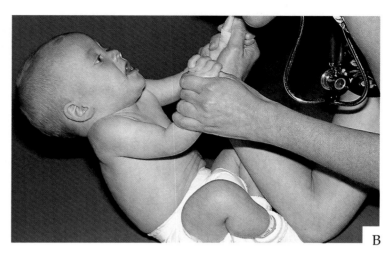

FIG. 3.5 Development of head control on the pull-to-sit maneuver. **A,** at 1 month of age, the head lags after the shoulders. **B,** at 5 to 6 months, the child anticipates the movement and raises the head before the shoulders.

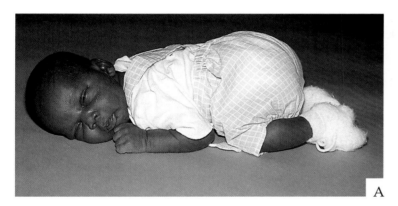
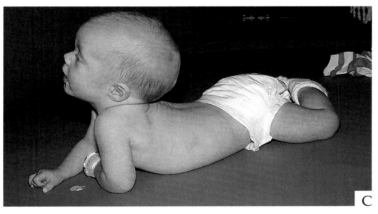

FIG. 3.6 Development of posture in prone. **A,** the newborn lies tightly flexed with the pelvis high and the knees under the abdomen. **B,** at 2 months of age, the infant extends the hips and pulls the shoulders slightly. **C,** at 3 to 4 months, the infant keeps the pelvis flat and lifts the head and shoulders.

to maintain a stable posture, even if they are rapidly moved or jolted. A timetable listing the expected emergence and disappearance of some of these early reflex patterns is presented in Figure 3.4.

Antigravity Muscular Control

HEAD CONTROL

The infant's earliest control task is to maintain a stable posture against the influence of gravity. This control develops in an organized fashion, from head to toe, or in a cephalocaudal progression, paralleling neuronal myelination. For example, neck flexors allow head control against gravity when a child is pulled from the supine to sitting position. Neonates show minimal control of the neck flexors, holding their heads upright only briefly when supported in a sitting position. When an infant is pulled to a sitting position, the head lags behind the arms and shoulders. As the infant reaches 5 to 6 months of age, she anticipates the direction of movement of the pull-to-sit maneuver, and flexes her neck before the shoulders begin to lift (Fig. 3.5).

TRUNK CONTROL/SITTING

In the prone position, a newborn remains in a tightly flexed position and can simply turn the face from side to side along the bed sheets. Progressive control of the shoulders and upper trunk in the first few months of life, plus a decrease in flexor tone, enables the young infant to hold the chest off the bed with the weight supported on the forearms (Fig. 3.6). Evolution of trunk control down the thoracic spine can also be

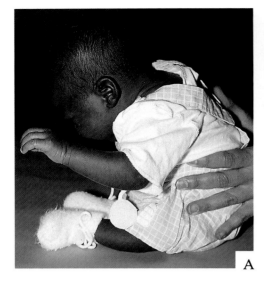

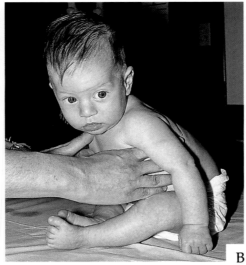

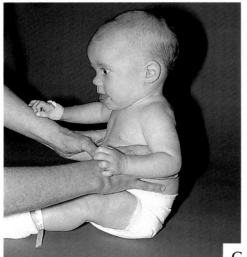

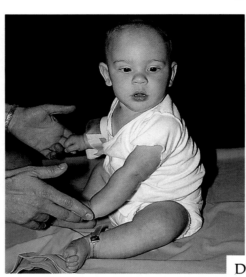

FIG. 3.7 Development of sitting posture. **A,** at 1 to 2 months of age, the head is held up intermittently but trunk control is lacking. **B,** at 2 to 3 months of age, the infant raises the head and shoulders well, but lacks control of the thoracolumbar area. **C,** at 3 to 4 months, support in the lumbar area is required to sit. **D,** at 5 to 6 months, the infant holds the head erect and the spine straight.

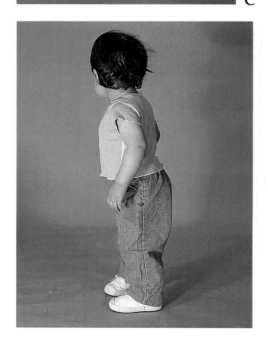

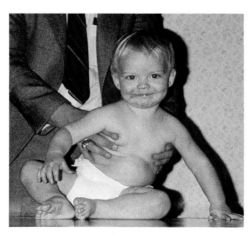

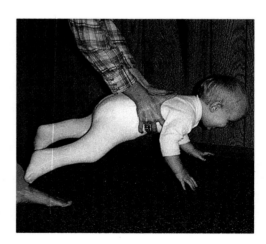

FIG. 3.9 Protective equilibrium response. As the child is pushed laterally by the examiner, he flexes his trunk toward the force to regain his center of gravity while one arm extends to protect against falling (lateral propping).

FIG. 3.10 Parachute response. As the examiner allows the child to free fall in ventral suspension, the child's extremities extend symmetrically to distribute his weight over a broader and more stable base upon landing.

FIG. 3.8 Standing. By 1 year of age, the lordotic curve, exaggerated here by a diaper, is evident.

EARLY GROSS MOTOR MILESTONE NORMALS

Task	Age Range (months)
Sits alone momentarily	4.0–8.0
Rolls back to stomach	4.0–10.0
Sits steadily	5.0–9.0
Gets to sitting	6.0–11.0
Pulls to standing	6.0–12.0
Stands alone	9.0–16.0
Walks three steps alone	9.0–17.0

Wide ranges in the attainment of these gross motor milestones in healthy children are the rule rather than the exception.

FIG. 3.11 (Reproduced from Bayley Scales of Infant Development, Psychological Corp., 1969)

observed with the infant in a sitting position (Fig. 3.7). As control reaches the lumbar area, the lumbar lordotic curve can be seen when the child is standing (Fig. 3.8).

HEAD RIGHTING/PARACHUTE RESPONSE

Balance and equilibrium reactions also emerge in a cephalocaudal sequence. Head righting refers to the infant's ability to keep the head vertical despite a tilt of the body. Four-month-old infants typically demonstrate this ability in vertical suspension, when they are gently swayed from side to side. As control moves downward, protective equilibrium responses can be elicited in a sitting infant by abruptly but gently pushing the infant's center of gravity past the midline in one of the horizontal planes. This reflex response, which involves increased trunk flexor tone toward the force and an outreached hand and limb away from the force, usually emerges by 6 months of age (Fig. 3.9). At 10 months, the child develops the parachute response, an outstretch of both arms and legs when the body is abruptly moved head first in a downward direction (Fig. 3.10). The acquisition of this equilibrium response demonstrates the integrity of the sensations and motor responses of the central nervous system, which allow independent sitting and standing in normal or motor-impaired children.

Development of Locomotion

Gross motor milestones can be described in terms of locomotion as well as antigravity muscular control (Fig. 3.11). Prone-to-supine rolling usually is accomplished by 3 to 4 months of age, after the child gains sufficient control of shoulder and upper trunk musculature to prop up on her arms. Supine-to-prone rolling requires control of the lumbar spine and hip region, as well as the upper trunk; this is usually present by 5 to 6 months of age. Early commando crawling, accomplished at 5 to 6 months of age (Fig. 3.12A), involves coordinated pulling with upper arms and passive dragging of the legs, akin to a soldier trying to keep his body out of the range of fire. By 6 to 9 months of age, as voluntary control moves to the hips and legs, the child is capable of getting up on hands and knees, assuming a quadruped position, and creeping (Fig. 3.12B). The next developmental milestone is supported standing. By 9 to 10 months of age, many children like to demonstrate this new skill either by holding on to a parent or by walking independently while holding on to furniture. This is called cruising (Fig. 3.12C). Increased control to the feet and disappearance of the plantar grasp reflex allow the child to walk independently. Walking three steps alone occurs at a median age of 11.7 months, with a range of 9 to 17 months of age (Fig. 3.12D).

Development of Complex Gross Motor Patterns

Further progress in gross motor skills continues throughout childhood. The developmental sequence beyond walking incorporates improved balance and coordination and progressive narrowing of the base of support. The sequence of milestones is as follows: running, jumping on two feet, balancing on one foot, hopping, and skipping. The child simultaneously learns to use muscle groups in timed sequences. By 13½ months, the child walks well, and by 36 months, he/she can balance on one foot for 1 second. Most children can hop by age 4. They can throw a ball overhead by 22½ months, but catching develops later, at almost 5 years.

Gross Motor Assessment During Health Maintenance Visits

The evaluation of gross motor skills can often begin when the pediatrician enters the office for a well-child visit. The typical 2-month-old infant is cradled in the parent's arms; the 6-month-old child is sitting with minimal support on the parent's lap or on the examination table next to the parent; the 12-month-old is cruising or toddling through the room. Though there is a wide age range in the onset and duration of each stage, nonetheless, the 6-month-old infant who lacks head control on the pull-to-sit maneuver, who cannot clear the table surface with his chest by supporting his weight on his arms when prone, who shows no head righting, or who has persistent primitive reflexes such as a complete Moro response or ATNR is at sufficient variance from his peers to warrant evaluation for a possible neuromuscular disorder. When gross motor delays are found in association with verbal/social delays, asymmetric use of one limb or one side of the body, or loss of previously attained milestones further diagnostic evaluation is indicated.

Evaluation of the older infant or toddler who has mastered walking can occur in the course of the physical and neurological evaluation. Many children enjoy showing off their abilities to jump, balance on one foot, hop, and skip. Some pediatricians use gross motor testing to establish rapport at the outset of a physical exam. However, since an aroused preschooler may not cooperate with a sedentary evaluation of heart or ears, many pediatricians hold off on motor evaluation until the conclusion of the examination. The Denver Developmental Screening Test includes basic milestones for assessment of children 2 to 6 years of age.

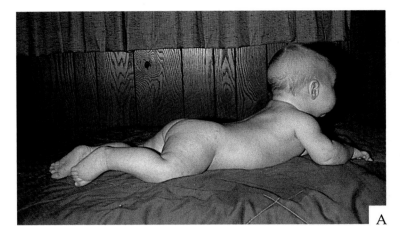

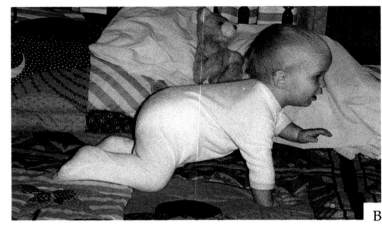

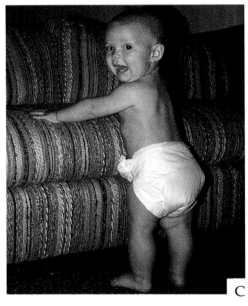

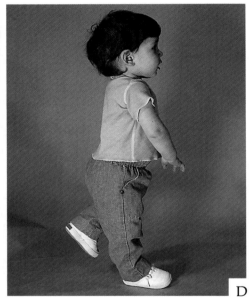

FIG. 3.12 Development of locomotion. *A*, crawling implies that the belly is still on the floor. *B*, creeping refers to mobility with the child on hands and knees (quadruped). *C*, cruising refers to standing with two-handed support on stationary objects before moving with steps. *D*, early free walking.

POTENTIAL CAUSES OF DELAYED GROSS MOTOR DEVELOPMENT

Global Developmental Delay

Genetic syndromes and
  chromosomal abnormalities
Brain morphologic abnormalities
Endocrine deficiencies—
  hypothyroidism, prolonged
  hypoglycemia
Neurodegenerative diseases
Congenital infections
Idiopathic mental retardation

Motor Dysfunction

Central nervous system
  damage—kernicterus, birth
  injury, neonatal stroke, trauma,
  prolonged seizures, metabolic
  insult, infection
Spinal cord dysfunction—
  Werdnig-Hoffmann disease,
  myelomeningocele, polio
Peripheral nerve dysfunction—
  brachial plexus injury,
  heritable neuropathies
Motor end-plate dysfunction—
  myasthenia gravis
Muscular disorders—
  muscular dystrophies
Other—benign congenital
  hypotonia

Motor Intact but Otherwise Restricted

Congenital malformations—
  bony or soft-tissue defects
Diminished energy supply—
  chronic illness, severe malnutrition
Environmental deprivation—
  casted, nonweight-bearing
Familial/genetic endowment—
  slower myelination
Sensory deficits—blindness
Temperamental effects—
  low activity level, slow to
  try new tasks
Trauma—child abuse

FIG. 3.13

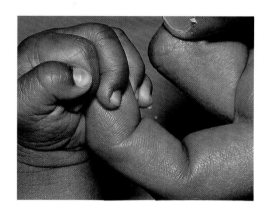

FIG. 3.14 Reflex hand grasp. A new-born reflexively grasps at a finger placed in the palm.

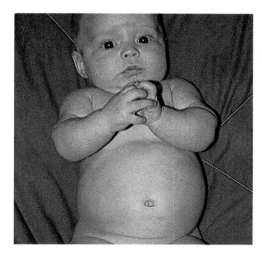

FIG. 3.15 Midline hand play. A 2-month-old infant brings hands together at the midline.

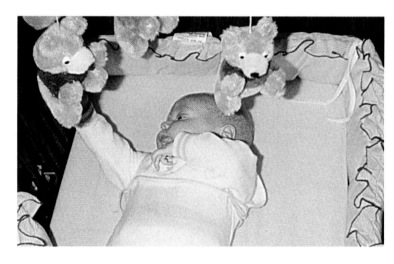

FIG. 3.16 Reaching and swiping. A 3-month-old infant uses his entire upper extremity as a unit in interacting with the toy.

At the discovery of delayed or atypical development, the pediatrician's first task is to develop a differential diagnosis and a plan to establish the specific diagnosis. Potential causes of delayed gross motor development are listed in Figure 3.13. Another equally important task is to recommend a treatment program. Physical therapy or infant stimulation programs should be actively considered for children with motor difficulties during infancy through preschool. Adaptive physical education programs are available for older children with mild problems that do not seriously impair function.

FINE MOTOR DEVELOPMENT

Involuntary Grasp

At birth, the neonate's fingers and thumb are typically tightly fisted. An infant grasps reliably and reflexively at any object placed in the palm (Fig. 3.14), and cannot release the grasp. Because of this reflex, the infant's range of upper extremity motion is functionally limited. Normal development leads to acquisition of a voluntary grasp.

Voluntary Grasp

The reflexive palmar grasp gradually disappears at about 1 month of age. From that point on, the infant gains control of fine motor skills in an orderly progression, from the midline to the periphery, or from proximal to distal. In the second or third month of life, the infant initially brings both hands together for midline hand play (Fig. 3.15). Shortly after that, he begins to swipe at objects held in or near the midline (Fig. 3.16). At this early stage, swiping is, in fact, a gross motor activity that involves the entire upper extremity as a unit. However, it is through swiping that the infant increases his exploratory range, and fine tunes the small muscles of the wrist, hand, and fingers.

Improvements in fine motor control increase sensory input from the hands, and permit greater hand manipulation through space. By 2 to 3 months of age, the hands are no longer tightly fisted, and the infant may begin sucking on a thumb or individual digit rather than the entire fist for self-comfort. A 3-month-old is usually able to hold an object in either hand if it is placed there, although he has limited ability to grasp voluntarily or to release that object. At approximately 4 to 5 months of age, infants begin to use their hands as entire units to draw objects toward them. Neither the hand nor the thumb functions independently at this point, and consequently, the child uses his hand like a rake.

Next, the child develops the ability to bend the fingers against the palm (palmar grasp), to squeeze objects, and to obtain them independently for closer inspection. Differentiation of the parts of the hand develops in association with differentiation of the two hands. Between 5 and 7 months of age, the infant can use hands independently to transfer objects across the midline. Further differentiation of the plane of movement of the thumb allows it to adduct as the fingers squeeze against the palm in a radial-palmar or whole hand grasp. With time, the thumb moves from adduction to opposition. The site of pressure of the thumb against the fingers moves away from the palm toward the fingertips in what is called an inferior

5 MONTHS RAKE	7 MONTHS RADIAL-PALMAR GRASP	9 MONTHS RADIAL-DIGITAL GRASP	10 MONTHS INFERIOR-PINCER GRASP	12 MONTHS FINE PINCER GRASP
Thumb adducted, proximal thumb joint flexed, distal thumb joint flexed	Raking object into palm with adducted totally flexed thumb and all flexed fingers, OR with two partly extended fingers	Between thumb and side of curled index finger, distal thumb joint slightly flexed, proximal thumb joint extended	Between ventral surfaces of thumb and index finger, distal thumb joint extended, beginning thumb opposition	Between fingertips or fingernails, distal thumb joint flexed

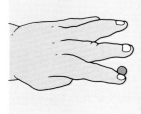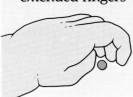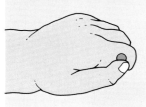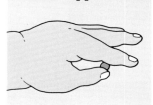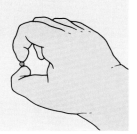

FIG. 3.17 *Development of prehension. (Adapted from Erhardt RP:* Developmental Hand Dysfunction. Theory, Assessment, Treatment. *Laurel, MD, RAMSCO Publishing, 1982, 61)*

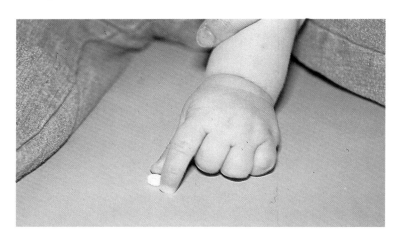

FIG. 3.18 *Fine pincer grasp. A 12-month-old child lifts a pill.*

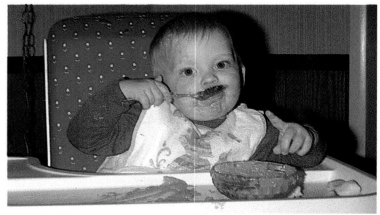

FIG. 3.19 *Independent feeding. A 15-month-old child uses fine motor skills to use a spoon independently.*

pincer or radial-digital grasp, seen around 9 months of age (Fig. 3.17). By 10 months of age, differentiated use of the fingers allows the child to explore the details of an object.

Between 9 and 12 months of age, the fine pincer grasp develops, allowing opposition of the tip of the thumb and the index finger (Fig. 3.17). This milestone enables the precise prehension of tiny objects (Fig. 3.18). The infant uses this skill in such tasks as self-feeding and exploration of small objects. By a year, the infant can position his hand in space to achieve vertical or horizontal orientation prior to grasping or releasing an object.

Development of Complex Fine Motor Skills

Early in the second year of life, the young child uses the grasp to master tools and to manipulate objects in new ways. Dropping and throwing, stacking, and putting objects in and out of receptacles become favorite pastimes. Mastery of the cup and spoon supplement finger feeding as a more efficient and less messy means of eating (Fig. 3.19).

Advancements in fine motor planning and control can be demonstrated through the child's ability to stack small cubes. After children master stacking, they show consistent patterns of improvement in reproducing structures that they have watched the examiner assemble (Fig. 3.20). The child's ability to copy a variety of drawings also improves during this period.

Fine Motor Evaluation and Testing

Fine motor testing can be incorporated readily into a physical examination, and may uncover problems with vision, neuromuscular control or perception, in addition to difficulties with attention or cooperation. The 4-month-old child usually can be encouraged to grasp a tongue depressor. By 6 to 9 months of age, the child should be offered two tongue depressors, one for each hand, since he can operate the hands independently. At 9 to 12 months, the child spontaneously points with an isolated index finger or picks up small objects with a fine pincer grasp. Children prior to 18 months of age generally use both hands equally well. Therefore, the child who develops consistent

FIG. 3.20

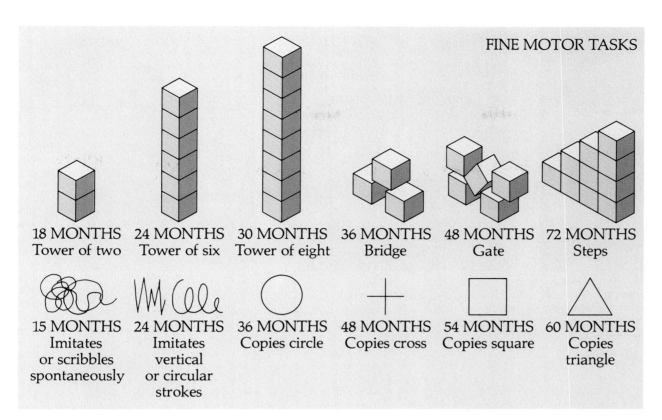

FINE MOTOR TASKS

18 MONTHS Tower of two	**24 MONTHS** Tower of six	**30 MONTHS** Tower of eight	**36 MONTHS** Bridge	**48 MONTHS** Gate	**72 MONTHS** Steps
15 MONTHS Imitates or scribbles spontaneously	**24 MONTHS** Imitates vertical or circular strokes	**36 MONTHS** Copies circle	**48 MONTHS** Copies cross	**54 MONTHS** Copies square	**60 MONTHS** Copies triangle

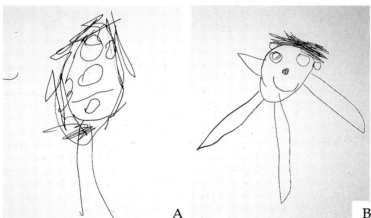

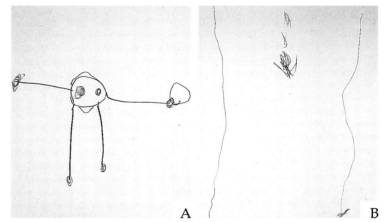

FIG. 3.21 *Development of skill at drawing a person.* **A,** *this drawing by a 4-year-old child includes five features: eyes, nose, mouth, hair, and legs. To calculate an age equivalent, the child earns ¼ year for each of the five features, added to a base age of 3 years. This drawing has an age equivalent of 4¼ years.* **B,** *a drawing by the same child at age 5. Note the inclusion of ears and arms as well as improvements in proportion. This drawing has an age equivalent of 4¾ years.*

FIG. 3.22 *Difficulties with visual-fine motor integration skills in a child with cerebral palsy.* **A,** *drawing by a bright 4-year-old who was born prematurely, but showed no developmental delays. Note the inclusion of seven features: eyes, hair, mouth, arms, hands, legs, and feet. The age equivalent for this drawing is 4¾ years.* **B,** *drawing by a 4-year-old child with spastic diplegia. Difficulties in organization appear related to visual-motor integration skills rather than to problems with fine motor skill.*

handedness with neglect of the other limb prior to that time should have a neurodevelopmental assessment. The child who has not developed use of the thumb and pincer grasp by 1 year of age deserves further evaluation, as does the child who is unable to copy vertical or horizontal lines by age 3 or circles by age 4.

Fine motor activities can be both engaging and nonthreatening to the preschool and school-age child; these activities allow the physician to make valuable observations and to establish a rapport. The physician can routinely request that the child use the waiting time or the period of history-taking to draw a self-portrait. These drawings provide a wealth of information not only on the child's capacities for fine motor control, but also on cognitive development and social/emotional functioning. A quick method for analyzing the age level of a drawing is to count the number of features in the drawing. The child receives one point for each of the following features: two eyes, two ears, a nose, a mouth, hair, two arms, two legs, two hands, two feet, a neck, and a trunk. Each point converts to the value of 1/4 year added to a base age of 3 (Fig. 3.21).

Children with brain damage are at particular risk for problems with perceptual-fine motor integration, even in the absence of visual problems and with minimal involvement of the upper extremities (Fig. 3.22).

Fine motor skills figure prominently in self-care activities. The child who lacks the dexterity to complete simple daily

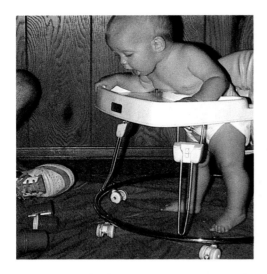

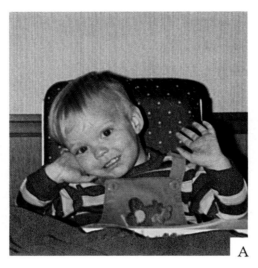

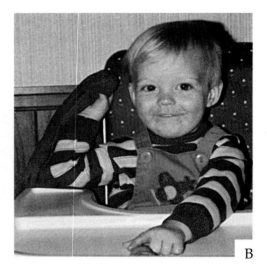

FIG. 3.23 Early object permanence: 6-month-old infant was able to track his toy through a vertical fall, and to search for it on the floor even after his gaze had been interrupted.

FIG. 3.24 Object permanence. **A** and **B**, 11-month-old child is able to locate a small hidden object even if no part of it remains visible. In doing so he is demonstrating his understanding that objects are permanent.

activities such as zippering, buttoning, or cutting with a knife may lack the self-esteem that accompanies independent self-care. Furthermore, the child who is continually dependent on parents or teachers may be viewed by peers, teachers, or perhaps, most damagingly, by himself as less mature. In the school-age child, inefficient fine motor skills can have a significant impact on the ability to compete with peers in timed tasks, even if the child is possessed of sound academic and conceptual skills. Occupational therapy and special education may enhance both fine motor skills and emotional development in these children.

COGNITIVE DEVELOPMENT
Early Sensory Processing

Innate sensory capabilities serve as the building blocks of cognitive development. Even at birth, the healthy neonate responds to visual and auditory stimuli. These responses, like the primitive reflexes, take the form of integrated patterns of activity.

The visual acuity of the full-term infant is estimated to fall between 20/200 and 20/400 and improves rapidly over the first year of life. Even at birth, it is possible to get the full-term infant to fix on faces 9 to 12 inches from her face and to track objects horizontally at least 30°. Some neonates, if assessed when calm and fully alert, can track objects 180° across the visual field. Newborns also respond to sound, typically quieting to a human voice or to gentle inanimate sounds such as rattles or music. In the first days of life, many children turn to the source of sound and search for it with their eyes. These maneuvers, found on the Brazelton Neonatal Behavioral Assessment Scale, are useful in demonstrating neurobehavioral characteristics of very young infants.

Examination must take place at optimal times, when the infant is alert; if the infant is drowsy or agitated, the ability to track visually or to search for sounds is severely compromised. If, when assessed under optimal circumstances and when fully alert, the infant does not show horizontal tracking of objects,

does not look at the toys or people he/she is involved with, or holds the head in an unusual position, the physician should recommend prompt evaluation for abnormal visual perception or central nervous system development.

Development of Sensorimotor Intelligence

During the first 2 years of life, the sensorimotor period of development, the young child's cognitive abilities can be surmised only through use of the senses and through the physical manipulation of objects. The nature of an infant's thinking is assessed through concrete interaction with the environment. During this period, the child develops an understanding of the concept of object permanence, the ability to recognize that an object exists even when it cannot be seen, heard, or felt. Simultaneously, he develops an understanding of cause-and-effect relationships. Progress in the child's development of these concepts is an important prerequisite to the development of pure mental activity, reflected in the ability to use symbols and language.

Early progress in the development of object permanence is indicated by the infant's continued though brief gaze at the site where a familiar toy or face has disappeared. At this point, the child also repeats actions that she has discovered will produce interesting results. Between 4 and 8 months of age, infants become interested in changes in the position and appearance of toys. They can track an object visually through a vertical fall (Fig. 3.23) and search for a partially hidden toy. They also begin to vary the means of creating interesting effects. In these early months, the child's play consists of exploring toys to gain information about their physical characteristics. Activities such as mouthing, shaking, and banging can provide sensory input about an object beyond its visual features. However, when mouthing of toys persists as the predominant mode of exploration after 12 to 18 months of age, assessment of cognitive function is warranted.

At approximately 9 to 12 months of age, infants are able to locate objects that have been completely hidden (Fig. 3.24). Not surprisingly, peek-a-boo becomes a favorite pastime at

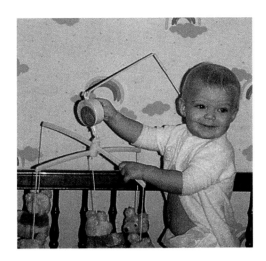

FIG. 3.25 Mature means-end reasoning: 15-month-old child turns the key of the music box atop the mobile to make it play. The child's understanding has advanced beyond that of direct causality, such as pulling a toy to bring it closer.

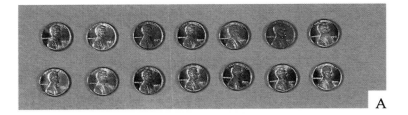

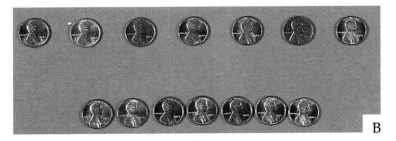

FIG. 3.26 Experimental design to demonstrate preoperational logic. The 3- or 4-year-old child agrees that the two rows in **A** have the same number of pennies. When the child sees the pennies moved into the configuration in **B**, he claims that the top row has more because it is longer.

this point. Later, the infant can crawl away from her mother and recall where to return to find her.

As children near 1 year of age, their interest in toys extends beyond their physical properties (color, texture, etc.). They may begin to demonstrate their awareness that different objects have different purposes. For example, a child might touch a comb to his hair in a meaningful non-pretend action, typical of the 9- to 12-month age range. Beyond 1 year of age, children begin to vary their behavior to create novel effects. They no longer need to be shown how to work dials or knobs on a busy box, nor do they need to hit something by accident to discover the interesting effect that will result.

By 18 months of age, children can deduce the location of an object even if they have not seen it hidden from view. They can maintain mental images of desired objects and develop plans for obtaining them. The child's understanding of causality also advances; cause-and-effect relationships no longer need to be direct to be appreciated (Fig. 3.25). These developments herald the beginning of a new stage in cognitive development, that of symbolic thinking. They also indicate the need for major changes in the parental approach to discipline.

Development of Symbolic Capabilities

In the second year of life, the child demonstrates mental activity independent of sensory processing or motor manipulation. For example, the child observes a television superhero performing a rescue mission and hours later reenacts the scene with careful precision. Clearly, the child has a mental image of the event and uses it to generate the delayed imitation.

As children develop the capacity for pure mental activity, they use objects to represent other objects or ideas. Genuine pretending begins; the child engages in playful representation of commonplace activities, using objects for their actual purpose but accompanied by exaggerated sounds or gestures. Pretend actions are combined into a series of events. For example, the child may hold a phone to her ear and then to a doll's ear, or may feed a teddy bear and then put the bear to bed.

The next stage in development allows the child to plan pretend activities in anticipation of the play theme to come, combining many steps into the play. Preparing for play indicates an advance in pretending beyond that of improvising with the objects at hand. For example, the child might be seen preparing the play area or searching for needed objects and announcing what the objects are meant to represent.

Development of Logical Thinking

The preschool child has well-developed capabilities for mental representation and symbolic thinking. However, limited life experience and lack of formal education lead to a unique and charming logic during this period. Preschoolers often assume that all objects are alive like themselves. A car and a tricycle, for example, may be seen as alive, perhaps because they are capable of movement. Similarly, the child claims that the moon follows her on an evening walk.

The logic of the preschooler is in large part influenced by the appearance of objects. Since an airplane appears to become smaller as it takes off, the preschooler may assume that all the people on the plane become smaller as well. Piaget demonstrated that preschoolers seem to think that number and quantity vary with appearance (Fig. 3.26). Under certain circumstances, a 4-year-old child may show understanding that a quantity remains invariant unless something is added or subtracted. That same child, however, may insist that two rows of pennies are different in number simply because of a compelling visual difference between them.

The idiosyncratic logic of the preschooler is gradually replaced by conventional logic and wisdom. School-age children follow a logic akin to adult reasoning, at least in so far as the stimuli are concrete. Faced with the same question about the pennies, they readily acknowledge that the two rows have the same number regardless of their visual appearance (see Fig. 3.26). They also know that the airplane just looks smaller because it has moved further from the viewer and they giggle at the suggestion that the people on the plane have shrunk. Their logical limitations become obvious only when they must reason about the hypothetical or the abstract.

Adolescents, at least those with the benefits of formal education, tend to extend logical principles to increasingly diverse problems. They can generate multiple logical possibilities systematically when faced with scientific experiments, and they can also consider hypothetical problems. These principles of

Findings Sometimes Present on History or Examination	Possible Disorder
Decreased vision or hearing	Specific sensory deficits
Startling spells, motor automatism	Seizure disorders
Lethargy, ataxia	Overmedication with anticonvulsants
Myxedema, delayed return on DTRs, thick skin and tongue, sparse hair, constipation, increased sleep, coarser voice, short stature, goiter	Hypothyroidism
Irritability, cold sweats, tremor, loss of consciousness	Hypoglycemia
Unexplained bruises of varying ages, failure to thrive	Child abuse and neglect
Short stature, weight below third percentile	Malnutrition or systemic illness producing failure to thrive
Poor purposeful attending in multiple settings	Attention deficit hyperactivity disorder
No specific findings	Environmental deprivation
Anemia	Iron deficiency or lead exposure
Absent venous pulsations or papilledema on funduscopic examination, morning vomiting, headaches, brisk DTRs in lower extremities	Increased intracranial pressure
Vomiting, irritability and seizures, failure to thrive	Some inborn errors of metabolism, e.g., methyl malonic acidemia
Hepatomegaly, jaundice, hypotonia, susceptibility to infection, cataracts	Galactosemia
Fair hair, blue eyes, "mousy" odor to urine	Phenylketonuria
Ongoing evidence of active or progressive disease	Chronic infection, inflammatory disease, malignancies

FIG. 3.27

reasoning are applied not only to school work but also to social situations. For example, the adolescent may think about who will go with whom to the school prom: "She thinks that I think that she wants to go with him, but I know that she wants to go with me."

Assessing Cognitive Development

Because the observations needed to assess cognitive abilities in the preverbal period are less well known by the general public than are the major motor milestones, parents often rely on physicians for guidance. Simple observation of the child's use of toys or objects can help determine cognitive progress. The pediatrician can induce the infant to look for a hidden toy or to play a game of peek-a-boo; the infant's anticipation of reappearance indicates his development of the concept of object permanence. Similarly, the toddler's ability to play with a toy telephone indicates the emergence of symbolic thought. Beyond the toddler stage, the physician typically relies on conversation and language ability to assess levels of cognitive skill.

For the parents, a delay in a child's attainment of a well-known milestone may create tremendous fear about ultimate learning potential. In many cases, such parental concerns are put to rest when the physician determines that the child's learning to date is age-appropriate. If a child does show delays in cognitive development, the physician should generate a differential diagnosis (Fig. 3.27) from knowledge of the child's level of functioning in multiple domains as well as aspects of history and physical examination.

Parents should be given information about their child's delay early enough to enable them to make informed decisions about early educational intervention. Pediatricians serve a critical role in referring children to such programs and in monitoring their progress. Active communication between the providers of early intervention and the physician facilitates a comprehensive and cohesive approach.

Physicians frequently need the consultation of colleagues in psychology and education to assess the cognitive abilities of their older preschool and school-age patients. A number of methods have been devised for formal assessment of mental achievement, and almost all parents are familiar with the terms "intelligence quotient" and "IQ." Though not a means of comprehensively assessing all mental capabilities, normal IQ scores are imperfect predictors of which children will have the attention, social skills, motivation, and intelligence to perform well in school. Low IQ scores may reflect a child's poor ability to grasp new concepts or they may indicate poor purposeful attending behaviors, as seen in depression or in attention deficit hyperactivity disorder. Low scores also may reflect poor social adjustment or limitations in test-taking capabilities, such as sitting in a chair at a table and applying maximal effort to a task requested by an unfamiliar authority figure. Frequently, low scores will result from a combination of difficulties in several areas.

TESTS USED IN THE ASSESSMENT OF COGNITIVE DEVELOPMENT

Type of Scale	Tests Used	Age Range
Standard intelligence scales	Stanford-Binet Intelligence Scale —4th edition	2–adult
	Wechsler Intelligence Scale for Children—Revised (WISC-R)	6–16 years
Nonverbal intelligence scales	Leiter International Performance Scale	2–18 years
Infant development tests	Bayley Scales of Infant Development	0–2 1/2 years
	Gesell Developmental Schedules	0–5 years
Developmental scales for the visually impaired	Reynell-Zinkin Scales	0–5 years
	Maxfield-Buchalty Social Maturity for Blind Preschool Children	0–6 years
Screening instruments	Denver Developmental Screening Test (DDST)	0–5 years
	Draw-a-Person Test (DAP-Goodenough-Harris Drawing Test)	3–adult

FIG. 3.28

If children with sensory or motor impairments are tested with instruments normed on able-bodied children, they will often obtain low scores. Different assessment techniques have been devised to circumvent specific disabilities while obtaining information about a child's cognitive abilities and these are typically administered by psychologists, child development specialists, or special educators (Fig. 3.28).

Assessment of a child's abilities to learn must go beyond standardized IQ tests. For example, some children who can score in the normal range on IQ tests will not be able to learn to read. A diversified and individualized assessment process should precede any educational recommendation. The pediatrician, in the role of advocate, should assure that assessments include information about the child's strengths and weaknesses, since educational planning should involve attention to all aspects of the child's abilities. Moreover, the pediatrician can encourage families to maintain an active, decision-making role in their child's education.

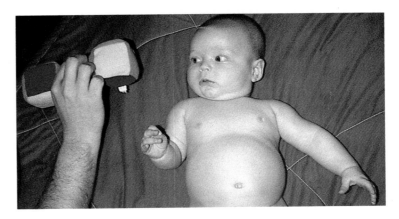

FIG. 3.29 Localizing sound: 3-month-old infant responds to interesting sounds by looking in the direction of the sound.

LANGUAGE DEVELOPMENT
Early Skills in Speech Perception and Production

The use of language—the ability to generate reproducible sounds or gestures that are recognized by others as representative of concepts—begins slowly and subtly in the first year of life. Language skills are subdivided into two realms: receptive skills—the ability to comprehend communication, and expressive skills—the ability to produce communication.

Neonates demonstrate skills that are useful in the eventual development of receptive language abilities. Even before birth, fetuses detect sounds and show preferences for some sounds over others. Pregnant women report that their unborn children may kick after sudden loud noises, and that they may kick harder with rock than with classical music. At birth, the infant is particularly attuned to the human voice and may turn

toward a parent who is gently whispering. Children remain interested in sounds as they grow older and turn toward the source of a sound by 3 to 4 months of age (Fig. 3.29).

Children also are able to differentiate speech sounds, even close to birth. Experimental paradigms, utilizing the fact that an infant's heart rate and sucking patterns change when they encounter new environmental stimuli, suggest that infants as young as 1 month of age can differentiate such similar speech sounds as /ba/ and /pa/.

By 2 to 3 months of age, children begin to *coo* or make musical sounds spontaneously. This is the first step toward the development of expressive verbal language.

By about 6 months of age, children place consonant sounds with vowel sounds creating what is known as babble. In this period, the infant says ma-ma or da-da without necessarily referring to the loving parent. By 9 to 12 months of age, they integrate babble with intonational patterns consistent with the parent's speech. This is called jargon.

RECEPTIVE AND EXPRESSIVE LANGUAGE MILESTONES

Age Range	Receptive Response	Expressive Response
0–1½ months	Startles or widens eye to sound	Shows variation in crying (hunger, pain)
1½–4 months	Quiets to voice, blinks eyes to sound	Makes musical sounds, coos, participates in reciprocal exchange
4–9 months	Turns head toward sound, responds with raised arms when mother says "up" and reaches for child, responds appropriately to friendly or angry voices	Babbles, repeats self-initiated sounds
9–12 months	Listens selectively to familiar words, begins to respond to "no," responds to verbal routine such as wave, bye-bye, or clap, turns to own name	Uses symbolic gestures and jargon, repeats parent-initiated sounds
12–18 months	Points to 3 body parts (eyes, nose, mouth), understands up to 50 words, recognizes common objects by name (dog, cat, bottle, ball, book), follows 1-step commands accompanied by gestures ("give me the doll," "hug your bear," "open your mouth")	Uses words to express needs, learns 20 to 50 words by 18 months, uses words inconsistently and mixed with jargon and/or echolalia
18 months–2 years	Points to pictures when asked "show me," understands "soon," "in," "on," and "under," begins to distinguish "you" from "me," can formulate negative judgments (a pear is not a cookie)	Uses telegraphic 2-word sentences ("go bye-bye," "up daddy," "want cookie"), 25% intelligibility
30 months	Follows 2-step commands, can identify objects by use	Uses jargon and echolalia infrequently, makes average sentence of 2½ words, adjectives and adverbs appear, begins to ask questions, asks adults to repeat actions ("do it again")
3 years	Knows several colors, knows what we do when we are hungry, thirsty, or sleepy, is aware of past and future, understands "today" and "not today"	Uses pronouns and plurals; can tell stories that begin to be understood; uses negative ("I can't," "I won't"); verbalizes toilet needs; can tell full name, age, and sex; forms sentences of 3 to 4 words, 75% intelligibility
3½ years	Can answer such questions as "do you have a doggie," "which is the boy," "what toys do you have," understands "little," "funny," "secret"	Can relate experiences in sequential order, can say a nursery rhyme, ask permission
4 years	Understands same versus different, follows 3-step commands, completes opposite analogies (a brother is a boy, a sister is a...), understands why we have houses, stoves, umbrellas	Tells a story, uses past tense, counts to 3, names primary colors, enjoys rhyming nonsense words, enjoys exaggerations, asks up to 500 questions a day
5 years	Understands what we do with eyes and ears, understands differences in texture (hard, soft, smooth) understands "if," "when," "why," identifies words in terms of use, begins to understand left and right	Indicates "I don't know," indicates "funny," "surprise," can define in terms of use, asks definition of specific words, makes serious inquiries ("how does this work," "what does it mean"); uses mature sentence structure and form

FIG. 3.30

PHONEMES AND INTELLIGIBILITY

Age Range*	Sounds Mastered	Percent Intelligibility (to a stranger)
2 years	. . .	50%
2½ years	. . .	75%
3 years	14 vowels and *p, b, m*	85%
4 years	10 vowel blends and *n, ng, w, h, t, d, k, g*	100%
5 years	*f, v, y, th, l, wh*	100%
6 years	*r, s, z, ch, j, sh, zh,* and consonant blends	100%

The ages presented here are to be viewed as general guidelines, as authorities will differ with regard to the specific ages associated with articulation and intelligibility.

FIG. 3.31

Later Development

In the second half of the first year, the child develops early skills in true receptive language. Milestones are listed in Figure 3.30. By 6 months of age, children reliably respond to their names, and at about 9 months they can follow verbal routines, such as waving bye-bye or showing how big they are. At about the same age, they also learn that pointing shares the focus of attention. The young infant looks at the point, while the older infant looks at the object to which the point is directed.

Receptive language can be demonstrated as children follow increasingly complex commands. For example, one-step commands such as "throw the ball" will be understood by approximately 1 year of age. The labeling of commonplace items in pictures is slightly more complex and begins after 1 year of age. The ability to choose between two pictures when asked "show me the..." should be consistent between 18 and 24 months of age.

By 2½ years of age, receptive language skills have advanced beyond the understanding of simple labels. The child is able to identify objects by their use. Continued advances in receptive language occur during the preschool years and are highly susceptible to environmental stimulation or deprivation.

Expressive language skills (see Fig. 3.30) lag behind receptive skills in the first year of life. But even before word production begins, a child's gestures have communicative intent. Many 9- to 10-month olds are able to communicate that their juice or cereal is "all gone" by placing their hands palms up, at shoulder height. Even older children gesture to make themselves better understood, as gross and fine motor skills develop faster than does the oropharyngeal musculature used in articulation.

Expressive language at first develops slowly. The child's first meaningful words are produced around the first birthday. Over the next 6 months, the child may master only 20 to 50 more words. These early words come and go from the child's vocabulary and tend to be idiosyncratic child-forms. After 18 to 24 months word usage increases rapidly, standard forms replace baby talk, and word combinations begin.

The child's earliest two-word sentences typically contain important content words but lack prepositions, articles, and verb-tense markings. This two-word phase has been called telegraphic speech. Once the child is capable of three- and four-word utterances, length limitations do not appear to be a significant barrier. By age 3, the child has developed complex language with the use of pronouns and prepositions. The child develops the ability to ask questions, though at age 3 the most frequently posed question is probably "why." The child also can use negation within a sentence. By age 5, the child uses all parts of speech, as well as clauses and complex sentences.

Mastering Intelligibility and Fluency

Sounds required in language are mastered at different rates. The child who is attempting to say a word containing sounds he cannot yet produce has a variety of choices on how to proceed: by omission of the difficult sound ("ba" for bottle), by substitution of a different sound ("fum" for thumb), or by distortion ("goyl" for girl). The information presented in Figure 3.31 provides an estimate of when mastery of particular sounds might be expected, along with estimates of overall intelligibility.

Assessing Language Development

In the early stages of prelinguistic and linguistic development, direct assessment by the pediatrician may be difficult. Children are likely to remain quiet in new situations, especially in the office where they received an injection. It is usually easy to engage a normally-developing child of age 3 in conversation. Before that age, the physician may need to rely on parental report.

The differential diagnosis for delayed expressive language development includes impaired hearing, global developmental delay or mental retardation, environmental deprivation, autism, and emotional maladjustment. Keeping this in mind, worrisome clinical situations include the 4- to 6-month-old infant who fails to coo responsively, the 9- to 10-month-old child who does not babble or whose cooing and babbling have diminished, and the 18-month-old child whose repertoire of words includes only "mama" or "dada." Beyond 18 months, a convenient rule of thumb is that children 2 years of age should use two-word utterances, at least half of which should be intel-

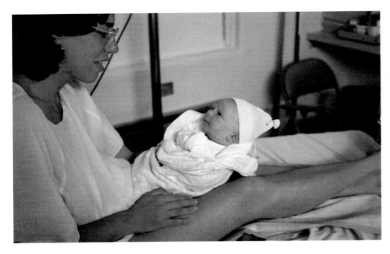

FIG. 3.32 *Early social skills. Newborn within an hour of birth fixates on the face of the mother.*

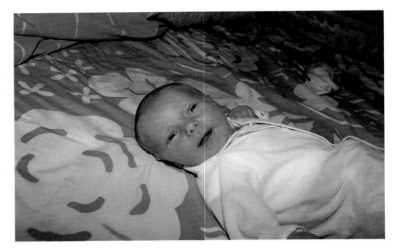

FIG. 3.33 *Early smiling. A 19-day-old infant smiles for her parents.*

ligible. By 3 years of age, children should use phrases of three or more words, three quarters of which should be intelligible. Children who fail to achieve these developmental milestones should undergo evaluation for hearing loss as well as for cognitive and emotional impairment.

Families often attribute language delays in their youngster to superficial and easily remediable physiological or social factors. "Tongue tie," for example, is sometimes associated with delayed speech. However, it may be the effect rather than the cause, as the frenulum of the tongue usually is tight because it has not been sufficiently exercised by early verbal practice. Similarly, children rarely delay language because "they don't need it." A toddler has tremendous motivation to improve his verbal skills, even if he has a loving family who is willing to try to meet his needs. When the toddler wants a particular food, a point toward the cupboard door will not specify precisely what he wants. His parents must offer him items one at a time and await his acceptance or rejection. The child's use of a verbal label will allow him to meet his needs efficiently.

Delays in the development of intelligibility might include any of the following:

1. Lack of intelligible speech by age 3.
2. Frequent omission of initial consonants after age 4.
3. Continued substitution of very easy sounds for harder ones after age 5.
4. Persistent articulation errors after age 7.

If any of these delays persists for 6 months or more, a referral should be initiated.

During the period in which articulation and vocabulary are being mastered, speech dysfluencies are common. Noticeable stuttering or rapid speech beyond age 4 should prompt further attention. The problems of nasality, inaudibility, and unusual pitch sometimes may be helped by a speech pathologist. Furthermore, the child of any age who is embarrassed by his or her speech is an appropriate candidate for referral.

Therapy for speech and language disorders has been shown to be helpful in improving the communication skills of children with language delays and problems of intelligibility. Keep in mind that a child whose unusual language pattern is destined to be outgrown will not suffer from monitoring by a communication disorders specialist; the child whose language impairment will not be outgrown has much to lose when help is delayed.

SOCIAL DEVELOPMENT

Early Capabilities: Social Responsivity

The earliest social-developmental task of newborns is to establish a mutually satisfying relationship with their care givers. Neonates begin the social-developmental process by fixing visually on faces in preference to other sights, a skill that is evident during the first few days of life (Fig. 3.32). The responsive smile develops soon thereafter (Fig. 3.33). The social smile is another innate behavior, although it may not appear until 4 to 6 weeks of life. Smiling appears in infants from all cultures at about the same time. Infants with visual impairment who cannot appreciate a smile on the faces of their care givers, nonetheless smile at ages comparable to sighted children.

Development of Attachment

During the first 6 months of life, infants are rather indiscriminate in their social behavior, laughing and giggling with anyone willing to play. Evidence of the special relationship between parent and child may be seen when the crying infant can be calmed only by a parents voice.

The infant develops a sense that her parent exists when out of sight sooner than she learns object permanence. By 6 to 8 months of age, children protest when their parents leave the room. As infants begin to recognize faces of familiar care givers, they may squirm and cling in the company of unfamiliar people, exhibiting stranger awareness. The severity of the reaction varies with the infant's temperament and with his or her previous experiences. Extreme reactions, known as stranger anxiety, are usually characteristic of children who have not had routine care from alternative care givers. Pediatricians are advised to refrain from holding the 9- to 12-month-old child at the well-child visit. A child who is securely in the parent's arms may remain playful and calm, but he may fret or cry when wrenched from that security.

By 1 year of age, most children have experienced periods of separation from a parent, whether it be for minutes or hours. Infants who have developed a secure attachment to their parents show signs of recognition and pleasure when they are reunited with them. As the child progresses in gross motor development, he initiates separation by walking away independently and exploring at greater distances from his parents.

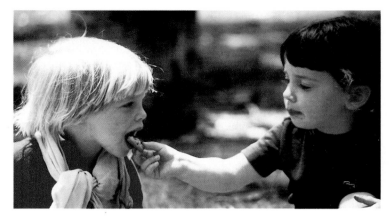

FIG. 3.34 Sharing. Two-year-old children with day-care experience share a special treat.

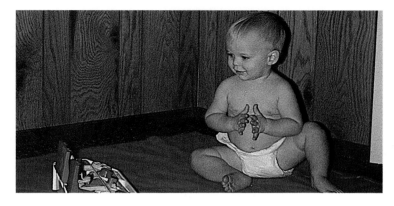

FIG. 3.35 Mastery smile. Thirteen-month-old boy demonstrates that toddlers beyond a year of age can take pride in their own accomplishments. This child is applauding his own success at having made the puppets appear.

Typically, the infant returns regularly for some verbal encouragement, eye contact, or hugging and then ventures farther. In contrast, infants who have not developed a secure attachment may show indifference, ambivalence, or disorganization at reunion with their parents. Their exploration of the environment during the toddler years is limited. These children are at risk for troubled social relationships as they become older.

Development of Social Play

Infants and young toddlers tend to line up and engage in similar activities simultaneously. Play in this age group typically is parallel. While parents often expect their young toddler to interact or share with peers, success in this age group is unusual. Sharing for a young toddler involves showing a prized toy to another or handing it to the other child only to take it back within seconds.

By 2 years of age, with the development of symbolic capabilities in cognitive development, children begin to pretend. They will seek to engage their parents in activities that satisfy their growing curiosity. They enjoy reading with care givers and having their labeling questions answered.

Near 3 years of age, children begin to include one another in their pretending games. At first both children may select the same role (two mothers, for example) while later, the roles will become more interactive. The young preschooler is especially interested in imitating the parent of the same sex but shows no preference for play partners to be boys or girls.

The child's abilities to share are shaped by his social experiences. Children who attend day care may share successfully at an earlier age than children raised at home (Fig. 3.34). Although it can be achieved through consistent experience, taking turns is also a challenge for the preschooler who possesses a limited concept of time. Impulse control is just developing in the preschool years. Active goals for this age group include learning to gain the cooperation of one's peers, learning to communicate ideas to new friends, and learning to handle conflicts.

By 4 to 5 years of age, peer interactions grow increasingly cooperative and complicated; pretend play involves themes requiring greater feats of imagination and experience, such as trips or parties. Older preschoolers enjoy helping with household tasks and frequently are more interested in participating in gender-specific activities than they were at an earlier age.

This interest may relate to cognitive as well as social development. As children understand that they are in the same category as their same-sex parent, they become interested in the implications of category membership. Strict adherence to the rules of category membership reflects the concrete and inflexible thinking of the preschooler.

Preschoolers do not often play games with rules. Rules are seen as variable, to be made and broken at the discretion of the players. It is often a challenge to get through a board game with a preschooler who decides not to follow the rules once he discovers that they are not working in his favor.

Children become capable of playing by rules when they reach school age. With superior logical capabilities, they realize that rules are invariant, and must be followed regardless of the personal implications. As they progress through the elementary school years, board games and sports become preferred activities for groups of peers.

Development of Sense of Self

Self-awareness and independence develop gradually throughout life. The earliest indications of an emerging identity occur at 6 to 9 months of age, when the infant displays interest in his own mirror image. The 7- to 8-month old may prefer to grab a cup and spoon rather than accept a passive role in eating. This same infant may resist pressure to do something that he would prefer not to do; for example, he may fuss to stand when he has been placed in a sitting position.

Beyond 1 year of age, toddlers rapidly expand their senses of self. They explore their environment with ease, and they are increasingly able to function independently. They can feed themselves and manage a cup and spoon, and they have clear ideas about what they want. Children at 1 to 2 years of age also enjoy their own accomplishments and can clap for their own successes (Fig. 3.35).

An emerging sense of self and the thrust for independence make discipline of the toddler a challenge. Parents may need help in viewing their child's refusals to eat, nap, or be washed as positive steps toward increased independence. They may also need support in setting limits on the child's behaviors.

As the child reaches 2 to 3 years of age, increased independence in verbal abilities, increased awareness of body sensations, and modest skills in donning and doffing clothing combine with the child's desire to imitate adults and to gain

THE LEVINE (POSTER) CRITERIA FOR DIAGNOSIS OF CEREBRAL PALSY

1. Posturing and abnormal movement patterns—extensor thrusts, blocks
2. Oropharyngeal problems—tongue thrusts, grimacing, swallowing difficulties
3. Strabismus
4. Tone—increased or decreased in muscles
5. Evolutional responses—persistent primitive reflexes or failure to develop equilibrium and protective responses
6. Reflexes—deep tendon reflex increased and plantar reflexes up going

FIG. 3.36

parental approval. This allows toilet training to begin. In fact, the developmental milestones mentioned here may be viewed as readiness signs. The pediatrician can review them with families at the 15- or 18-month visit so that parents can time their toilet-training efforts to the child's developmental rate and style. Children differ substantially in their interest in achieving bladder and bowel control, and parents may benefit from counseling to maintain a relaxed approach.

In other areas as well, children need support in their attempts to initiate and control their own activities. Toward this end, parents can be encouraged to allow their child to practice emerging self-care skills, such as zippering or buttoning a coat, even when the practice costs precious time in a rushed schedule. Should the child become frustrated or disappointed, a response of empathy is likely to soothe more effectively than a response of reason, since rational reasoning is limited during this preoperational cognitive period.

By mid to late elementary school, cognitive development has progressed toward abstract and hypothetical thinking, such that children are able to reflect self-consciously about themselves and others. First- or second-graders struggle to understand the causes of conflict or their emotional reactions to it. Older elementary-school children and adolescents are able to analyze situations, reasons, and reactions. They begin to understand their own motivations as well as the environmental triggers of their responses.

Throughout childhood, the desire to grow up is in continued conflict with the desire to remain a child. The young preschooler is just beginning to address this issue. Families frequently report that a child's accomplishments in social-emotional functioning backslide when unexpected stresses challenge household equilibrium or when the child becomes ill. As a result, temporary regressions to earlier, safer levels of functioning may occur in some children. It is important that parents learn to view these lapses as expected components of development rather than as intentional lapses on the part of the child. However, if the regression is prolonged and significant, the physician may initiate an evaluation of the child's emotional status.

During elementary-school years, at least in Western cultures, the child's self-image is strongly influenced by success or failure in school. Difficulties with learning not only put additional pressures on the child; they also may damage the child's sense of self-worth. Parents and teachers of children with learning problems should be especially willing to praise the child for accomplishments and good behavior. Physicians should be particularly sensitive to the higher risk of emotional and behavioral problems in children with learning difficulties so that they can make timely referrals to colleagues in the mental health professions.

Evaluation of Social Development

Subtle indicators of social-developmental status can be gleaned in the course of a routine pediatric visit. The physician has the opportunity to note not only how the infant behaves but also the style of parental care giving and the nature of the parent-child relationship. The young infant typically shows social responsiveness to both the parent and the pediatrician, although at 9 months of age, there is a definite preference for the familiar parent. Also at this age, particularly in times of stress, the infant turns to the parent for support and comfort. Children of limited responsiveness, who avoid physical contact, who avert their gaze, or who in other ways fail to contribute to a mutually satisfying reciprocal exchange are of concern. Of equal concern are parents who are harsh, unresponsive, or threatening in response to the infant's needs.

Given the nature of social-developmental change, the assessment of possible problems must rely largely on history. Parents tend to be frank and open about the nature of their relationship with their child if questions are asked in a direct but nonjudgmental way. Difficulties in social development may relate to constitutional and temperamental characteristics of the child as well as to philosophy and practices of the parent. By remembering the bidirectional nature of causality in social development, the physician can avoid slipping into criticisms or judgments.

The older preschool or school-age child may be able to give, independently, direct information about social development. For example, the child may be able to name special friends and the activities that he enjoys with those friends. Young preschoolers might name both boys and girls, and list rough-and-tumble or fantasy play as favorite activities. Older preschoolers might name same-sex friends but similar activities. School-age children might add board games and sports to their list of activities.

VARIATIONS IN DEVELOPMENTAL PATTERNS

The presence or absence of a single skill at a particular age is rarely sufficient to determine developmental status. Developmental progress is highly dependent on multiple factors: the general health of the child, opportunities for learning, temperamental characteristics, willingness to try new experiences, genetic endowments, coordination and strength, and socioeconomic factors. Only if delays occur in more than one domain, and persist over time, are they considered significant. The challenge for the pediatrician is to differentiate variation from deviation.

Sometimes it is the parents who raise developmental concerns. These concerns must be addressed freely and openly. Parents are rarely comforted by superficial evaluation and pat reassurance, and while prudent waiting may serve some fami-

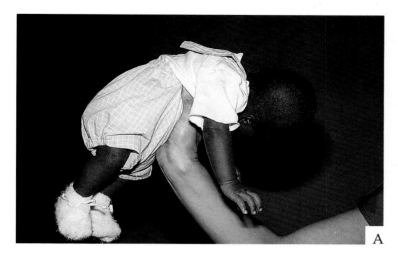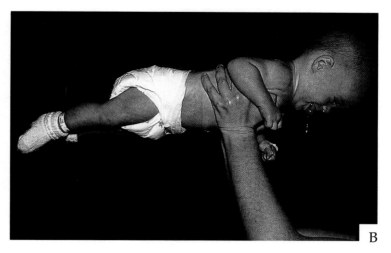

FIG. 3.37 Ventral suspension. **A,** this infant's posture is normal for a 1- to 3-month-old child held in ventral suspension. The head, hips, and knees are flexed. **B,** for a child 4 months of age or older held in ventral suspension with normal posture, the head, hips, and knees may be extended. This finding is abnormal in a child less than 3 months of age.

lies well, it may arouse anxiety and anger in others. If a comprehensive evaluation of a given problem is beyond the capabilities of the pediatrician, early referral should be considered.

Evaluation of developmental problems proceeds in the same manner as evaluation of other medical concerns: history, physical examination (including neurological and developmental evaluation), and laboratory testing. Important in establishing a diagnosis is consideration of the pattern of development across all domains. For example, findings of hypotonia and selective problems in gross motor skills along with normal development in cognition, language, and social skills are suggestive of a neuromuscular disorder or benign congenital hypotonia. In contrast, hypotonia found along with global developmental delay is suggestive of a central nervous system problem. It is also important to differentiate delayed behavior from deviant behavior. For example, since even neonates are able to make good eye contact with their care givers, the toddler who avoids eye contact is showing deviancy rather than delay. The combination of sustained deviant social behavior and delayed language development is suggestive of childhood autism.

In the following sections, specific primary developmental disorders are described. Each includes a discussion of physical findings, diagnostic criteria, etiology if known, and general issues of management and prognosis.

CEREBRAL PALSY
Definition

Cerebral palsy is a disorder of movement and posture resulting from injury to the motor areas of the brain. The type of cerebral palsy varies according to the location of the injured area. Injury may occur prenatally, during labor and delivery, or postnatally, up through the preschool years. The majority of affected patients have a history of perinatal complications. However, in 20 to 30 percent of cases, no etiology can be established. The key to making the diagnosis is to establish that motor problems are static rather than progressive. Regression of motor skills suggests a different set of diagnostic possibilities, including surgically treatable lesions of the brain or spinal cord, or inherited neurodegenerative diseases.

Physical Examination

A diagnosis of cerebral palsy and a determination of its subtype can be established through physical examination. However, physical findings over the first year of life are highly variable and nonspecific. Early signs may include decreased passive tone in the presence of elicitable, brisk, deep tendon reflexes without concomitant weakness. Early problems with sucking and swallowing may predate evidence of motor delays.

Because the findings may change, the definitive diagnosis of cerebral palsy should not be made until the child is at least 1 year of age. Beyond that point, the diagnosis is based on abnormal findings in four out of six major motor areas: posture, oral-motor functioning, visual-motor functioning, tone, evolution of primitive reflexes, or muscle-stretch reflexes (Fig. 3.36).

ABNORMALITIES OF TONE
Because damage to the central nervous system prevents the inhibition and balance of the inherent tone of the muscles, abnormalities of tone are particularly significant in the diagnosis of cerebral palsy. After initial hypotonia, a child may well develop increased tone between 12 and 18 months of age, showing clearly rigid or spastic hypertonia by age 2.

The child who demonstrates increased extensor tone beginning in early infancy also is at risk for cerebral palsy. Under normal circumstances, infants less than 3 months of age, when supported ventrally, maintain their heads in slight flexion with the trunks mildly convex (Fig. 3.37A). However, with exaggerated tone in the antigravity muscle group, the infant may elevate his head above the horizontally level trunk (Fig. 3.37B). Similarly, with the infant in the prone position on a mat, unknowing parents may be pleased by their child's apparent precocious development of head control or of early belly-to-back rolling in the first 2 months of life, when, in fact, both of these findings are suggestive of excessive extensor posturing.

Further evidence of abnormally increased tone will be found when the supine child is pulled to an upright position and extends at the hips and knees, coming to stand on pointed toes rather than ending up in the appropriate sitting posture. This child, when placed in vertical suspension, will not right his head as expected, and will later scissor the lower extremi-

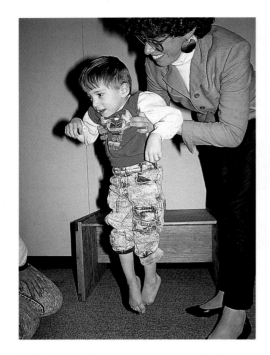

FIG. 3.38 Scissoring. Excessive pull of the hip adductors and internal rotators in this child of 3 years results in his legs crossing in a scissorlike pattern while he is supported in vertical suspension.

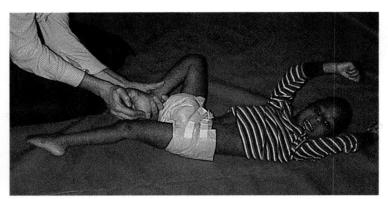

FIG. 3.39 Marie-Foix maneuver. By flexing the child's toes, the therapist can reduce extensor tone enough to obtain abduction of the hip and knee flexion in this child with spastic quadriplegia.

FIG. 3.40 Asymmetric Moro response. Note one hand is fisted and one open. This child warrants a complete neurologic examination and close followup.

ties as a result of hypertonia of the leg adductors and internal rotators (Fig. 3.38). Parents may find it difficult to position these infants for diapering and feeding; knowledge of the Marie-Foix maneuver, used to break up excessive extension in the lower extremities (Fig. 3.39) will help them.

ABNORMALITIES IN DEVELOPMENT OF PRIMITIVE REFLEXES AND EQUILIBRIUM RESPONSES

Abnormal persistence of primitive reflexes is helpful in making a diagnosis of cerebral palsy. Damage to the central nervous system prevents high levels of control from superseding and inhibiting the influence of the early reflexes. Thus, obligate or persistent primitive reflexes are signs of cerebral palsy. For example, in the normal variant of the asymmetric tonic neck reflex (ATNR), the infant can move out of the posture if the gaze is directed to the other side of the body. In an obligate ATNR, however, the infant remains in the fencer position until the head is passively moved. This finding is not normal in a child of any age, and is highly suggestive of the static encephalopathy and motor deficit characterizing cerebral palsy.

Also strongly suggestive of cerebral palsy is the non-obligate ATNR that persists beyond 6 months of age. This is one possible explanation for a consistent preference in a 6- to 12-month-old child to sleep or lie with the head turned in a particular direction. Similarly, persistence of the Moro response beyond 6 months of age is associated with cerebral palsy, as is a lack of development of lateral protective equilibrium reactions by 7 to 8 months or of the parachute reaction by 10 months of age.

Sub-Types of Cerebral Palsy

HEMIPARESIS

Hemiparesis is caused by asymmetrical damage to the motor control areas of the central nervous system. In children with hemiparesis, functional discrepancies often predate asymmetric changes in tone or reflexes. The upper extremities may be affected more severely than the lower extremities. Asymmetric use of the upper or lower extremities is rare during the first 4 months of life. When seen in the resting state, or when elicited with the ATNR or the Moro response (Fig. 3.40), it is more likely related to lower motor neuron disease than to cerebral injury (see Chapter 2, Neonatology). At 4 to 6 months, during the development of early reaching and grasping, signs of hemiparesis include the presence of one hand that is fisted, the child's arm getting caught beneath him when he tries to prop himself up on elbows or hands, and evidence that the arm is not used in simple tasks. Increased resistance to supination at the wrist, limited flopping of one wrist when the upper extremities are gently shaken, or extra beats of unilateral clonus at the ankle are other clues.

Later, during the first year of life, abnormal findings include a failure to develop the protective response of lateral propping, or the development of an asymmetric parachute response. In addition, crawling may be uneven, with propulsion coming from one side while the opposite arm and leg are dragged behind.

Children with hemiparesis will have sufficient difficulty compensating for their lack of protective responses, their uneven strength, and poor balance. Walking is typically de-

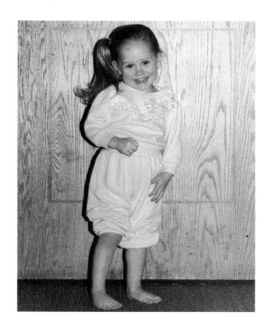

FIG. 3.41 *Note the arm held in flexion and internal rotation, and the leg circumducted on the involved side in this child with hemiplegic cerebral palsy.*

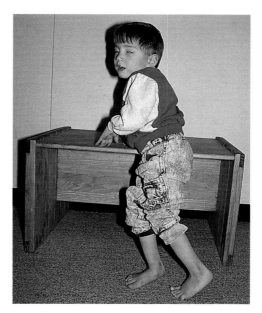

FIG. 3.42 *Toe walking. Four-year-old child with cerebral palsy cruising on furniture. Notice that the child is crouched due to hamstring tightness and is toe walking due to gastrocnemius tightness.*

layed until 2½ to 3 years of age. In mildly affected children, walking may be almost normal, but when asked to run, the child may show posturing of the upper extremity in flexion and internal rotation. Usually, the lower limb will rotate internally and the foot may be held in equinus, making it functionally longer on the swing-through part of the gait. To clear the foot from the floor, the child will compensate by swinging the leg farther out in abduction or by circumducting the affected side. These patterns, in some cases, also can be observed in standing (Fig. 3.41).

Children with hemiparesis may neglect the visual field on their affected side. Parents should position their infant so that visual stimulation is provided to the intact visual field. Another consideration is that of abnormal bony stresses caused by asymmetric muscle strength. In children with hemiparesis, unequal spinal stresses predispose them to scoliosis, especially during growth spurts.

SPASTIC DIPLEGIA/QUADRIPLEGIA
Spastic diplegia implies dysfunction of the lower extremities, with normal or limited involvement of the upper extremities. Spastic quadriplegia implies dysfunction of both upper and lower extremities. The child with spasticity may present with delayed sitting, crawling or walking, or with toe walking (Fig. 3.42). In the supine position, children with spastic diplegia may keep their lower extremities in the "frog" position, with the hips and knees flexed and the hips externally rotated. In the erect position, the child may internally rotate and adduct the legs, leading to scissoring (see Fig. 3.38). The ankles assume the equinus position. The child who toe-walks will have brisk, deep tendon reflexes, limited range of ankle motion, Babinski reflexes, and a normally proportioned muscle mass.

The differential diagnosis of toe walking includes the muscular dystrophies, tethered spinal cords and spinal tumors, peripheral neuropathies, and fixed bony deformities of the feet. Unilateral or asymmetric toe walking may indicate leg-length discrepancy or a dislocated hip as an isolated finding or in conjunction with spasticity.

DYSTONIC-ATHETOID CEREBRAL PALSY
In children with athetoid or ataxic cerebral palsy, involuntary movements do not present until after the first year of life. However, affected infants tend to be hypotonic and normoreflexic from the outset, and motor milestones are delayed. Between 1 and 2 years of age, hypotonia is usually replaced by spasticity, and involuntary movements appear. Exaggerated tone and dyskinetic movements reach maximal intensity around age 3. Athetoid cerebral palsy has been associated with bilirubin encephalopathy and damage to the basal ganglia.

HYPOTONIC CEREBRAL PALSY
Some hypotonic infants with exaggerated reflexes do not progress to hypertonicity. The putative explanation is cerebellar dysfunction with pyramidal track involvement. The child with hypotonic cerebral palsy usually exhibits severe motor and intellectual disability. The prognosis for independent functioning is quite poor. Hypotonic cerebral palsy must be differentiated from benign congenital hypotonia, an isolated disorder of tone, which spares other developmental areas.

Associated Findings with Cerebral Palsy

As many as 75 percent of children with diplegia or quadriplegia have strabismus (see Chapter 19, Ophthalmology). Refractive errors are found in 25 to 50 percent of children with cerebral palsy. Clumsiness due to motor imbalance of the lower extremities may be exaggerated by altered depth perception resulting from impaired visual function. Ophthalmologic referral for phorias and tropias that persist beyond 4 months of age is important to prevent amblyopia.

Hearing loss is also associated with cerebral palsy. While clinical evaluation may suggest hearing loss, a definitive diagnosis requires an audiological assessment. Brainstem auditory responses can be obtained to assess hearing capabilities in infants less than 6 months of age and in older children unable perform in conditioned play audiometry because of motor or intellectual problems.

Approximately 50 percent of children with cerebral palsy have intellectual limitations or mental retardation. Learning disabilities and attentional weaknesses are more prevalent in this population than in the general population. Furthermore, behavioral problems may develop as a result of the frustration encountered in trying to adjust to motor disabilities.

Prognosis

Overall, the ability of individuals with cerebral palsy to live and work independently depends on the severity of the motor handicap and associated cognitive impairments. If a child is 4 years of age or older and has not achieved sitting balance, independent walking with or without crutches is rarely possible. A child 2 to 4 years of age who cannot sit and has three or more primitive reflexes is also unlikely to walk.

As cerebral palsy affects multiple systems, children with the disorder are best served by an interdisciplinary team including not only medical professionals but also social workers, psychologists, occupational and physical therapists, speech and communication therapists, and educational and vocational specialists. In many cases, children will require educational support for both physical and intellectual problems. They may also require behavioral management training or pharmacological intervention for attentional weaknesses. Some of the behavioral problems can be prevented by matching developmental expectations to the child's functional capacities. These children and their families benefit enormously from the support of a primary care physician who offers routine health-care maintenance, diagnostic and preventative procedures such as referrals to audiology and ophthalmology specialists, and advice and counseling on the interpretation of team evaluations.

MENTAL RETARDATION
Definition

According to the American Association on Mental Deficiency, mental retardation is defined as "significantly subaverage general intellectual functioning existing concurrently with deficits in adaptive behavior and manifested during the developmental period." Significantly subaverage functioning refers to scores, obtained on standardized intelligence tests, that are at least 2 standard deviations below age-group norms; adaptive behaviors refer to the broader areas of functioning such as self-care, community survival skills (such as using the telephone, making change, and using public transportation), and social interactions; and the developmental period refers to the period from birth to 18 years of age.

The ability to predict intellectual performance and academic achievement from developmental testing during infancy is quite limited. Only in children falling far behind age expectations should one estimate permanent intellectual disability. Nonetheless, if an infant shows delayed cognitive development, the parents' reasonable concerns can be met with a referral to an early intervention program.

As the child approaches school age, particularly if he has had optimal educational support, the ability to predict later difficulties improves. The rate of developmental progress during the preschool years is often a good predictor of later intellectual performance. After initial cognitive developmental delays, if a child is able to achieve 6 months' progress in 6 months' time, the prognosis for normal intellectual capacity is good. However, if the child achieves, for example, 4 months' progress in 6 months' time, the rate of development is 67 percent of the expected rate, and the prognosis for later intellectual functioning is poor. By the time a child is 6 to 7 years of age, limitations as measured on an IQ test typically characterize the individual's abilities throughout his lifetime. At that point, the term mental retardation is more specific and accurate than developmental delay.

Physical Examination

Physical examination can be helpful in determining the cause of mental retardation. Most children classified as mentally retarded function in the mildly retarded range. These children often have a normal physical examination, with no apparent evidence of malformation or deformity. In contrast to children with severe mental retardation, who will be readily identified, children with mild retardation are likely to present with normal motor milestones and delays only in adaptive areas such as self-care, language acquisition, or play. The detection of disability in these mildly affected youngsters may not be possible until the child experiences school performance difficulties.

The average IQ of parents of children with mild mental retardation is lower than the population norm. Thus, many of these parents also show limitations in intellectual abilities. For this reason, the etiology of mild mental retardation is generally felt to be multi-factorial, including both multiple genetic contributions and limited social enrichment.

The more significant the degree of retardation, the more likely that a specific etiologic factor will be found. Children who score in the moderate, severe, or profound ranges are likely to have congenital malformations of the central nervous system, severe neurological insults in the prenatal or perinatal period, an inherited disorder, or another specific diagnosis. A systematic approach to the physical examination may reveal clues to the nature of the underlying disorder.

GROWTH PATTERN AND VITAL SIGNS

Aberrant growth patterns which are in and of themselves the cause for assessment, may be associated with developmental delays and mental retardation. Obesity appears as part of a number of syndromes associated with mental deficiency, such as Laurence-Moon syndrome and Prader-Willi syndrome (see Chapter 1, Genetics). Children who are exceptionally large may have cerebral giantism (Soto syndrome). Small-for-date infants deserve close study for evidence of anomalies or infection; they are also at risk for abnormal development. Extreme to moderate short stature, with or without skeletal dysplasia, is associated with many dysmorphic syndromes that include mental retardation as an associated finding. Growth curves have been prepared for children with Down syndrome since they tend to be shorter than the general population (Fig. 3.43). However, if children are shorter than expected even for the population of children with Down syndrome, or if children fall off of their own curve after following a percentile, then endocrine-function abnormalities such as hypothyroidism should be investigated.

SKIN FINDINGS

Hemangiomas, multiple café au lait spots, and sebaceous adenomas may be evidence of an underlying neurocutaneous abnormality, thereby providing a constitutional basis for a developmental delay. Von Recklinghausen's disease and tuberous sclerosis, both examples of neurocutaneous disorders, are inherited as autosomal dominant, although there is a high rate of spontaneous mutation. If these disorders are diagnosed or suspected, examination of the immediate family is warranted (see Chapter 15). Hirsutism occurs in both fetal alcohol and fetal hydantoin syndromes (see Chapter 1). Abnormal fingernail formation can signal teratogenic influences or ectodermal dysplasias (see Chapter 8).

CRANIAL ABNORMALITIES

Head circumference provides an obvious clue to the cause of mental retardation; undergrowth of the cranium may indicate central nervous system damage or dysgenesis; overgrowth may indicate hydrocephalus. Abnormal skull shape may indicate that the underlying nervous system has undergone unusual physical stresses.

Transillumination will aid in the diagnosis of porencephalic cysts or of other structural defects in young infants (see Chapter 15). The presence of an intracranial bruit may indicate an arteriovenous malformation, although such bruits are sometimes heard in normal infants. Even in the absence of these signs, children with moderate, severe, and profound mental retardation may warrant an imaging study of the central nervous system because of the high incidence of identifiable abnormalities.

FACIAL ABNORMALITIES

The presence of certain facial characteristics may suggest a specific etiology of mental retardation. Minor malformations including hypotelorism or hypertelorism, epicanthal folds, colobomata, and auricles that are large, abnormally formed, or set low in comparison to the plane of the eyes are rare in the general population. In isolation, one dysmorphic feature may be insignificant. However, the presence of three or more of these features correlates highly with a major malformation, often of heart, kidney, or brain. Patterns of dysmorphic features may suggest a specific diagnosis such as a genetic syndrome, chromosomal abnormality, or prenatal exposure. For example, flat facies, upturned palpebral fissures, epicanthal folds, single palmar creases, and clinodactyly are associated with trisomy 21 (Down syndrome) (Fig. 3.44). Likewise, a lengthened philtrum, a thin vermilion border, and microcephaly are clinical features of the fetal alcohol syndrome.

Some of these unusual features themselves are clues to the etiology of the intellectual disability or are the result of abnormal functioning, even in prenatal life. For example, aberrant patterning of scalp hair may indicate abnormal cerebral morphology. The pattern of hair growth is affected by pressures from the developing brain on the overlying scalp in early gestation. The absence of a posterior hair whorl or the presence of multiple hair whorls is suggestive of abnormal prenatal brain growth. Small palpebral fissures also result from abnormal brain growth; the eye is an extension of the brain and small eyes are suggestive of abnormal early brain development. Similarly, a high-arched palate may be secondary to abnormal motor activity of the tongue in utero, suggesting a prenatal origin of motor problems.

OTHER PHYSICAL ABNORMALITIES

Hepatosplenomegaly in the neonatal period may suggest congenital infection, or, in childhood, may indicate a heritable storage disease affecting central nervous system and developmental functioning. Large testes are found in youngsters with fragile X chromosomal abnormalities, while hypogonadism is a concomitant of the Prader-Willi syndrome. About one half of the patients with this syndrome will be found to have an abnormality on chromosome 15 (see Chapter 1).

Changes in the long bones of the limbs may show evidence of congenital infection; disproportionate bone length may suggest metabolic disorders such as homocystinuria or the osteochondrodysplasias. Errant toe proportions or changed crease patterns on the hands or soles of the feet may suggest early morphogenetic changes associated with certain defined syndromes. Lethargic or pale children may prompt an examination for iron deficiency or lead intoxication, which also may contribute to subnormal intellectual progress.

Prognosis

Some 3 percent of newborns will be classified as mentally retarded at some point in their lives. In a society that prizes intellectual accomplishment, the identification of cognitive delays is upsetting for a family. Findings of unusual features in any aspect of the physical examination may help to provide an explanation for abnormal or delayed cognitive development. In evaluating the cause of developmental delay, the greatest need beyond that of assessing the possibility of remediation, is that of providing parents with appropriate genetic, behavioral, and educational counseling. Evidence that a child's lack of developmental progress is related to constitutional factors can help relieve parents of guilt feelings.

In the past, physicians have often underestimated the capabilities of children with mild to moderate retardation. Similarly, families often interpret a diagnosis of mental retardation to mean that their child will make no further developmental progress. Estimates of functional abilities for children who are classified as mentally retarded are variable. Children with mild mental retardation (IQ scores 2–3 standard deviations below the mean; 69–55) can be taught to read and write and to do simple mathematics. As adults they often live independently and hold jobs. The extent of their disability will be most prominent during the school years or during times of life crisis beyond school age. Children with moderate mental retardation (IQ scores 3–4 standard deviations below the mean; 54–40) probably will not learn to read and write. Nonetheless, their abilities in language, self-care, and adaptation skills may allow them to live and work in semi-independent supervised settings. Children with severe and profound mental retardation (4–6 standard deviations below the mean; 39–24 and below) require substantial lifelong support.

The benefits of early intervention will be maximized by early identification. Careful historical documentation of the child's opportunities for interaction with parents, other children, and stimulating environments will help in determining the type and degree of intervention needed. The importance of careful screening of infant and preschool development by informed health professionals and of close collaboration between physicians and early intervention personnel cannot be overemphasized.

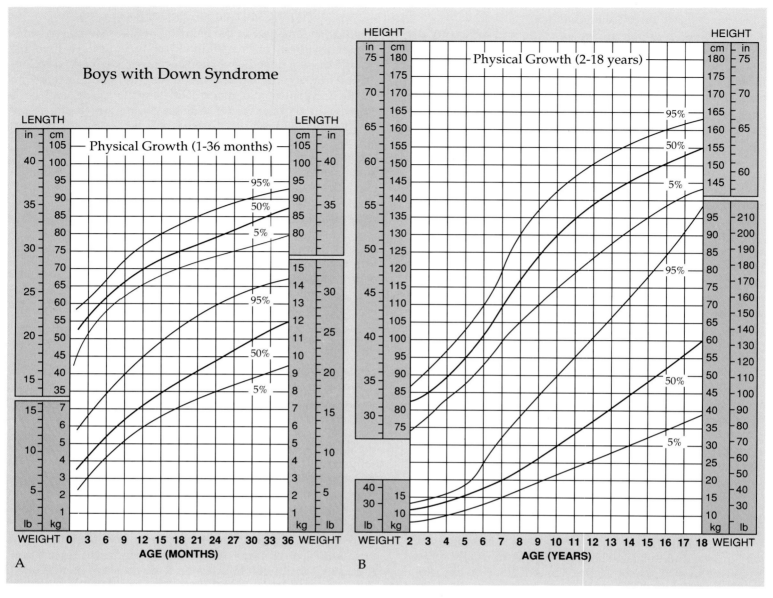

FIG. 3.43 (Reproduced by permission from Cronk C, Crocker AC, Pueschel SM, et al: Growth charts for children with Down syndrome. Pediatrics, 1988;81:108)

SPECIFIC LANGUAGE AND READING DISORDERS

Definition

Delays and disturbances in language development are most frequently associated with mental retardation, hearing impairment, childhood autism, and environmental deprivation. However, language difficulties may occur in an otherwise normal child; in such cases, they are referred to as specific language disabilities, usually of unknown etiology. Some theories stress difficulties with high-level concepts and symbolic capabilities, and others stress auditory perceptual impairments as the root of specific language disorders.

Physical Examination

There are no specific physical signs associated with specific language disorders. The physician's role is, in large part, to rule out other disorders with different etiologies and prognoses. Hearing assessment is indicated for any child with delays or deviancies in language development, since hearing loss is treatable. In early infancy, this requires use of brainstem auditory-evoked response, an electrophysiological measure that records brain waves as a function of sound exposure. In older infants and toddlers we typically utilize conditioned play techniques. The child is rewarded for turning toward the source of a sound. In preschoolers, conventional audiometry

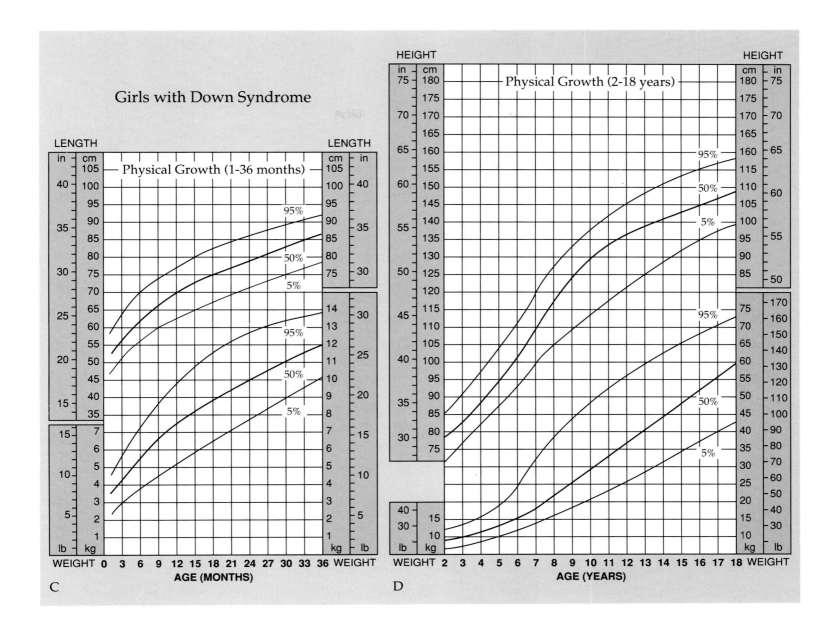

Girls with Down Syndrome

Physical Growth (1-36 months)

Physical Growth (2-18 years)

C

D

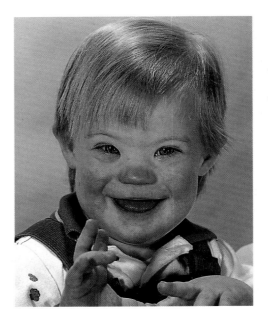

FIG. 3.44 Down syndrome. Note the upslanting palpebral fissures, flat nasal bridge, epicanthal folds, small ears, and small hands.

with the use of headphones allows for evaluation of each ear independently (Fig. 3.45).

Hearing should be assessed in all children with syndromes known to be associated with hearing loss. These include Treacher-Collins, osteogenesis imperfecta, Waardenburg, and congenital rubella syndromes. Evaluation should not await delays in language acquisition. Abnormalities of the external ear including preauricular tags and pits also may be associated with abnormalities of the ossicular chain and conductive, as well as sensorineural hearing loss. Again, early hearing assessment is advisable for children with abnormalities of the external ear, the palate, or facial structures, or for chil-

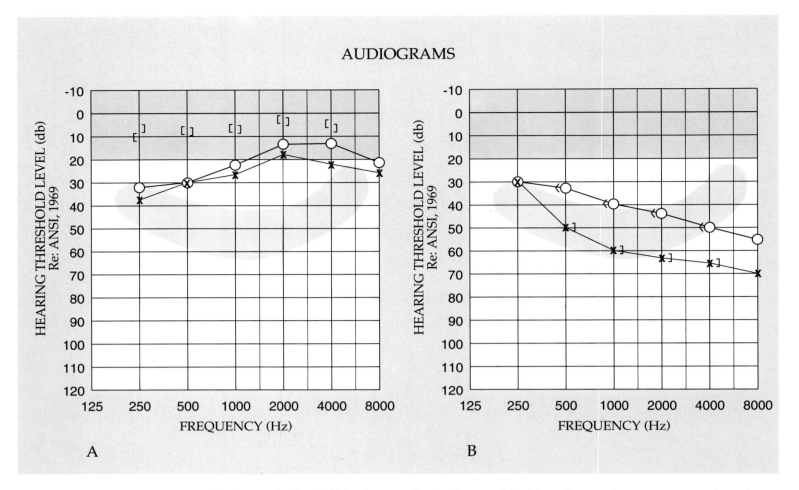

A

B

FIG. 3.45 Audiograms. The letter "X" indicates the threshold for the left ear and the letter "O" indicates the threshold for the right ear. Brackets indicate bone conduction. A, this audiogram indicates mild conductive hearing loss in both ears. Notice that more energy is required for detection of sound in the low-frequency range. Bone con-

duction is normal. B, this audiogram demonstrates sensorineural hearing loss. The left ear shows a sloping pattern with mild to moderate loss in the low-frequency range and severe loss in the high-frequency range. The right ear shows mild to moderate loss throughout the frequency range.

CONDITIONS ASSOCIATED WITH SENSORINEURAL HEARING LOSS

Family history of childhood hearing impairment
Congenital perinatal infection (CMV, rubella, herpes, toxoplasmosis, syphilis)
Anatomical malformations of head or neck
Birth weight less than 1,500 grams
Hyperbilirubinemia above levels indicated for exchange transfusion
Bacterial meningitis
Severe asphyxia
Exposure to ototoxic medications

FIG. 3.46

dren who are otherwise at risk for hearing impairment (Fig. 3.46). Conditions associated with varying degrees of hearing loss, their disabling effects, and the interventions required for children with these conditions are listed in Figure 3.47.

Some 60 percent of all cases of sensorineural hearing loss in preverbal children will be of undetermined etiology. For these

children, an absence of expected hearing behaviors is the best clue to the presence of a hearing problem. Healthy newborns react to sounds with startle responses and with changes in their level of alertness. In the neonatal period, and then again after 3 months of age, the infant should be able to turn toward the source of a sound (see Fig. 3.29). Qualitative differences in the early behaviors of children with hearing impairment in comparison to their peers without hearing impairment have been observed in sensorimotor functioning, receptive and expressive language, and social functioning. These abnormalities include indifference to the spoken word, decreased vocalization and sound production, increased visual attentiveness, altered social rapport, and frustrations in communicating.

The relationship between language development and otitis media with effusion is unclear. Chronic otitis media with effusion may be associated with a variable, mild to moderate conductive hearing loss (see Fig. 3.47). Some studies have found an association between frequent bouts of otitis media and delays in speech and language, presumably a consequence of variable hearing loss. However, other studies have found no such relationship. In the absence of a straightforward correlation between the appearance of the tympanic membrane or the results of tympanometry and the degree of hearing loss in otitis media with effusion, one sensible approach is to evaluate the hearing status of affected children through audiometry. If hearing loss is documented, or if the child shows a delay in

DISABLING EFFECTS OF HEARING LOSS

Average Hearing 500–2000 Hz (ANSI)	Description	Condition	Sounds Heard Without Amplification	Degree of Disability (if not treated in first year of life)	Probable Needs
0–15 dB	Normal range	Serous otitis, perforation, monomeric membrane, tympanosclerosis	All speech sounds	None	None
15–25 dB	Slight hearing loss	Serous otitis, perforation, monomeric membrane, sensorineural loss, tympanosclerosis	Vowel sounds heard clearly; may miss unvoiced consonant sounds	Mild auditory dysfunction in language learning	Consideration of need for hearing aid; lipreading; auditory training, speech therapy, preferential seating
25–40 dB	Mild hearing loss	Serous otitis, perforation, tympanosclerosis, monomeric membrane, sensorineural loss	Hears only some louder-voiced speech sounds	Auditory learning dysfunction, mild language retardation, mild speech problems, inattention	Hearing aid, lipreading, auditory training, speech therapy
40–65 dB	Moderate hearing loss	Chronic otitis, middle ear anomaly, sensorineural loss	Misses most speech sounds at normal conversational level	Speech problems, language retardation, learning dysfunction, inattention	All the above, plus consideration of special classroom situation
65–95 dB	Severe hearing loss	Sensorineural or mixed loss from sensorineural loss plus middle ear disease	Hears no speech sounds of normal conversation	Severe speech problems, language retardation, learning dysfunction, inattention	All the above; plus probable assignment to special classes
More than 95 dB	Profound hearing loss	Sensorineural or mixed loss	Hears no speech or other sounds	Severe speech problems, language retardation, learning dysfunction, inattention	All the above; plus probable assignment to special classes

FIG. 3.47 *(Reproduced by permission from Stewart JM, Downs MP: Medical management of the hearing-handicapped child, in Northern JL (ed):* Hearing Disorders, *ed 2. Boston, Little Brown, 1984, 271)*

language development, aggressive medical or surgical management may be warranted.

Prognosis

Many toddlers with specific language disorders will develop adequate speech, language, and communication skills by the middle of elementary school. At present, there are no variables consistently associated with a good prognosis; however, the prognosis for communication is clearly improved through early communication therapy. Physicians should not hesitate to refer children with speech and language delays for assessment and treatment.

Many toddlers and preschoolers with selective problems in language acquisition develop reading difficulties during the school-age years. Difficulty in a specific aspect of learning that is greater than that expected for the child's overall intellectual functioning qualifies as a learning disability. Reading disorder

Age of Infant	Behavior
Term	Focus on face, briefly tracks vertically and horizontally, turns toward diffuse light source, widens eyes to object or face at 8-12 inches
1 month	Blinks at approaching object, tracks 60° horizontally, 30° vertically
2 months	Tracks across midline, follows movement 6 feet away, smiles to a smiling face, raises head 30° in prone
3 months	Eyes and head track 180°, looks at hands, looks at objects placed in hands
4-5 months	Reaches for object (12-inch cube) 12 inches away, notices raisins 1 foot away, smiles at familiar adult
5-6 months	Smiles in mirror
7-8 months	Rakes at raisin
8-9 months	Notes visual details, pokes at holes in peg board and at elevator buttons
9 months	Neat pincer grasp
12-14 months	Stacks blocks, places peg in round hole

FIG. 3.48

or dyslexia is a frequent finding in a child with an early history of language delay and a positive family history of reading disability. With increasing age, children with reading difficulties tend to improve. However, in many cases, reading will remain an area of relative weakness in comparison to other cognitive and academic skills.

Children with reading disorders show abnormal or inefficient eye movements in the course of reading. This observation has led to visual training as a treatment strategy. However, the literature supports the notion that in most cases, a reading problem is a high-level language difficulty, not a visual or visual-motor problem.

VISUAL IMPAIRMENT

Visual experience facilitates the learning of many important concepts of space and form that are important in the development of motor skills, perception, cognition, and social skills (Fig. 3.48). Thus, in situations of congenital blindness or visual impairment, developmental patterns may be altered and delayed, demonstrating the close interrelationships that exist among developmental domains. Children with visual impairments can learn to increase the use of residual visual functioning and of other sensory modalities. The physician's understanding of the impact of visual impairment is important to evaluate whether developmental progress is being achieved as expected in this population and to assure that unexpected delays and deviancies are appropriately diagnosed and treated.

Gross and Fine Motor Development

Apparently, much of the motivation for the infant with normal vision to raise his head 90° when he is in the prone position is to increase his visual field. Without the feedback of interesting sights, the infant with severe visual impairment may not attain this milestone until 11 to 12 months of age. In contrast, rolling occurs in infants who are blind at close to the same age as in infants with normal vision. If sitting independently is an active goal, it can occur by 6 to 7 months of age. However, transitional movements from lying to sitting or from sitting to standing will occur several months later in infants without sight than in infants able to see.

Protective reactions develop more slowly in infants with severe visual impairment, and these are expected to appear in the 10- to 12-month age range. This delay, as well as the inability to integrate visual cues in attaining balance and equilibrium, and the lack of a visual impetus to explore distant toys, may contribute to a typical delay in crawling or walking. Paired auditory-tactile cues presented to children with severe visual impairment may stimulate their interest in objects beyond their reach, thus accelerating gross motor development.

Regarding fine motor development, information gathering by index finger and manual manipulation may be more accurate in the child who is blind than in the child with normal vision. However, the youngster who is blind may experience a delay in the acquisition of precise prehension, which sometimes never develops, with raking favored as a more efficient means of exploration.

Cognitive Development

The development of cognitive skills in the child with visual impairment must, of necessity, depend on use of the other sensory modalities. For this reason, careful global evaluation of the child with severe visual impairment should be conducted early in infancy to assure that the other senses are intact.

A child with normal vision develops the understanding that objects are permanent even when they cannot be seen, felt, heard, sniffed, or tasted. For the child with severe visual impairment, the opportunities for object perception are fewer and thus, the understanding of object permanence typically develops later, stimulated by encouragement of the infant to reach for sound cues. Similarly, this child's understanding of conservation of continuous quantity, that a cup of water contains the same volume of liquid in a tall thin container as it does in a short fat one, also develops later than in the child with normal vision.

Haptic perception, the acquisition of information about objects or spaces by exploration with the hands, appears to be more important in the cognitive development of the child with severe visual impairment than in that of the child with normal vision. For this reason, tactile exploration in the child who is blind cannot be promoted at too early an age. In fact, without such encouragement, these children may be fearful and resistant to unfamiliar new feelings.

Language and Intellectual Development

Verbal imitation and receptive language skills may develop normally in healthy children who are blind. As one might expect, these children may have difficulty with words relating to visual concepts, such as "light," "dark," or "color." They also may have problems with words referring to large things that cannot be touched ("sky" or "stars"), things that change slowly ("age" or "growth"), or the concept "I." However, some children with severe visual impairment show accurate use of all of these concepts and even make the distinction between the words "look" and "see." In these cases, the child probably uses available linguistic information to substitute for visual information.

While standard IQ tests cannot be used to assess intellectual capabilities of children with severe visual impairment, standardized instruments have been developed to assess their cognitive development. Receptive and expressive language skills figure prominently in these assessments. In addition, interview schedules of adaptive behavior in communication and self-help skills have been normed for children with visual impairment.

Social Development

Infants who are blind lack the opportunity to benefit from face-to-face contact with their care givers, from the visual reinforcement of smiling, from the use of facial expressions to assist in the interpretation of voices or actions, and from the experience of tracking parents across the room to know that even when they cannot be heard or felt they are still there. These differences in sensory input affect their social and emotional development. Parents of infants with severe visual impairment frequently need to be coached to use touch and sound to reinforce smiling and other desired behaviors in their child.

At about the same time that children with normal vision smile at familiar faces, children who are blind will smile in response to familiar touching and kinesthetic handling. Smiling in response to a familiar voice, however, may occur inconsistently up to 1 year of age. The infant who is blind will demonstrate attachment by calming to the tactile exploration of the care giver's familiar face or hands.

Blind children of about 1 year of age may present with stranger awareness, although a greater hurdle will be their reaction to separation. Because these children have a limited capacity to track their care givers, separations from them may induce panic states even among older ones. Similarly, the development of independent care giving and play may be delayed, and may require specific interventions.

Parents should be advised that, without purposeful stimulation, children who are blind may engage in nonpurposeful motor activities such as eye rubbing or rocking, and that these stereotypic behaviors, referred to as blindisms, are difficult to extinguish. Blindisms can often be channeled to purposeful stimulation by directing the child's hands to exploration of a toy or by distracting the child with conversation or music. These efforts will serve to channel the child's activities in a more socially adaptive direction.

SUMMARY

The tasks of routine developmental surveillance, identification of children with variations, and referral for appropriate developmental services, especially during infancy and in the preschool years, fall largely, and often exclusively, to the primary care physician. Although we have provided estimates regarding the expected chronology of development, these developmental milestones are guidelines rather than fixed time frames within which behavior acquisition may be judged as normal or abnormal. In evaluating a child, the physician must employ these guidelines in the light of his or her own clinical judgment, taking into account the child's own personality traits, experiences, and degree of cooperation.

Recommendations for further assessment and treatment should be made in consultation with the family

BIBLIOGRAPHY

American Academy of Pediatrics Joint Committee on Infant Hearing: Position statement 1982. *Pediatrics* 1982;70:496-497.

Diagnostic and Statistical Manual of Mental Disorders, ed 3. Washington, DC, American Psychiatric Association, 1980.

Dixon SD, Stein MT (eds): *Encounters with Children.* Chicago, Year Book Medical Publishers, 1986.

Fraiberg S: *Insights from the Blind.* New York, Basic Books, 1977.

Illingsworth RS: *The Development of the Infant and Young Child Abnormal and Normal,* ed 7. New York, Churchill Livingstone, 1980.

Knobloch H, Pasamanick B (eds): *Gesell and Amatruda's Developmental Diagnosis,* ed 3. New York, Harper & Row, 1974.

Levine M, Carey W, Crocker A, Gross R: *Developmental-Behavioral Pediatrics.* Philadelphia, WB Saunders, 1983.

Louick D, Baland T: Psychological tests: a guide for pediatricians. *Pediatr Ann* 1978;7(12):86-101.

Northern JL, Downs MP: *Hearing in Children.* Baltimore, Williams & Wilkins, 1974.

Opitz JM: Mental retardation: biological aspects of concern to pediatricians. *Pediatr Rev* 1980;2(2):41-40.

Scheiner AP, Moomaw M: Care of the visually handicapped child. *Pediatr Rev* 1982;4(3):74-81.

Smith D: *Recognizable Patterns of Human Malformation.* Philadelphia, WB Saunders, 1976.

Smith DW, Simons FER: Rational diagnosis evaluation of the child with mental deficiency. *Am J Dis Child* 1975;129:1285.

PEDIATRIC ALLERGY AND IMMUNOLOGY

David P. Skoner, M.D. ◆ Andrew H. Urbach, M.D. ◆ Philip Fireman, M.D.

CLASSIFICATION OF HYPERSENSITIVITY DISORDERS

		Interval Between Exposure and Reaction	Effector Cell or Antibody	Target or Antigen	Examples of Mediators	Examples
Type I	Anaphylactic a. Immediate b. Late phase	 <30 minutes 2 to 12 hours	IgE	Pollens, foods, drugs, insect venoms	 a. Histamine b. Leukotrienes	Anaphylaxis Allergic rhinitis Allergic asthma Urticaria
Type II	Cytotoxic	Variable (minutes to hours)	IgG, IgM	Red blood cells Lung tissue	Complement	Immune hemolytic anemia Rh hemolytic disease Goodpasture syndrome
Type III	Immune complexes	4–8 hours	Antigen with anti body	Vascular endothelium	Complement Anaphylatoxin	Serum sickness Poststreptococcal glomerulonephritis
Type IV	Delayed type	24–48 hours	Lymphocytes	*Mycobacterium tuberculosis* Chemicals	Lymphokines	Contact dermatitis Tuberculin skin test reactions

FIG. 4.1 *(Reproduced from Gell PGH, Coombs RRA:* Clinical Aspects of Immunology, *ed 2, Philadelphia, FA Davis, 1968)*

FIG. 4.1

Disorders of the immune system are diverse and range from mild to severe in their manifestations and impact on normal function. This chapter emphasizes physical findings and characteristic symptoms of children with disorders of hypersensitivity and immunodeficiency, as well as diagnostic techniques and radiographic findings. Topics have been chosen on the basis of (1) their prevalence and importance in the pediatric population and (2) their association with characteristic physical findings.

IMMUNOLOGICAL HYPERSENSITIVITY DISORDERS

Hypersensitivity disorders of the human immune system have been classified by Gell and Coombs into four groups (Fig. 4.1) based on the different mechanisms by which immune reactions may initiate tissue inflammation. Type I reactions occur promptly after the sensitized individual is exposed to antigen and are mediated by specific IgE antibody. This mechanism is

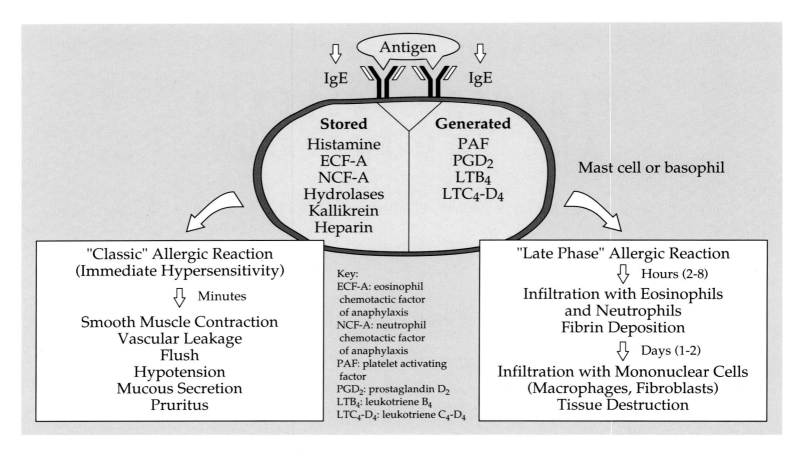

FIG. 4.2 Mechanism of antigen-induced mediator release in Type I hypersensitivity. Note that both an early (classic) and late phase reaction can follow antigen exposure.

responsible for the common disorders of immediate hypersensitivity, such as allergic rhinitis and urticaria. Type II reactions involve antibodies directed against antigenic components of peripheral blood or tissue cells, resulting in cell destruction. Examples of this type include autoimmune hemolytic anemia, and Rh and ABO hemolytic disease of the newborn, which will be discussed in Chapter 15. In Type III reactions, antigen-antibody complexes are deposited in or near blood vessels, stimulating tissue inflammation mediated by complement or toxic leukocyte products. Examples of this type of reaction are hypersensitivity pneumonitis, serum sickness, and the immune-complex-mediated renal diseases. Type IV reactions occur 24 to 48 hours after antigen exposure and involve cell (T-lymphocyte)-mediated tissue inflammation. Examples of this type are tuberculin and fungal delayed cutaneous hypersensitivity reactions, and contact dermatitis (see Chapter 8).

Type I Disorders

Development of Type I or immediate hypersensitivity depends on hereditary predisposition, sensitization, and subsequent reexposure to specific antigens, known as allergens. The mechanism of antigen-induced mediator release in Type I hypersensitivity reactions is shown in Figure 4.2. Type I reactions may occur in one or more target organs, including the upper and lower respiratory tracts, the skin, conjunctivae, and gastrointestinal tract. Manifestations depend on the system(s) involved, as shown in Figure 4.3. Acuteness or chronicity of target organ manifestations depends on the particular allergen(s) to which the individual is sensitized. Inhalation of pollens produces seasonal symptoms, and inhalation of indoor molds,

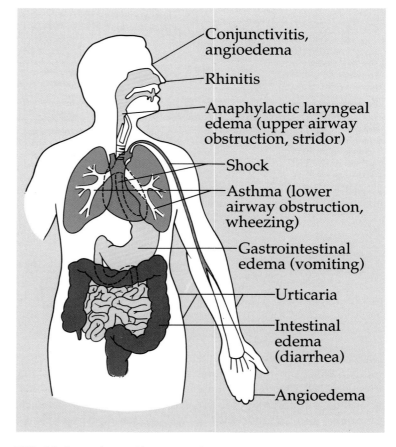

FIG. 4.3 Systemic manifestations of Type I hypersensitivity disorders. Note the characteristic physical findings of each affected organ system.

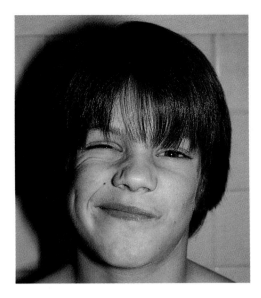

FIG. 4.4 Facial grimacing and twitching caused by nasal itching in patient with allergic rhinitis. These are frequently repeated and easily noted during patient evaluation.

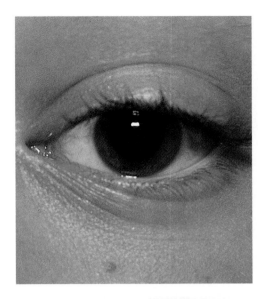

FIG. 4.6 Dennie's lines originate in the inner canthus and traverse one-half to two-thirds the length of the lower lid margin, in an arc nearly parallel to it.

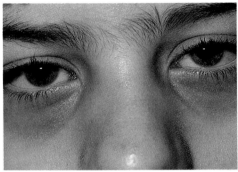

FIG. 4.5 "Allergic shiners" or dark circles beneath the eyes in patient with allergic rhinitis.

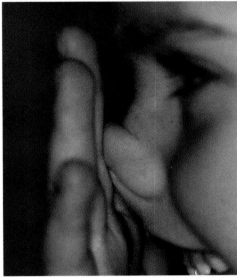

FIG. 4.7 The "allergic salute" is characteristic of children with allergic rhinitis and nasal itching, and is usually noticed by parents.

house dust, mite fragments, or animal danders produces year-round or perennial symptoms. Foods, insect venoms, and drugs produce intermittent symptoms depending on time of exposure.

ALLERGIC RHINITIS

Allergic rhinitis, characterized by inflammation, edema, and weeping of the nasal mucosa, is the most common of all allergic disorders and occurs in 10 to 20 percent of the population. Diagnosis is based on characteristic history, physical findings, and laboratory (skin test) results. Common presenting symptoms include nasal congestion and pruritus, clear rhinorrhea, and paroxysms of sneezing. Congestion may be bilateral or unilateral or may alternate from side to side. It is generally more pronounced at night. While older children blow their noses frequently, younger children do not. Instead, they sniff, snort, and repetitively clear their throats. Nasal pruritus stimulates grimacing and twitching (Fig. 4.4) and picking or rubbing the nose (allergic salute). Picking and repetitive sneezing and blowing may produce enough irritation to cause epistaxis. In the case of allergy to seasonal pollens, the symptoms may be acute, have an explosive onset, and be confined to the period during which the particular airborne pollen is detectable. Trees and grass typically pollinate in the spring, while ragweed (classic "hay fever") pollinates in the fall. In contrast, symptoms may be chronic and more indolent in the case of allergy to perennial allergens, including molds, dust, mite and animal danders.

Many patients have prominent itching and watering of the eyes in conjunction with nasal symptoms, and some experience pruritus of the throat or ears. Associated symptoms include (1) disturbed sleep and snoring; (2) morning dryness and irritation of the throat as a result of mouth breathing; (3) lassitude, fatigue, and irritability from sleep interruption; (4) early-nighttime cough; and (5) if maxillary, frontal, and ethmoidal sinuses are affected, a sensation of pressure over the cheeks, forehead, and bridge of the nose.

Many children with long-standing allergic rhinitis can be recognized by their facial characteristics. Ocular manifestations of the allergic disposition include cobblestoned conjunctivae (see Fig. 4.28), the allergic shiner, and Dennie's lines. Allergic shiners, bluish discolorations or dark circles beneath the eyes, are commonly observed in patients with allergic rhinitis (Fig. 4.5). This finding may represent chronic melanocyte stimulation due to repeated rubbing in response to itching. Dennie's lines are prominent folds or creases on the lower eyelid (Fig. 4.6), running parallel to the lower lid margin. While these lines were originally thought to indicate a predisposition to allergy, current data suggest that these signs may be present in any condition associated with periocular pruritus and scratching, and/or chronic nasal congestion. Frequent upward rubbing of the nose with the palm of the hand to alleviate itching (the allergic salute, Fig. 4.7) promotes development of a transverse

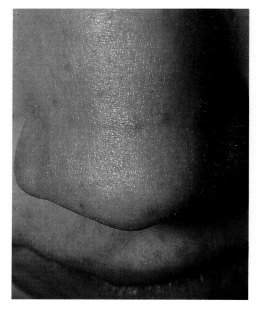

FIG. 4.8 The nasal crease across the lower third of the nose results from chronic upward rubbing of the nose with the hand (allergic salute). (Courtesy of Dr. Meyer B. Marks)

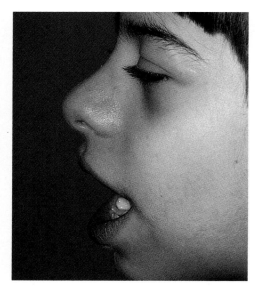

FIG. 4.9 Characteristic adenoid-type facies in a patient with long-standing allergic rhinitis. Note the open mouth and gaping habitus.

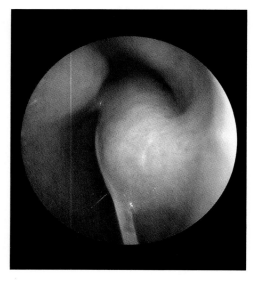

FIG. 4.10 Pale, edematous, inferior nasal turbinate of patient with allergic rhinitis, as seen through a fiberoptic rhinoscope. Even though this tool is not routinely used in evaluations, the physical findings are well illustrated, including watery nasal secretions.

nasal crease across the lower third of the nose (Fig. 4.8). Chronic obstruction produced by nasal mucosal edema may result in the typical open-mouthed, adenoid-type facies (Fig. 4.9).

On rhinoscopy, attention should be focused on position of the nasal septum, nasal patency, mucosal appearance, and presence and character of secretions, polyps, or foreign bodies (see Chapter 22). Use of a vasoconstrictor spray may be necessary to decrease edema and improve the examiner's view. The typical rhinoscopic findings in allergic rhinitis include a marked decrease in nasal patency due to swollen inferior turbinates, which appear wet and blue-gray in color (Fig. 4.10). Degree of nasal obstruction may be estimated by digitally occluding one nostril and maintaining normal breathing through the other with the mouth closed. It will be roughly proportional to the intensity of inspiratory nasal sounds, except when there is complete occlusion (no sounds). The mucosa appears edematous, and secretions are clear and watery or white. Examination of a Wright-stained smear of this discharge typically reveals eosinophils (see Fig. 4.69).

Depending on the specific allergies, allergic rhinitis may be acute, recurrent, or chronic, and must be distinguished from a number of nonallergic conditions. This necessitates a thorough medical and family history and careful examination. In some instances, response to a trial of medication and/or observations over time may be necessary to confirm the diagnosis. When symptoms are seasonal or regularly associated with exposure to specific allergens, the distinction is generally clear. In evaluating patients with perennial or recurrent but nonseasonal symptoms, allergy, recurrent infection, eosinophilic nonallergic rhinitis, and vasomotor rhinitis must be considered.

Children with frequent upper respiratory infections and/or persistent nasal congestion can present a major diagnostic challenge. In some cases the phenomenon is due to frequent or heavy exposure to pathogens. This is particularly true of children in their first year of day care or nursery school. In other patients, tonsillar and adenoidal hypertrophy provides favorable conditions for recurrent infections (see Chapter 22).

Atopic children may have increased risk of infection by virtue of impaired flow of secretions stemming from mucosal edema, and infectious symptoms may be more protracted. They often have a history of frequent colds (more than the average of six to eight per year) which are unusually prolonged, lasting 1 to 2 weeks rather than the typical 3 to 5 days. During the course of infections, nasal eosinophilia disappears and the character of the nasal discharge often changes. With viral infections nasal discharge tends to be clear or white, but with bacterial infection it is often cloudy and yellow or green in color. Diagnosis of underlying atopy in these children is facilitated by obtaining a thorough past medical and family history with questions specifically directed at possible allergic symptoms and environmental allergens. Having the parents keep a symptom record with the patient on and off antihistamine therapy and reexamination at a time when the child is not acutely infected can be valuable as well.

Other forms of rhinitis that must be distinguished from allergic rhinitis are enumerated in Figure 4.11. While characterized by eosinophilia, eosinophilic nonallergic rhinitis does not produce nasal pruritus, and patients lack specific IgE antibodies as measured by skin testing or serum RAST. Patients with vasomotor rhinitis do not complain of pruritus, have a clear discharge without eosinophils, and also lack specific IgE antibodies. Vasomotor rhinitis is thus considered a form of noninflammatory rhinitis, the etiology of which is unknown. The condition is diagnosed most frequently in adults, but may affect children. A vasocongestive form, characterized by marked nasal congestion but not secretion, and a vasosecretory form, characterized by a chronic, profuse, clear rhinorrhea, but minimal congestion, have been identified. Nonspecific precipitants of symptoms, like sudden changes in environmental temperature and humidity, should be avoided in these patients, because pharmacologic management frequently is unsuccessful. Rhinitis medicamentosa is a condition seen in patients who have been using alpha-adrenergic vasoconstrictor nose drops as decongestants for more than a few days. The disorder is

COMPARISON OF ALLERGIC AND NONALLERGIC RHINITIS

	Allergic	Nonallergic	
		ENR*	Vasomotor
Usual onset	Childhood	Childhood	Adulthood
Family history of allergy	Usual	Coincidental	Coincidental
Collateral allergy	Common	Unusual	Unusual
Symptoms			
Sneezing	Frequent	Occasional	Occasional
Itching	Common	Unusual	Unusual
Rhinorrhea	Profuse	Profuse	Profuse
Congestion	Moderate	Moderate to marked	Moderate to marked
Physical examination			
Edema	Moderate to marked	Moderate	Moderate
Secretions	Watery	Watery	Mucoid to watery
Nasal eosinophilia	Common	Common	Occasional
Allergic evaluation			
Skin tests	Positive	Coincidental	Coincidental
IgE antibodies	Positive	Coincidental	Coincidental
Therapeutic response			
Antihistamines	Good	Fair	Poor to Fair
Decongestants	Fair	Fair	Poor to Fair
Corticosteroids	Good	Good	Poor
Cromolyn	Fair	Unknown	Poor
Immunotherapy	Good	None	None

*ENR = eosinophilic nonallergic rhinitis

Reproduced from Fagin J, Friedman R, Fireman P: Allergic rhinitis. Pediatr Clin North Am 28 1981; (4):802.

FIG. 4.11

characterized by rebound vasodilation which produces an erythematous, edematous mucosa in association with profuse clear nasal discharge.

Some children with perennial allergic rhinitis have congestion that is so constant and severe as to produce signs of chronic nasal obstruction. This must be distinguished from other causes both acquired and congenital (see Chapter 22). Again history, physical findings, and results of nasal smears and therapeutic trials of antihistamine are major clues to diagnosis, which may then be confirmed by IgE testing.

The majority of patients with allergic rhinitis have mild symptoms which are easily controlled by intermittent antihistamine administration and/or environmental control. In many of these the pattern of symptoms suggests the probable responsible allergens, obviating the need for specific IgE testing. Those with severe symptoms only partially alleviated by antihistamines and those with perennial symptoms who require daily therapy should be referred for specific IgE testing and possible desensitization therapy.

RESPIRATORY DISTRESS

Respiratory distress in children (tachypnea with or without grunting, flaring, retractions, and cyanosis) of any etiology (allergic, infectious, anatomic) must be promptly evaluated and treated, since failure to do so may result in progression to respiratory failure, apnea, coma, and death. The first step in approaching respiratory distress is to differentiate upper from lower airway disorders. Once the level of involvement has been established, the cause can be promptly assigned on the basis of specific symptoms and signs. Appropriate therapy must be initiated without delay, based on the severity of distress and the type of disorder. At times, various degrees of upper and lower airway obstruction may coexist, as in laryngotracheobronchitis.

An algorithm for determining the etiology of respiratory distress in children is shown in Figure 4.12, demonstrating differences in physical findings between upper and lower airway obstructive disorders. Upper airway obstruction causes difficulty in moving air into the chest, whereas lower airway obstruction causes difficulty in moving air out of the chest. This difference results in the characteristic physical findings in each type. In general, lower airway obstruction produces prolongation of the expiratory phase of respiration and typical expiratory wheezing, whereas upper airway obstruction prolongs the inspiratory phase. Wheezing is defined as musical or whistling auscultatory sounds, heard more often on expiration

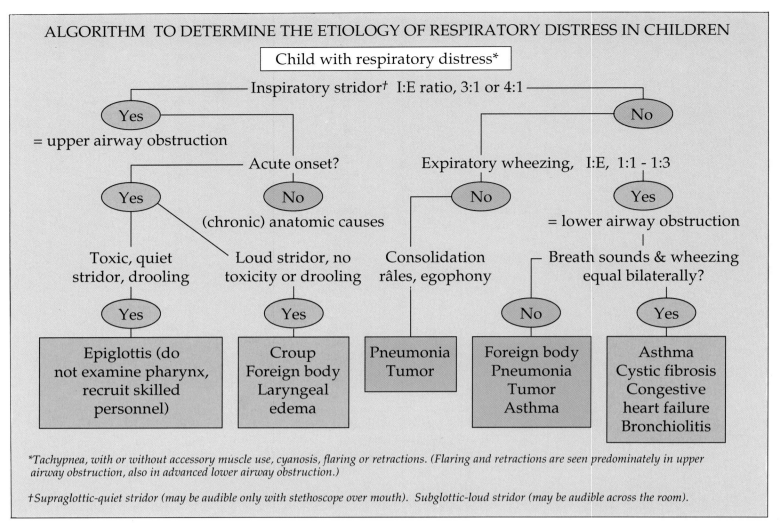

FIG. 4.12

than on inspiration. Inspiratory stridor, seen with upper airway obstruction, can mimic wheezing or both can be detected concomitantly, but their differentiation is seldom confusing to the experienced observer. Stridor is defined as a crowing sound, usually heard during the inspiratory phase of respiration. It tends to be loud when the obstruction is subglottic and quiet when obstruction is supraglottic.

All forms of acute upper airway obstruction present with suprasternal, supraclavicular, and subcostal retractions, which increase as the obstruction progresses. Mild to moderate increases in respiratory and heart rates are common. In lower airway disorders such as pneumonitis and asthma, retractions are primarily intercostal, and when present usually indicate a significant degree of obstruction. Respiratory rate and heart rate are often markedly increased. Retractions are usually generalized in severe airway obstruction of any etiology.

In this chapter we will concentrate on disorders in which respiratory distress stems from hypersensitivity. These include anaphylactic laryngeal edema, in which upper airway obstruction is the result of an acute allergic reaction, and three lower airway disorders: asthma, hypersensitivity pneumonitis, and allergic bronchopulmonary aspergillosis. Infectious causes of acute upper airway obstruction and foreign body aspiration are discussed in Chapter 22.

Anaphylactic Laryngeal Edema
Anaphylactic (Type I hypersensitivity) laryngeal edema typically presents with symptoms and signs of subglottic obstruction such as tightness or pressure in the upper chest, stridor, dyspnea, and retractions. Onset is immediate and explosive following bee stings, drug administration, or food ingestion. Asphyxiation may result from delays in diagnosis or treatment. Frequently, other organ systems are also involved. Facial angioedema is common, and many patients have associated urticaria. Wheezing reflecting pulmonary involvement and vomiting due to gastrointestinal reaction may also be seen. In severe cases there is massive third spacing of fluid resulting in cardiovascular shock, with an initial phase of flushing and warm extremities due to vasodilation. This phase is superseded by pallor and cold due to vasoconstriction. Therapy depends on severity, and ranges from administration of antihistamines to use of epinephrine, steroids, volume expansion, and pressor agents.

Acute and Chronic Asthma
Type I hypersensitivity reactions can occur in large and small airways of the lungs and result in the disorder termed "asthma." Asthma is characterized by inherent hyperreactivity of the airways to one or more of several stimuli, including aller-

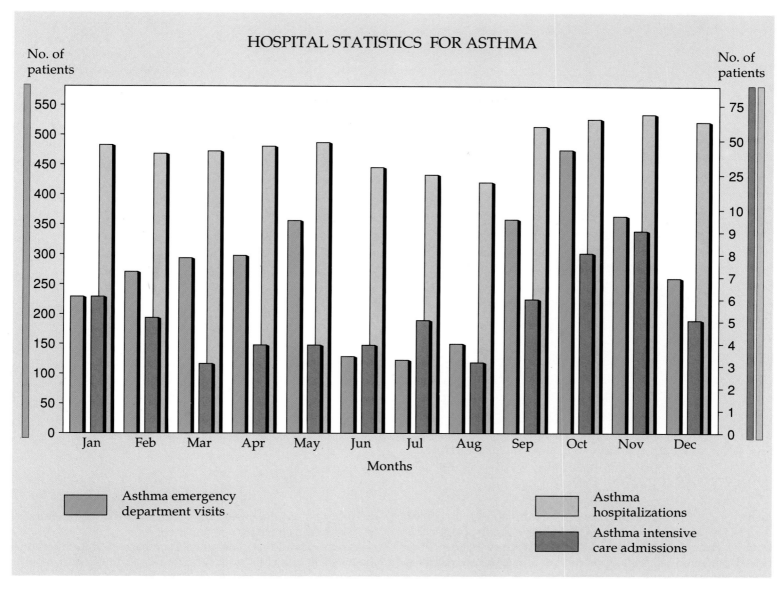

FIG. 4.13 Number of emergency department visits for wheezing (1986–1987) and number of asthma admissions (1982–1985) to Children's Hospital of Pittsburgh, and number of asthma intensive care unit admissions to Children's Hospital of Los Angeles (1969–1977) by month of year. (Adapted with permission from Friday GA, Fireman P: Morbidity and mortality of asthma. Pediatr Clin North Am 1988; 35(5):1153; Richards W, Lew C, Carney J, et al: Review of intensive care unit admissions for asthma. Clin Pediatr 1979; 18(6):346; and Fireman P, Slavin RG: Atlas of Allergies. New York, Gower, 1990)

gens, infections, exercise, chemical agents, cold or dry air, emotions, and weather changes. Hence in some cases asthma has an atopic basis and in others it does not. Specific allergens which have been implicated in atopic patients are pollens, molds, house dust, animal danders, drugs, food, and insect venoms. On exposure, these allergens, via Type I hypersensitivity, produce the characteristic features of asthma: mucosal edema, increased mucous production, and smooth muscle contraction which results in bronchoconstriction. These responses combine to produce obstruction of both large and small airways which, if recurrent and reversible with bronchodilator drugs, is the hallmark of asthma.

Affected individuals are usually aware of the specific stimuli that trigger their asthma. Viruses are the most common precipitants of asthma in children, especially respiratory syncytial virus, parainfluenza viruses, and rhinoviruses. These infections usually affect both upper and lower airways, producing rhinorrhea, nasal congestion, and fever in addition to wheezing, which tends to develop insidiously. In contrast, allergytriggered episodes typically lack fever and have a more explosive onset of wheezing.

Asthma is one of the leading causes of pediatric morbidity. Peak incidence of onset is before the age of 5 years. In childhood, males are affected 30 percent more often than females and tend to have more severe disease. Beyond puberty, the sex distribution is equal. Asthmatic children with respiratory allergy and eczema usually have a more severe course than those who wheeze only with upper respiratory infections.

Emergency department visits, hospitalization, and intensive care unit admissions for asthma usually peak in the late fall or early winter months and, to a lesser extent, in the spring (Fig. 4.13). These seasonal patterns may be related to environmental temperature and humidity changes, allergen exposure, or respiratory infections.

The diagnosis of asthma is frequently based on historical findings alone, indicating the importance of taking a thorough

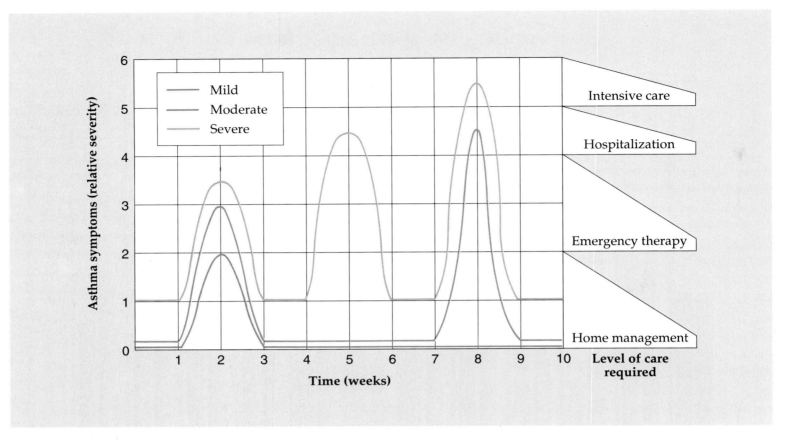

FIG. 4.14 *Grading of asthma severity by symptoms and levels of care required. (Reproduced with permission from Fireman P, Slavin RG:* Atlas of Allergies. *New York, Gower, 1990)*

history. Even though asthma is a familial disorder, its clinical expression requires not only a hereditary predisposition but specific environmental factors as well. Family history often reveals affected siblings, parents, or first-degree relatives. Environmental survey can determine possible provocative factors, especially allergens, infections, occupational exposures, smoking, exercise, stress, climate, and medication use (aspirin, propranolol). The history should emphasize frequency, duration, and intensity of suspected episodes. A description of symptoms between acute episodes aids in determination of chronicity (night cough, exercise intolerance, fatigue, school absenteeism, social function). Individuals with asthma most commonly present with recurrent episodes of wheezing which, depending on the severity, may require emergency treatment. Episodes may be infrequent and/or seasonal, but may occur as frequently as every day. The spectrum of presenting complaints, however, is broad, and affected individuals may complain only of mild, occasional wheezing or shortness of breath with exercise and/or colds, or persistent dry hacking cough. The condition is diagnosed after three or more episodes have been successfully treated with bronchodilators. The frequency and severity of acute asthma episodes and the level of symptoms between episodes can be used to grade asthma severity and guide therapy (Fig. 4.14).

The early stages of an asthma exacerbation in children are characterized by the onset of cough, rhinorrhea, and chest tightness, as well as chest retractions or audible wheezing. The parents should be educated to critically and accurately observe their child for the warning signs and, in collaboration with the managing physician, identify the onset of asthmatic exacerbation at home. The institution of appropriate therapy can halt

the progression of airway obstruction and reduce the number of visits to the emergency department.

Asthma should be considered as part of the differential diagnosis in any child with recurrent or chronic lower respiratory symptoms or signs. Even though a high index of suspicion must be maintained, excessive or erroneous diagnoses may result if they are made hastily without appropriate supportive evidence; normal children or those with potentially more severe disorders may be mistakenly labeled with the stigma of asthma and inappropriately treated. Parents must be instructed that physician assessment is essential during suspected episodes of asthma, so that wheezing or other signs of lower airway obstruction and reversibility may be documented. If the diagnosis is unclear on clinical grounds, then specific laboratory studies must be performed to document asthma and rule out disorders that mimic asthma. Pulmonary function tests in asthmatic children older than 5 years show airways obstruction at baseline or after appropriate challenge with methacholine, exercise, or cold air, and document reversibility after administration of an aerosolized bronchodilator. (Fig. 4.15A,B). In children younger than 5 years, or those in whom testing is unreliable, the diagnosis must be made on the basis of historical and physical findings, in conjunction with clinical response to bronchodilators. Lack of an immediate response to a bronchodilator does not eliminate asthma as a diagnostic consideration, however.

A thorough physical examination provides valuable information regarding the diagnosis of asthma and its severity and chronicity. The physical findings in asthma vary with the chronicity and state of activity of the disease process at the time of examination. The findings of acute asthma are marked-

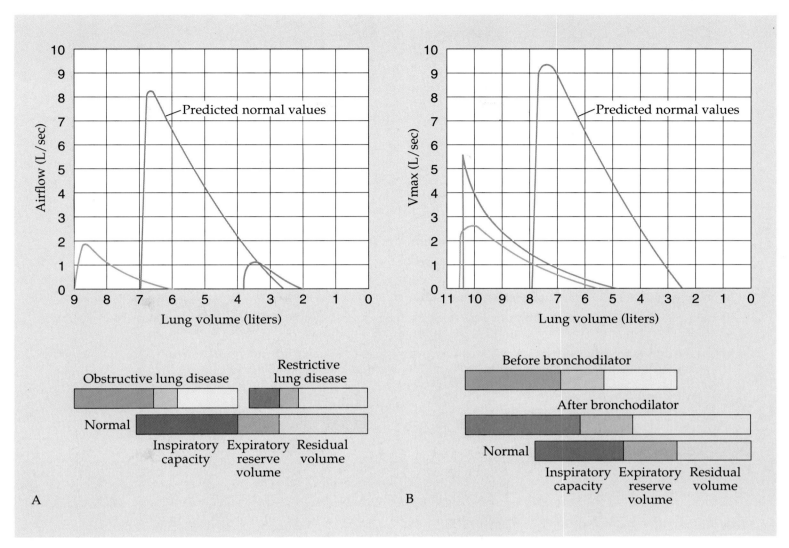

FIG. 4.15 **A**, maximum expiratory flow rates are reduced in both obstructive lung diseases such as asthma and restrictive lung disease. However, in asthma, the airflow is limited at high lung volumes, in contrast to restrictive lung disease, in which airflow is limited because lung volume is decreased. **B**, bronchoconstriction characteristic of hyperreactive airways is generally reversible. Indices of expiratory airflow in asthmatic patients thus improve after inhalation of a nebulized bronchodilator (e.g., a beta-adrenergic agonist). (Reproduced with permission from Cherniack RM: Continuity of care in asthma management. Hosp Pract 1987; 22(9):119-143)

ly different from those of chronic and latent or quiescent asthma. Between episodes, the examination usually is entirely normal. Often, however, gentle compression of the anterior chest with the hand, at the end of the expiratory phase, will elicit auscultatory wheezing over the posterior chest. If a patient with prolonged obstruction has not received appropriate therapy, signs of chronic lung disease may be present. These include a paucity of subcutaneous fatty tissue and a barrel-chest configuration (Fig. 4.16). Râles, wheezing, rhonchi, and decreased intensity and duration of the inspiratory phase of respiration are commonly noted on auscultation. Clubbing as a sign of chronic asthma is rare, and if present in a wheezing child suggests another chronic pulmonary disease.

During acute asthma, the following historical features should be noted: time of onset, possible triggers, present medications, comparison with previous episodes, and presence of complicating factors (vomiting, fever, chest pain). Examination should document the presence and degree of (1) dyspnea (the patient's own assessment of breathlessness), wheezing, accessory muscle use (visible contractions of the scalene and/or

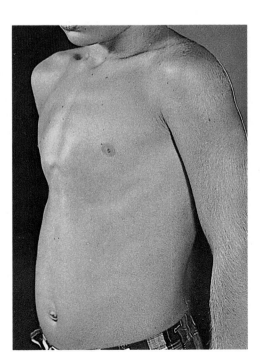

FIG. 4.16 The barrel-chest configuration of chronic asthma. Physical findings include an increased anteroposterior diameter of the chest and decreased respiratory excursion of the chest wall. (Courtesy of Dr. Meyer B. Marks)

THE MEASUREMENT OF PULSUS PARADOXUS

	Blood Pressure in Relation to Time and Respiratory Phase (mmHg)				
	Expiration	**Inspiration**	**Expiration**	**Inspiration**	**Expiration**
Normal (no airway obstruction)	125/70	120/70	125/70	120/70	125/70
Asthma (airway obstruction)	125/70	100/70	125/70	100/70	125/70

Method

1. Pump sphygmomanometer cuff to occlude the peripheral pulse.
2. As the cuff pressure falls, listen carefully for the onset of the first Korotkoff sound.
3. Note the pressure at which the first Korotkoff sound is detected. This should be heard only during expiration. (In above example, 125 = normal and asthma.)
4. Continue to slowly decrease the cuff pressure until the first sound is detected during both inspiration and expiration. Note this pressure. (In above example, 120 = normal; 100 = asthma.)
5. When the difference between the two pressures is greater than or equal to 10, pulsus paradoxus is present. (In above example, 5 = normal, no pulsus paradoxus and 25 = asthma, pulsus paradoxus.)

FIG. 4.17

ASTHMA SCORING SYSTEM

Score	0	1	2	3
Color	Normal	Normal (0 score)	Normal (0 score)	Dusky or cyanotic
Retractions	None	Mild intercostal only	Moderate intercostal to generalized	Generalized, with marked use of accessory muscles
Air Entry*	Normal	Slight to mild decrease	Moderate decrease	Severe decrease to nearly absent breath sounds
I/E Ratio	1.5/1	<1.5/1 but >1/2	1/2 to 1/3	>1/3
Level of Consciousness	Normal	Restless or agitated only when disturbed	Restless or agitated when undisturbed	Lethargic, tiring, or depressed
Wheezing	None, with good air entry	Scattered or mild generalized wheezes with mild decrease of air entry	Moderate generalized wheezing with moderate decrease of air entry	Severe generalized wheezing or absent with poor air entry

*If air entry is asymmetric, the worst area is the one to score.

FIG. 4.18

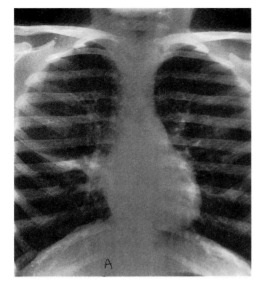

FIG. 4.19 Anteroposterior chest radiograph of child with acute asthma. Note the flattened diaphragms, hyperinflation, peribronchial thickening, and right middle lobe atelectasis.

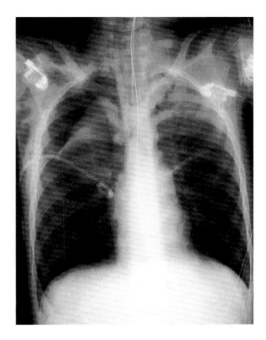

FIG. 4.20 Chest radiograph showing right-sided pneumothorax in intubated patient with acute asthma and respiratory failure. Clinical manifestations include pleuritic chest pain, dyspnea, cyanosis, tachypnea, and cough. Also, note the marked hyperinflation of the lungs which can result in cardiac compression (narrow cardiac shadow) and compromise of cardiac venous return, and the extensive right-sided subcutaneous emphysema. (Courtesy of Dr. Beverly Newman, Children's Hospital of Pittsburgh)

sternocleidomastoid muscles), and suprasternal, intercostal, or substernal retractions (visible depression in the chest wall during inspiration), all of which are graded as absent, mild, moderate, or severe; (2) cyanosis (central, involving the lips, and/or peripheral, involving the nail beds); (3) inspiratory breath sounds (normal or decreased); (4) air exchange (normal, decreased, or absent); and (5) abnormalities of the inspiration/expiration (I:E) ratio. In addition, râles are often heard, and pulse, respiratory rate and blood pressure are frequently elevated. Pulsus paradoxus, an exaggerated decrease in systolic blood pressure during inspiration (Fig. 4.17), correlates highly with the degree of airway obstruction and can serve as an indicator of severity and a guide to therapy. This phenomenon may result from physical forces on the pericardium that impede venous return and reduce cardiac output during forced inspiration. Normally, the inspiratory decrease in systolic blood pressure is less than 10 mmHg and not discernible during routine sphygmomanometry. In acute asthma, it is usually greater than 10 (up to 30 and 40) and easily detectable. The presence of pulsus paradoxus is correlated with a forced expiratory volume in 1 second of less than 20 percent predicted.

Individuals with asthma may be distinguished by their characteristic symptoms and signs during acute episodes, which typically change as the degree of airway obstruction increases. Symptoms usually consist of progressively increasing shortness of breath and difficulty breathing, with or without rhinorrhea, low-grade fever, and vomiting. On examination, expiratory wheezing or a prolonged expiratory phase may be the only manifestations of mild asthma. However, as the obstructive process progresses, the expiratory phase becomes longer and the wheezing louder. Eventually, airways collapse and signs of hyperinflation develop (low diaphragms, decreased lateral excursions of the chest wall with breathing, and hyperresonance to percussion). There are visible sternocleidomastoid contractions; increased anteroposterior chest diameter; circumoral cyanosis; and suprasternal, intercostal, and substernal retractions. Subjectively, the patient experiences chest tightness and anxiety, and works harder to breathe.

Accessory muscle use and retractions develop with or without a marked degree of wheezing on auscultation. To maximize air exchange, the child assumes a characteristic sitting posture, bending slightly forward. Frequent examinations are warranted, and any change in sensorium requires prompt evaluation. As respiratory muscles tire, the patient becomes lethargic and cyanotic, even with supplemental oxygen. Maximum effort to breathe produces feeble air exchange, manifested by decreased intensity and duration or lack of inspiratory breath sounds. This is due to the decrease in audible sounds associated with respiration as air exchange decreases. Consequently, a patient with severe obstruction and impending respiratory failure may not be wheezing because he is moving too little air to do so. With extreme fatigue, respiratory muscles fail, retractions decrease, and respiratory failure is imminent unless appropriate therapy is promptly initiated. Following initial examination, serial assessment of the degree of respiratory distress, using the parameters outlined in Figure 4.18, facilitates determination of response to therapy.

Histopathologic features of acute asthma include airway infiltration with inflammatory cells, increased intraluminal mucus with plugging of small airways, edema, bronchoconstriction, and smooth muscle hypertrophy. Because asthma has both bronchoconstrictive and inflammatory components, the ideal therapeutic regimen should incorporate a combination of bronchodilator and anti-inflammatory agents.

The radiographic features of the hyperinflation, peribronchial cuffing, and atelectasis, characteristic of uncomplicated acute asthma, are illustrated in Figure 4.19. Complications are generally diagnosed radiographically (Fig. 4.20), but may be suggested by symptoms and signs. Pneumothorax should be suspected in any asthmatic who develops pleuritic chest pain associated with dyspnea, cyanosis, tachypnea, and occasionally cough. Examination reveals respiratory distress, marked hyperinflation and decreased chest wall excursion, and decreased or absent breath sounds on the affected side. With tension pneumothorax, the trachea, mediastinum, and cardiac landmarks may be

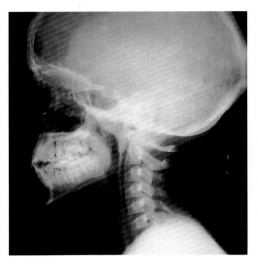

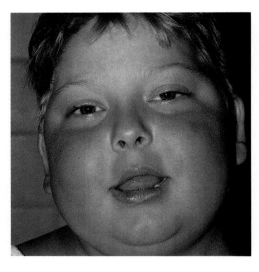

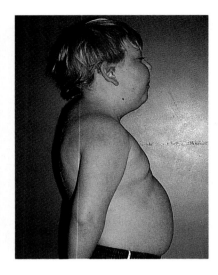

FIG. 4.21 Spontaneous pneumomediastinum in a child with asthma. Note the dissection of air in soft tissues just anterior to the vertebrae. Clinical manifestations include dysphagia. (Courtesy of Dr. Beverly Newman, Children's Hospital of Pittsburgh)

FIG. 4.22 Complications of corticosteroid therapy for chronic asthma. "Moon-type"

facies (left) and buffalo hump (right), both due to abnormal fat distribution.

DIFFERENTIATING FEATURES OF ASTHMA AND BRONCHIOLITIS IN CHILDREN

	Asthma	Bronchiolitis
Primary etiologies	Viruses, allergens, exercise, etc.	Respiratory synctial virus, other viruses
Age of onset	50% by 2 years of age 80% by 5 years of age	<24 months
Recurrent wheezing	Yes (characteristic)	70% (≤2 episodes) 30% progress to asthma (≥3 episodes)
Onset of wheezing	Acute if allergic or exercise-induced	Insidious
Concomitant symptoms of upper respiratory infection	Yes, if infectious	Yes
Family history of allergy and asthma	Frequent	Infrequent in children with ≤2 episodes
Nasal eosinophilia	With allergic rhinitis	Absent
Chest auscultation	If viral, as in bronchiolitis Nonviral: high-pitched expiratory wheezes	Fine, sibilant râles, and coarse inspiratory and expiratory wheezes
Concomitant allergic manifestations	If allergic asthma	Usually absent
IgE level	Elevated (if allergic)	Normal
Responsive to bronchodilator	Yes (characteristic)	Unresponsive or partially responsive

FIG. 4.23

shifted to the opposite side. Pneumomediastinum (Fig. 4.21) and subcutaneous emphysema, usually involving the neck and supraclavicular areas, are more common than pneumothorax. When mild they may be asymptomatic and detected inci-

dentally on chest radiograph. With more extensive air dissection the patient may complain of neck and chest pain, and the subcutaneous emphysema may be visibly evident as a soft-tissue swelling of the neck and chest which is crepitant (has a

ASSOCIATED SYMPTOMS AND SIGNS IN THE WHEEZING CHILD WHICH ARE HELPFUL IN DIFFERENTIAL DIAGNOSIS

Symptoms/Signs	Diseases Associated with Wheezing	
	In Infants	In Older Children
Positional changes	Anomalies of great vessels, gastroesophageal reflux	Gastroesophageal reflux
Failure to thrive	Cystic fibrosis, tracheoesophageal fistula, bronchopulmonary dysplasia	Cystic fibrosis, chronic hypersensitivity pneumonitis, alpha$_1$-antitrypsin deficiency, bronchiectasis
Associated with feeding	Tracheoesophageal fistula, gastroesophageal reflux	Gastroesophageal reflux
Environmental triggers	Allergic asthma	Allergic asthma, allergic bronchopulmonary aspergillosis, acute hypersensitivity pneumonitis
Sudden onset	Allergic asthma, croup	Allergic asthma, foreign body aspiration, croup, acute hypersensitivity pneumonitis
Fever	Bronchiolitis, pneumonitis	Infectious asthma, acute hypersensitivity pneumonitis, croup
Rhinorrhea	Bronchiolitis, pneumonitis	Infectious or allergic asthma, croup
Concomitant stridor	Tracheal or bronchial stenosis, anomalies of the great vessels, croup	Foreign body aspiration, croup
Clubbing		Cystic fibrosis, bronchiectasis, bronchopulmonary dysplasia

FIG. 4.24

crunching sensation) on palpation. Pneumothorax and pneumomediastinum can produce characteristic auscultatory findings, including a crackling "mediastinal crunch" at the base of the heart, and a systolic crunch or knock. The latter sound has been referred to as "noisy pneumothorax," and frequently is audible to both patient and physician without the aid of a stethoscope.

Other complications which are diagnosable on physical examination include those induced by chronic steroid use, such as weight gain, "moon-type" facies, hirsutism, polycythemia (red, ruddy complexion) (Fig. 4.22), and short stature (see Chapter 9, Endocrinology). Such side effects of excessive steroid therapy for chronic asthma should be avoidable complications.

In children with recent onset of wheezing, asthma must be differentiated from other disorders associated with wheezing. In infants, this differentiation includes bronchiolitis, features of which are listed in Figure 4.23 (see Chapter 16). Many asthmatic exacerbations are triggered by infection; 30 to 50 percent of children with recurrent bronchiolitis will later be diagnosed as having asthma. Even though these two entities may be dif-

ferent manifestations of the same or a similar disease, the distinction remains a clinically useful one for the following reasons: (1) the children with bronchiolitis who do not develop asthma may be inappropriately labeled with the stigma of asthma; and (2) children less than 2 years of age frequently may not respond to inhaled or injected bronchodilators. Depending on response to a trial dose, the ongoing bronchodilator therapy characteristic of asthma management may or may not be indicated in children with bronchiolitis. While children with pneumonia (particularly of viral origin) may wheeze, they are more likely to have râles or normal findings on auscultation, with the diagnosis suggested by tachypnea in association with retractions, nasal flaring, or expiratory grunting. Other causes of wheezing are listed in Figure 4.24. Airway compression by anomalous vessels (see Chapter 5) or mass lesions is often distinguishable from bronchiolitis by virtue of absence of signs of infection, and from asthma by failure to respond to bronchodilators. History and presence of infiltrates help in diagnosis of aspiration which can mimic asthma closely, often responding to bronchodilator therapy. Radiographic studies such as barium swallow with fluoroscopy can be very

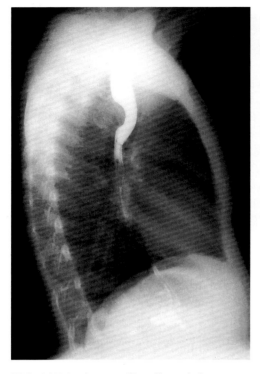

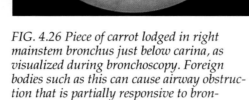

FIG. 4.26 Piece of carrot lodged in right mainstem bronchus just below carina, as visualized during bronchoscopy. Foreign bodies such as this can cause airway obstruction that is partially responsive to bron-

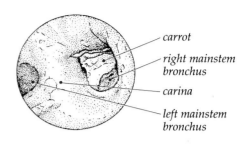

chodilator. (Courtesy of Dr. Sylvan Stool, Children's Hospital of Pittsburgh. Reproduced from Fireman P, Slavin RG: Atlas of Allergies. New York, Gower, 1990)

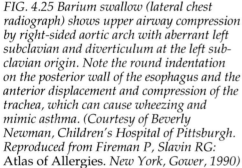

FIG. 4.25 Barium swallow (lateral chest radiograph) shows upper airway compression by right-sided aortic arch with aberrant left subclavian and diverticulum at the left subclavian origin. Note the round indentation on the posterior wall of the esophagus and the anterior displacement and compression of the trachea, which can cause wheezing and mimic asthma. (Courtesy of Beverly Newman, Children's Hospital of Pittsburgh. Reproduced from Fireman P, Slavin RG: Atlas of Allergies. New York, Gower, 1990)

helpful in distinguishing among these entities (Fig. 4.25). pH-probe testing may be required to identify gastroesophageal reflux (see Chapter 10).

In older children who have sudden onset of wheezing and respiratory distress, the differential diagnosis includes respiratory infections, left ventricular failure, and aspiration. Respiratory infections such as croup may be distinguished by their characteristic histories and tendencies to involve the upper airways (see Chapter 22). Lower respiratory infections (pneumonia) generally produce fever and more localized findings of rales, decrease and change in quality of breath sounds, and egophony. Left ventricular failure, especially with pulmonary edema, may present with acute respiratory distress and wheezing. A history of cardiac disease and diffuse crackles or basilar rales and a third heart sound on auscultation help to distinguish this condition from asthma. Aspiration of a foreign body with lodgment in a mainstem bronchus may produce wheezing (Fig. 4.26). A history of a choking episode and physical findings of unilateral wheezing and hyperresonance aid in distinguishing aspiration from asthma, but do not confirm the diagnosis. It is important to remember that wheezing due to foreign body aspiration may respond at least in part to bronchodilator therapy.

In the older child or adult with mild, infrequent episodes of wheezing that respond to bronchodilator therapy, asthma is readily diagnosed. However, with daily wheezing, frequent exacerbations, lack of response to bronchodilators, or poor growth, other diagnoses must be considered, including chronic obstructive pulmonary disease, cystic fibrosis, alpha$_1$-antitrypsin deficiency, carcinoid syndrome, and an associated immunological deficiency. Chronic obstructive pulmonary diseases, which include chronic bronchitis, emphysema, bronchiectasis, and bronchopulmonary dysplasia, are distinguished by their lack of significant reversibility with bronchodilator therapy. Cystic fibrosis may present with chronic cough, wheezing, and recurrent infections. Additionally, malabsorption with bulky, foul-smelling stools, failure to thrive, and clubbing of the nail beds are common. Alpha$_1$-antitrypsin deficiency, an inherited autosomal-recessive disorder, is characterized by the onset of progressive emphysema in a young adult, and is one cause of neonatal hepatitis.

OCULAR ALLERGY

Ocular allergic reactions may involve the eyelid, the conjunctiva, or both. The eyelids have a rich blood supply and loose connective tissue. This facilitates edema collection in response to inflammation generated by histamine release in allergic conditions or by trauma. Immediate hypersensitivity reactions that produce eyelid angioedema may be triggered by a vast number of stimuli, including pollens, dusts, insect stings or bites, foods or drugs. They are characterized by sudden onset of periorbital edema, pruritus, and erythema following exposure to an allergen (Fig. 4.27). The disorder is distinguished from cellulitis by lack of induration, absence of tenderness and fever, and the fact that involvement is usually bilateral (see Chapter 22).

Allergic conjunctivitis may be acute or chronic and seasonal or perennial, depending on the allergen(s) to which the individual is sensitized. Commonly implicated allergens include weed, tree, and grass pollens; molds; dust; and animal dander. In the acute, seasonal form, onset may be explosive and coincident with the beginning of ragweed pollination. This condition frequently accompanies seasonal allergic rhinitis, and most commonly is due to ragweed and grass pollen. Itching and excessive tearing are the most prominent symptoms.

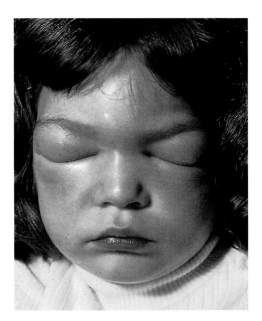

FIG. 4.27 Eyelid angioedema in child with venom allergy. Onset was explosive following exposure to the bee sting. (Reproduced from Fireman P, Slavin RG: Atlas of Allergies. New York, Gower, 1990)

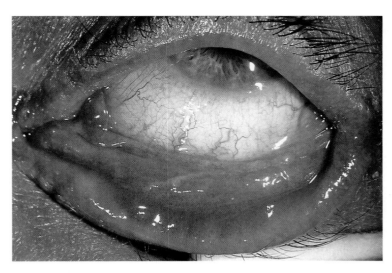

FIG. 4.29 Atopic keratoconjunctivitis with chronic papillary conjunctivitis. Note the stringy mucopurulent discharge often seen in this disorder. (Reproduced from Fireman P, Slavin RG: Atlas of Allergies. New York, Gower, 1990)

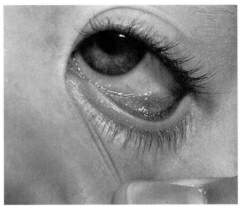

FIG. 4.28 Allergic cobblestoning of the conjunctivae in chronic allergic conjunctivitis. This granular appearance is due to edema and hyperplasia of the papillae.

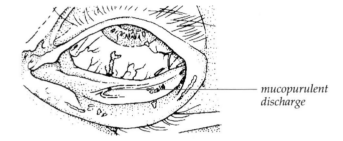

mucopurulent discharge

Pruritus often interferes with sleep, and vision may be impaired by excessive discharge.

Physical findings depend on the degree of chronicity. In the acute form, these findings consist of diffuse bilateral conjunctival edema and hyperemia. Photophobia, profuse tearing, and mild lid swelling are commonly associated. In the chronic form, the conjunctivae appear pale, with mild edema and hyperplasia of the papillae. This may result in a fine, granular appearance of the conjunctivae, which is termed "allergic cobblestoning" (Fig. 4.28). More prominent cobblestoning is seen in vernal conjunctivitis. The clinical diagnosis may be confirmed by finding eosinophilia on smear of conjunctival secretions, and skin testing to the suspected allergen(s).

The differential diagnosis of allergic conjunctivitis includes atopic conjunctivitis, atopic keratoconjunctivitis, and vernal conjunctivitis. Individuals with *atopic conjunctivitis* have a history of asthma, allergic conjunctivitis, or infantile eczema. Serum IgE levels are elevated during the active phase of the disease, but there is no seasonal variation in severity. The disease usually begins in the late teens, and many patients experience a remission during adulthood. The eyelids manifest a thickened, lichenified, red, exudative or dry rash. *Atopic keratoconjunctivitis* occurs in patients with atopic dermatitis, and is characterized by erythema and thickening of the conjunctivae (Fig. 4.29). This may progress to scarring and vascularization of the cornea in severe cases. Ocular disease activity parallels that of cutaneous disease.

Vernal conjunctivitis is uncommon and chronic in nature. Its typical occurrence during the spring and summer is sugges-

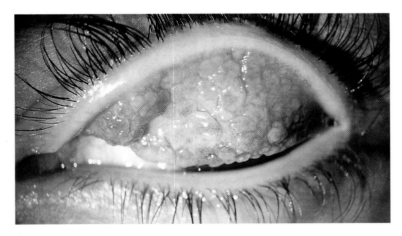

FIG. 4.30 Vernal conjunctivitis, palpebral form. The giant papillary elevations are easily seen without magnification. (Reproduced from Fireman P, Slavin RG: Atlas of Allergies. New York, Gower, 1990)

tive of an allergic etiology, but this is unproven. Young, atopic males are affected most frequently. Symptoms include severe itching, photophobia, blurring of vision, and lacrimation. Physical examination reveals white, ropy secretions containing many eosinophils. A palpebral form manifests hypertrophic nodular papillae that resemble cobblestones on the upper eyelids (Fig. 4.30). The papillae consist of dense fibrous tissue with eosinophilic infiltrates. In the bulbar form, nodules appear as gelatinous masses called Trantas' dots, usually found at the

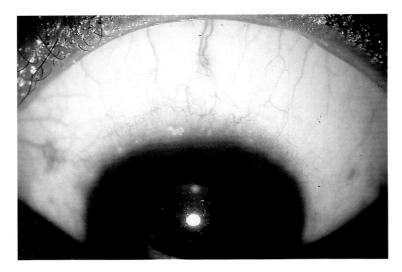

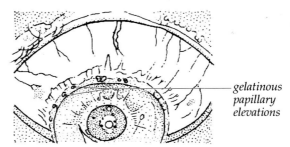

FIG. 4.31 Vernal conjunctivitis, limbal form. Note the gelatinous papillary elevations of the limbal tissue. (Reproduced from Fireman P, Slavin RG: Atlas of Allergies. New York, Gower, 1990)

— gelatinous papillary elevations

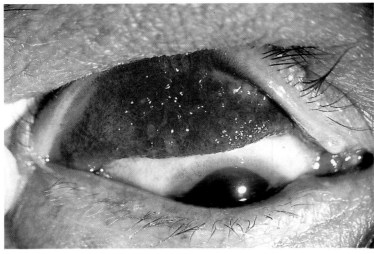

FIG. 4.33 Urticarial lesions. Note the well-demarcated borders, redness, elevation, and occasional confluence of the palpable lesions. (Courtesy of Dr. Michael Sherlock)

FIG. 4.32 Characteristic lesions of giant papillary conjunctivitis. These hobnail-like elevations of the upper tarsal conjunctiva, evident on eversion of the upper eyelid, occur when the upper lid meets a foreign body such as a contact lens, prosthesis, or exposed suture. (Reproduced from Fireman P, Slavin RG: Atlas of Allergies. New York, Gower, 1990)

corneal-scleral junction (Fig. 4.31). This disease usually remits with maturity, and is rarely seen in adults. *Giant papillary conjunctivitis*, which appears clinically and histologically to be a mild form of vernal conjunctivitis, is associated with the use of hard and soft contact lenses (Fig. 4.32). The stimulus is believed to be foreign material that accumulates on the surface of the contact lenses. Whether this material is antigenic and this represents an immune-mediated disease is not known.

URTICARIA/ANGIOEDEMA

Hypersensitivity reactions in which the skin is the major target organ are manifest clinically as diffuse erythema, urticaria, or angioedema. Type I hypersensitivity to inhalants, foods, insect venoms, and drugs is the most common mechanism, but urticaria and angioedema may also accompany Type II (transfusion reaction) or Type III reactions (cutaneous vasculitis, serum sickness). These disorders result from increased vascular permeability. The resultant edema collects in the dermis in urticaria, and primarily in the subcutaneous tissues in angioedema. While frequently seen in combination, urticaria

and angioedema may also appear individually. Urticaria is most frequently an acute disorder that resolves spontaneously. When duration of recurrences exceeds 6 weeks, the condition is arbitrarily termed "chronic urticaria." In contrast to acute urticaria, extensive evaluations frequently do not reveal the cause(s) of chronic urticaria.

Urticarial lesions are well circumscribed, raised, palpable wheals that blanch with applied pressure (Fig. 4.33). They are usually erythematous, but may be pale or white with a red halo. Typically, the lesions are intensely pruritic; however, in some instances pruritus is mild. Angioedema is characterized by diffuse subcutaneous tissue swelling with normal or erythematous overlying skin. Itching is usually intense. The face, hands, feet, and perineum are the most commonly involved sites (Fig. 4.34).

Skin involvement may be generalized or localized to body parts exposed to a provoking stimulus. Careful history-taking concerning recent exposures and medications is often rewarding. In cases with associated fever and respiratory and/or gastrointestinal symptoms, infectious diseases due to viruses (including enterovirus, hepatitis B, and Epstein-Barr virus), group A beta-hemolytic streptococcus, and helminth infection should be considered. Generalized urticaria with or without angioedema may also be the initial manifestation of erythema multiforme or Henoch-Schönlein purpura. Thus, in cases in which a specific etiology is unclear, parents should be informed of possible evolution and instructed regarding observation of signs and symptoms.

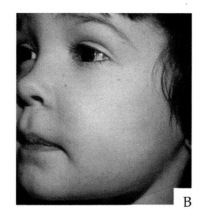

A

B

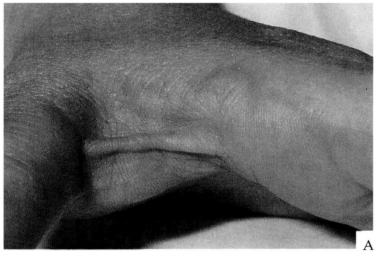

A

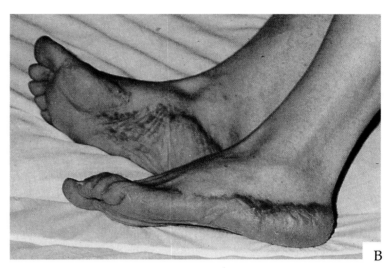

B

FIG. 4.35 Cutaneous eruptions on the sides of the hands and feet of patients with serum sickness. **A**, the finger web of a patient is shown in the early stages of serum sickness; a scalloped band of erythema can be seen on the side of the finger at the margin of palmar skin. **B**, the feet of a thrombocytopenic patient are shown at the clinical peak of serum sickness. At the margin of plantar skin is a band of purpura. The purpura was preceded by a band of erythema. (Reproduced with permission from Lawley TJ, Bielory L, Gascon P, et al: Prospective clinical and immunologic analysis of patients with serum sickness. N Engl J Med 1984; 311:1409)

The urticaria associated with serum sickness is due to a necrotizing vasculitis involving small venules. Histamine release associated with both IgE-dependent reactions and complement activation may contribute to the pathophysiology of this form of urticaria. Typically, Type I hypersensitivity produces intense pruritus, while Type II and III hypersensitivity reactions may be associated with a burning sensation. In addition to urticarial lesions, patients with serum sickness may present with fever, malaise, arthralgias, gastrointestinal disturbances, and lymphadenopathy. These patients also may present with a characteristic serpiginous erythematous and purpuric eruption on the hands and feet at the junction of palmar and plantar skin (Fig. 4.35A,B), which is considered a cutaneous marker for the disease. The most common cause of serum sickness is a hypersensitivity reaction to drugs. Erythema multiforme, a cutaneous hypersensitivity disorder, also can be caused by drugs and involves the surfaces of the palms and soles. The cutaneous lesions associated with erythema multiforme can be distinguished from those due to serum sickness by their symmetrical distribution and by the characteristic appearance of the initial lesion. This lesion is a dusky red macule or erythematous wheal that evolves into an iris or target lesion, which is the hallmark of erythema multiforme (see Dermatology, Chapter 8).

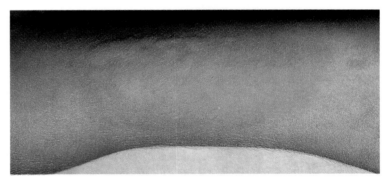

FIG. 4.36 Positive ice cube test in child with cold urticaria. An ice cube placed on the arm for 10 minutes results in urticaria of the exposed skin. Onset is usually immediate, but may be delayed for up to 4 hours after cold exposure.

A subgroup of urticarial disorders results from hypersensitivity to physical and mechanical factors. These include cold urticaria, pressure-induced urticaria and angioedema, aquagenic and solar urticaria, and exercise-induced urticaria. History and distribution of lesions are often helpful in identifying the source, which can then be confirmed by challenge (Fig. 4.36).

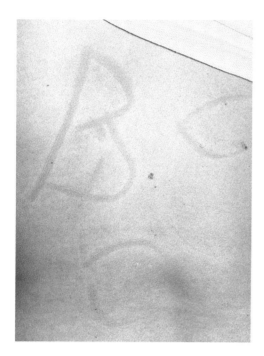

FIG. 4.37
Dermographism or writing on the skin is the most common type of urticaria induced by physical or mechanical factors. Firm stroking of the skin with fingernail or tongue blade will result in urticaria of the traumatized skin.

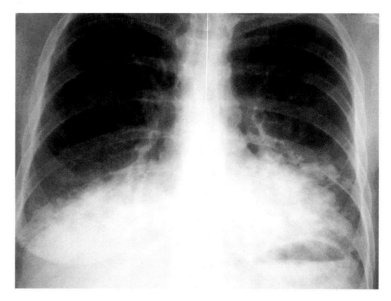

FIG. 4.38 Chest radiograph of patient with acute hypersensitivity pneumonitis. Note the soft, patchy coalescent infiltrates in both lower lung fields.

Dermographism, translated literally as the `ability to write on the skin' (Fig. 4.37), is a form of trauma-induced pressure urticaria. It is elicited by stroking the skin with a fingernail or tongue blade. The initial white line secondary to reflex vaso-constriction is supplanted by pruritic, erythematous linear swelling, as seen in a classic wheal and flare reaction. The condition is chronic and the etiology unclear. Patients with dermographism suspected of having an atopic disorder cannot be skin tested for specific IgE antibody because all tests appear positive.

Type III Disorders

HYPERSENSITIVITY PNEUMONITIS

Although IgE-mediated allergic respiratory diseases (allergic rhinitis, asthma) are the most common manifestations of inhalant sensitivities in humans, other immunological respiratory diseases, involving non-IgE immune mechanisms, may result from the inhalation of antigens present in the susceptible individual's environment. A wide variety of inhaled biological dusts may induce an inflammatory lung disease involving the interstitium, alveoli, and airways. The most common form of hypersensitivity pneumonitis is caused by inhalation of thermophilic actinomycetes (Micropolyspora faeni), antigens present in moldy vegetable compost, and is termed farmer's lung. Other forms (and their causative dusts and antigens) include malt-worker's lung (moldy malt, Aspergillus species) and bird-breeder's lung (avian dust, avian proteins). The disorder is termed "hypersensitivity pneumonitis" or "extrinsic allergic alveolitis," and appears to be immune-complex-mediated.

Hypersensitivity pneumonitis is a syndrome with a broad spectrum of presenting symptoms and signs. The clinical features depend on several factors: (1) the nature of the inhaled dust, (2) the intensity and frequency of inhalation exposure, and (3) the immunological responsiveness of the exposed individual. A concomitant upper respiratory infection or other pulmonary insult may be an important factor in induction.

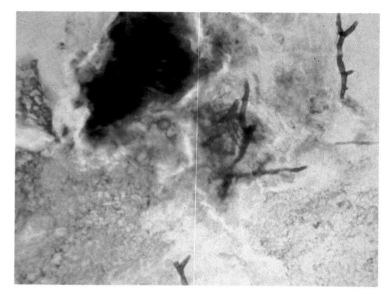

FIG. 4.39 Sputum smear from patient with allergic bronchopulmonary aspergillosis. Note the fungal mycelia characteristic of this disorder. (Reproduced by permission from Slavin RG, Laird TS, Cherry JD: Allergic bronchopulmonary aspergillosis in a child. J Pediatr 1970; 76:416–421)

Development of sensitization to the inhaled organic dust requires several months to years.

In the acute form, systemic and respiratory symptoms usually develop explosively, within 4 to 6 hours of exposure. These consist of cough, dyspnea, fever as high as 104°F, chills, myalgia, and malaise. Symptoms may persist up to 18 hours, subside spontaneously, and recur with each subsequent exposure. During such attacks, the patient appears acutely ill and dyspneic on physical examination. On chest auscultation, bibasilar end-inspiratory râles may be noted, and these may persist for weeks after the episode subsides. Chronic disease results from mild, continuous exposure. Progressive dyspnea,

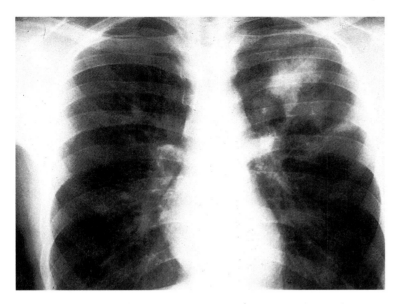

FIG. 4.40 Chest radiograph of patient with allergic bronchopulmonary aspergillosis. These patients are frequently asymptomatic despite extensive areas of consolidation. (Courtesy of Dr. Raymond G. Slavin, St. Louis University)

decreased exercise tolerance, productive cough, anorexia, and weight loss develop insidiously. Episodes of chills and fever are much less common than in the acute form. Physical findings in these patients include wheezing, cyanosis, and clubbing. Evidence of cor pulmonale develops as pulmonary inflammation and fibrosis progress.

Chest radiographs may be normal if attacks are widely spaced, but more commonly show characteristic findings which include fine, sharp nodulations, reticulation, and coarsening of bronchovascular markings. During an attack, soft, patchy, ill-defined parenchymal densities that tend to coalesce may be seen bilaterally (Fig. 4.38). Diffuse fibrosis with parenchymal contraction or honeycombing is a sign of end-stage disease. Pulmonary function tests reveal restrictive lung disease, especially in the chronic form, and challenge with the offending antigen may result in an immediate and a delayed response.

The differential diagnosis of hypersensitivity pneumonitis should include other conditions that cause interstitial lung disease and intermittent, explosive, and progressive pulmonary and systemic symptoms (drug-induced lung disease, recurrent pneumonias, allergic bronchopulmonary aspergillosis, sarcoidosis, collagen vascular diseases). Environmental (history, collection of antigenic materials) and immunological (serum IgG precipitins to thermophilic actinomycetes, Aspergillus species, or avian protein) studies, along with close observation of the patient during periods of exposure and avoidance, are useful in diagnosing this disorder.

ALLERGIC BRONCHOPULMONARY ASPERGILLOSIS

Aspergillus species, in addition to being one cause of hypersensitivity pneumonitis and allergic asthma, also cause a disorder termed "allergic bronchopulmonary aspergillosis." This entity is characterized by migrating pulmonary infiltrates and peripheral blood and sputum eosinophilia. Both Type I and Type III hypersensitivity are thought to be involved in pathogenesis. Most affected individuals are young; several under 2 years. Affected individuals are usually atopic and have a history of asthma. They present with anorexia, headache, generalized myalgias, loss of energy, temperature elevation, and acute episodes of wheezing and dyspnea. Sputum production is prominent and parents often report that their child's cough is productive of solid mucoid lumps of different sizes, shapes, and colors, ranging from dirty green to brown or beige. Physical findings include the general signs of lower airway obstruction (see section on asthma). On auscultation, crepitant râles are frequently heard over areas of pulmonary consolidation.

Laboratory studies that assist in diagnosis include:

1. Direct examination of sputum plugs reveals fungal mycelia (Fig. 4.39) and large numbers of eosinophils in most patients. Cultures are not considered diagnostic, as they may be negative during episodes of pulmonary consolidation and positive at other times.
2. Peripheral blood examination reveals eosinophilia, generally greater than $1,000/mm^3$.
3. Serum IgE level (A. fumigatus specific and nonspecific) is markedly elevated and may be as high as 78,000 ng/ml.
4. Skin testing: Even though a positive immediate wheal and flare reaction to A. fumigatus is not considered diagnostic of allergic bronchopulmonary aspergillosis, a negative reaction makes the diagnosis unlikely. Most patients will also experience a secondary skin reaction (Arthus-type) at the injection site, first noted at 3 to 4 hours, consisting of erythema and poorly defined edema, reaching a peak at 8 hours and resolving by 24 hours.
5. Serum precipitating antibody (IgG) to A. fumigatus is found in most patients, but titer has a poor correlation with disease activity and intensity of the clinical picture.
6. Chest radiography most commonly shows a massive homogenous consolidation without fissure displacement. The upper lobes are most commonly involved, and infiltrates characteristically shift rapidly from one site to the other. Remarkably, radiographic findings do not correlate well with clinical severity, and patients with extensive consolidation may be asymptomatic (Fig. 4.40).
7. Bronchography reveals the distinctive findings in allergic bronchopulmonary aspergillosis. These include saccular bronchiectasis of proximal bronchi with normal filling of distal ones, in distinct contrast to usual forms of bronchiectasis.

Allergic bronchopulmonary aspergillosis is being recognized with greater frequency as awareness increases. The diagnosis requires a high index of suspicion and should be considered in any asthmatic who has pulmonary infiltrates or suddenly uncontrollable disease. Allergic bronchopulmonary aspergillosis and hypersensitivity pneumonitis are frequently confused. Early diagnosis and corticosteroid treatment are necessary to prevent progression to severe, irreversible, end-stage lung disease.

IMMUNOLOGICAL DEFICIENCY DISORDERS

Normal Development of the Immune System

Integrity of the immune system is essential to maintain appropriate host defense mechanisms, which consist of humoral antibody, cell-mediated immunity, phagocytic, and comple-

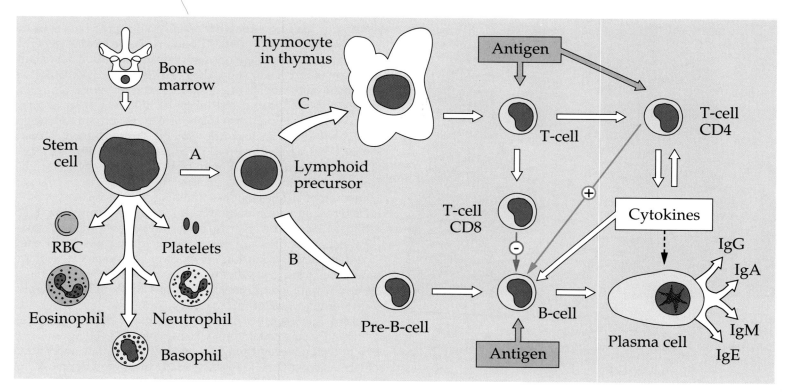

FIG. 4.41 *Schematic representation of T- and B-cell ontogeny. Defects along pathway A result in combined immune deficiencies. Pathway B is responsible for normal antibody production, while normal cell-medi-* *ated immunity requires the integrity of pathway C. Cytokines are soluble products of activated lymphocytes and include interleukins and interferons.*

ment systems. Defects of one or more of these host defense mechanisms result in immunodeficiency disorders. In addition, skin and mucosal surface abnormalities may result in breakdown of the physical barriers that ordinarily prevent invasion of microorganisms.

Cellular and humoral immunity is dependent on the maturation of two distinct lymphoid cell lines, the T- and B-lymphocytes, both originating from a common bone-marrow stem cell. Both T- and B-lymphocytes undergo a complex series of maturational changes before arriving at a stage where they are capable of antigen-stimulated differentiation (Fig. 4.41). The thymus-dependent T-lymphocytes are responsible for cell-mediated immune responses directed against viruses, fungi, or less common pathogens, such as *Pneumocystis carinii*. Other functions of T-lymphocytes include graft rejection and tumor cytotoxicity. Subpopulations of T-lymphocytes also collaborate in immunoregulation by expression of helper and suppressor functional activities. On the other hand, the thymus-independent B-lymphocytes are precursors of plasma cells. Plasma cells produce the various classes of immunoglobulins that serve as functional antibodies for antigen recognition. Deficiencies of one or more of the immunoglobulin classes

(IgG, IgA, IgM) constitute humoral or serum antibody immunodeficiency. Some patients, despite having normal numbers of B-cells and plasma cells and normal serum immunoglobulin levels, are nonetheless immunodeficient because they lack functional antibodies. Many of the immunodeficiency disorders described below are a result of either an arrest in cell maturation or a defect in the immunoregulatory cell interactions necessary for antigen recognition. Abnormalities in maturation of B- or T-lymphocytes result in humoral or cellular immunodeficiency, respectively. Abnormalities in maturation of both cell lines result in combined immunodeficiency.

Abnormal Function of the Immune System: Suspicion and Evaluation

Deficiencies of the immune system can involve lymphocytes (humoral and/or cellular immunodeficiency), phagocytes (chronic granulomatous disease), the complement system (heredity angioedema), and the mucosal barrier (immotile-cilia syndrome). Humoral (antibody) deficiency disorders are characterized by recurrent infections with high-grade extracellular encapsulated bacterial pathogens and chronic sinopulmonary

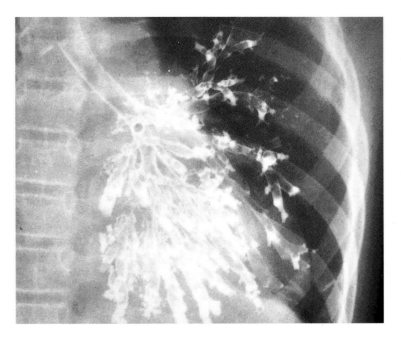

FIG. 4.42 Bronchogram reveals bronchiectasis of the left lower lobe in an older child with hypogammaglobulinemia. Symptoms consisted of chronic cough and sputum production.

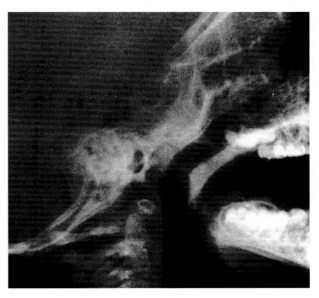

FIG. 4.43 Lateral neck radiograph shows absent adenoids in patient with congenital hypogammaglobulinemia.

infections. In contrast, cellular deficiencies are manifested by recurrent infections with low-grade or opportunistic infectious agents such as fungi, viruses, or *Pneumocystis carinii,* and associated with growth retardation, wasting, and diarrhea. These patients are susceptible to graft-versus-host disease if given fresh blood and can have fatal reactions from live virus vaccination.

Other immune deficiencies, such as mucosal barrier defects, may present in a more subtle fashion, with few life-threatening infections and normal growth. Thus, the clinician frequently is confronted with the question of whether or not a patient should be evaluated for immunodeficiency. In general, children with infections that are frequent, recurrent or chronic, and are caused by unusual organisms or respond poorly to therapy, should be evaluated for immunodeficiency. Moreover, growth retardation or a family history of early death should raise the clinician's level of suspicion. In screening for immunodeficiency, both quantitative and functional aspects of the components of the immune system are considered. A simple office evaluation for immunodeficiency should include quantitation of serum IgG, IgA, and IgM, and specific functional antibody titers to tetanus (or other antigens) for evaluation of humoral immunity, delayed hypersensitivity skin testing for cellular immunity, a nitroblue tetrazolium (NBT) test for phagocyte function, and levels of C_3, C_4, and total hemolytic complement for evaluation of complement component quantity and function. These screening tests can be performed in most laboratories and will identify most severe immune deficiency disorders.

Humoral Immunodeficiency (B-Lymphocyte)

CONGENITAL HYPOGAMMAGLOBULINEMIA
Congenital hypogammaglobulinemia may be X-linked (Bruton-type) or autosomal-recessive. Affected infants are clinically well for the first few months of life, due to placentally acquired maternal antibodies, but subsequently develop recurrent or chronic infections with virulent bacterial pathogens such as gram-positive cocci and *Haemophilus influenzae.* The infections may localize in the upper and lower respiratory tracts resulting in sinusitis, otitis media, and pneumonia. Sepsis, meningitis, and skin infections are also common. One of the complications of the chronic lower respiratory infections to which they are predisposed is bronchiectasis. This is characterized clinically by chronic cough with increased sputum production and by abnormal chest radiographs (Fig. 4.42). In the absence of chronic lung disease, growth is usually unimpaired and survival to adulthood is common with appropriate gammaglobulin and antibiotic therapy.

The physical findings are those of localized infection, with specific signs depending on the particular structure(s) infected. In addition, these children frequently manifest a paucity of adenoidal, tonsillar, and other lymphoid tissues (Fig. 4.43). The diagnosis of hypogammaglobulinemia should be considered in any child who has recurrent infections with virulent bacterial pathogens, and is confirmed by finding markedly decreased levels of the immunoglobulin classes (IgG, IgA, IgM) in the serum.

FIG. 4.44

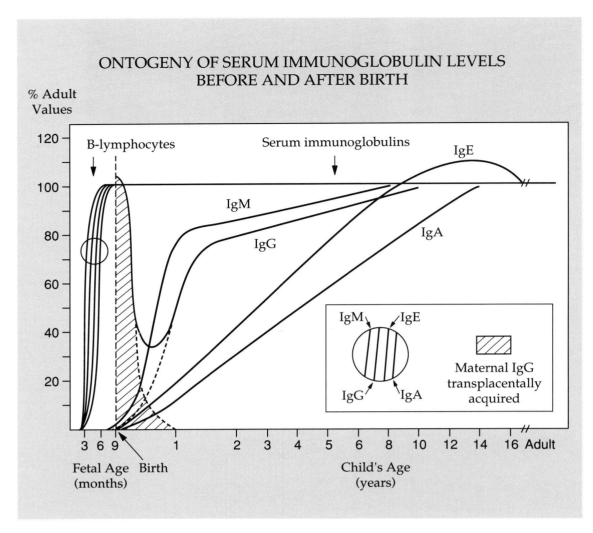

ONTOGENY OF SERUM IMMUNOGLOBULIN LEVELS
BEFORE AND AFTER BIRTH

TRANSIENT HYPOGAMMAGLOBULINEMIA OF INFANCY

As shown in Figure 4.44, term infants are born with high levels of serum IgG, due to active placental transport of maternal IgG. The serum IgG level normally declines during the first 7 months of life until the infant attains the ability to actively synthesize IgG. The diagnosis of transient hypogammaglobulinemia is applied to infants in whom the low serum IgG concentration observed during the first 7 months of life is prolonged. Serum IgG levels in these infants usually attain age-appropriate values by 18 to 24 months of age. Despite the low levels of serum IgG, these infants can synthesize specific antibodies to tetanus and other antigens. Gamma globulin replacement therapy is generally not indicated for this condition.

IgG SUBCLASS DEFICIENCY

Serum IgG immunoglobulin is comprised of four subclasses termed IgG1, IgG2, IgG3, and IgG4. Normal serum values for each are age-related (Fig. 4.45). IgG1 is the most plentiful of the subclasses and is considered the subclass which responds immunologically to foreign protein antigens such as tetanus toxoid. Conversely, polysaccharide antigens of the encapsulated *Haemophilus influenzae* or *pneumococcus* are considered to stimulate antibody synthesis predominantly in the IgG2 subclass.

Clinical immunologists have recently defined a role for quantitation of IgG subclasses in the evaluation of immunode-ficiency. IgG subclass deficiency is defined by a low IgG subclass concentration combined with a deficient antibody response of that subclass. These patients usually present with a history of chronic sinopulmonary infections, but have a normal growth pattern. Gamma globulin replacement therapy is indicated in this condition.

SELECTIVE IgA DEFICIENCY

Selective IgA deficiency, which affects 1:500 to 1:700 of the population, is the most common humoral antibody deficiency. Even though these patients are deficient in mucosal secretory IgA, only half of affected individuals manifest symptoms. Synthesis of IgG and IgM immunoglobulins is usually normal. Most cases are sporadic, but siblings with IgA or other immunodeficiencies have been frequently reported.

IgA deficiency has been associated with a variety of clinical syndromes. Chronic infections of the sinuses and middle ear are common, but severe or recurrent lower respiratory disease is unusual unless another form of immunodeficiency coexists with the IgA deficiency. Individuals with selective IgA deficiency may have severe malabsorption manifesting as chronic diarrhea, and have an increased incidence of autoimmune syndromes (collagen vascular disease) and of atopy. Therefore, the patient with a history of recurrent upper respiratory or sinopulmonary infections, malabsorption, or arthritis should be investigated for serum IgA deficiency.

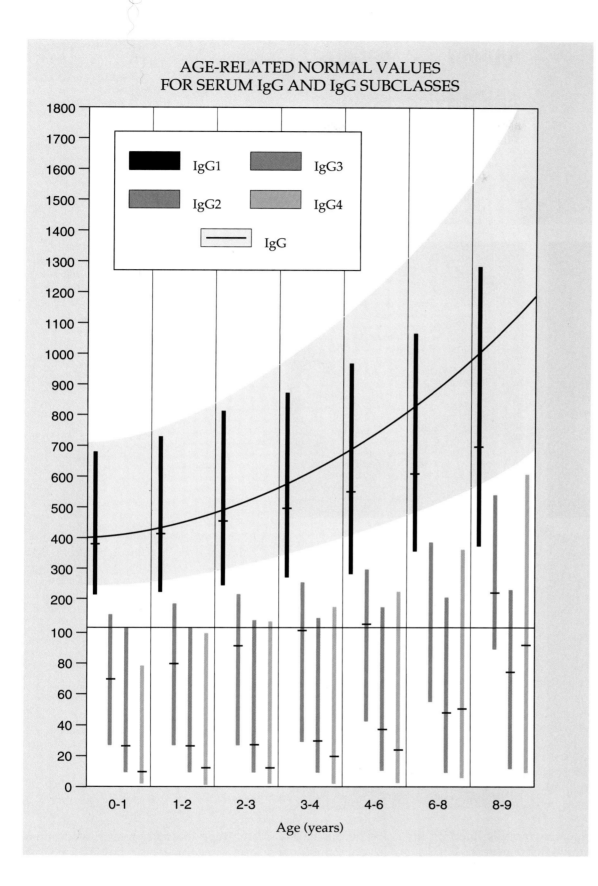

AGE-RELATED NORMAL VALUES
FOR SERUM IgG AND IgG SUBCLASSES

FIG. 4.45 (Reproduced with permission from Smith TF: Immunodeficiency in chronic pediatric respiratory illness. Hosp Pract 1986; 21(8):145)

Cellular Immunodeficiency (T-Lymphocyte)

Isolated defects of T-lymphocyte, or cell-mediated immunity, are rare. Since normal T-cell function is necessary for regulation of antibody production, many cellular immunodeficien-cies are also associated with humoral immunodeficiencies. Patients with T-cell deficiencies experience an increased frequency of severe infections with viral agents such as herpes simplex and cytomegalovirus, certain fungi, intracellular parasites, and other organisms of relatively low virulence. Figure

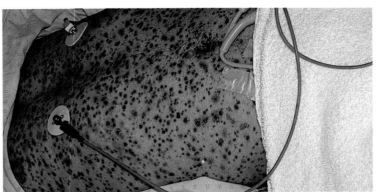

FIG. 4.46 Adolescent with abnormal T-cell function and disseminated varicella, in whom pneumonia resulted in respiratory failure.

FIG. 4.47 Characteristic facial features of child with DiGeorge syndrome, frontal (left) and lateral (right) views. Note the micrognathia, hypertelorism, low-set malformed ears, and the midline sternotomy scar following repair of a congenital heart defect.

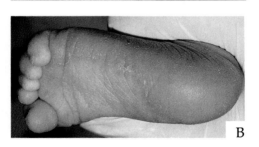

FIG. 4.48 Widespread fungal dermatitis with C. albicans over the trunk **A**, and foot **B**, of child with SCID. Note the dystrophic changes of the nails secondary to chronic infection **C**. Normal immune surveillance usually prevents persistent infection with this ubiquitous organism.

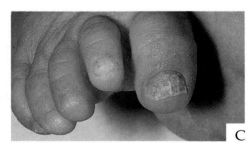

B

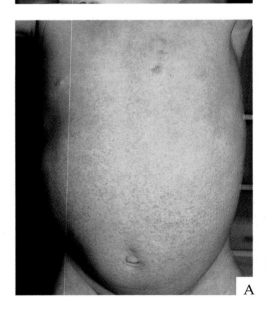

A

C

4.46 demonstrates a severe disseminated varicella infection in a child with congenital cellular immunodeficiency.

DIGEORGE SYNDROME

DiGeorge syndrome is a pure T-cell immunodeficiency disorder characterized by absent T-lymphocytes with normal or near-normal B-lymphocyte numbers and function. Thymic hypoplasia, which results from abnormal development of the third and fourth branchial pouches during embryogenesis, is the hallmark of DiGeorge syndrome. The thymus provides the necessary microenvironment for maturation of lymphoid precursors into functioning T-lymphocytes. When the thymus is absent, this normal maturation does not proceed, resulting in cellular immunodeficiency. Since major cardiovascular structures and the parathyroid glands are derived from the same branchial pouches, affected children frequently present with signs of congenital heart disease and hypocalcemic tetany or seizures within the first few days of life. Associated abnormalities include unusual facies (Fig. 4.47), esophageal atresia, and hypothyroidism.

Even though the T-cell defect may be transient and resolve spontaneously, many of these infants succumb to overwhelming infections with bacteria, viruses, and fungi unless reconstituted with fetal thymus transplantation.

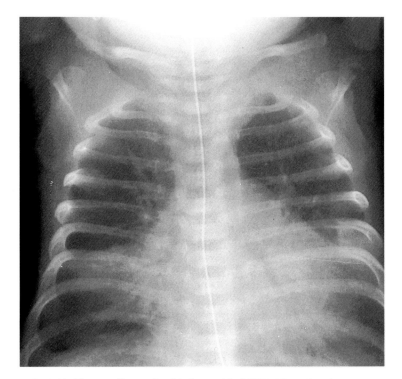

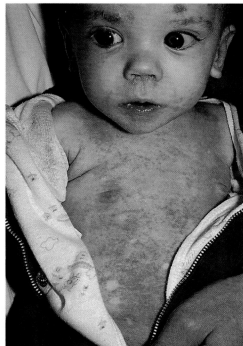

FIG. 4.50 Child with Wiskott-Aldrich syndrome. The skin eruptions on the trunk and face are eczematoid and pruritic, but not always similar to atopic dermatitis in flexural distribution. Many of these patients have thrombocytopenia which results in petechiae of varying distribution and intensity. (Reproduced from Fireman P, Slavin RG: Atlas of Allergies. New York, Gower, 1990)

FIG. 4.49 Chest radiograph of infant with SCID. Note the absent thymic shadow and bilateral pulmonary infiltrates.

Combined T- and B-Lymphocyte Disorders

SEVERE COMBINED IMMUNODEFICIENCY DISORDERS

Severe combined immunodeficiency disease (SCID) is a heterogeneous group of disorders with varying etiologies. The consequent defects in stem cell maturation ultimately result in abnormalities of both humoral and cellular immunity (see Fig. 4.41). Inherited deficiency of the enzyme adenosine deaminase (ADA) is also associated with combined immunodeficiency. The mechanism involves the accumulation of metabolic substrates that are toxic to both T- and B-lymphocytes. ADA deficiency may be responsible for up to 25 percent of all cases of SCID.

Having deficiencies of both cell-mediated (T-lymphocyte) and humoral (B-lymphocyte) immunity, these infants present with recurrent, severe bacterial, viral, fungal, and protozoan infections. Manifestations typically appear in the first few months of life and are often associated with failure to thrive, diarrhea, and candidiasis (Fig. 4.48). Affected infants may be distinguished from normal babies by virtue of frequency and severity of infections, and of their recalcitrance to appropriate antimicrobial therapy. Presenting symptoms usually involve the respiratory tract, since pneumonia due to *P. carinii* or virulent bacterial pathogens is common. In addition to the clinical findings of infection, examination discloses hypoplastic or absent tonsils and lymph nodes. Laboratory abnormalities include peripheral blood lymphopenia; decreased serum IgG, IgA, and IgM; and defective lymphocyte responses to mitogens such as phytohemagglutinin. Histological examination of tonsillar, adenoidal, and lymph node remnants reveals immature lymphoid tissue. The thymus is typically dysplastic histologically and radiographically (Fig. 4.49); normal lobulation and corticomedullary differentiation are lacking and the number of lymphocytes is decreased.

Once the diagnosis of SCID is considered, the child must be placed in protective isolation and given appropriate supportive therapy. All administered blood products must be irradiated to prevent the potential development of severe graft-versus-host disease.

PARTIAL COMBINED IMMUNODEFICIENCY DISORDERS
Congenital Disorders

Wiskott-Aldrich syndrome is an X-linked recessive disorder characterized by eczema, thrombocytopenia with cutaneous petechiae, and recurrent infections which begin in infancy (Fig. 4.50). The immunodeficiency may result in infectious complications later in life. Inability to form antibody to bacterial capsular polysaccharide antigens is the most commonly reported immunological defect, but some patients also manifest a partial defect in T-lymphocyte responses.

Ataxia-telangiectasia is a complex and intriguing immunodeficiency disorder with autosomal-recessive inheritance. The pathogenesis is unclear, since no theory has been developed that explains the hallmark multisystem involvement characteristic of this disorder: telangiectasia, progressive ataxia, and variable immunodeficiency. Most patients develop ocular telangiectasia and ataxia during the first 6 years of life (see Fig. 15.18, Chapter 15, Neurology). The ataxia is cerebellar in nature and characteristically progressive. Neurological involvement may be extensive, including abnormalities of speech, movement, and gait and mental retardation. The progressive, variable immunodeficiency consists most commonly of selective IgA deficiency and depressed T-cell function. Selective IgG subtype and IgG deficiencies have also been reported. Recurrent sinus and pulmonary infections, which may lead to bronchiectasis, are common and may be responsible for early death. These patients, in addition to those with other forms of immunodeficiency, have a higher incidence of neoplasia.

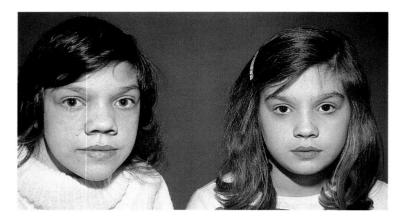

FIG. 4.51 Coarse facial features of female with hyper-IgE syndrome (left). Her sister (right) has IgA deficiency. Although distinct in etiology, these illustrate the frequency with which immune deficiencies are observed in family members of IgA-deficient individuals.

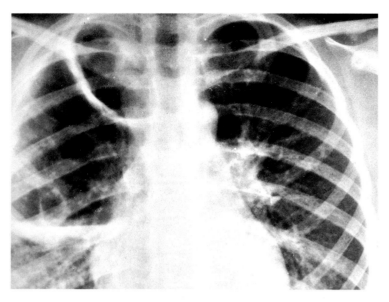

FIG. 4.52 Clearly outlined pneumatocele in the right lung of patient with hyper-IgE syndrome. This encapsulated lesion frequently complicates S. aureus pneumonia.

The hyper-IgE syndrome is a disorder of autosomal-recessive inheritance characterized by marked elevation of serum IgE. Clinical features include recurrent staphylococcal infections, a pruritic eczematoid dermatitis, and coarse facial features (Fig. 4.51). Recurrent staphylococcal skin infections, including impetigo and furuncles, are especially common and typically quite resistant to therapy. Staphylococcal pneumonia complicated by pneumatocele formation (Fig. 4.52) and lung abscesses are not infrequent. Other organisms of relatively low virulence, including *Candida albicans,* may cause infection. Immunological findings include markedly elevated IgE levels (often greater than 10,000 IU/ml), eosinophilia, abnormal cell-mediated immunity, and, in certain patients, abnormal polymorphonuclear leukocyte chemotaxis.

Short-limbed dwarfism is an autosomal-recessive disorder associated with metaphyseal or spondyloepiphyseal dysplasia and immunodeficiency usually involving T-cell function. Since the immunodeficiency is variable, many affected children have no increase in frequency or severity of infections, while others develop fatal, overwhelming infections. At birth, the head size is normal, the hands and limbs are short, and elbow extension is limited. Radiographic abnormalities include flaring of ribs, sclerosis, and cystic changes of the widened metaphyses (Fig. 4.53). A variant consists of short-limbed dwarfism and cartilage hair hypoplasia in which fine, sparse hair is characteristic.

Acquired Disorders

Acquired immunodeficiency syndrome (AIDS) results from the most severe form of infection by human immunodeficiency virus (HIV). As of 1990, approximately 2,000 children in the United States have been reported to the Center for Disease Control (CDC) with HIV infection that fulfills their definition of AIDS (see Bibliography, Falloon J, et al). Estimates suggest that the true number of children infected with the virus is five to eight times greater. Of these children, the vast majority are infected prenatally by HIV-infected mothers. Studies suggest a 20 to 60 percent risk of an HIV-positive mother transmitting the virus to her offspring in utero. Transmission by exposure to HIV-tainted blood products comprises the bulk of remaining cases, but has decreased due to blood bank screening procedures. Like the adults, adolescents encounter HIV through high-risk behaviors such as unprotected sexual activity and needle sharing during intravenous drug use. Transmission by casual contact with an HIV-infected individual in normal living conditions and school settings has not been reported to date. However, transmission of HIV by way of breast milk and organ donation has been reported.

HIV is an RNA virus which is tropic for T-helper lymphocytes and macrophages. The virus becomes integrated into the host genome during cell replication and hence persists in the infected individual for life. Humans are the only known reservoir for this virus. Following viral exposure, a subset of HIV-infected individuals will develop acute HIV infection. This illness occurs weeks after exposure and may mimic mononucleosis with fevers, sweats, malaise, lethargy, anorexia, nausea, myalgia, arthralgia, headaches, sore throat, diarrhea, lymphadenopathy, and rash. Others will bypass this clinical entity and seroconvert asymptomatically. In both groups of patients, incubation and replication of virus occurs for a variable time period. Many infected individuals will then proceed to develop a spectrum of clinical presentations ranging from mild symptoms to the most severe form of HIV infection, AIDS.

In children, HIV is often suspected by a history of maternal high-risk behaviors or by the clinical presentation. A broad

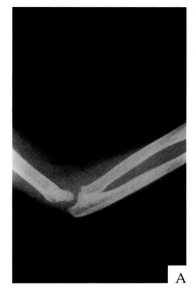
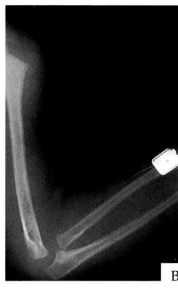

FIG. 4.53 **A**, forearm radiograph of a 3-year-old child with short-limbed dwarfism. Stenosis of the medullary cavity is evidenced by increased density. Bones are also of increased caliber and length. **B**, forearm radiograph of normal 3-year-old child.

A   B

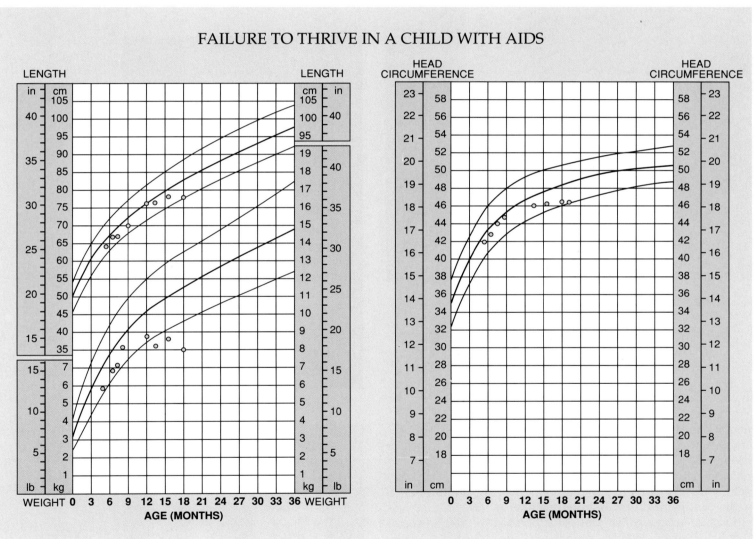

FIG. 4.54 Failure to thrive. Note deceleration of growth parameters for length, weight, and head circumference.

range of clinical manifestations have been described in individuals infected with HIV. Many of these symptoms are nonspecific, necessitating a high index of suspicion. Because most children are infected congenitally, HIV tends to be an illness of young children in which 50 percent present with the infection by the age of 1 year and 82 percent present by 3 years of age. In perinatally acquired HIV, the mean age of diagnosis of AIDS by CDC definition is 17 months, with a median age of 9 months. Infants infected prenatally or during the birthing process present with failure to thrive (Fig. 4.54), develop-

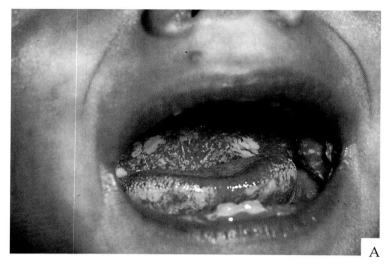

A

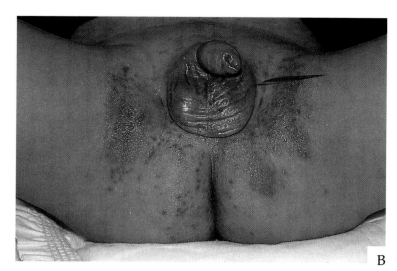

B

FIG. 4.55 *Child with AIDS.* **A**, *oral thrush.* **B**, Candida *diaper dermatitis.* (**A**, *courtesy of Drs. G. B. Scott, M. T. Mastrucci, U. of Miami School of Medicine*)

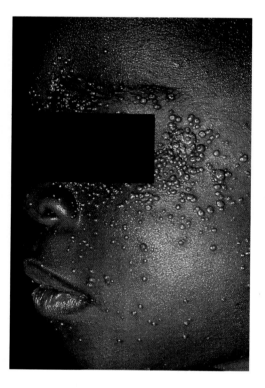

FIG. 4.57 *Severe molluscum contagiosum in a patient with AIDS. (Courtesy of Drs. G. B. Scott and M. T. Mastrucci, University of Miami School of Medicine)*

FIG. 4.56 Pneumocystis carinii *pneumonia in a child with AIDS. Note diffuse bilateral haziness. (Courtesy of Drs. G. B. Scott and M. T. Mastrucci, University of Miami School of Medicine)*

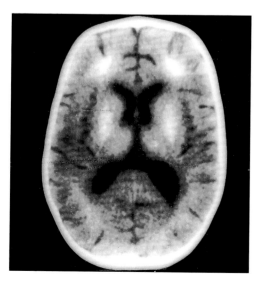

FIG. 4.58 *CT scan in infant with AIDS. Note frontal lobe and basal ganglia calcification, and increased ventricular size secondary to cerebral parenchymal volume loss.*

mental delay or loss of developmental milestones, hepatosplenomegaly, lymphadenopathy, thrush, or *Candida* skin infections (Fig. 4.55), diarrhea, chronic pneumonitis, and recurrent or particularly severe bacterial infections. The latter include meningitis, sepsis, pneumonia, abscess, cellulitis, otitis media, and sinusitis. Common pathogens are *Streptococcus pneumoniae, Haemophilus influenzae, Salmonella, Staphylococcus aureus* and gram-negative organisms. The repeated bacterial infections which characterize perinatally acquired AIDS usually develop during the first 2 to 5 months of life.

Although bacterial infections are often seen in HIV-infected infants, opportunistic infections related to defects in cell-mediated immunity also occur. The most common of these is *Pneumocystis carinii* pneumonia (Fig. 4.56), occurring in half the children who fit the formal CDC definition for AIDS. Other opportunistic infections include Mycobacterium avium-intracellulare, *Candida* esophagitis, cytomegalovirus (CMV), cryp-

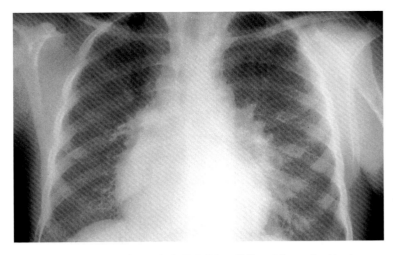

FIG. 4.59 LIP in a child with AIDS. Note diffuse bilateral reticulo-nodular infiltrates.

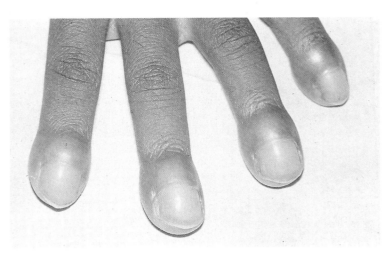

FIG. 4.60 Clubbing in patient with LIP and AIDS. (Courtesy of Drs. G. B. Scott and M. T. Mastrucci, University of Miami School of Medicine)

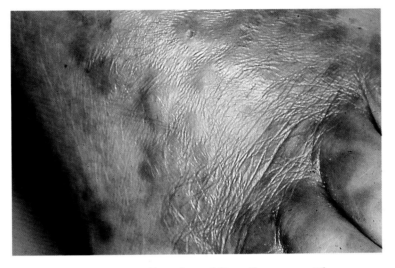

FIG. 4.61 Cutaneous manifestations of Kaposi's sarcoma. The purplish, hyperpigmented plaques and nodules are characteristic.

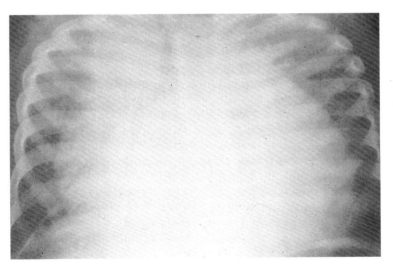

FIG. 4.62 Cardiomyopathy in a patient with AIDS. Note massively increased heart size. (Courtesy of Drs. G. B. Scott and M. T. Mastrucci, University of Miami School of Medicine)

tosporidiosis, herpes simplex virus, cryptococcosis, toxoplasmosis, and a variety of other organisms (Fig. 4.57).

A particularly devastating feature of HIV infection is the encephalopathy which leads to development delay, loss of developmental milestones, and behavioral alterations. Also seen are pyramidal tract signs, paresis, ataxia, pseudobulbar palsy, and decreased tone. The computerized tomographic scans and magnetic resonance imaging studies often show severe brain atrophy with increased ventricular size, and calcium in the basal ganglia and frontal lobes (Fig. 4.58). The course of HIV-related neurologic disease is variable and may be intermittent, static, or unrelentlessly progressive.

Lymphoid interstitial pneumonitis (LIP) and pulmonary lymphoid hyperplasia (PLH) leading to chronic interstitial pneumonitis occur in approximately 50 percent of AIDS patients (Fig. 4.59). These two forms of chronic lung disease present insidiously with clubbing of the fingers (Fig. 4.60),

hypoxemia, a diffuse reticulonodular infiltrate and, at times, hilar and mediastinal adenopathy. Children with LIP-PLH often have lymphadenopathy, salivary gland enlargement, high immunoglobulins, and a longer survival than children who present primarily with opportunistic infections.

As with many immunodeficiencies, malignancies also occur in children with AIDS, though at rates significantly lower than in adults. Kaposi sarcoma (Fig. 4.61), which occurs primarily in Haitian children, and lymphoma have been reported.

Other clinical manifestations of HIV include salivary gland enlargement, diarrhea, hepatitis, pancreatitis, cardiomyopathy (Fig. 4.62), eczema, nephrotic syndrome, and pancytopenia. HIV infection, therefore, presents with a multitude of clinical patterns. The clinical pattern of disease reflects direct HIV infection as well as immune system deregulation, including both evidence of immune deficiency and autoimmune disease. A variety of immunologic abnormalities occur with HIV infec-

FIG. 4.63

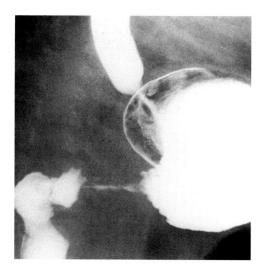

FIG. 4.64 Barium contrast radiogram demonstrating the "string sign," a thin line of barium which represents narrowing of the gastric antrum secondary to granuloma formation. This child presented with persistent vomiting, but none of the usual stigmata of chronic granulomatous disease.

tion (Fig. 4.63). Recently, a variety of diagnostic techniques have been developed to assist the clinician in confirming clinical suspicion. The ELISA (enzyme-linked immunosorbent assay) test is the most ubiquitous screening test for HIV infection. It detects the presence of antibody to HIV in the serum of the patient signifying viral infection. It also may indicate passively transmitted antibody from mother to offspring. The time from viral exposure to detection of antibody is variable, but most patients will be seropositive within several months of exposure. Occasionally, patients seroconvert later, and in rare instances seroconversion never occurs. The Western Blot test is a more specific antibody test which detects the presence of specific antibodies to various HIV antigens. The p24 antigen capture technique is a serologic test to detect the presence of the p24 antigen of HIV. Its presence is one step closer to the detection of the virus itself. Viral culture of leukocytes remains the gold standard for detection of HIV infections, but new techniques such as polymerase chain reaction (PCR) hold promise for viral detection. This test utilizes a gene amplification technique to detect the presence of the HIV DNA genome. The aforementioned core of blood tests provides the clinician with valuable tools for confirming the presence of HIV in their patients.

Prognosis remains poor but, with new therapies for HIV itself, the importance of early diagnosis and aggressive management are heightened.

Chronic mucocutaneous candidiasis is a T-cell disorder typified by superficial candidal infections of mucous membranes, skin, and nails. This illness may be sporadic or familial. The disorder is often associated with an endocrinopathy, and variants of this syndrome may include hypoparathyroidism, hyperthyroidism, and polyendocrinopathy. Candidal infections typically begin in early childhood, but may be delayed for up to 20 years. Other manifestations of chronic mucocutaneous candidiasis result from the associated endocrinopathies, of which hypoparathyroidism is the most common. Abnormalities of the immune system include absent cutaneous delayed hypersensitivity to Candida and lack of lymphokine production by Candida-stimulated lymphocytes. Other mechanisms of host defense, including immunoglobulins, are normal. Treatment of chronic mucocutaneous candidiasis involves long-term antifungal therapy. Local application of nystatin and clotrimazole may prevent progression, but is rarely curative. Ketaconazole given orally has resulted in dramatic clinical improvement and decreased morbidity in affected patients.

Phagocytic Disorders

Polymorphonuclear leukocytes and mononuclear cells play vital roles in the defense against acute infections. Normal neutrophil numbers, intact neutrophil chemotaxis, phagocytosis, and killing are all necessary for the rapid elimination of microorganisms that invade skin or mucous membranes. Patients with neutropenia are highly vulnerable to bacterial infections, as are patients with disorders of phagocyte function. The neutropenias and Chediak-Higashi syndrome are discussed in Chapter 11.

Chronic granulomatous disease of childhood is one example of neutrophil dysfunction. Neutrophil chemotaxis and phagocytosis are intact, but killing of ingested microorganisms is defective. The responsible biochemical defect results in abnormal leukocyte oxidative metabolism, and inability to kill microorganisms. Intracellular survival of ingested bacteria, even those not typically associated with granuloma formation, can lead to development of granulomatous lesions. Because of its X-linked recessive inheritance, the disorder predominantly affects males; females are affected less frequently. Clinically, children with chronic granulomatous disease become symptomatic early in life. The most common presenting problems are severe, recurrent infections of the skin and lymph nodes with *Staphylococcus aureus*. The skin infections often become chronic and heal slowly. Suppurative lymphadenitis often requires surgical drainage. Pneumonitis may progress to produce pneumatoceles (see Fig. 4.52). Osteomyelitis of the small bones of the hand and foot is common. Hepatosplenomegaly is a constant physical finding and presumably represents involvement of the reticuloendothelial system. Granulomas may also develop in other organ systems as well, and may or may not be palpable on examination. In the patient whose radiograph is seen in

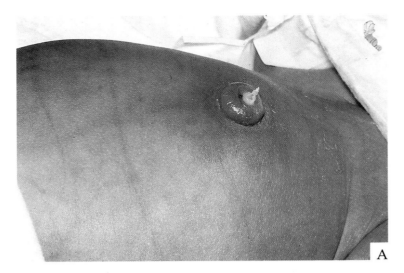

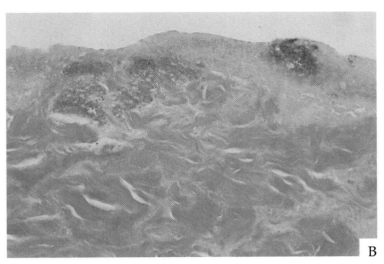

FIG. 4.65 *A, infection involving and surrounding the umbilical cord in infant with intercellular adhesion molecule (ICAM) deficiency. (Courtesy of Dr. Kenneth Schuit, Children's Hospital of Pittsburgh.) B, histopathologic appearance of scalp abscess in infant with intercel-* *lular adhesion molecule (ICAM) deficiency. Note the presence of bacterial colonies (purple staining) and distinct lack of host cellular inflammatory response. (Courtesy of Drs. Kenneth Schuit and William Robichaux, Children's Hospital of Pittsburgh)*

Figure 4.64, the diagnosis of chronic granulomatous disease was suggested by the finding of antral narrowing secondary to granulomatous involvement of the gastric antrum.

Intercellular adhesion molecule (ICAM) deficiency is a recently defined, rare syndrome which is due to deficiency of one or more of a group of cell-membrane glycoproteins termed intercellular adhesion molecules (ICAM) and normally used by phagocytes to move and adhere to surfaces. The patients present with a variety of symptoms and signs, all of which are related to the inability of phagocytes to adhere and move toward a chemoattractant. These include delayed umbilical cord severance (Fig. 4.65A), persistent peripheral blood granulocytosis (lack of vascular margination), recurrent soft tissue infections, and impaired wound healing. Since these patients do not mobilize neutrophils in response to infection, many aspects of the normal inflammatory response are lacking, including the formation of pus (Fig. 4.65B). This may confound the diagnosis when infection is suspected. ICAM deficiency should be suspected in any infant with periumbilical problems and persistent peripheral blood leukocytosis (frequently >50,000 cells/mm³).

Complement System Disorders

The complement system is a complex system of nine distinct serum proteins, designated C1 through C9, which require serial activation, via either the classical or alternative complement pathways. Complement mediates and amplifies many of the biological functions of the immune system. These functions include: (1) enhancement of phagocytosis (opsonization) and viral neutralization; (2) mediation of inflammation via chemotaxis and alteration of vascular permeability; (3) cell lysis; and (4) modulation of the immune response. Defects of the complement system result from decreased levels of or absence of components, or from production of components which function abnormally. Although rare, inherited deficiencies of most complement components have been reported. Clinical presentation varies, depending on specific complement protein involved. Frequent modes of presentation for complement component deficiencies are collagen vascular diseases for C1–C4, dissemi-

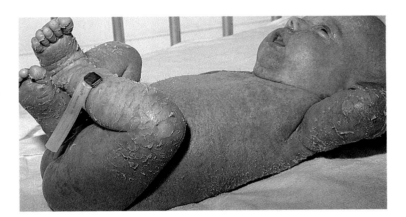

FIG. 4.66 *Exfoliative dermatitis characteristic of severe seborrhea in an infant with Leiner syndrome.*

nated infections with pyogenic bacteria for C3, and disseminated neisserial infections for C5–C8.

LEINER SYNDROME

Shortly after the turn of the century, Leiner described an infantile syndrome characterized by recurrent infections, severe seborrheic dermatitis, intractable diarrhea, and failure to thrive (Fig. 4.66). These children were subsequently observed to have a functional abnormality of C5 and an inability to opsonize yeast particles. Yeast opsonization has been used to identify individuals with Leiner syndrome, as other functional and antigenic assays of C5 are normal in these patients. Mothers of these children lack functional C5 in their breast milk; therefore, this disease occurs almost exclusively in breast-fed babies and not those fed cow milk formulas, which do contain functional C5. The disorder is self-limited, tending to resolve by age 2 months, coincident with appearance of endogenous functional C5.

HEREDITARY ANGIOEDEMA

Hereditary angioedema is an autosomal-dominant disorder characterized by absence or abnormal function of a protein in the complement cascade known as C1 esterase inhibitor.

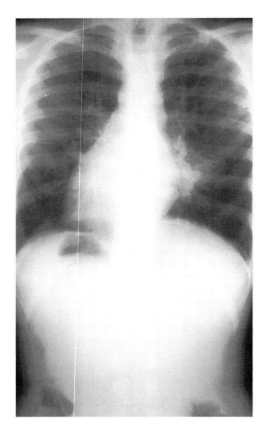

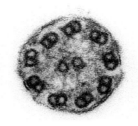 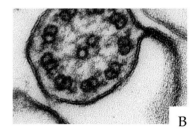

A B

FIG. 4.67
Dextrocardia and situs inversus of abdominal organs in patient with Kartagener syndrome. Abnormal ciliary motion is thought to result in malrotation during embryogenesis.

FIG. 4.68 **A**, *electron micrograph of cilia from patient with immotile cilia syndrome. Note the absence of dynein arms from the outer doublets.* **B**, *normal cilia with dynein arms. (Reproduced from Bluestone C, Stool S: Pediatric Otolaryngology. Philadelphia, WB Saunders, 1983, vol 1)*

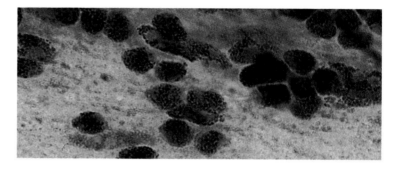

FIG. 4.69 *Eosinophilia on nasal smear from patient with allergic rhinitis.*

Inhibitors of the complement system are naturally occurring and are capable of blocking activated complement components. C1 esterase inhibitor binds to activated C1 and thereby prevents further activation of the classical pathway. In the absence of C1 inhibitor, complement activation proceeds unchecked. This results in increased vascular permeability and the observed clinical features of angioedema. Many clinicians do not consider hereditary angioedema an immunodeficiency disorder because these patients do not have recurrent infections. Nevertheless, a defect in the complement system is responsible for the clinical manifestations. This disorder is characterized by recurrent bouts of swelling that involve any part of the body, but which most typically involve the face, extremities, and the respiratory and gastrointestinal tracts. The swelling is generally self-limited and episodic. Laryngeal edema is a frightening, life-threatening complication that may result in asphyxiation. Involvement of the gastrointestinal tract is characterized by severe abdominal pain, bloating, vomiting, and rarely intestinal obstruction due to intussusception.

Mucosal Barrier Disorders

Intact mucosal barriers are of crucial importance in preventing the entrance of ubiquitous microorganisms into the host. The respiratory and gastrointestinal mucosa aid in host defense by secreting antibodies (predominantly IgA) into their lumina. Also, physical factors such as saliva flow in the oral cavity, intestinal peristalsis, and the coughing reflex are important in the "washing out" effect on potential pathogens.

Immotile cilia syndrome is characterized by a defect in mucociliary transport, another component of the mucosal barrier. This disorder was first described as Kartagener syndrome, which consists of a triad of situs inversus viscerum (Fig. 4.67), chronic sinusitis, and bronchiectasis. These patients were also

noted to be infertile, because their spermatozoa were poorly motile as a result of lack of dynein arms in the ultrastructure of their tails. Studies revealed similar defects in mucosal cilia and led to recognition of the fact that the phenomenon could exist in the absence of situs inversus viscerum. The resultant ciliary dysfunction impedes mucous clearance and produces a combination of the following signs and symptoms: (1) early onset of chronic rhinorrhea; (2) chronic otitis media; (3) chronic sinusitis with opaque sinuses on radiography; (4) chronic productive cough; (5) bronchiectasis; (6) digital clubbing; and (7) nasal polyps. The disorder should be suspected in any child with chronic or recurrent upper or lower respiratory tract infections. When situs inversus viscerum is not present, the diagnosis of immotile cilia syndrome requires confirmation by electron microscopic analysis of cilia obtained from biopsy of the nasal or tracheobronchial mucosa (Fig. 4.68)

DIAGNOSTIC TECHNIQUES IN ALLERGY AND IMMUNOLOGY

Skin Testing: Immediate Hypersensitivity

For over 100 years, hypersensitivity skin tests have been used to confirm the diagnosis of allergy. This in vivo method detects the presence of IgE antibody specific to the test antigen. The prick skin test is the safest and most specific test, and correlates best with symptoms. It involves placing a drop of antigen solution on cleansed skin. A blunt needle is passed through the drop, punctures the skin, and is rapidly withdrawn without scratching the skin. The test site is "read" in 15 to 20 minutes by recording the presence or absence of a wheal and surrounding flare (erythema) their sizes. A typical scoring system is listed below.

Although the prick skin test is very specific, it is less sensitive than intradermal skin tests. If prick tests are negative, then intradermal tests should be performed. This test involves injecting 0.02 ml of antigen solution intradermally and is also read in 20 minutes. The scoring system used for interpretation is:

Grade 0(-)(wheal <3 mm, erythema 0–5 mm)
Grade 1+ (wheal 3–5 mm, erythema 0–10 mm)
Grade 2+ (wheal 5–10 mm, erythema 5–10 mm)
Grade 3+ (wheal 10–15 mm, erythema >10 mm)
Grade 4+ (wheal >15 mm or with pseudopods, erythema >20 mm).

Although more sensitive, the results of intradermal tests do not correlate as well with symptoms as do those of prick testing. Appropriate antigen solutions must be used to assure reliability, and results must be correlated with clinical symptoms. In addition, drugs that inhibit or suppress histamine action or release, such as antihistamines and cromolyn, must be discontinued 24 to 48 hours prior to skin testing. An in vitro correlate of skin testing is the serum RAST, which correlates well with history but is less sensitive than skin testing.

Nasal Smear

The nasal smear is another helpful tool in diagnosing allergic and nonallergic nasal disease. Mucus is obtained by having the patient sneeze into wax paper or by swabbing the posterior nares. The secretions are then applied in a thin layer onto a microscope slide. The slide is stained with either Wright's or Hansel's stain and the percentage of eosinophils is noted (Fig. 4.61). The presence of eosinophilia (greater than 25 percent), along with positive skin tests, is very suggestive of allergic disease. When skin tests are negative, the presence of nasal eosinophilia can differentiate eosinophilic nonallergic rhinitis from vasomotor rhinitis. This distinction has important therapeutic implications.

Skin Testing: Delayed Hypersensitivity

Traditionally, cell-mediated immunity has been assessed by the delayed hypersensitivity skin test. Intradermal injection of 0.1 ml of antigen solution in a sensitized individual is followed by the development of an indurated erythematous reaction over several hours. This reaction peaks at 24 to 48 hours and is recorded at 48 hours. A positive test occurs when 10 mm or more of induration and erythema is present. Using an antigen such as *C. albicans*, the majority of children with intact cellular immunity will have positive tests after 6 to 12 months of age. Other antigens such as diphtheria and tetanus, if tested within 6 to 12 months of booster immunization, will frequently show delayed hypersensitivity. Purified protein derivative (PPD) is used to document exposure and sensitization to the tubercle bacillus. If delayed hypersensitivity skin tests are negative in a child with suspected immunodeficiency, a thorough evaluation of the T-lymphocyte system is indicated. For diagnosis of patients with contact dermatitis, delayed hypersensitivity skin testing is performed by the patch test technique (see Chapter 8).

REFERENCES

Buckley RH: Immunodeficiency. *J Allergy Clin Immunol* 1983; 72:627–644.

Burrows B, Martinez FD, Halonen M, et al: Association of asthma with serum IgE levels and skin-test reactivity to allergens. *N Engl J Med* 1989;320:271–277.

Cooper DA, Maclean P, Finlayson R, et al: Acute AIDS retrovirus infection. *Lancet* 1985;1:537–540.

DeVita VT, Hellman S, Rosenberg SA (eds): *AIDS—Etiology, Diagnosis, Treatment, and Prevention*, ed 2. Philadelphia, JB Lippincott, 1988.

Ellis EF: Asthma in childhood. *J Allergy Clin Immunol* 1983; 72:526–539.

Ellis EF (ed): Pediatric allergy. *Pediatr Clin North Am* 1983; 30(5):773–974.

Falloon J, Eddy J, Wiener L: Human immunodeficiency virus infection in children. *J Pediatr* 1989;114:1–30.

Heiss R: Immunology of AIDS. *Pediatr Ann* 1987;16:495–503.

Henderson FW, Clyde WA, Collier AM, et al: The etiologic and epidemiologic spectrum of bronchiolitis in pediatric practice. *J Pediatr* 1979;95:183.

Howard WA: Differential diagnosis of wheezing in children. *Pediatr Rev* 1980;1:239.

Kaliner M: Mast cell mediators and asthma, in Herzog H, Perruchoud AP (eds): *Progress in Respiration Research–Asthma and Bronchial Hyperreactivity*. Basel, Switzerland, S Karger, 1985.

Kozinetz CA, Crane MM, Reves RR: Pediatric infection and AIDS: epidemiology. *Semin Pediatr Infect Dis* 1990; 1:6–16.

Laurence J: The immune system in AIDS. *Sci Am* 1985; December:84–93.

Lawley TJ, Bielory L, Gascon P, et al: A prospective clinical and immunologic analysis of patients with serum sickness. *N Engl J Med* 1984;311:1407–1413.

Middleton E Jr, Reed CE, Ellis EF (eds): *Allergy: Principles and Practice*. St. Louis, CV Mosby, 1983.

Peter G (ed): *Report of the Committee on Infectious Diseases* ("The Red Book"), ed 21. Elk Grove, IL, American Academy of Pediatrics, 1988, 91–115.

Primer on Allergic and Immunologic Disease. *JAMA* 1982; 20:248.

Rosen FS, Cooper MD, Wedgewood RJ: The primary immunodeficiencies (Part 1). *N Engl J Med* 1984; 311:300–310.

Rubinstein A: Pediatric AIDS. *Curr Probl Pediatrics* 1986; 16:362–409.

Rubinstein A, Morecki R, Silverman B: Pulmonary disease in children with AIDS and ARC. *J Pediatr* 1987; 108:498–503.

Scott GB, Buck BE, Leterman JG, et al: Acquired immunodeficiency syndrome in infants. *N Engl J Med* 1984;310:76–81.

Shearer WT: Pediatric acquired immunodeficiency disease: an overview. *Semin Pediatr Infect Dis* 1990;1:3–5.

Skoner DP, Caliguiri L: The wheezing infant. *Pediatr Clin North Am* 1988;35(5):1011–1030.

Steihm ER, Fulginiti VA (eds): *Immunologic Disorders in Infants and Children*. Philadelphia, WB Saunders, 1980.

PEDIATRIC CARDIOLOGY

F. Jay Fricker, M.D. ◆ Sang C. Park, M.D. ◆ Cora C. Lenox, M.D

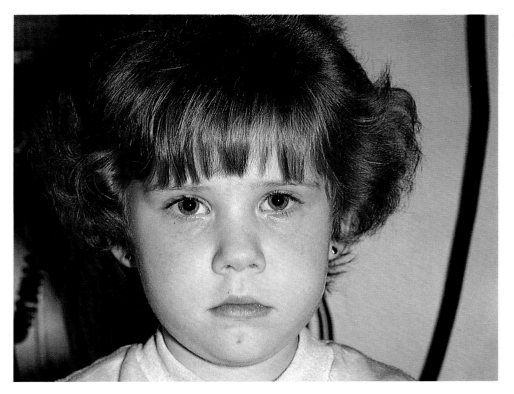
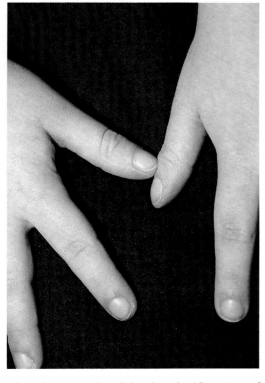

FIG. 5.1 *This child shows no obvious cyanosis of the face and lips, although the photograph at right demonstrates clubbing: loss of nail* *angle and curvature of nails, especially of the thumb. (Courtesy of Dr. L.B. Beerman)*

The practice of cardiology as a pediatric subspecialty continues to evolve with new imaging technology. Complex structural congenital anomalies previously delineated only at autopsy can now be defined in great detail by a combination of techniques that include echocardiography, angiography, and nuclear magnetic resonance imaging. The medical cost associated with these new technologies is significant, but a proper initial assessment of the child with suspected congenital heart disease helps avoid the expense of unnecessary testing. The emphasis of this chapter remains the physical examination, chest x-ray, and electrocardiogram. In addition, we cover 2-dimensional echocardiography and color flow Doppler imaging of common congenital heart lesions to reflect their important contribution to the practice of pediatric cardiology in the 1980s.

The three prerequisites to a good cardiovascular examination are a proper environment, a cooperative child, and the conviction on the part of the physician that the examination is important. The heart murmur is not the only, and often not even the most important part of the cardiac physical examination. Blood pressure determination, character of the pulse and precordial activity, observation of cyanosis, clubbing, and dysmorphic facial features may provide clues to the diagnosis and nature of congenital heart lesions before auscultation is even performed.

PHYSICAL DIAGNOSIS OF CONGENITAL HEART DISEASE
Cyanosis and Clubbing

Even before mild desaturation is detectable, early clubbing and cyanosis may be seen (Figs. 5.1 and 5.2). The base of the nail, especially the thumbnail, may show loss of angle as

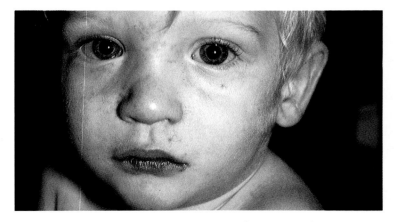

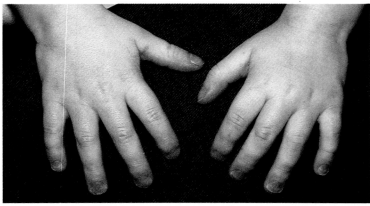

FIG. 5.2 This child demonstrates moderate cyanosis of the lips (top) and nails (bottom). Note also the reddish discoloration of the eyes due to conjunctival suffusion.

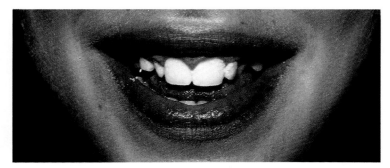

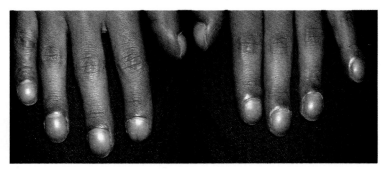

FIG. 5.3 Severe cyanosis of the lips, tongue, and mucous membranes can be noted on top, associated with marked clubbing and cyanosis of the nails on bottom.

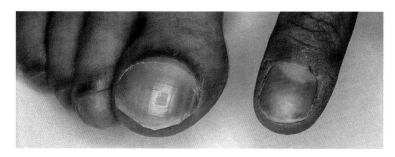

FIG. 5.4 Differential cyanosis and clubbing due to reverse shunting through a patent ductus arteriosus in a patient with pulmonary vascular disease. Note marked cyanosis and clubbing of the toes, while the finger appears to be normal. (Courtesy of Dr. J.R. Zuberbuhler)

early as 3 months of age (see Pediatric Pulmonary Disorders, Chapter 16). Elevated hemoglobin and hematocrit, and loss of nail angle indicate hypoxemia and the presence of a right-to-left intracardiac shunt (Fig. 5.3).

Observation of the lips and mucous membranes for the presence of cyanosis is best done in good daylight, since fluorescent light may produce a false cyanotic tinge. In the presence of polycythemia with hemoglobin in the l8- to 20-g range and hematocrit over 60 percent, the conjunctival vessels become engorged and plethoric (Fig. 5.2). Differential cyanosis between the upper and lower extremities is an unusual clinical finding. If the patient has pulmonary vascular disease, reverse flow through a patent ductus arteriosus, and no right-to-left intracardiac shunting, cyanosis and clubbing should be found in the lower extremities but not in the hands (Fig 5.4).

Blood Pressure and Pulse

Blood pressure determination in infants and children is an integral part of the cardiac physical examination. Attention to proper cuff size will prevent the misdiagnosis of systolic hypertension from an undersized cuff. In general, it is better to use an oversized cuff because reduction in systolic blood pressure will be minimal. Blood pressure can be tracked in children over time and tables depicting normal blood pressure range for age have been published. Blood pressure determination in both arms and a lower extremity will detect coarctation of the aorta, lend support for the diagnosis of su-

pravalvular aortic stenosis (blood pressure higher on the right arm than on the left arm), and help assess the severity of aortic valve disease—including aortic valve stenosis (narrow pulse pressure) and aortic regurgitation (wide pulse pressure).

Heart Murmur Evaluation

In the newborn, a common innocent heart murmur originates from the branch pulmonary arteries taking off at an acute angle from the main pulmonary artery. Characteristically, this murmur is early systolic and loudest over both axillae and back. The murmur of branch pulmonary artery stenosis has the same distribution as the structural lesions that cause increased pulmonary blood flow. Pathologic systolic murmurs in the newborn are caused by restrictive ventricular septal defects and lesions producing left and right ventricular outflow tract obstruction (i.e., tetralogy of Fallot and valvular aortic or pulmonic stenosis). In the newborn it can be difficult to distinguish the murmur of a small restrictive ventricular

INNOCENT MURMURS MIMICKING CONGENITAL HEART DISEASE	
Innocent Heart Murmur	**Structural Congenital Heart Disease**
Systolic Ejection Murmur Heard at the Base of the Heart	
High left sternal border	Pulmonic valve stenosis *Ejection click *Transmission to back Atrial septal defect *Parasternal lift *S2 wide split *Diastolic murmur of tricuspid flow
High right sternal border	Aortic valve stenosis *Ejection click *Radiation to neck
Still's Murmur	
Vibratory quality Location-left mid sternal border	Ventricular septal defect *Character of murmur Discrete subaortic stenosis *Radiation to aortic area
Venous Hum	
Continuous Locaton-neck and under clavicles Disappears in supine posture	Patent ductus arteriosus *Location under left clavicle *No change with position Coronary AV malformation *Accentuated in diastole
Carotid and Cranial Bruits	
Murmur over carotids and head	Aortic stenosis AV malformation *Continuous murmur would support AV malformation

Distinguishing features

FIG. 5.5

SYNDROMES AND TRISOMIES, WITH ASSOCIATED CARDIOVASCULAR ABNORMALITIES	
Syndrome	**Common Cardiac Defect**
Down	Atrioventricular septal defects, patent ductus, anomalous subclavian artery
Ellis-van-Creveld	Atrial septal defect or single atrium
Holt-Oram	Atrial and ventricular septal defects, arrhythmias
Marfan	Dilatation and aneurysm of aorta, aortic and mitral insufficiency, mitral valve prolapse
Noonan	Dysplastic pulmonic valve, atrial septal defect
Turner	Coarctation of the aorta, bicuspid aortic valve
Williams	Supravalvular aortic stenosis, pulmonary artery stenosis
Trisomy	
13	Patent ductus, septal defects, pulmonic and aortic stenosis (atresia)
18	Ventricular septal defect, polyvalvular disease, coronary abnormalities

FIG. 5.6

septal defect from that of a severe right ventricular outflow tract obstruction in tetralogy of Fallot. The implications of this differential diagnosis are such that an echocardiogram is recommended in infants with this clinical presentation.

In contrast to popular belief, the presence of a continuous murmur from a patent ductus arteriosus is extremely rare in a full-term newborn infant. In fact, if a continuous murmur is heard in the newborn, you should always think of patent ductus-dependent pulmonary blood flow and complex pulmonary atresia.

It is common for preschoolers and school-age children to be referred for evaluation of a heart murmur. Innocent murmurs of childhood fall into four major categories: systolic ejection murmurs at the base, vibratory or Still's murmur, venous hum, and carotid and cranial bruits. In most instances there are associated clinical and laboratory studies which can distinguish the innocent from the pathologic murmur. Figure 5.5 summarizes the distinguishing features and differential diagnosis.

Syndrome-Associated Physical Findings

Dysmorphology of face and habitus suggests certain syndromes associated with congenital heart disease (Fig. 5.6).

The typical features in *Down syndrome* (trisomy 21) were demonstrated in Chapter 1. About 40 percent of children with this syndrome have structural lesions, such as atrioventricular septal defects, isolated ventricular septal defects, patent ductus arteriosus, or anomalous origin of the subclavian arteries.

Although many infants with Down syndrome present with chronic congestive heart failure and growth failure,

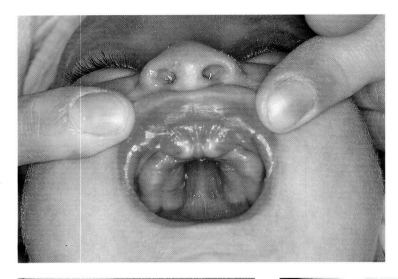

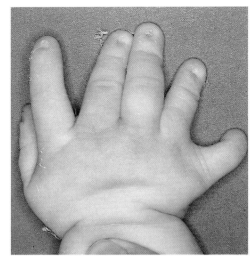

FIG. 5.7 This infant with Ellis-van Creveld syndrome demonstrates characteristic facial features (left) and multiple digits (polydactyly) (right).

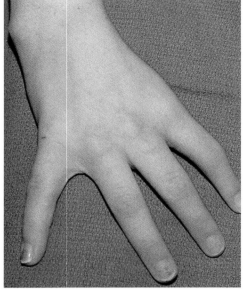

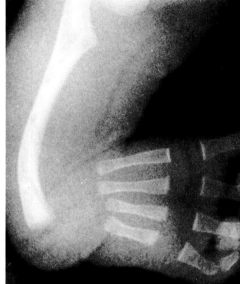

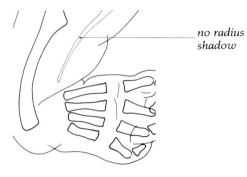

no radius shadow

FIG. 5.8 Clinical photograph (left) reveals the absence of the radius and thumb in a patient with Holt-Oram syndrome. The associated cardiovascular abnormality is an atrial septal defect. Radiographic examination (right) demonstrates the absence of a radius shadow; the missing thumb is apparent. (Clinical photograph courtesy of Dr. L.B. Beerman)

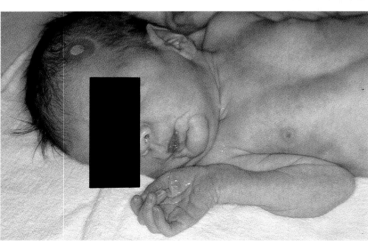

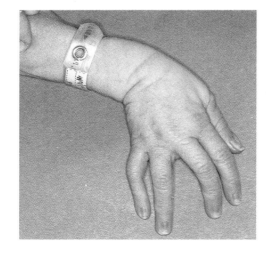

FIG. 5.9 Infant with Marfan syndrome. Note the narrow face, pectus, laxity, and long arms and fingers (left). At right is a close-up view of the infant's hand.

there is a subset that grows and develops appropriately. Pulmonary vascular resistance does not decrease in the usual fashion in this group, and these children develop early pulmonary vascular disease. Because this presentation may be silent, it is important that all children with Down syndrome be thoroughly evaluated during infancy. The evaluation should include an echocardiogram to rule out congenital heart disease.

Ellis-van Creveld syndrome is an autosomal recessive disorder characterized by multiple oral frenula, natal teeth, and polydactyly (Fig. 5.7). The patient with this syndrome frequently has an atrial septal defect or a common atrium.

Holt-Oram syndrome, an autosomal-dominant disorder, is associated with upper limb deformities consisting of narrow shoulders, hypoplasia of the radius, and phocomelia (Fig. 5.8). Absence of both radius and thumb or proximal displacement of the thumb are the most frequent findings. Commonly associated cardiovascular abnormalities include an

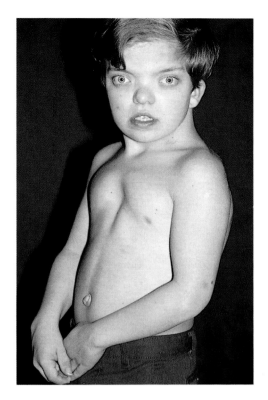

FIG. 5.10 Child displays characteristic features of Noonan syndrome: widely spaced eyes, low-set ears, webbing of the neck, shield chest, pectus, and increased carrying angle of the arms.

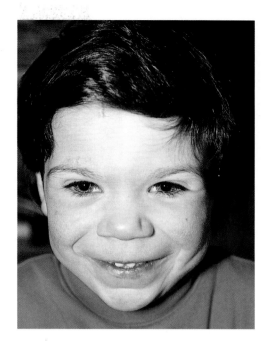

FIG. 5.11 Child with elfin facies (Williams syndrome). Note the wide-set eyes, upturned nose, large maxilla, prominent philtrum and pointed chin. (Courtesy of Dr. R.A. Mathews)

GENETIC SYNDROMES AND INBORN ERRORS OF METABOLISM, WITH THEIR ASSOCIATED CARDIOVASCULAR FINDINGS

Genetically Determined Diseases	Cardiac Findings
Metabolic – storage	
Pompe disease (glycogen storage)	Cardiomyopathy (storage of glycogen in myocardium)
Mucopolysaccharidosis	Storage of MPS in arteries, coronaries, and valves with insufficiency and stenosis
	Hurler MPS IH, Hunter II, Scheie IS, IHS, Morquio IV
Hyperlipoproteinemia, familial type II	Premature atherosclerosis of arteries, including coronaries
Neurologic	
Friedreich's ataxia	Cardiomyopathy (congestive or hypertrophic)
Muscular dystrophies	Myocardial degeneration and fibrosis

Inborn Error of Metabolism (no proven genetic basis)	Cardiac Findings
Progeria	Hypercholesterolemia, atherosclerotic changes in arteries, including coronaries

FIG. 5.12

atrial septal defect, ventricular septal defect, and dysrhythmias (atrial and ventricular ectopy, and atrioventricular block).

Marfan syndrome also has an autosomal dominant inheritance; it manifests as a connective tissue disorder in which the elastic fibers are disrupted, causing cystic medial necrosis of the aorta as well as joint laxity and subluxation of the ocular lens. Affected patients are tall, with increased limb length compared with the trunk. In fact, their arm span exceeds their height. The cardiovascular abnormalities consist of aneurysms of the aorta and aortic sinuses with dissection. Associated aortic and mitral valve regurgitations are common (Fig. 5.9).

Patients with *Noonan syndrome* have features characteristic of Turner syndrome, but possess normal chromosomes. Clinically, these children have phenotypic findings of Turner, including webbing of the neck, pectus, shield chest with widely spaced nipples, short stature, epicanthal folds, low-set ears, and increased carrying angle of the arms (Fig. 5.10). Commonly seen cardiovascular defects include pulmonary stenosis in association with a dysplastic pulmonary valve and an atrial septal defect. Occasionally, there may be dysplasia of all cardiac valves and later development of myocardial hypertrophy. The syndrome appears as an autosomal dominant disorder; multiple members of a family often are affected.

The most common cardiac defects in *Turner syndrome* are coarctation of the aorta and a bicuspid aortic valve (see Chapters 1 and 9 for a detailed discussion of Turner syndrome).

Patients with *Williams syndrome* characteristically have "elfin" facies: a broad maxilla, a small mandible with full mouth and large upper lip (philtrum), upturned nose and a full forehead (Fig. 5.11). This syndrome has been associated with hypercalcemia in infants and may have a genetic but undefined hereditary basis. Supravalvular aortic stenosis and pulmonary artery branch stenosis are common cardiovascular abnormalities.

In addition there are many genetically determined diseases and inborn errors of metabolism with cardiac involvement, the most common of which are listed in Figure 5.12.

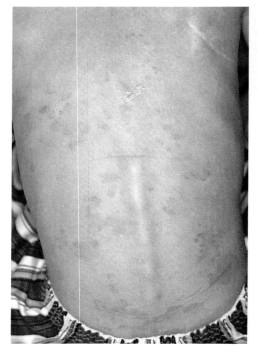

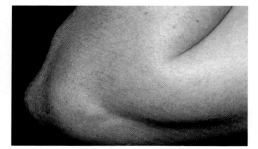

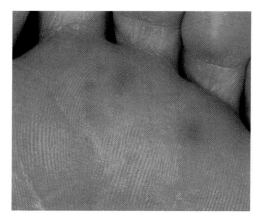

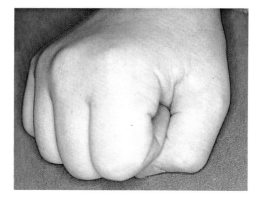

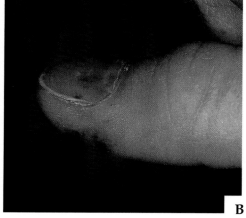

FIG. 5.15 *Janeway lesions, small painless nodules in the sole of a patient with bacterial endocarditis.*

FIG. 5.13 *Erythema marginatum rash in a child with acute rheumatic fever. Note the wavy margins in the distribution on the trunk.*

FIG. 5.14 *Subcutaneous nodules over bony prominences of the elbow (top) and knuckles of the hand (bottom) in a patient with chronic rheumatic heart disease.*

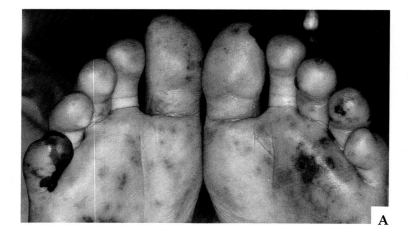

A

B

FIG. 5.16 **A,** *hemorrhagic lesions in a patient with acute bacterial endocarditis. (Courtesy of Dr. W.H. Neches.)* **B,** *subungual splinter hemorrhages.*

Visible Clues in Acute Rheumatic Fever

Examination of the skin in a patient with acute rheumatic fever may reveal the typical rash of erythema marginatum, though this rash is not specific for rheumatic fever. It is nonpruritic, has sharp serpiginous margins, and is found on the inner aspects of the upper arms, thighs, and on the trunk (Fig. 5.13). The differential diagnosis includes: (l) drug rash, which is papular and pruritic; (2) rash of glomerulonephritis, which is macular and has no sharp margins; (3) rash of juvenile rheumatoid arthritis, which is pink, macular, and lacks wavy margins, and which may be transient; and (4) the cutaneous findings of Kawasaki disease (see Chapter 7).

Subcutaneous nodules are rare in chronic rheumatic heart disease, but if found, they are almost always associated with severe carditis. These movable, nontender, cartilage-like swellings vary in size from 2 mm to 1 cm and are never transient. They are seen over the bony prominences of the large joints and external surfaces of the elbows and knuckles of the hands, knees, and ankles. They also may be felt along the spine and over the skull. While difficult to photograph, they are easily palpated (Fig. 5.14).

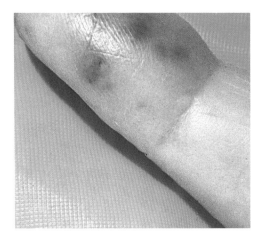

FIG. 5.17 Osler nodes, painful erythematous nodular lesions resulting from infective endocarditis. (Courtesy of Dr. J.F. John, Jr.)

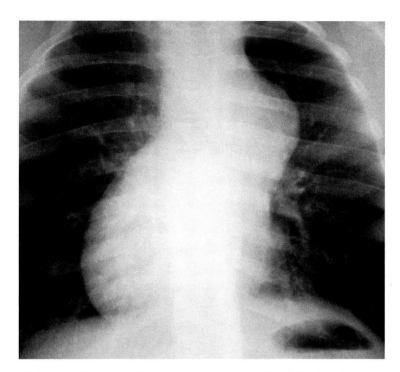

FIG. 5.18 Dextrocardia (heart in the right side of the chest) associated with situs solitus. This pattern is commonly associated with ventricular inversion (corrected transposition of the great arteries). The prominent vascular shadow noted along the right-sided cardiac border is the aorta.

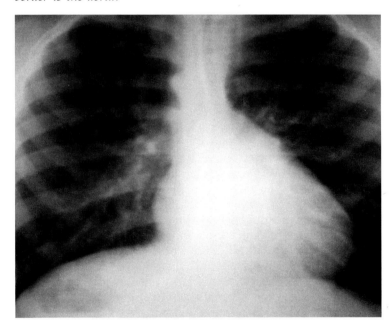

FIG. 5.19 Levocardia with situs inversus. Discordance of the apex of the heart and visceral situs often is associated with structural congenital heart defects. The hepatic portion of the inferior vena cava is absent in this patient, and there is azygous vein continuation. Note the prominence of the shadow at the high right-sided cardiac border.

Signs of Bacterial Endocarditis

Although the clinical presentation of bacterial endocarditis varies according to the infecting organism, it should be suspected in any patient with congenital or acquired heart disease who has prolonged fever without apparent cause. The classic skin lesions include petechiae, splinter hemorrhages of the nails, conjunctival hemorrhages and Janeway lesions (Fig. 5.15), all of which are manifestations of vasculitis. Vegetations occasionally dislodge and embolize in an end artery, which results in hemorrhagic or gangrenous lesions (Fig. 5.16). Osler nodes, which present as small tender erythematous nodules, are found in both the intradermal pads of the fingers and toes or in the thenar or hypothenar eminences (Fig. 5.17). All the above findings are often associated with a new heart murmur, splenomegaly, spiking fever, and positive blood culture. Clubbing of the fingers may occur in chronic cases.

LABORATORY AIDS IN THE DIAGNOSIS OF CONGENITAL HEART DISEASE

In addition to a comprehensive physical examination, the chest roentgenogram, electrocardiogram and, particularly, cross-sectional echocardiography have provided valuable information concerning specific congenital heart lesions and allowed therapeutic decisions to be made without cardiac catheterization.

Chest Roentgenogram

The chest x-ray is useful to screen patients with suspected congenital heart disease. It will exclude apparent pulmonary problems such as pneumothorax, pneumomediastinum, or parenchymal lung disease mimicking cyanotic congenital heart disease. The review of any chest roentgenogram requires a systematic approach.

Cardiac Apex and Visceral Situs

The location of the cardiac apex and visceral situs provides important diagnostic clues. Discordance of the situs and cardiac apex (i.e., apex to the right with situs solitus or apex to the left with situs inversus) often is associated with structural congenital heart disease (Figs. 5.18, 5.19). Dextrocardia (apex to the right) with situs solitus is a frequent presentation of

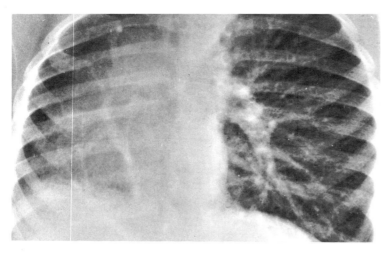

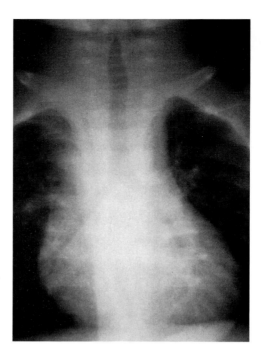

FIG. 5.21 Atrial isomerism should be suspected when the heart is midline on the chest x-ray and with situs ambiguus. The best radiographic sign of right or left atrial isomerism pertains to the symmetry of bronchial anatomy, with right atrial isomerism being related to bilateral right bronchi and left atrial isomerism to bilateral left bronchi.

FIG. 5.20 Radiographic appearance of scimitar syndrome with a hypoplastic right lung. The scimitar-shaped shadow is formed by pulmonary veins draining the sequestered segment and connecting to the inferior vena cava. Note also the systemic artery coursing diagonally upward from the abdominal aorta to the sequestered lobe.

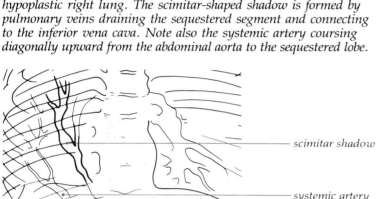

ventricular inversion or corrected transposition of the great arteries (Fig. 5.18). Dextrocardia also can be seen with primary pulmonary problems. *Scimitar syndrome* comprises dextrocardia with hypoplasia of the right lung (Fig. 5.20). In this case, a major portion of the right lung (usually the right lower lobe) has its arterial supply by way of a systemic artery from the descending aorta and the pulmonary venous return from that lung drains abnormally into the inferior vena cava, forming a scimitar (Fig. 5.20). Patients with levocardia (apex to the left) with either situs inversus or situs ambiguus have complex congenital heart diseases, such as transposition of the great arteries, pulmonary atresia, and atrioventricular septal defects. Atrial isomerism can be recognized as bilateral symmetrical short or long bronchi. This is best demonstrated with a magnified penetrated chest x-ray focusing on bronchial anatomy (Fig. 5.2l). Almost all patients with this anomaly have complex congenital heart disease.

Shape and Size

Cardiac size is important, but the shape of the cardiac image may provide a clue as to which heart chambers are enlarged and the likely structural diagnosis. In the cyanotic newborn with transposition of the great arteries the cardiac image appears as an "egg on a string" (Fig. 5.22). If the thymic shadow does not obscure it, the mediastinal shadow shows a narrow waist due to the posterior medial position of the main pulmonary artery. This produces the "string." Pulmonary vascular markings usually are increased, although vascularity may be normal in the immediate newborn period.

In tetralogy of Fallot with pulmonic stenosis the heart appears "boot-shaped," because right ventricular hypertrophy causes the apex (toe of the boot) to turn upward (Fig. 5.23). The concavity of the left upper cardiac border is due to the small right ventricular outflow tract and pulmonary artery segment.

In tetralogy of Fallot with pulmonary atresia the heart is shaped like an "egg on its side" (Fig. 5.24). The pulmonary blood flow to the lungs may be supplied by either a patent ductus arteriosus or systemic arterial collateral vessels. The pulmonary vascular markings are decreased if pulmonary blood flow is patent ductus-dependent, and increased if large systemic collaterals supply pulmonary blood flow.

In corrected transposition of the great arteries, the heart has a "valentine or heart shape" with the apex pointing downward just to the left of the midline, as shown in Figure 5.25. The fullness in the left upper border is due to the ascending aorta.

Massive cardiac size is typical in patients with Ebstein's malformation of the tricuspid valve. In this anomaly there is displacement of the inferior and septal leaflets of the tricuspid valve into the ventricle causing severe tricuspid valve regurgitation or stenosis. As a result the right atrium becomes

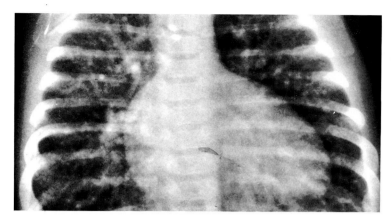

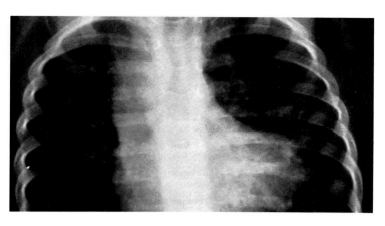

FIG. 5.22 "Egg on a string" heart shadow due to transposition of the great arteries. The main pulmonary artery is posterior and slightly to the left of the aorta, contributing to the narrow waist (the "string").

FIG. 5.23 Tetralogy of Fallot with pulmonic stenosis produces this "boot-shaped" heart. Due to right ventricular hypertrophy, the apex is tilted upward, and the small right ventricular infundibulum and small main pulmonary artery cause the concavity in the left upper border of the heart. Right aortic arch is present.

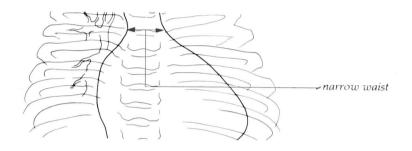

narrow waist

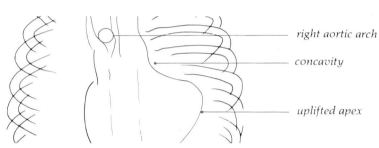

right aortic arch

concavity

uplifted apex

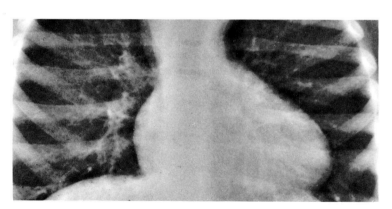

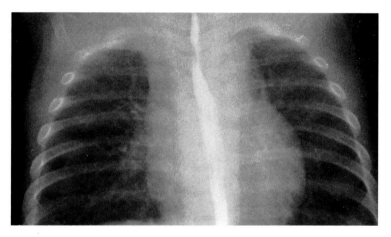

FIG. 5.24 Tetralogy of Fallot with pulmonary atresia produces this "egg on its side" appearance. Note the uplifted apex due to the right ventricular hypertrophy. There is concavity due to the absence of right ventricular outflow and small main pulmonary artery segment. Note also the right aortic arch.

FIG. 5.25 Radiograph shows the "valentine-shaped" heart characteristically found in transposition of the great arteries. Note the ascending aorta on the left side.

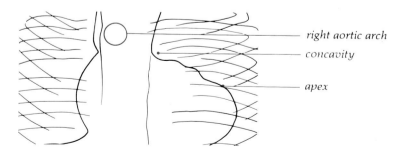

right aortic arch

concavity

apex

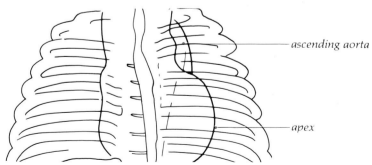

ascending aorta

apex

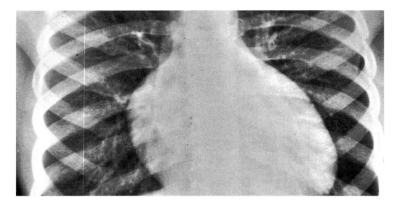

FIG. 5.26 Radiograph demonstrates the "box-shaped" heart associated with Ebstein's anomaly of the tricuspid valve. Note the enlarged right atrium and right ventricular outflow tract.

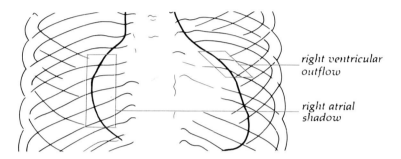

right ventricular outflow

right atrial shadow

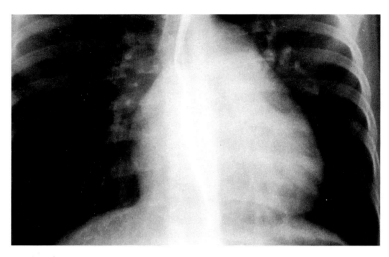

FIG. 5.27 X-ray of a child with an atrial septal defect. Note the enlarged right atrium, right ventricle, and pulmonary artery, as well as the increased pulmonary vascular markings.

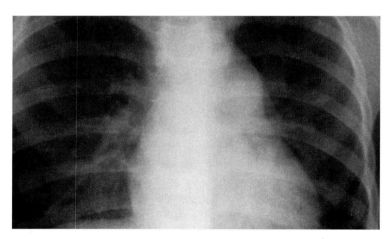

FIG. 5.28 Prominence of the main and left pulmonary arteries is the only radiographic abnormality in this child with pulmonic valve stenosis.

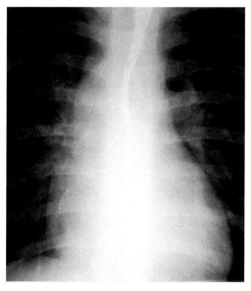

FIG. 5.29 The only radiographic sign of aortic valve stenosis in children is dilatation of the ascending aorta.

FIG. 5.30 Radiograph of a 5-year-old child reveals the characteristic signs of coarctation of the aorta. The site of the stenosis can be observed at the center of the "3" sign with pre- and poststenotic dilatation of the aorta.

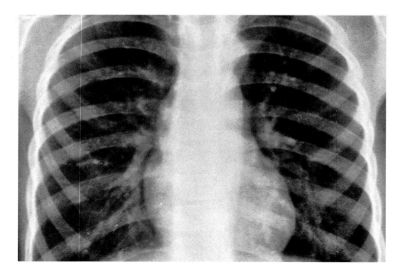

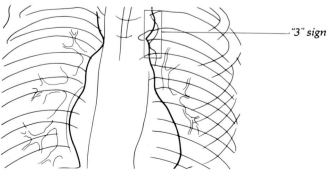

"3" sign

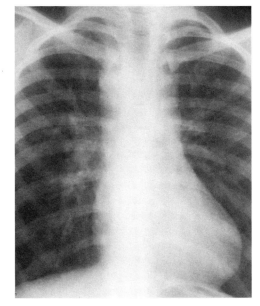

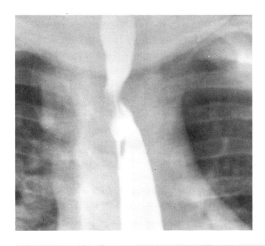

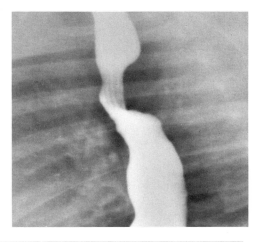

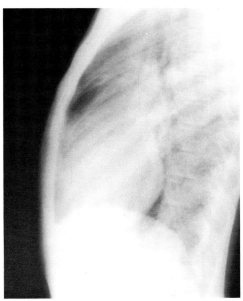

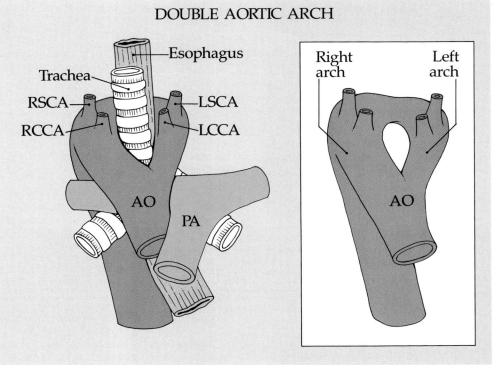

DOUBLE AORTIC ARCH

Esophagus

Trachea

RSCA — — LSCA

RCCA — — LCCA

AO

PA

Right arch   Left arch

AO

FIG. 5.31 Right aortic arch in a child with truncus arteriosus is demonstrated by deviation of the tracheal air column to the left.

FIG. 5.32 A barium esophagram is essential when infants with stridor are evaluated. In this child, the bilateral compressions and

marked retroesophageal indentation are caused by a double aortic arch.

markedly enlarged and, along with the right ventricle, contributes significantly to a cardiac image of a box-shaped heart (Fig. 5.26).

Left-to-right shunt lesions from atrial septal defects, ventricular septal defects, or a patent ductus arteriosus demonstrate specific chamber enlargement as well as increased pulmonary vascular markings. A significant atrial defect will show enlargement of all right-sided cardiac chambers, including right atrium, right ventricle, and pulmonary artery Fig (5.27). A patent ductus arteriosus shows enlargement of all left-sided cardiac chambers, including the aorta. In patients with a ventricular septal defect, the right atrium is the only heart chamber that is not enlarged.

Great Vessels

The radiographic appearance of the great arteries also may suggest a specific structural congenital heart defect. The main and left branch pulmonary arteries usually are enlarged in

patients with pulmonary valve stenosis (Fig. 5.28). The characteristic radiographic finding of congenital aortic valve stenosis is dilatation of the ascending aorta, best seen as an overlapping shadow with a superior vena cava along the right upper cardiac border (Fig. 5.29). Coarctation of the aorta not diagnosed in a timely fashion may show the distinct radiographic finding of a reversed "E" or "3" sign caused by poststenotic dilatation of the descending aorta (Fig. 5.30).

The normal left aortic arch causes a shift of the tracheal air column to the right, while a right arch causes a similar deviation to the left (Fig. 5.31). A right aortic arch has been associated with tetralogy of Fallot or truncus arteriosus in about 30 percent of patients with those lesions.

The addition of a barium swallow to the chest x-ray is an important diagnostic tool in the assessment of patients with upper airway obstruction from vascular rings. If a bilateral indentation is noted on the barium esophagram, a double aortic arch should be suspected (Fig. 5.32). A right aortic arch with distal origin of the left subclavian or a left aortic arch

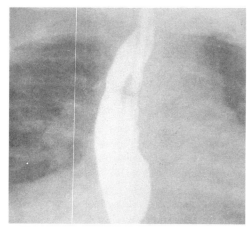

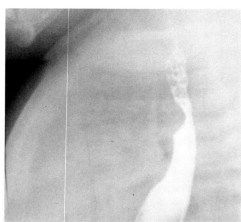

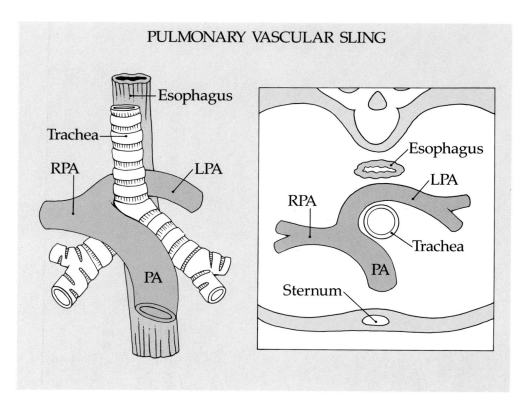

FIG. 5.33 Anomalous left pulmonary artery (the pulmonary artery sling) can be observed as a rounded indentation between the barium-filled esophagus posteriorly and the air-filled trachea anteriorly.

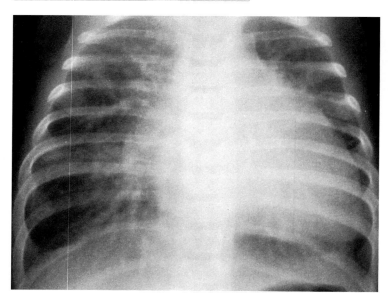

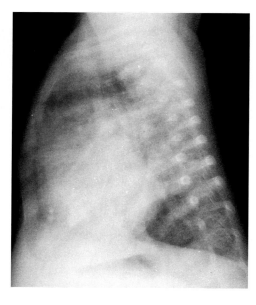

FIG. 5.34 Postero-anterior and lateral radiographs from a 2-month-old infant with a large left-to-right shunt from a ventricular septal defect. The lung hyperinflation with flattened hemidiaphragms is clearly seen on the lateral projection. This finding is predictive of associated pulmonary hypertension.

with distal origin of the right subclavian also produces posterior indentation on the barium esophagram, but usually it is not associated with airway compromise. An anterior esophageal indentation is almost always due to distal origin of the pulmonary artery coursing between the trachea and esophagus, and causing a pulmonary sling (Fig. 5.33).

Pulmonary Vascularity

Left-to-right shunt lesions are associated with increased pulmonary blood flow that cause primarily arterial or a combination of arterial and venous markings on the chest radiograph. Hyperinflation seen on the chest x-ray is a characteristic finding in infants with large left-to-right shunt associated with pulmonary hypertension (Fig. 5.34). Patients with pulmonary venous obstruction, such as infradiaphragmatic total anomalous pulmonary venous return, show a fine reticular pattern of pulmonary venous obstruction which may mimic respiratory distress syndrome in the neonate (Fig. 5.35). It should be cautioned that the interpretation of pulmonary vascularity can be quite difficult and should always be interpreted within the context of other clinical findings.

Skeletal Abnormalities

Attention also should be given to the thoracic cage, including the spine and ribs. Although abnormal fusions of ribs and hemivertebrae are not pathognomonic for specific congenital

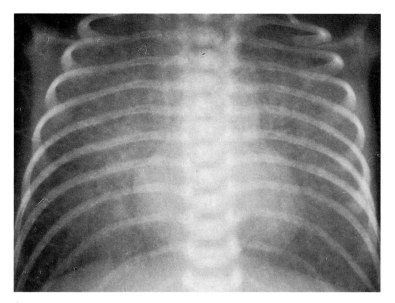

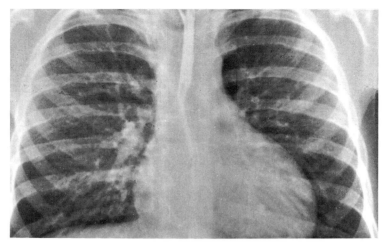

FIG. 5.36 *Rib notching can be observed here, resulting from coarctation of the aorta in the older child.*

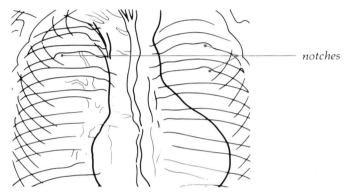

notches

FIG. 5.35 *A total anomalous pulmonary venous return below the diaphragm leads to a radiographic finding of severe pulmonary venous obstruction and pulmonary edema, mimicking a respiratory distress syndrome.*

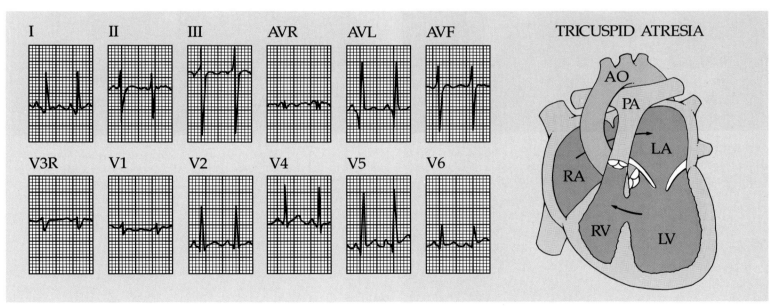

FIG. 5.37 *Electrocardiogram of a child with tricuspid atresia. Note the left axis deviation, left atrial enlargement, and left ventricular*

hypertrophy. AO = aorta; LA = left atrium; LV = left ventricle; PA = pulmonary artery; RA = right atrium; RV = right ventricle.

heart lesions, there is a higher incidence when these findings are present. Rib notching is a distinct radiographic finding in patients with coarctation of the aorta (Fig. 5.36). Scoliosis is a rather common finding in teenage patients with cyanotic congenital heart disease. Pectus excavatum may cause a false impression of cardiac enlargement due to a "pancaking" effect on the heart from a narrow anterior posterior thoracic diameter.

Electrocardiography

The electrocardiogram remains an important tool for the pediatric cardiologist to assess arrhythmias and ventricular hypertrophy. It is not useful for diagnosing specific congenital heart lesions. There are "classic" electrocardiograms that point to specific congenital heart lesions. Tricuspid atresia in the newborn is invariably associated with left axis deviation and left ventricular enlargement (Fig. 5.37) that is abnormal

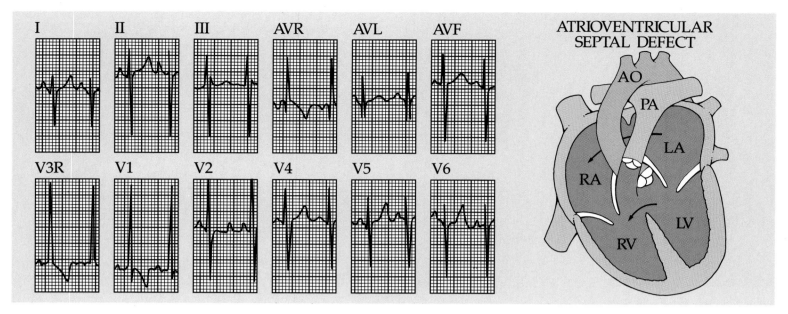

ATRIOVENTRICULAR SEPTAL DEFECT

FIG. 5.38 *Typical electrocardiogram of a child with an atrioventricular septal defect. Note the superior (northwest) axis deviation and right ventricular hypertrophy.*

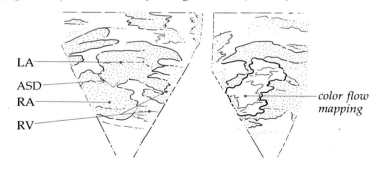

FIG. 5.39 *A large secundum atrial septal defect (left) is seen in the fossa ovale area on the subcostal view (arrow). Color flow mapping (right) confirms marked left-to-right shunt (dotted).*

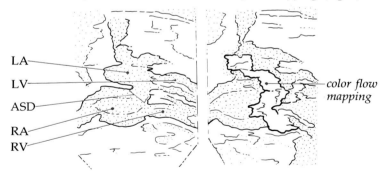

FIG. 5.40 *A partial form of an atrioventricular septal defect (left) is seen in the inferior portion of the atrial septum (arrow). Significant left-to-right shunt is shown on color flow mapping (right).*

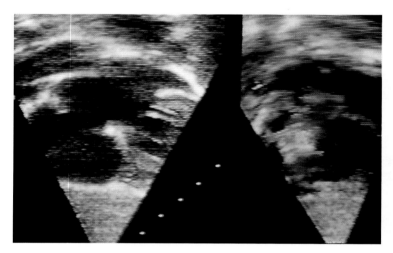

for a newborn infant. Similarly, an abnormal superior axis may be associated with an atrioventricular septal defect (Fig. 5.38), single ventricle, or other complex cardiac anomalies. Electrocardiograms with these patterns should alert the physician to the presence of structural congenital heart disease.

Echocardiography

Cross-sectional echocardiography has been the most important advance in the investigation of congenital heart defects in the 1980s. The echocardiographic image in various cross-sectional views can accurately identify common and complex

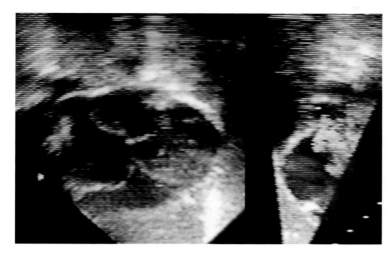

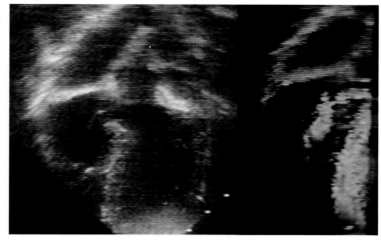

FIG. 5.41 *Sinus venosus defect* (left) *appears in the posterosuperior portion of the atrial septum, where the right upper pulmonary vein (RUPV, arrow) opens directly into the superior vena cava (SVC, arrow). Shunts from the anomalous drainage from the right upper pulmonary vein as well as from the left atrium are seen on color flow mapping* (right).

FIG. 5.42 *On this apical four-chamber view, a perimembranous ventricular septal defect* (left) *is seen in the ventricular septum (arrow). Significant left-to-right shunt through the defect is confirmed by color flow mapping* (right).

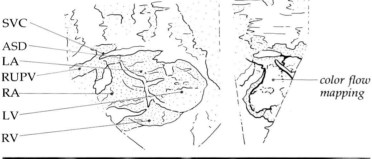

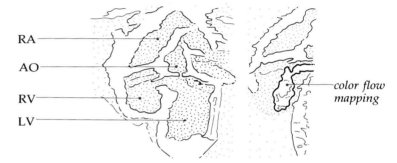

FIG. 5.43 *Muscular ventricular septal defect. No apparent defect in the ventricular septum could be visualized on 2-dimensional imaging* (left). *However, color flow mapping* (right) *confirmed a tiny defect in the muscular septum near the apex by showing a jet (yellowish-red jet). In addition, a trivial tricuspid valve regurgitation is noted (blue jet).*

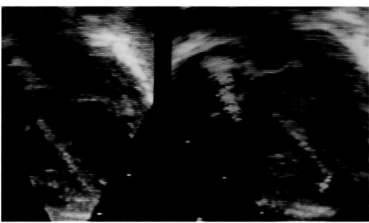

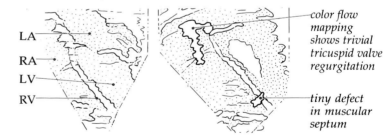

structural congenital heart defects. The addition of Doppler and color flow mapping provides another dimension to the accuracy of anatomic diagnosis and noninvasive hemodynamic assessment. Thus, cross-sectional echocardiography and Doppler imaging have provided invaluable assistance to the management of patients with congenital heart disease and represent a complementary tool to cardiac catheterization and angiography.

All types of septal defects can be readily visualized by cross-sectional echocardiography. The atrial septal defects are reliably demonstrated by the subcostal approach and views. The most common type is the secundum defect which involves the mid portion of the atrial septum (Fig. 5.39). An ostium primum defect known as a partial form of an atrioventricular septal defect is seen in Figure 5.40. The sinus ve-

nosus type of atrial septal defect is located in the posterosuperior portion of the atrial septum at the opening of the superior vena cava and is associated with partial anomalous pulmonary venous return of the right upper pulmonary vein (Fig. 5.41).

Similarly, a ventricular septal defect can be accurately diagnosed by utilizing the apical four-chamber view as shown in Figure 5.42. The most common defect is in the perimembranous septum located in the subaortic area bordered by the atrioventricular valves. However, a defect located in the muscular septum can be difficult to image, particularly if it is located near the apical trabecular area of the ventricle. Recently, color flow mapping techniques have been facilitating the detection of even the smallest defect when imaging of the defect is not possible (Fig. 5.43).

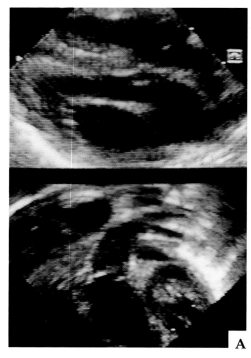

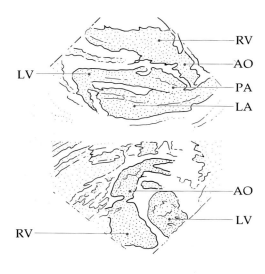

FIG. 5.44 Transposition of the great arteries. **A,** the parasternal long axial view shows a parallel arrangement of the great vessels (top). Origination of the aorta from the right ventrical is confirmed in the apical four-chamber view (bottom). **B,** connection of the pulmonary artery with the left ventricle (left) confirms the diagnosis. The color flow map (right) shows left-to-right shunt through a small patent duct (PDA) appearing as a yellowish-red jet.

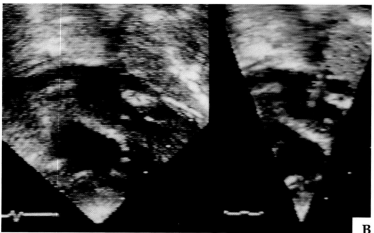

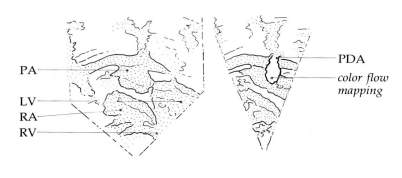

Accurate diagnosis of most structural congenital heart diseases, whether simple or complex, can be made by echocardiography. A systematic approach to define major intracardiac connections is a useful starting point: (l) venoatrial connection (systemic or pulmonary venous return to the right or left atrium); (2) atrioventricular; and (3) ventriculoarterial connection (ventricle to the great vessels).

If the pulmonary veins are not communicated with the left atrium, total anomalous pulmonary venous return should be suspected. Corrected transposition is the most likely diagnosis when the atrioventricular connection is not concordant, whereas transposition of the great arteries is suspected when the ventriculoarterial connection is discordant. The rather characteristic finding of parallel takeoff of the great vessels from both ventricles is seen in transposition of the great arteries, which is characterized by anteriorly located aorta from the right ventricle and posteriorly positioned, and by the pulmonary artery originating at the left ventricle (Fig. 5.44).

Typical findings in another common cyanotic heart lesion, tetralogy of Fallot, are a dilated aortic root which overrides the ventricular septum, a large perimembranous ventricular septal defect, and a right ventricular outflow obstruction (Fig. 5.45). The aortic arch also can be visualized by a suprasternal approach, and the diagnosis of interrupted aortic arch or coarctation of the aorta can be readily diagnosed in most cases (Fig. 5.46).

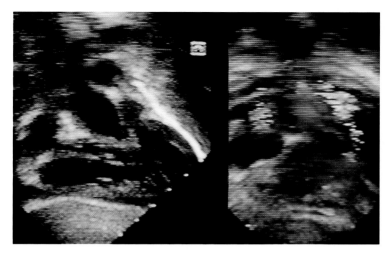

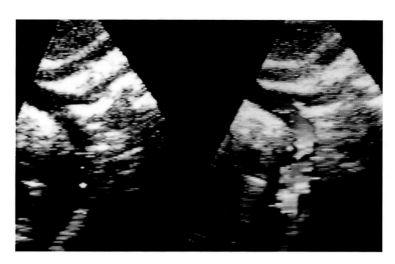

FIG. 5.45 *Tetralogy of Fallot. This subcostal view shows both val-vular pulmonic as well as infundibular stenotic components* (left). *Color flow map* (right) *confirms formation of turbulence (mosaic color) across the stenotic area.*

FIG. 5.46 *Coarctation of the aorta. This suprasternal view* (left) *demonstrates a discrete narrowing* (arrow) *in the proximal portion of the descending aorta. Color flow map* (right) *confirms the turbu-lent flow pattern* (aliasing) *across the coarctation. LCCA = left common carotid artery; LSCA = left subclavian artery.*

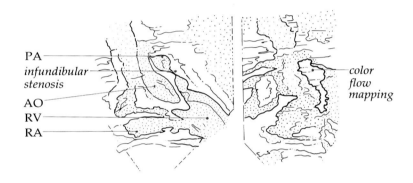

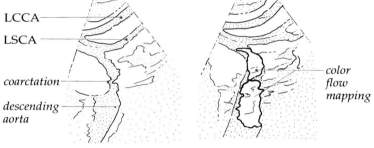

BIBLIOGRAPHY

French JW, Guntheroth WG: An explanation of asymmetric upper extremity blood pressures in supravalvular aortic stenosis. The coanda effect. *Circulation* 1970;42:31-36.

Greenwood RD: Cardiovascular malformations associated with extra cardiac anomalies and malformation syndromes. *Clin Pediatr (Phila)* 1984;23(3):145-151.

National Heart, Lung, and Blood Institute Task Force on Blood Pressure Control in Children: Report. *Pediatrics* 1977:59(suppl):797-820.

Spicer RL: Cardiovascular disease in Down syndrome. *Pediatr Clin North Am* 1984;31(6):1331-1343.

Zuberbuhler JR: *Clinical Diagnosis in Pediatric Cardiology*. Edinburgh, Churchill-Livingstone, 1981.

CHILD ABUSE AND NEGLECT

Holly W. Davis, M.D. ◆ Mary Carrasco, M.D.

Child abuse and neglect constitute a pediatric public health problem of enormous magnitude. Their relative contribution to morbidity and mortality is especially prominent in developed nations where sanitation, immunization, and high standards of medical care have substantially reduced the sequelae of infectious diseases.

Although the true incidence of abuse and neglect appears to have increased within the last century, improved reporting must also be considered. Caffey, in the late 1940s, and then Kempe and coworkers in the early 1960s, fostered a marked increase in the recognition of the physical manifestations of abuse and of the real needs and problems of child abuse victims. Subsequent passage of legislation mandating reports of suspected cases has further improved the incidence and accuracy of reporting. Thus, while some of the increasing incidence is real, much is probably due to these developments. Additionally, societal standards have changed, for much of what is presently regarded as abuse was once sanctioned as discipline.

Four major forms of abuse have been delineated: physical abuse, sexual abuse, physical neglect, and emotional abuse. Not infrequently, an individual child is found to be the victim of more than one form. For purposes of reporting under abuse laws, the abuse or neglect generally must result from the acts or omissions of a parent, guardian, custodian, or other caretaker of the child.

Statistics (National Committee for Prevention of Child Abuse) for the United States in 1989 underline the extent of the problem: 2.4 million cases were reported, representing an increase of 10 percent over 1988. Of these, 55 percent involved neglect, 27 percent physical abuse, 16 percent sexual abuse, and 8 percent emotional maltreatment. There were 1,237 reported fatalities, and 50 percent of these were under 1 year of age. These figures may significantly underestimate actual numbers; it is estimated that for every case reported, two go unreported. Furthermore, recent investigations suggest that many fatal cases are listed as being due to natural causes or accident, because many coroners and pathologists have not received thorough training in the manifestations of abuse and neglect. Obtaining full skeletal surveys on all unexplained infant death victims can uncover a significant percentage who were victims of abuse.

EPIDEMIOLOGY

The incidence of child abuse, per capita, is greatest in lower socioeconomic groups, probably due in part to chronic stress and problems of socialization. Nevertheless, abuse is a phenomenon found in all socioeconomic, cultural, racial, and religious subsets of society.

Parental Risk Factors

1. Past history of being an abused child.
2. Poor socialization and lack of trust in others. Such people have difficulty with relationships, and are thus poorly able to develop and utilize support systems. A common pattern involves an unmarried mother, living with a series of paramours each of whom stays for a short period and then leaves to be replaced by another. These men have no investment in the woman's children, and tend to have little patience with them.
3. Limited ability to cope with stress, anger, and frustration, and a tendency to lash out physically in response to negative feelings.
4. Alcoholism, addiction, or psychosis. The recent increase in crack addiction has had a particular impact, resulting in a disturbing rise in cases of gross neglect and unusually brutal physical abuse.
5. Membership in fringe group cults or sects.

Child Risk Factors

1. Age less than 3 years. Young children are unable to escape attack, are incapable developmentally of meeting many expectations, and frequently are negativistic and stubborn.
2. Infants separated from their mothers at birth because of illness or prematurity (perhaps due in part to impaired bonding).
3. Infants born with congenital anomalies, and children with chronic illness (possibly due to parental grieving and guilt compounded by the chronic stress of caring for a handicapped child).
4. Foster children and, less commonly, adopted children.

A common thread underlying all of these risk factors appears to be one of unmet expectations; either unrealistic

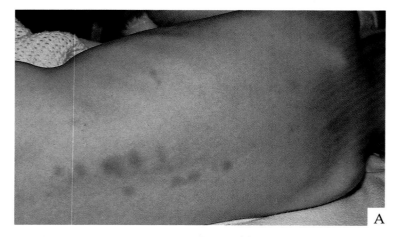
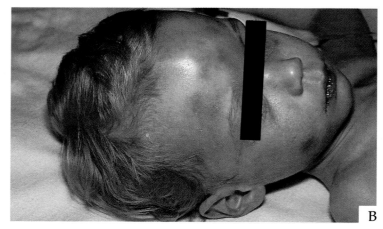
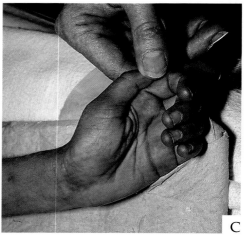
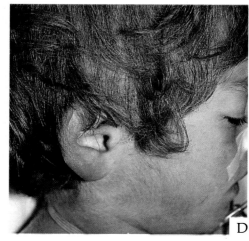
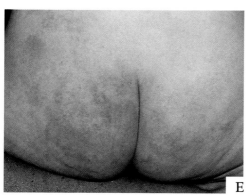

FIG. 6.1 *Inflicted bruises found in unusual locations. **A**, multiple ecchymoses are evident over the back and upper chest of this child who presented poorly nourished but with normal coagulation studies. **B**, the same patient with multiple bruises of the face and forehead. **C**, this child had severe contusions over the hands and feet which were inflict-* *ed with a ruler. **D**, the same child had a markedly swollen and contused ear as well. **E**, at first glance this toddler appeared to have a diaper rash, but on closer inspection the lesions were found to be petechiae and purpura due to a severe spanking.*

parental expectations of the child or the child's inability to meet realistic expectations due to developmental delay, hyperactivity, or inconsistent discipline.

The increasing incidence of fatal cases has led to an effort to detect identifiable risk factors that might be predictive of fatal outcome. All perpetrators studied were severely abused themselves as children. Poverty, unemployment, a long history of family violence, drug and alcohol abuse, and adolescent parenthood were common threads. Crying and toilet training accidents were the most common triggering events. Victims frequently had histories of prior suspicious injuries before the final beating.

With the preceding as background, the approach to diagnosis of the major forms of abuse can now be addressed more specifically.

PHYSICAL ABUSE

Physical abuse is usually repetitive, and tends to escalate in severity over time. Given this, early recognition, reporting, and intervention are essential to preventing future, more severe injuries. The diagnosis of inflicted injury is based on a constellation of factors including historical, physical, and behavioral observations. Radiographs and laboratory studies are often useful in confirming injuries, and in ruling out other differential possibilities.

Historical Factors

In many instances, one or more of the following historical red flags provides the first clue to the possibility of abuse.

1. *The history is incompatible with the type or degree of injury;* e.g., the distribution of lesions or type of injury doesn't fit the mechanism reported, or the history suggests a minor injury but major trauma is found.
2. The history of how the injury occurred is vague, or the parent has no idea of how it happened.
3. The history changes each time it is told to a different health care worker.
4. The parents, when interviewed separately, give contradictory histories.
5. The history is not credible. The child may be said to have done something developmentally impossible; e.g., having climbed and fallen when yet unable to sit.

Behavioral Factors

1. *There is often a significant delay between the time of injury and the time of presentation.*
2. The parent may not show the degree of concern appropriate to the severity of the child's injury.

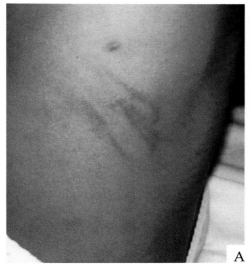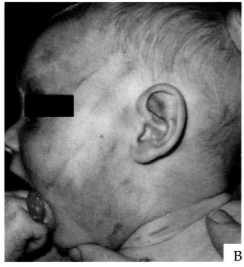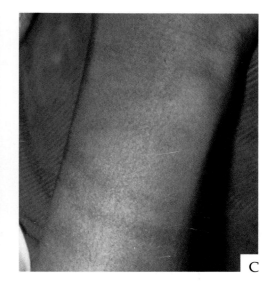

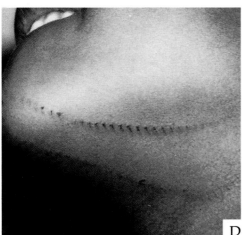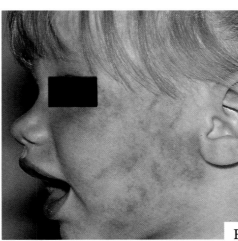

FIG. 6.2 *Imprint marks reflecting the weapons used to inflict them. A, fresh looped cord marks. B, characteristic parallel lines seen as a result of being beaten with a leather belt. C, multiple linear contusions inflicted with a switch. D, chain imprints on the neck and chin. E, handprint contusion of the face.*

3. A pathologic parent-child interaction is observed. Here unrealistic expectations, inappropriate demands, or angry impulsive behavior are expressed by the parent towards the child.Such parents are often unaware of their child's needs andinsensitive to behavioral cues.

Miscellaneous Observational Red Flags

1. History or evidence of repeated visits for accidents or injuries.
2. History or evidence of repeated fractures.
3. History of evidence of repeated ingestions.

While some victims of physical abuse are brought in with a chief complaint of abuse, many (if not most) are not. The latter may come with a chief complaint of an accidental injury or may have an unrelated or somewhat peripheral chief complaint. Whenever one's index of suspicion is aroused by historical or observational findings, the physician should seek more detailed information concerning the family's current living situation, stresses, and emotional support systems. Particular attention should be paid to personal (ill health, job loss, separation) and environmental (pending eviction, heat or utilities discontinued) crises, degree of isolation (no family supports, no phone), and prior problems with family violence, alcohol, or drugs. Asking questions about methods of discipline and parental reactions to common triggering events such as stubborn behavior, prolonged crying, and toilet training accidents can be most illuminating. This and the medical history should be obtained in a supportive, nonjudgmental manner, as interrogation will only serve to alienate the parent, limiting the value of the data obtained. Bear in mind that many of these parents truly want help. Typically, they feel very alone, guilt-ridden, and inadequate as persons and parents, their own abusive behavior often evoking painful memories of having been abused themselves.

In approaching the child, one must recognize that his parents are the only ones he knows, that he loves them, and may feel in some way deserving of abuse. Young children rarely acknowledge that a parent has injured them, especially when questioned directly, and may have been sworn to secrecy. If they can be interviewed alone (when old enough to give a history) in pleasant, nonthreatening surroundings, helpful historical information can often be obtained via indirect questions, and through drawings or play.

Physical Findings and Patterns of Injury

SURFACE MARKS: BRUISES, WELTS, AND SCARS
Inflicted injuries are often found in unusual locations such as the back, buttocks, upper arms and thighs, chest, face (other than the chin or forehead), ears, hands, and feet (Figs. 6.1 and 6.2). Particular attention should be paid to checking children with hand prints or bruises over the upper medial thighs for

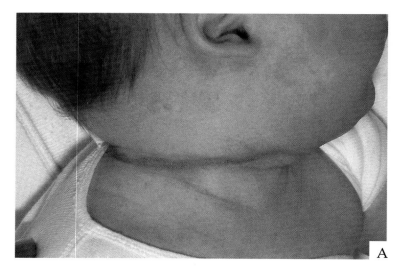

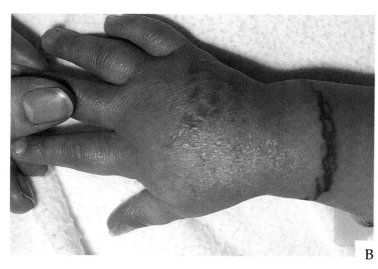

FIG. 6.3 Strangulation and restraint marks. *A,* this circumferential cord burn was the result of an attempted strangulation. *B,* a deep circumferential rope burn of the wrist with considerable edema and early skin breakdown are seen in this infant who was tied to the side rails of her crib.

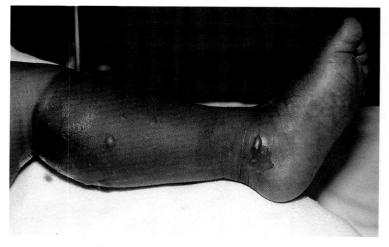

FIG. 6.4 Tourniquet injury. This toddler was brought in with severe skin, soft tissue and muscle necrosis of his entire lower leg. His mother reported finding a strap wrapped tightly around the leg below the knee on checking him in the morning. She did not know how it had gotten there and denied hearing his cries of pain which surely lasted for hours.

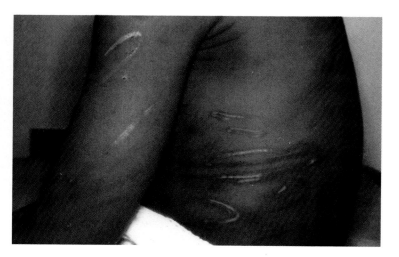

FIG. 6.5 Multiple scars produced by a prior whipping with a looped cord.

evidence of concurrent sexual abuse. This is in contrast to the "usual" small bruises found on the shins, extensor surfaces of the forearms, and the forehead of a normally active child (see Fig. 6.25). In order to avoid errors in diagnosis, children presenting with multiple bruises in unusual locations should be thoroughly examined for evidence of an underlying coagulopathy, and screening coagulation studies should be performed before arriving at a final diagnosis.

In many instances, the surface marks are recognizable imprints of the weapon used to inflict injury. Those most commonly seen include looped-cord marks; belt, buckle, or switch marks; finger, thumb, and hand prints (Fig. 6.2). Strangulation and restraint marks are a result of attempted hanging, choking or, in some instances, of tying the child to a crib, bed or chair

(Fig. 6.3A,B). On rare occasions, bizarre tourniquet injuries are encountered (Fig. 6.4). These are more likely in children of psychotic or addicted parents, and can result in severe ischemia and necrosis.

The resolution time of a bruise varies widely, depending on the degree of force used to produce it. It is therefore difficult to determine accurately the ages of ecchymotic lesions other than to say that they are fresh or old and to clearly document their size, color, and configuration. Bear in mind that the presence of old scars reflecting prior use of a weapon in a child with acute injuries can be helpful in identifying abuse or confirming prior abuse (Fig. 6.5).

All external signs of trauma should be carefully documented both in writing and by photography.

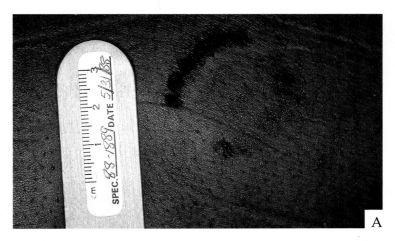
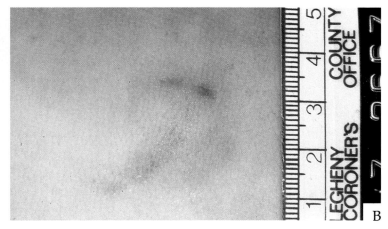
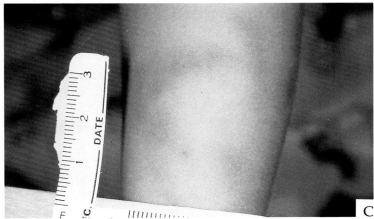
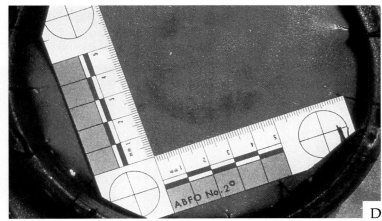

FIG. 6.6 *Bite marks.* **A,** *this adolescent was bitten by another teenager. Deep abrasions, left especially by the upper arch, clearly reflect the imprint of the incisors.* **B,** *in this bite mark inflicted on a toddler by a 6-year-old, the configuration of the upper central incisors is clearly seen (note the diastema). The lower arch has left indistinct abrasions and contusions.* **C,** *at first glance this bite mark could be mistaken for a bruise; however, on close inspection, the outline of the dental arch*

becomes evident. The size of the arch is clearly that of an adult or adolescent. **D,** *viewed under ultraviolet light, bite marks that are weeks to months old can still be identified, even though the skin overlying the site has returned to normal. (**A, B,** and **C,** courtesy of Dr. Michael N. Sobel, Pittsburgh, PA;* **D,** *courtesy of Dr. Thomas J. David, Atlanta, GA)*

BITE MARKS

Bite marks can be yet another manifestation of physical abuse. In cases where the resulting imprint is distinct, it is as identifiable as a fingerprint, and its size enables the examiner to clearly distinguish between that of another child and that of an adult (Fig. 6.6A–C). Each bite mark should be carefully photographed in its entirety, and then photos should be taken perpendicular to the plane of the imprint of each arch, with a ruler or measuring tape in each photo. Such evidence can enable a forensic dentist to make a model of the perpetrator's dentition, which can specifically reveal his or her identity. Ultraviolet photography can disclose a clear image of bite marks weeks or months after all surface marks have disappeared (Fig. 6.6D). This has proven highly useful in identifying abusers of children with a past history of being bitten, but who

have no acute lesions. Finally, if the patient has not bathed or washed the bite wound since it was inflicted, swabbing the area with a saline-soaked cotton-tipped applicator is indicated, to obtain a sample of the perpetrator's saliva. Crime lab analysis of this material can positively identify the perpetrator.

BURNS

While generally accidental, burns are a fairly common mode of abusive injury. Here too, inconsistency of history, the pattern of injury, and delay in seeking medical attention are valuable clues.

Immersion scalds are among the more common forms of inflicted burns. Typical patterns include symmetrical burns of both hands (Fig. 6.7A), of both feet, or of the lower legs and perineum, produced by dipping the infant or child in scalding

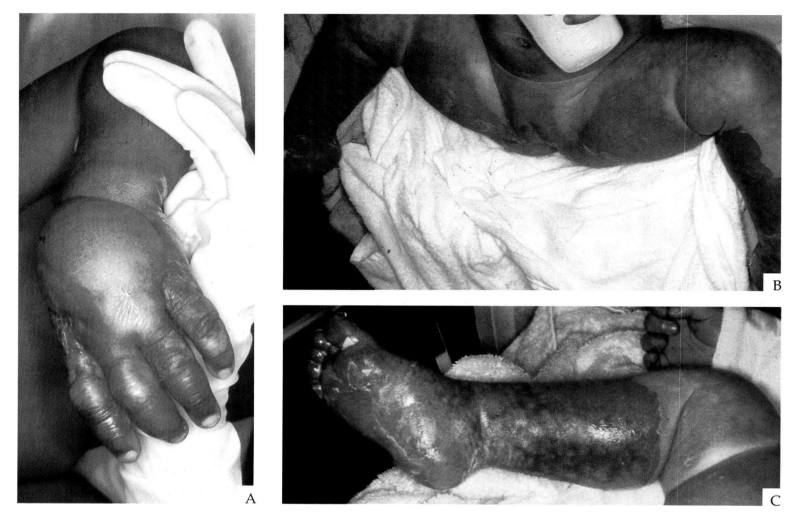

FIG. 6.7 Inflicted scalds. **A,** this child suffered severe second-degree dip burns on both hands and wrists. **B,** patient seen 2 days after receiving dip burns to the lower extremities and perineum. **C,** close-up of severe second-degree burn of the foot and lower leg. (Courtesy of Dr. Thomas Layton, Mercy Hospital, Pittsburgh)

DURATION OF EXPOSURE REQUIRED TO PRODUCE FULL THICKNESS BURN IN WATER AT VARIOUS TEMPERATURES	
Water Temperature	**Duration of Exposure**
120°F	10 minutes
130°F	30 seconds
140°F	5 seconds
150°F	2 seconds
158°F	1 second

FIG. 6.8

water (Fig. 6.7B,C). Despite claims to the contrary, such burns are rarely accidental. Figure 6.8 shows the duration of time required to produce a full-thickness burn in adult skin at different water temperatures. While the time may be slightly shorter for a child's skin, normal children would, if accidentally putting a hand or foot into water over 120°, tend to withdraw it in a fraction of a second, after the tips of their fingers or toes made contact with the water.

Other types of burns may reflect the instruments used to inflict them. For example, one may see the full thickness imprint of a hot iron or of the grill of a space heater (Fig. 6.9). No child with normal sensation would remain in contact with these objects long enough to incur such a burn. Burns inflicted with a curling iron produce second-degree or full-thickness imprints in unusual locations such as the extensor surfaces of the arms or legs, the back, chest, abdomen, or buttocks (Fig. 6.10). Accidental curling iron injuries usually occur when an older infant or toddler grabs a hot curling iron. Hence, they involve the palmar surface of one hand and its fingers.

Inflicted cigarette burns leave sharply circumscribed, full-thickness imprints approximately 7 to 8 mm in diameter (5 mm if a slim cigarette is used), over which a thick, black eschar soon forms (Fig. 6.11A,B). If this eschar is removed, one sees full-thickness skin loss. Subacutely, these lesions fill in with granulation tissue (Fig. 6.11B), and on completion of healing, the child is left with a deep, punched-out scar (Fig. 6.11C). Accidental cigarette burns, occurring when the child brushes against the lit end of an adult's cigarette, tend to be superficial, tangential, and usually involve one hand, cheek, and forearm. This presentation is in contrast to some impetiginous lesions which may appear to have a thick brown eschar. When the latter eschar is lifted off, the lesion will be found to be very superficial (see Fig. 6.33).

CHILD ABUSE AND NEGLECT

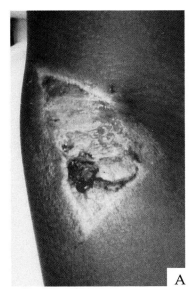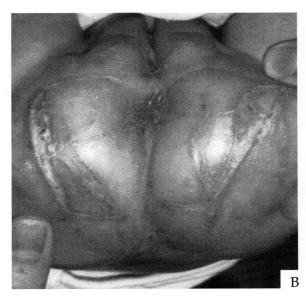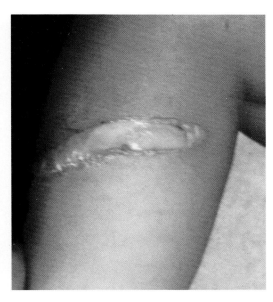

FIG. 6.9 **A,** the pattern of this full-thickness burn to the arm reflects that a hot iron was used on this patient. **B,** this infant received multiple, linear, full-thickness burns when she was forced to sit on the hot grill of a space heater.

FIG. 6.10 A deep imprint of the hot wand of a curling iron is seen over the lateral aspect of this child's lower leg.

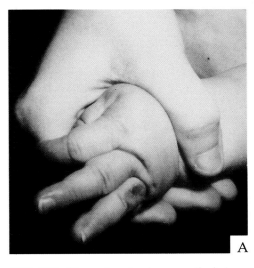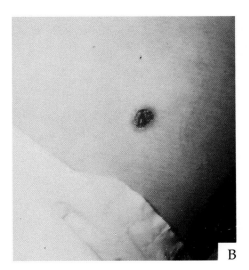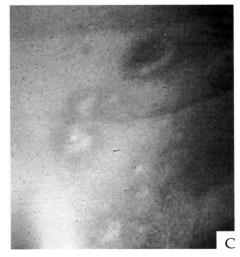

FIG. 6.11 These sharply circumscribed cigarette burns are relatively acute. **A,** the eschar has been removed revealing full-thickness skin

loss. **B,** the lesion has begun to granulate in. **C,** full-thickness, punched-out scars are characteristic of healed cigarette burns.

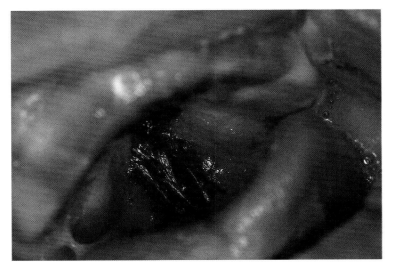

FIG. 6.12 Inflicted palatal lacerations. This infant's soft palate was shredded by repeated stabs with a sharp object. He presented with a complaint of spitting up blood and no history of trauma.

ORAL INJURIES

Occasionally, child abuse results in oral bruises and lacerations. One of the most typical patterns is that of bruising of mucosa of the upper lip or the maxillary gingiva associated with tearing of the frenulum. This is produced when the perpetrator holds a hand tightly over the child's mouth to silence screaming. On rare occasions, bizarre intraoral lacerations are found (Fig. 6.12). The usual mode of presentation is with a complaint of spitting or vomiting blood.

SKELETAL INJURIES

Children with abuse-related skeletal injuries may have a history of minor injury or a reported mechanism of injury that does not fit the fracture pattern. Frequently, the chief complaint is one of unexplained irritability; sometimes it is totally unrelated (e.g., a rash, vomiting, or URI) with no history of injury given. Since presentation is often delayed, fractures identified on radiographs commonly show signs of healing, e.g., callus and/or subperiosteal new bone formation. The degree of callus formation and the extent of periosteal new bone and

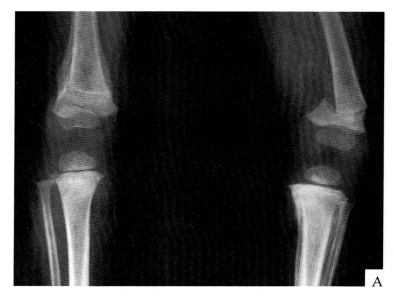

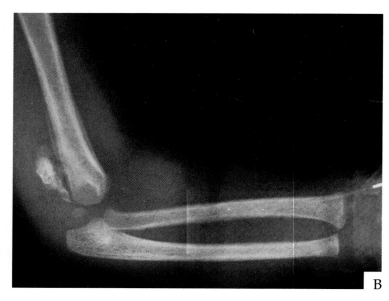

FIG. 6.13 Multiple fractures of varying ages. This child presented with a chief complaint of refusing to bear weight. On examination, he had marked swelling, tenderness, and crepitance over the distal left femur. Radiographic examination confirmed the acute fracture and also revealed multiple additional fractures in various stages of healing. **A,** there are old fractures of the distal right femur with callus and subperiosteal new bone formation. Relatively new metaphyseal chip frac-

tures are seen in the right proximal tibia, and vigorous subperiosteal new bone formation encompasses the left tibia. **B,** on skeletal survey, he was also found to have a healing fracture of the distal humerus with vigorous callus formation, subperiosteal new bone, and considerable soft tissue swelling. (Courtesy of the Department of Radiology, Children's Hospital of Pittsburgh)

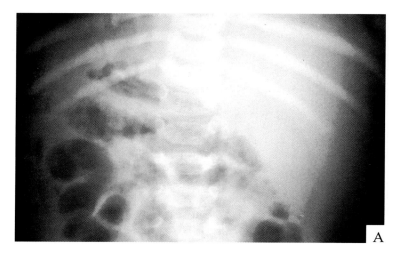

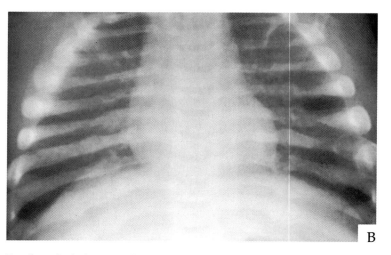

FIG. 6.14 Rib fractures. **A,** this infant presented with a history of vomiting and irritability. An abdominal film obtained to rule out intestinal obstruction showed a normal bowel gas pattern but revealed multiple rib fractures in various stages of healing which were missed.

B, when the infant was finally tracked down 2 months later, her chest x-ray demonstrated in excess of 20 healing rib fractures. (Courtesy of the Department of Radiology, Children's Hospital of Pittsburgh)

remodeling are clues to the ages of the various fractures. The periosteum in infants and very young children resists tearing and has great osteogenic potential; consequently, many non-displaced fractures are no longer tender or only subtly tender at the time of examination.

Two radiographic fracture patterns are pathognomonic for abuse. The first is multiple, unexplained fractures (often symmetrical) of varying ages involving the long bones and ribs of an infant or young child who has otherwise normal bones (Fig. 6.13). Often, these fractures are transverse, from a blow delivered perpendicularly to the long axis of the bony shaft, or oblique, as a result of twisting. Rib fractures are most common over the posterior portion of the ribs near the costovertebral articulations, although they can be found anterolaterally as well (Fig. 6.14).

The second pathognomonic fracture type is sometimes termed a metaphyseal chip or corner fracture. Perhaps it is more appropriately described as a bucket handle fracture. This is because the fracture line actually traverses the primary spongiosa of the metaphysis, just beneath the junction with the epiphysis. The fracture then crosses the outer aspects of the metaphysis. In many cases, the central portion of the fracture is radiographically invisible, and only the metaphyseal chips are seen on x-ray (Fig. 6.15; see Fig. 6.13A). In some cases, a thin metaphyseal lucency may be evident, although this often requires special oblique views (Fig. 6.15B). This fracture type is due to violent shaking while holding the child by the trunk, the hands, or feet.

Long bone fractures, particularly transverse and oblique fractures of the humerus and femur without a clear history of

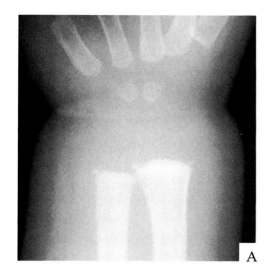

A

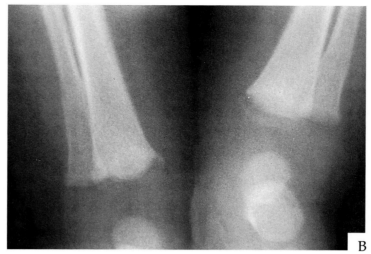

B

FIG. 6.15 **A,** metaphyseal chip fractures of the distal radius and ulna produced by vigorous shaking. **B,** bucket handle fractures of both distal tibias. The fracture lines traverse the entire width of the distal metaphyses. (**A,** courtesy of the Department of Radiology, Children's Hospital of Pittsburgh. **B,** courtesy of Dr. Bruce Rosenthal, The Mercy Hospital of Pittsburgh)

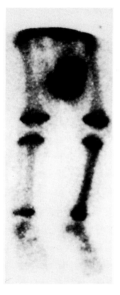

FIG. 6.16 Bone scan of a child abuse victim. This 14-month-old child presented with low-grade fever and refusal to walk. Radiographs were normal. The scan, obtained because of suspicion of infection, revealed increased uptake throughout the entire left tibia. Workup for infection was negative, and repeat radiographs 2 weeks later revealed healing fractures and extensive subperiosteal new bone formation.

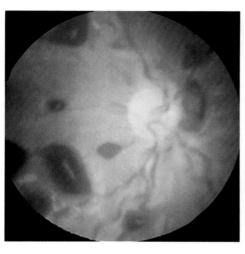

FIG. 6.17 Multiple retinal hemorrhages are seen on funduscopic examination of this infant who was a victim of "the shaken baby syndrome." Subdural hematoma and multiple metaphyseal "shake" fractures are typical associated findings. (Courtesy of Dr. Stephen Ludwig, Children's Hospital of Philadelphia)

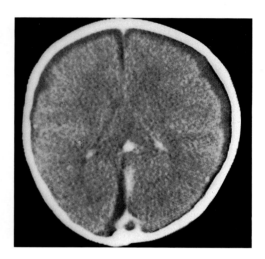

FIG. 6.18 Subdural hematomas in the shaken baby syndrome. This CT scan reveals subdural hematomas along the falx and over the cerebral convexities. These are seen as a dark rim along the falx and between the bony calvarium and the brain substance. (Courtesy of the Division of Neuroradiology, University Health Center of Pittsburgh)

a consistent major mechanism of injury, are highly suspect, as are any rib fractures in infants or toddlers. In fact, the ribs of children under 5 years of age are so flexible that accidental fractures are rarely found, even after major motor vehicle accidents and falls.

The frequency of skeletal injury in young abused children necessitates that examination of the suspected abuse victim include careful palpation of *all* bones for evidence of tenderness, crepitus, or callus formation. Because of the greater probability of multiple occult fractures in the infant and toddler, a skeletal survey is advisable when the child is less than 2 years of age. In older children, careful physical examination should reveal areas requiring radiographic evaluation.

Bone scans can reveal occult (radiographically invisible) fractures within hours of injury (Fig. 6.16), and they can be particularly helpful in detecting acute posterior rib fractures in infants. However, while more sensitive than standard radiographs, they are less specific. Radiographs have to be taken of sites detected by scan to help distinguish fractures from other lesions, and help determine mechanism of injury.

Bone scans are also less available, more time-consuming and expensive, usually require sedation, involve more radiation, and their accuracy is highly dependent on the technician and interpreter.

SHAKEN BABY SYNDROME

Another classic constellation of findings is that seen in the "shaken baby syndrome." Victims are usually less than 1 year of age; frequently, they are younger than 6 months. In addition to the metaphyseal chip or bucket handle fractures described above (see Fig. 6.15A,B), they show retinal hemorrhages (Fig. 6.17) and subdural hematomas (Fig. 6.18) resulting from shearing forces which tear fragile bridging veins between the dura and the cortex. This was thought to be the result of violent shaking of infants who have weak neck muscles and relatively large heads. However, recent work has demonstrated that shaking alone probably does not produce forces adequate to cause the shearing. Rather, it appears that the act of throwing the infant down (even on a soft surface such as a mattress) following the shaking, is what produces the G-forces required to

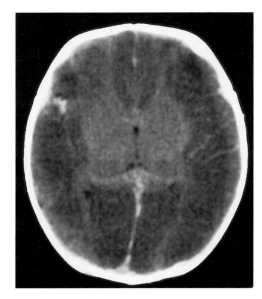

FIG. 6.19 *Cortical hypodensities suggestive of infarction are seen on computed tomography in this infant who was shaken and then thrown against a wall. (Courtesy of the Division of Neuroradiology, University Health Center of Pittsburgh)*

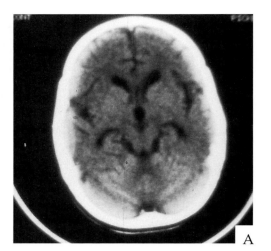

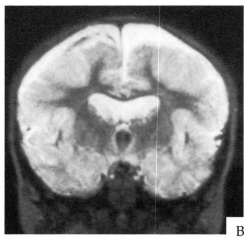

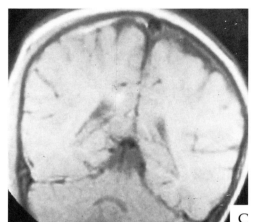

FIG. 6.20 *A and B, this 3-year-old abuse victim presented with lethargy, vomiting, hyporeflexia and acute onset of blindness. The CT scan reveals ventricular enlargement and cortical atrophy but no hemorrhage. The MRI demonstrates small bilateral subdural hemorrhages as well. C, this 5-month-old infant with head and facial bruises, bilateral retinal hemorrhages, and multiple rib fractures was found to have subdural hemorrhages of differing ages on MRI. The white subdural on the right is between 0 and 14 days of age, while the gray subdural on the left is older than 14 days. (Courtesy of Dr. Randell Alexander, University of Iowa)*

produce these CNS injuries. Many such episodes result in loss of consciousness, frightening the perpetrator who then leaves the baby to rest, hoping that he or she will improve. During the ensuing interval, intracranial pressure may increase, and seizures may occur, resulting in hypoventilation or respiratory arrest and adding hypoxic injury to the physical trauma.

Modes of presentation vary depending on the severity of the CNS injury and include unrelated chief complaints, a history of a minor fall, seizures, respiratory distress, choking, or apnea. Unless the infant is thrown down on a hard object or against a wall following the shaking, there will be little or no evidence of external injury. As noted earlier, posterior rib fractures may also be present if the infant was held by the trunk while being shaken.

Physical findings may include lethargy, increased or decreased tone, rhythmic eye opening, and bicycling movements of the extremities. Decreased ability to follow the examiner's face, decreased responsiveness to pain, and poor suck and grasp are important findings. The fontanelle is usually full, but may or may not be tense.

Retinal hemorrhages are seen in between 50 and 100 percent of victims (see Fig. 6.17). Some controversy has arisen with regard to the uniqueness of retinal hemorrhage to this syndrome. However, studies of children with severe documented accidental head injuries and studies in progress following cardiopulmonary resuscitation are not finding retinal hemorrhages, suggesting that they may well be unique to shaking.

One of the most common findings on computed tomography in the shaken baby syndrome is that of a subdural hematoma along the falx in the parieto-occipital area. This may be accompanied by a midline shift due to hemorrhage and/or concomitant cerebral injury, as well as by subdural blood over the convexities (see Fig. 6.18). In more severe cases, one may see an infarction pattern consisting of hypodensities of the cortex and underlying white matter, or even loss between gray and white matter differentiation (Fig. 6.19). These changes result in part from hypoventilation and hypoxia which, in turn, are due to increased intracranial pressure. They indicate a poor prognosis for neurologic recovery. When cerebral swelling is severe, it can compress the ventricles and sulci, obscuring small subdural hematomas. Recent studies utilizing magnetic resonance imaging have demonstrated the superior sensitivity of this technique in detecting small subdural hematomas, especially over the convexities (Fig. 6.20). MRI can also detect hemorrhages of differing ages, because image intensity changes as the blood begins to break down.

OTHER CNS INJURIES

Blunt head injuries with varying degrees of central nervous system insult are also common following abuse. This is especially true for infants who have been thrown to the floor, against a wall, or into other objects, as their heads are relatively large and they tend to land head first. Injuries range from surface hematomas and linear fractures to complex skull fractures, subdural and epidural hematomas, diffuse cerebral

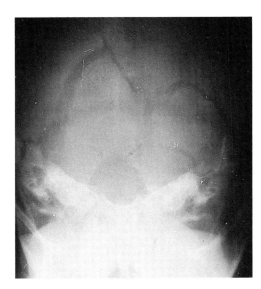

FIG. 6.21 Multiple occipital fractures are seen in a child who presented with a history of a minor fall and scalp swelling. It was later acknowledged that he had been thrown against a brick wall. (Courtesy of the Department of Radiology, Children's Hospital of Pittsburgh)

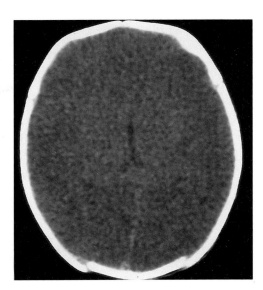

FIG. 6.22 Massive cerebral edema. This CT scan of an infant who presented with altered level of consciousness and seizures reveals occipital fractures and diffuse cerebral swelling causing ventricular compression. (Courtesy of the Division of Neuroradiology, University Health Center of Pittsburgh)

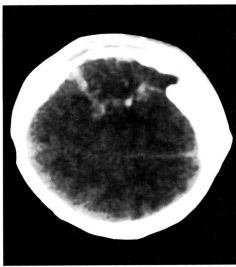

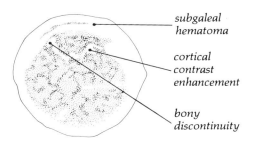

subgaleal hematoma

cortical contrast enhancement

bony discontinuity

FIG. 6.23 Cerebal contusion. Computed tomography of a 4-week-old infant (who allegedly rolled out of his crib while the side rails were up) shows a large subgaleal hematoma obscuring an underlying fracture, severe cerebral swelling with a shift of the midline, and cortical contrast enhancement indicative of a cerebral contusion. (Courtesy of the Division of Neuroradiology, University Health Center of Pittsburgh)

swelling and cerebral contusions with attendant cerebral edema (Fig. 6.21–23).

Children with moderate and severe degrees of injury tend to present acutely, with one or more of the following complaints: bump on the head, vomiting and irritability, altered level of consciousness, seizures, or abnormal posturing. On occasion, they may present in shock due to massive subgaleal and/or intracranial hemorrhage, or with a history of respiratory arrest. History of trauma may be vague or nonexistent. The reported mechanism of injury may be inconsistent with the type and/or severity of injuries found. Patients who have incurred milder trauma tend to present subacutely with one or more of the following: intermittent vomiting and irritability, rapidly increasing head circumference with split sutures and a full fontanelle, failure to thrive, and developmental delay typically affecting social more than motor development.

Careful external, general, neurologic, and funduscopic examinations are warranted in evaluating these patients. Neurologic examination may reveal altered level of consciousness, signs of increased intracranial pressure, alterations in tone, or, on occasion, focal abnormalities. While routine skull radiographs are best for detecting fractures, computed tomography (CT) is indicated when there is any suspicion of possible intracranial injury, as it clearly delineates most intracranial

hemorrhages and cerebral edema, as well as subgaleal hematomas and many fractures. It is especially good at revealing interhemispheric subdural hematomas along the falx. Recent experience with MRI has shown it to be superior to CT in detecting very small parenchymal hemorrages and in delineating posterior fossa and spinal injuries.

ABDOMINAL AND CHEST INJURIES

While less common than surface injuries, skeletal and head trauma, chest and abdominal injuries do occur in child abuse and can be quite severe. Typically, they result from being punched and/or kicked forcefully, or from being thrown to the floor or against a wall or piece of furniture. External findings are often minimal or absent; trauma often goes unreported or is ascribed to a minor mechanism. Presentation often is delayed, but may be prompt if signs and symptoms are severe.

The major types of abdominal pathology are duodenal hematomas, small intestinal and/or mesenteric tears, pancreatic and renal contusions, and lacerations of the liver or spleen. Patients with duodenal hematoma typically present with signs of intestinal obstruction (e.g., vomiting and abdominal pain). Plain radiographs may reveal an air-fluid level in a dilated duodenal loop proximal to the hematoma, while an upper GI series and sonar studies reveal narrowing of the lumen and

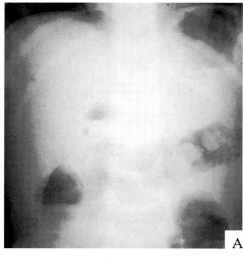

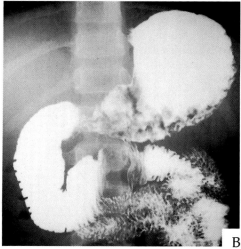

FIG. 6.24 Duodenal hematoma. **A,** abdominal film reveals an air fluid level in the dilated duodenal loop proximal to the duodenal hematoma. **B,** this upper GI series shows narrowing of duodenal lumen and widening of duodenal wall at the site of hematoma. Obstruction is partial, as some barium has passed through the narrowed segment. (Courtesy of the Department of Radiology, Children's Hospital of Pittsburgh)

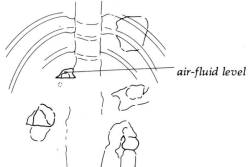

air-fluid level

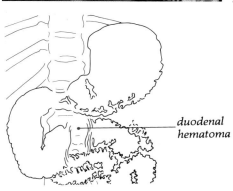

duodenal hematoma

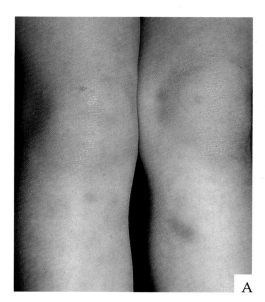

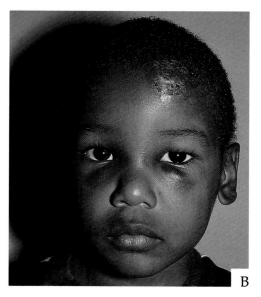

FIG. 6.25 Normal bruises. **A,** a number of small, nonspecific bruises are present over the knees and shins of this active youngster. **B,** black eyes following a forehead contusion. This boy had fallen from a slide 3 days before. Blood from his forehead hematoma had tracked down through the facial soft tissues creating these shiners.

thickening of the duodenal wall (Fig. 6.24). Children with small intestinal or mesenteric tears generally complain of diffuse abdominal pain and have signs of diffuse tenderness, distention, and peritoneal irritation. Splenic and hepatic lacerations may present similarly or may produce signs of hypovolemia, shock, or even sudden collapse which is often unexplained by history. In most instances of inflicted abdominal trauma, abuse is not confirmed until special radiographic studies including sonography and CT scans have been obtained or surgery has been performed.

Inflicted thoracic injuries include pulmonary and myocardial contusions, pulmonary lacerations, and thymic or subpleural hemorrhages. Rarely, a severe blow causes myocardial or aortic rupture and the child is dead on arrival following sudden collapse. The chief complaint on presentation may be one of respiratory distress, chest pain, or sudden collapse. Typically, there is no history of injury or a report of only minor trauma.

Differential Diagnosis of Inflicted Injuries vs Findings Due to Accident or Illness

While it is highly important to detect injuries due to abuse in order to protect children from future and potentially more serious trauma, it is also most important to avoid unjustly accusing parents of abuse. This subjects them to the ordeal of a child protective services investigation, causing tremendous emotional stress. Accurate diagnosis requires clear knowledge not only of patterns of injury seen following abuse, but also of mechanisms of injury and their resulting findings, the types of

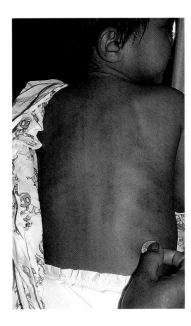

FIG. 6.26 Coin rubbing. Vigorous stroking of the skin of a febrile child with a coin produces a peculiar bruising pattern. Here the father, a Vietnamese immigrant, demonstrates the technique.

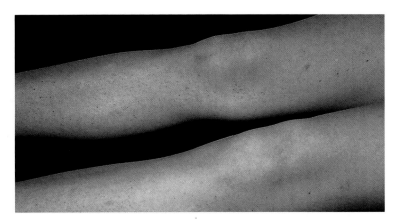

FIG. 6.27 ITP. This school-age child was seen with a chief complaint of a rash following a viral upper respiratory infection. Examination revealed diffuse petechiae and scattered purpuric lesions. Her hemoglobin and white blood cell count and differential were normal, but her platelet count was markedly reduced.

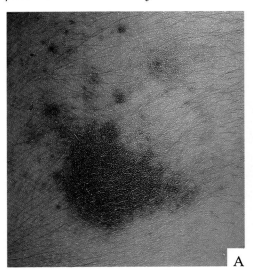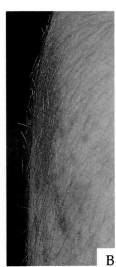

FIG. 6.28 A, dramatic bruises with thick round centers can be seen in children with aplastic anemia or clotting factor deficiencies. B, this view from the side demonstrates the elevation of the central portion of the ecchymosis.

accidental injuries commonly seen at various ages, and of diseases and congenital disorders that predispose to bleeding or increased bony fragility. Where doubt exists, the services of experienced clinicians with expertise in the fields of child abuse, orthopedics and pediatric surgery should be sought.

DIFFERENTIAL DIAGNOSIS OF SURFACE BRUISES
Accidental Bruises

Ordinary, play-related bruises can be distinguished from those due to abuse by virtue of the fact that they tend to be small and non-specific in configuration. They are typically located over the bony prominences of the shins, knees, elbows, extensor forearms, chin, or forehead (Fig. 6.25A). Larger bruises, and even those with configurations suggesting an object, can also be accidental or the result of an altercation with another child. In such cases, however, presentation for care is prompt, the mechanism of injury is consistent with the findings, and in most instances, the incident was witnessed.

Black eyes following forehead contusions may be mistaken for inflicted bruises. If the initial injury produces a large forehead hematoma, subsequent tracking of blood through the facial soft tissues is likely over the ensuing 24 to 72 hours, producing ecchymotic discoloration along the sides of the nose and under the lower eyelids (Fig. 6.25B). This gives the illusion of direct periorbital trauma. The history and lack of tenderness in the periorbital area help confirm the true origin of these findings.

Bruises Due to Subcultural Healing Practices

The influx of immigrants from Southeast Asia to the United States and Canada since the late 1970s has made it important to be aware of non-abusive healing practices which produce unusual bruising patterns. The most common of these is coin rubbing in which the skin of the trunk and back are rubbed vigorously with the edge of a coin as a means of treating fever. This leaves a pattern of bruises resembling the branches of a fir tree (Fig. 6.26). In another practice termed cupping, a candle is lit and the flame placed under a small cup to create a vacuum. The cup is then applied to the forehead or trunk. On removal, a round imprint is left on the skin. As the indentation resolves, a characteristic circular ecchymosis remains.

Purpura Due to Bleeding Disorders or Vasculitis

Purpuric lesions associated with coagulopathies and acute vasculitic disorders must also be recognized and distinguished from inflicted bruises.

Thrombocytopenia

Patients with acute idiopathic thrombocytopenic purpura (ITP) and acute leukemia can have purpuric lesions located anywhere in the body. Being due to thrombocytopenia, these are usually associated with petechiae (Fig. 6.27). Patients with chronic aplastic anemia can have bruises with round thick centers similar to those seen in children with clotting factor deficiencies (Fig. 6.28). These hematologic abnormalities usually are readily detectable by obtaining a complete blood count with differential and platelet count

Clotting Factor Deficiencies

Children with clotting factor deficiencies—the hemophilias and von Willebrand's disease—tend to bruise easily, and their bruises are often much more impressive than one would ordi-

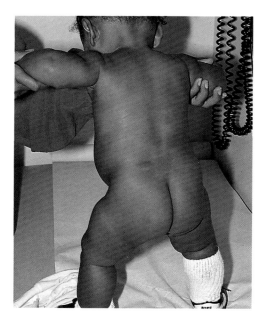

FIG. 6.29 This toddler, referred from day care for multiple bruises, had an unusual number of hyperpigmented Mongolian spots.

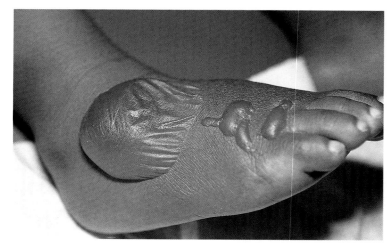

FIG. 6.30 The splash-and-droplet pattern of an accidental scald is evident on the foot of a toddler who grabbed a hot cup of tea from the table.

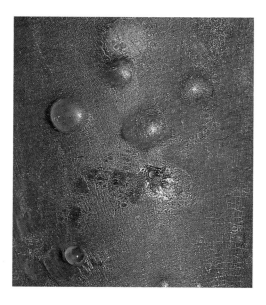

FIG. 6.31 Vesiculation due to mite bites. These pruritic vesicles are relatively thick-walled, almost perfectly round, and with no evidence of splash.

appearance of the exanthem. In many, the initial lesions are urticarial, although pruritus is mild or absent. The purpuric lesions appear in crops, with the first being distributed below the waist. Subsequent crops tend to involve the extensor forearms, cheeks, and ears. Periarticular swelling and stocking glove angioedema, which wax and wane, are common, as is crampy or colicky abdominal pain (see Chapters 7 and 8, Rheumatology and Dermatology).

Hyperpigmented Spots
Most dark-skinned infants have patchy areas of hyperpigmentation ("Mongolian spots") in which the epithelial cells contain increased amounts of melanin. These are most commonly located over the sacrum and buttocks, although they may be found elsewhere on the trunk and extremities. These areas are flat, nontender, and typically a bit more blue or green than true acute ecchymotic lesions (Fig. 6.29).

DIFFERENTIAL DIAGNOSIS OF ACCIDENTAL VS INFLICTED BURNS
All children incur accidental burns in the course of growing up, and it is important to be able to distinguish these from inflicted burns. Many are so small and minor that no medical care is sought. Children with accidental burns usually present soon after the incident, and the history is consistent with the physical findings.

Accidental Scalds
Accidental scalds typically occur when a hot liquid is spilled, producing a splash-and-droplet pattern (Fig. 6.30). The child usually has grabbed a cup of hot coffee, tea, or cocoa, or the handle of a pot on the stove. In some instances, a parent or older sibling has stumbled while carrying a pan of hot liquid or food. Such burns commonly involve the chest, a hand or foot, or occasionally the head.

Vesicular Reactions to Insect Bites
Some mites inject a blistering agent to which the patient responds with vesiculation. Such vesicles and blisters have been mistakenly attributed to sprinkling the child with scalding water. On close inspection, however, the lesions (which are pruritic rather than painful) tend to be almost perfectly round

narily expect from the reported mechanism of injury. While most males with severe hemophilia are detected in early infancy (frequently following circumcision), those with mild disease and children with von Willebrand's disease may escape detection for years, and this can be a source of confusion. Clues to an underlying factor deficiency include (1) bruises with round, thick centers (see Fig. 6.28); (2) a clear mechanism of injury consistent with the configuration but not the severity of the bruise; (3) a family and child who seem well adjusted and interact appropriately. There also may be a positive family history for bleeding problems, especially following surgery or delivery of a baby. Whenever any question exists about possible factor deficiency, a full coagulation profile is recommended; many patients with von Willebrand's disease will have a normal PT and PTT.

Vasculitis
Patients with vasculitis disorders may develop diffuse purpuric lesions which can be mistaken for inflicted bruises. In the pediatric population, Henoch-Schoenlein purpura is by far the most common of these. Affected children often have a history of antecedent viral or streptococcal infection, followed by

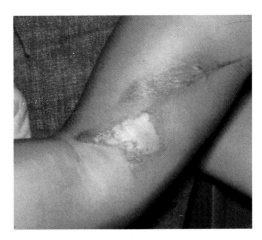

FIG. 6.32 These linear and patchy burns are characteristic of an accidental iron burn. In this case, the patient's brother pulled the iron down while she had her back turned.

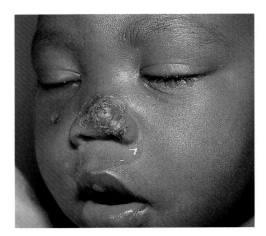

FIG. 6.33 Impetigo. This infant was initially suspected of having a cigar burn, but close inspection revealed a new peripheral bullous rim. This and the presence of another early impetigenous lesion on the cheek enabled the correct diagnosis to be made.

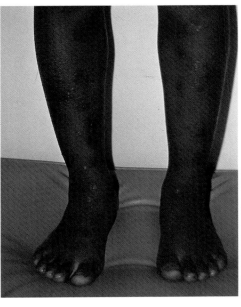

FIG. 6.34 Post-inflammatory hyperpigmentation following insect bites. When this child was seen for a followup visit for flea bites, he had a multitude of round, hyperpigmented spots at the sites of the original bites. The fact that they are macular and their distribution distinguish these from cigarette burn scars. (Courtesy of Dr. Michael Sherlock)

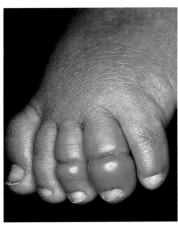

FIG. 6.35 The mild erythema and edema of the third and fourth toes are the result of constriction by hairs that accidentally became wrapped around them. (Courtesy of Dr. Thomas J. Daley, Bronx-Lebanon Hospital, New York)

with no evidence of splash, and the roof of each blister or vesicle has a thicker wall than that of the blister of a second-degree burn (Fig. 6.31).

Accidental Iron Burns
Pulling an iron down from the ironing board by yanking on its cord is the classic scenario for an accidental iron burn in a young child. The iron being heavier at one end falls end over end, producing a configuration of two or three linear or patchy first- or second-degree burns separated by gaps (Fig. 6.32). In older children and adolescents, burns are more often acquired in the course of ironing and usually consist of small linear burns of the hand or fingers.

Impetigo and Insect Bites
On occasion, impetigenous lesions have been mistaken for cigarette or cigar burns. This is often the case with bullous impetigo, in which the initial central bulla has ruptured and crusted over. On careful inspection, one can detect formation of a bullous rim around the more central crusts, and other lesions usually can be found nearby (Fig. 6.33). Removal of the crust will reveal that the lesion is very superficial in contrast to the full-thickness depression seen when the eschar is removed from an inflicted cigarette or cigar burn.

Following resolution of the acute inflammatory phase of insect bites, children are often left with round, hyperpigmented or hypopigmented areas that have been mistaken for healed cigarette burns (Fig. 6.34). However, their usual distribution is over the lower legs above the sock line. The fact that these are macular and not punched out scars should enable the clinician to make the distinction between these and the scars left by cigarette burns.

ACCIDENTAL TOURNIQUET INJURIES
Perhaps the most common form of accidental tourniquet injury is that due to a hair that becomes tightly wrapped around the toe of an infant (Fig. 6.35). The constriction causes pain and irritability which prompts the parent to seek the cause. Hence, such patients are brought in promptly before circulatory compromise occurs. We have also seen young children with mild hand edema as a result of putting rubber bands around their wrists for bracelets.

DIFFERENTIATION OF ACCIDENTAL AND PATHOLOGIC FRACTURES FROM INFLICTED FRACTURES
Accidental Fractures
In most instances, it is relatively easy to recognize a truly accidental fracture: the incident is usually witnessed, and the mechanism of injury is clearly reported. Care is typically sought promptly, although occasional exceptions occur, especially when the patient is a stoic athlete with a minor fracture who avoids complaining in order not to miss an important game. Accidental fractures are usually single or isolated, or involve both bones of the forearm or lower leg.

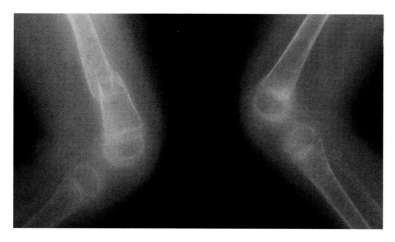

FIG. 6.36 Demineralization from disuse. Severe osteopenia and a femur fracture incurred during physical therapy are evident in this child who was left quadriplegic after an earlier injury. (Courtesy of the Department of Radiology, Children's Hospital of Pittsburgh)

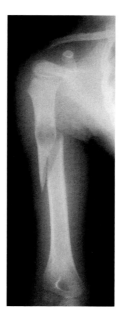

FIG. 6.37 Fracture through a unicameral bone cyst. This boy presented with intense pain and swelling of his upper arm after a relatively minor fall. The radiograph reveals a pathologic fracture through a unicameral bone cyst which has caused considerable cortical thinning. (Courtesy of the Department of Radiology, Children's Hospital of Pittsburgh)

Conditions Associated with Pathologic Fractures

Three relatively unusual conditions account for the majority of pathologic fractures seen in the pediatric population: osteogenesis imperfecta, demineralization from disuse, and bone cysts.

Osteogenisis Imperfecta (OI). The term osteogenesis imperfecta refers to a group of heritable conditions in which abnormal collagen formation results in osteoporosis and increased susceptibility to fractures (see Chapter 21, Orthopedics). Children with OI Types II (10 percent of cases) and III (18 percent of cases) are born with multiple fractures and deformities, have blue sclerae, and extreme osteoporosis, making the diagnosis evident at the time of delivery. Patients with OI Types I (66 percent of cases) and IV (6 percent of cases) have milder involvement, although those with fractures tend to have clear radiographic evidence of cortical thinning. They also tend to have mild, short stature, with lower extremity bowing and dentinogenesis imperfecta (see Chapter 20, Oral Disorders). Most patients with OI Type I have blue sclerae, lax ligaments, and many have a family history of hearing impairment. They also have wormian bones on skull x-rays. When these children do incur fractures, they present early, as do normal children with accidental fractures, and the mechanism of injury fits the fracture pattern described, although the force of impact may be less than ordinarily required to produce a fracture. Their injuries usually involve the shafts of the long bones of the forearms or legs, as is true of most accidental fractures.

The greatest difficulty in differential diagnosis may occur in an infant or young child with OI Type IV, at which time osteopenia may not be apparent. These patients do not have blue sclerae, and may not have abnormal teeth. In these cases, a skull x-ray can be of great help, as wormian bones usually will be present in this form of the disorder as well. Family history may also be helpful. The incidence of OI Type IV in the population is extremely low, being 1 in 1 to 3 million.

Demineralization From Disuse. Children with severe cerebral palsy, severe neuromuscular diseases, para- or quadriplegia that essentially leaves them confined to bed or a wheelchair develop muscular atrophy and bony demineralization due to disuse. Cortical thinning is frequently marked (Fig. 6.36) and makes the patient vulnerable to fractures following application of even minor forces.

Bone Cysts. Benign bone cysts are seen in pediatric patients usually near the metaphyseal ends of long bones. As they enlarge, they cause cortical thinning, leaving the bone vulnerable to fracture (Fig. 6.37). Similar pathologic fractures may occur at sites of osteomyelitis or in portions of bone replaced by tumor.

Conditions Associated with or Mimicking Fractures

Rickets. Radiographic changes seen in rickets include metaphyseal irregularities, periosteal reaction, and fractures. However, cupping and fraying of the metaphyses and cortical thinning are evident, thus helping to distinguish these findings from fracture healing in an infant with a normal skeleton. Clinically, widened metaphyses and costochondral beading also help to make the diagnosis (see Chapter 10, Nutrition and Gastroenterology).

Premature infants who, because of severe illness or lung disease have prolonged nutritional problems necessitating total parenteral nutrition (TPN), are particularly vulnerable to rickets with attendant bony fragility. Because these infants often require chest physiotherapy, they may incur multiple rib fractures. When these are detected on chest x-rays obtained in evaluating a respiratory illness following discharge from the nursery, abuse is often suspected. Given a history of prematurity and prolonged hospitalization, it is wise to contact that hospital and review prior films before diagnosing abuse. Careful inspection of the current films will often show residual metaphyseal and costal changes characteristic of rickets.

Copper Deficiency. This is an exceptionally rare phenomenon that should be readily distinguishable from abuse. It occurs in nutritional and inherited forms. Prematurity; a change in early infancy to whole, powdered or evaporated milk; severe malabsorption syndromes; and prolonged TPN are the major predisposing factors. Clinically, affected infants have pale skin, hypopigmented hair, edema, enlarged scalp veins and seborrhea, with or without failure to thrive or developmental delay. All have neutropenia and a hypochromic microcytic anemia

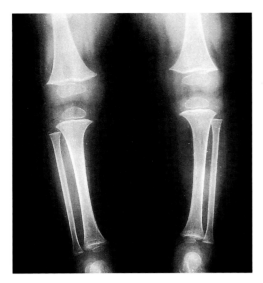

FIG. 6.38 Scurvy. Note the increased density of the zones of provisional calcification and the lucency of the underlying spongiosa. The metaphyses are also widened, and early spur formation is seen. (Courtesy of the Department of Radiology, Children's Hospital of Pittsburgh)

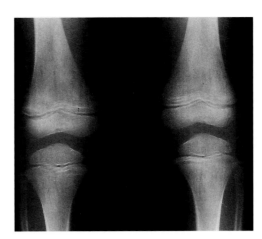

FIG. 6.39 Leukemic lines. These lucent metaphyseal bands can be seen in some children with acute leukemia or other severe systemic illnesses. However, they are rarely associated with fractures. (Courtesy of the Department of Radiology, Children's Hospital of Pittsburgh)

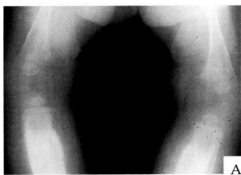

A

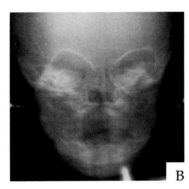

B

FIG. 6.40 Caffey's disease. A, intense periosteal reaction and cortical thickening are seen in the lower extremities. B, mandibular involvement has resulted in dramatic thickening. These findings, associated symptoms, and absence of fractures distinguish this condition from the skeletal changes of abuse. (Courtesy of the Department of Radiology, Children's Hospital of Pittsburgh)

that is resistant to iron therapy; their bones are grossly abnormal radiographically. Findings include overt osteoporosis, cupped metaphyses, metaphyseal spurs, widened anterior ribs, periosteal reaction and, at times, soft tissue calcification (see Chapter 10, Nutrition and Gastroenterology).

Menkes' kinky hair syndrome is the inherited form due to an x-linked recessive defect in copper absorption. These children are markedly pale, and have a characteristic facies with pudgy cheeks; horizontal, twisted eyebrows; and little facial expression. Their hair is dull or lusterless, sparse, and kinky with pili torti (see Chapter 8, Dermatology). Affected infants are also grossly abnormal neurologically, with hypertonia, decreased movement, lethargy, myoclonic seizures, and difficulty maintaining normothermia being major findings.

Scurvy. Although children with vitamin C deficiency (now exceedingly rare) tend to bruise easily because of vascular fragility, their diagnosis should be readily distinguishable from findings of abuse when radiographs are taken. While periosteal reaction is seen due to subperiosteal hemorrhage, and while there may be fractures through the zone of provisional calcification and through metaphyseal spurs, their cortices are thin, and the ends of the long bones show characteristic changes consisting of increased density of the zone of provisional calcification and increased lucency of the underlying spongiosa (Fig. 6.38). These infants are irritable, tend to move little because of bone pain and often have gingival bleeding as well.

Hypervitaminosis A. Chronic vitamin A intoxication produces a thick, wavy periosteal reaction which most commonly involves the ulnas and metatarsals, although other long bones can be affected. Hard, tender swellings may be evident on palpation. Absence of fractures and of metaphyseal abnormalities should help distinguish this from abuse. The history, and findings of papilledema and/or split sutures on skull x-ray due to concomitant pseudotumor cerebri, also aid in differentiation.

Leukemia. Children with acute leukemia may develop diffuse demineralization, periosteal reactions and osteolytic lesions. Lucent metaphyseal bands termed leukemic lines are also seen (Fig. 6.39). The relative osteopenia and typical lack of fractures, combined with the antecedent history; physical findings which may include adenopathy, visceromegaly and sternal tenderness; and the results of hematologic tests should distinguish these findings from those of abuse.

Caffey's Disease. A rare disorder of unknown etiology, Caffey's disease is characterized by cortical thickening and painful periosteal reaction (Fig. 6.40). Bones are otherwise normally mineralized, and fractures are not seen. Involvement of the mandible seen in 75 percent of affected patients results in dramatic thickening. The clavicle and ulna are other common sites, although other bones can be involved. Most patients are under 6 months of age and all have fever, anorexia, and marked irritability.

DIFFERENTIAL DIAGNOSIS OF ACCIDENTAL VS INFLICTED HEAD INJURIES

Accidental head injuries are common in childhood as a result of falls and other accidents, and the vast majority are minor. Presentation is usually prompt because a head injury, no matter how minor, tends to provoke considerable parental anxiety. Again, the history is usually clear, and the mechanism is consistent with the physical findings. Mild forehead and scalp contusions with or without small lacerations or abrasions are by far the most common injuries seen. Linear skull fractures can result from relatively mild falls onto hard surfaces, but these do not tend to be associated with significant changes in consciousness level. More severe injuries are incurred as a result of more serious mechanisms of injury, including major falls, bicycle and sports accidents, and motor vehicle accidents.

DIFFERENTIATION OF ACCIDENTAL FROM INFLICTED ORAL INJURIES

Falls, sporting and bicycle accidents are the usual sources of accidental oral injuries which include lip and chin lacerations; loosened or avulsed teeth; and gingival, palatal or retropharyngeal lacerations from falls with an object in the mouth (see Chapters 20 and 22, Oral Disorders and Otolaryngology). These injuries, like head injuries, provoke considerable parental anxiety, and result in prompt presentation for care with a clear history and consistent mechanism of injury.

DIFFERENTIAL DIAGNOSIS OF ACCIDENTAL VS INFLICTED CHEST AND ABDOMINAL INJURIES

Accidental chest and abdominal injuries in children are predominantly the result of blunt force trauma, and are similar in nature to those caused by abuse. However, victims of accidental injuries have a clear history of a major mechanism of injury that was often witnessed. Immediate care is sought and findings are consistent with the history.

SEXUAL ABUSE

Krugman has defined sexual abuse as the engaging of a child in sexual activities that the child does not understand, to which the child cannot give informed consent, or which violate the social taboos of society. In such incidents, the child is used to provide sexual gratification to the perpetrator and/or other person(s) present.

Of all the forms of abuse, sexual abuse has been and probably remains the most underreported. However, in the last few years (in part as a result of increased media attention) there has been a dramatic increase in cases referred to child protective service agencies. In 1989, there were 384,000 such cases, a figure nearly three times that recorded in 1988. Nevertheless, as prevalence studies suggest that as many as 20 to 30 percent of all women have experienced at least one episode of sexual abuse by age 18, it is clear that underreporting remains considerable. While females are more frequently victimized, males are by no means immune to the problem. Studies suggest that between 5 and 15 percent of boys will be victimized at least once by the age of 18.

Sexual abuse may involve visual exposure to exhibitionist or masturbatory behavior; fondling, masturbation, and digital manipulation; oral/genital contact; and direct genital contact, including penetration or attempted penetration of the vagina or anus. Previous studies of perpetrators suggest that between 30 and 37 percent are parents, parent surrogates, or close relatives; between 26 and 60 percent are known to the victim but are unrelated (neighbors, babysitters, nursery school or day care personnel); and between 11 and 37 percent are strangers. U.S. statistics for 1988 suggest some changes in this pattern. Forty-two percent of reported perpetrators were the child's nat-

ural parent or stepparent, and 25 percent were other relatives. When the perpetrator is a family member or acquaintance, the encounter is generally nonviolent, with persuasion, bribery or threats used to enlist the victim's cooperation and ensure secrecy. Not infrequently, these experiences are repetitive and occur over long periods of time. There is also a well described pattern of escalating levels of involvement, with initial fondling and digital manipulation progressing to actual penetration over time. The victim bears both the guilt of engaging in unwanted sexual activity and the pressure of keeping it a secret. Lack of violence or physical injury does not imply consent, as the offender is usually in a position of power over the victim, making it difficult for the child to refuse to engage in the activity or disclose it. Episodes involving strangers are more likely to be isolated incidents and frequently involve physical violence, adding the emotional stress of being in a potentially life-threatening situation.

Forensic requirements for a detailed history, physical examination, and multiple laboratory specimens (all carefully documented) necessitate a lengthy evaluation which, if not sensitively handled, can compound the existing emotional trauma. This can be minimized if the physician approaches the patient and family with patience, gentleness, and tact.

Because physical findings are often normal and when present are frequently nonspecific, the history is often the key aspect of the evaluation. Hence, it is essential that historical information be documented meticulously (and where possible, verbatim), since many of these cases have the potential for legal prosecution. It is also important to avoid leading questions, although in certain situations they may be necessary in order to elicit enough information to ensure protection of the child. The parent or parents accompanying the child should be interviewed first, if possible, apart from each other. They should also be interviewed separately from the child. During this interview one can obtain information about the child's emotional status and recent behavior; present and past history; family psychosocial situation; household members or other persons caring for the child, or people who live in or visit the home who might have unwitnessed access to the child; the events that appear to have led to the disclosure; and terms used by the child for body parts.

In approaching the child, one should convey an understanding that he or she may have been sworn to secrecy, but that the person who asked this has a serious problem and can't be helped to stop unless the child tells you just what has happened. Kindness, empathy, and gentleness in questioning are essential. If the child is willing and able to give a history, it, as well as the exact phrasing of the questions asked, should be documented verbatim. Begin by talking about favorite subjects such as friends, favorite toys, games, and activities. Thereafter, it is best to ask general questions, reserving more specific questions for situations in which the child is unable to disclose and there is a very strong suspicion of sexual abuse. If the child is unwilling to discuss the episode or episodes and there is a strong suspicion of sexual abuse, a return visit or referral for a play therapy session with a trained clinician is recommended.

When children give spontaneous detailed descriptions of sexual experiences, these are usually accurate and not imagined. Asking non-directive questions to ascertain the site in which the activity occurred and the number of times it happened, and questions related to clothing worn, etc., can be useful in documenting the child's credibility. It is also important to determine the patient's understanding of the need for accuracy

MOST COMMON SUBSTITUTE COMPLAINTS IN SEXUAL ABUSE CASES*

Any Age	Preschool Age	School Age	Adolescence
Abdominal pain	Excessive clinging	Decreased school	Same as school age plus:
Anorexia	Thumbsucking	performance	Runaway behavior
Vomiting	Speech disorder	Truancy	Suicide attempts
Constipation	Encopresis/enuresis	Lying, stealing	Perpetration of
Sleep disorders	Excessive masturbation[†]	Tics	sexual offenses[†]
Dysuria		Anxiety reaction	
Vaginal discharge[‡]		Phobic and obsessional	
Vaginal bleeding[‡]		states	
Rectal bleeding		Depression	
		Conversion reaction	
		Encopresis/enuresis	

*Note that most of these complaints are also symptomatic of disorders more prevalent than sexual abuse.
†Symptoms highly suspicious of sexual abuse.
‡ Symptoms somewhat suspicious of sexual abuse

FIG. 6.41

in relating the history and of the difference between telling the truth and telling a lie. Yet another problem has arisen in that many children who are required to repeat the history to the multiple authorities begin to sound robotic and may become so traumatized that they recant to avoid further questioning.

Recent recognition of the problem of false accusations of sexual abuse made in the heat of child custody battles has raised questions regarding the veracity of many such claims. Ongoing research suggests that when the child's disclosure is made without benefit of leading questions and is reported with feeling and often some hesitancy and in age-appropriate terms, the report is accurate. In contrast, children coached to make false claims tend to relate a history in a rote manner and often use adult-oriented words.

A thorough and complete physical examination is warranted for all patients suspected of being sexually abused, with examination of the genitalia and rectum deferred until last. Each part of the examination should be explained as the examiner proceeds. When possible, and if the child so chooses, a parent or supportive adult should be present. As the parents are usually anxious, it is important that details of the exam be described to them before it is begun. If an attempt to inspect the perineum provokes anxiety which cannot be allayed, the procedure should be deferred, unless there is gross bleeding, pain and discharge, or evidence of venereal disease. Under these circumstances, the patient should be admitted and examined, and specimens collected under general anesthesia. If the patient is asymptomatic and there is no evidence of violence, trauma or discharge, the procedure can be deferred and performed at a followup visit. It is most important that the child not feel that he/she is being assaulted yet again during the examination and interview process.

In our experience with prepubertal patients, external inspection of the genitalia suffices in the vast majority of cases, and the insertion of a speculum is rarely indicated. The procedure is painful, provides little in the way of useful information, and usually provokes much parental anxiety. In the few instances in which internal examination is required, it should be performed under general anesthesia.

Modes of Presentation

As most cases of sexual abuse do not involve physical violence, most patients have no signs of physical injury, and physical findings are completely normal. In cases of sexual assault involving violence and resulting in injury, a significant proportion of victims seek medical care promptly, most acknowledge the nature of the problem at the time of presentation, and physical findings are more often positive.

While there has been a significant increase in the percentage of patients who have disclosed inappropriate touching prior to presentation, it continues to be true that many victims of long-term sexual abuse present with vulvovaginitis with vaginal discharge due to a sexually transmitted pathogen, or with substitute complaints generated by physical and/or emotional sequelae (Fig. 6.41). While there is a wide range of differential diagnostic possibilities in patients presenting with these problems, sexual abuse should be considered and addressed among the diagnostic considerations. It is appropriate to ask questions about the possibility of inappropriate touching, and if there is any suspicion of this, a more detailed psychological assessment by a specially trained clinician is warranted. It is of note that a significant proportion of sexual abuse victims do not disclose immediately. This, in our experience, seems to be particularly true of children presenting with sexually transmitted disease. However, after repeated visits with a single clinician during a stepwise evaluation, they can develop enough trust to be able to disclose.

Examination Techniques

PERINEAL EXAMINATION

Several techniques may be used for examination of the genital and perianal areas in different age groups. In the post-pubertal age group, a standard gynecologic examination usually can be performed with the patient in the lithotomy position (see Chapter 18, Gynecology). In cases of acute injury, consideration must be given to the severity and extent of the injuries before proceeding. If examination and specimen collection are

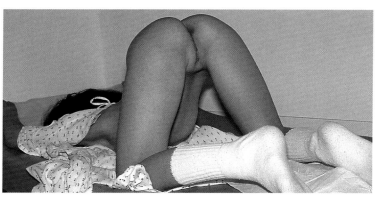

FIG. 6.42 Knee-chest position. Having the knees widely separated facilitates visualization. Note the sway-back position needed.

DOCUMENTATION REQUIRED IN SEXUAL ABUSE EVALUATION

Interview

Record exact questions
asked (may be used
in court)
Avoid leading questions
if possible

Physical Exam

General exam
Tanner staging
Scarring/bruising

Past History

Especially of
ano-genital symptoms
Behavioral changes

Genital Exam

Magnification used
Position/Technique
Supine with labial
separation
Supine with labial
traction
Knee-chest, sway-back
Degree of relaxation

Perianal Exam

Position
Degree of relaxation

Perineum/Labia

Lacerations
Abrasions
Erythema
Bruising
Discharge

Vestibule

Erythema
Urethra

**Posterior
Fourchette**

Labial adhesions
Neovascularization
Friability

Hymen

Configuration
(annular,
crescentic,
redundant)
Edges
Thin and sharp
Thickened
Rolled
Projections
Notching
Vascularity

Hymenal Orifice

Horizontal diameter
Vertical diameter

Vagina

Visualized
Not visualized
Ridges
Rugae
Discharge

Perianal Area

Pigmentation
Erythema
Venous congestion
Anal wink/reflex
Paradoxical
relaxation/dilatation
(timing, measurments)
Presence of stool
Fissures
Skin tags
Lacerations
Sphincter folds
Sphincter tone

FIG. 6.43

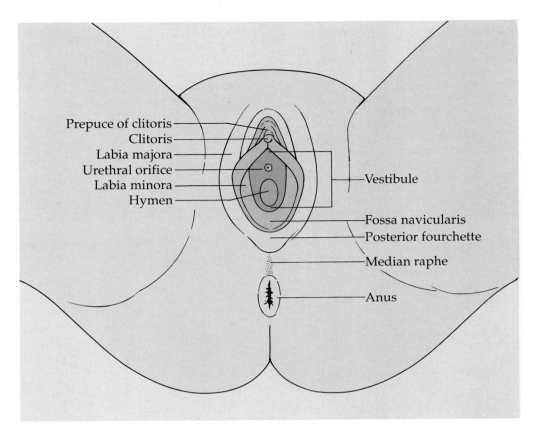

FIG. 6.44 Normal anatomy. Location of the genital structures of the prepubertal female.

Prepuce of clitoris
Clitoris
Labia majora
Urethral orifice
Labia minora
Hymen

Vestibule

Fossa navicularis
Posterior fourchette

Median raphe

Anus

likely to cause extreme physical pain or emotional distress, or if internal injuries are likely, consideration should be given to examination under anesthesia.

The purposes of the perineal examination in the prepubertal child are: (1) to obtain full visualization of the patient's perineal and perianal anatomy; (2) to detect any evidence of acute injury, infection, or scarring indicative of prior injury; (3) to determine the size and configuration of the hymenal orifice; and (4) to collect specimens as indicated. As noted earlier, internal speculum examination is not necessary unless there is evidence of internal extension of injury and, in such cases, the examination, specimen collection, and repair should be done in the operating room under general anesthesia.

In examining prepubertal patients, any one of three positions may be used to achieve good visualization of the genital area. The one most commonly used is the supine frog-leg position with the patient lying supine on the examining table. This position can also be used with the child semi-reclining on the parent's lap—semi-supine frog-leg position. We have also had good success with the semi-supine lithotomy position (both are illustrated in Chapter 18, Gynecology). The latter is accomplished by having the parent sit on the examining table leaning back against the wall. The child then sits on her lap with buttocks resting just above the parent's knees, and leans back. The parent then places her/his hands under the patient's knees, flexing them and abducting the hips. The third position used is the knee-chest position (Fig. 6.42), which probably provides the best exposure of the perineum. In using this, it is important that the child's shoulders and chest touch the table, achieving a "sway-back" posture. This position is difficult to use in children under 2 years of age, and some older children object to it.

To facilitate visualization of the introitus in the supine or semi-supine frog-leg or lithotomy positions, the labia must be manually separated. In the labial separation method, the examiner places the index fingers over the lower portion of the labia majora and gently presses downward and laterally. In the labial traction technique, the labia majora are grasped between the thumb and index fingers and gently pulled outward and upward. The latter usually achieves better visualization of the hymen and its orifice and the greatest hymenal transverse di-ameter. It is also generally possible to see the lower third of the vagina using this technique (see also Chapter 18, Gynecology).

In the knee-chest position, exposure of the introitus is facilitated by placing the thumbs over the edge of the gluteus muscles at the level of the introitus and lifting them upward. Because abnormal widening of the hymenal opening can be an important finding in some sexual abuse victims, the horizontal diameter should be carefully measured. However, this diameter does vary with position; hence, it is important to document not only the diameter, but also the position of the patient when the measurement was obtained. Measurements are best noted using the supine or semi-supine frog-leg position or the supine or semi-supine lithotomy position with labial traction.

Good lighting and magnification are also important. Use of the colposcope is ideal, but this device is not readily available to most practitioners. Alternatively, a magnifying halogen lamp or an otoscope may be used.

It is very important that a complete description of the appearance of the genitalia be documented on the chart (Fig. 6.43), and if possible, magnified photographs of the genital area should be taken. These obviate the need for reexamination when a second opinion is requested. Such documentation requires knowledge of basic gynecologic anatomy and terminology, which are shown in Figure 6.44 (see also section on Differential Diagnosis; and section on Normal Developmental Changes in the Gynecology chapter).

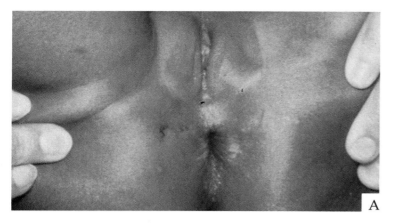

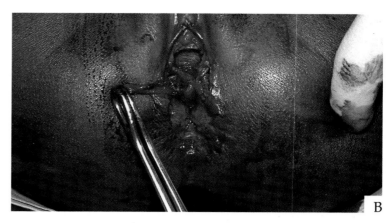

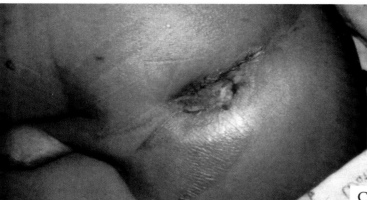

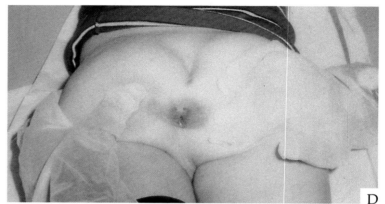

FIG. 6.45 *Acute traumatic findings of sexual abuse and assault.* ***A,*** *abrasions, contusions, and punctate tears of the perineum and perianal areas can be seen in this prepubertal girl.* ***B,*** *severe genital trauma in a prepubertal girl following rape. Inspection reveals a hymenal tear at 6 o'clock extending posteriorly through the perineal body to the rectum. Under anesthesia, a 1-inch vaginal tear was discovered along* *with a rectal tear and complete disruption of the external anal sphincter.* ***C,*** *perianal lacerations, abrasions, and burns are apparent in this prepubertal boy. It is suspected that the burns were inflicted to cover up the evidence of sodomy.* ***D,*** *prominent, perianal ecchymoses were found in this 3-year-old boy who had been sodomized.* (***B,*** *courtesy of Dr. Kamthorn Sukarochana, Children's Hospital of Pittsburgh)*

PERIANAL EXAMINATION

Sodomy is a common form of sexual abuse in both boys and girls. To achieve optimal visualization, the perianal exam should be conducted in the knee-chest position. Care should be taken to look for evidence of abrasions, tears, fissures or other lesions, and for evidence of rapid dilatation of the external sphincter. The absence of physical findings is the norm and does not make the history any less credible. Following specimen collection, a digital rectal examination should be performed to assess sphincter tone.

Physical Findings

ACUTE TRAUMATIC FINDINGS OF SEXUAL ASSAULT AND SEXUAL ABUSE

Victims of sexual assault often show evidence of physical trauma other than genital injuries. Bruises and abrasions of the head, face, neck, chest, forearms, knees, and thighs are common. Occasionally, even more severe non-genital injuries are encountered.

Genital and rectal examination may reveal contusions, erythema, abrasions or lacerations (Fig. 6.45A–D; see Figs. 18.17-18.20). Perineal lesions tend to be located in the posterior portion of the introitus as opposed to lesions caused by straddle injury, which are usually more anterior or located over the labia majora and inner thighs (see Fig. 18.18). It is also important to note that perineal injuries often heal very quickly and

completely, with no residual scarring. At times, evidence of seminal products in the form of a vaginal discharge will be observed if the patient is seen within 24 to 72 hours of the latest incident and has not bathed (Fig. 6.46). Seminal fluid has been reported to fluoresce under Wood's lamp, but in our tests, we found only weak fluorescence when wet and none when dry. Under normal light, the seminal products are practically invisible after drying. If a history of ejaculation is obtained, and the area has not been washed, swabbing the perineum and inner thighs with saline-moistened cotton swabs may yield a sample of dried seminal fluid which can be identified by the crime lab. Swabs should be air-dried following the collection process.

When external contusions or tears are seen, internal injury must be suspected. The prepubescent girl is particularly vulnerable to severe internal trauma as a result of forceful penetration of either the vagina or the rectum (see Fig. 6.45). This stems from the fact that the structures are relatively small, and the tissues more delicate and rigid. Young children with mild external injuries may in fact have major internal tears including perforation of the peritoneum and damage to pelvic vessels, mesentery, and intestine (see Chapter 18, Gynecology). Signs of internal pathology may be subtle, but such patients will have evidence of vaginal bleeding, vaginal hematoma, lower abdominal rebound tenderness, or evidence of occult blood loss. Therefore, when such findings are present, examination under general anesthesia (EUA) is indicated. The post-

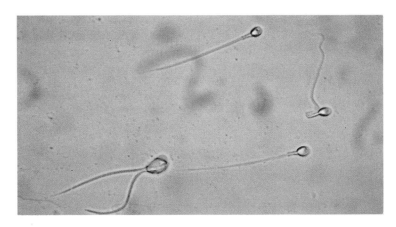

FIG. 6.46 *Microscopic appearance of seminal fluid removed from a young rape victim. When a vaginal discharge is found in a patient presenting within 72 hours after sexual abuse, a wet mount may reveal sperm. A portion of the discharge should also be collected for acid phosphatase, blood grouping, and enzyme studies.*

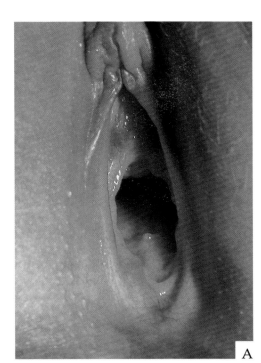

FIG. 6.47 *Abnormal hymenal findings as a result of chronic sexual abuse. A, the hymen is almost completely absent, and the remaining edges are thickened. B, the hymenal rim has markedly thickened and rolled margins and is notched in the 5 o'clock position. C, scarring, edema and excoriation of the perineal body, extending to the anterior anal rim. (B and C, courtesy of Dr. Pat Bruno, Sunbury Community Hospital, Sunbury, PA)*

A

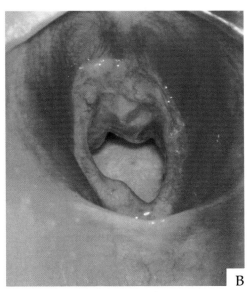

B

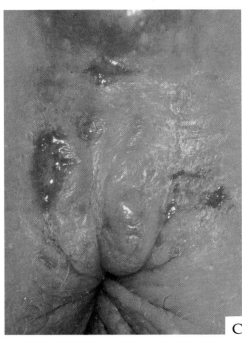

C

pubescent female can usually be adequately assessed by careful pelvic examination, unless she is emotionally unable to tolerate the procedure, in which case an EUA would also be advisable.

Rectal examination is necessary for assessment of internal tears, pelvic tenderness, sphincter tone, and for bimanual palpation.

ABNORMAL AND SUSPICIOUS FINDINGS IN CASES OF SEXUAL ABUSE
Perineal Abnormalities

While physical findings are normal in up to 80 percent of victims, abnormal and/or suspicious findings can be detected on careful inspection in the rest; however there is considerable controversy over the significance of some findings. One of these is enlargement of the hymenal orifice. A general rule of thumb for normal transverse diameter in the supine frog-leg or lithotomy position with labial traction is 1 mm per year of age. This is not an absolute, however, and deviations of 2 to 3 mm are probably within the normal range. Hence, mild widening in the absence of other abnormal findings should not be used in isolation as evidence for sexual misuse. For unknown reasons, obese children may have an increased hymenal diameter. The significance of this is unclear. Marked enlargement is highly suspicious, however (see Fig. 6.47A). Other physical findings associated with chronic sexual misuse include a thickened, rolled hymenal rim with little remaining hymenal tissue (Fig. 6.47A) and notching of the rim, especially between 3 and 9 o'clock (Fig. 6.47B). Presence of bumps along the rim between 3 and 5 o'clock and 7 and 9 o'clock; the presence of abnormal blood vessels over the posterior portion of the hymenal membrane; and excoriations and scarring of the perineal body (Fig. 6.47C) are also seen as a result of sexual abuse. We have also seen lichenification due to chronic abrasive action. Erythema is a common but totally nonspecific finding (see Fig. 18.30).

Male victims may have evidence of urethral discharge and mild abrasions and contusions of the penis, scrotum or median raphe.

Oral Abnormalities

Forceful orogenital contact may result in perioral and intraoral injuries. These may include fissuring or tears at the corner of the mouth and gingival and palatal contusions. Such oral

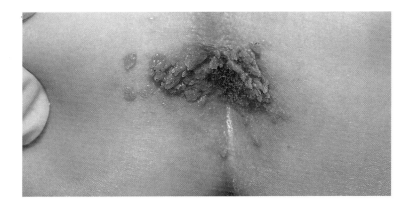

FIG. 6.48 *Condylomata accuminata. Coalescent and discrete condylomata are seen in the perianal area of a 4-year-old boy with a history of being sodomized.*

lesions are unusual, however. In contrast, asymptomatic gonococcal infection of the pharynx is relatively common.

Anal and Perianal Abnormalities

Patients who have been repetitively sodomized may manifest paradoxical anal sphincter relaxation on gluteal stroking to assess for an anal wink reflex, or immediate dilatation of the anal sphincter to greater than 2 cm when placed in the knee-chest position. When the latter is seen in the absence of stool in the rectal vault, the findings are highly suspicious. Repeated sodomy also is said to result in funnelling "of the perianal area." This rare finding occurs from loss of fatty tissue in the gluteal area. The presence of tears in the perianal area and fissures are suspicious, although the latter are not specific to sexual abuse, being seen frequently in children with chronic or recurrent constipation. Tears that extend beyond the hair follicle-bearing areas are thought to be more characteristic of abuse. Evidence of perianal burns is strongly suggestive of abuse, and infliction of burns may be used in an attempt to obscure injuries due to sodomy (see Fig. 6.45C).

Evidence of Sexually Transmitted Disease

The presence of sexually transmitted diseases in the prepubertal child is strongly suggestive of sexual abuse, except in occasional instances when other modes of transmission can be documented. In fact, many victims are identified upon presenting with a vaginal or urethral discharge that is positive for a venereal pathogen. In females, this usually is manifest by vulvovaginitis with a vaginal discharge, with *Neisseria gonorrhea* and *Chlamydia trachomatis* being the most commonly identified pathogens (see Chapter 18, Gynecology). Males may have overt urethritis or asymptomatic urethral infection.

Vulvovaginal, urethral, oral and rectal infections with the gonococcus are almost always acquired via sexual contact, as is vulvovaginal *Chlamydia* in the child over 2 to 3 years (see below), and *Trichomonas* in the peripubertal child. Development of *Condylomata accuminata* after infancy is highly suspicious, though not diagnostic for abuse (Fig. 6.48). Genital herpes infections may be acquired via sexual contact, but are more often the result of spread from oral or hand lesions as a result of poor attention to hand-washing (see Fig. 18.38A). The major mode of acquisition of *Gardnerella vaginalis* remains unclear Nonspecific vaginal discharges, especially when chronic or recurrent, are also suspect. All should be tested for the presence of sperm.

Nonsexual transmission of the gonococcus, *Chlamydia*, *Trichomonas*, and HPV occurs primarily during the process of vaginal delivery. Gonococcal infections tend to produce symp-

toms early in the neonatal period. Perinatally acquired Trichomonas causes a copious vaginal discharge in the neonate which can abate even without treatment, although the organism can persist for months. In contrast, neonatal acquisition of Chlamydia may persist for 18 months to 3 years. Hence, finding this organism in the very young child cannot be considered diagnostic of sexual abuse. Because of its prolonged incubation period, the human papilloma virus may not produce lesions until several months after delivery despite being transmitted at birth.

Finally, it must be noted that in some instances children develop sexually transmitted diseases as the result of sexual contact with other infected children. In such cases, aggressive case finding can result in identification of the index child who is an abuse victim.

Specimen Collection

Laboratory studies are designed to augment the physical assessment of injury, identify sexually transmitted pathogens, and document the presence or absence of seminal fluid. The likelihood of finding the latter is so small after 72 hours that these studies can be omitted if the patient seeks attention 3 or more days after the last incident. Cultures should be obtained regardless of time of presentation or lack of symptoms, as infections may be asymptomatic (although asymptomatic vaginal infection in prepubertal girls is rare). This is particularly true of oral and rectal gonorrhea.

In the prepubertal child with vaginal discharge, all cultures may be obtained from the discharge on the perineum except for *Chlamydia*, which necessitates swabbing the vaginal wall. (Note: The ELISA or Chlamydiazyme® test is not indicated in prepubertal patients, both because it is inaccurate and because it does not constitute adequate legal evidence of infection in court.) In the absence of discharge, vaginal specimens are needed for all cultures. It is important to note that the hymen is extremely sensitive, and that touching it with the swab will induce a significant amount of pain in most patients. Saline-moistened calcium alginate swabs on thin metal wires are the easiest to insert atraumatically. Instillation of saline via an 18- or 19-gauge soft rubber catheter is an alternative method sometimes useful for patients with very small hymenal orifices. The saline is instilled with the child in the semi-supine lithotomy position, and allowed to remain for 20 to 30 seconds. It then can be aspirated back as the mother lowers the child's legs and the saline bubbles out. Application of topical xylocaine ointment to the hymenal area prior to collection of specimens can help to reduce discomfort, and is

DOCUMENTATION REQUIRED IN SEXUAL ABUSE EVALUATION: GUIDELINES FOR SPECIMEN COLLECTION IN SEXUAL ABUSE EXAMINATION AT CHILDREN'S HOSPITAL, PITTSBURGH

Orogenital Contact	Genital Contact		Anal Contact
	No Evidence of Penetration	**Evidence Consistent with Vaginal Penetration**	

1. Swabs: use two at a time‡
  a. For wet mount for sperm*
  b. For two air-dried slides*
  c. For GC culture
  d. Consider *Chlamydia* culture if patient older than 3 years
2. Consider baseline RPR (repeat in 4-6 weeks if initial test is negative)
	1. Urinalysis for occult blood
	2. Vaginal swabs or aspirate†‡
	  a. For wet mount for sperm*, *Trichomonas*, *Gardnerella*, and *Candida*
	  b. For two air-dried slides*
	  c. For GC and routine culture
	  d. *Chlamydia* culture if patient older than 3 years
	  e. For Gram stain if vaginal discharge is present
	3. Consider baseline RPR (repeat in 4-6 weeks if initial test is negative)
		1. Urinalysis for occult blood
		2. If external tears seen:
		  a. Consult surgeon for possible EUA
		  b. If EUA done, collect specimens then
		3. Vaginal swabs or aspirate†‡
		  a. For wet mount for sperm,* *Trichomonas*, *Gardnerella*, and *Candida*
		  b. For two air-dried slides*
		  c. For GC and routine cultures
		  d. *Chlamydia* culture if patient older than 3 years
		  e. For Gram stain if vaginal discharge present
		4. Consider RPR (repeat in 4-6 weeks if initial test is negative)
			1. If external tears seen:
			  a. Consult general surgeon for possible EUA
			  b. If EUA done, collect specimens then
			2. Swabs: use two at a time and insert no more than 1 cm‡ (must be done before rectal examination)
			  a. For wet mount for sperm*
			  b. For two air-dried slides*
			  c. For GC and routine cultures
			  d. *Chlamydia* culture if patient older than 3 years
			3. If no tears:
			  a. Rectal exam
			  b. Stool guaiac: if positive consult general surgeon
			4. Consider baseline RPR (repeat in 4-6 weeks if initial test is negative)

*Omit if seen >72 hours after the last incident, except in patients with vaginal discharge.
†In postpubertal patients cervical swabs must be obtained for GC and Chlamydia cultures and for Gram stain.
‡Two of the swabs used to obtain specimens should be air-dried and placed in a sterile test tube for acid phosphatase, blood group, and enzyme studies. When specimens are obtained by vaginal aspirate, a small amount of aspirate should be applied to two swabs which should then be processed in the same manner.

FIG. 6.49

probably wise for girls with small hymenal openings or redundant hymenal tissue. As the knee-chest position produces maximal hymenal opening, this is the optimal position if the child will tolerate it.

In the post-menarchal patient, cervical cultures for gonorrhea and *Chlamydia* in addition to cultures of the vaginal pool are indicated. The possibility of pregnancy must also be considered in all such patients.

In obtaining rectal specimens for gonorrhea and *Chlamydia*, the swab should be inserted no more than 1 to 2 cm to avoid fecal contamination which interferes with culture results.

Patients with evidence of trauma need urinalysis and rectal examination to check for evidence of bleeding, and may require sonography or computerized tomography if physical findings suggest internal extension of injury. Prepubertal girls with evidence of vaginal bleeding or a vaginal hematoma must have an internal examination under anesthesia. In such instances, specimen collection is deferred until that time.

Figure 6.49 presents guidelines for specimen collection in sexual abuse cases, and Figure 6.50 enumerates the additional

ADDITIONAL SPECIMENS NEEDED IN RAPE CASES
(Seen within 72 hours)

Specimens may be obtained by the physician or nurse. All containers used in evidence collection should be paper and must be labeled with:

Patient's name	Body site	Initials of collector
Type of specimen	Date and time	

Clothing If the patient is wearing the same clothes, they should be collected along with debris, as this may provide valuable clues regarding the assailant. The patient should disrobe while standing on a towel or sheet. Each article including the towel or sheet should then be placed in a separate paper bag. Avoid shaking the articles. Each bag is then labeled and sealed.

Fingernail scrapings* These may provide bits of skin, fiber, and debris from the assailant. Scraping from beneath the nails or nail clippings should be obtained. Specimens from each hand should be collected over separate sheets of paper, and placed in separate paper envelopes, sealed, and labeled.

Hair samples* Any loose or suspected foreign hairs should be collected, placed in an envelope, and labeled. If patient is postpubescent, comb pubic hairs onto a sheet of clean paper, fold, place in an envelope with the comb, label "combed pubic hair," and seal. Then, gently pull a small clump of the patient's pubic hair (12 hairs are needed), place on clean paper, fold, put in envelope, label "standard pubic hair," and seal. Then, comb and obtain head hairs in this same manner.

Blood sample 5 cc of blood should be drawn for blood grouping and enzyme typing, and placed in a purple top tube.

Saliva sample This enables testing of the patient's secretory status. The specimen should be obtained either by wiping the patient's oral mucosa with a gauze pad or by having the patient expectorate onto a gauze pad. The pad is then placed in an envelope, sealed, and labeled.

Destination of Specimens

The following specimens are handled by the hospital laboratories or performed in the ER:

Urinalysis	Gram stains	RPR
Wet preps	Stool guaiac	Cultures

All other specimens are to be signed over to police custody for transport to the crime laboratory.

Maintaining an Unbroken Chain of Evidence

Evidence should be packaged and labeled upon collection. All evidence should be kept together and must remain under the direct supervision of the physician, the nurse, or the security guard until signed over to the police. Receipt for release of evidence to police should be signed before evidence is given over to the police.

*Omit if patient has already bathed and shampooed.

FIG. 6.50

specimens required by law enforcement authorities in rape cases. Each specimen for the crime lab should be packaged and labeled immediately after collection. All evidence should then be kept together, and must remain under the direct supervision of the physician or nurse who was present at the time of collection until it is handed over to the authorities. Finally, police should sign a receipt for release of evidence upon accepting the specimens. Commercially available rape assessment kits greatly facilitate this process. Failure to adhere to these procedures breaks the chain of evidence and invalidates its use in legal proceedings. When rape has been perpetrated by a stranger (e.g., not a caretaker), the patient or parent must sign a consent form prior to collection of evidence.

Differential Diagnosis of Sexual Abuse

Not only are there a wide range of non-abusive causes of the physical and behavioral symptoms which serve as presenting complaints of many sexual abuse victim's but, in addition, physical findings (when present) are variable, often nonspecific, and many have a variety of other causes as well. Furthermore, as the result of McCann's pioneering work, the wide variation in normal findings is only beginning to be appreciated. Erythema of the vaginal vestibule is seen commonly in asymptomatic non-abused prepubertal girls. It can also be seen in abuse victims, and in children with irritant and other forms of vulvovaginitis.

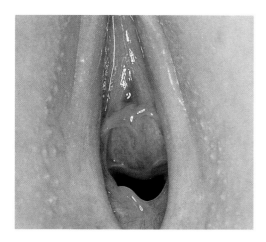

FIG. 6.51 *Hymenal septal remnant. A small tag or mound of tissue is seen near the midline of the posterior portion of the hymen and has smooth, sharp edges. This is thought to be a normal variant and a remnant of the hymenal septum. (Courtesy of Dr. John McCann, University of California at San Francisco)*

A number of normal anatomic variants are now recognized as well. Septal remnants seen as tags near the midline on either the anterior or posterior portion of the hymenal membrane (Fig. 6.51 and see Chapter 18, Gynecology) and even anterolateral hymenal flaps are normal findings, as are periurethral bands. These and intravaginal ridges were once erroneously thought to be the result of scarring. Thin labial adhesions are a common finding in normal children, as well. There is a wide variation in normal hymenal configuration and shape of orifice (see Figs. 18.3 and 18.6), and some degree of variation in diameter that must be appreciated by the examining physician.

Vulvovaginitis has a wide variety of etiologies, many of which are noninfectious, including chemical irritation, poor perineal hygiene and/or aeration, nonabusive frictional trauma, and contact dermatitis (see Chapter 18, Gynecology). Many infectious cases are due to respiratory or gastrointestinal pathogens or are seen concurrently with urinary tract infections (see Chapter 18, Gynecology). Thus, vulvovaginitis due to sexually transmitted disease probably constitutes a minority of vulvovaginal complaints in prepubertal children. In order to avoid misdiagnosis of abuse, it is wise to defer diagnosis until definitive culture results are obtained.

The clinical findings of urethral prolapse have been mistakenly attributed to sexual abuse because the bleeding, purplish-red prolapsed mucosal tissue which protrudes between the labia minora often overlies the vaginal orifice simulating edematous traumatized redundant hymenal folds. The condition is often first discovered when blood or serosanguinous discharge is found on the diaper or underwear, as dysuria is unusual and urination is not impeded. With magnification, the urethral orifice can be seen at the center of the mass, which is soft and markedly tender. Following application of topical Xylocaine®, the prolapse can be lifted, revealing the hymen underneath. The condition is unusual, tends to occur only in children under 12 years, and two thirds of affected girls are black. The cause is unknown. Treatment requires surgical excision (see Chapter 14, Urologic Disorders).

Lichen sclerosis et atrophicus has often been mistakenly attributed to sexual abuse. The perineal skin is paper thin and hypopigmented and tears easily. Its etiology remains unknown.

As noted earlier, sexually inflicted trauma in the course of attempted or actual penetration generally results in contusions and tears of the posterior portion of the hymen and introitus. In contrast, straddle injuries produce lesions of the anterior and anterolateral portions as these are tissues most likely to be crushed between the pubic ramus and the object on which the child falls. Findings include contusions, abrasions and superficial lacerations, the latter being frequently found at the junction of the labia majora and minora. Finally, anal fissures and skin tags are most commonly sequelae of constipation. The fissures do not extend beyond the perianal skin bearing hair follicles, whereas tears produced by sodomy usually exceed this limit. Spontaneous sphincter relaxation occurring 30 seconds to 3 or 4 minutes after adopting the knee-chest position is also normal, while immediate relaxation is suspicious. Perianal erythema, hyperpigmentation, and venous engorgement also are common findings in normal children.

PASSIVE ABUSE OR NEGLECT

This type of abuse is by far the most commonly reported, accounting for over 50 percent of cases each year (55 percent in 1989). In its mildest form, this may be seen as a lack of vigilance and safeguarding of the young child who is thereby at greater risk for accidents and ingestions. In its more severe form, the patient presents with failure to thrive and developmental delay as a result of inadequate or ineffective nurturing. Typically, in infancy, the patient has been fed irregularly and inadequately, given little interactional attention, and received minimal basic care. In some cases it appears that the infant may have picked up on maternal anxiety and depression and developed secondary anorexia and autonomic disturbances of intestinal motility. Some of these infants actually begin to resist contact and become difficult to feed.

Risk factors are similar to those seen in cases of active physical abuse, with a few additions. More of these infants were unwanted, and often little or no prenatal care was sought during pregnancy. Mothers of such infants are more likely to be frankly depressed or mentally dull and to have difficulty caring for the children they already have. The incidence of maternal drug abuse as a predisposing factor has increased substantially over the past decade. Frequently, the parent appears relatively unconcerned about the child's failure to thrive, having brought the child for a minor unrelated problem such as a cold or rash, or for vomiting or constipation. Some present with a history of colic, crying "all the time," or a feeding problem. There are often glaring inconsistencies in the feeding history (e.g., "he takes 6 ounces every 4 hours" and "he takes 16 ounces in 24 hours"). Many mothers readily acknowledge that they often do not hold the baby for feedings, but instead prop the bottle on a towel or against the side of the bed. When they do hold the infant during a feeding, they put him/her down immediately afterward. A high percentage of these infants

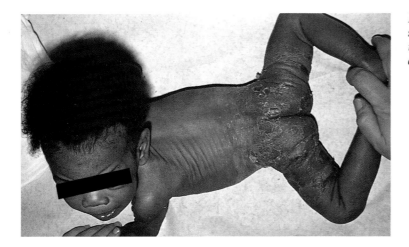

Fig. 6.52 Findings of severe neglect. Note decreased subcutaneous tissue, particularly those over the thighs and buttocks, but also over the thorax and upper arm. The patient also manifests a serious worried expression and severe diaper rash. (Courtesy of Dr. Michael Sherlock)

have received little or no professional well-child care and are behind on their immunizations.

On examination, the child is usually found to be significantly undergrown. Weight may be below the 3rd percentile, or there may be evidence of plateauing of weight gain. In long-standing cases, height and head circumference are abnormally low as well. Comparison with birth parameters and measurements made at prior visits (if any) reveal that the child has "fallen off the curve." The more severe case presents with decreased subcutaneous tissue (most notable over the buttocks and thighs), a pinched face, and sunken prominent eyes (Fig. 6.52). These children tend to look serious, smiling infrequently, appearing apathetic and withdrawn when left alone, and often lying on their backs with their arms up beside their heads. They show more interest in inanimate objects than in people, and while they appear vigilant toward people at a distance, they tend to become upset when someone approaches. They tend to avoid making eye contact, and often object to being touched, held, or cuddled. Vocalization is sparse, and development is delayed and uneven, with social milestones being behind motor development. We have even seen some who have had abnormal tone, scissoring, and posturing suggestive of a neurologic problem, which promptly abated within a few days of hospitalization. Poor hygiene, dirty clothes, and badly neglected diaper rashes are common additional findings suggestive of neglect.

The easiest, least traumatic way to confirm the diagnosis of psychosocial failure to thrive is to remove the infant from his home environment and observe his growth in a nurturing situation. Milder cases will gain weight promptly, while marasmic infants may take 1 to 2 weeks before resuming growth.

While pure psychosocial failure to thrive is the most common form of growth failure in infancy, accounting for 40 to over 50 percent of cases, up to 25 percent of cases are of purely organic origin, and in another 25 percent, growth failure is due to a combination of organic and psychosocial factors. In the latter instances, affected infants often have suffered pre- or perinatal insults that have resulted in growth retardation, chronic pulmonary disease, and/or neurologic deficits that complicate feeding and care provision. Neurologic dysfunction also may impair the infants' ability to provide interactive feedback to their mothers.

Given the frequency of psychosocial failure to thrive and combined psychosocial and organic failure to thrive, and given the stresses of caring for infants with severe organic disorders, it is essential in evaluating the infant with poor growth to obtain a thorough psychosocial and family history

as well as a detailed medical history. The latter should include information regarding duration of the problem, mode of onset, and pattern of growth. It is also helpful to inquire about how easy or difficult the parents find taking care of this child to be. A complete review of systems—gastrointestinal, cardiorespiratory, neurologic, genitourinary, and endocrine—emphasizing intake and output is often helpful. A thorough general physical examination will reveal gross abnormalities in patients with underlying CNS, cardiopulmonary, and genetic problems. A few basic screening tests (CBC and differential; urinalysis and culture; sedimentation rate; stool pH, reducing substance, and fat stain; and urea nitrogen, electrolytes, and creatinine) will rule out most other organic causes of failure to thrive. Figure 6.53 summarizes the most common causes of infantile growth failure and their major findings on evaluation.

EMOTIONAL ABUSE

This form of abuse accompanies all of the others previously described, but can also occur in isolation and can range from inattentiveness to frank rejection, scapegoating, or even terrorization. Because emotional abuse is very difficult to document since it leaves no visible stigmata, it accounts for the smallest proportion of reported cases (8 percent in 1989). Victims may present with chronic severe anxiety, agitation, hyperactivity, depression, or frank psychotic reactions. Many are socially withdrawn, have trouble relating with peers, and generally perform poorly in school. Low self-esteem is the rule. When suspected, psychological testing and psychiatric examination may prove helpful.

CONCLUSION

While treatment and follow-up are beyond the scope of an atlas of physical diagnosis, a few additional points bear emphasis. Use of a team approach including physicians, nurses, and social workers greatly facilitates evaluation of victims of abuse and their families, and reduces the burden of any one health care worker. Reporting requirements necessitate only *reasonable* grounds for suspicion, and place the onus of full investigation on state agencies. Close followup, while highly important, is often neglected, especially when patients get caught up in large bureaucratic systems. Having improved our performance on identification and documentation of cases, we must increasingly address ourselves to facilitating better long-term outcome.

Cause	Approximate Percent of All Cases	History	System-Specific Physical Findings	System-Specific Laboratory Studies
Psychosocial	50% or more	Vague inconsistent feeding history, history of bottle propping	None. May have soft neurologic signs	None
Central nervous system	13%	Poor feeding, gross developmental delay, vomiting	Grossly abnormal neurologic examination	Frequent gross abnormalities on EEG and CT scan or grossly abnormal neuromuscular function testing
Gastrointestinal	10%	Chronic vomiting and/or diarrhea, abnormal stools	Often negative, may have abdominal distention	Abnormal barium or endoscopic studies, abnormal stool examination (pH-reducing substances, fat stain, Wright stain
Cardiac	9%	Slow feeding, dyspnea and diaphoresis with feeding, restlessness and diaphoresis during sleep	Often cyanotic, or have signs of congestive heart failure	Abnormal echocardiogram, ECG, catheterization
Genetic	8%	May have positive FH or developmental delay	Often have facies typical of a syndrome, skeletal abnormalities, or neurologic abnormalities, visceromegaly	May have typical radiographic findings, chromosomal abnormalities, abnormal metabolic screens
Pulmonary	3.5%	Chronic or recurrent dyspnea with feeding, tachypnea	Grossly abnormal chest examination	Abnormal chest radiograph
Renal	3.5%	May be negative or may have history of polyuria	Often negative, may have flank masses	Abnormal urinalysis, frequently elevated BUN and creatinine, signs of renal osteodystrophy on x-rays
Endocrine	3.5%	With hypothyroidism, constipation and decreased activity level; with diabetes, polyuria, polydipsia	With hypothyroidism, no wasting but mottling, umbilical hernia, often open posterior fontanelle. With diabetes, often without specific abnormality, but may have signs of dehydration, ketotic breath, and hyperpnea. With hypopituitarism and isolated GH deficiency, growth normal until 9 months or later, then plateaus, but normal weight for height; delayed tooth eruption	Decreased T4, increased TSH; glucosuria and hyperglycemia; abnormal pituitary function studies

FIG. 6.53

BIBLIOGRAPHY

Ablin DS, Greenspan A, Reinhart M, Grix A: Differentiation of child abuse from osteogenesis imperfecta. *Am J Radiol* 1990;154:1035–1046.

Alexander RC, Schor DP, Smith WL: Magnetic resonance imaging of intracranial injuries for child abuse. *J Pediatr* 1986;109:975–979.

Bauer CH (ed): Failure to thrive.*Pediatr Ann* 1978;7(11):737-795

Bays J, et al: Changes in hymenal anatomy during examination of prepubertal girls for possible sexual abuse. *Adolesc Pediatr Gynecol* 1990;3:42–46.

Bays J: Substance abuse and child abuse: impact of addiction on the child. *Pediatr Clin North Am* 1990;37:881–904.

Berdon WE, et al: *Caffey's Pediatric X-ray Diagnosis*, ed 2. Chicago, Year Book, 1985.

Bruce DA, Zimmerman RA: Shaken impact syndrome. *Pediatr Ann* 1989;18(8):482–494.

Chadwick DL, et al: *Color Atlas of Child Sexual Abuse*. Chicago, Year Book, 1989.

Duhaime AC, Gennarelli TA, et al: The shaken baby syndrome: a clinical, pathological and biomechanical study. *J Neurosurg* 1987;66:409–415.

Green FC (ed): Incest and sexual abuse. *Pediatr Ann* 1979; 8(5):1–103.

Hammerschlag MR, et al: False positive results with the use of chlamydial antigen detection tests in the evaluation of suspected sexual abuse in children. *Pediatr Infect Dis J* 1988;7:11.

Helfer RE: The neglect of our children. *Pediatr Clin North Am* 1990;37:923–942.

Helfer RE, Kempe HC (eds): *The Battered Child*, ed 3. Chicago, University of Chicago Press, 1980.

Helfer RE, Kempe HC (eds): *Child Abuse and Neglect: the Family and the Community*. Cambridge, MA, Ballinger, 1976.

Homer MD, Ludwig S: Categorization of etiology of failure to thrive. *Am J Dis Child* 1981;135:848–851.

Huffman JW: *Gynecology of Childhood and Adolescence*, ed 2. Philadelphia, WB Saunders, 1981.

Johnson CF: Inflicted injury versus accidental injury. *Pediatr Clin North Am* 1990;37:791–814.

Kleinman PK: *Diagnostic Imaging of Child Abuse*. Baltimore, Williams & Wilkins, 1987.

Kleinman PK, Blackbourne BD, et al: Radiologic contributions to the investigation and prosecution of cases of fatal infant abuse. *N Engl J Med* 1989;320:507–511.

Kleinman PK, Marks SC, et al: The metaphyseal lesion in abused infants: a radiologic-histopathologic study. *Am J Radiol* 1986;146:895–905.

Krugman RD: Recognition of sexual abuse in children. *Pediatr Rev* 1986;8:25.

Lavy U, Bauer CH: Pathophysiology of failure to thrive and gastrointestinal disorders. *Pediatr Ann* 1978;7(11):10–33.

Levin AV, Magnusson MR, et al: Shaken baby syndrome diagnosed by magnetic resonance imaging. *Pediatr Emerg Care* 1989;5:181–186.

McCann J, et al: Perianal findings in prepubertal children selected for non-abuse: a descriptive study. *Child Abuse Negl* 1989;13:179–193.

McCann J, et al: Comparison of genital examination techniques in prepubertal girls. *Pediatrics* 1990;85:182–187.

McCann J: Use of the colposcope in childhood sexual abuse examinations. *Pediatr Clin North Am* 1990;37:863–880.

Merten DF, Carpenter BLM: Radiologic imaging of inflicted injury in the child abuse syndrome. *Pediatr Clin North Am* 1990;37:815–838.

Muram D: Child sexual abuse: genital tract findings in prepubertal girls. I. The unaided medical examination. *Am J Obstet Gynecol* 1989;160:328–332.

Neinstein LS, et al: Non-sexual transmission of sexually transmitted diseases: an infrequent occurrence. *Pediatrics* 1984;74:67–76.

Newberger EH: Pediatric interview assessment of child abuse: challenges and opportunities. *Pediatr Clin North Am* 1990;37:943–954.

Paradise JE: The medical evaluation of the sexually abused child. *Pediatr Clin North Am* 1990;37:839–862.

Reece RM: Unusual manifestations of child abuse. *Pediatr Clin North Am* 1990;37:905–922.

Rosenn DW, Loeb LS, Jura MB: Differentiation of organic from nonorganic failure to thrive syndrome in infancy. *Pediatrics* 1980;66:698–704.

Sills RH: Failure to thrive. *Am J Dis Child* 1978;132:967–969.

Thoennes N, et al: The extent, nature and validity of sexual abuse allegations in custody/visitation disputes. *Child Abuse Negl* 1990;14:151–163.

West MH, Billings JD, Frair J: Ultraviolet photography: bite marks on human skin and suggested technique for exposure and development of reflective ultraviolet photography. *J Forensic Sci* 1987;32:1204–1213.

Woodlong BA, Kossosis PD: Sexual misuse. *Pediatr Clin North Am* 1981;28:481–499.

PEDIATRIC RHEUMATOLOGY

Andrew H. Urbach, M.D.

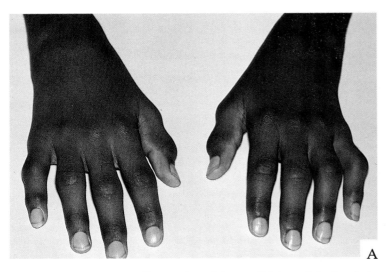

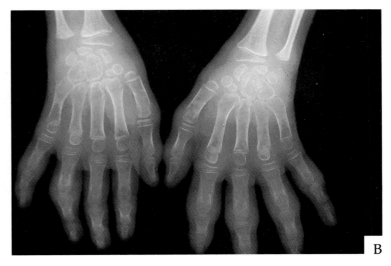

FIG. 7.1 Swelling and inflammation of the small joints of the hands in a patient with polyarticular juvenile rheumatoid arthritis (JRA). **A**, note the inability to fully extend the fingers. **B**, on x-ray, fusiform swelling of the proximal interphalageal (PIP) joints with demineralization, and diffuse soft-tissue swelling are seen.

The collagen vascular diseases are a diverse group of disorders associated with inflammation of the connective tissues. Their etiologies and pathogenesis remain largely unknown at this time. Despite advances in the laboratory diagnosis of these entities, many of the collagen vascular diseases are still diagnosed by the clinical constellation of physical findings with which they present.

Most of the collagen vascular diseases manifest themselves as distinct clinical entities and can be diagnosed as such; however, overlap occurs. This chapter illustrates the more distinctive clinical features of these rather unique disorders.

JUVENILE RHEUMATOID ARTHRITIS

Juvenile rheumatoid arthritis (JRA) is the most common of the collagen vascular diseases in children. Its true incidence is not known, though it is estimated that there are approximately 250,000 affected persons in the United States alone.

The first clear description of this entity was presented by George Still in 1897. He postulated multiple etiologies for JRA, and this concept is still supported today. JRA can present as systemic, polyarticular, or pauciarticular disease, all having inflammation of the synovial tissue as one of their cardinal features. Synovium is usually hypertrophied and joint effusions may occur. On physical examination one may note joint swelling (Fig. 7.1), with loss of normal anatomical landmarks, tenderness, decreased joint mobility, warmth, erythema, and joint deformity (Fig. 7.2). It is typical for the child with JRA to present with constant and daily pain. Symptoms often develop gradually over a period of weeks or months before evaluation occurs. "Morning stiffness" is often reported with the loosening up of the "gel phenomena" as the day progresses. Similar symptoms occur after inactivity such as napping and prolonged sitting. Weather changes may exacerbate symptoms, though they have no impact on the underlying pathology of the disease. Arthralgia without actual joint swelling is a common presentation of JRA. Extreme pain, intense erythema, and extremely warm joints should suggest not JRA, but rather an infectious etiology for this dramatic presentation. The child with acute rheumatic fever often presents with exquisitely tender migratory joint findings with very acute onset. Again, this presentation should direct the clinician away from the diagno-

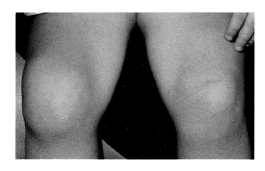

FIG. 7.2 This toddler with pauciarticular JRA has unilateral knee swelling with slight erythema. The right knee demonstrates loss of the normal anatomical landmarks.

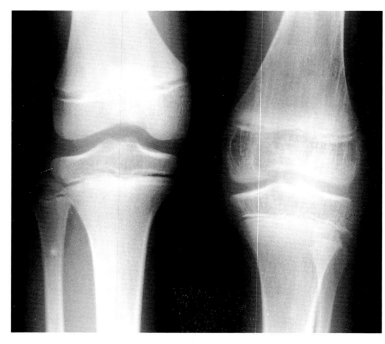

FIG. 7.3
Demineralization of the left femur and tibia with soft-tissue swelling and hypertrophy of the epiphyses secondary to hyperemia.

CLASSIFICATION OF JRA

Type	%	Characteristics	Sex Ratio	Rheumatoid Factor/ANA	Iridocyclitis	Severe Arthritis
Systemic	20	Systemic symptoms; large (L) & small (S) joints affected	M > F	– /–	–	25%
Polyarticular						
RF –	25	Early or late onset of symptoms; L/S	F > M	– / 25%	–	10–15%
RF +	10	Late onset of symptoms; L/S Rheumatoid nodules	F > M	+ / 50–75%	–	Majority
Pauciarticular						
Early onset	25	Few joints; hips & SI joints not involved	F > M	– / 60%	50%	Not usually severe
Late onset	15	Few joints; SI, hips involved, HLA B27 75%	M > F	– / –	Occasional	Ankylosing spondylitis sometimes present

FIG. 7.4 (Adapted from Schaller JG:Juvenile rheumatiod arthritis.Pediatr Rev 1980;2(6):163-174)

sis of JRA. Despite objective arthritis, the JRA patient may not present with pain. When inflammation persists for a long enough period of time, destruction of the articular surface and bony structures may occur (Fig. 7.3). Due to the poor regenerative properties of articular cartilage, these deformities may be permanent. Fortunately, most cases of JRA do not have permanent joint deformity associated with them.

The group of diseases placed under the rubric JRA combines diverse entities, generally divided into three categories:

1. Systemic onset disease.
2. Polyarticular disease: rheumatoid factor negative and positive.
3. Pauciarticular disease: early childhood onset and late childhood onset.

This classification of disease is based on its presentation during the first 6 months of illness (Fig. 7.4).

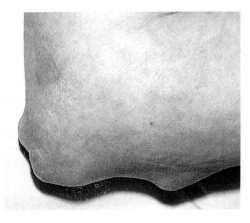

FIG. 7.6 Subcutaneous nodules over the pressure points of the elbow.

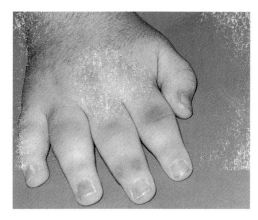

FIG. 7.7 Swelling of the PIP and MCP joints in this patient with polyarticular JRA produces spindle-shaped fingers.

FIG. 7.5 Rash of systemic onset JRA is erythematous, macular, and often evanescent. It can be more prominent during periods of fever. The rash was pruritic in this patient.

Systemic Onset JRA

Systemic onset JRA (Still disease) represents 20 percent of all children with JRA. Fever, rash, irritability, arthritis, and visceral involvement dominate the clinical presentation. The fever usually spikes greater than 39°C and often can occur twice daily. Chills are associated with fever, but rigors do not occur. Though the late afternoon is a typical time for a temperature spike, many other patterns may occur. Other manifestations of systemic onset JRA such as rash and joint symptoms may wax and wane during febrile periods.

The rash of JRA is macular, 2 to 6 mm in diameter, evanescent, salmon, or red with slightly irregular margins (Fig. 7.5). There is often an area of central clearing. The rash usually occurs on the trunk and proximal extremities, but may also be distal in distribution with palms and soles affected. Though the rash generally does not produce discomfort, some patients report pruritus. Superficial mild trauma to the skin or exposure to warmth and stress may precipitate the rash. While rash is seen with polyarticular JRA, it does not occur with pauciarticular disease.

Arthritis and arthralgia almost invariably occur at some time during the presentation and often will secure the already suspected diagnosis. When fever of unknown origin is the sole initial presentation of systemic onset JRA, the diagnosis must remain tentative. Myalgia can be prominent early, as can hepatosplenomegaly and lymphadenopathy. Serositis, pleuritis, pericarditis, hyperbilirubinemia, liver enzyme elevations, leukocytosis, and anemia have also been seen with this illness. Only 25 percent of this group of JRA patients progress to have chronic joint symptoms.

Polyarticular Onset JRA

Polyarticular onset of disease accounts for 35 percent of all children with JRA. Five or more joints need to be involved in the absence of prominent systemic signs and symptoms. There appear to be two subgroups within this category: rheumatoid factor seronegative and seropositive. The seropositive group is felt to be nearly identical to the adult entity of rheumatoid arthritis (RA). Onset usually occurs after age 8 and, as with seronegative disease, females predominate; 80 percent of all adult RA patients are seropositive.

In addition to the joint findings of warmth, swelling, erythema, and tenderness seen in both subgroups, seropositive disease provides some additional clues to diagnosis. The subcutaneous nodules which occur in seropositive disease are firm, nontender nodules on the skin surface with a predilection for pressure points (Fig. 7.6). The most common location is the elbow, but the nodules also occur on the heels, hands, knees, ears, scapulae, sacrum, and buttocks. Other features of seropositive disease may include cutaneous vasculitis, Felty syndrome (leukopenia and splenomegaly), and Sjögren syndrome (keratoconjunctivitis sicca and parotitis).

The onset of polyarthritis may be either insidious or acute. While the seropositive group progresses to destructive synovitis and a prolonged chronic course in more than half of the patients, children with seronegative disease often have remarkably little permanent joint destruction relative to their duration of symptoms. Any synovial joint may be involved in the inflammatory process, including the knees, wrists, elbows, ankles, the small joints of the feet, the proximal interphalangeal (PIP) joints, and the metacarpophalangeal (MCP) joints (Fig. 7.7). The lumbosacral spine is usually spared.

Pauciarticular Onset JRA

Pauciarticular onset JRA is strictly defined as onset of disease in fewer than five joints, though clearly children with additional joints may informally belong in this category. The large joints (knees, ankles, and elbows) are often asymmetrically involved. Two subgroups seem to exist under this heading:

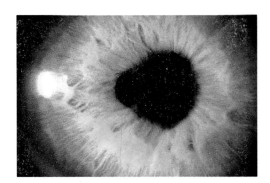

FIG. 7.8 Iridocyclitis with an irregular pupil in a patient with pauciarticular JRA. Note synechiae projecting posteriorly toward the lens.

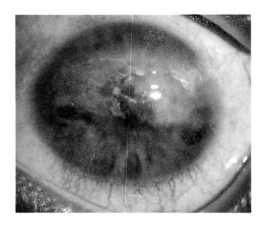

FIG. 7.9 Band keratopathy in a patient with JRA. Note the calcium deposits in Bowman's layer.

FIG. 7.10 Ankylosing spondylitis with fusion of C2, C3, C4 occurring during an 18-month period between **A** and **B**.

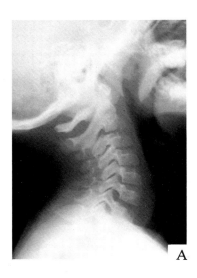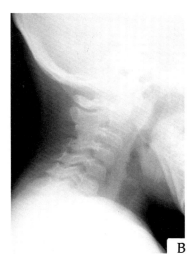

A
B

early and late onset. In early-onset pauciarticular disease there is female predominance, the ANA is positive in 25 percent, and onset is usually before the fifth birthday. As with polyarticular disease, systemic symptoms do not dominate the clinical picture. If the disease does not progress to polyarticular involvement within the first half-year of illness, the patient often will maintain the pauciarticular pattern. While joint disease may be visible, pain is rarely severe. This disease entity is particularly unique because of its 50 percent association with chronic iridocyclitis. In its earliest stages, diagnosis often depends on slit-lamp examination, though photophobia, eye pain, and erythema can occur. The first clinical sign is cellular exudate in the anterior chamber. If the uveitis is left untreated, synechiae (adhesions) between the iris and lens may develop, leading to an irregular and poorly functioning pupil (Fig. 7.8). Further along in the clinical course, band keratopathy (calcium deposits in the cornea) (Fig. 7.9) may occur, as well as cataracts or glaucoma. For these reasons eye examinations three to four times yearly are recommended early in the disease's course for high-risk patients, so that visual handicap does not result. Ophthalmologic complications may not parallel the activity of the arthritis.

While fulfilling the criteria of JRA, late onset pauciarticular disease may be more logically placed among the spondyloarthropathies (Fig. 7.10). Affected patients are generally males, older than 8 years, and there is involvement of hips, knees, ankles, and foot joints. Onset can be acute and of a

more prolonged nature in children with a family history of spondyloarthropathies or associated conditions. In the child who progresses to lumbar and sacral joint disease, the designation spondyloarthropathy is appropriate. Other children will manifest findings of Reiter syndrome (a seronegative asymmetric arthropathy associated with urethritis, cervicitis, dysentery, inflammatory eye disease, or other mucocutaneous disease) and some will go on to have limitation of spinal flexion. Still others will never progress to a spondyloarthropathy, and hence the designation of JRA will continue to be more appropriate.

Extra-Articular Manifestations of JRA

Many extra-articular features of JRA have been reported. The more common ones are listed in Figure 7.11. Linear growth retardation is well known to occur in the child with active JRA. The degree of retardation and the ultimate prognosis for reaching adult height are related to the severity and duration of inflammation. During early illness, bony development may be advanced while later in the course of the illness the opposite may be true. Premature epiphyseal fusion may occur. In addition, steroids themselves may inhibit linear growth. Careful use of standardized growth curves will assist in the early detection of growth failure. This may, in turn, guide one's long-term therapeutic approach.

EXTRA-ARTICULAR MANIFESTATIONS OF JRA

	Polyarticular (%)	Pauciarticular (%)	Systemic Disease (%)
Fever	30	0	100
Rheumatoid rash	10	0	95
Rheumatoid nodules	10	0	5
Hepatosplenomegaly	10	0	85
Lymphadenopathy	5	0	70
Chronic uveitis	5	20	0
Pericarditis	5	0	35
Pleuritis	1	0	20
Abdominal pain	1	0	10

FIG. 7.11 (Adapted from: Cassidy JT: Textbooks of Pediatric Rheumatology New York, John Wiley, 1982)

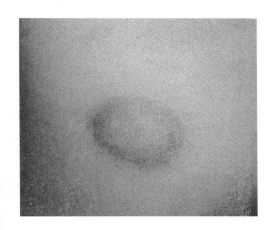

FIG. 7.12 Erythema chronicum migrans in a patient with Lyme arthritis. The lesion may be a large erythematous macule with central clearing, occurring singly or multiply.

Cardiac involvement occurs in over one-third of systemic onset JRA patients. Pericarditis, myocarditis, and endocarditis all occur, with pericarditis being the most common. The presence of chest pain, a friction rub, tachycardia, dyspnea, and supportive x-ray findings may all occur. These episodes may last for weeks to months and are usually associated with a generalized flare of disease.

A variety of other extra-articular manifestations, including hepatosplenomegaly and lymphadenopathy are particularly common in systemic disease. Tenosynovitis and myositis (without enzyme elevation) occur, as does a generalized vasculitis. Many clinicians report hematuria and proteinuria as well.

Differential Diagnosis

Because JRA is largely a clinical diagnosis, very strict clinical criteria have been set to make the diagnosis of JRA. Most authors suggest the presence of objective joint findings (arthritis) for a minimum of 6 consecutive weeks coupled with the exclusion of other causes of arthritis in children. The extra-articular features of JRA, as discussed earlier, may solidify the diagnosis purely because of their distinctiveness, that is, uveitis and rheumatoid nodules.

Because of its destructive nature, pyogenic arthritis (Staphylococcus, Streptococcus, Haemophilus influenzae, etc.) must be ruled out in any child with active joint disease. The intensely red and tender joint, well beyond the degree one usually sees with JRA, should raise one's suspicion of a bacterial pathogen. This, combined with systemic symptoms of infection (fever, chills, malaise) should prompt one to perform an arthrocentesis early in the course of the illness. If the joint in question is the hip, one's suspicion should be even higher because of the rarity with which the hip is the first affected joint in JRA. Other infectious etiologies include Lyme arthritis. This spirochetal form of arthritis is tick-borne, and usually affects the knee, elbow, or wrist. Malaise, fever, myalgia, lymphadenopathy, headache, meningismus, and weakness may also occur in the first phase of the illness. The distinctive rash, known as erythema chronicum migrans (Fig. 7.12), begins as an erythematous macule or papule. After this clears, the borders of the lesion expand to form an erythematous circular lesion which can be as large as 30 cm in diameter. Other manifestations of Lyme disease include neurologic complications such as seventh nerve palsy, meningitis, radiculoneuritis, and the cardiac manifestations of heart block and myopericarditis. Salmonella, Shigella, Yersinia, and Campylobacter should also be considered. A multitude of viruses are known to cause arthritis. These include rubella; hepatitis B; adenovirus; the herpes viruses, including Epstein-Barr virus, cytomegalo-virus, varicella-zoster, and herpes simplex; parvoviruses; mumps; and enteroviruses as echovirus and coxsackievirus Some have been directly recovered from joints, while others cause a "reactive" arthritis and may not directly affect the joint.

Malignancies such as neuroblastoma and leukemia may appear to present with joint disease. More careful evaluation will generally reveal bone pain. Sickle cell disease, particularly in the form of dactylitis, can have prominent digit involvement. Inflammatory bowel disease, acute rheumatic fever, hemophilia, trauma, hypermobility syndrome, psoriasis, and Henoch-Schönlein purpura must also be thought of in the patient with arthritis. All of the collagen vascular diseases can have significant joint disease; however, their clinical features and laboratory tests can usually distinguish them from JRA.

DERMATOMYOSITIS

Dermatomyositis (DM) is an uncommon but distinctive disease which accounts for approximately 5 percent of all collagen vascular diseases in children. Though it was first described in 1887, its etiology remains largely unknown. The hallmarks of this entity are various skin manifestations coupled with nonsuppurative inflammation of muscle. Dermatomyositis affecting the adult generally carries a worse prognosis than if encountered in the pediatric age group. There is no association with malignancy in pediatric DM patients, as there is in adults. Nevertheless, vasculitis of varying severity is often seen earlier in the course of the illness in children and

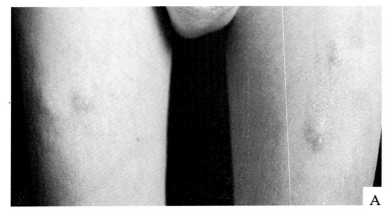

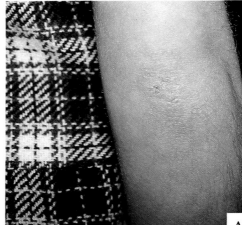

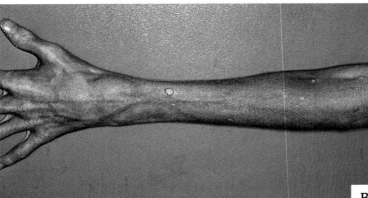

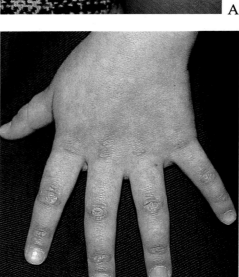

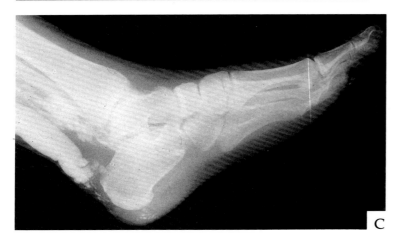

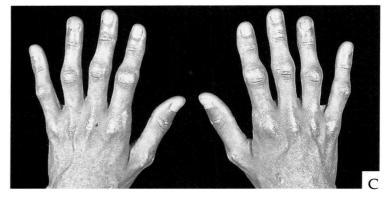

FIG. 7.13 **A,** nodular calcific densities in thighs of patients with dermatomyositis (DM). **B,** atrophy, hyperpigmentation, and subcutaneous calcium deposits in the arm of a patient with "burned-out" DM. **C,** radiologic evidence of soft-tissue calcification in a patient with DM.

there is a relatively high incidence of calcinosis (nodular calcium deposits) in nonvisceral tissues such as muscle (Fig. 7.13). Pressure points and severely affected soft tissues are particularly susceptible.

Though the age range for DM is broad, the 5- to 14-year-old child is particularly at risk. Females predominate by a 2:1 ratio. There is no racial bias nor is there any evidence of a familial predisposition.

Clinically, patients usually present with fatigue and symmetrical proximal muscle weakness, particularly affecting the hip girdle and legs. Though shoulders and arms are often involved, this may not be as easily detected in the child. The first complaints are often inability to climb stairs and distur-

bances of gait. Dysphagia, dysphonia, and dyspnea may occur if the respective muscles for these functions are affected. The involved muscles may be tender and indurated, with a superficially edematous appearance. A pathognomonic rash seen in three-quarters of DM patients can confirm the diagnosis. Even in the absence of this distinctive rash, all patients will have some degree of cutaneous disease. The rash is symmetrical and erythematous, with atrophic changes located over the extensor surfaces of the knees, elbows, PIP and MCP joints, and Gottron's papules (Fig. 7.14). Other features of the rash include a violaceous discoloration of the eyelids, eyelid edema, a scaly red rash in a malar distribution, and telangiectasia (Fig. 7.15), and the characteristic dystrophic skin changes.

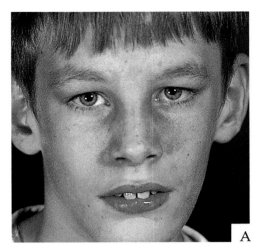

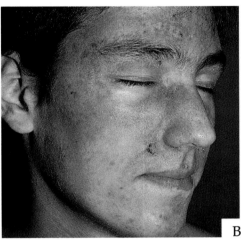

FIG. 7.15 **A**, facial rash of DM with a violaceous color around the eyes and malar region. **B**, more severe, erythematous, scaly rash involving almost the entire face. Note involvement of nasolabial folds.

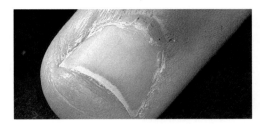

FIG. 7.16 Nail bed telangiectasia. Erythema can be seen around the nail edge. The pinpoint telangiectasia may require a magnifying lens to identify.

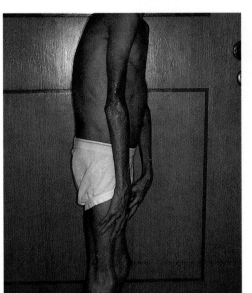

FIG. 7.17 "Burned-out" chronic DM. Limbs are thin, with muscle and skin atrophy. Diffuse contractures have occurred.

As opposed to systemic lupus erythematosus, which also has a malar rash, the nasolabial folds are not spared in dermatomyositis. One also sees nail bed telangiectasia (Fig. 7.16), digital ulceration, and hyper- or hypopigmentation of the skin. Sunlight may worsen the rash and the myositis. The rash may precede muscle disease. However, because of the pathognomonic features of the rash, the diagnosis of DM can often be suspected before other overt symptoms occur. Constitutional symptoms such as anorexia, malaise, weight loss, and fever may be present with this entity. The illness may progress at variable rates in different patients; however, the majority of patients have a more insidious rather than acute course. Unfortunately, long delays in diagnosis can occur, particularly in the insidious group. Other more uncommon findings are mouth ulcers, retinitis, hepatosplenomegaly, pulmonary infiltrates, myocarditis, and pericarditis. Although calcinosis occurs in 40 percent of children with dermatomyositis, it does not occur during the acute phase of the illness. On the other hand, in chronic indolent disease, it may be the presenting complaint.

The clinical diagnosis of DM can be supported by an abnormal EMG, muscle biopsy, elevated muscle enzymes [creatine kinase (CK), aspartate aminotransferase (AST, SGOT), aldolase], elevated ESR, and a positive ANA. Steroids are the mainstay of therapy and their early use will often preserve muscle function and minimize the potentially destructive nature of this illness (Fig. 7.17).

SYSTEMIC VASCULITIS

The vasculitides are a broad group of disorders with a common pathology characterized by blood vessel inflammation. The type of inflammation, organ systems affected, and size of the vessels vary with each disease entity. Henoch-Schönlein purpura (HSP) is an example of small-vessel involvement. Polyarteritis nodosa, infantile polyarteritis nodosa, and Kawasaki syndrome represent medium- and small-vessel disease. Cranial arteritis and Takayasu's arteritis are examples of giant-cell arteritis. Immunologic markers often are associated with vasculitic disorders. Circulating immune complexes, rheumatoid factor, antinuclear antibodies, elevated immunoglobulins, and depressed complement are examples of frequently seen immunologic markers.

Henoch-Schönlein Purpura

Henoch-Schönlein syndrome consists of nonthrombocytopenic purpura, arthritis and arthralgia, gastrointestinal symptomatology, and a variety of renal findings. Seventy-five percent of cases occur in children less than 10 years of age with the median age being 5 years. Most authors report that this syndrome occurs after an upper respiratory infection or other viral illness, though HSP has been reported following insect bites, dietary allergens, and numerous drugs. There does not appear to be a familial predilection, and all races have been affected.

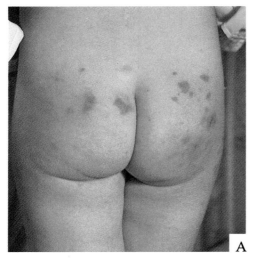

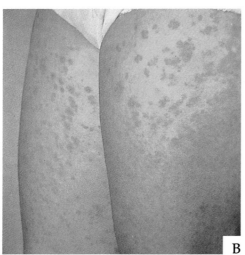

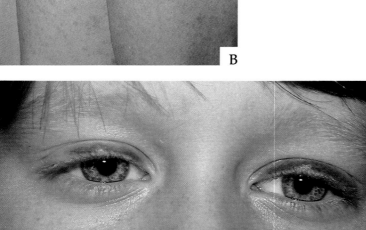

FIG. 7.18 The distinctive rash of Henoch-Schönlein purpura (HSP). *A* and *B*, it characteristically involves the buttocks and lower extremities, with purpuric coalescent lesions. Note the striking waist-down distribution. *C*, eyelid involvement has been reported.

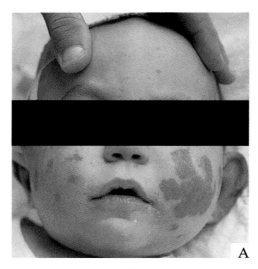

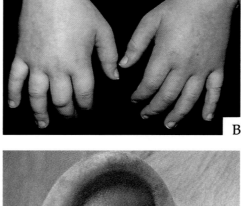

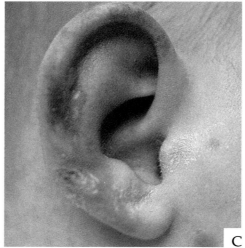

FIG. 7.19 An infant with HSP. *A*, the rash may occur on the face along with edema. *B*, rash and edema may be present in the extremities. *C*, ulceration and vesicles are an unusual manifestation of HSP.

The clinical picture of HSP is that of a previously well child who acutely develops a distinctive skin rash, arthritis, and abdominal pain. The skin rash allows for definitive diagnosis and hence it is said to occur in all patients with HSP. Fifty percent of patients present with the rash, which usually involves the buttocks, lower extremities, and the hands (waist-down distribution) with the trunk and face generally being spared (Fig. 7.18). The lesions begin as petechial or approximately 0.5-cm purpuric areas which coalesce and become confluent with nearby lesions. They begin as red macules or papules and progress with time to purplish and then brownish areas. Typically, varying stages of eruption are simultaneously pres-

ent. On occasion, ulceration and vesicles will occur. Some patients will have lesions that mimic urticaria and about 25 percent will have subcutaneous edema (Fig. 7.19). The edema is nonpitting, painless, evanescent, and most commonly affects the hands (Fig. 7.19B) and feet. The child less than 2 years of age is most likely to have edema as a feature of this illness. The younger child is also more likely to display facial involvement (Fig. 7.19A,C).

Approximately 85 percent of patients will display some form of gastrointestinal symptomatology. Simple colicky abdominal pain can be the only symptom, but its severity can raise physician concerns about more threatening abdominal complica-

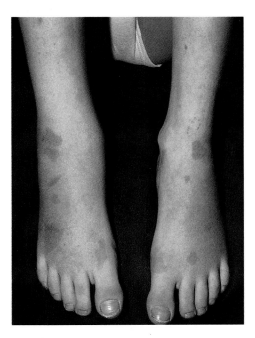

FIG. 7.20 The arthritis of HSP. Note the swelling of the right ankle in addition to the purpuric rash.

FIG. 7.21 (Adapted by permission from Center for Disease Control: Kawasaki disease New York. MMWR 1980;29:61–63)

tions. Massive gastrointestinal hemorrhage or intussusception occurs in 5 percent of patients and complete perforation rarely occurs. Melanotic stools, vomiting, ileus, and hematemesis may be present as well. In rare circumstances abdominal pain can precede the other features of HSP, making diagnosis impossible until the characteristic rash appears.

The periarticular swelling that occurs presents as arthritis or arthralgia and is a part of HSP in three-quarters of reported cases. Knees and ankles are the most common sites of involvement (Fig. 7.20). Warmth and erythema are not usually associated with the pain and swelling that occur. The joints are never affected permanently and this feature of HSP generally resolves in several days. As with the gastrointestinal symptoms, arthritis can precede the rash. For this reason, one needs to consider HSP in the child with acute onset of arthritis.

While renal involvement is detected in only half of HSP patients, it is important because the degree of renal pathology generally affects the patient's ultimate prognosis. Renal manifestations can be as mild as hematuria or proteinuria, but they may be as severe as nephrotic syndrome, nephritis, and, in 5 percent of patients, end-stage renal disease. Patients will usually declare themselves within several months, but cases of renal failure and hypertension have occurred many years after the initial illness. Berger's disease (IgA glomerulonephritis) is felt by many to be HSP without rash and, hence, an alternative manifestation of the same pathologic process.

Other features of HSP include low-grade fever, malaise, scrotal swelling with pain, cerebral vasculitis, CNS bleeding, seizures, nosebleeds, parotitis, pancreatitis, and cardiopulmonary disease.

The course of the illness varies with age. The majority of patients are over their initial illness in 4 weeks; however, 50 percent will have at least one recurrence. Recurrences generally are limited to cutaneous and mild abdominal symptomatology.

Clotting functions and platelet counts in these patients are normal. The presence of IgA complexes in the glomeruli, skin, and serum of infected individuals may be a clue to diagnosis. Elevated serum IgA levels are found in about half of affected patients. Since there are no diagnostic laboratory examinations for this syndrome, the history and physical examination provide clues to the successful recognition of HSP.

Kawasaki Syndrome

Although the exact etiology of Kawasaki syndrome has eluded investigators, the clinical features and natural history of this distinctive vasculitic entity are very well described. The need to rapidly recognize the presentation of this disease is heightened by its potentially devastating cardiac sequelae. New developments in treatment appear to alter the incidence of these sequelae; therefore, the early recognition of Kawasaki syndrome may favorably impact on morbidity and mortality.

Kawasaki syndrome, first described in 1967 by Tomisaku Kawasaki, describes a unique constellation of clinical findings labeled as mucocutaneous lymph node syndrome. This multisystem syndrome was independently described by Melish in 1974 in Hawaii. Since that time the syndrome has been recognized in all racial groups worldwide. Individuals of Asian ancestry are most commonly affected, and Japanese children have a particularly high incidence within this group. The risk to black children is greater than the risk to white children. Males are more commonly affected than females by a ratio of 1.6 to 1. The peak age is 6 months to 2 years, with 75 percent of cases occurring in children younger than 5 years. Middle and upper socioeconomic classes are over-represented. A variety of etiologies have been suggested as the cause of Kawasaki syndrome, but all have fallen short of complete acceptance. Currently, many investigators suspect a microbial agent as the most likely culprit.

The clinical features of the syndrome are remarkably constant. The Center for Disease Control currently defines the entity as illustrated in Figure 7.21. However, cases of incom-

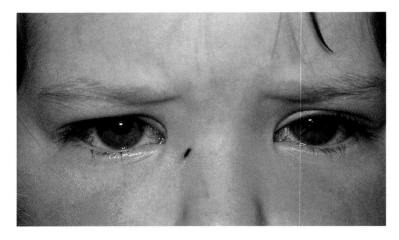

FIG. 7.22 Nonexudative, nonulcerative, bulbar conjunctivitis.

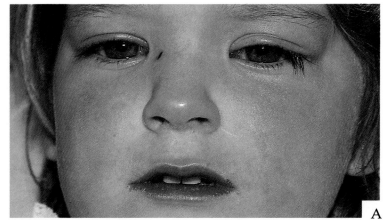

A

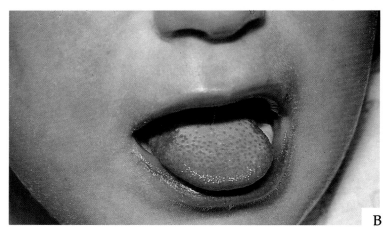

B

FIG. 7.23 **A**, erythematous, cracked lips and **B**, "strawberry tongue" are oral findings of Kawasaki syndrome.

plete Kawasaki syndrome have been encountered recently, adding uncertainty to the clinician's approach to diagnosis. As the ability to diagnose Kawasaki syndrome improves, one would expect a broadening of the clinical spectrum of the disease. For now, the shrewd clinician must consider this diagnosis when any of the diagnostic criteria are met, particularly in children under the age of 1 year. The importance of appropriate clinical suspicion in the *forme fruste* of the disease cannot be overemphasized in the current climate of new and encouraging therapeutic modalities geared to prevent cardiac sequelae.

The course of the illness is triphasic: acute (up to 11 days), subacute (11 to 21 days), and convalescent (21 to 60 days). The acute phase is characterized by fever, irritability, conjunctivitis, oropharyngeal erythema, rash, lymphadenopathy, and distal extremity edema and erythema. The onset of fever is sudden, often spiking as high as 40°C. It is remitting in character, with a mean duration of 12 days in the untreated individual. Some patients may continue to be febrile for 30 days or more without therapy. Fever generally precedes other clinical signs and symptoms by 1 to 2 days. The conjunctivitis appears early in the progression of the illness. It is nonexudative, nonulcerative with bulbar predominance, and can persist for 3 to 5 weeks (Fig. 7.22). Additional eye findings include anterior uveitis or acute iridocyclitis reported in 83 percent of patients during the first week of illness and 66 percent after the first week. The anterior uveitis is self-limited. Because it is not seen in many entities in the differential diagnosis of Kawasaki syndrome, its presence may be a helpful diagnostic tool. Oral findings include red, cracked, fissured lips, "strawberry tongue," and diffuse mouth erythema (Fig. 7.23). These findings may last for several weeks as well. The rash of Kawasaki syndrome may manifest itself in many forms: scarlatiniform, morbilliform (Fig. 7.24), macular and papular erythema, urticarial plaques, or even pustular. It can be pruritic, but the presence of vesicles, erythroderma, petechiae, or purpura should suggest another diagnosis. A predilection for involvement of intertriginous areas, particularly the perineum, has been noted (Fig. 7.25). Peeling generally occurs several days prior to the desquamation of fingers and toes. A particularly striking feature of the acute phase of the syndrome is erythema and edema of the hands (Fig. 7.26) and feet, often associated with refusal to walk. The characteristic desquamation of fingers and toes beginning at the nail-fingertip junction occurs between 11 and 21 days during the subacute phase (Fig. 7.27). Fingertip peel-

FIG. 7.24 Morbilliform rash is one possible manifestation.

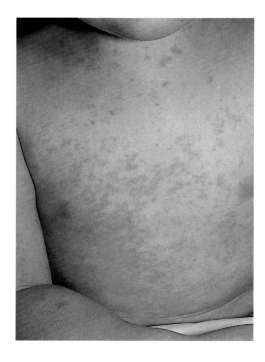

ing precedes toetip peeling, but only during a brief interval. In its most dramatic form the entire distal extremity can peel. Several months after the acute phase of illness, transverse grooves called Beau's lines are noted in the fingernails (Fig. 7.28). Although the initial syndrome was named mucocutaneous lymph node syndrome, the presence of a 1.5-cm or

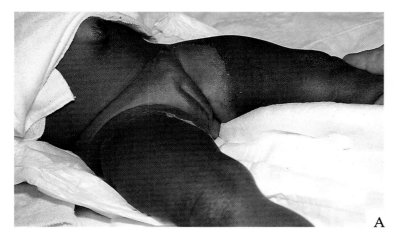

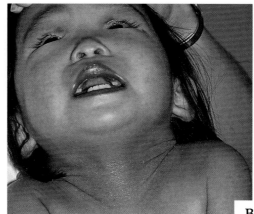

FIG. 7.25 **A,** perineal rash with peeling and **B,** neck rash with peeling. Note that peeling of intertriginous rash occurs prior to extremity peeling.

A

B

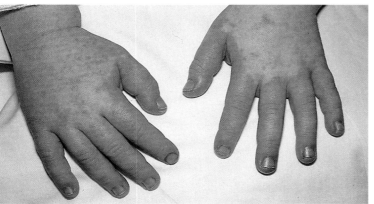

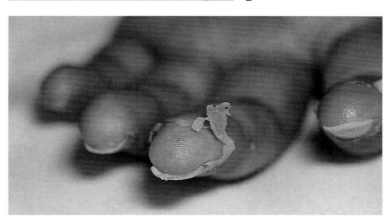

FIG. 7.26 Swollen, erythematous hands. Note fusiform appearance.

FIG. 7.27 Fingertip and toetip peeling in subacute phase of Kawasaki syndrome. (Adapted by permission from Center for Disease Control: Kawasaki disease New York. MMWR 1980;29:61–63)

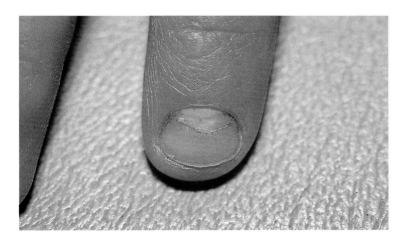

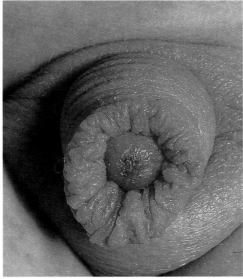

FIG. 7.29 Inflammation of the urethral meatus (often associated with sterile pyuria).

FIG. 7.28 Beau's lines of fingernails in the convalescent phase of Kawasaki syndrome.

greater cervical lymph node is the least consistent feature, occurring in only 50 percent of children.

While many of the aforementioned features are considered central to the diagnosis of Kawasaki syndrome, it is often the associated features of the disease that add credence to the diagnosis. During the acute phase, an "early" form of arthritis (20 percent) and arthralgia (40 percent) occur. Both the small and large joints are affected. Urethritis and inflammation of the urethral meatus occur and generally are accompanied by pyuria (Fig. 7.29). Central nervous system changes such as lethargy, meningismus, aseptic meningitis, facial nerve palsy, and paralysis of extremities have been described. Diarrhea, vomiting, abdominal pain, and hepatitis are frequent gastrointestinal features seen early in the illness. Acute cardiac features include pericarditis, pericardial effusion, myocarditis, mitral insufficiency, and congestive heart failure. Because of the dynamic nature of this syndrome, meticulous and frequent physical examinations are essential.

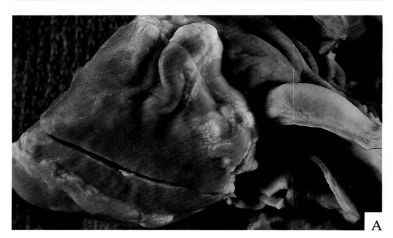

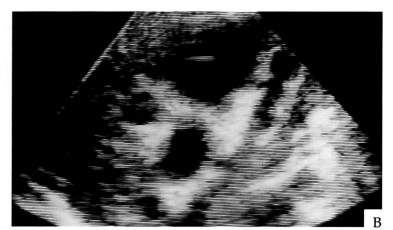

FIG. 7.30 Transient dilatation of the gallbladder noted by ultrasonography.

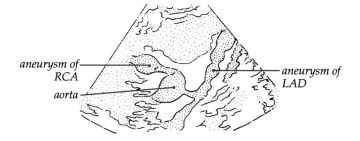

FIG. 7.31 **A,** coronary artery aneurysms. **B,** cross-sectional echocardiogram in the short-axis view of the aortic root in a patient with Kawasaki syndrome shows multiple large saccular aneurysms in the left anterior descending artery (LAD), as well as in the right coronary artery (RCA).

As alluded to earlier, the subacute phase of Kawasaki syndrome witnesses the distinctive fingertip and toetip peeling (see Fig. 7.27). Additionally, pancreatitis, transient gallbladder dilatation (Fig. 7.30), late-onset arthritis, and thrombocytosis also occurs. It is also a time when arterial aneurysms occur in axillary, iliac, renal, hepatic, cerebral, brachial, femoral, and, most notably, coronary arteries.

The combination of coronary artery aneurysms (Fig. 7.31) and thrombocytosis places patients in the subacute phase at particular risk for myocardial infarction. Approximately 20 percent of untreated patients develop coronary artery aneurysms. Although many regress spontaneously, 1 or 2 percent of affected individuals will die from related complications. Eighty-five percent of these deaths occur during the first 10 to 40 days of illness. The natural history of these aneurysms results in thromboembolism and vessel occlusion, and leads to myocardial infarction in a small group of patients. Others develop coronary artery stenosis or persistent asymptomatic

aneurysms of varying sizes. Particularly worrisome indicators for the development of aneurysms include male gender, age younger than 12 months, fever lasting more than 2 weeks, recurrent fever after defervescence, recurrence of rash, exaggerated leukocytosis and sedimentation rate, and cardiac rhythm disturbances. Current therapeutic interventions with aspirin and intravenous immunoglobulins appear to have significantly decreased the risk of cardiac complications.

The convalescent phase is apparently a period of relatively low risk, though the long-term impact of coronary artery vasculitis, and the incidence and severity of atherosclerotic heart disease remain a concern.

In addition to the clinical features described above, laboratory studies also may be helpful in the diagnosis of Kawasaki syndrome.

Differential diagnosis includes scarlet fever (both streptococcal and staphylococcal), staphylococcal scalded skin syndrome, toxic shock syndrome, leptospirosis, disseminated yersiniosis,

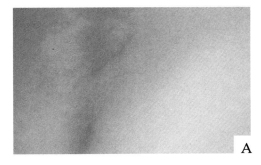

FIG. 7.32 Forms of morphea. **A,** hypopigmented plaque of scleroderma with skin atrophy. **B,** "salt and pepper" appearance of a plaque in a patient with scleroderma. Note the hyperpigmentation within the hypopigmented lesion.

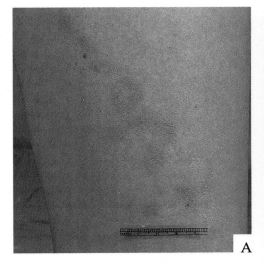

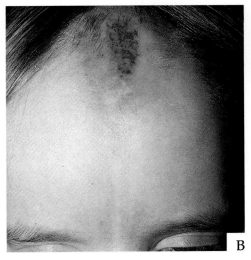

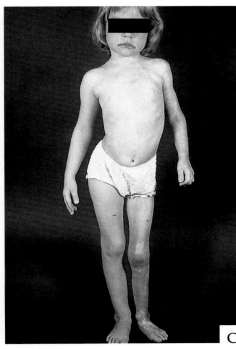

FIG. 7.33 **A,** linear scleroderma. Localized involvement of a dermatome with hyperpigmentation. **B,** an unusual form of local scleroderma affecting the scalp, termed "en coup de sabre" (stroke of the saber). **C,** linear scleroderma affecting the left side of the body.

Rocky Mountain spotted fever, rubeola, enteroviral infection, Reiter's disease, juvenile rheumatoid arthritis, and systemic lupus erythematosus. Cultures, serologic tests, patient age, and clinical course of disease will help in distinguishing these other disorders.

Polyarteritis nodosa is an example of small- and medium-sized vessel disease. Its infantile form is felt to be synonymous with Kawasaki syndrome. Polyarteritis nodosa in children is characterized by fever, hypertension, abdominal pain, rash, neurologic disease, arthritis, arthralgia, and cardiomegaly. Laboratory abnormalities include elevated WBC, anemia, hematuria, proteinuria, azotemia, and antistreptococcal antibodies. Although a pathologic diagnosis is often needed for definitive diagnosis, the features described above should increase the clinician's suspicions very considerably. Polyarteritis nodosa in young infants may be clinically and pathologically indistinguishable from Kawasaki syndrome.

SCLERODERMA

Scleroderma is an uncommon collagen vascular disease which involves the skin, gastrointestinal tract, heart, lungs, and kidneys as well as a variety of other organ systems. Scleroderma, or "tight skin," remains an enigmatic entity with no known etiology and no consistently effective therapy. In recent years, increasing numbers of patients with scleroderma have been presented in the pediatric literature; however, prior to 1960, only 12 children with generalized scleroderma were described. Presently less than 5 percent of patients with collagen vascular disease carry this diagnosis. There appears to be a female predominance, but no racial or genetic predisposition has been reported.

The cutaneous manifestations and the presence or absence of systemic involvement guide the clinician in classifying scleroderma. Local disease is classified in three categories: morphea, linear scleroderma, and "en coup de sabre" (stroke of the saber). Morphea may present in the form of plaques, drops (the "guttate" variety), or with diffuse cutaneous involvement (Fig. 7.32). Linear scleroderma affects a single dermatome. When linear scleroderma affects a limb, poor growth and deformity of the extremity may occur. The form of scleroderma known as "en coup de sabre" affects the face and scalp, with potential involvement of all structures beneath the superficial lesion including the bone and brain (Fig. 7.33). Systemic scleroderma or progressive systemic sclerosis is notable because visceral organ involvement occurs. Variants of systemic scleroderma are the CREST syndromes, which are comprised of *c*alcinosis cutis, *R*aynaud's phe-

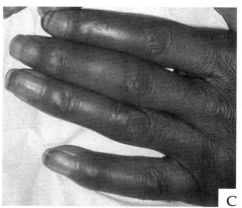

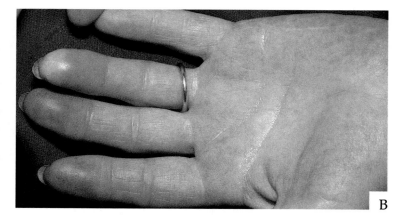

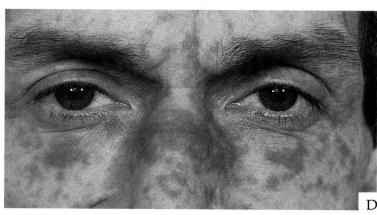

A

B

C

D

FIG. 7.34 CREST syndrome: **A,** cutaneous calcinosis. **B,** Raynaud's phenomenon (note cyanosis as well as pallor of the fingertips). **C,** sclerodactyly. **D,** telangiectasia. Esophageal dysmotility may also occur.

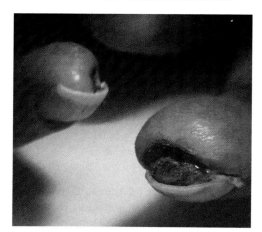

FIG. 7.35 Digital pitting ulcers, one of the three minor diagnostic criteria for scleroderma.

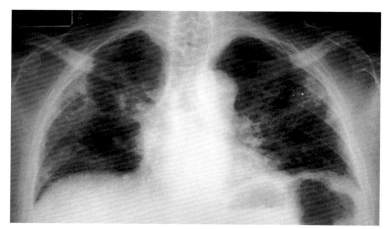

FIG. 7.36 Bilateral pulmonary fibrosis in a patient with scleroderma.

nomenon, *e*sophageal abnormalities, *s*clerodactyly, and *t*elangiectasias (Fig. 7.34). Often, mixed connective tissue disease (MCTD) is considered under the same classification.

In 1980, the American Rheumatism Association developed criteria for the clinical diagnosis of scleroderma. The single major criterion is the presence of proximal scleroderma or the typical cutaneous manifestations of the disease proximal to the wrists. The three minor criteria decided upon are sclerodactyly, digital pitting ulcers (Fig. 7.35), and, lastly, bilateral pulmonary fibrosis (Fig. 7.36). In order to diagnose scleroderma one must confirm the presence of one major and two minor criteria.

Many organ systems may be involved in the child afflicted with scleroderma. Cutaneous manifestations frequently bring children to medical attention, but, because of the insidious and subtle onset of skin lesions, there is often a delay in diagnosis. Early in the clinical course, the skin is edematous with a particular predilection for the distal extremities; rarely, more proximal limb, face, and trunk involvement is present. The induration phase, for which scleroderma is named, is characterized by loss of the natural pliability of the skin and the presence of a palpable skin thickness. The skin will take on a shiny, tense appearance, with distal tapering of the fingers (see Fig. 7.34C). The visual impression that movement might be impaired is, in fact, supported by the lack of flexibility in the hands (Fig. 7.37) and the typical scleroderma facies. Tight skin and skin atrophy produce the appearance of a fixed stare, pinched nose, thin pursed lips, small mouth, prominent teeth, and characteristic grimace (Fig. 7.38). Early in the clinical course, the skin lesions may appear erythematous or viola-

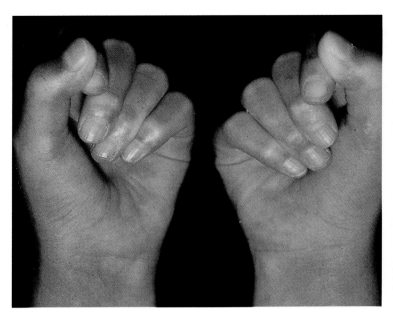

FIG. 7.37 Lack of flexibility in the hands is another characteristic of scleroderma.

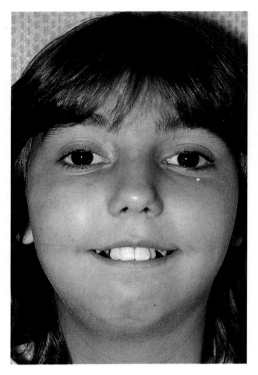

FIG. 7.38 Facial features of scleroderma. The skin appears tight and drawn, without evidence of wrinkles. (Courtesy of Dr. J. Jeffrey Malatack, Children's Hospital of Pittsburgh)

ceous; later they progress to become soft and atrophic, with a visible indentation. Subcutaneous calcium deposits (calcinosis cutis) may occur at pressure points and will occasionally extrude through the skin in a fashion similar to DM (see Fig. 7.13). These lesions may be painful and not uncommonly may ulcerate. Often, generalized hyperpigmentation occurs with punctuated areas of hypopigmentation or vitiligo (complete depigmentation) (see Figs. 7.32 and 7.33). Telangiectasias of three varieties are known to occur: linear telangiectasias of the cuticles, well-defined macules of various sizes and shapes, and the reddish-purple papules typical of Osler-Weber-Rendu disease (tiny circular lesions positioned eccentrically from their telangiectatic spokes) (see Fig. 7.34D).

Because of the involvement of the digital arteries in scleroderma, patients often develop the clinical picture of Raynaud's phenomenon (see Fig. 7.34B). Patients will develop intense pallor secondary to cold or emotional stress. This is followed by cyanosis and erythema, and is often associated with pain or paresthesias. In its most severe form, ischemia may lead to necrosis and eventual gangrenous destruction of tissue.

Gastrointestinal symptoms occur in approximately half of the children, though more detailed investigation often indicates the presence of abnormalities in a larger percentage. Esophageal dysmotility associated with gastroesophageal reflux often leads to dysphagia and symptoms of esophagitis. In more severely affected individuals, aspiration and cough may occur while esophageal strictures can develop if the process of reflux is chronic. If the small bowel is involved, cramps, diarrhea, and constipation may result from peristaltic dysfunction. Bacterial overgrowth, steatorrhea, weight loss, volvulus, and even perforation can occur. Colonic disease occurs in the form of wide-mouth diverticula and a loss of the normal colonic architecture.

As might be expected, mortality and morbidity are often the results of the cardiorespiratory complications of the disease. In addition to pulmonary fibrosis, one may see tachypnea, cough, dyspnea with exertion, findings of pulmonary hypertension,

ANTIBODIES FOUND IN PATIENTS WITH SCLERODERMA AND CREST

Antibody	Percentage of Patients
SCL-70	10 to 20 PSS
Antinuclear antibody (ANA)	90 PSS
Anti-centromere	80 to 90 CREST syndrome
Anti-ribonuclear protein (RNP)	25 PSS
Anti-nucleolar	40 to 50
SS-A (Ro)	Occasionally positive
SS-B (La)	Occasionally positive
Rheumatoid factor (RF)	33 local scleroderma

FIG. 7.39 (Adapted from Tan EM: Antinuclear antibodies in diagnosis and management Hosp Pract 1983;18:74-79)

and pleural effusion. Cardiac involvement includes heart block, congestive heart failure, ECG changes, and pericardial effusion. These abnormalities appear to be a result of myocardial fibrosis, vascular insufficiency, and inflammation.

Other manifestations of disease are arthritis, arthralgia, proximal muscle weakness, systemic hypertension, proteinuria, azotemia, renal failure, Sjögren syndrome, and various CNS findings such as sensory cranial nerve dysfunction, and decreased vibratory sensation. A variety of antibodies are found in scleroderma, and these are outlined in Figure 7.39.

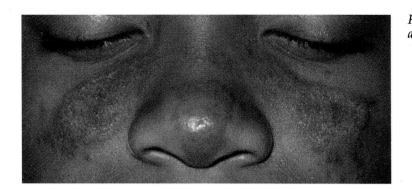

FIG. 7.40 *Typical malar rash of SLE. Erythema, erosion, and atrophy are present. Note sparing of nasolabial folds.*

SYSTEMIC LUPUS ERYTHEMATOSUS

Systemic lupus erythematosus (SLE) is a complex autoimmune disease with a myriad of clinical presentations. SLE may present in an insidious fashion and hence, escape early diagnosis, or it may present acutely and progress rapidly, leading to the patient's demise. As with other collagen vascular diseases, its etiology is unknown. The disease may involve just one organ system or, more commonly, it may be a multisystem disease. Because of the large number of serologic markers known to occur in SLE, it is considered by many to be the prototype of autoimmune disease. To increase diagnostic accuracy, the American Rheumatism Association revised its classification criteria. This classification is highly sensitive and specific for the diagnosis of this disease. The main diagnostic criteria include malar and/or discoid rash, photosensitivity, oral ulcers, arthritis, serositis, renal disorders, neurologic disorders, hematologic disorders, immunologic abnormalities, and the presence of antinuclear antibody.

The word "lupus," which means wolf, alludes to the erosive nature of the rash of SLE—"wolf bite" (Fig. 7.40). This feature of the disease was critical to the diagnosis of SLE until the discovery of the LE (lupus erythematosus) cell in 1948. The LE cell represents a healthy neutrophil which has phagocytized the nuclear debris of a nonliving cell that has been coated with antibody. This antibody is directed against deoxyribonucleoprotein (DNP), which is made up of both DNA and histones. The presence of this serologic marker for lupus greatly expanded the recognized clinical entity of SLE. With the recognition of milder cases of SLE and the advent of new therapies, the prognosis has improved substantially.

While SLE comprises 10 percent of the group of patients with collagen vascular disease, its incidence is approximately 1 in 200,000 in children, with teenage girls predominating. Females are affected five times more often than males, and black patients are more commonly affected than white patients. The disease is very rare in children under 5 years of age. The incidence of other connective tissue diseases is higher among family members of patients with SLE. Hematologic malignancies and immunodeficiencies are also reported in increased frequency among SLE relatives. These well-described phenomena may reflect a genetic alteration of immunity or, as some researchers suggest, the effects of a transmissible agent. Drugs are known to induce a lupus-like reaction, and their withdrawal leads to a resolution of this syndrome. Among the more common offenders are the anticonvulsants, hydralazine, oral contraceptives, and antibiotics. The high incidence of disease in females, SLE's common exacerbation during pregnancy, and the induction of disease by birth control pills support the role of hormonal factors as contributing to the pathogenesis of SLE. Other investigators suggest the influence of viruses, sunlight, and emotional stress on those developing lupus.

While immunologic markers have made the diagnosis of SLE considerably easier, one must still have a high index of suspicion to obtain these studies. The early symptoms are often nonspecific and sometimes go unrecognized as harbingers of serious disease. Fever, fatigue, malaise, anorexia, and weight loss may be the only symptoms that the clinician has to suspect the diagnosis. In the adolescent population, these symptoms may be all the more difficult to interpret. Conversely, this multisystem disease may present with a plethora of physical findings, and the presentation may be so dramatic that clues to diagnosis are quite readily apparent. Among the more commonly involved organ systems are skin, joints, reticuloendothelial, renal, cardiac, and pulmonary.

Cutaneous manifestations of SLE are present at some time during the course of the disease in 80 percent of affected individuals. The classic butterfly rash in the malar distribution is seen about one-third of the time (see Fig. 7.40). In contrast to patients with dermatomyositis (see Fig. 7.15), patients with SLE have nasolabial-fold sparing. The rash of lupus is often reddish-purple, raised, with a whitish scale (Fig. 7.41). When the scale is removed, the underlying skin often shows "carpet tack"-like fingers on the unexposed side of the scale itself. Carpet tacking is caused by the contouring of the scale into the skin follicles. These fingerlike projections on the scale strongly suggest the diagnosis of lupus. Purplish-red urticarial lesions also occur, but these do not produce scale and do not cause atrophy as other lupus lesions do. If the skin manifestations are left untreated, the patient's appearance will be marred by hypo- and hyperpigmentation. Mucosal erosions and ulcers of both the oral cavity and nasal mucosa are part of lupus as well (Fig. 7.42). Alopecia (Fig. 7.43) is seen in 20 percent of patients, and may occur as broken hair shafts or patchy, red, scaling areas on the scalp which may eventually scar and cause permanent hair loss. Other reported mucocutaneous findings are livedo reticularis (blotchy cyanotic areas in a lacy pattern), urticaria, atrophy, and telangiectasia. Though rare in children, discoid lupus refers to the absence of systemic disease in the presence of typical lupus dermatologic pathology.

The vasculitis of lupus, a small-vessel vasculitis, is responsible for a number of easily recognized clinical findings. The skin may be purpuric, or in more severe instances, necrotic

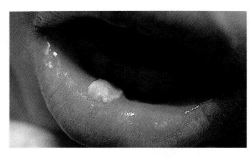

FIG. 7.42 *Mucosal ulceration of the lip as evidence of vasculitis in SLE.*

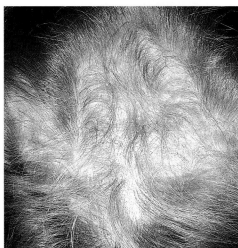

FIG. 7.43 *Scarring alopecia seen in SLE.*

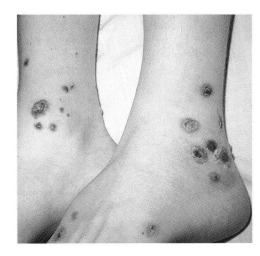

FIG. 7.44 *Cutaneous vasculitis in SLE. Purpuric, ulcerative, and necrotic skin lesions of active disease.*

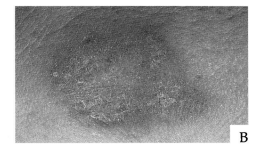

FIG. 7.41 **A,** *the localized erythematous rash of SLE in a nonmalar distribution.* **B,** *the rash of SLE often has a slight white scale.*

lesions may result (Fig. 7.44). The vasculitic component of lupus may also present with full-blown Raynaud's phenomenon. With repeated tissue injury, one may see glossy, atrophic, ulcerated skin and distorted nail architecture.

The heart is often significantly involved in patients with lupus. While the pericardium is most commonly involved, the myocardium and the endocardium may also be of clinical importance. Pericarditis can be nonpainful and may present only as cardiomegaly on chest radiograph or as pericardial effusion on echocardiogram. However, one might also see chest pain or auscultate a friction rub. The myocardium, when affected, can lead to the life-threatening complications of arrhythmia, heart failure, and infarction. "Libman-Sacks endocarditis" is the term given to the verrucous projections of fibrinoid necrosis in the endocardium. These lesions rarely cause clinical symptoms, though the presence of a murmur should

raise one's suspicion of endocardial disease. The mitral valve is most commonly involved, although aortic and tricuspid valves may be similarly affected.

Pulmonary manifestations of lupus are particularly difficult to diagnose noninvasively. Migrating pneumonitis, particularly involving the lung bases, suggests "lupus lung;" however, distinguishing these densities from infection may be impossible without invasive procedures. Typically, patients have atelectasis, pleural effusions, interstitial pneumonitis, or hemorrhage (Fig. 7.45). These sequelae may present as cyanosis, dyspnea, or almost any other form of respiratory distress.

Unlike the destructive arthritis of JRA, lupus arthritis is more transient and episodic, and rarely results in loss of function. The fact that arthralgia is more predominant than arthritis has been noted consistently. Any joint may be involved, but the fingers are particularly susceptible. Myalgia and weakness

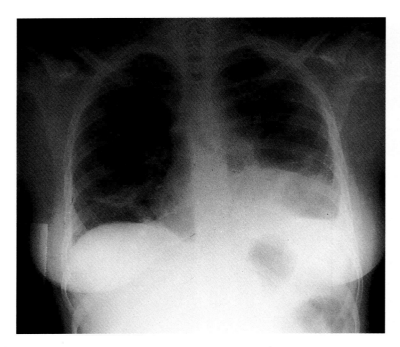

FIG. 7.45 *Atelectasis, pleural effusions, and pulmonary infiltrates in a teenage girl with SLE.*

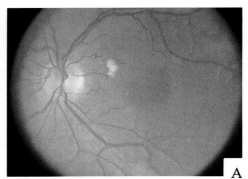

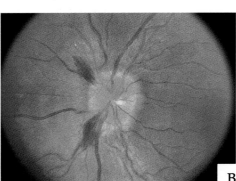

FIG. 7.46 **A,** *a white exudate (cotton-wool spot) between the disc and macula.* **B,** *papilledema with flame hemorrhages.*

also occur as a feature of lupus, but do not dominate the clinical picture as they do in DM.

CNS signs and symptoms of lupus present a great challenge to physicians. A wide range of neurologic and psychiatric manifestations of the disease have been described. Further complicating the spectrum of CNS lupus is the difficulty in distinguishing the disease itself from side effects of therapy (particularly steroids), emotional response to the disease, and a non-CNS etiology for CNS pathology (e.g., hypertension). It is estimated that approximately one-quarter of all lupus patients have some form of CNS disease. The findings range from mononeuritis multiplex (inflammatory lesions of multiple nerves located in anatomically unrelated parts of the body) to chorea, ataxia, peripheral neuropathy, seizures, headaches, psychosis, pseudomotor cerebri, and intellectual impairment. In fact, the thorough investigation of a large number of neurologic disorders mandates screening serologies for lupus. As a direct extension of the brain, the retina, not surprisingly, may also show evidence of disease. Best known of the ocular manifestations is the cotton-wool spot, an exudative whitish lesion of the retina. Hemorrhage and papilledema are also seen (Fig. 7.46). As might be expected, the CNS effects of lupus are responsible for much morbidity as well as mortality.

At least as important as CNS disease in determining ultimate prognosis is the degree of renal involvement. Approximately three-quarters of all children with SLE will have some degree of clinically apparent renal disease. This often manifests itself in the first 2 years of illness, but can also appear many years after the initial diagnosis. The type of pathology seen largely relates to the nature of immune complex deposition at various sites in the kidney. At a histologic level, renal involvement may be classified as membranous nephritis, focal or diffuse nephritis, or mesangial nephritis. Other than the glomeruli, the tubules, interstitium, and blood vessels may be involved. From the clinician's point of view, these lesions are difficult to distinguish. More importantly, one must search for the presence of renal involvement at frequent intervals. This is

best accomplished by urinalysis for protein, hematuria, red cell casts, and abnormalities in the specific gravity patterns over time. One must also obtain BUN and creatinine, 24-hour urine for creatinine clearance and protein at periodic intervals. Hypertension may also direct the clinician to the presence of renal disease. To complicate the clinical picture, histologic evidence of renal pathology may be present even when all the above clinical parameters are normal. Early biopsy is advocated by many rheumatologists, as is the careful serologic evaluation of these patients.

Additional clinical findings in SLE include lymphadenopathy with or without hepatosplenomegaly, hepatitis, anemia, leukopenia, thrombocytopenia, disorders of esophageal motility, pancreatitis, malabsorption, diarrhea, and abdominal pain. Lupus is also reported in infants of mothers with the disease. IgG is passed by the placenta to the fetus, leading to positive serologies and findings of lupus. The presence of rash (Fig. 7.47), thrombocytopenia, Coombs-positive hemolytic anemia, and congenital heart block should suggest the diagnosis. Half of infants with diagnosis of congenital heart block will be found to have mothers with SLE, though only a small percentage of mothers with lupus will have affected infants. Fortunately, neonatal lupus is transient, lasting only a few months.

Perhaps more than any other collagen vascular disease, the clinical diagnosis of lupus can be confirmed serologically. The ANAs represent a group of antibodies found in serum which are directed against antigens within the cellular nuclei of lupus patients. These antibodies combine with their respective nuclear antigens to form immune complexes. Many of these immune complexes go on to cause the histopathology and symptomatology of lupus. The well-described lupus erythematosus (LE) cell is simply a reflection of this pathologic mechanism. Because the ANA test can now directly detect DNP, the LE cell is only significant from a historical perspective.

Other antibodies found in SLE patients are listed in Figure 7.48. Anti-native DNA antibodies are detected in 50 to 60 percent of lupus patients, but of note is the fact that they are rarely found in non-lupus patients. Antibodies to single-stranded DNA are also present in SLE; however, their presence in many other entities limits their clinical utility. Ribonucleoprotein (RNP), while better known for its presence in high titers in mixed connective tissue disease, is also seen in low titers in 30 to 40 percent of lupus patients. Other SLE antibodies include SS-A and SS-B (Sjögren syndrome), also known as Ro and La, respectively. Anti-Ro antibodies are associated with heart block in infants of mothers with SLE. Lastly, one finds antibodies to Sm antigen, a nonhistone antigen which appears to be very specific for lupus.

In summary, SLE is a chronic disease with a variable course and with periods of varying activity. While the mortality and morbidity remain high, marked improvement in prognosis has occurred in recent years.

ACKNOWLEDGMENTS

Thanks to Drs. Bernard Cohen, John Zitelli, A'Delbert Bowen, Basil Zitelli, J. Carlton Gartner, Jr., J. Jeffrey Malatack, Joseph McGuire, Holly Davis, Virginia Steen, Joseph Warnicki, Albert Biglan, Cora Lennox, Sang Park, Chester Oddis, Susan Gelnett, and Mary Killian for their valuable assistance with photographs and text.

BIBLIOGRAPHY

Bell DM: Kawasaki update: more answers, fewer questions. *Contemp Pediatr* 1985;2:20–36.

Brewer EJ, Gedalia A: The child with joint pain: an algorithmic approach. *Contemp Pediatr* 1985;2:18–34.

Brewer EJ: Pitfalls in the diagnosis of juvenile rheumatoid arthritis. *Pediatr Clin North Am* 1986;33(5):1015–1032.

Burns JC, Wiggins JW Jr, Toews WH, et al: Clinical spectrum of Kawasaki disease in infants younger than 6 months of age. *Pediatrics* 1986;Nov:759–763.

Cassidy JT: Miscellaneous conditions associated with arthritis in children. *Pediatr Clin North Am* 1986;33(5):1033–1052.

Eichenfield AH: Diagnosis and management of Lyme disease. *Pediatr Ann* 1986;15(9):583–594.

Emery H: Clinical aspects of systemic lupus erythematosus in childhood. *Pediatr Clin North Am* 1986;33(5):1177–1190.

Lohr JA, Rheuban KS: Kawasaki syndrome. *Infect Dis Clin North Am* 1987;1(3):559–574.

Meadow SR, Scott DG: Berger disease: Henoch-Schönlein syndrome without the rash. *J Pediatr* 1985;106:27–32.

Melish ME: Kawasaki syndrome. *Pediatr Rev* 1980:2(4):107–114.

Pachman LM: Juvenile dermatomyositis. *Pediatr Clin North Am* 1986;33(5):1097–1117.

Rennebohm RM: Rheumatic diseases of childhood. *Pediatr Rev* 1988;10(6):183–190.

Rowley AH, Gonzalez-Crussi F, Gidding SS, et al: Incomplete Kawasaki disease with coronary artery involvement. *J Pediatr* 1987;110:409–413.

Silber DL: Henoch-Schönlein syndrome. *Pediatr Clin North Am* 1972;19(4):1061–1070.

Singsen BH: Scleroderma in children. *Pediatr Clin North Am* 1986;33(5):1119-1140

Smith LEH, Burns JC: Kawasaki disease and the eye. *Resident Staff Phys* 1988;34:48–52.

Smith LEH, Newburger JW, Burns JC: Kawasaki syndrome and the eye. *Pediatr Infect Dis J* 1989;8:116–118.

Tan EM, Cohen AS, Fries JF, et al: The 1982 revised criteria for the classification of SLE. *Arthritis Rheum* 1982;25(11):1271–1277.

Urbach AH, McGregor RS, Malatack JJ, et al: Kawasaki disease and perineal rash. *Am J Dis Child* 1988;142:1174–1176.

Wedgewood RJ, Schaller JG: The pediatric arthritides. *Hosp Pract* 1977;June:83–97.

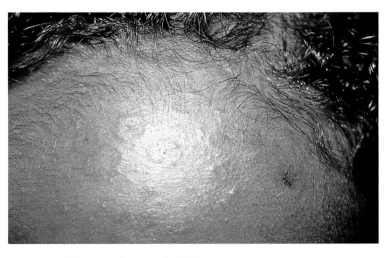

FIG. 7.47 The rash of neonatal SLE.

ANTIBODIES FOUND IN SLE PATIENTS

Antibody	Percent of Patients
Native DNA (doubled-stranded)	50 to 60
DNP (DNA and histone protein)	Up to 70 (usually high titer)
RNP (RNA and non-histone protein)	30 to 40
Histones	
All SLE patients	60
Drug-induced lupus patients	95
SS-A (Ro)	30 to 40
SS-B (La)	15
Sm	30

FIG. 7.48 (Adapted from Tan EM: Antinuclear antibodies in diagnosis and management Hosp Pract 1983;18:74-79)

PEDIATRIC DERMATOLOGY

Bernard A. Cohen, M.D. ◆ Holly W. Davis, M.D. ◆ Susan B. Mallory, M.D. ◆ John A. Zitelli, M.D.

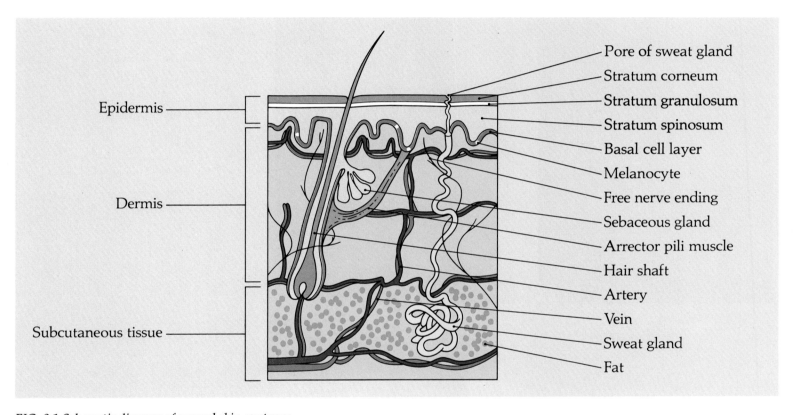

Epidermis

Dermis

Subcutaneous tissue

Pore of sweat gland
Stratum corneum
Stratum granulosum
Stratum spinosum
Basal cell layer
Melanocyte
Free nerve ending
Sebaceous gland
Arrector pili muscle
Hair shaft
Artery
Vein
Sweat gland
Fat

FIG. 8.1 Schematic diagram of normal skin anatomy.

INTRODUCTION

Most of us think of our skin as a simple, durable covering for our skeleton, muscles, and internal organs. However, the skin is actually a very complex organ, consisting of many parts and appendages (Fig. 8.1). The outermost layer, the stratum corneum, is an effective barrier to the penetration of irritants, toxins and organisms, as well as a membrane that holds in body fluids. The remainder of the epidermis manufactures this protective layer. Melanocytes within the epidermis are important in protecting us from the harmful effects of ultraviolet light, and Langerhans cells are one of the body's first lines of immunologic defense.

The dermis, consisting largely of fibroblasts and collagen, is a tough, leathery, mechanical barrier against cuts, bites, and bruises. Its collagenous matrix also provides structural support for a number of cutaneous appendages. Hair, which grows from follicles deep within the dermis, is important for cosmesis as well as protection from sunlight and particulate matter. Sebaceous glands arise as outgrowths of the hair follicles. Oil produced by these glands helps to lubricate the skin and contributes to the protective epidermal barrier. The nails are specialized organs of manipulation that also protect sensitive digits. Thermoregulation of the skin is accomplished by eccrine sweat glands as well as by changes in cutaneous blood flow, regulated by glomus cells. The skin also contains special-

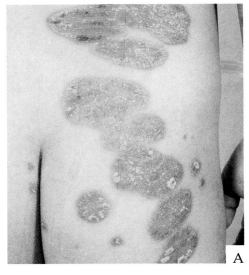

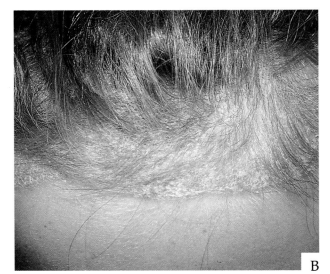

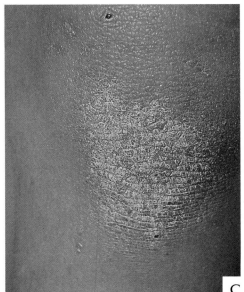

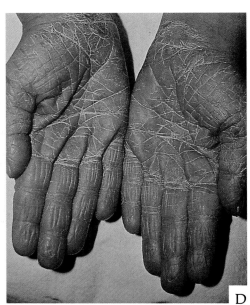

FIG. 8.2 Psoriasis. **A,** typical erythematous plaques are topped by a silver scale. **B,** thick tenacious scale on a red base extends from the forehead onto the scalp of this 10-year-old girl. **C,** this large plaque is located over the pressure point of the knee. **D,** skin of the palms is markedly thickened, with silvery fissuring of the palmar creases. (**C** and **D**, courtesy of Dr. Michael Sherlock)

ized receptors for heat, pain, touch, and pressure. Sensory input from these structures helps to protect the skin surface against environmental trauma. Beneath the dermis, in the subcutaneous tissue, fat acts as stored energy and as a soft, protective cushion.

Defects or alteration in any component of the skin may result in serious systemic disease or death. Each and every part of the skin can be affected by congenital, inflammatory, infectious, and degenerative disorders and tumors. For example, an altered stratum corneum is seen in ichthyosis, melanocytes are selectively destroyed in vitiligo, the epidermis proliferates in psoriasis, excess collagen is produced in the connective tissue nevus of tuberous sclerosis, hair is preferentially infested by certain fungi, and so on. In addition, the skin is affected by many systemic diseases and may thus provide readily visible markers for internal disorders. A skin examination may demonstrate lesions of vasculitis, explaining a child's hematuria. The white macules of tuberous sclerosis may give insight into the cause of seizures.

Examination and Assessment of the Skin

The skin is the largest, most accessible, and easily examined organ of the body, and is the organ of most frequent concern to the patient. Therefore, all physicians should be able to recognize basic skin diseases and dermatologic clues to systemic disease.

Optimal examination of the skin must be performed in a well-lit room. The physician should inspect the entire skin surface including hair, nails, scalp, and mucous membranes. This may present particular problems in infants and teenagers, since examination of the skin in small segments may be necessary to prevent cooling or embarrassment. Although no special equipment is required, a hand lens and side lighting do aid in the assessment of skin texture and small discrete lesions.

Despite the myriad conditions affecting the skin, a systematic approach to the evaluation of a rash or exanthem facilitates and simplifies the process of developing a manageable differential diagnosis. After assessing the general health of the patient, the practitioner should obtain a detailed history of the

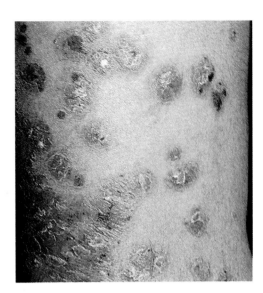

FIG. 8.3 Guttate psoriasis. Small plaques with typical scales quickly developed in a generalized distribution after a streptococcal pharyngitis.

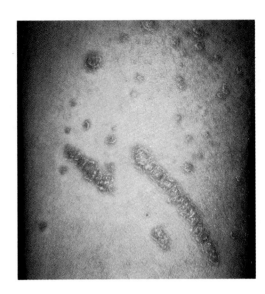

FIG. 8.4 Koebner phenomenon in psoriasis. Lesions are often induced in areas of local trauma such as these scratches.

skin symptoms including date of onset, inciting factors, evolution of lesions, and the presence or absence of pruritus. Recent immunizations, infections, drugs, and allergies may be directly related to new rashes. The family history may suggest a hereditary or contagious process, and the clinician may need to examine other members of the family. Review of nursery records and photographs will help to document the presence of congenital lesions. Attention should then turn to the distribution and pattern of the rash. The *distribution* refers to the location of the skin findings, while the *pattern* defines a specific anatomic or physiologic arrangement. For example, the distribution of a rash may include the extremities, face or trunk, while the pattern could be flexural or intertriginous. Other common patterns include sun-exposed sites, acrodermatitis, pityriasis rosea, clothing-covered sites, and dermatomal configurations.

Next, the clinician should consider the local *organization* of the lesions, defining the relationship of primary and secondary lesions to one another in a given location. Are the lesions scattered or clustered (herpetiform)? Are they linear, serpiginous, confluent, or discrete?

Finally, the practitioner may develop a differential diagnosis using the morphology of the cutaneous lesions. Primary lesions (macules, papules, wheals, plaques, vesicles, pustules, bullae, comedones, milia, nodules, tumors) arise *de novo* in the skin. Secondary lesions (erosions, ulcers, crusts, excoriations, fissures, lichenification, atrophy, scars) evolve from primary lesions or result from manipulation of primary lesions by the patient.

As an outline of specific pediatric dermatoses defies any one scheme of organization, we have selected what we find to be a clinically practical format. First, we will cover common papulosquamous and vesiculopustular eruptions which account for a large majority of rashes seen in children. This will be followed by sections covering reactive erythemas, insect bites and infestations, tumors and infiltrations of the skin, neonatal dermatology, vascular lesions, congenital and acquired nevi, and disorders of pigmentation. The chapter will conclude with a discussion of disorders of the hair, the nails, and complications of topical therapy.

PAPULOSQUAMOUS DISORDERS

Papulosquamous eruptions share the morphologic features of papules and scales. However, it is important for the clinician to understand that the diverse papulosquamous disorders are produced by a variety of different mechanisms. In psoriasis, increased production of keratinocytes by the basal cell layer results in a markedly thickened epidermis and stratum corneum (scaly surface layer). In dermatitic processes such as atopic dermatitis, contact dermatitis, seborrheic dermatitis, pityriasis rosea, and fungal infections, inflammation results in both increased production and abnormal maturation of epidermal cells, with subsequent scale production. Increased adherence of cells in the stratum corneum may result in the retention hyperkeratosis characteristic of ichthyosis vulgaris which is frequently seen in association with atopic dermatitis.

Psoriasis

Psoriasis is a common disorder characterized by red, well-demarcated plaques, with dry, thick, silvery scales. These tend to be located on the extensor surfaces of the extremities, the scalp, and the buttocks (Fig. 8.2A and B). In some patients, the distribution consists of large lesions over the knees and elbows (Fig. 8.2C). Thickening and fissuring of the skin of the palms may also be seen (Fig. 8.2D). In other children, many drop-like (guttate) lesions are scattered all over the body (Fig. 8.3). In infants, psoriasis may present as a persistent diaper dermatitis (see Fig. 8.41). Lesions of psoriasis are often induced in areas of local injury, such as scratches, surgical scars, or sunburn, a response termed the Koebner phenomenon (Fig. 8.4). Nail changes include red-brown psoriatic plaques in the nail bed (oil-drop changes), surface pitting, and distal hyperkeratosis (see Fig. 8.120).

The factors initiating the rapid turnover in epidermal cells that produce the psoriatic plaques are unknown, although an inherited predisposition is suspected, and upper respiratory tract and streptococcal infections are known to precipitate lesions. Though the increased epidermal growth causes a thickening of the skin in the psoriatic plaque, there are also

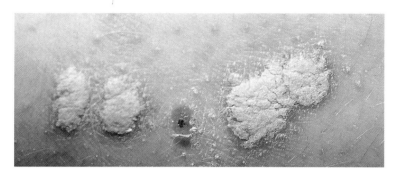

FIG. 8.5 Auspitz sign. Removal of the thick scale from a psoriatic plaque produces small points of bleeding from tortuous capillaries.

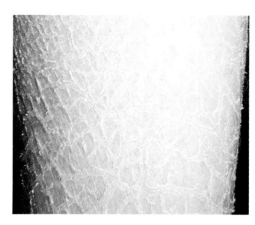

FIG. 8.6 Ichthyosis vulgaris. The typical fish-scale appearance is seen in this closeup of the shin of a fair-skinned patient.

areas between the epidermal ridges where the skin is very thin and the scale is close to the subepidermal vessels. Thus, when the scale is removed, small bleeding points are often seen. This is called the Auspitz sign, and it is the hallmark of psoriasis (Fig. 8.5).

The course of psoriasis is chronic and unpredictable, marked by remissions and exacerbations. Although psoriasis is thought to be rare in childhood, 37 percent of adults with the disorder first develop lesions before the age of 20.

The Ichthyoses

Ichthyosis refers to a group of inherited dermatoses characterized by dry, scaly skin. Various types have been identified according to clinical course, histopathology, and biochemical markers.

ICHTHYOSIS VULGARIS

Ichthyosis vulgaris is transmitted as an autosomal dominant trait and affects about 0.5 percent of the population. Although the rash is not present at birth, by 3 months of age, thick, fish-like scales may be apparent on the shins and extensor surfaces of the arms (Fig. 8.6). Occasionally, scales become more generalized, involving the trunk, but the flexures are usually spared. Lesions tend to flare during the winter months (because of the drying effect of central heating) and improve during the summer, particularly with increasing age. Biopsy of involved skin shows retention hyperkeratosis and a thinned granular layer in the epidermis. Topical emollients usually keep pruritus and scaling under control.

SEX-LINKED ICHTHYOSIS

Sex-linked ichthyosis occurs in 1 in 6,000 males, although findings are occasionally present in hemizygous female carriers. Infants may begin with a collodion membrane (see Fig. 8.83) which peels during the first several weeks of life and is followed by the development of generalized "dirty" brown scales, particularly on the abdomen, back, and anterior legs and feet (Fig. 8.7). The central face and flexures are spared. Skin biopsy demonstrates an increased granular layer and stratum corneum, and biochemical studies demonstrate decreased or absent steroid sulfatase in the serum and skin.

LAMELLAR ICHTHYOSIS

Lamellar ichthyosis is a rare autosomal dominant disorder occurring in less than 1 in 250,000 births. Infants are usually born with a collodion membrane (see Fig. 8.83). During the first month of life, thick, brownish-gray, sheet-like scales with raised edges appear. Scaling is prominent over the face, trunk

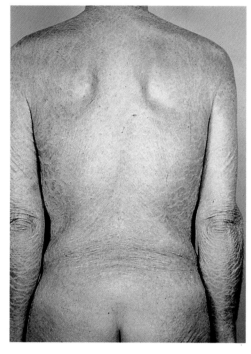

FIG. 8.7 Sex-linked ichthyosis. "Dirty" brown scales persist on the flanks, elbows, and shoulders despite the use of topical lubricants.

and extremities (Fig. 8.8). In contrast to ichthyosis vulgaris, the flexural areas are involved in the lamellar form. Eversion and fissuring of the eyelid margins (ectropian) and lips (eclabium) are common complications. The palms and soles show thick keratoderma with fissuring. Some improvement of the scaling occurs with age, and topical keratolytics such as lactic acid and salicylic acid may provide some benefit. Severe cases may respond to oral administration of retinoids such as 13-cis-retinoic acid (Accutane®).

EPIDERMOLYTIC HYPERKERATOSIS

Epidermolytic hyperkeratosis is a rare autosomal dominant form of ichthyosis, characterized by the development of generalized, thick, warty scales and intermittent blistering with severe involvement of the flexures (Fig. 8.9). In the newborn period, blisters may be widespread, suggesting a diagnosis of herpes simplex or epidermolysis bullosa. Histologically, massive hyperkeratosis is associated with ballooning of squamous cells and formation of microvesicles. Epidermal turnover is also markedly increased. The mainstay of treatment includes use of keratolytics, lubricants, and antibiotics for secondary infection, which is common and usually due to *Staphylococcus aureus*. Oral retinoids may also produce significant improvement in scaling.

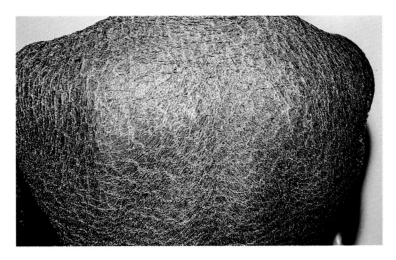

FIG. 8.8 Lamellar ichthyosis. Note the thick brown scales covering the entire skin.

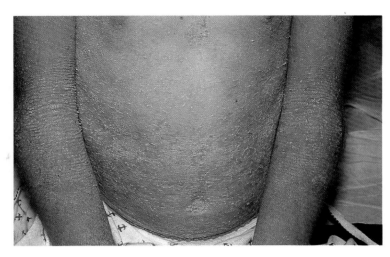

FIG. 8.9 Epidermolytic hyperkeratosis is characterized by thick, warty scales, and intermittent blistering. The flexural creases are particular sites of involvement.

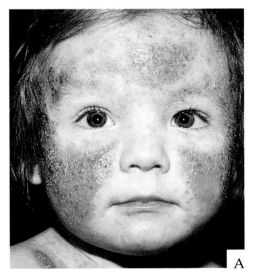

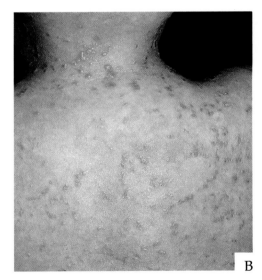

FIG. 8.10 Infantile atopic dermatitis or eczema. **A,** this infant has an acute, weeping dermatitis on the cheeks and forehead. Involvement of **B,** the trunk; and **C,** the extremities, with erythema, scaling and crusting are evident. Usually, the diaper area is the only portion of the skin surface that is spared (**B** and ,**C** reproduced with permission from Fireman P, Slavin RG: Atlas of Allergies, Gower, New York, 1991, 15.16).

A

B

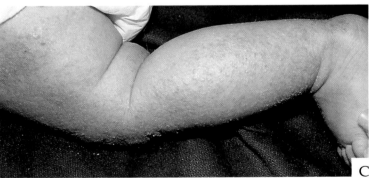

C

The Dermatitides

Depending on duration of involvement, the dermatitides are characterized clinically by acute changes (including redness, edema, and vesiculation) and/or chronic changes (such as scaling, lichenification, increased and decreased pigmentation) in the skin. Microscopically, these disorders are characterized by infiltration of the dermis with inflammatory cells, variable thickening of the epidermis, and scaling.

ATOPIC DERMATITIS (ECZEMA)

Atopic dermatitis or eczema is one of the most common and annoying skin disorders in children. This entity can be divided into three phases based on the age of the patient, each having a different distribution.

The *infantile phase* of atopic dermatitis begins between 1 and 6 months of age, and lasts about 2 or 3 years. Characteristically, the rash is manifest by red, itchy papules and plaques, many of which ooze and crust. Lesions are distributed over the cheeks, forehead, scalp, trunk, and the extensor surfaces of the extremities, and patches are often symmetrical (Fig. 8.10).

The *childhood phase* of atopic dermatitis occurs between ages 4 and 10 years. The dermatitis is typically dry, papular, and intensely pruritic. Circumscribed scaly patches are distributed

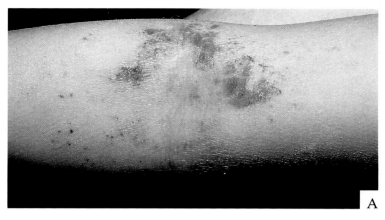

A

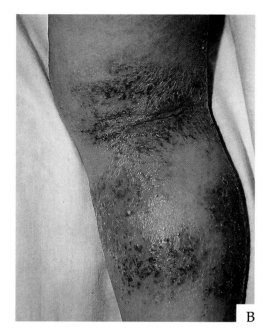

B

FIG. 8.11 Childhood atopic dermatitis with lesions on the arms (**A**) and the legs (**B**). In childhood, eczema involves the flexural surfaces of the upper and lower extremities. The neck, ankles, wrists and posterior thighs also may be severely affected. (**A**, reproduced with permission from Fireman P. Slavin RG: Atlas of Allergies. Gower, New York, 1991, 15.7; **B**, courtesy of Dr. Michael Sherlock)

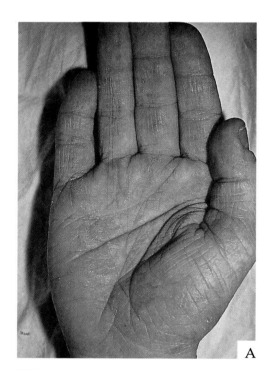

A

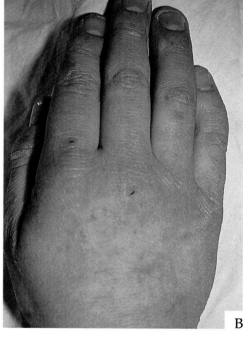

B

FIG. 8.12 Involvement of the hand in eczema. **A,** cracking, dryness, and scaling of the palmar surface is typical. **B,** excoriations and lichenification are also found over the dorsum of the hand and fingers. (Courtesy of Dr. Michael Sherlock)

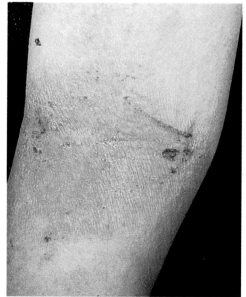

FIG. 8.13 Adult atopic dermatitis. Erythematous excoriated plaques with indistinct borders are seen in the antecubital areas. Note the dried blood from recent excoriation.

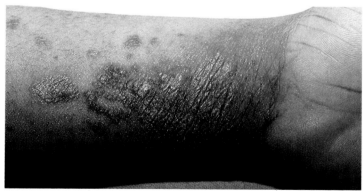

FIG. 8.14 Lichenification. Marked thickening of the skin in an area of chronic scratching. In addition, this patient shows post-inflammatory hyperpigmentation.

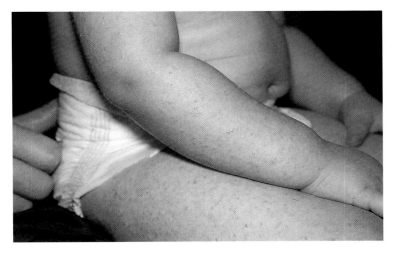

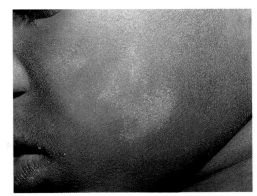

FIG. 8.16 Pityriasis alba. In some atopic individuals, subtle inflammation may result in development of poorly demarcated, hypopigmented patches that are covered by a fine superficial scale.

FIG. 8.15 Keratosis pilaris. Fine follicular papules are symmetrically distributed over the extensor surfaces of the arms and legs of this toddler.

on the wrists, ankles, and antecubital and popliteal fossae (Fig. 8.11); these frequently become secondarily infected, probably as a result of organisms introduced by intense scratching. Cracking, dryness, and scaling of the palmar and plantar surfaces of the hands and feet are also common (Fig. 8.12). Remission may occur at any time, or the disorder may evolve into a more chronic type of adult dermatitis. Seventy-five percent of children with atopic dermatitis improve between the ages of 10 to 14; the remaining children may go on to develop chronic dermatitis.

The *adult phase* of atopic dermatitis begins around age 12, and continues indefinitely. Major areas of involvement include the flexural areas of the arms, neck, and legs (Fig. 8.13). Eruptions are sometimes seen on the dorsal surfaces of the hands and feet, and between the fingers and toes. Lichenification may be marked (Fig. 8.14).

Other associated findings include xerosis (dryness); ichthyosis vulgaris (see Fig. 8.6); keratosis pilaris (keratin plugging of hair follicles and formation of perifollicular scales over the extensor surfaces of the extremities) (Fig. 8.15); hyperlinearity of the palms (see Fig. 8.12A); Dennie-Morgan folds (double skin creases under the lower eyelid [see Chapter 4]); and altered cellular immunity, which is manifested by an unusual susceptibility to certain cutaneous infections such as warts, herpes simplex, and molluscum contagiosum. Hyper- and hypopigmentation may be marked and, at times, may be the predominant findings (see Figs. 8.103 and 8.104).

In the rash of *pityriasis alba*, which is seen often in patients with atopic dermatitis, inflammatory changes are minimal. Poorly-defined, hypopigmented, scaly patches measuring 2 to 4 cm in diameter, are noted most commonly on the face and extremities (Fig. 8.16), although they may involve the trunk as well.

The cause of atopic dermatitis remains elusive. An immunologic etiology is suggested by the chronic elevation of immunoglobulin E (IgE) seen in a majority of patients. Some investigators have proposed an aberrant cutaneous response to histamine and other mediators of inflammation as a primary mechanism. However, laboratory findings vary from patient to patient and in the same patients at different times in the course of their disease. Atopic dermatitis seems to occur in families, in association with other atopic conditions including asthma, allergic rhinitis, and food allergies, suggesting some degree of genetic predisposition. Pathophysiologically, a number of external factors including dry skin, soaps, wool fabrics, foods, infectious agents, and environmental antigens may act in concert to produce pruritus, which is universal in atopics. The resultant scratching leads to the acute and chronic changes typical of atopic dermatitis. On occasion, patients with scabies may develop classic eczema as a result of intense scratching, though on close inspection the primary lesions usually can be identified.

The differential diagnosis of atopic dermatitis includes seborrhea, contact dermatitis, pityriasis rosea, psoriasis, fungal infections, histiocytosis X, and acrodermatitis enteropathica. It can be distinguished from seborrhea based on distribution of lesions, as atopic dermatitis spares moist, intertriginous areas such as the axillae and perineum, where seborrhea is prominent. Exposure history and distribution help distinguish contact dermatitis, and discreteness of lesions and distribution distinguish pityriasis. The thick, silvery scale and Koebner phenomenon help distinguish psoriasis, and central clearing with an active microvesicular border helps differentiate tinea corporis. The rash of histiocytosis is greasier and more generalized. It is associated with petechiae and often accompanied by chronicly draining ears and hepatosplenomegaly (see Fig. 8.75; see Chapter 11, Hematology). The acral distribution of lesions and gastrointestinal symptoms help in distinguishing acrodermatitis (see Chapter 10, Nutrition and Gastroenterology).

The mainstays of treatment of atopic dermatitis are elimination or avoidance of predisposing factors; hydration and lubrication of dry skin; use of antipruritic agents to relieve itching and break the itch/scratch cycle; and topical steroids. As secondary infection is common, this should be looked for carefully and treated promptly with systemic antibiotics.

Dyshidrotic eczema, nummular eczema, juvenile plantar dermatosis, and lip-licking and thumb-sucking eczema are conditions often seen in association with atopic dermatitis. However, they may present as independent entities.

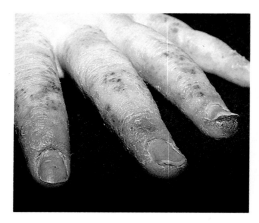

FIG. 8.17 Dyshidrosis. Chronic cracking, oozing, and scaling develop after the tiny pruritic vesicles have been scratched.

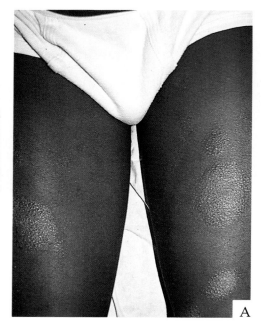

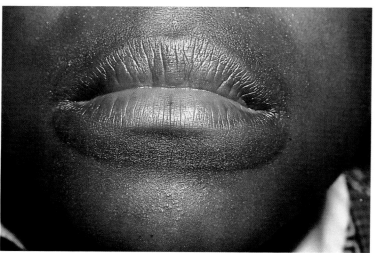

FIG. 8.18 Nummular eczema. **A,** these round to oval-shaped lesions are typically located over the extensor thighs or abdomen. **B,** on close inspection, they are seen to be studded with tiny vesicles. These lesions do not show central clearing. (Courtesy of Dr. Michael Sherlock)

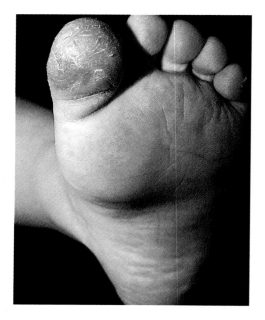

FIG. 8.19 Juvenile plantar dermatosis. This variant of atopic dermatitis is localized to the plantar surfaces of the toes and feet. Note the erythema, scaling, and cracking.

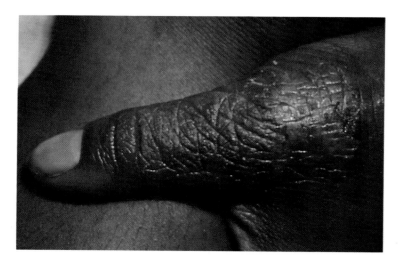

FIG. 8.20 Lip-licking eczema. The perioral skin is inflamed and thickened as a result of repetitive licking of the lips. (Courtesy of Dr. Michael Sherlock)

DYSHIDROTIC ECZEMA

Dyshidrosis is a severely pruritic, chronic, recurrent, vesicular eruption affecting the palms, soles, and lateral aspects of the fingers and toes. Characteristically, the vesicles are symmetrical, multilocular, and 1 to 3 mm in diameter. These rupture, leaving scales and crust on an erythematous base (Fig. 8.17). Pathologically, this eruption demonstrates spongiotic vesicles and normal eccrine sweat glands. The cause is unknown; however, frequent exposure to water, wet or sweat-soaked shoes, or chemicals (on the hands) may trigger or exacerbate the condition. Treatment is similar to that for acute atopic dermatitis. Use of charcoal-impregnated foam insoles can significantly help foot symptoms.

NUMMULAR ECZEMA

Nummular eczema is an acute papulovesicular eruption named for its coin-shaped configuration. Lesions are intensely pruritic, well circumscribed, round to oval, red, scaly patches studded with 1 to 3 mm vesicles (Fig. 8.18A and B). They are usually located on the extensor thighs or abdomen of children

FIG. 8.21 Thumb-sucking eczema. Repeated wetting and drying from persistent thumb-sucking have resulted in the eczematoid changes with cracking, fissuring, and lichenification. (Courtesy of Dr. Michael Sherlock)

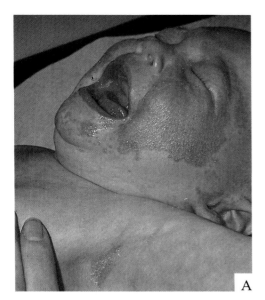

A

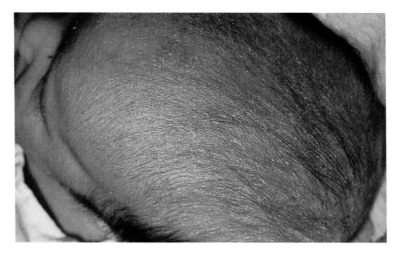

FIG. 8.22 Seborrhea. The slightly greasy, red, scaling eruption involves the hair-bearing areas of the face and axilla (A), and prominently affects the diaper area (B). Post-auricular lesions are common, and often become secondarily infected as in this case (C). (Courtesy of Dr. Michael Sherlock)

FIG. 8.23 Scalp seborrhea.Greasy scaling of the scalp, known as cradle cap is typical and varies in severity. (Courtesy of Dr. Michael Sherlock)

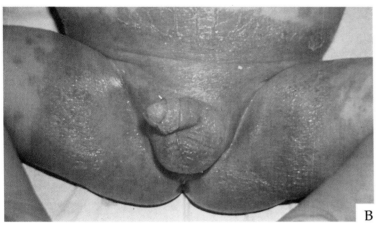

B

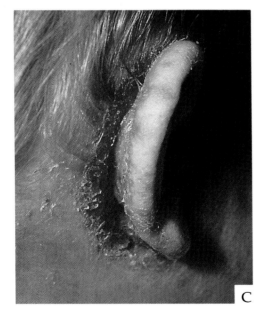

C

JUVENILE PLANTAR DERMATOSIS

Juvenile plantar dermatosis ("sweaty sock syndrome") is seen commonly in toddlers and school-age children. Chronic, red, scaly patches with cracking and fissuring typically begin in the fall or winter on the anterior plantar surfaces of the feet and great toes (Fig. 8.19). Although the cause is unknown, the condition is triggered by excessive sweating and/or repeated wetting of the skin inside the child's shoes (especially those made of synthetic materials that do not breathe), followed by drying of the skin at night. Consequently, the mainstay of treatment consists of lubricating and covering the feet at night. Topical steroids may be necessary in severe cases. The eruption tends to subside in the summer, and resolution in adolescence is common. Use of charcoal-impregnated foam insoles is also helpful in this condition.

LIP-LICKING AND THUMB-SUCKING ECZEMA

The repeated wetting and drying from persistent lip-licking (especially in winter) or thumb-sucking can produce eczematoid changes of the perioral skin (Fig. 8.20) or of the skin of the involved thumb (Fig. 8.21).

SEBORRHEA

Seborrheic dermatitis is characterized by a red and scaling eruption that occurs predominantly on hair-bearing and intertriginous areas, e.g., the scalp, eyebrows, eyelashes, perinasal, presternal, and postauricular areas, and the neck, axilla, and groin (Fig. 8.22). In affected infants, scalp lesions consist of a greasy, salmon-colored, scaly dermatitis called cradle cap (Fig. 8.23). A severe type may be more generalized. In adolescents, the dermatitis may manifest itself as dandruff or flaking of the eyebrows, postauricular areas, or flexural areas.

Although the pathogenesis of seborrheic dermatitis is unknown, Pityrosporum and Candida species have been implicated as causative agents. A role for neurologic dysfunction is suggested by the increased incidence and severity in neurologically impaired individuals.

The dermatitis of seborrhea is usually non-pruritic and mild in nature. Most cases respond to topical steroids, and many clear spontaneously. Antiseborrheic shampoos may also be helpful. In infants and young children, atopic dermatitis can have a greasy, scaly appearance and may be confused with

who also may have atopic dermatitis and/or keratosis pilaris and dry skin. Lack of central clearing helps distinguish these lesions from tinea corporis (see Fig. 8.31). Although the rash is often resistant to therapy, it may respond to the treatment for acute dermatitis outlined above. Application of occlusive dressings (e.g., Duoderm®, Comfeel®) may be useful in recalcitrant cases.

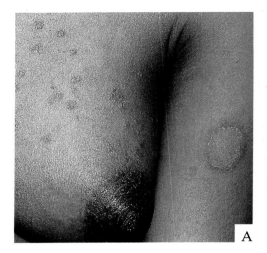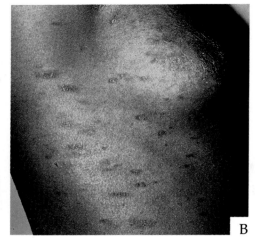

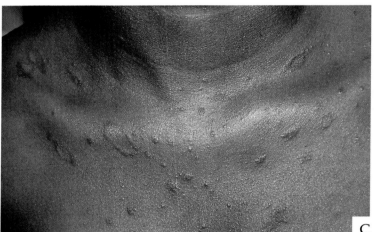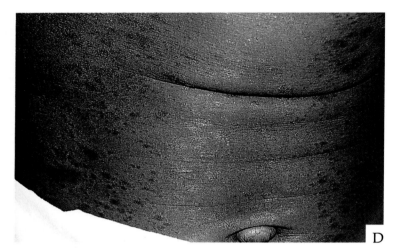

*FIG. 8.24 Pityriasis rosea. **A**, the large herald patch on the arm of this adolescent girl shows evidence of central clearing, mimicking tinea corporis. **B**, numerous oval lesions are seen on the trunk, which can appear in a fir tree distribution on the back. **C** and **D**, the orientation of the long axes of the oval lesions along lines of skin cleavage are seen in association with variations in appearance of lesions. In **B**, scaling is prominent; in **C**, lesions are quite raised and only slightly scaly; in **D**, the ovals are macular. (**A**, **C**, and **D** courtesy of Dr. Michael Sherlock)*

seborrhea. However, atopic dermatitis in infants produces intense pruritus and invariably spares moist sites such as the diaper area and axillae. The differential diagnosis of seborrhea also includes histiocytosis X (in which the rash is generalized and usually associated with chronic draining ears and hepatosplenomegaly) and tinea corporis (in which lesions usually are more circumscribed, with an active border and central clearing). Scalp lesions may be difficult to differentiate from psoriasis.

PITYRIASIS ROSEA

Pityriasis rosea is a benign, self-limited disorder which can occur at any age, but is more common in adolescents and young adults. A prodrome of malaise, headache, and mild constitutional symptoms occasionally precedes the rash. The typical eruption begins with the appearance of a "herald patch" (Fig. 8.24A), which is a large, isolated, oval lesion, usually pink in color and slightly scaly; it may occur anywhere on the body. Occasionally, it clears centrally, simulating tinea corporis. From 5 to 10 days later, other smaller lesions appear on the body, frequently concentrated on the trunk. These begin as small, round papules which then enlarge to ovals up to 1 to 2 cm in size, with a scaly surface. They are usually somewhat raised, but can be macular as well. The long axes of the ovals often run parallel to the skin lines of the thorax, creating a "Christmas tree" pattern (Fig. 8.27C and D). The rash reaches its peak in several weeks, and then slowly fades

over 4 to 6 weeks. The average total duration is 2 to 3 months. Ultraviolet light may hasten the disappearance of the eruption. Although the cause is unknown, the peak incidence in late winter and the low recurrence rate favor an infectious, probably viral, etiology.

Other eruptions that can resemble pityriasis rosea include guttate psoriasis, viral exanthems, measles-like (morbilliform) drug eruptions, and secondary syphilis. As noted above, the appearance of the herald patch may simulate tinea corporis, but a KOH prep will be negative.

CONTACT DERMATITIS

Contact dermatitis refers to a group of conditions in which a dermatitic or inflammatory reaction in the skin is triggered by direct contact with environmental agents. In the most common form, *irritant contact dermatitis*, changes in the skin are induced by caustic agents such as acids and alkalis, hydrocarbons, and other primary irritants. Anyone exposed to these agents in a high enough concentration for a long enough period of time will develop a contact dermatitis. The rash is usually acute, with well-demarcated erythema, crusting, and/or blister formation.

In contrast, allergic contact dermatitis is a T-cell-mediated immune reaction to an antigen coming into contact with the skin. Although it frequently presents with acute onset of erythema, vesiculation, and pruritus, the rash may become chronic with scaling, lichenification, and pigmentary changes. Often,

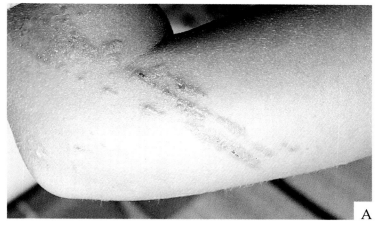

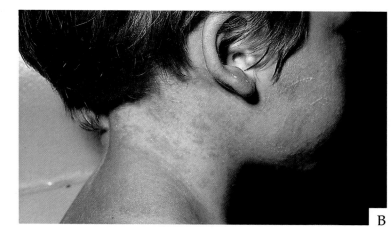

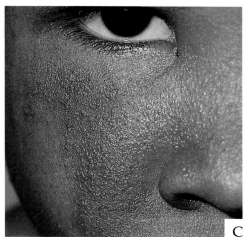

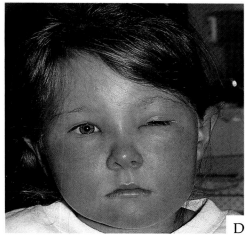

FIG. 8.25 Poison ivy or rhus dermatitis. *A, linear streaks of pruritic vesicles are typical of contact dermatitis to a plant. B and C, with more heavy exposure, however, the eruption can develop in relatively large patches. Also note the microvesicular appearance of the facial lesion in the child shown in C. D, reactions involving the face and genitalia can provoke impressive swelling.*

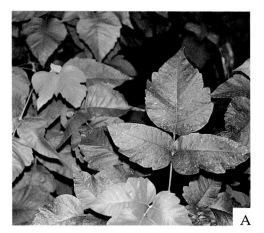

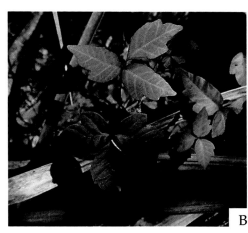

FIG. 8.26 *A, poison ivy. The plant has characteristic shiny leaves in groups of three. It may resemble a vine or a low shrub or bush. B, poison oak. This too has leaves in groups of three, although the edges tend to be more scalloped than those of poison ivy. (B, courtesy of Dr. Mary Jelks)*

the allergen is obvious, as is the case with poison ivy or nickel jewelry. However, in other cases careful questioning may be re-quired to detect the inciting agent.

The initial reaction occurs after a 7- to 14-day period of sensitization in susceptible individuals. Once sensitization has occurred, re-exposure to the allergen will provoke a more rapid reaction, sometimes within hours. This is a classic example of Type IV (delayed) hypersensitivity (see Chapter 4).

Rhus Dermatitis (Poison Ivy)

The most common allergic contact dermatitis in the United States is poison ivy or rhus dermatitis. This typically appears as linear streaks of erythematous papules and vesicles (Fig.

8.25A); however, with heavy exposure, the rash may appear in relatively large patches (Fig. 8.25B and C). When lesions involve the skin of the face or genitalia, impressive swelling can occur (Fig. 8.25D).

Direct contact with the sap of poison ivy, poison oak, or poison sumac, whether from leaves, stems, or roots is necessary to produce the dermatitis (Fig. 8.26). Contact with clothing that has brushed against the plant, with logs or railroad ties on which the vine has been growing, or with smoke from a fire in which the plant is being burned are other means of exposure. Areas of skin exposed to the highest concentration of plant oil will develop changes first. Other sites that have received lower doses will then vesiculate in succession, giving an illusion of

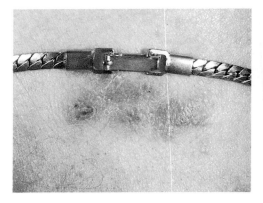

FIG. 8.27 Nickel contact dermatitis. The location of the rash is helpful in determining the cause of a contact dermatitis.

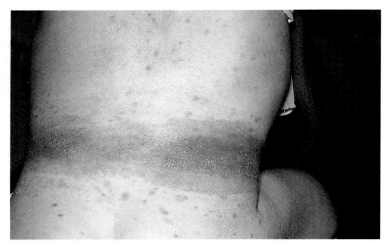

FIG. 8.28 Rubber contact dermatitis. This child had become sensitized to the elasticized waist bands of his underpants.

spreading. However, within about 20 minutes after contact, the rhus oil becomes tissue fixed to the epithelial cells and cannot be spread further. Thorough washing within minutes of exposure can prevent the eruption.

Other common offending agents are nickel (Fig. 8.27), rubber (Fig. 8.28), glues and/or dyes in shoes (Fig. 8.29), ethylenediamine in topical lotions, neomycin, and topical anesthetics.

Photocontact Dermatitis

Some allergens, known as photosensitizers, require sunlight to become activated. Photocontact dermatitis caused by drugs (e.g., tetracyclines, sulfonylureas, and thiazides) characteristically erupts in a symmetric distribution on the face, the "V" of the neck, and the arms distal to the end of the shirt sleeves. Topical photosensitizers (dyes, coal tar, furocoumarins and halogenated salicylanilides) produce localized patches of dermatitis when applied to sun-exposed sites (Fig. 8.30). These allergens are found in cosmetics, sunscreens, dermatologic products, and germicidal soaps.

"Id" Reaction

Occasionally, the local reaction in a contact dermatitis is so severe that the patient develops a widespread secondary eczematous dermatitis. When the dermatitis appears at sites which have not been in contact with the offending agent, the reaction is referred to as autoeczematization or an "id" reaction.

Basic Principles of Management

Although localized patches of contact dermatitis are best treated topically, widespread reactions require a 2-week tapering course of systemic corticosteroids beginning at 0.5 to 1.0 mg/kg/day. Patients may experience rebound of the rash if treated with a shorter course. Response is usually seen within 48 hours. Oral steroids also may be indicated in localized reactions involving the eyelids, extensive areas of the face, genitals, and/or hands, where swelling and pruritus may become incapacitating.

Fungal Infections

Two types of fungal organisms produce clinical cutaneous disease: dermatophytes and yeasts. Dermatophytes include the tinea or ringworm fungi, while yeasts include *Candida* species, which are associated with diaper dermatitis, and *Pityrosporum* species which cause tinea versicolor.

TINEA CORPORIS

Tinea corporis is a superficial fungal infection of the non-hairy or glabrous skin. It has been labeled "ringworm" because of its characteristic configuration consisting of pruritic, annular lesions with central clearing, and an active vesicular border made up of microvesicles which rupture and then scale (Fig. 8.31A and B). Lesions, which may be single or multiple, typically begin as red papules or pustules which rupture and evolve to form papulosquamous lesions. These then spread out from the periphery as new vesicles form and begin to clear centrally (Fig. 8.31C). Over a period of several weeks, the patches may expand up to 5 cm in diameter. Tinea corporis can be found in any age group, and it is usually acquired from an infected domestic animal (*Microsporum canis*), or through direct human contact (*Trichophyton tonsurans*).

Clinically, tinea may be differentiated from atopic dermatitis by its propensity for autoinoculation from the primary patch to other sites on the patient's skin, by spread to close contacts, and by the central clearing noted in many lesions. Moreover, the rash of atopic dermatitis tends to be symmetric, chronic, and recurrent in a flexural distribution. Unlike tinea, patches of nummular eczema are self-limited and do not clear centrally. The herald patch of pityriasis rosea is often mistaken for tinea. However, it is KOH-negative, and the subsequent development of the generalized rash with its characteristic truncal distribution is distinctive (see Fig. 8.24A). The clinical pattern, findings, and chronic nature of psoriasis and seborrhea help differentiate them from tinea. Though granuloma annulare produces a characteristic ringed eruption, on palpation, the lesions are firm, and they do not usually show epidermal changes (scales, vesicles, pustules) unless scratching has been intense. Lesions of granuloma annulare usually are only slightly pruritic or asymptomatic (see Fig. 8.76).

The diagnosis of tinea corporis is confirmed by potassium hydroxide examination of the skin. The first step is to obtain material by scraping the loose scales at the margin of a lesion (Fig. 8.32A). These should be mounted onto the center of the slide, with one or two drops of 20 percent KOH added. Next, a glass coverslip is applied and gently pressed down with the eraser end of a pencil to crush the scales (Fig. 8.32B). The slide is then heated, taking care not to boil the KOH solution, and

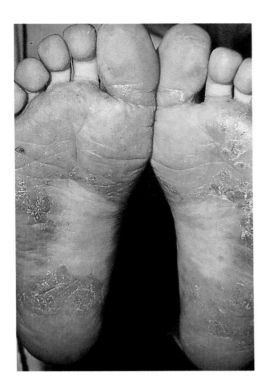

FIG. 8.29 Contact dermatitis of the foot. This adolescent became sensitized to the glue under the insoles of his shoes. Note the sparing of the instep. (Courtesy of Dr. Michael Sherlock)

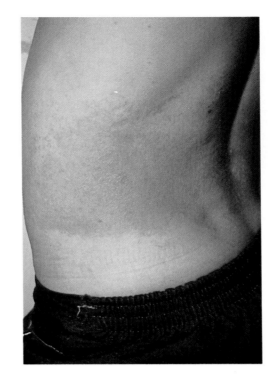

FIG. 8.30 Photocontact dermatitis. This boy developed contact dermatitis following sun exposure while out swimming. The offending agent was found to be in his soap. (Courtesy of Dr. Michael Sherlock)

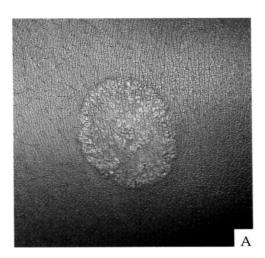

A

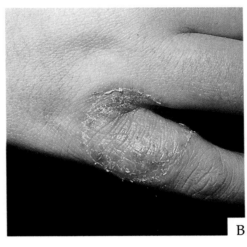

B

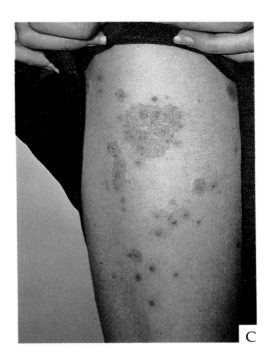

C

FIG. 8.31 Tinea corporis. The characteristic annular lesions show many variations in appearance. **A,** this lesion has a very raised, active border, and shows central clearing. **B,** sharply circumscribed lesion shown here is macular and is more prominently erythematous and scaly. **C,** the evolution of lesions from papules and pustules into larger papulosquamous patches is seen on this girl's leg. (**B** and **C,** courtesy of Dr. Michael Sherlock)

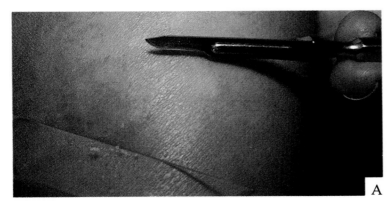

A

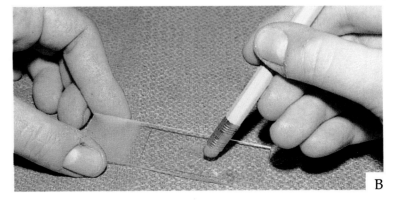

B

FIG. 8.32 Potassium hydroxide (KOH) preparation. **A,** small scales should be scraped from the edge of the lesion onto a microscope slide. **B,** crush the scales to make a thin layer of cells in order to easily visualize the fungus.

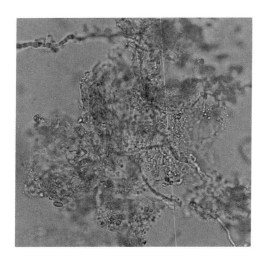

FIG. 8.33 Positive KOH prep of skin scrapings. Fungal hyphae are seen as long septate branching rods at the margins and center of the scales.

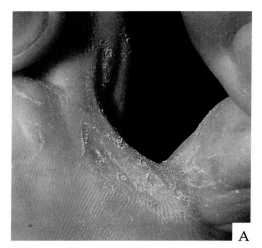

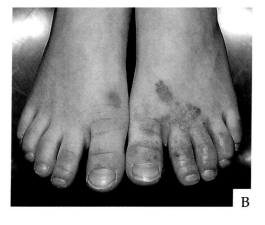

FIG. 8.34 Tinea pedis. **A,** scaling, cracking, and peeling rims of ruptured vesicles are seen predominantly in the web spaces. **B,** in this patient, lesions extend from the web spaces over the dorsum of the foot. **C,** the instep and ball of the foot are other common sites of involvement. (**A,** courtesy of Dr. Michael Sherlock)

again, the coverslip is pressed down. When viewing the slide under the microscope, the condenser and light source should be set at low levels, to maximize contrast, with the objective at 10x. On focusing up and down, true hyphae are seen as long, branching, often septate rods of uniform width, that cross the borders of epidermal cells (Fig. 8.33). Cotton fibers, cell borders, or other artifacts may be falsely interpreted as positive findings.

Tinea infections on glabrous skin respond readily to topical antifungal creams (e.g., imidazoles such as miconazole, clotrimazole, econazole, naftifine, ketoconazole, and tolnaftate). When lesions are multiple and widespread, oral therapy with griseofulvin is indicated.

TINEA PEDIS

Commonly referred to as athlete's foot, tinea pedis is a fungal infection of the feet with a predilection for the web spaces between the toes. It is quite common in adolescence, somewhat less so in prepubertal children. The infecting organisms are acquired from contaminated shower, bathroom, locker room, and gym floors, and their growth is fostered by the warm, moist environment of shoes.

In some cases, scaling and fissuring predominate; in others, vesiculopustular lesions and maceration are found. The infection begins between and along the sides of the toes, where it may remain (Fig. 8.34A). However, lesions can extend over the dorsum of the foot (Fig. 8.34B), and may involve the plantar surface as well, particularly the instep and the ball of the foot. Patients complain of a combination of burning and itching which are frequently intense.

This diagnosis often can be made on clinical grounds, and is confirmed by KOH preparation of skin scrapings. The mainstays of treatment are topical antifungal creams or powders, and adopting measures designed to reduce foot moisture. The latter include careful drying of the feet after bathing, wearing cotton rather than synthetic socks, and shoes that do not promote sweating, or better still, sandals. In patients with severe inflammatory lesions, oral antifungal agents may be required. Secondary bacterial infection (particularly with gram-negative organisms) may be a problem.

Tinea pedis is distinguished from contact dermatitis of the feet by virtue of the fact that the latter spares the interdigital web spaces. Dyshidrosis can have a similar distribution, but KOH preparation will be negative.

TINEA VERSICOLOR

Tinea versicolor is a common dermatosis characterized by multiple small, oval, scaly patches measuring 1 to 3 cm in diameter, usually located in a guttate or raindrop pattern on the upper chest, back, and proximal portions of the upper extremities of adolescents and young adults (Fig. 8.35A and B). However, all ages may be affected, including infants. Facial involvement is seen occasionally. The eruption is caused by a dimorphous form of *Pityrosporum*. Warm, moist climates, pregnancy, immunodeficiency, and genetic factors predispose people to the development of infection.

The rash is usually asymptomatic, although some patients complain of mild pruritus. Typically, they go to the physician because they are bothered by the cosmetic appearance of the lesions. Lesions may be light tan, reddish, or white in color, giving rise to the term versicolor. They are darker than surrounding skin in non-sun-exposed areas (Fig. 8.35C), and lighter in areas that have tanned on exposure to sunlight (Fig. 8.35A and B).

The diagnosis of tinea versicolor can generally be made on the basis of the clinical appearance of lesions and their distribution. It can be confirmed by examining the lesions under Wood's lamp, which reveals a characteristic tan to salmon-

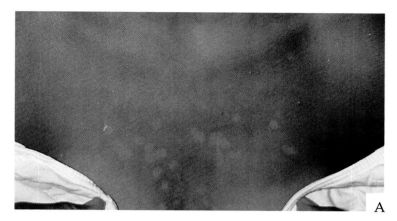

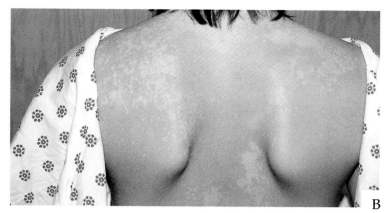

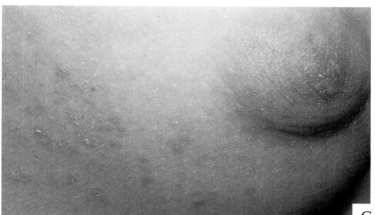

FIG. 8.35 Tinea versicolor. **A** and **B,** multiple oval patches are seen in a guttate or raindrop pattern over the upper chest and back of two patients. **C,** in areas not exposed to sunlight, lesions are darker than surrounding skin, while in **A** and **B** sun-exposed lesions fail to tan, remaining lighter than surrounding skin. (Courtesy of Dr. Michael Sherlock)

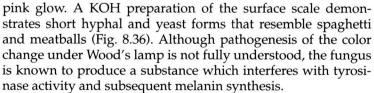

FIG. 8.36 Positive KOH preparation for tinea versicolor. The combination of hyphal and yeast forms of the fungus simulates the appearance of spaghetti and meatballs.

inflammatory hypopigmentation; the presence of fine superficial scaling and some residual pigmentation (even in hypopigmented areas) help rule out vitiligo.

Topical desquamating agents such as selenium sulfide and propylene glycol produce rapid clearing of the superficial lesions. Localized eruptions may be treated with topical antifungal creams such as miconazole, and recalcitrant cases will respond to oral ketoconazole. Patients must be counseled about the high risk of recurrence and reminded that pigmentary changes may take months to clear, even after eradication of the fungus.

Diaper Dermatitis

Because the diaper area is warm, often moist, and frequently contaminated by feces which are laden with organisms, diaper dermatitis is one of the most common skin disorders of infancy and early childhood.

IRRITANT DIAPER DERMATITIS

The diaper area is a prime target for irritant dermatitis because it is bathed in urine and feces and occluded by plastic diaper covers. Failure to change diapers frequently is a major predisposing factor, as this provides time for fecal bacteria to form ammonia by splitting the urea in urine. Harsh soaps, irritant chemicals, and detergents contribute to the process. Irritant diaper dermatitis is usually confined to the convex surfaces of the perineum, lower abdomen, buttocks, and proximal thighs,

pink glow. A KOH preparation of the surface scale demonstrates short hyphal and yeast forms that resemble spaghetti and meatballs (Fig. 8.36). Although pathogenesis of the color change under Wood's lamp is not fully understood, the fungus is known to produce a substance which interferes with tyrosinase activity and subsequent melanin synthesis.

The differential diagnosis of tinea versicolor includes postinflammatory hypopigmentation and vitiligo. The history and distribution help to distinguish tinea versicolor from post-

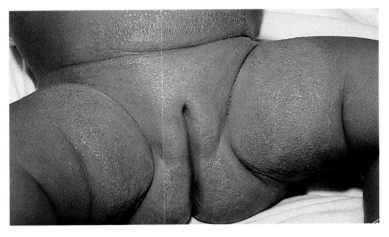

FIG. 8.37 *Irritant or ammoniacal diaper dermatitis. Note the involvement of the convex surfaces, and the sparing of the intertrigenous creases.*

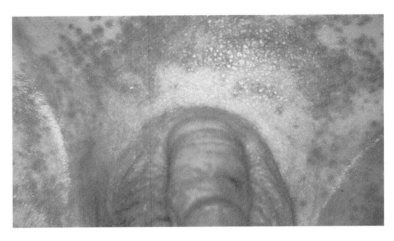

FIG. 8.38 *Candidal diaper dermatitis. The eruption is bright red with numerous pinpoint satellite papules and pustules. Intertrigenous areas are prominently involved.*

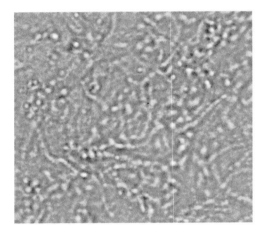

FIG. 8.39 *KOH preparation of skin scrapings from an infant with candidal diaper dermatitis demonstrating pseudohyphae and spores.*

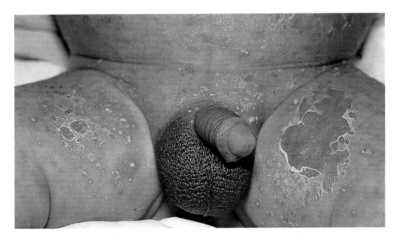

FIG. 8.40 *Staphylococcal diaper dermatitis. There are numerous intact thin-walled pustules surrounded by erythematous halos, as well as multiple areas in which pustules have ruptured, leaving a collarette of scale around a denuded erythematous base.*

sparing intertriginous areas (Fig. 8.37). When neglected, this may progress with further skin breakdown and ulceration. Frequent diaper changes, gentle, thorough cleansing of the area, and application of lubricants and barrier pastes usually result in clearing of the dermatitis. A short course of low-potency steroids may hasten resolution.

Persistent diaper dermatitis that does not resolve with conservative therapy may be due to other disorders such as candidiasis, seborrheic dermatitis, and psoriasis. These should be suspected, particularly when intertriginous areas are involved.

CANDIDAL DIAPER DERMATITIS

Candidal diaper dermatitis appears as a bright red eruption, with sharp borders and pinpoint satellite papules and pustules (Fig. 8.38). Examination of pustule contents by KOH preparation reveals the typical budding yeasts and pseudohyphae of *Candida* (Fig. 8.39). Candidal diaper dermatitis is occasionally associated with oral thrush, and it is a common sequela of oral or parenteral antibiotic therapy. One should suspect a secondary invasion by *C. albicans* whenever intertriginious areas

are involved or a diaper rash fails to respond to symptomatic treatment. Most cases respond well to topical antifungal therapy.

STAPHYLOCOCCAL DIAPER DERMATITIS

Irritant diaper dermatitis is frequently complicated by secondary staphylococcal infection or pustules may appear as primary lesions, especially in the first few weeks of life. The presence of thin-walled pustules on an erythematous base (larger than those seen with *Candida*) should alert the clinician to the diagnosis. Typically, these rupture rapidly and dry, producing a collarette of scaling around the denuded red base (Fig. 8.40). A Gram stain of pustule contents demonstrates neutrophils and clusters of gram-positive cocci. Bacterial cultures are confirmatory, but are rarely necessary. Early diagnosis and treatment with oral and topical antibiotics result in rapid resolution.

SEBORRHEIC DIAPER DERMATITIS

Seborrheic diaper dermatitis is characterized by salmon-colored, greasy lesions with a yellowish scale. The rash is particu-

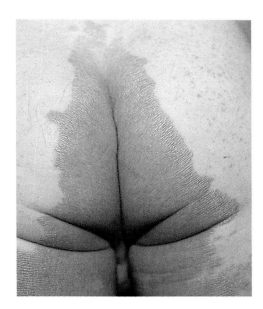

FIG. 8.41 Psoriatic diaper dermatitis. This child had a persistent diaper rash which did not respond to routine therapy. Note that scaling is not as intense as in psoriatic lesions seen elsewhere on the body.

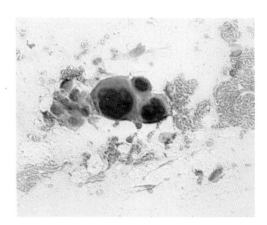

FIG. 8.42 Tzanck preparation. Note the multinucleated giant cells characteristic of viral infection with herpes simplex and varicella/zoster.

larly prominent in the intertriginous areas (see Fig. 8.22B). Unless secondarily infected with *Candida* (which is common), satellite lesions are not seen. Typically, seborrheic dermatitis of the scalp, face, and postauricular areas is seen in association with this form of diaper dermatitis.

PSORIATIC DIAPER DERMATITIS

Psoriasis occasionally begins as an erythematous, scaling eruption in the diaper area (Fig. 8.41). Although lesions may develop subsequently on the trunk and extremities, the rash may persist for months in the diaper area alone. Failure of a diaper rash to respond to empiric therapy over several weeks should raise this as a diagnostic possibility. Skin biopsy is the only way to confirm the diagnosis.

VESICULOPUSTULAR DISORDERS

Vesiculopustular eruptions range from benign, self-limited conditions to life-threatening diseases. Early diagnosis, especially in the young child, is mandatory. Systematic evaluation of the clinical findings and few rapid diagnostic techniques allow these various disorders to be readily differentiated from one another.

Viral Infections

Viral infections, including Herpes simplex and varicella/zoster, produce characteristic vesiculopustular exanthems that are presented in Chapter 12, Infectious Diseases. However, we will describe here the technique of confirming the suspicion of an herpetic lesion by preparing a Tzanck smear.

The Tzanck smear is obtained by removing the roof of the blister with a scalpel or scissors and scraping its base to obtain the moist, cloudy debris. This is then spread onto a glass slide with the scalpel blade, air dried, and stained with Giemsa or Wright's stain. The diagnostic finding in viral blisters is the multinucleated giant cell (Fig. 8.42). This is a syncytium of epidermal cells with multiple, overlapping nuclei; hence, it is much larger than other inflammatory cells. Unfortunately, a positive Tzanck smear cannot be used to differentiate one blis-

tering viral exanthem from another, and a viral culture should be obtained when the clinical situation dictates.

Bacterial Infections

Several common cutaneous bacterial infections present with vesiculopustular reactions as well. In impetigo, the eruption tends to be discrete and localized, whereas in staphylococcal scalded skin syndrome (SSSS) tends to be associated with a diffuse erythroderma. Gram staining of material aspirated from bullae or removed from the base of an impetiginous lesion will be positive for organisms. However, in patients with SSSS, the organism must be sought from non-cutaneous sources (nasopharynx, conjunctivae, sinuses, lungs, bone, etc.), as the diffuse cutaneous blistering is due to elaboration of epidermolysin by the infecting organism and not to the organism's direct action within individual lesions (see Chapter 12).

Toxic Epidermal Necrolysis

Toxic epidermal necrolysis (TEN) is a serious vesicuopustular disorder in which generalized erythroderma is followed by widespread necrosis and sloughing of the epidermis. Although the cause may be unclear, hypersensitivity reactions to medications, antecedent viral infections, connective tissue disorders, and malignancy have been implicated. A prodrome of fever, malaise, and sore throat usually precedes the appearance of the erythroderma, which is then superceded in 24 to 48 hours by diffuse cleavage at the dermal-epidermal junction (in contrast to SSSS, in which the plane of cleavage is high in the epidermis). The Nikolsky sign is present as in SSSS. TEN is also characterized by diffuse mucous membrane involvement including the oral mucosa, conjunctivae, airway, urethra, vagina, and anus. Erythema, hemorrhage, and crust formation are marked, and healing may be associated with the development of ectropion and formation of scars. This also helps distinguish TEN from SSSS, in which the nose and conjunctivae tend to be the only mucous membranes involved and in which Gram stain and culture of the exudates from these sites are usually positive for the offending organism.

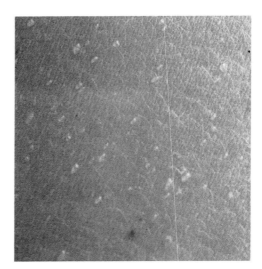

FIG. 8.43 Miliaria crystallina. Seen primarily over the head, neck and upper trunk, these tiny thin-walled sweat-retention vesicles rupture readily, then quickly desquamate.

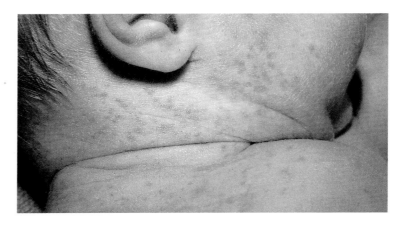

FIG. 8.44 Miliaria rubra. Numerous tiny papulopustular lesions dot the skin around the folds of this infant's neck.

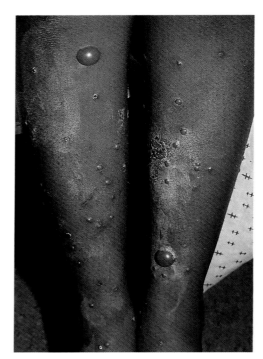

FIG. 8.45 Vesicular reaction to insect bites. This child's lower legs are studded with numerous thick-walled vesicles and bullae which have formed in response to insect bites.

Because the line of cleavage is so deep in TEN, fluid and electrolyte losses are proportionately greater, and recovery takes considerably longer (up to 1 month). Intensive supportive therapy is required to prevent complications from these losses, and to prevent secondary bacterial infection which is an ever-present danger.

Although the initial target lesions are characteristic, bullous erythema multiforme or Stevens-Johnson syndrome may progress to a clinical picture indistinguishable from TEN. Triggering factors and course are also similar (see section on Reactive Erythemas).

Miliaria

MILIARIA CRYSTALLINA

Miliaria crystallina is a condition in which obstruction of the eccrine sweat ducts in the outer layer of the epidermis results in the formation of multiple 2 to 3 mm sweat-retention vesicles. Being thin-walled, these are readily ruptured (Fig. 8.43). In infants, lesions form over the head, neck, and upper trunk. In older children, they are more commonly seen in areas of desquamating sunburn.

MILIARIA RUBRA

Sweat duct obstruction deeper in the epidermal or dermal layers produces an erythematous papulopustular eruption known as miliaria rubra (prickly heat) (Fig. 8.44). This rash occurs commonly in infants and children, especially over the face, upper trunk, and the intertriginous area of the neck, as a result of tight-fitting clothing or use of occlusive lubricants, particularly during hot, humid weather. Wearing lightweight, loose-fitting clothing, elimination of greasy topical agents, and the use of corn starch or powder facilitates clearing of the rash.

Vesiculation Following Insect Bites

Inflammatory reactions to insect bites, though often beginning as edematous papules, may evolve into pruritic vesicles and bullae on red bases (see Fig. 8.45). This is particularly true of the bites of grass and sand mites. The eruption is frequently misdiagnosed as chickenpox or bullous impetigo. The lack of systemic complaints, localization to exposed areas (especially the lower legs), and seasonal occurrence tend to point to the diagnosis. Furthermore, the vesicles have thicker walls than those of bullous impetigo, and they do not rapidly umbilicate and crust as is true of varicella lesions. Tzanck smears and Gram stains also are negative in bullous insect bite reactions (See section on Bites, Stings, and Infestations).

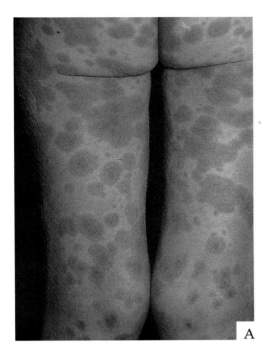

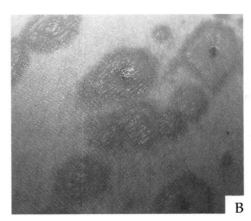

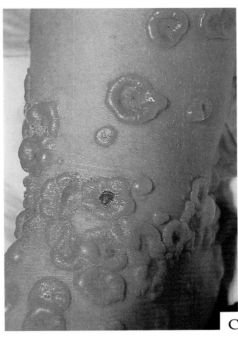

FIG. 8.46 Erythema multiforme. **A,** the characteristic target lesions are symmetrically distributed. **B,** in these typical target lesions with central dusky areas, the peripheral rims are beginning to vesiculate. **C,** in this case, the peripheral rims have become frankly bullous. (*A* and *C*, courtesy of Dr. Michael Sherlock)

THE REACTIVE ERYTHEMAS

The term reactive erythema refers to a group of disorders characterized by erythematous patches, plaques, and nodules which vary in size, shape, and distribution. Unlike other specific dermatoses, they represent cutaneous reaction patterns triggered by a variety of endogenous and environmental agents. In children, the most common reactive erythemas include erythema multiforme, erythema nodosum, urticaria, vasculitis, and drug eruptions.

Erythema Multiforme

Erythema multiforme (EM) is a distinctive, acute hypersensitivity syndrome that may be caused by many different types of agents including drugs, viruses, bacteria, foods, and immunizations. It may also arise in association with connective tissue disorders. Infectious diseases and medications are the most common causes in children.

The classic eruption is symmetrical, and may occur on any part of the body, although it typically appears on the dorsum of the hands and feet, and the extensor surfaces of the arms and legs. Involvement of palms and soles is typical. The initial lesions are dusky, red macules or erythematous

wheals that evolve into iris- or target-shaped lesions, the hallmark of EM (Fig. 8.46A and B). In many instances, the initial crop of lesions closely simulates diffuse urticaria, although EM lesions are typically much less pruritic. The target configuration is due to formation of a central depression which may be blue, violaceous, or white, while the elevated periphery tends to remain erythematous. In some cases, vesicles or bullae develop centrally, and in others, the peripheral rings may vesiculate or become bullous (Fig. 8.46C). The eruption continues in crops which last from 1 to 3 weeks. In most patients, the disease is self-limited, and systemic manifestations are limited to low-grade fever, malaise, and myalgia.

STEVENS-JOHNSON SYNDROME (BULLOUS ERYTHEMA MULTIFORME)

Rarely, erythema multiforme progresses to become Stevens-Johnson syndrome, with large areas of epidermal and mucous membrane necrosis and shedding. Hence, Stevens-Johnson syndrome is thought to represent the most severe end of the spectrum of erythema multiforme. In this disorder, constitutional symptoms are prominent, including high fever, cough, sore throat, vomiting, diarrhea, chest pain, and arthralgias. Vesiculation occurs early and is often hemorrhagic and exten-

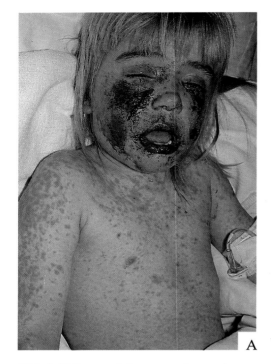

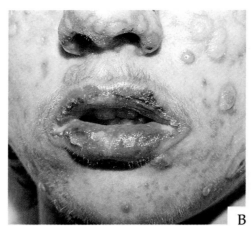

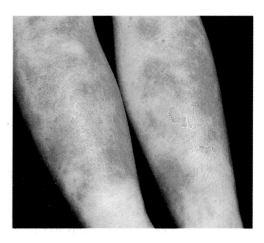

FIG. 8.48 Erythema nodosum. Note the typical, red, raised, tender nodules overlying the pretibial surfaces of the legs.

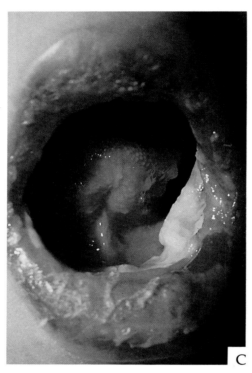

FIG. 8.47 Stevens-Johnson syndrome. **A,** severe bullous and erosive lesions cover the face, neck and extremities. **B,** typical bullae, target lesions, and erosions of the lips are seen in this boy. **C,** this child has numerous vesicles and bullae of the oral mucosa along with formation of a shaggy white membrane consisting of sloughed debris. (**C,** courtesy of Dr. Michael Sherlock)

sive (Fig. 8.47A and B). Mucous membrane involvement, particularly of the oral, conjunctival, and urethral mucous membranes, is routine and often severe. It consists of formation of fragile, thin-walled bullae that rupture early, leaving shallow ulcerations, which are rapidly covered by a gray, yellow, or white membrane (Fig. 8.47C). Conjunctival involvement can progress to involve the cornea, resulting in scarring unless aggressive ophthalmologic treatment is instituted early on. Fluid and electrolyte imbalances due to losses from ruptured bullae, and secondary infection are major risks in this disorder, which has a mortality ranging between 5 and 25 percent.

Erythema Nodosum

Erythema nodosum is characterized by symmetrical, red, tender nodules, 1 to 5 cm in diameter, which are usually located over the pretibial surfaces (Fig. 8.48). Most likely, it represents a hypersensitivity reaction in response to streptococcal infection, medication, sarcoidosis, tuberculosis, or other bacterial or fungal infections. Noninfectious disorders such as ulcerative colitis and regional ileitis have also been implicated.

Erythema nodosum is most often seen in children older than

10 years. The lesions begin as red, tender, slightly elevated nodules that develop into brownish-red or purplish-red lesions within a few days. The disorder usually lasts between 2 and 6 weeks, although recurrences are common.

Differential diagnosis includes cellulitis, insect bites, thrombophlebitis, ecchymoses, and vasculitis. The fact that lesions are symmetric, recurrent, and persistent helps exclude cellulitis and ecchymoses. Their pretibial and extensor location helps differentiate them from thrombophlebitis. Insect bite reactions are typically pruritic, and other exposed sites such as the arms, head, and neck may be involved. The deep-seated nature of the nodules in erythema nodosum should allow differentiation from the smaller, more superficial palpable lesions of cutaneous vasculitis.

Treatment should be directed toward the underlying cause. Nonsteroidal anti-inflammatory agents may be effective in reducing pain, and bed rest is beneficial.

Urticaria

Urticaria, commonly known as hives, is characterized by the sudden appearance of transient, well-demarcated wheals that

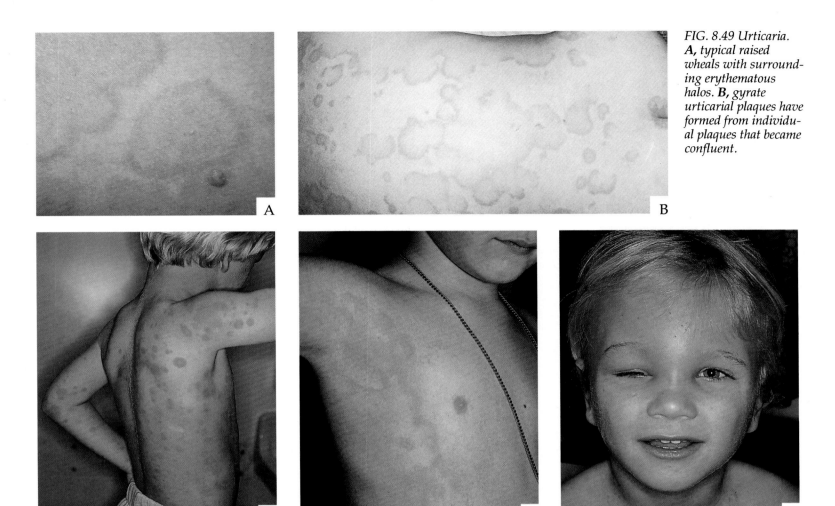

FIG. 8.49 Urticaria. A, typical raised wheals with surrounding erythematous halos. B, gyrate urticarial plaques have formed from individual plaques that became confluent.

FIG. 8.50 Urticarial/Erythema multiforme-like reaction to cefaclor. **A** and **B,** extensive urticarial, target and gyrate lesions are seen over the back, arms, and trunk. **C,** facial edema involving the forehead was prominent in this child.

are usually intensely pruritic, especially when arising as part of an acute IgE-mediated hypersensitivity reaction (Fig 8.49A). Individual lesions usually last 1 to 2 hours, but they may persist up to 24 hours. They may have an edematous white center and macular red halo, or the reverse—a red center with an edematous white halo. Size can vary from a few millimeters to giant lesions of over 20 cm in diameter. Central clearing with peripheral extension may lead to the formation of annular, polycyclic, and arcuate plaques, simulating erythema multiforme and erythema marginatum (Fig. 8.49B). The reaction may involve the mucous membranes and can spread to the subcutaneous tissue producing woody edema known as angioedema.

Urticaria can be caused by a variety of immunologic mechanisms, including IgE antibody response, complement activation, and abnormal levels of or sensitivity to vasoactive amines. Most commonly, acute urticaria (lasting less than 6 weeks) is caused by a hypersensitivity reaction to food, drugs, insect bites, contact allergens, inhaled substances, or acute infections (especially ß-streptococcal infections and viral infections, including mononucleosis). Chronic urticaria (last-

ing more than 6 weeks) can be a sign of an underlying disorder such as occult infection (of the urinary tract, sinuses, or dentition), hepatitis B, or connective tissue disease (see also Chapter 4).

URTICARIAL/ERYTHEMA MULTIFORME-LIKE REACTION

One relatively common, acute clinical picture involves a constellation of urticarial lesions, periarticular swelling, and extremity angioedema in conjunction with acute upper respiratory infection or following use of sulfa-containing antibiotics or cefaclor. The urticaria is typically either nonpruritic or only mildly pruritic, and lesions evolve into target shapes or gyrate plaques simulating erythema multiforme, although they do not vesicate (Fig. 8.50A,B). With this eruption, painful migratory periarticular swelling is seen, especially involving wrists and ankles, and often associated with bluish discoloration of overlying skin. Migratory stocking-glove angioedema, which is also painful, is common; occasionally, facial edema is seen as well (Fig. 8.50C). Symptoms tend to wax and wane over 1 to 3 weeks until the condition resolves. This appears to be a

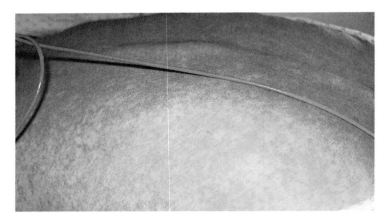

FIG. 8.51 Morbilliform drug eruption. This fine maculopapular exanthem developed in a child taking ampicillin. It was mildly pruritic and generalized rapidly.

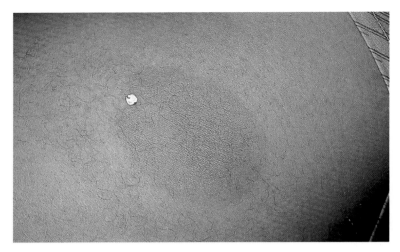

FIG. 8.52 Fixed drug eruption. This hyperpigmented patch with an erythematous border developed on the flank of an adolescent taking tetracycline.

delayed hypersensitivity or "serum sickness-like" reaction, although some of the clinical features resemble those of vasculitic eruptions.

Drug Eruptions

MORBILLIFORM DRUG ERUPTIONS

Many different types of drug eruptions are seen in children. Morbilliform or maculopapular exanthems account for more than half of all cutaneous drug reactions. The rash is reminiscent of measles or other viral exanthems (see Chapter 12). Erythematous macules and papules, which may range from fine to blotchy, begin to erupt on the face and trunk within 5 to 14 days after starting a medication. They then spread to the extremities over 1 to several days (Fig. 8.51). The rash, which may be pruritic, is occasionally restricted to the extremities or appears acrally (distally) and spreads centrally. Lesions may become confluent and generally resolve over 1 to 2 weeks with the development of mild purpura and fine desquamation.

FIXED DRUG ERUPTIONS

Fixed drug eruptions occur repeatedly in the same cutaneous site after re-exposure to the offending drug. Post-inflammatory hyperpigmentation is usually marked and may be the only manifestation of the rash during remissions. Morphologically and histologically, the target and bullous lesions of fixed drug reactions may be indistinguishable from erythema multiforme and may, in fact, represent a localized form of EM (Fig. 8.52).

Henoch-Schönlein Purpura

Henoch-Schönlein purpura (HSP) is an inflammatory disorder with multiple predisposing conditions, characterized by a diffuse vasculitis involving the small, nonmuscular blood vessels of the skin, gastrointestinal tract, kidneys, joints, and, rarely, the lungs and central nervous system. Although the exact etiology is unclear, the frequent history of antecedent upper respiratory or gastrointestinal infection suggests a hypersensitivity phenomenon resulting in a localized or widespread vascular insult. Other factors including drugs, food, immunizations, and chemical toxins have been implica-ted, as well. Histologically, immune complex deposition in capillaries and post-capillary venules is associated with a leukocytoclastic vasculitis in the skin and other involved organs.

Following a prodrome of headache, anorexia, and fever lasting 1 to a few days, patients may develop one or more of the following in any order: rash, abdominal pain, and arthritis. Cutaneous lesions consist of erythematous macules, urticarial papules, and purpuric papules and plaques which tend to appear in crops (Fig. 8.53A), each resolving over 5 to 7 days, although the total duration of this waxing and waning eruption may last anywhere from 1 to 8 weeks (average 2 to 3). Fifteen to 40 percent of affected children have one or more recurrences, usually within 6 weeks of resolution of the first episode.

While in most children the initial crop consists of purpuric lesions distributed symmetrically below the waist (over the buttocks, lower abdomen, and lower extremities), in some this may be preceded by a generalized urticarial eruption which is minimally pruritic and waxes and wanes over 1 to several days before the appearance of purpura. Subsequent crops of purpura usually involve the extensor surfaces of the arms, cheeks, and tips of the ears. The rash may also involve the trunk and genitalia. In unusually severe cases, skin necrosis may occur, heralded by the appearance of bullae.

Joint involvement consists of painful, tender periarticular swelling, especially involving wrists, ankles, and knees. The overlying skin tends to be ecchymotic. Stocking-glove edema of the hands and feet is also common (Fig. 8.53B). In young children, nonpruritic angioedema of the face, scalp, sacral

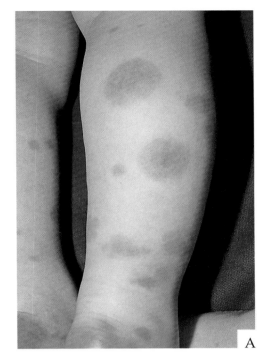

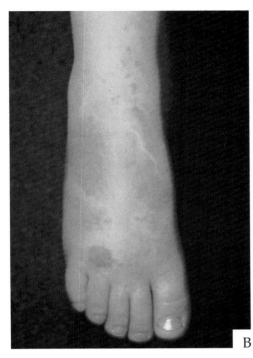

A

B

FIG. 8.53 Henoch-Schönlein purpura. A, palpable purpuric macules, papules, and plaques are seen over the legs and heels of this toddler. B, stocking angioedema of the foot with overlying purpuric skin changes. (B, courtesy of Dr. Michael Sherlock)

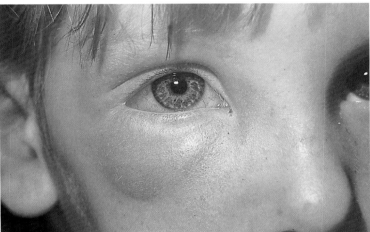

FIG. 8.54 Facial swelling due to a mosquito bite. The area was pruritic, non-tender and non-indurated. (Courtesy of Dr. Michael Sherlock)

and progressive (see Chapter 13, Nephrology). Central nervous system involvement is extremely rare, and its presence is usually heralded by severe headache, altered level of consciousness, and/or seizures following meningeal hemorrhage.

Treatment of Henoch-Schönlein purpura is generally supportive, although gastrointestinal, renal, and central nervous system vasculitis may respond to systemic corticosteroids.

The cutaneous lesions of HSP must be differentiated from acute bacterial, viral, and rickettsial infections (see Chapters 5 and 12). Negative blood cultures and classic findings on cutaneous examination and skin biopsy will define HSP. Purpuric rashes associated with thrombocytopenia are more likely to be associated with petechiae and can be ruled out by a normal platelet count. Finally, vasculitic rashes may also be seen in collagen vascular disorders such as lupus erythematosus, mixed connective tissue disease, and dermatomyositis (see Chapter 7). These disorders can usually be excluded by the absence of other findings.

BITES, STINGS, AND INFESTATIONS

Insect and spider bites may be associated with a number of cutaneous and systemic reactions. Lesions are found on exposed areas of skin, particularly the lower legs, arms, head, and neck. During the warm summer months they may also appear on the trunk. Protected areas (including the buttocks, groin, and axillae) are invariably spared. When bites involve the face, they can cause significant pruritic swelling which, though erythematous, is non-tender and non-indurated (Fig. 8.54).

Insect Bites

Insect bites, most commonly caused by mosquitoes, fleas, mites, and flies, tend to produce mild acute local reactions including erythema, edema, and urticarial papules which are

and/or genital area may be prominent. These phenomena wax and wane as does the exanthem (see Chapter 7, Rheumatology).

Gastrointestinal symptoms can precede, coincide with, or follow the appearance of cutaneous lesions. Segmental edema of the intestinal tract can cause crampy to colicky abdominal pain and may even serve as the lead point for an intussusception. Mucosal hemorrhage can be the source of gastrointestinal bleeding which can range from occult loss to massive hematochezia or hematemesis (see Chapter 10, Nutrition and Gastroenterology).

Up to 25 percent of patients develop nephritis between 1 and 8 weeks after onset of symptoms (peak 1 to 3 weeks). This is more common in older children, and it is usually mild and self-limited. It is first detected by finding evidence of hematuria and proteinuria on urinalysis. Occasionally, nephritis is severe

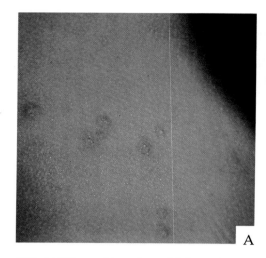

FIG. 8.55 Insect bites. **A,** *multiple erythematous papules with central puncta were the result of flea bites.* **B,** *another child had an intense hemorrhagic reaction to flea bites.* (**A,** *courtesy of Dr. Michael Sherlock*)

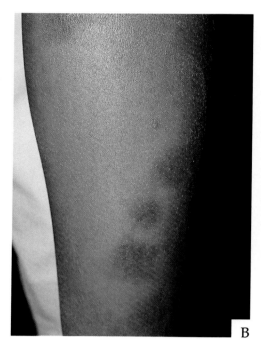

FIG. 8.56 Spider bites. *A marked inflammatory response consisting of a central wheal with a wide erythematous halo is seen in this child.*

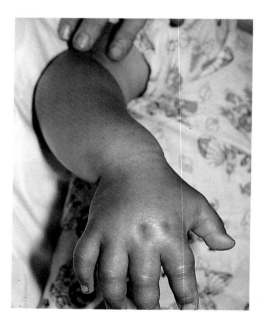

FIG. 8.57 Delayed hypersensitivity response to a bee sting. *Marked swelling of the hand and fingers developed over 24 hours following a sting between the fingers.*

typically pruritic (Fig. 8.55A). A tiny central crust or hemorrhagic punctum may be apparent on close inspection. Occasionally, patients develop more intense hemorrhagic reactions (Fig. 8.55B).

Mosquito and mite bites occur only during the warm months of spring, summer, and fall. Flea bites occur year round, typically in households with pets. They are usually found on the lower legs above the sock line, but can be more diffusely distributed on crawling infants and toddlers. Excoriation caused by scratching makes them prone to secondary impetiginization. On occasion, the bites of grass or sand mites can produce frank blistering as the venom they inject contains a blistering agent (see Fig. 8.45).

Biting flies include sand flies, blackflies, horseflies, and gnats. The bite itself causes immediate pain, and is usually followed by the development of a painful papule which sometimes vesiculates centrally.

Spider Bites

Spider bites tend to provoke more intense inflammatory reactions than those of most insects. Commonly, this consists of an area of erythema and induration which frequently becomes ecchymotic and is simultaneously painful and pruritic (Fig. 8.56). Less often, the lesions may vesiculate or even progress to develop central necrosis with eschar formation. The latter is particularly typical of the bite of the brown recluse spider.

Hymenoptera Stings

Bee, wasp, hornet, and yellow jacket stings typically produce a mild local reaction consisting of pain, erythema, and edema appearing within 2 hours after the sting. The honey bee leaves its stinger behind, embedded in the skin. As this may continue to release venom for up to an hour, it should be removed as soon as possible using a horizontal scraping motion with a knife or fingernail. Grasping the stinger between forceps or two fingernails can actually inject more venom. There is some evidence that topical application of a paste of papain (meat tenderizer) mixed with water within minutes of the sting may reduce the severity of local reactions.

Hymenoptera stings commonly produce a late-onset increase in swelling which is more diffuse than the initial reaction, and which tends to peak in 48 to 72 hours. This is the result of a delayed hypersensitivity reaction, and it is described by patients as being both pruritic and painful (Fig. 8.57). Treatment is symptomatic.

In approximately 0.5 to 0.8 percent of the population, hymenoptera stings cause severe, acute, anaphylactic reactions within 15 minutes of the sting (see Chapter 4).

Papular Urticaria

Papular urticaria is a delayed hypersensitivity reaction to the bites of mosquitoes, fleas, bedbugs, or other insects. It usually occurs in infants and children in the spring and summer

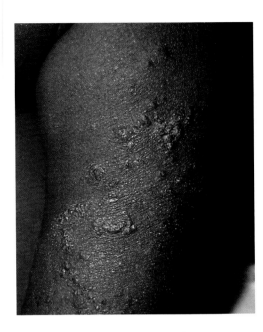

FIG. 8.58 Papular urticaria. This severe excoriated papular reaction developed in response to recurrent flea bites. (Courtesy of Dr. Michael Sherlock)

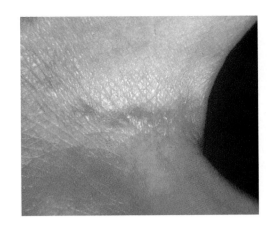

FIG. 8.59 Scabies burrow. This linear lesion in the finger web is characteristic of an itch mite burrow.

months. Lesions consist of 3- to 10-mm urticarial wheals with a central punctum and are intensely pruritic. They tend to be grouped in clusters (Fig. 8.58), and are often excoriated or secondarily infected. They recur in crops, and each may persist for 2 to 10 days or longer.

General principles of therapy for insect bites consist of insect control, use of insect repellents, and application of topical corticosteroids supplemented by oral antihistamines for symptomatic relief. Parenteral administration of epinephrine, antihistamines, and corticosteroids combined with intensive supportive care may be lifesaving in anaphylactic reactions.

Infestations

SCABIES

Scabies is a highly contagious infestation caused by the itch mite *Acarus scabiei*, which burrows under the skin. It is contracted by direct contact with other infested humans. The characteristic eruption appears 4 to 6 weeks after initial contact, and it is thought to represent a hypersensitivity reaction to the mites. Intensely pruritic papules, vesicles, pustules, and linear burrows appear in the finger and toe webs, the axillae, over the flexor surfaces of the wrists and elbows, around the nipples and waist, and over the groin and buttocks. The burrow, which is produced by the female mite, is the pathognomonic sign of scabies. It consists of a small, scaly linear papule with pinpoint vesicles at the ends (Fig. 8.59). In infants and toddlers the distribution differs, with the head, neck, trunk, palms, soles, dorsa, and instep portions of the feet, and lateral aspect of the wrists being more prominently involved (Fig. 8.60A and B). They also are more prone to developing an intense nodular reaction to the mite (Fig. 8.60C).

In many patients, excoriation, secondary infection, or even development of a widespread secondary eczematous eruption (as a result of scratching) alters the appearance of or masks the primary lesions, making diagnosis more difficult. Therefore, scabies must be considered in any individual who has no antecedent history of atopic dermatitis but presents with severe pruritus and recent onset of an eczematous rash. The distribution of scabies in intertriginous areas as well as over the palms, the dorsa, and the soles of the feet helps to differentiate it from other insect bite reactions.

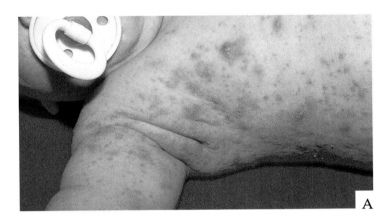

A

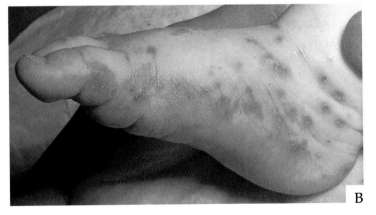

B

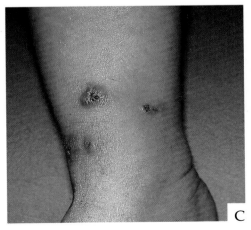

C

FIG. 8.60 Infantile scabies. Widespread, pruritic, red papules, pustules, and vesicles are seen (**A**) over the trunk and axilla and (**B**) the dorsa and instep portions of the feet, where burrows are also evident. **C**, infants are also more likely to develop an intense nodular reaction to the mite.

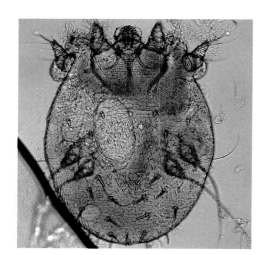

FIG. 8.61
Microscopic appearance of adult scabies mite. Note the small oval egg within the body.

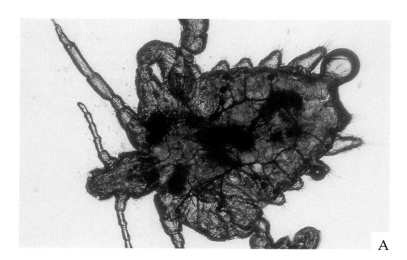

A

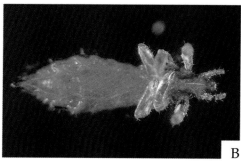

B

FIG. 8.62
Microscopic appearance of lice. **A,** the crab louse has a short, broad body, with claws spaced far apart. **B,** the head louse has a long, thin body, with claws spaced close together.

While scabies can often be diagnosed clinically, an unequivocal diagnosis can be made with a skin scraping that shows a mite, mite eggs, or feces. The most important factor in obtaining a successful scraping is choice of site. Burrows and papules are most likely to be identified on the wrists, finger webs, feet, or elbows. A fresh burrow can be identified as a 5- to 10-mm raised mound with a small dark spot resembling a fleck of pepper at one end. This spot is the mite, and it can be lifted out of the burrow with a needle or the point of a scalpel blade. If a scalpel is used to scrape the burrow, it is worthwhile to place a drop of mineral oil onto the skin to ensure adherence of the scrapings to the scalpel. The scrapings are placed on a slide, another drop of mineral oil is added, and a coverslip is applied.

Mites are eight-legged arachnids easily seen under the scanning power of the microscope (Fig. 8.61). Care must be taken to focus through thick areas of skin scrapings so as not to miss camouflaged mites. The presence of eggs (smooth ovals, approximately one-half the size of an adult mite) or feces (red-brown pellets, often seen in clusters) is also diagnostic.

Eradication of scabies necessitates topical application of lindane lotion to all household members (for varying periods of time, depending on age), and thorough cleansing of all dirty clothing and bedding. Permethrin 5% cream (Elimite®) is a new product with similar efficacy and a superior safety profile, particularly in young children. Symptomatic therapy with oral antipruritic agents and topical steroids may be required long after the mites have been killed, e.g., until the secondary reaction has subsided.

LICE

Three varieties of lice produce clinical disease in humans, and all can involve the scalp hair in children. Crab lice (*Phthirus pubis*) are transmitted primarily by sexual contact. They are short and broad, with claws spaced far apart to grasp the sparse hairs on the trunk, pubic area, and eyelashes (Fig. 8.62A). They are typically found inhabiting the pubic hair and, occasionally, axillary hair and other body hair in adolescents and adults. Their bites produce bluish, pruritic papules which are distributed over the lower abdomen and upper thighs. Pruritus is intense, and a secondary eczematous rash may develop, particularly in the pubic area, as a result of scratching. Young children lacking pubic and axillary hair may develop scalp or eyelash infestations after close contact with infested adults. Body lice (*Pediculus humanus corporis*) generally live in bedding or clothing, and their eggs may be found in the seams of trousers or underwear. Bites produce urticarial papules, seen primarily over the waist, neck, shoulders, and axillae, which are usually obliterated by excoriations and secondary bacterial infection.

Head lice (*Pediculus humanus capitis*) represent the most common infestation in children. The lice are acquired by close physical contact, or by sharing hats, combs, brushes, or scarves with an infested person or by rubbing against upholstered furniture recently used by such a person. Head lice are long and thin, with claws spaced close together to grasp the more densely distributed scalp hairs (Fig. 8.62B). Pruritus is the principal symptom, and the resultant scratching produces scalp excoriations which are vulnerable to secondary infection. Occipital adenopathy is common.

Nits are seen as oval, white 0.5-mm dots glued onto the hair shafts about 1 to 3 cm from the scalp (Fig. 8.63A), particularly above and behind the ears. These are firmly attached to the hair and do not move along the hair shafts as do the hair casts for which they are frequently mistaken. While nits may be seen along the entire length of the hair, they are deposited by the lice only near the scalp. Those far from the root indicate a span of perhaps months between infestation and examination.

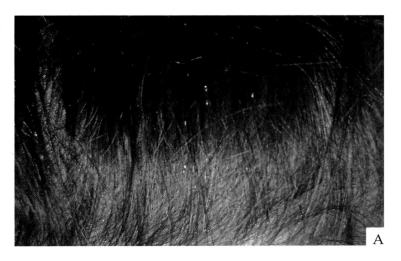

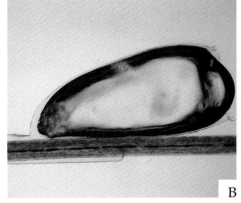

FIG. 8.63 Head lice. **A,** nits appear as tiny white dots that adhere to the hair shafts. They are typically found 1 to 3 cm from the scalp above and behind the ears. **B,** microscopic appearance of the nit of a head louse attached to a scalp hair. Microscopic examination distinguishes nits from hair casts and other artifacts. (**A,** Courtesy of Dr. Michael Sherlock)

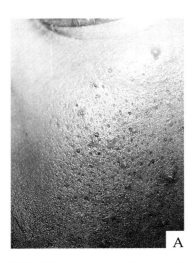

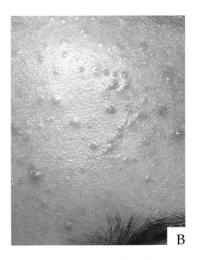

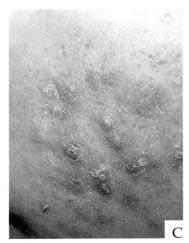

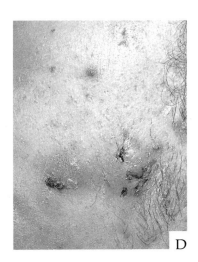

FIG. 8.64 **A,** comedonal acne with open comedones or blackheads are seen over the cheek. **B,** comedonal acne with closed comedones or whiteheads on the forehead, accentuated by side lighting. **C,** papulo-pustular acne with inflamed papules and pustules over the cheeks, which responded well to antibiotics. **D,** cystic acne shows deep cysts with marked erythema that can cause severe scarring after the acne has resolved.

Nits are difficult to remove and may, in fact, be nonviable shells. Patients adequately treated for lice will still have nonviable shells attached to the hair. Removal is facilitated by use of a weak vinegar rinse (which is left on under a shower cap or towel for 15 to 20 minutes), followed by combing with a fine-toothed comb or by cutting the hair close to the scalp. This is important because the persistence of dead nits is a common cause of misunderstanding by school health care workers who insist on re-treating the children or sending them home from school. New or viable nits rarely recur in a previously treated child, and reports of lice resistant to treatment are rare and poorly documented. Active disease is present only if a viable organism or new nits attached close to the scalp are identified.

Diagnosis of pediculosis must be considered in patients with unexplained scalp pruritus. A careful search for the organism may permit a specific diagnosis. Lice are six-legged insects visible to the unaided eye; they are commonly found on the scalp, eyelashes and pubic areas. They are best identified close to the skin or scalp, where they can be seen moving around and where their eggs are more numerous and more obvious. Diagnosis can be made either by identifying a louse or by plucking hairs and confirming the presence of nits by microscopic examination (Fig. 8.63B).

Eradication of lice requires application of lindane shampoo to infested hair-bearing areas of all household members and cleaning measures similar to those specified for ridding the house of scabies. Special attention should also be given to hats, scarves, and coat collars.

ACNE

Acne vulgaris, a disorder of the pilosebaceous apparatus, is the most common skin problem of adolescence. Lesions may appear on the face as early as age 8, although they usually begin to develop in the second decade of life with the onset of puberty. Other areas with prominent sebaceous follicles including the upper chest and back may be involved as well.

The exact pathogenesis of acne is unknown. However, abnormalities in follicular keratinization are thought to produce the earliest acne lesion, the microcomedone. In time, microcomedones may grow into clinically apparent open comedones (blackheads) (Fig. 8.64A) and closed comedones (whiteheads) (Fig. 8.64B). The entire process is driven by

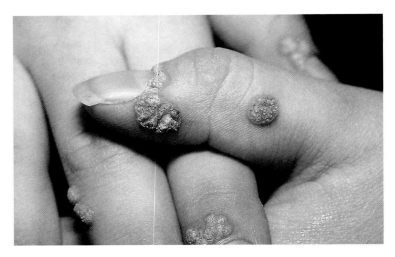

FIG. 8.65 Verruca vulgaris. Dry, rough, and crusty, these common warts usually involve the hands. The periungual distribution in this girl was due, in part, to her habit of picking at her cuticles.

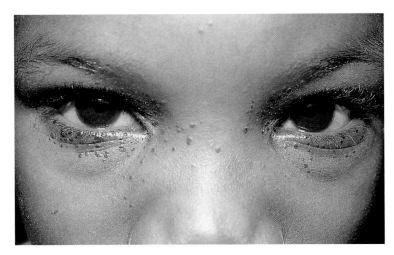

FIG. 8.66 Flat warts or verruca plana. These tiny, light brown warts are spread by scratching.

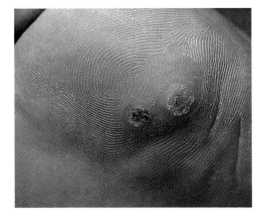

FIG. 8.67 Plantar warts. Two painful lesions are seen over the ball of the foot. Note how they interrupt the normal skin lines.

androgens, which stimulate sebaceous gland differentiation and growth, and the production of sebum. The proliferation of *Propionibacterium acnes* in noninflammatory comedones, and the rupture of comedone contents into the surrounding dermis may trigger the development of inflammatory papules, pustules, and cysts (Fig. 8.64C). Cystic acne is typified by nodules and cysts scattered over the face, chest, and back (Fig. 8.64D). This form frequently leads to scarring.

Although therapy must be individualized, patients with mild to moderate comedonal and/or inflammatory acne respond well to a combination of topical retinoic acid, benzoyl peroxide, and antibiotics. Moderate to severe papulopustular acne warrants the use of oral antibiotics in combination with topical agents. Oral 13-cis retinoic acid (Accutane®) should be reserved for patients with severe, scarring cystic acne recalcitrant to conservative measures.

TUMORS AND INFILTRATIONS

Persistent lumps and bumps in the skin often raise fears of skin cancer. Fortunately, primary skin cancer is extremely rare in childhood, and most tumors and infiltrated lesions are benign. Hemangiomas and nevi, which can be regarded as tumors, will be discussed in subsequent sections later in this chapter.

Warts

Warts are benign tumors produced by human papilloma virus (HPV) infection of the skin and mucous membranes. In children, they are seen most commonly on the fingers, hands, and feet. The incubation period for warts varies from 1 to 6 months, and the majority of lesions disappear spontaneously over a period of 5 years. Local trauma promotes inoculation of the papilloma virus. Thus, periungual lesions are common in children who bite their nails or pick at hangnails.

Investigators have identified over 50 human papilloma viruses capable of producing warts, and many of these organisms produce characteristic lesions in specific locations. For

instance, the discrete, round, skin-colored papillomatous (roughened) papules typical of verruca vulgaris (common warts) are produced by HPV Types 2 and 4 (Fig. 8.65). The subtle, minimally hyperpigmented, flat warts (verruca plana) which are caused by HPV 3 are frequently spread by picking and scratching and thus may become widespread on the face, arms, and legs (Fig. 8.66).

Plantar warts (Fig. 8.67) are associated with HPV Type 1. Although not proven, the spread of these warts probably occurs by contact with contaminated, desquamated skin in showers, pool decks, and bathrooms. Being much larger below the skin surface than is apparent from their external appearance, they often cause pain when the patient walks. While lesions can be confused with corns, calluses, or scars, they can be distinguished by their interruption of the normal skin lines (dermatoglyphics). Characteristic black dots in the warts are thrombosed superficial capillaries.

Warts can also be found on the trunk, oral mucosa, and conjunctivae. Anogenital lesions (condylomata acuminata) are usually associated with HPV Types 6 and 11, and the possibility of sexual abuse must be considered in children with lesions in this site (see Chapter 6).

Molluscum contagiosum is characterized by sharply circumscribed single or multiple skin-colored, dome-shaped papules with a waxy surface. They usually have umbilicated centers, although some lesions have protruding white centers (Fig.

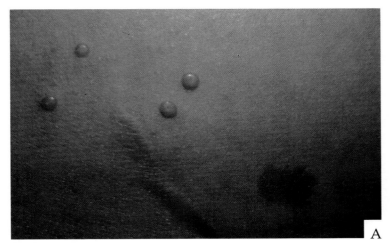

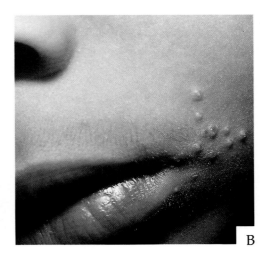

FIG. 8.68 Molluscum contagiosum. **A,** four sharply circumscribed waxy papules with umbilicated centers surround this child's appendectomy scar. **B,** lesions have spread on the face of this boy as a result of scratching. Note that some of these lesions have protruding white centers. (**A,** courtesy of Dr. Michael Sherlock)

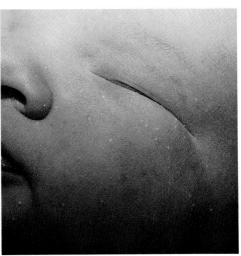

FIG. 8.69 Milia. Small, white-yellow papules found close to the skin surface, are particularly common around the eyes and midface.

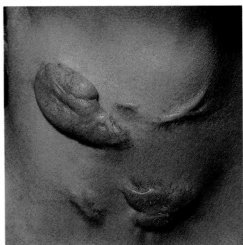

FIG. 8.70 Keloids. An abnormal reparative reaction to skin injury, keloids are characterized by proliferation of fibroblasts and collagen that extends beyond the margins of the original wound.

8.68A,B). This contagious disease is caused by a poxvirus. Lesions are found on the trunk, axillae, face, and genitals. They usually begin as pinpoint elevations of the skin and rapidly increase in size to 5 mm. The lesions are spread by scratching, and thus, are often arranged in a linear configuration (Fig. 8.73B). Frequently, a curd-like core can be expressed from the center; microscopic examination of this material reveals typical molluscum bodies. Destruction of lesions by curetting their cores or by application of a blistering agent and plastic tape which is peeled off in 3 days is curative, although many patients undergo spontaneous remission.

Although warts are self-limited in most children, persistent, widespread lesions should suggest the possibility of congenital or acquired immunodeficiency. In fact, warts may become a serious management problem in oncology and transplant patients who are chronically immunosuppressed.

Milia

Milia (Fig. 8.69) are small (1 to 2 mm), whitish-yellow papules commonly seen on the face in neonates. They are firm and, unlike pustules, not easily removed by pressure. Milia consist of epithelial-lined cysts arising from hair follicles. They are persistent, although they may resolve spontaneously after months to years. They usually arise without any apparent cause, although they are often seen after skin injury, such as that caused by blistering eruptions or dermabrasion. They are a characteristic feature of the dystrophic form of epidermolysis bullosa (see Fig. 8.86A).

Keloids

Keloids are rubbery nodules or plaques that result from the proliferation of fibroblasts and deposition of collagen following injury to the skin (Fig. 8.70). They can be pruritic or tender, especially during the active growing phase, and they may extend well beyond the margins of the original wound. This latter trait distinguishes keloids from hypertrophic scars which remain confined to the wound margins and flatten spontaneously within 6 months of the injury. Keloids may arise spontaneously or occur in a familial form. They are most common in blacks, and occur most often on the ear lobes, upper trunk, and deltoid areas. Fortunately, they are not seen on the midface. Keloids regress with intralesional steroid injections, alone or in combination with surgical excision. However, recurrences are common.

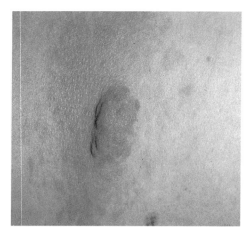

FIG. 8.71 Neurofibromatosis. Soft pink neurofibroma arising within a café au lait spot. Usually, neurofibromas arise from normal skin.

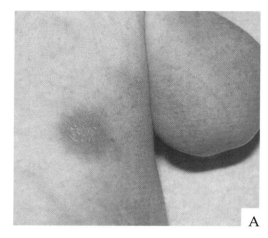

FIG. 8.72 Mastocytoma. **A,** the solitary brown plaque on this infant's back contained numerous mast cells on histopathologic examination.

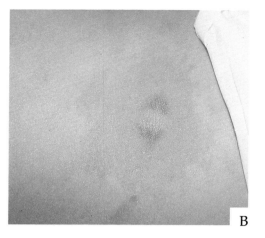

B, Darier's sign. Following firm stroking, a wheal and flare appears. This is diagnostic for mastocytoma.

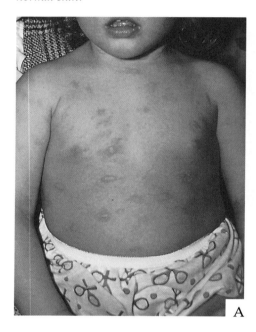

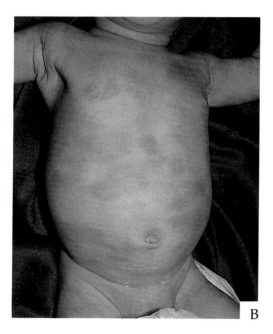

FIG. 8.73 Urticaria pigmentosa. **A,** numerous hyperpigmented macules are seen over the trunk of this preschool girl. **B,** more extensive lesions are evident in this infant who also has a wheal and flare reaction after accidental rubbing. (**A,** courtesy of Dr. Michael Sherlock)

Neurofibromas

Neurofibromas are solitary or multiple growths of neural tissue, presenting as soft, skin-colored or pink dermal nodules (Fig. 8.71). The central portion of an early lesion is particularly soft, and fingertip pressure creates the illusion of pressing in a buttonhole. Von Recklinghausen's disease (neurofibromatosis) is a syndrome characterized by the presence of multiple neurofibromas, café au lait spots, and various systemic disorders. When considering this diagnosis, it is important to remember that the neurofibromas usually appear after puberty, whereas in prepubertal children, café au lait spots are the most important cutaneous marker of von Recklinghausen's disease (see Chapter 15). Solitary neurofibromas without other stigmata of neurofibromatosis occasionally develop in normal individuals.

Mastocytosis

Cutaneous mastocytosis refers to a group of disorders characterized by dermal infiltrations of mast cells.

MASTOCYTOMA

Isolated mastocytomas may be seen in neonates and infants. They usually appear as skin-colored or light brown, slightly indurated plaques, 1 to 2 cm in size (Fig. 8.72A). Development of a wheal-and-flare following firm stroking of the lesion (Darier's sign) confirms the diagnosis (Fig. 8.72B). This is a response to the vascular effects of histamine released from infiltrating mast cells. Occasionally, enough histamine will be released from a large mastocytoma to cause localized blistering or systemic symptoms of flushing, wheezing, or diarrhea. Mastocytomas can be located anywhere on the body, and usually resolve by puberty.

URTICARIA PIGMENTOSA

Urticaria pigmentosa is another form of cutaneous mastocytosis that presents with numerous small, brownish papules or plaques, most commonly on the trunk (Fig. 8.73A). These may be present at birth or they may appear later in childhood. The hyperpigmented macules overlying mast cell infiltrates also typically react to stroking with a wheal and flare (Fig. 8.73B).

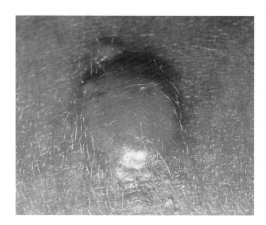

FIG. 8.74 Juvenile xanthogranuloma. This 1-cm yellowish nodule located on the back of a 3-month-old infant is the result of infiltration and proliferation of histiocytes.

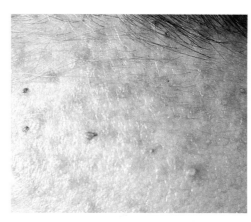

FIG. 8.75 Letterer-Siwe disease. The skin manifestations of the histiocytosis syndrome are similar and show infiltrated scaling papules with petechiae, resembling seborrheic dermatitis.

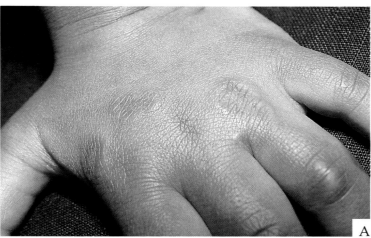

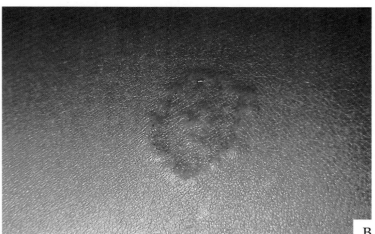

FIG. 8.76 Granuloma annulare. **A,** three raised, indurated rings with intact overlying skin are seen on this child's hand. **B,** this segmented ring is slightly excoriated due to scratching. (**B,** courtesy of Dr. Michael Sherlock)

Urticaria pigmentosa in children is usually limited to the skin, and often resolves by adolescence. However, the bone marrow, gastrointestinal tract, and other organs may be involved. Rare systemic findings in children with urticaria pigmentosa include chronic diarrhea, gastric ulcers, flushing reactions, headaches, and failure to thrive. In infancy, there is a tendency for lesions to blister and, rarely, widespread erosions may result in dehydration and sepsis.

Juvenile Xanthogranuloma

Infiltration of the skin by other types of cells can also occur. An example is juvenile xanthogranuloma (JXG), in which local infiltration and proliferation of histiocytes forms an isolated plaque or nodule or groups of small nodules (Fig. 8.74). These asymptomatic red or yellow-brown lesions grow very rapidly in infants and young children, but resolve spontaneously later in childhood. They are not associated with abnormalities of circulating lipids. In cases with multiple lesions, there may be an associated ocular involvement; this is the most common cause of non-traumatic hyphema in children. Hence, ophthalmologic evaluation is important in patients with multiple or diffuse xanthogranulomas.

The Histiocytoses

The histiocytosis syndromes are more serious proliferative disorders of Langerhans cells. The group includes Letterer-Siwe disease, Hand-Schüller-Christian disease and eosinophilic granuloma. Skin infiltration is most common in Letterer-Siwe disease. This entity begins in infancy with a diffuse papular, scaly eruption that differs from the usual seborrheic dermatitis by virtue of its associated infiltrated, crusted papules and petechiae (Fig. 8.75). Diagnosis is suggested by the presence of associated systemic manifestations such as hepatosplenomegaly and chronically draining ears. It is confirmed by skin biopsy, which shows characteristic Langerhans granules within the cytoplasm of infiltrating mononuclear cells (see Chapter 11).

Granuloma Annulare

When fully evolved, granuloma annulare is an annular eruption histologically characterized by dermal infiltration of lymphocytes around altered collagen. The lesion begins as a nodule or papule which gradually extends peripherally to form a ring. The initial papule and subsequent ring are raised and indurated, and in some cases, the ring is broken up into segments. The overlying epidermis is usually intact and the same color as the adjacent skin. However, it may be slightly erythematous or even hyperpigmented (Fig. 8.76A). Most lesions are asymptomatic, although a few are reported to be mildly pruritic. In the latter instance, superficial excoriation due to scratching may be noted (Fig. 8.76B). Lesions are most commonly found on the extensor surfaces of the lower legs, feet, fingers, and hands, but other areas may be involved. They

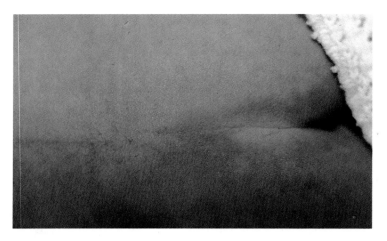

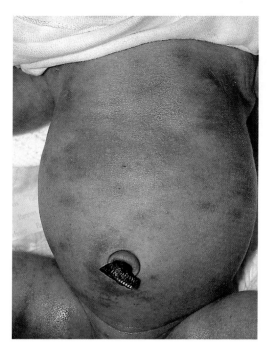

FIG. 8.78 Erythema toxicum neonatorum. Numerous yellow papules and pustules are surrounded by large intensely erythematous rings on the trunk of this infant.

FIG. 8.77 Mongolian spot. Typical slate-gray lesion located over the lumbosacral area of this black infant.

resolve spontaneously within a few months to several years, and no treatment is required. Their origin is unclear.

Granuloma annulare is most commonly confused with tinea corporis or ringworm (see Fig. 8.31). However, the thickened indurated character of the ring and the lack of an active microvesicular and scaling border enable clinical distinction.

NEONATAL DERMATOLOGY

The skin of a newborn differs from that of an adult in several ways: it is thinner, less hairy, has fewer sweat and sebaceous gland secretions, and has weaker intercellular attachments. During the neonatal period, common rashes or skin abnormalities may develop which need to be differentiated from more serious cutaneous disorders. Transient phenomena include erythema toxicum neonatorum, and transient neonatal pustular melanosis. More serious diseases include Letterer-Siwe disease (because it involves other organ systems) and staphylococcal scalded skin syndrome (because of potential fluid and electrolyte disturbances and life-threatening infection).

Mongolian Spots

Mongolian spots are flat, slate-gray to blue-black, poorly circumscribed macules. They are most commonly located over the lumbosacral area and buttocks (Fig. 8.77), although they can appear anywhere on the body. The spots range in size from 1 to 10 cm and may be single or multiple (see Fig. 6.29). Ninety percent of black infants, 81 percent of Oriental infants, and 9.6 percent of white newborns have these macules, which contain accumulations of melanocytes deep within the dermis. There is no known risk of malignancy, and Mongolian spots usually fade without therapy by age 7.

Erythema Toxicum Neonatorum

This is a benign, self-limited asymptomatic disorder of unknown etiology. It occurs in up to 50 percent of term infants and has no racial or sexual predisposition. Lesions usually begin 24 to 48 hours after birth, but may appear up to the tenth day of life. The disorder has been described as "flea-bite" dermatosis of the newborn, owing to the intense erythema with a central papule or pustule that resembles a flea bite (Fig. 8.78). Lesions are typically 2 to 3 cm in diameter, and there may be a few to several hundred on the back, face, chest, and extremities. The palms and soles are usually spared. A smear of material from a central pustule reveals numerous eosinophils; concomitant circulating eosinophilia is present in up to 20 percent of patients. The eruption fades spontaneously within 5 to 7 days. No treatment is necessary.

Differential diagnosis includes transient neonatal pustular melanosis, staphylococcal folliculitis, milia neonatorum, miliaria rubra and herpes simplex (see Chapter 12). Infections can be excluded with a Gram stain, Tzanck smear, and cultures, when necessary.

Transient Neonatal Pustular Melanosis

Transient neonatal pustular melanosis (TNPM) is a self-limited dermatosis of unknown etiology. The rash usually presents at birth with 1- to 2-mm vesiculopustules or ruptured pustules that disappear in 24 to 48 hours, leaving pigmented macules with a collarette of scale (Fig. 8.79A and B). Lesions may appear anywhere on the body, but are most often seen on the neck, forehead, lower back, and legs. Wright stain of a pustular smear shows numerous neutrophils; Gram stain and culture are negative for bacteria. The hyperpigmentation fades in

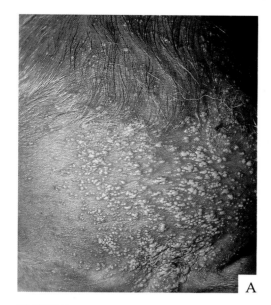

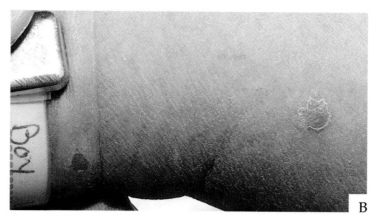

FIG. 8.79 Transient neonatal pustular melanosis. **A,** a myriad of tiny pustules dot the forehead and scalp of this neonate. **B,** when the pustules rupture, a pigmented macule surround by a collarette of scale remains.

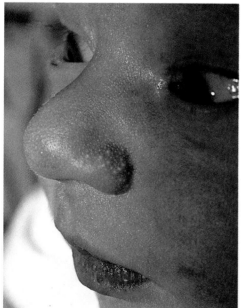

FIG. 8.80 Sebaceous gland hyperplasia. Note the yellowish papules on the nose of this infant.

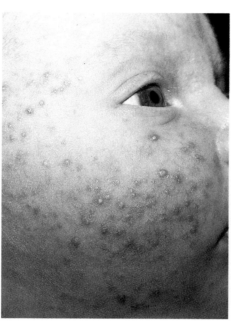

FIG. 8.81 Neonatal acne. Red papules and pustules are present over the nose and cheeks of this infant.

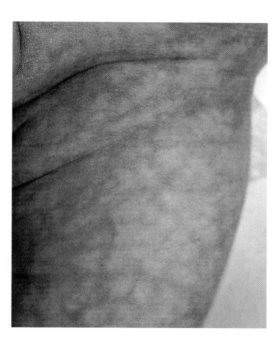

FIG. 8.82 Cutis marmorata. Note the reticulated bluish-purple mottling of this infant's thigh.

3 weeks to 3 months. TNPM is a benign disorder and requires no therapy. Differential diagnosis is similar to that of erythema toxicum neonatorum.

Sebaceous Gland Hyperplasia and Neonatal Acne

Sebaceous gland hyperplasia is a common entity consisting of multiple 1- to 2-cm papules, usually located over the nose and cheeks of term infants (Fig. 8.80). It is a normal physiologic response to maternal androgenic stimulation of sebaceous gland growth. Lesions resolve spontaneously by 4 to 6 months.

Neonates can, however, develop acne vulgaris in the first few weeks of life. This condition is also thought to be secondary to stimulation of the sebaceous glands and induction of abnormal keratinization of the hair follicles by maternal androgens. Lesions consist of comedones, papules, and pus-

tules usually located over the cheeks, forehead, and upper chest (Fig. 8.81). Neonatal acne usually resolves spontaneously over 4 to 8 weeks as the effects of maternal hormones dissipate. Though therapy is rarely required, use of 2.5% benzoyl peroxide and avoidance of topical oils may hasten resolution. The likelihood that these children will develop adolescent acne is unknown.

Cutis Marmorata

Cutis marmorata (Fig. 8.82) is a transient, net-like, reddish-blue mottling of the skin due to variable vascular constriction and dilatation. It is a normal response to chilling, and upon rewarming, normal skin color returns. The discoloration is seen primarily over the trunk and extremities in infants. In neonates, the condition is benign. However, if mottling persists beyond 6 months of life, it may be a sign of congenital hypothyroidism.

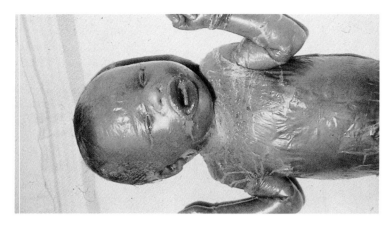

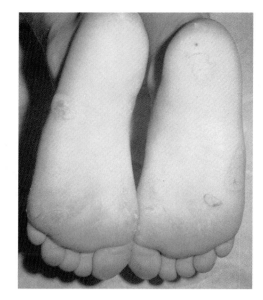

FIG. 8.84
Epidermolysis bullosa simplex. Numerous non-scarring blisters form easily in pressure areas. Scarring does not occur.

FIG. 8.83 Collodion baby. A shiny, tansparent membrane covered this baby at birth; she later developed lamellar ichthyosis. Note the ectropion and eclabium (eversion and fissuring of the eyelid margins and lips).

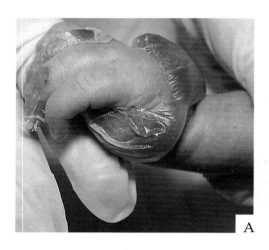

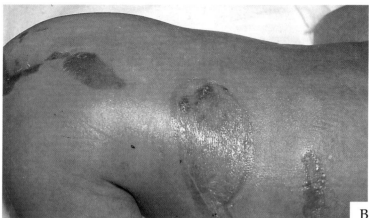

A

B

FIG. 8.85 Junctional epidermolysis bullosa. Widespread involvement was seen in this infant at birth. **A,** note the erosions and the large, intact blister over the thumb and dorsum of the hand. **B,** large denuded areas are evident over the back and buttocks.

Collodion Baby

In several variants of ichthyosis, particularly lamellar ichthyosis, the infant is born encased in a thick, parchment-like scale known as a collodion membrane (Fig. 8.83). This dries and is shed in large sheets within 7 to 14 days. Significant secondary fluid, electrolyte, and heat losses can occur. Although scaling may resolve completely in some infants, most go on to develop cutaneous findings typical for the underlying ichthyosis (see Figs. 8.7 and 8.8).

Epidermolysis Bullosa

Epidermolysis bullosa (EB) is a group of inherited mechano-bullous disorders characterized by the development of blisters following mild friction or trauma. There are three general types: simplex, junctional, and dystrophic (scarring). These types are classified according to the level at which blister formation takes place. Each type has several subgroups, and all typically present with blistering in the newborn period.

EPIDERMOLYSIS BULLOSA SIMPLEX

In epidermolysis bullosa simplex, blister formation takes place in the basal cell layer of the epidermis. On presentation, blistering can be mild or marked, generalized over the entire body, or localized to the hands and feet (Fig. 8.84). The disorder is inherited as an autosomal-dominant trait. While there is no scarring, secondary infection is a common complication.

JUNCTIONAL EPIDERMOLYSIS BULLOSA

Junctional epidermolysis bullosa, inherited as an autosomal-recessive trait, usually presents at birth with bullae and erosions in a generalized distribution. Blisters form at the junction of the epidermis and dermis (Fig. 8.85). The most common form is usually fatal within the first year, due to sepsis and fluid loss. A milder subtype resembles generalized EB simplex.

DYSTROPHIC EPIDERMOLYSIS BULLOSA

The scarring forms of EB are divided into dominant and recessive types. The plane of cleavage is in the upper portion of the dermis. In both, scarring occurs as the blisters heal, and milia are common (Fig. 8.86A). The dominant form results in much less scarring than the recessive form; patients with the latter show retardation in growth and development, severe oral blisters, loss of nails and, sometimes, syndactyly (Fig. 8.86B).

Skin biopsies are helpful in distinguishing among the three general types of epidermolysis bullosa in neonates, and they are also helpful in determining prognosis. Treatment is symptomatic and supportive. Genetic counseling is advisable.

Incontinentia Pigmenti

Incontinentia pigmenti (IP) is an X-linked, dominant disorder that affects the skin and may also involve the central nervous system, eyes, and skeletal system. It is seen predominantly in females, and thus, is thought to be fatal to males *in utero*. Clinically, the disorder may present in any of three general

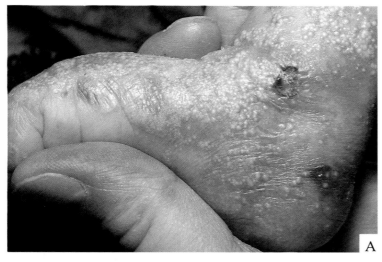
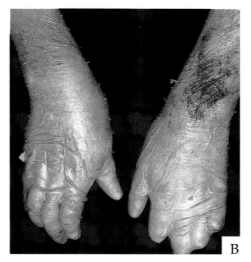

FIG. 8.86 Dystrophic epidermolysis bullosa. **A,** blisters, erosions, and hundreds of milia are seen on the foot and ankle of this newborn. **B,** in this child with the recessive form of EB dystrophica, severe scarring encased the fingers, resulting in syndactyly.

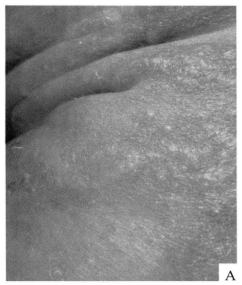
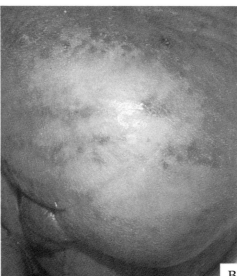
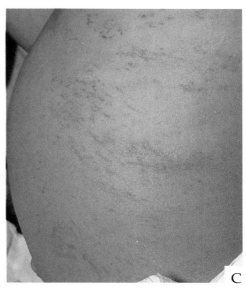

FIG. 8.87 **A,** incontinentia pigmenti (bullous phase). Inflammatory blisters and crusts are characteristic. **B,** in the papular phase, linear streaks of red papules often overlap the bullous and hyperpigmented phase. **C,** in the hyperpigmented phase, swirled, hyperpigmented swirls and streaks appear, as seen on the trunk of this older girl.

phases, with some overlap. In the first phase, inflammatory vesicles or bullae appear initially on the trunk and extremities usually within the first 2 weeks of life (Fig. 8.87A). New blisters then develop over the ensuing 3 months. At this stage, a skin biopsy shows characteristic inflammation with intraepidermal eosinophils. Before the blistering phase ends, the second phase, marked by development of irregular, warty papules, supervenes (Fig. 8.87B). These lesions resolve spontaneously within several months. A characteristic swirling or streaking pattern of brown to blue-gray pigmentation on the trunk or extremities marks the third phase (Fig. 8.87C). These pigmented whorls are usually located in different areas from those involved in the first two phases. The pigmentation lasts for many years and then gradually fades, leaving subtle, streaky, hypopigmented scars that may be the only residual cutaneous findings seen in affected mothers, who should be carefully examined for these markers of IP.

A number of other systemic manifestations affecting various other body systems are seen in patients with IP. Thirty percent have central nervous system abnormalities such as seizures, mental retardation, and spasticity. Ophthalmic complications,

including strabismus, cataracts, blindness, and microphthalmia are seen in 35 percent of IP patients. Pegged teeth and delayed dentition are seen in 65 percent. Cardiac and skeletal malformations have also been reported.

Differential diagnosis of IP in the blistering stage includes herpes simplex, bullous impetigo, and EB. Warts or epidermal nevi may mimic the warty phase. The swirled pigmentation of the third phase is very characteristic and not likely to be confused with other hyperpigmentation disorders. No specific therapy is required for IP, but genetic counseling is advisable.

HEMANGIOMAS

Congenital vascular malformations termed hemangiomas are the most common neoplasms of childhood, occurring in 10 to 40 percent of all newborns. These lesions arise when islands of angioblastic tissue fail to re-establish normal communication with the vascular system. Hemangiomas can be divided into two groups—raised and flat—depending on their architecture. Although family members may be affected, hemangiomas are not thought to be inherited.

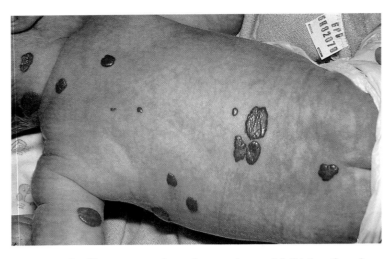

FIG. 8.88 Capillary or strawberry hemangiomas. Multiple soft, red, raised lesions dot the back and arms of this otherwise healthy 1-month-old.

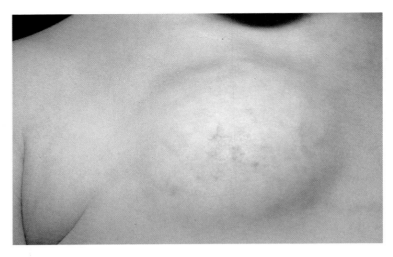

FIG. 8.89 Cavernous hemangioma. The vessels that make up this large, partially compressible lesion are deep beneath the skin surface but still impart a bluish hue to the overlying skin. Note the indistinctness of the margins.

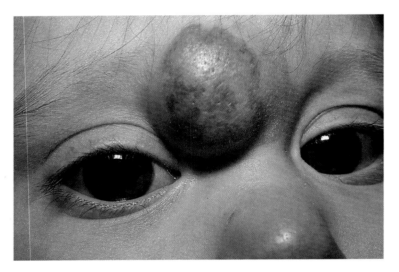

FIG. 8.90 Mixed hemangioma. The hemangioma on this child's nasal bridge has both capillary and cavernous components.

Raised Hemangiomas: Capillary and Cavernous

The skin overlying a *capillary hemangioma* (sometimes called a "strawberry hemangioma") is usually normal or slightly red at birth. However, within the first few months of life, there is marked vascular overgrowth resulting in bright red discoloration and definite elevation above the surrounding skin surface (Fig. 8.88). Lesions are soft, compressible, and usually range in size from 0.5 to 4 cm, although they can be much larger.

The vessels that comprise *cavernous hemangiomas*, another of the palpable forms, are located deep beneath the surface of the skin and appear bluish in color (Fig. 8.89). The borders of the lesion are usually indistinct, and it feels like a doughy mass that is only partially compressible. When placed in a dependent position, cavernous hemangiomas enlarge as they fill with blood—a finding that helps differentiate them clinically from lymphangiomas. Combined capillary and cavernous hemangiomas are common, as well (Fig. 8.90).

The natural history of raised hemangiomas is one of rapid growth for approximately 1 year, followed by a plateau period during which the lesion remains the same size. This is then followed by a period of slow involution (Fig. 8.91). Fifty percent of raised hemangiomas disappear by age 7, and 90 percent by age 9. In 40 percent of patients, the skin overlying the resolved lesion shows mild redundancy with telangiectasis.

Given the natural history of involution, watchful waiting is the best clinical approach unless the hemangioma involves a vital structure. Steroids or surgical intervention may be indicated if the lesion is life threatening (e.g., involves the airway) or if it interferes with vital functions (e.g., vision). Yellow pulsed dye laser therapy shows promising results. Complications such as ulceration, bleeding or infection occur infrequently. Ulceration, which frequently hastens resolution of the lesion as it heals, can be treated with wet compresses and topical antibacterial ointments.

Flat Hemangiomas

PORT WINE STAINS

Port wine stains, named for their purplish-red color, are flat hemangiomas present at birth. Unlike capillary and cavernous hemangiomas, these lesions do not enlarge but tend to remain stable and flat. However, in adults, small angiomatous papules may develop within the lesion over time. The discoloration is due to permanent dilatation of mature capillaries. Most commonly, these lesions are located unilaterally on the face (Fig. 8.92). Port wine stains involving an extremity may be associa-

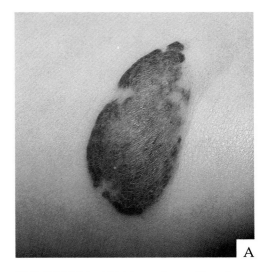 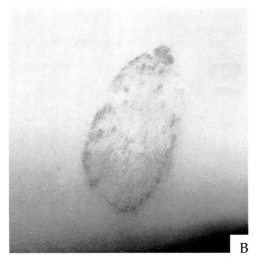 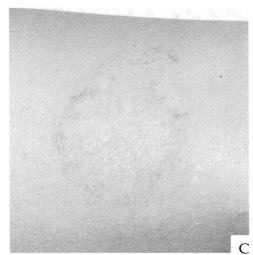

FIG. 8.91 Natural history of a capillary hemangioma. After growing for approximately 1 year, raised hemangiomas gradually involute. **A,** appearance at 5 months. **B,** at 2 years. **C,** almost total resolution at 5 years.

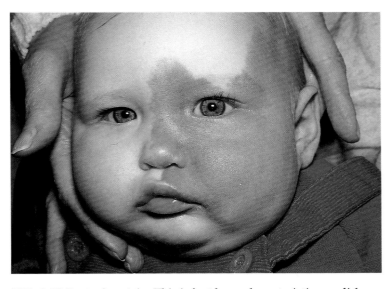

FIG. 8.92 Port wine stain. This infant has a characteristic purplish-red lesion covering nearly half of his face.

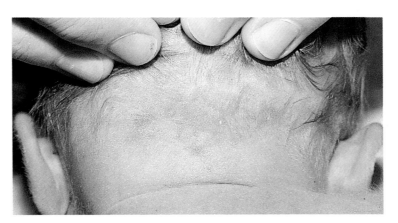

FIG. 8.93 Nevus flammeus or salmon patch. A typical, light red splotchy area is seen at the nape of the neck.

ted with local overgrowth of soft tissue and bone due to the abnormally rich blood supply. This results in hemihypertrophy, a phenomenon called the Klippel-Trenaunay-Weber syndrome. When a port wine stain involves the first branch of the fifth cranial (trigeminal) nerve, it can be associated with vascular malformations of the ipsilateral meninges and cerebral cortex, a constellation termed the Sturge-Weber syndrome. Seizures, mental retardation, hemiplegia and glaucoma are associated features (see Chapter 15).

NEVUS FLAMMEUS

Another type of flat hemangioma is the nevus flammeus, or "salmon patch" (Fig. 8.93). This lesion is a normal variant seen in 40 percent of newborns, and is usually located at the nape of the neck, the glabella, forehead, or upper eyelids. The patches represent distended capillaries and tend to fade within the first year of life. They may become more apparent during episodes of crying, breath-holding, or physical exertion.

Pyogenic Granuloma

Pyogenic granuloma is a common, benign, vascular tumor that resembles a small hemangioma. It is thought to be due to vascular overgrowth of granulation tissue following trauma or reaction to a foreign body such as a thorn, splinter, or piece of glass. It is seen in children and young adults, usually located on the face or an extremity, although on occasion the trunk and mucous membranes may be involved. Lesions are solitary, bright red, soft nodules which are often pedunculated. They

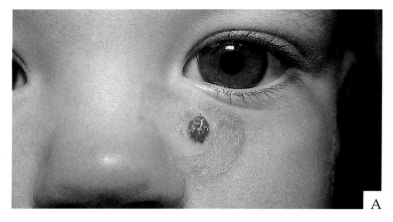

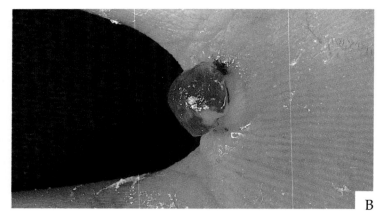

FIG. 8.94 Pyogenic granuloma. **A,** a raised hemorrhagic papule. Developed on this infant's cheek **B,** another rapidly growing, friable lesion is present between his fingers.

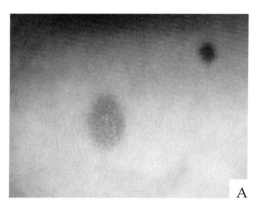

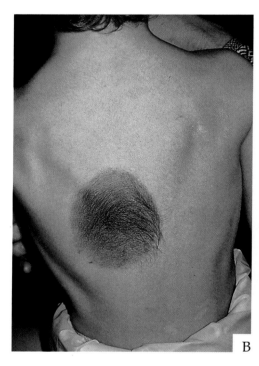

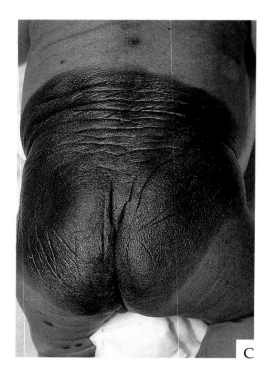

FIG. 8.95 Congenital nevomelanocytic nevi. **A,** two small nevi with differing degrees of hyperpigmentation seen on the thigh of this infant. **B,** the large nevus on the back of this adolescent has become more prominently hairy. Also note the darker areas within the plaque. **C,** the giant nevus seen in this infant covering the lower back and buttocks is uniformly pigmented and has smaller satellite nevi. (**B,** courtesy of Dr. Michael Sherlock)

average 5 to 6 mm in diameter, the surface is friable and bleeds easily (Fig. 8.94A,B). The rapid growth characteristic of these tumors can cause them to be confused with malignancies such as melanomas. Treatment consists of electrodesiccation of the blood vessels at the base. The lesion will occasionally recur, in which case repeat surgery is recommended.

NEVI AND MELANOMAS

"Nevomelanocytic nevus" is a term used to describe a group of congenital and acquired pigmented lesions located in the dermis which contain nevus cells derived from the neural crest. These nevus cells, like melanocytes in the epidermis, have the ability to synthesize melanin. The term "nevus" also refers to a group of congenital skin lesions composed of mature or nearly mature cutaneous elements organized in an abnormal fashion. Also known as hamartomas, these may be comprised of almost any epidermal or dermal structures.

Nevomelanocytic Nevi

CONGENITAL NEVOMELANOCYTIC NEVI
Congenital forms of nevomelanocytic nevi (CNN) consist of pigmented plaques often associated with dense hair growth. At birth, lesions may be tan or light pink, with only soft vellus hairs (Fig. 8.95A). During infancy and childhood, the nevus darkens, the hair becomes more prominent, and small, dark macules or nodules may appear within the larger plaque (Fig. 8.95B).

Giant CNNs covering large areas of skin (usually greater than 20 cm) are associated with a 2- to 15-percent lifetime risk of progression to melanoma (Fig. 8.95C). Early treatment is

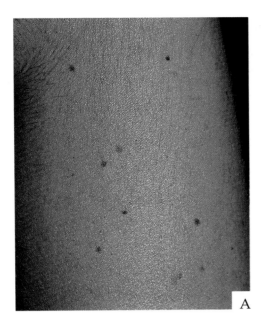

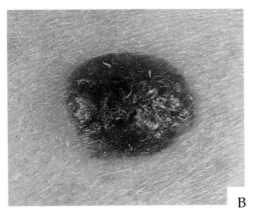

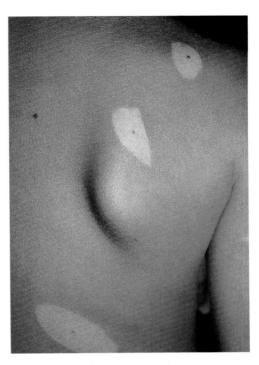

FIG. 8.96 Acquired nevomelanocytic nevi. **A,** junctional nevi. These brown macules are flat on palpation. **B,** this typical compound nevus is raised, with a regular border and uniform pigmentation.

FIG. 8.97 Large, hypopigmented halos surround three relatively small nevi on the back of this boy.

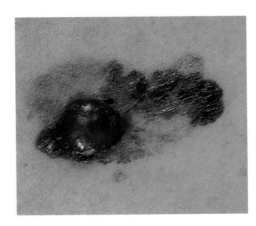

FIG. 8.98 Melanoma. This lesion shows the irregularity of outline, color, and thickness, typical of a melanoma.

recommended and consists of full-thickness excision followed by grafting. Some very large nevi may not be amenable to surgical management, however, and thus require impeccably close observation (facilitated by regular comparative photographs at 6- to 12-month intervals). Regular examinations should include careful palpation of the entire lesion because melanomas may arise deep within the nevus without visible surface change.

Small CNNs may also be associated with a higher than normal risk of developing melanoma, but the actual incidence is unknown. To date, there are no uniformly accepted guidelines for treatment. However, all CNNs must be differentiated from other congenital pigmented spots such as urticaria pigmentosa, lentigines, café au lait spots, and Mongolian spots.

ACQUIRED NEVOMELANOCYTIC NEVI
Nevomelanocytic nevi acquired after birth are often referred to as "moles." These begin to develop in early childhood as small, pigmented macules 1 to 2 mm in diameter, which are flat on palpation. At this stage, the nevus cells are limited to the epidermal-dermal junction and are called junctional nevi (Fig. 8.96A). They then enlarge slowly and become papular or even pedunculated. In such elevated nevi, the nevus cells have proliferated into the dermis to become either intradermal or compound nevi (Fig. 8.96B). During puberty, these lesions may darken noticeably and increase in size. However, normal nevomelanocytic nevi rarely exceed 1 cm in diameter. They tend to be located on sun-exposed areas and are seen less frequently on the soles, palms, legs, genitalia, and mucous membranes. Generally, nevi change slowly over months to years and warrant observation only.

Sudden enlargement of a nevus with redness and tenderness may occur because of infection of a hair follicle within the nevus or the rupture of a follicular cyst with acute foreign body

inflammation. This may alarm the patient and necessitate dermatologic evaluation. Another, slower change causing concern in patients is the appearance of a hypopigmented ring and mild local pruritus around a benign nevus. This is called a halo nevus (Fig. 8.97), and it is caused by a cytotoxic T-lymphocyte reaction against both the nevus cells and the innocent melanocytic bystanders. As a result, the nevus tends to disappear partially or completely, and the halo eventually repigments.

NEVI AND MELANOMAS
As long as the clinical appearance of a nevus is typical, excision is unnecessary. However, a number of changes in pigmented lesions may portend the development of melanoma (Fig. 8.98). These include:

1. A change in size, shape, or outline, with scalloped, irregular borders.

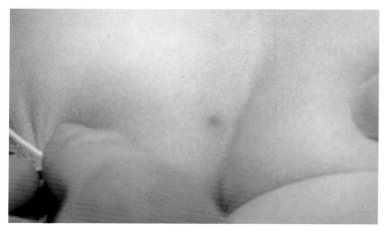

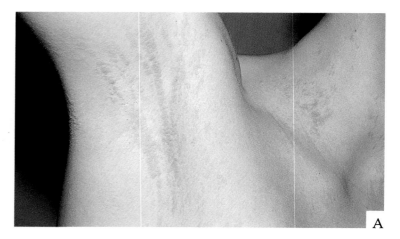

FIG. 8.99 *Blue nevus. This blue nodule was made up of deep nevus cells; it was firm on palpation.*

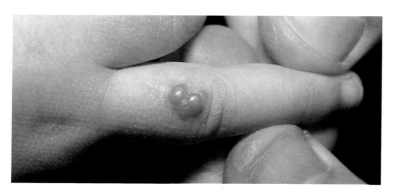

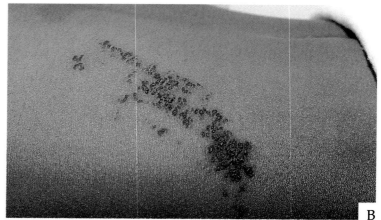

FIG. 8.100 *Spitz nevus. This raised, red nevus grows rapidly.*

FIG. 8.101 *Epidermal nevi.* **A,** *light color in whites.* **B,** *darker color in blacks. More extensive nevi may be associated with systemic abnormalities (epidermal nevus syndrome).*

2. A change in the surface characteristics, such as development of a small, dark, elevated papule or nodule within an otherwise flat plaque; flaking, scaling, ulceration, or bleeding.

3. A change in color, with the appearance of black, brown, or mixing of red, white or blue.

4. Burning, itching, or tenderness, which may be an indication of the body's immune reaction to malignancy.

Fortunately, melanomas are still very rare in children. However, their incidence is increasing, and curative treatment is contingent on early diagnosis and prompt excision. A keen awareness of diagnostic features is important.

Melanomas in children may occur *de novo*, or they may develop within a giant congenital nevus, the latter being the most common source of this condition in children. Another cause of melanoma in the pediatric age group is transplacental transfer of maternal melanoma. Thus, neonates born to mothers with a history of melanoma should be examined and followed carefully. Conversely, mothers of infants born with melanoma should be examined thoroughly for signs of the malignancy.

Differential diagnosis of childhood melanoma includes congenital and acquired nevocytic nevi; the blue nevus, a small, firm, blue papule consisting of deep nevus cells (Fig. 8.99); traumatic hemorrhage, especially under the nails or in mucous membranes; vascular lesions, such as pyogenic granuloma or angiokeratoma; and the Spitz nevus (benign juvenile melanoma), a red and rapidly growing nevocytic nevus (Fig. 8.100) that can be confused, both clinically and histologically, with melanoma.

Hamartomatous Nevi

Hamartomatous nevi can be comprised of epidermal structures, hair follicles (nevus pilosis), apocrine and eccrine glands (apocrine and eccrine nevi), fibroblasts (connective tissue nevi), blood vessels (nevus flammeus, see Fig. 8.93), and multiple components (nevus sebaceous).

Epidermal nevi are not rare in pediatric patients. They are composed of epidermal structures only and must be distinguished from nevus sebaceous (see below). The lesion may be present at birth or may develop during childhood and appears as a slightly hyperpigmented papillomatous or verrucous growth (Fig. 8.101). Verrucous changes are particularly likely at puberty. It may be small and localized, linear, dermatomal or generalized. The numerous clinical presentations are reflected in the number of descriptive synonyms: nevus verrucosus for localized disease, nevus unius lateralis for linear or unilateral involvement, and ichthyosis hystrix for bilateral involvement with irregular geometric patterns. Important associations with extensive epidermal nevi are seizures, mental retardation,

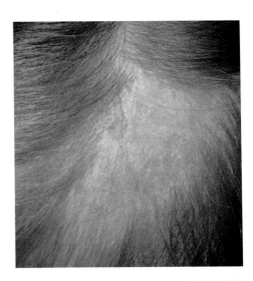

FIG. 8.102 Nevus sebaceous of Jadassohn. This yellowish hairless plaque was present at birth.

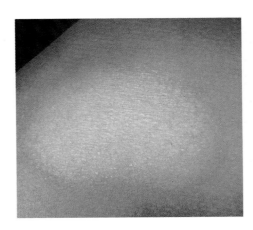

FIG. 8.104 Post-inflammatory hypopigmentation. This reaction followed chronic dermatitis. Note the narrow rim of hyperpigmentation at the margin.

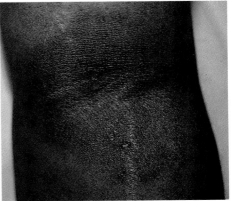

FIG. 8.103 Post-inflammatory hyperpigmentation. This arose following chronic atopic dermatitis and trauma from persistent scratching.

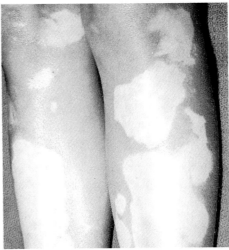

FIG. 8.105 Vitiligo. Completely depigmented patches are seen on the legs. Occasionally, macules of repigmentation arise from epidermal appendages within the white patches. A characteristic distribution helps to distinguish vitiligo from other causes of hypopigmentation.

ocular and skeletal defects (for epidermal nevus syndrome, see Chapter 15).

Nevus sebaceous of Jadassohn is characterized by a hairless, well-circumscribed, skin-colored or yellowish plaque located on the scalp, face, or neck (Fig. 8.102). The lesion is usually solitary and may be linear or round. It is present at birth, although at puberty, the plaque may become more verrucous, raised, and nodular (see Chapter 15, Neurology). Histologically, epidermal proliferation is seen along with abortive hair follicles, sebaceous glands and apocrine structures. Approximately 10 to 15 percent of these nevi develop into secondary neoplasms, the most common being basal cell carcinoma, although other appendageal tumors have been reported. Long-term regular observation or prophylactic full-thickness excision is necessary.

DISORDERS OF PIGMENTATION

Childhood disorders of pigmentation are usually of cosmetic importance only, although some pigmented lesions are markers of multisystem disease.

Post-Inflammatory Pigmentary Changes

The most common pigmentation disorder is post-inflammatory hyper- (Fig. 8.103) or hypopigmentation (Fig. 8.104). This follows inflammatory disorders of the skin, such as dermatitis, infection, or injury, and usually resolves spontaneously over a few months. Histologically, melanocytes are normal in these areas, although the dispersion of melanin and pigment to other cells is disturbed. Tinea versicolor may also present as hypopigmented patches covered with a fine scale, but KOH examination will confirm the correct diagnosis by demonstrating typical "spaghetti and meatballs" organisms (see Figs. 8.35, 8.36). Post-inflammatory hypopigmentation must be distinguished from vitiligo, in which there is a complete absence of pigment and usually no associated scaling or history of prior inflammation.

Vitiligo

In vitiligo (Fig. 8.105), there is a complete loss of pigmentation. Lesions are macular and usually are seen in a characteristic distribution around the eyes, mouth, genitals, elbows, hands, and feet. Spontaneous but slow repigmentation may occur in areas beginning around the openings of hair follicles, resulting in a speckled appearance. Histologically, melanocytes are absent in areas of vitiligo, and evidence suggests that they are destroyed by an autoimmune mechanism.

Ash Leaf Spots

White oval macules, termed ash leaf spots because of their shape, are a valuable early marker of tuberous sclerosis. These appear at birth or shortly thereafter as 1- to 3-cm macular lesions on the trunk. They are not as sharply demarcated or

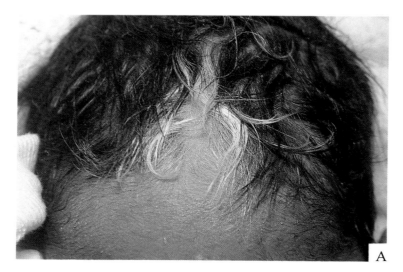

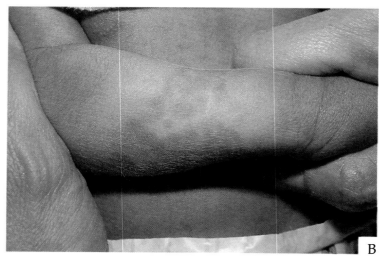

FIG. 8.106 Piebaldism. **A,** a white forelock overlies a depigmented patch of scalp and forehead. **B,** this infant also has a hypopigmented patch on his arm in which smaller areas of hyperpigmentation are seen.

ivory white as the lesions of vitiligo, and their truncal distribution is different (see Chapter 15).

The identification of ash leaf macules may be enhanced, particularly in lightly pigmented individuals, by the use of a Wood's light; this method of examination should be part of the assessment of any child who presents with idiopathic seizures in infancy. The visible purple light emitted is absorbed by normal melanin in the skin. In a darkened room, areas of hypopigmentation or depigmentation appear bright violet, whereas normally melanized skin reflects little visible light and appears dull purple or black. In addition to tuberous sclerosis, Wood's light examination may also be helpful in delineating the full extent of pigmentary changes in vitiligo and post-inflammatory hypopigmentation.

Albinism

The term albinism refers to a heterogenous group of inherited disorders characterized by congenital hypopigmentation of the skin, eyes, and hair. It occurs in an X-linked ocular form (in which the skin appears clinically normal) and an autosomal recessive oculocutaneous form. In oculocutaneous albinism (OCA), both sexes and all races are affected equally. This form of the disorder is subdivided into a number of variants based on clinical findings and biochemical markers. Tyrosinase-negative and tyrosinase-positive subtypes have been identified based on the ability of plucked hairs to produce pigment when incubated in tyrosine. In classic tyrosinase-negative OCA, children are born without any trace of pigment. Affected individuals have snow-white hair, pinkish-white skin, and translucent or blue irises. Nystagmus is common, as is moderate to severe strabismus and poor visual acuity (see Chapter 19, Ophthalmology). Although children with tyrosinase-positive OCA may be clinically indistinguishable from their tyrosinase-negative counterparts at birth, they usually develop variable amounts of pigment with increasing age. Eye color may vary from gray to light brown, and hair may change to blond or light brown. Most black patients will acquire as much pigment as light-skinned whites.

Because they lack the protection of melanin, patients with OCA are at high risk for early development of basal cell and squamous cell skin cancers. Hence, they should be instructed in use of sunscreens and avoidance of excessive sun exposure.

PIEBALDISM

Piebaldism (partial albinism) is a rare autosomal dominant disorder characterized by a white forelock and a circumscribed congenital leukoderma. The typical lesions include a triangular patch of depigmentation and white hair on the frontal scalp. The apex of this patch points toward the nasal bridge (Fig. 8.106A) and the patient may also show hypopigmented or depigmented macules on the face, neck, ventral trunk, flanks, or extremities (Fig. 8.106B). Within areas of decreased pigmentation, scattered patches of normal pigmentation or hyperpigmentation may be seen. The lesions are stable throughout life, although some variability in pigmentation may occur with sun exposure. Special variants of piebaldism include Waardenburg's syndrome, in which leukoderma is associated with lateral displacement of the inner canthi and inferior lacrimal ducts, a flattened nasal bridge, and sensorineural deafness; and Wolf's syndrome, an autosomal recessive disorder associated with neurologic deficits.

Other Pigmentary Disorders

Café au lait spots are tan macules that can be an indication of neurofibromatosis (von Recklinghausen's disease, see Chapter 15) or of Albright syndrome, in which they are associated with polyostotic dysplasia. Most café au lait spots, however, occur in otherwise healthy individuals and vary from a few millimeters to over 10 cm in size. Borders are discrete but may be smooth or irregular. Swirled hyperpigmentation may be a marker of incontinentia pigmenti (see Fig. 8.87C), and diffuse hyperpigmentation may be seen in Addison's disease and hemochromatosis. Peutz-Jeghers syndrome is manifest by lentigo-like pigmentation of the lips (see Chapter 17), oral

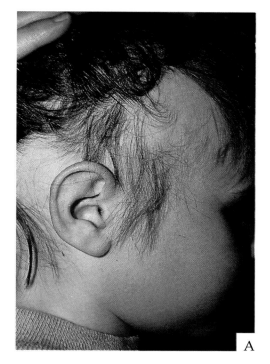

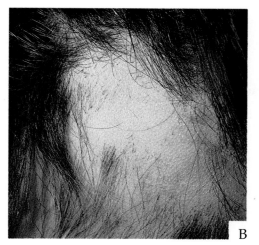

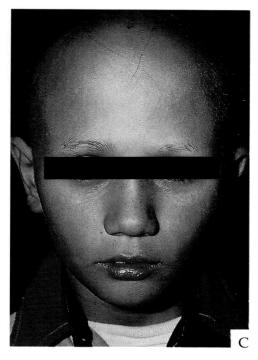

FIG. 8.107 Alopecia areata. **A,** patches of complete hair loss with otherwise normal scalp are typical of this disorder. **B,** in this closeup, small broken hairs which pull out easily are seen at the margins. **C,** in this boy, the disorder has progressed to alopecia totalis. Note that his eyebrows are involved as well. (**A** and **C,** courtesy of Dr. Michael Sherlock)

mucosa, hands and fingers, and benign, small-intestinal polyps in children (see Chapter 10).

DISORDERS OF HAIR AND NAILS

Diseases of the hair and nails make up an integral part of pediatric dermatology. Both hair and nails are composed of keratin, produced by the epidermal hair follicles and the nail matrix. Some diseases are specific to these structures, while others affect the skin as well. In many cases, important diagnostic clues to skin disease can be found in related abnormalities of the hair and nails.

The Alopecias

The most common diseases of the hair result in some degree of hair loss or alopecia. Evaluation begins by determining whether scarring is present. Non-scarring alopecia can be caused by growth defects causing the hair to be lost by the roots (effluvium) or by defects of the hair shaft causing breakage.

ALOPECIA DUE TO SYSTEMIC INSULT:
TELOGEN AND ANAGEN EFFLUVIUM

Normal hair cycles through a growth phase lasting 3 years or more (anagen phase) and a resting phase of 3 months (telogen phase), after which the hair is shed. The cycle then begins again. Telogen effluvium is one form of partial, temporary alopecia seen 3 months after a severe illness, surgery, or high fever. It rarely causes more than 50 percent hair loss. The initial systemic insult induces more than the usual 20 percent of hairs to enter the telogen phase, and 3 months later, these hairs are shed simultaneously, producing marked thinning of scalp hair until new anagen hairs regrow. Anagen effluvium is the sudden loss of the growing hairs (80 percent of normal scalp hairs), caused by the abnormal cessation of the anagen phase. The hair shafts taper and lose adhesion to the follicle. This type of hair loss is most common after systemic chemotherapy.

ALOPECIA AREATA

Alopecia areata is a form of localized anagen effluvium, presenting with round patches of alopecia which may be located anywhere on the scalp, eyebrows, lashes, or body. Occasionally, hair loss is diffuse or generalized. The injury causing cessation of growth is thought to be of immunologic origin. Clues to diagnosis include absence of inflammation and scaling in the involved areas of scalp, and the presence of short (3 to 6 mm), easily epilated hairs at the margins of the patch (Fig. 8.107A,B). Under magnification, these hair stubs resemble exclamation points as the hair shaft narrows just before its point of entry into the follicle. Another finding in many patients with alopecia areata is Scotch plaid pitting of the nails consisting of rows of pits crossing in a transverse and longitudinal fashion (see Fig. 8.119). The clinical course of alopecia areata is difficult to predict. The disorder may resolve spontaneously; it may persist, with the appearance of new patches while the old patches regrow; or it may progress to total scalp or even generalized alopecia (alopecia totalis) that can be permanent (Fig. 8.107C).

TRAUMA-INDUCED ALOPECIA
Trichorrhexis Nodosa

Alopecia caused by hair shaft breakage is due to a structural defect of the hair, and it is easily diagnosed by microscopic examination. The most common structural defect is acquired trichorrhexis nodosa. This presents at any age as brittle, short hairs that are perceived by the patient as nongrowing. By gently pulling, one can demonstrate that many hairs are easily

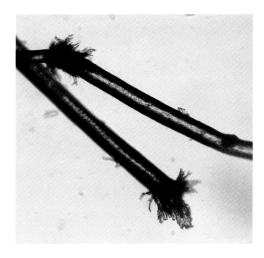

FIG. 8.108 Trichorrhexis nodosa. A brittle hair shaft defect usually caused by over-manipulation of the hair or chemical use. The frayed broom appearance is typical.

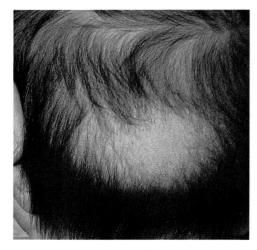

FIG. 8.109 Friction alopecia. Hair loss of the occiput resulted from rubbing of the head on sheets and pillows.

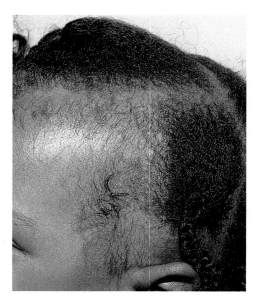

FIG. 8.110 Traction alopecia. The hair thinning and loss is due to excessive traction on the hairs as a result of tight braiding.

broken. Microscopically, the distal ends of the hairs are frayed, resembling a broom (Fig. 8.108). Other hairs may have nodules resembling two brooms stuck together. The fragility is caused by damage to the outer cortex of the hair shaft, resulting in a loss of structural support. Without this support, the weaker fibrous medulla frays like an electrical cord with broken insulation. This disorder is most common in blacks, arising from the trauma of combing tightly curled hairs. It is also seen after repeated or severe chemical damage to the cortex from hair straighteners, bleaches, and permanents. Since hair growth is normal, the disorder is self-limited, and normal hairs regrow when the source of the damage is eliminated.

Other common causes of hair loss associated with shaft abnormalities include friction alopecia, traction alopecia, and trichotillomania. All are caused by external trauma and breakage of an otherwise normal hair shaft.

Friction Alopecia

Friction alopecia (Fig. 8.109) is common on the posterior scalp of neonates and infants, where the head rubs on the pillow or bed clothes. Although worrisome to parents, this disorder is self-limited. When severe or longstanding, it should raise the question of neglect, suggesting that the infant is being left to lie in his crib for extended periods of time.

Traction Alopecia

Traction alopecia (Fig. 8.110) is common in young girls whose hairstyles, such as ponytails, pigtails, braids, or cornrows, maintain a tight pull on the hair shafts. This traction causes shaft fractures, as well as follicular damage; if prolonged, permanent scarring alopecia can result.

Trichotillomania

Trichotillomania is a fairly common disorder seen in school-aged children and adolescents that mimics many other types of alopecia. It presents with bizarre patterns of hair loss, often in broad, linear bands on the vertex or sides of the scalp where the hair is easily twisted and pulled out (Fig. 8.111). Rarely, the entire scalp, eyebrows, and eyelashes are involved. The most important clue is the finding of short, broken-off hairs along

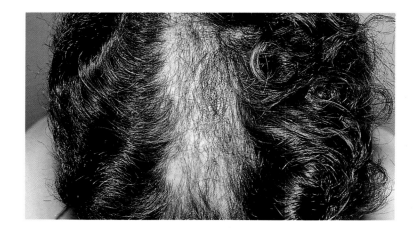

FIG. 8.111 Trichotillomania. This linear patch of short broken hairs is typical of hair pulling.

the scalp, with stubs of different lengths in adjacent areas. This is caused by repetitive pulling and/or twisting of the hair which fractures the longer shafts. Once broken, the hairs are too short to be rebroken until they grow longer.

Trichotillomania is often confused with alopecia areata because there are patches of hair loss with short hairs and involvement of the eyebrows and eyelashes. However, in trichotillomania, patches of hair loss are never completely bald, and the hair shafts are normal anagen hairs that are usually difficult to remove from the scalp. In addition, there are no associated nail abnormalities.

Parents and children usually deny vigorously that the alopecia could be caused by the child, and thus diagnosis rests on a high index of suspicion and recognition of the clinical findings. Although trichotillomania may occur in children with severe psychiatric disease, most cases are associated with situational stress (e.g., school phobia, marital or social problems) or habitual behavior.

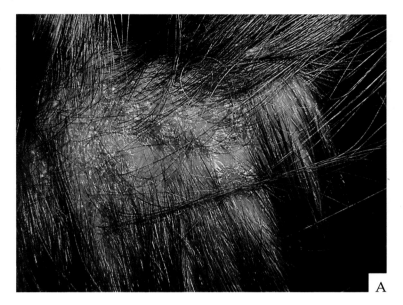

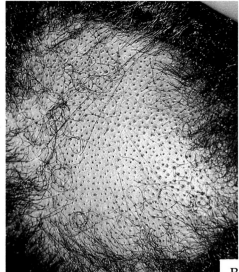

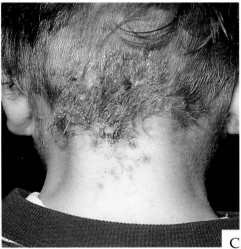

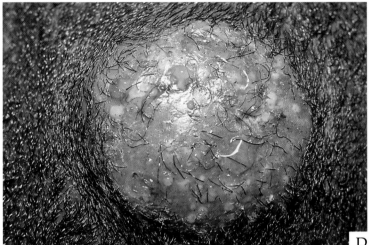

FIG. 8.112 Tinea capitis can present in many guises. **A**, in this child, mild erythema and scaling of the scalp were associated with partial alopecia. **B**, infiltration of hair shafts by endothrix has resulted in widespread breakage at the scalp, producing a "salt-and-pepper" appearance. **C**, superficial papules and pustules have ruptured, producing a weeping, crusting lesion simulating impetigo. **D**, kerion. A boggy mass has formed as a result of an intense inflammatory response. This child, seen relatively late in the course, had total alopecia over the involved area. Note that the lesion is studded with pustules. (**A**, courtesy of Dr. Michael Sherlock)

SCARRING ALOPECIA

Scarring alopecia in children is less common than non-scarring alopecia and may be caused by a number of disorders. Aplasia cutis congenita is an ulceration of the vertex of the scalp of a newborn that heals with a hairless scar. Morphea (localized scleroderma) may involve the scalp with indurated, hairless plaques. Scarring alopecia may also result from severe infection (e.g., inflammatory tinea capitis) or trauma, such as oil burns from hot-comb straightening of the hair. A scalp biopsy is often helpful in determining the cause of scarring alopecia.

Tinea Capitis Infections of Hair and Scalp

Fungal infection of the hair weakens the shaft, causing breakage. This typically results in the development of multiple patches of partial alopecia. *Trichophyton tonsurans* is the organism responsible for over 95 percent of the scalp ringworm in the United States. For unknown reasons, infection is endemic among black school children, although it is occasionally found in whites. *Microsporum canis* (the dog and cat ringworm) accounts for a few cases of tinea capitis and shows no racial predilection.

There are a variety of clinical presentations of tinea capitis. In some patients, mild erythema and scaling of the scalp are seen in association with partial alopecia (Fig. 8.112A). In other cases, infection by endothrix, which invades the hair shafts, causes widespread breakage at the scalp creating a "salt-and-pepper" appearance, with the short residual hairs appearing as black dots on the surface of the scalp (Fig. 8.112B). Occasionally, scalp lesions are annular, simulating tinea corporis. In yet other children, sensitization to the infecting organism results in more erythema, edema, and pustule formation. As the latter rupture, the area weeps and golden crusts form, simulating impetigo (Fig. 8.112C). Less commonly, intense inflammation causes formation of raised, tender, boggy plaques or masses studded with pustules that simulate abscesses, termed kerions (Fig. 8.112D). Unless treated promptly and aggressively with oral antifungal agents and, in severe cases, steroids, the latter may produce scarring and per-

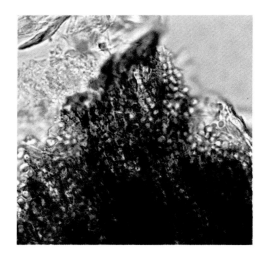

FIG. 8.113
Microscopic appearance of hair shafts infected with fungi. Note the tight packing of fungal arthrospores that cause hair shaft fragility and breakage (KOH mount for endothrix).

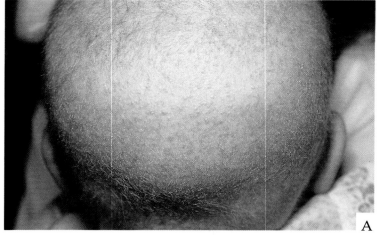

A

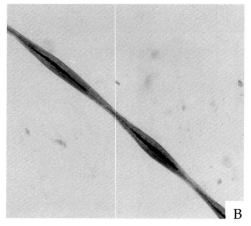

B

FIG. 8.114
Monilethrix. *A,* short broken hairs give the appearance of diffuse alopecia. *B,* microscopically, one can see periodic narrowing of this hair shaft. Hairs are brittle, and break off at constricted points near the scalp.

manent hair loss. Incision and drainage are not indicated as loculations are small and septae thick. The more inflammatory forms are often associated with occipital, post-auricular, and posterior cervical adenopathy. It is important to remember that when pustules, weeping and crusting lesions involve the scalp or hairline, the infection is far more likely to be of fungal than bacterial origin.

Fungal infection of the scalp is readily confirmed by a KOH examination of infected hairs (Fig. 8.113). Hairs should be pulled from the scalp rather than cut so that the root is available for examination as well. A Wood's light may also be useful in certain patients. Formerly, its most common use was in screening patients for fungal alopecia because the then-most-common causative organism, *Microsporum audouinii,* was easily identified by its fluorescence under Wood's light. Today, *Trichophyton tonsurans,* which does not fluoresce, is the most common causative organism in the United States. Currently, only *M. canis,* which causes 5 percent of cases, fluoresces bright blue-green.

Topical antifungal agents do not penetrate deeply enough to be effective in treatment of tinea capitis. Hence, oral antifungal agents (griseofulvin or ketoconazole) are administered over 2 to 4 months. This usually eradicates the infection. However, the risk of recurrence is high. Concurrent use of selenium sulfide shampoo (2.5 percent) reduces spore formation and shedding, and thus may help minimize risk of spread to siblings and classmates until oral treatment is complete.

Congenital and Genetic Disorders

Some structural defects of the hair shaft are congenital in origin or associated with heritable syndromes.

MONILETHRIX AND PILI TORTI

Monilethrix is a developmental hair defect that produces brittle, beaded hair. The condition is autosomal dominant and clinical manifestations usually appear after 2 to 3 months of age, when the fetal/neonatal vellus hairs are replaced by abnormal beaded hairs (Fig. 8.114A). The scalp is most severely affected, although hair on any part of the body can be involved. The disease is generally permanent. Microscopically, there is regular, periodic narrowing of the hair shafts (Fig. 8.114B). Breakage occurs in the constricted areas close to the scalp. Care must be taken not to confuse monilethrix with pili

torti, another structural defect in which the hair shaft is twisted on its own axis. Pili torti may be localized or generalized, and also appears with the first terminal hair growth of infancy. It may be associated with Menkes' kinky hair syndrome, an inherited defect of copper absorption, which also affects the central nervous, cardiovascular, and skeletal systems.

Disorders Affecting the Nails

Patients may seek the advice of a physician for nail disorders because of pain or cosmetic concerns. For the physician, knowledge of nail disorders is helpful in detecting clues to systemic disease.

PARONYCHIA

Paronychia is a common childhood disorder. It presents as a red, swollen, tender nail fold, usually on the side or at the base of the nail. The acute form, with sudden swelling and marked tenderness, is often caused by bacterial invasion after trauma to the cuticle or after a dermatitis that has damaged the stratum corneum barrier (see Chapter 12). Chronic paronychia may involve one or several nails. There is usually an associated history of chronic dermatitis or frequent exposure to water. Tenderness is mild, and a small amount of pus can sometimes be extruded. There is often some degree of associated nail dystrophy (Fig. 8.115). The causative organisms are Candida species, usually *C. albicans.* This form resolves with the use of topical antimycotics and avoidance of water.

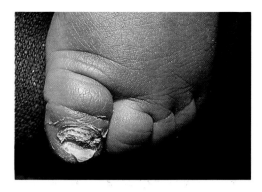

FIG. 8.115 Chronic paronychia with nail dystrophy due to Candida infection.

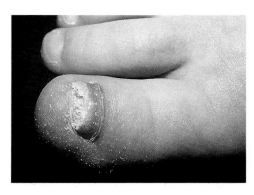

FIG. 8.116 Onychomycosis due to a chronic dermatophyte infection of the nail plate in a 4-year-old boy. This is rare in prepubertal children.

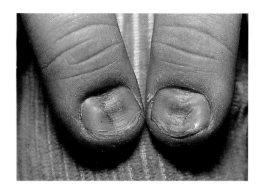

FIG. 8.117 Traumatic nail dystrophy. This teenager developed median nail dystrophy as a result of chronically picking at his nails.

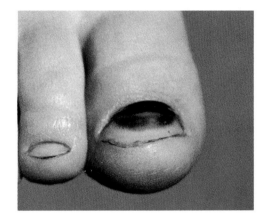

FIG. 8.118 Traumatic subungual hemorrhage. Discoloration due to traumatic hemorrhage under the toenail is common in children and athletic adults. It is a result of jamming the toe into the end of the shoe while running or stopping (turf toe).

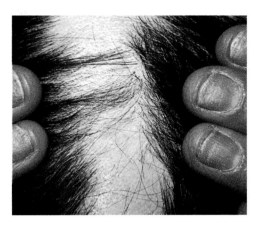

FIG. 8.119 Broad, shallow Scotch-plaid pitting of the nails associated with alopecia areata.

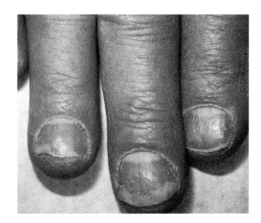

FIG. 8.120 Psoriatic nails. Psoriasis affecting the nails results in onycholysis and pitting.

ONYCHOMYCOSIS AND NAIL DYSTROPHY

Onychomycosis, or fungal infection of the nail plate (Fig. 8.116), is very rare in children before puberty. Thus, nail dystrophy should not be treated as a fungal infection unless proven by microscopic examination or fungal culture. Dystrophic nails (Fig. 8.117) occur frequently as a complication of trauma or underlying dermatosis, such as psoriasis or atopic dermatitis.

TRAUMA

Trauma to the nail may cause subungual hemorrhage, resulting in a brown-black discoloration. This is particularly likely following crush injuries. Usually, the diagnosis is simple, unless trauma is subtle. When a large, painful hematoma is produced, this should be evacuated using electrocautery to relieve pain and reduce risk of infection. Pigmentation at the base of the great toenail, caused by jamming the toe into the end of the shoe at a sudden stop, is called "turf toe" and results in mild subungual hemorrhage (Fig. 8.118). This must be distinguished from melanoma. Hemorrhage can be identified by the presence of purple-brown pigment in the distal nail and normal proximal outgrowth of the nail.

NAIL FINDINGS IN OTHER DERMATOLOGIC DISORDERS

Nail disorders may provide clues to other dermatologic or pediatric syndromes. For example, alopecia areata is associated with a characteristic Scotch-plaid pitting of the nails (Fig. 8.119). Similarly, psoriasis affects the nails in a number of ways that may help to distinguish it from other scaling disorders. Psoriasis in the nail matrix results in scattered pits that are larger, deeper, and less numerous than those found in alopecia areata (Fig. 8.120). Psoriasis of the nail bed, especially under the distal nail, causes separation of the nail from the underlying skin (onycholysis), and oil-drop discoloration with heaped-up scaling. Onycholysis alone, without pits or discoloration, may be caused by trauma, infection, nail-polish hardeners, or phototoxic reactions to drugs such as tetracycline.

COMPLICATIONS OF TOPICAL SKIN THERAPY

An important rule in medicine is "do no harm." To follow that rule, the physician must recognize the adverse effects of the therapies prescribed.

Topical Steroids

The most commonly used topical medications are steroids. These may be classified as high or low potency, according to their biological activity. Generally, fluorinated steroids are more potent than nonfluorinated steroids, and those in ointment bases are more active than those in cream or lotion bases. High-potency steroids should be used only for short periods of time or major side effects may develop. These include skin atrophy (Fig. 8.121), telangiectases, and increased skin fragility; acneiform eruptions; permanent skin striae (Fig. 8.122); and masking or delayed recognition of infections and infestations such as tinea corporis and scabies.

Use of fluorinated steroids should be avoided on the face, genitals, or intertriginous areas because absorption is greater and side effects are more common. Accidental injection of steroids into fat on attempted intramuscular injection may cause permanent subcutaneous atrophy (Fig. 8.123). If the medication is applied to large areas, if the treated area is occluded, or if therapy is continued for a long period, adrenal suppression may result.

Secondary bacterial infections and viral infections such as chickenpox may also progress with unusual rapidity in children on widespread topical or systemic corticosteroids. Hence, patients should be instructed to look for early signs of secondary infection and return promptly if they develop. Further, all patients placed on high-dose steroids who have no past history of varicella should be alerted to return immediately for zoster immune plasma if they discover that they have been exposed to chickenpox.

Other Agents

Other complications from topical medications, such as contact dermatitis, can be easily prevented. Allergic contact dermatitis is frequently seen as a reaction to both prescribed and over-the-counter drugs. The most common allergens are neomycin, "-caine" topical anesthetics or antipruritics, and ethylenediamine (a preservative in many topical preparations). It is important to remember that anaphylaxis can occur even in response to topical medications, especially if applied to broken skin. Hence, obtaining a history of drug allergies is important before prescribing topical agents.

Fortunately, most complications of therapy can be avoided if the physician has clear knowledge of the disease, of its treatment, and of the pharmacologic agents being prescribed.

REFERENCES

Hurwitz S: *Clinical Pediatric Dermatology.* Philadelphia, WB Saunders, 1981.

Meneghini CL, Bonifazi E: *An Atlas of Pediatric Dermatology.* Chicago, Year Book Medical Publishers, 1986.

Ruiz-Maldonado R, Parish LC, Beare JM: *Textbook of Pediatric Dermatology.* Philadelphia, Grune and Stratton, 1989.

Schachner LA, Hansen RC: *Pediatric Dermatology.* New York, Churchill Livingstone, 1988.

Weinberg S, Leider M, Shapiro L: *Color Atlas of Pediatric Dermatology*, ed 2. London, McGraw-Hill, 1990.

Weston WL: *Practical Pediatric Dermatology.* Boston, Little Brown, 1985.

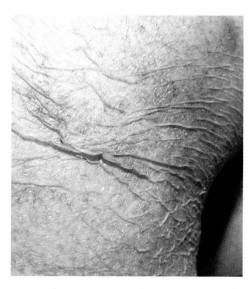

FIG. 8.121 *Steroid-induced skin atrophy. Topical steroids may cause marked atrophy and fragility of the skin, especially if used under occlusion regularly for more than 1 month.*

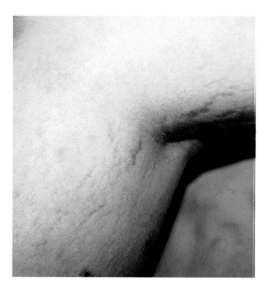

FIG. 8.122 *Steroid-induced striae distensae. Prolonged use of potent fluorinated steroids may cause permanent striae distensae.*

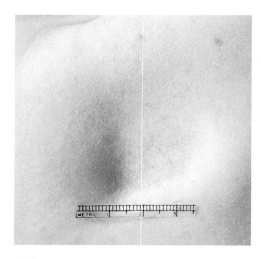

FIG. 8.123 *Steroid-induced subcutaneous atrophy. Injection of steroids into fat instead of muscle often produces subcutaneous atrophy. While in some cases this may resolve in 6 to 12 months, in others it can be permanent.*

PEDIATRIC ENDOCRINOLOGY

David Finegold, M.D.

Clinical presentations of endocrine disease vary widely such that alterations in hormonal balance can result in children who are too fat, too thin, too short, or too tall. While the molecular explanations for states of excessive or insufficient hormone secretion constantly become more sophisticated with improvements in our understanding of the physiology and biochemistry, the clinical presentations of abnormal endocrine states remain constant. Recognition of the physical signs associated with these states is important as our ability to treat and correct these imbalances advances. The following descriptions will emphasize the physical signs associated with normal endocrine maturation and with states of hypo- and hypersecretion of hormones.

THE ANTERIOR PITUITARY GLAND

The pituitary gland in humans contains anterior and posterior sections that have substantially different functions. In this chapter we will concentrate on the anterior section and on its relationship to the release of hormones in endocrine glands. The anterior pituitary contains cells that secrete three types of hormones: corticotropin-related peptide hormones, glycoprotein hormones, and somatomammotropins. These compounds have great biologic potency and, with the exception of prolactin, are regulated through closed feedback loops as well as through specific agonists and antagonists.

The **corticotropin-related peptide hormones** consist of adrenocorticotropic hormone (ACTH), α-melanocyte-stimulating hormone (α-MSH), and γ- and β-lipotropins (γ-LPH, β-LPH). These hormones are derived from a common precursor molecule, proopiomelanocortin, within whose amino-acid structure are contained their sequences. Within the subunit structure of β-LPH also are contained the important neuroendocrine molecules α, β-, and γ-endorphin, and enkephalin. After posttranslational processing from this large precursor molecule, the secretion of ACTH is regulated by the level of corticotropin-releasing factor (CRF) in the pituitary portal plasma and by the level of plasma cortisol secreted from the adrenal gland, which then has a negative feedback effect on further secretion of ACTH (Fig. 9.1). While the relationship between ACTH and cortisol secretion has been well studied, less is known about β-lipotropin secretion, along with secretion of its subunits α, β-, and γ-endorphin, and about enkephalin and β-MSH secretion.

The **glycoprotein hormones** of the pituitary include follicle-stimulating hormone (FSH), luteinizing hormone (LH), and thyroid-stimulating hormone (TSH). Each of these hormones is composed of two dissimilar peptide subunits. The α chain is highly similar in structure among the three hormones. However, the β chain is unique and confers specificity from one hormone to another. These three hormones also contain significant amounts of carbohydrate and sialic acid residues along with their basic amino acid structures. As the corticotropin-related peptide hormones are stimulated by hypothalamic secretion, similarly, LH and FSH secretions are positively stimulated by gonadotropin-releasing hormone (GnRH).

The control of LH and FSH secretion is sensitive to the periodic nature of GnRH release. If GnRH periodicity is perturbed—either by increasing or decreasing the frequency of GnRH pulses, or by continuously exposing the gonadotrophs to GnRH stimulation—LH and FSH secretion may be shut off. This knowledge has permitted the development of potent GnRH agonist analogues which are effective in the treatment of disorders such as central precocious puberty.

The primary action of FSH and LH is on the gonads. FSH directly stimulates gametogenesis in the testes and supports follicular development in the ovary. LH stimulates Leydig cell function of the testes, producing testosterone, and acts to promote luteinization of the ovaries (Fig. 9.2). The negative feedback effect of sex steroids on LH and FSH production is dramatically emphasized in the postmenopausal woman or in the young girl with Turner syndrome in whom marked elevations of these hormones occur. Inhibin is another recently discovered glycoprotein produced by the gonads which appears to inhibit FSH release.

TSH stimulates many aspects of thyroid function. These aspects include increasing the size of thyroid cells and also the vascularity of the gland. Specific increases in the size of follicular epithelial cells and in the amount of colloid may easily be determined. Moreover, TSH increases radioactive iodide uptake, thyroglobulin synthesis, and thyroxine and triiodothyronine release from the thyroid gland. Basic alterations in thyroid cell biochemistry also may occur following TSH administration. The rate of TSH section appears to be determined by the level of circulating thyroid hormone as well as by the hypothalamic hormone, thyrotropin-releasing hormone (TRH). However, negative feedback of TSH secre-

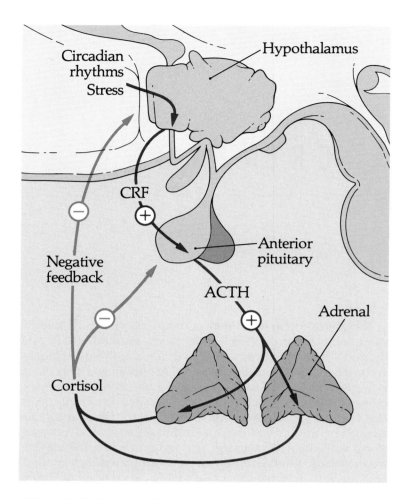

FIG. 9.1 Feedback regulation of adrenocorticotropic hormone (ACTH) at the level of the hypothalamus, pituitary, and adrenal glands.

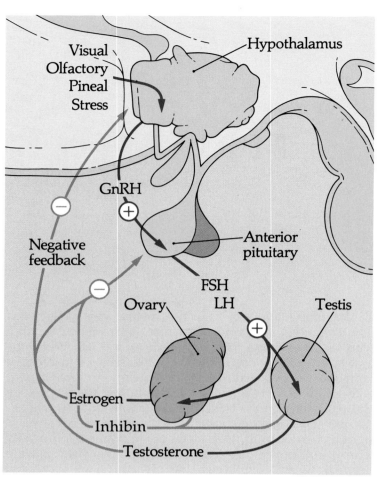

FIG. 9.2 Feedback regulation of luteinizing hormone (LH) and follicle-stimulating hormone (FSH) at the level of the hypothalamus, pituitary, and gonads.

tion by circulating thyroid hormone occurs mainly at the pituitary level (Fig. 9.3).

The somatomammotropin hormones, **prolactin** (PRL) and **growth hormone** (GH), have similar chemical structures as well as some overlap of their biologic activity. The amino acid sequences of both contain two or three disulfide bridges.

PRL acts directly on its target organs and does not require an intermediary secondary endocrine gland. PRL's only major function in humans is the initiation and maintenance of lactation. In contrast to the other anterior pituitary hormones, prolactin appears to be under tonic stimulation. Chronic inhibition through hypothalamic secretory mechanisms appears to be the major regulator of unrestrained prolactin secretion. Dopaminergic pathways and dopamine have potent prolactin inhibitory properties and, in fact, dopamine appears to fit many criteria for the physiologic prolactin inhibiting factor. Bromocriptine, a potent dopaminergic agonist compound, has been used to treat states characterized by prolactin hypersecretion.

GH modulates complex metabolic processes. Although the molecular basis of GH action continues to remain obscure, its obvious effects can be seen in hypopituitary children in whom it has been used for treatment. GH stimulates an increase in lean body mass as well as a marked increase in the size of the heart, pancreas, liver, and kidneys. It also has positive effects on carbohydrate, fat and protein metabolism, and causes a decrease in body fat. GH inhibits carbohydrate uptake by muscle. This diabetogenic effect of GH action has been well demonstrated and is a known complication of GH hypersecretion. On the other hand, hypoglycemia may be seen in patients who are GH-deficient.

GH appears to mediate some of its effects on bone and linear growth via the somatomedins. These peptides have some structural similarity to proinsulin. Somatomedin C appears to mediate sulfate and phosphate incorporation into cartilage. Somatomedin C is identical to the peptide originally called insulin-like growth factor I (IGF-I). GH is regulated on chronic and acute levels through a variety of mechanisms. A

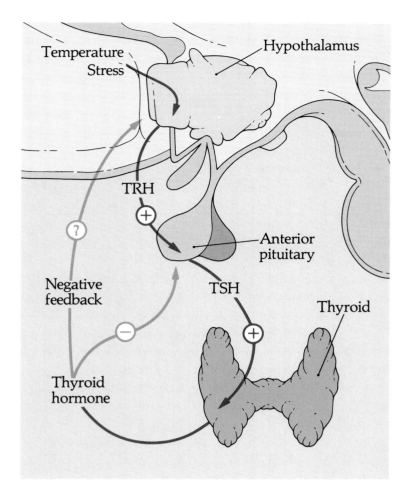

FIG. 9.3 Feedback regulation of thyroid-stimulating hormone (TSH) at the level of the hypothalamus, pituitary, and thyroid gland.

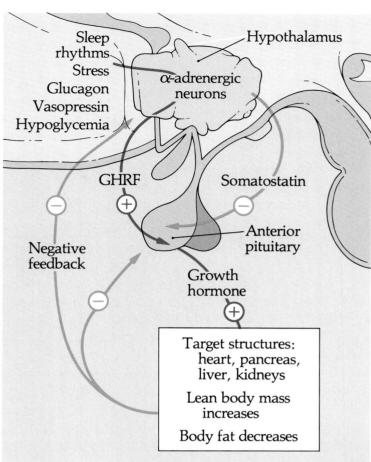

FIG. 9.4 Feedback regulation of growth hormone (GH) at the level of the hypothalamus, pituitary, and target organs.

rapid fall in plasma glucose concentration may elicit a brisk rise in GH secretion. However, hypoglycemia of slow onset may not activate GH secretion. Neural factors such as sleep, stress, and α-adrenergic agonists may result in augmentation of GH secretion. Glucagon and vasopressin appear to cause hormonal augmentation of GH secretion. A fall in plasma somatomedin also may result in GH elevations. Recently, the hypothalamic GH-releasing factor (GHRF) has been identified and appears to be an important physiologic stimulant of GH secretion, just as the hypothalamic peptide somatostatin appears to be important in the inhibition of GH secretion. The physiologic regulation of growth hormone secretion appears to be closely related to the balance of somatostatin secretion and GHRF secretion. When somatostatin predominates, growth hormone is suppressed, and when somatostatin secretion is low and GHRF secretion active, GH levels increase in the plasma (Fig. 9.4).

The anterior pituitary, with its diverse cell types and hormonal secretory patterns, controls many important biologic processes. Anterior pituitary hormone deficiencies cause subsequent deficiencies in the output of secondary endocrine glands. Consequently, specific aspects of growth and development are consistently disturbed by oversecretion or undersecretion of the pituitary. Particular alterations in physical appearance should alert physicians to an abnormality in the anterior pituitary, and to subsequent secondary deficiencies (e.g., in the thyroid or adrenals).

NORMAL GROWTH

Normal growth occurs at a varying rate, through the process of normal development. Moreover, wide variability exists in growth rates between individual children at different ages. Incremental growth rate is one of the most important ele-

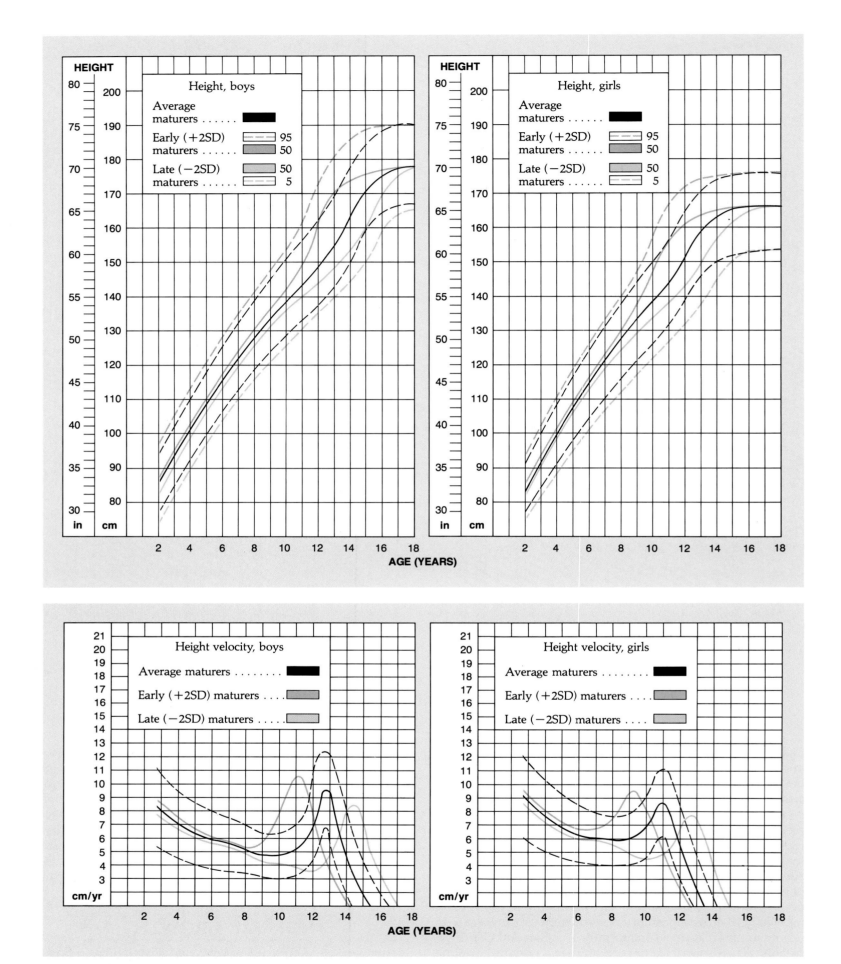

FIG. 9.5 Linear growth and growth velocity curves for boys and girls. (Adapted from Tanner JM, Davies PSW: Clinical longitudinal standards for height and height velocity for North American children. J Pediatr 107:317–329, 1985)

DIFFERENTIAL DIAGNOSIS OF CHILDREN WITH SHORT STATURE

Familial short stature (genetic)
Constitutional delay of sexual development
Malnutrition and psychosocial factors
Systemic disease
   Pulmonary
      Cystic fibrosis
      Asthma
   Cardiac and circulatory
      Congenital heart disease (cyanotic and acyanotic)
      Acquired heart disease
   Renal
      Renal insufficiency
      Pyelonephritis (chronic)
      Renal tubular acidosis
   Gastrointestinal and hepatic
      Malabsorption
      Inflammatory bowel disease
      Hepatic insufficiency
   Neurological
      Mental retardation with growth delay
   Musculoskeletal and connective tissue
      Chondrodystrophies
      Storage diseases
      Rickets
      Skeletal dysplasias
   Immunologic
      Immune deficiencies

Syndromes associated with short stature
   Chromosomal abnormalities
      Trisomies 13, 18, 21
      Turner syndrome
   Other syndromes
      Noonan
      Progeria
      Silver
      Cockayne
      Seckel
States of endocrine hypo- or hypersecretion
   Hypopituitarism
   Hypothyroidism
   Hypoadrenalism
   Hyperadrenalism

FIG. 9.6

ments in assessing whether a child has a pathologic abnormality of growth. As seen in Figure 9.5, the growth velocity curve may be calculated as the first derivative of the linear growth curve. This manipulation graphically illustrates the wide variability in growth rates at different ages. The curve also illustrates that in the first 2 to 3 years of life, growth is constantly decelerating. The growth velocity during infancy rapidly decelerates. Most children find their percentile track by 15 to 18 months of age. During the first 36 months of life, children who fall across percentiles in a downward fashion must be followed closely and a decision made as to whether a detailed investigation regarding the cause is appropriate. The hand x-ray for bone age is uninformative before 18 months of life. Hence, if a delayed bone age is suspected in the first 36 months of life, epiphyseal development should be estimated by way of a hemiskeleton radiographic examination. During the latency years, a long period of constant growth occurs and is followed by a sharp acceleration in growth velocity during adolescence. A growth rate below 4 to 5 cm/yr for both girls and boys between 4 years of age and the adolescent growth spurt is abnormal and should be investigated. This sharp increase in growth velocity is the harbinger of puberty. The growth velocity of adolescence also is the only time during which the rapid growth of the infant is recapitulated.

It is important to remember that of those children with short stature and normal body proportions who are brought to their pediatrician for evaluation, only a few will have growth failure of an endocrine origin. The differential diagnosis of children with short stature may be noted in Figure 9.6. In fact, the vast majority of short children who have organic illness suffer from major systemic diseases of cardiac, pulmonary, gastrointestinal, or renal origin. The most common etiology of short stature in children is short parents. The genetic potential of a child is heavily determined by the growth achieved by both parents and by their relatives, and this information should be part of a careful history taken in evaluating short children. Determination of epiphyseal maturation, or bone age, is often helpful in evaluating children with short stature. Children who have genetically determined short stature generally will have a bone age equivalent to their chronologic age. Those who have constitutional delay as a cause of short stature usually are of normal length at birth, but develop mild growth deceleration in early childhood. Growth velocity is usually in the 3 to 25 percentile for age. Puberty is delayed, as is the pubertal growth acceleration. A family history of "late bloomers" or delayed puberty is common. Bone age in constitutional delay is delayed, being more consistent with the child's height age rather than chronologic age.

Genetic syndromes (such as Turner syndrome or Down syndrome) provide examples of cases in which chromosomal abnormalities limit physical growth. Congenital disorders of bone mineralization and bone growth, such as the chondro-

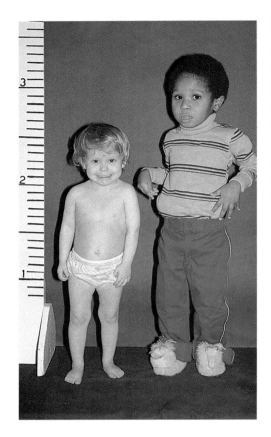

FIG. 9.7 The normal 3½-year-old boy is in the 50th percentile for height. The short 3-year-old girl exhibits the characteristic "Kewpie" doll appearance, suggesting a diagnosis of GH deficiency.

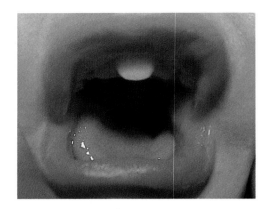

FIG. 9.8 The presence of a single central maxillary incisor should alert the clinician to investigate the possibility of GH deficiency. (Courtesy of Dr. P. Lee)

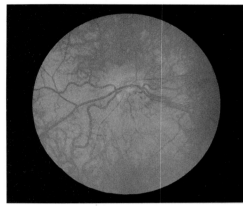

FIG. 9.9 Pale optic discs, suggesting optic atrophy, often are seen with septo-optic dysplasia. This finding also suggests pituitary endocrine deficiencies ranging from isolated GH deficiency to panhypopituitarism. (Courtesy of Dr. D. Hiles)

dystrophies, also represent an important cause of short stature. An aggressive endocrine investigation should be undertaken to ascertain the presence or absence of hypopituitarism and GH deficiency only after these other diseases have been eliminated from consideration.

While deficiencies of other anterior pituitary hormones, such as TSH or ACTH, may result in secondary hypothyroid and hypoadrenal states, these states tend to be milder than those of primary hypothyroidism or Addison's disease and hence their clinical signs are not as striking. The most striking feature of the panhypopituitary patient remains that of growth retardation.

SPECIFIC HORMONAL IMBALANCES
Growth Hormone Deficiency

The phenotypic features of a child with GH deficiency are most striking. GH deficiency tends to be recognized by the characteristic features of normal body proportion and increased adiposity around the trunk and extremities. As seen in Figure 9.7, GH-deficient children have delicate features, and, in males with this disorder, the genitalia frequently are small. Children with hypopituitarism tend to have high-pitched voices compared with other children of the same age. In GH deficiency, the height age is delayed along with a significant delay in the bone age.

Children with a variety of midline defects have a higher incidence of hypopituitarism when compared with normal children. The child seen in Figure 9.8 has a single central maxillary incisor—an example of a midline abnormality consistently associated with GH deficiency. Other physical findings suggestive of pituitary endocrine abnormalities include the syndrome of septo-optic dysplasia with pale optic discs (Fig. 9.9), and children with cleft lip and cleft palate. These

embryologic defects, presenting in infancy, also may be associated with significant risks of hypoglycemia. Recurrent protracted hypoglycemia may be an early presentation of hypopituitarism. The hypoglycemia is effectively treated with GH replacement therapy.

Thyroid Gland Disorders

The thyroid gland is situated in the neck or, rarely, at the base of the tongue or in the mediastinum. Both overactivity and underactivity of the thyroid gland may be associated with goiter; however, the signs of hyperthyroidism and hypothyroidism are dramatically different. Examination of the thyroid gland is an important step in the evaluation of a suspected abnormality in thyroid hormone release.

As seen in Figure 9.10, the thyroid gland usually can best be palpated with the examiner behind the patient. After identification of the cricothyroid cartilage, the second and third fingers are moved laterally along the trachea just medial to the sternocleidomastoid muscles. Two distinct lobes are palpable, the right lobe usually greater in size than the left lobe. With goiter present, these lobes may be quite easily identified. The texture of the gland will vary in hyperthyroidism and hypothyroidism; the former usually being soft and fleshy, and the latter usually firm or bosselated. Since the thyroid is directly supported by the trachea, having the patient swallow several mouthfuls of water will elevate and depress a palpable gland along with the trachea during the swallowing motion.

Most physicians are familiar with the symptoms associated with hyperthyroidism, or Graves' disease. An acceleration in basal metabolism with concomitant tachycardia, weight loss, heat intolerance, and nervousness are characteristic. Exophthalmus, a characteristic eye finding of Graves' disease, usually is less dramatic in children than in adults, but the

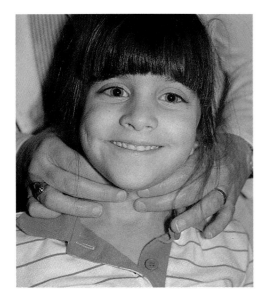

FIG. 9.10 Correct palpation of the thyroid gland is performed from behind the child.

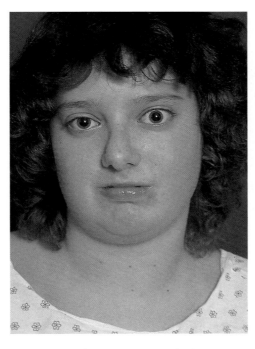

FIG. 9.11 These patients with Graves disease illustrate mild thyromegaly and proptosis or ophthalmopathy. Ophthalmopathy

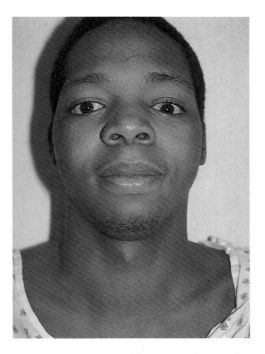

is less dramatic in children than the eye disease seen in adult patients with Graves disease.

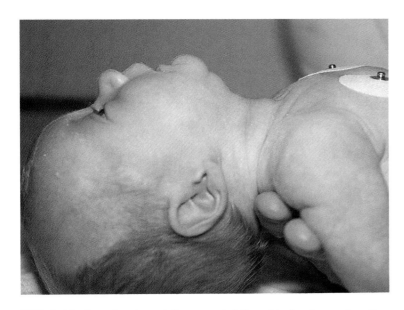

FIG. 9.12 Examination of the neonatal thyroid gland may be effectively performed by elevating the infant's trunk and allowing the head to drop back gently, as shown.

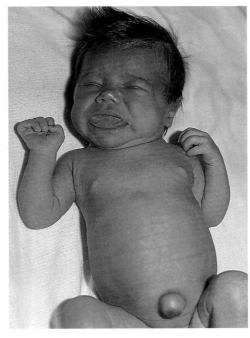

FIG. 9.13 A child with cretinism. (Courtesy of Dr. T.P. Foley, Jr.)

appearance of proptosis can easily be appreciated (Fig. 9.11). The hyperthyroid gland can become quite large, as much as 3 to 4 times normal size, and it is quite warm during palpation. A bruit often may be heard over a hyperthyroid gland.

Either congenital or acquired hypothyroidism may also produce goiter. Goiter in an infant with congenital hypothyroidism is suggestive of an enzymatic defect in thyroid hormone biosynthesis. To demonstrate goiter in a newborn infant, the examiner's hand is placed gently under the back and shoulder blades of the infant, and the infant's trunk is raised from the bed (Fig. 9.12). As the head falls backward, the neck is elevated and a goiter, if present, will be displayed prominently. Because of neonatal thyroid screening, the coarse features of the congenital hypothyroid baby referred to as a cretin (Fig. 9.13) hopefully are now a thing of the past. However, the broad nasal bridge, thick lips, and dull appearance characteristic of a cretin were seen regularly in endocrine clinics and pediatric offices not long ago because of the difficulty of making this diagnosis in early life. Careful retrospective evaluation of hypothyroid babies identified through neonatal thyroid screening has made clear that all such physical findings may be absent or too subtle to diagnose with certainty in the neonatal period. This uncertainty, in combination with the success of early treatment of congenital hypothyroidism, mandates continued neonatal thyroid screening.

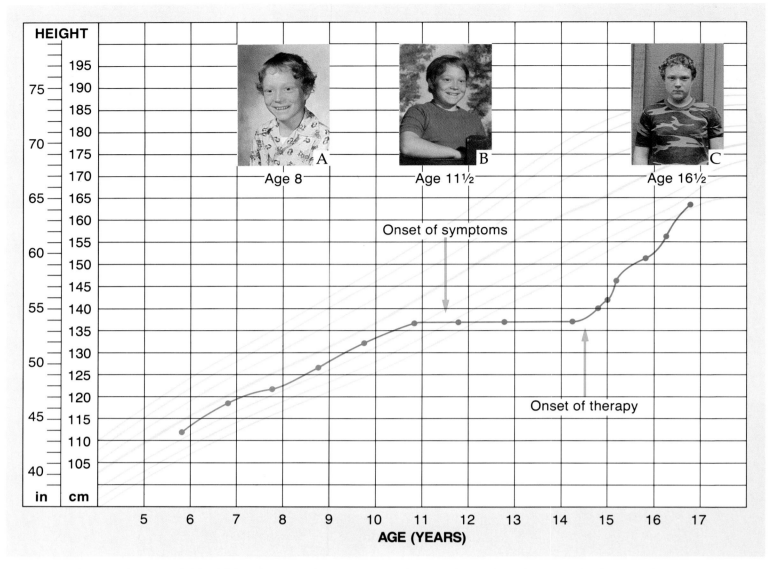

FIG. 9.14 The growth curve of this child with acquired hypothyroidism shows marked growth deceleration. Following thyroid replacement, significant catch-up growth occurs. The inserted photographs illustrate: **A,** the child prior to the onset of acquired hypothyroidism. **B,** the change in body habitus associated with acquired hypothyroidism, and **C,** resolution following thyroid replacement at the indicated times.

Acquired hypothyroidism, most frequently caused by Hashimoto's thyroiditis, may also present in a subtle fashion. Despite the subtlety of these clinical findings, the astute clinician will still take note of dry skin, constipation, hair loss, depressed or delayed relaxation phase of deep tendon reflexes, and weakness of the child with acquired hypothyroidism. The most dramatic expression of acquired hypothyroidism may be a sharp deceleration in growth, as seen in the growth curve shown in Figure 9.14. Following institution of thyroid hormone therapy, rapid catch-up growth occurs, returning the child to normal growth percentiles.

Turner Syndrome

Although genetic in origin (see Chapter 1), Turner syndrome must be included in any discussion of short stature. While its nature need not be solely endocrine, Turner syn-

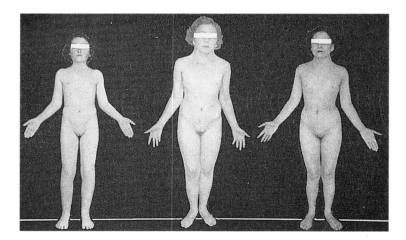

FIG. 9.15 Turner used this photograph to describe the syndrome that bears his name. Note the clinical heterogeneity within the syndrome.

COMMON CLINICAL FINDINGS IN TURNER SYNDROME

Skeletal growth disturbances
  Short stature
  Short neck
  Abnormal upper- to lower-segment ratio
  Cubitus valgus
  Short metacarpals
  Madelung's deformity
  Scoliosis
  Genu valgum
  Characteristic facies: micrognathia,
    high-arched palate

Lymphatic obstruction
  Webbed neck
  Low posterior hairline
  Rotated ears
  Edema of hands, feet
  Nail dysplasia
  Characteristic dermatographics
Germ cell defects
  Gonadal failure
  Infertility

Miscellaneous defects
  Strabismus
  Ptosis
  Multiple pigmented nevi
  Cardiovascular anomalies
  Hypertension
  Renal and renovascular anomalies
  Hearing abnormalities
Associated disorders
  Hashimoto's thyroiditis
  Hypothyroidism
  Alopecia
  Vitiligo
  Gastrointestinal disorders
  Carbohydrate intolerance

Adapted from Lippe BM: Primary ovarian failure, in Kaplan SA (ed):
Clinical Pediatric and Adolescent Endocrinology. *Philadelphia, WB Saunders, 1982, p 275.*

FIG. 9.16

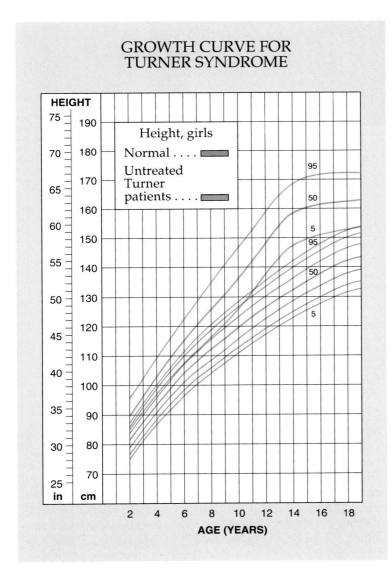

GROWTH CURVE FOR TURNER SYNDROME

FIG. 9.17

drome is a common diagnosis in short women seen in endocrine clinics. Some of the clinical presentations of Turner syndrome are shown in the pictures of young women reported in the original article by Turner (Figure 9.15). The wide carrying angle (cubitus valgus), shield-like chest, and webbed neck may be easily appreciated. A more comprehensive list of physical findings in patients with Turner syndrome is listed in Figure 9.16. Turner syndrome should be suspected in any short girl presenting with pubic and/or axillary hair, and absence of breast development and menses. Karyotyping is diagnostic in a clinical picture suggestive of Turner syndrome. Recent studies suggest that growth hormone treatment with or without weak androgenic steroids may significantly augment ultimate adult growth in girls with Turner syndrome. Growth charts for untreated girls with this syndrome are shown in Figure 9.17.

Parathyroid Gland Dysfunction

Dysfunction of the parathyroid glands usually does not present a unique phenotype. Chvostek's sign (distortion of the face when the seventh nerve is stimulated with a reflex hammer) or Trousseau's sign (cramping of the hand when a blood pressure cuff is elevated significantly above the systolic blood pressure) may be the only significant sign seen in an individual with hypocalcemia. However, Albright's hereditary osteodystrophy, one specific form of hypoparathyroidism, is associated with a very characteristic phenotype. These patients may have a round facies, short stature, obesity, skin

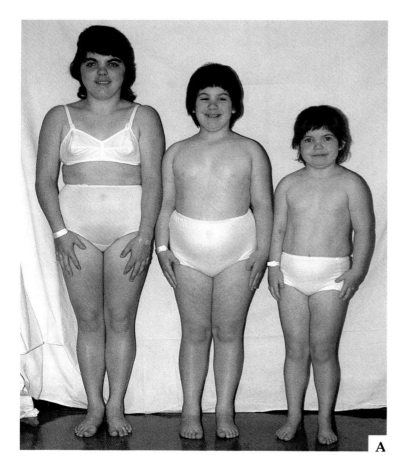

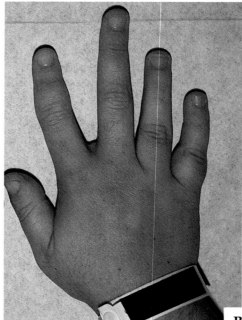

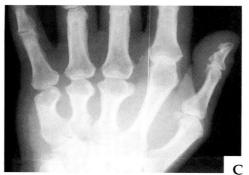

FIG. 9.18 **A**, sisters with Albright's hereditary osteodystrophy (pseudohypoparathyroidism). **B**, the short fourth metacarpal may easily be appreciated in this photograph. **C**, radiograph of the hand illustrates the short fourth metacarpal seen in pseudohypoparathyroidism as well as in other syndromes such as Turner syndrome. This child also has a short third metacarpal, as well. (**A** and **B**, courtesy of Dr. J. Parks. **C**, courtesy of Dr. J. Medina)

hyperpigmentation with irregular margins, and a short thick neck (Fig. 9.18A). Shortening of the metacarpals and metatarsals is seen most commonly in the fourth digit, and less commonly in the other digits (Figs. 9.18B and C). These patients may have decreased intelligence as well as subcutaneous calcification, may present with hypocalcemia and hyperphosphatemia, and characteristically have reduced phosphaturia when given exogenous parathyroid hormone. This disorder is hereditary and is passed with an inheritance suggestive of an X-linked dominant gene. Albright's hereditary osteodystrophy should be suspected in a short child who is having difficulty with hypocalcemia and whose history reveals similarly affected family members.

Adrenal Gland Dysfunction

Hyperfunction or hypofunction of the adrenal glands results in some of the most dramatic physical alterations of any endocrinologic disorder. Cushing syndrome, the phenotype resulting from excess glucocorticoid action, is seen in endogenous as well as in exogenous steroid exposure. Rounded facies, plethora, and a central obesity are characteristic of Cushing syndrome (Fig. 9.19). The so-called buffalo hump behind the neck has been described frequently. These children often may show centripetal obesity. Because of their excessive metabolism, muscle weakness and muscle wasting occur, resulting in comparatively thin extremities (see Fig.

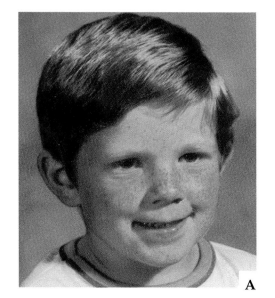

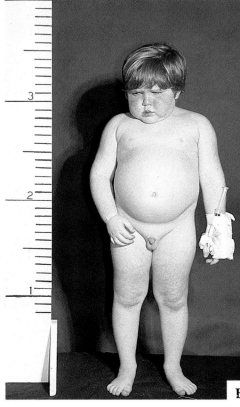

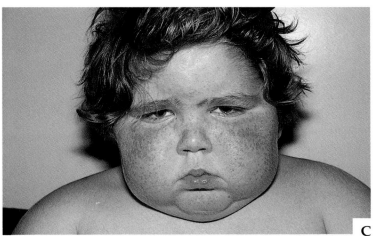

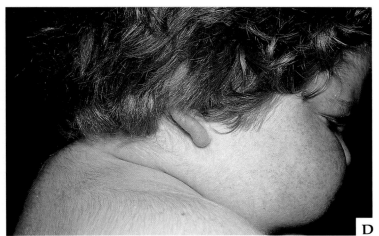

FIG. 9.19 *Cushing syndrome. These photographs show how dramatic the changes associated with Cushing syndrome are, and how rapidly they can occur.* **A**, *patient prior to the onset of Cushing syndrome.* **B**, *patient 4 months after* **A** *was taken. Note the centripetal obesity of the trunk compared with the extremities after the onset of Cushing syndrome.* **C**, *moon facies is clearly demonstrated and should raise the diagnostic index of Cushing syndrome. In diagnosing Cushing syndrome, equally important to the physical manifesta tions shown here is the presence of growth failure.* **D**, *buffalo hump. Excessive adipose tissue over the lower cervical and upper thoracic spine is characteristic of Cushing syndrome.*

9.19B). These children frequently are irritable and quite miserable. The skin is usually thinned and easily bruised. Hypertension and, ultimately, loss of bone mineral and osteoporosis occur with long-standing glucocorticoid exposure.

Endogenous Cushing syndrome may be caused by adrenal tumors, pituitary adenoma, or ectopic ACTH production. The high- and low-dose dexamethasone suppression test remains the most important diagnostic study for differentiating between the etiologies of Cushing syndrome. The develop-

ment of effective ACTH assays and of urinary free-cortisol measurement has added new diagnostic power to this classic study. Following two days of baseline studies, dexamethasone is administered in a "low dose" of 0.005 to 0.006 mg/kg, or 0.25 mg, every 6 hours for three days in the older child or adult. Following the low-dose administration, a "high dose" of 0.02 to 0.025 mg/kg, or 2 mg, every 6 hours is administered for the last three days of the tests. The differential findings in the specific etiology of Cushing syndrome are listed

THE DIFFERENTIAL DIAGNOSIS OF CUSHING SYNDROME AS INTERPRETED FROM THE DEXAMETHASONE SUPPRESSION TEST

	Normal	Adrenal Tumor	Pituitary Hypersecretion
	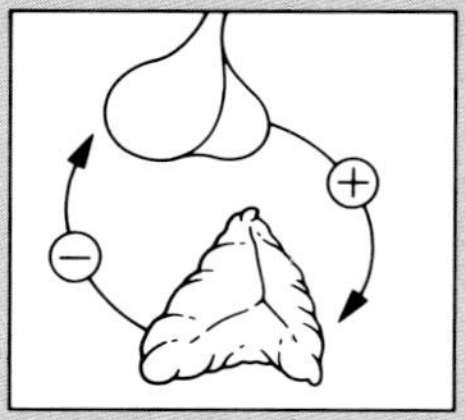	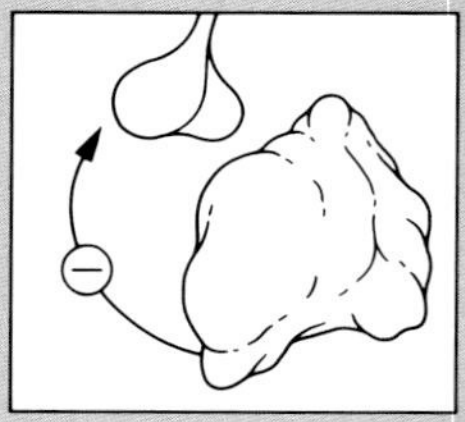	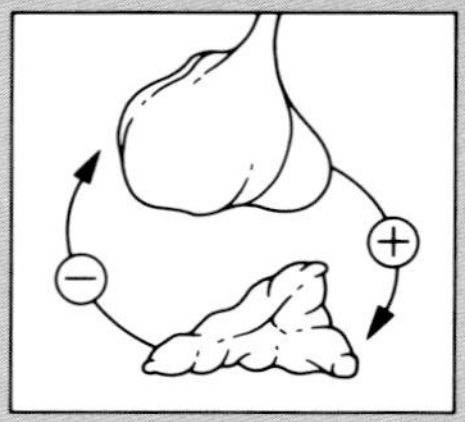
Plasma cortisol diurnal rhythm	10–25 μg% rhythmic	High no rhythm	High no rhythm
Plasma ACTH	Normal	Low	High
Plasma ACTH after adrenalectomy, on normal cortisol replacement	Normal	Low	High
Plasma glucocorticoid response to ACTH	3–5 fold rise	+, 0	+
Urinary glucocorticoid response to metyrapone	2–4 fold rise	0	+
Plasma glucocorticoid response to dexamethasone	Suppressed	No fall	Partial fall

FIG. 9.20 The differential diagnosis of Cushing syndrome as interpreted from the dexamethasone suppression test. (Adapted from Williams RH: Textbook of Endocrinology, 6th ed. WB Saunders, Philadelphia, 1981, p 272)

in Figure 9.20. Improvement in surgical technique has been responsible for an improved outcome in the treatment of pituitary Cushing syndrome. Medical therapy for adrenal tumors or to supress pituitary ACTH production is still inadequate.

In striking contrast to the obesity seen with glucocorticoid excess, patients with Addison's disease (glucocorticoid and mineralocorticoid deficiency) present with a thin body habitus and wasting of subcutaneous tissue (Fig. 9.21A). There is little change seen in overall growth rate. Frequently a striking hyperpigmentation or bronzing of the skin occurs, with emphasis of this pigmentary change in flexor creases and in scars, and over the areolae of the nipples (Fig. 9.21B through D). Vitiligo may occur as well. Frequently patients may be confused and weak. In far-advanced Addison's disease vascular collapse is common. The decreased circulating plasma volume is reflected by the thinned narrow heart shadow seen on a chest radiograph (Fig. 9.21E). If untreated, patients with Addison's disease gradually weaken and die. However, replacement of glucocorticoid with cortisol, and of mineralocorticoid with a compound such as 9-α-fludrocortisone (Florinef) allows the patient with Addison's disease to lead a normal life. Tuberculosis was formerly the most common cause of Addison's disease. Autoimmune destruction of the adrenal gland has now replaced tuberculosis as the most common cause of Addison's disease. The clinical manifestations of Addison's disease are less fully expressed in individuals who have either isolated ACTH deficiencies or hypothalamic alterations in corticotropin-releasing factor kinetics. This is well demonstrated in the girl with isolated ACTH deficiency seen before and after treatment (Fig. 9.21F, G.) Although she has the clinical wasting associated with Addison's disease, her skin is pale as opposed to bronzed.

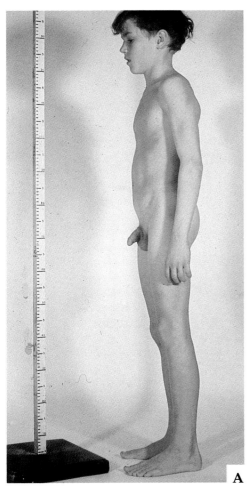

A

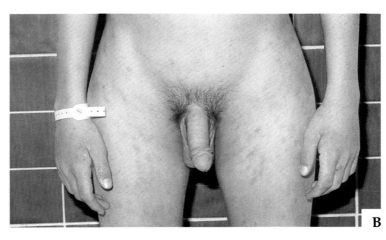

B

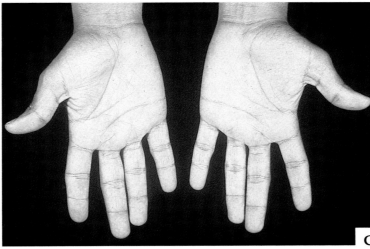

C

FIG. 9.21 **A**, this patient shows the thin habitus and ill appearance characteristic of Addison's disease. **B–D**, hyperpig-mentation may be marked. **E**, microcardia is characteristically seen on chest radiograph. **F**, young girl with isolated ACTH deficiency shows wasting and pallor rather than ex-cessive bronzing. **G**, the same girl after therapy. (**A** through **D**, courtesy of Dr. M. New. **E**, courtesy of Dr. J. Medina)

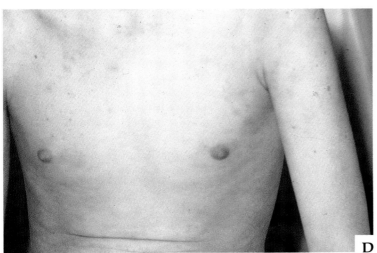

D

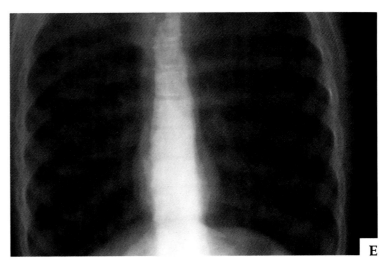

E

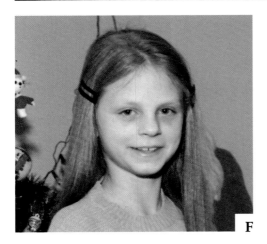

F

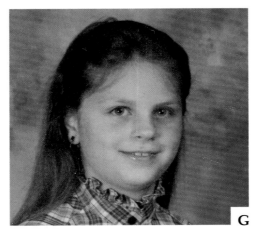

G

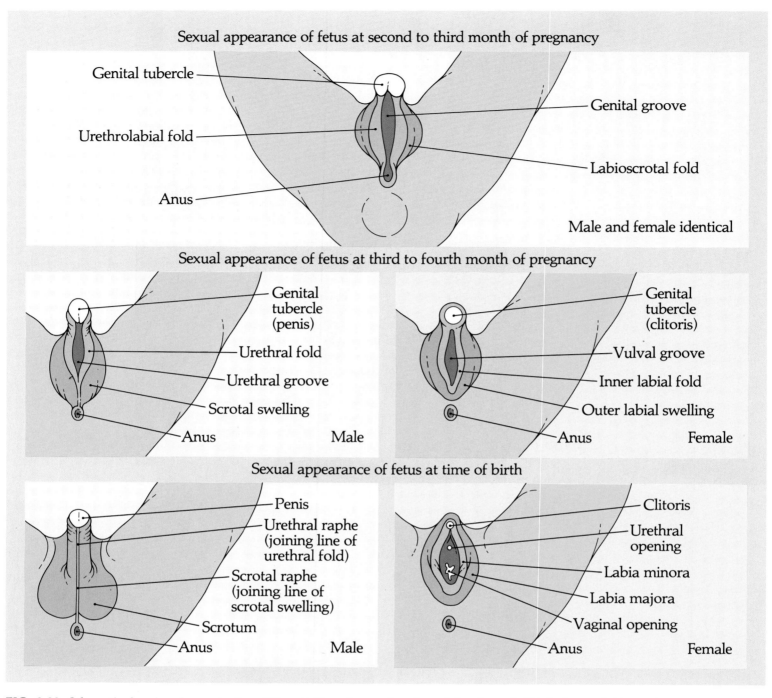

Sexual appearance of fetus at second to third month of pregnancy

Genital tubercle

Urethrolabial fold

Anus

Genital groove

Labioscrotal fold

Male and female identical

Sexual appearance of fetus at third to fourth month of pregnancy

Genital tubercle (penis)

Urethral fold

Urethral groove

Scrotal swelling

Anus   Male

Genital tubercle (clitoris)

Vulval groove

Inner labial fold

Outer labial swelling

Anus   Female

Sexual appearance of fetus at time of birth

Penis

Urethral raphe (joining line of urethral fold)

Scrotal raphe (joining line of scrotal swelling)

Scrotum

Anus   Male

Clitoris

Urethral opening

Labia minora

Labia majora

Vaginal opening

Anus   Female

FIG. 9.22 *Schematic drawing demonstrating differentiation of normal male and female genitalia during embryogenesis.*

SEXUAL MATURATION

Anomalies of Early Sexual Development

Sexual maturation begins in fetal life. With normal progression, a normal internal and external male or female genital anatomy is formed (Fig. 9.22). If normal progression of sexual development fails, however, children may be born with ambiguous genitalia (Fig. 9.23), which presents a difficult and urgent diagnostic problem for the obstetric/pediatric team. Children with ambiguous genitalia must be evaluated with

urgency and a diagnosis determined as quickly as possible. This provides the basis for an appropriate recommendation to parents regarding the sex of rearing, and also for the rapid and appropriate institution of therapy in cases where medical intervention is necessary.

The classification of anomalous sexual development can be based on gonadal development. Some disorders of gonadal differentiation (such as Klinefelter syndrome, Turner syndrome, and their variants) may not necessarily present with anomalous external genitalia. True hermaphroditism, while

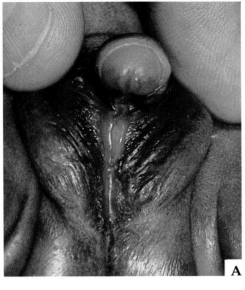

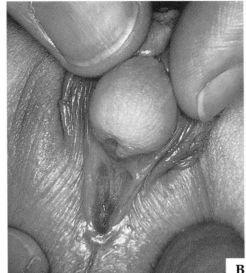

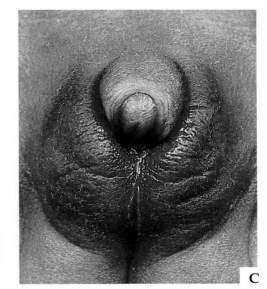

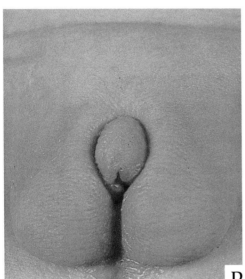

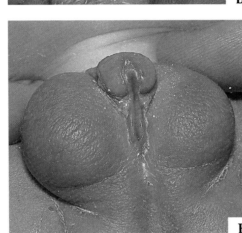

FIG. 9.23 Examples of ambiguous genitalia. These cases include (A) a true hermaphrodite, and (B–E) congenital virilizing adrenal hyperplasia. (B through D courtesy of Dr. D. Becker)

rare, frequently may present with ambiguous genitalia at birth. Female pseudohermaphrodites (genotype, XX) are those individuals who have ovaries, although they present with ambiguous external genitalia. The most common cause of female pseudohermaphroditism is virilizing adrenal hyperplasia. However, any androgen or synthetic progestin transferred from the maternal circulation, either exogenously administered to the mother or endogenously produced by the mother, may result in virilization of the fetal genitalia. Teratogenic factors also may have an effect on the development of the external genitalia. These factors are constantly being elucidated as new drugs are introduced into the environment. Male pseudohermaphroditism is the term applied to individuals (genotype, XY) who have testes and ambiguous external genitalia. The etiologies of male pseudohermaphroditism are multiple and complex, and reflect the complex biosynthetic and hormonal processes required to induce

normal development of the male external genitalia. Testicular unresponsiveness to either human chorionic gonadotropin (HCG) or LH is an early developmental error that will affect external genital development. Inborn errors of testosterone biosynthesis at both adrenal and testicular levels also will interfere with external genital development, since the development of external genitalia in the male is induced by the effects of both testosterone and dihydrotestosterone. A deficiency in the hormone may induce these abnormalities, or a defect in the hormone receptor may affect development, with inadequate recognition of androgenic hormones resulting in feminization of normal males. This is seen in its most dramatic form in the syndrome of testicular feminization, where the genitalia show no ambiguity, although the gonads are testes, and the individual's karyotype is XY. Karyotypic abnormalities, especially variants of the mixed or XY gonadal dysgenesis syndrome, also may be associated with ambiguous genita-

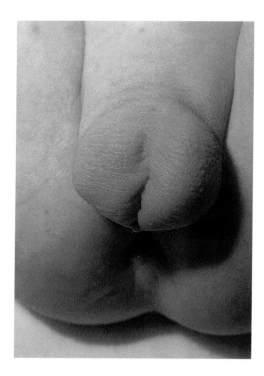

FIG. 9.24 Agenesis of the phallus. (Courtesy of Dr. D. Becker)

lia. Rare cases of ambiguous genitalia are unclassifiable and the mechanisms associated with these disorders remain to be elucidated.

It is important to remember that some children born with anatomic variants such as agenesis of the phallus (Fig. 9.24) may have neither a karyotypic nor a biochemical defect, but rather a simple developmental anomaly. These also may outlie the classification of ambiguous genitalia described above. Regardless, any child seen at birth with ambiguous genitalia should not receive a sex assignment until such time as the appropriate sex of rearing may be properly assessed and assigned. An appropriate sex assignment must be based on the following considerations: potential for mature sexual function, potential fertility, and the long-term psychological and intellectual impact on the child and family.

Development in Puberty

The pattern of timing of pubertal events for males and females is generally predictable (Fig. 9.25). However, for both males and females, the age of puberty varies in different regions of the world. In the United States, the onset of breast development and pubic hair growth occurs at approximately 10½ years of age, with menarche occurring at approximately 12½ years of age. However, considerable variations exist in these numbers for any individual patient.

THE TANNER STAGES

Because the onset and progression of puberty is so variable, Tanner has proposed a scale, now uniformly accepted, to describe the onset and progression of pubertal changes (Fig. 9.26). Males and females are rated on five-point scales. Males

are rated for both genital development and pubic hair growth, while females are rated for breast development and also for pubic hair growth. The stages for male genital development are as follows (see Fig. 9.26A): STAGE I (Preadolescent). The testes, scrotal sac, and penis have a size and proportion similar to that seen in early childhood. STAGE II. There is enlargement of the scrotum and testes, and a change in the texture of the scrotal skin. The scrotal skin also may be reddened, a finding not obvious when viewed on a black and white photograph. STAGE III. Further growth of the penis has occurred, initially in length, although with some increase in circumference. There also is increased growth of the testes and scrotum. STAGE IV. The penis is significantly enlarged in length and circumference, with further development of the glans penis. The testes and scrotum continue to enlarge and there is distinct darkening of the scrotal skin. Again, this is difficult to evaluate on a black and white photograph. STAGE V. The genitalia are adult with regard to size and shape.

The stages in male pubic hair development are as follows (see Fig. 9.26B): STAGE I (Preadolescent). Vellous hair appears over the pubes with a degree of development similar to that over the abdominal wall. There is no androgen-sensitive pubic hair. STAGE II. There is sparse development of long pigmented downy hair, which is only slightly curled or may be straight. The hair is seen chiefly at the base of the penis. This stage may be difficult to evaluate on a photograph especially if the subject has fair hair. STAGE III. The pubic hair is considerably darker, coarser, and more curly. The distribution of hair has now spread over the junction of the pubes, and at this point the hair may be recognized easily on black and white photography. STAGE VI. The hair distribution is now adult in type but still is considerably less than that seen in adults. There is no spread to the medial surface of the thighs. STAGE V. Hair distribution is adult in quantity and type, and is described as an inverse triangle. There can be spread to the medial surface of the thighs.

In young women, the Tanner stages for breast development are as follows (see Fig. 9.26C): STAGE I (Preadolescent). Only the papilla is elevated above the level of the chest wall. STAGE II (Breast Budding). Elevation of the breasts and papillae may occur as small mounds along with some increased diameter of the areolae. STAGE III. The breasts and areolae continue to enlarge, although they show no separation of contour. STAGE IV. The areolae and papillae elevate above the level of the breasts and form secondary mounds with further development of the overall breast tissue. STAGE V. Mature female breasts have developed. The papillae may extend slightly above the contour of the breast, due to recession of the areolae.

Pubic hair growth in females is staged as follows (see Fig. 9.26B): STAGE I (Preadolescent). Vellous hair develops over the pubes in a manner not greater than that over the anterior abdominal wall. There is no sexual hair. STAGE II. Sparse, long pigmented downy hair, which is straight or only slightly curled, appears. These hairs are seen mainly along the labia. This stage is difficult to quantitate on black and white photography, particularly when pictures are obtained of fair-haired subjects. STAGE III. Considerably darker, coarser, and more curled sexual hair appears. The hair has now spread sparsely over the junction of the pubes. STAGE IV. The hair distribution is adult in type but decreased in total quantity. There is no spread to the medial surface of the thighs. STAGE

PEDIATRIC ENDOCRINOLOGY

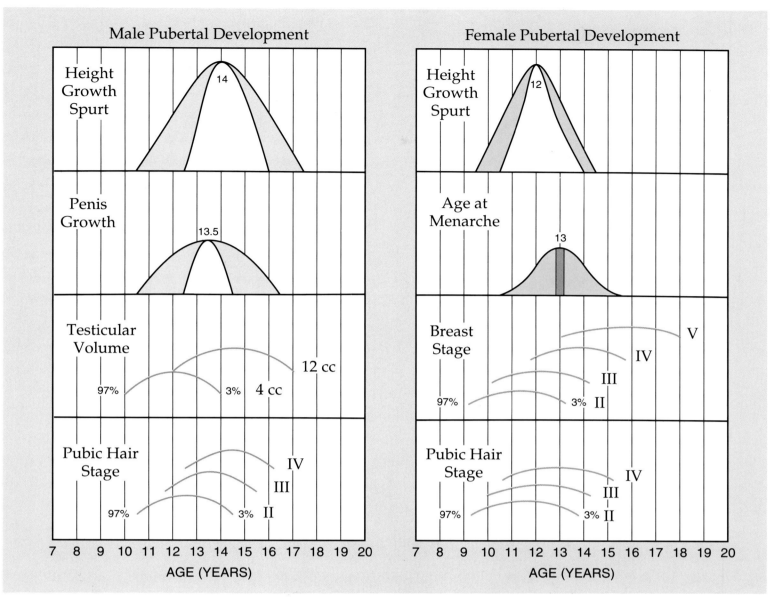

FIG. 9.25 Schematic representation of the onset of male and female puberty. (Adapted from Johnson TR, Moore WM, Jeffries JE: Children are Different: Development Physiology, ed 2. Columbus, OH, Ross Laboratories, Division of Abbott Laboratories, 1978, pp 26–29)

v. Hair is adult in quantity and type, and appears in an inverse triangle of the classically feminine type. There is spread to the medial surface of the thighs but not above the base of the inverse triangle.

PRECOCIOUS PUBERTY

The Tanner classification has become an important instrument for communication among physicians, allowing a semi-quantitative description of the pubertal progression of both boys and girls. However, variations in the timing and normal progression of puberty often are associated with specific pathologic entities. A diagnosis of precocious or early development may be made if sexual maturation begins under age 8 for girls and under 9 for boys. In girls, the causes of isosexual precocity (development along lines of the same sex) are related to alterations in gonadal or central nervous system function. True precocious puberty follows an early onset of secretion of pulsatile LH and of FSH, and the subsequent response of the ovary. Estrogen-secreting tumors of the ovary, however, will suppress development of normal LH and FSH secretion. The McCune-Albright syndrome, polyostotic fibrous dysplasia with sexual precocity, has been associated with either central or peripheral etiologies for precocious puberty.

Long-standing hypothyroidism in girls may be associated with isosexual precocity and inappropriate secretion of gonadotropins. Galactorrhea also may occur in association with elevated prolactin levels.

Isosexual precocity in young boys also may be caused by central nervous system abnormalities or by peripheral dysfunction. However, intracranial neoplasms are more com-

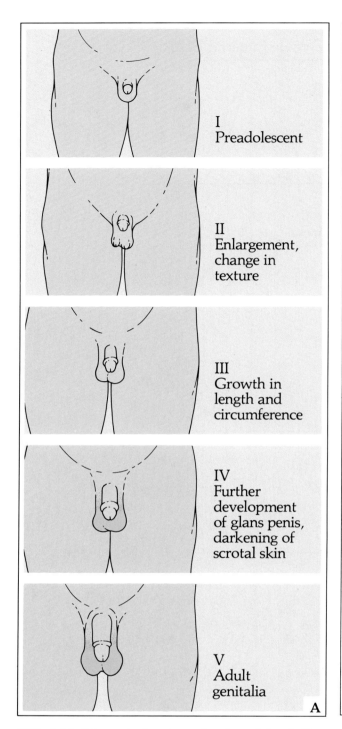

FIG. 9.26 Schematic drawings of male and female Tanner stages, show: **(A)** male genital development. **(B)** pubic hair development. **(C)** breast development. (Adapted from Johnson TR, Moore WM, Jefferies JE: Children are Different: Development

monly associated with precocious puberty in boys as compared with girls. Adrenal or testicular neoplasms in young boys are unusual but do occur. Late-onset congenital virilizing adrenal hyperplasia also may result in isosexual precocity in males.

PREMATURE THELARCHE AND ADRENARCHE

Premature Thelarche

This condition may occur before expected pubertal development (Fig. 9.25). The breast tissue may appear unilaterally or bilaterally and may regress or persist (Fig. 9.27). Premature

thelarche is a diagnosis of exclusion, and cannot be made in the presence or progression of other pubertal signs. The ingestion of exogenous estrogens, such as oral contraceptives, should always be suspect in cases of breast enlargement. Neonatal breast enlargement secondary to maternal hormones may occur in either sex. This condition regresses with time, and may be confused with premature thelarche and/or precocious puberty.

Premature Adrenarche

In contrast to premature thelarche, the appearance of pubic and/or axillary hair prior to expected pubertal development

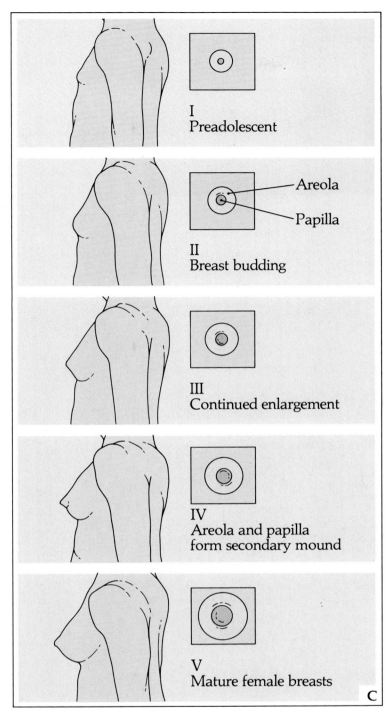

I
Preadolescent

II
Breast budding

Areola

Papilla

III
Continued enlargement

IV
Areola and papilla form secondary mound

V
Mature female breasts

C

Physiology, *ed 2. Columbus, OH, Ross Laboratories, Division of Abbott Laboratories, 1978, pp 26–29)*

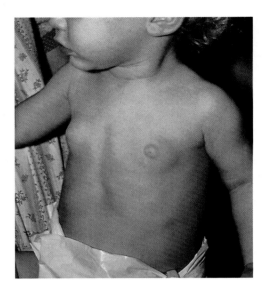

FIG. 9.27 Isolated breast enlargement in a toddler with premature thelarche.

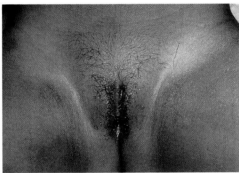

FIG. 9.28 Pubic hair development in a prepubertal girl with premature adrenarche.

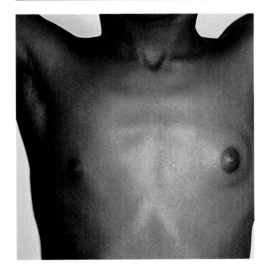

FIG. 9.29 Adolescent male with asymmetrical breast enlargement.

often is associated with a pathologic diagnosis (Fig. 9.28). Late-onset forms of adrenal hyperplasia and, more uncommonly, adrenal and/or gonadal tumors, are seen in patients with premature adrenarche. Patients with late-onset forms of adrenal hyperplasia may be differentiated with ACTH stimulation testing. The presence of adrenal or gonadal tumors is best defined by imaging procedures, as well as blood and urine steroid level determination.

ADOLESCENT MALE GYNECOMASTIA
Adolescent gynecomastia in the male is common, occurring in up to 40 percent of boys (Fig. 9.29). Breast development usually is mild and regresses with advancing puberty. However, in some cases breast development progresses to a female breast contour that corresponds to Tanner stage III or greater. This may become a profound psychologic burden and require surgical intervention. The differential diagnosis includes Klinefelter syndrome and estrogen-secreting tumors. Small testes are associated with both conditions. Additionally, patients with Klinefelter syndrome exhibit a eunuchoid body habitus. Karyotyping and measuring of estrogen and gonadotropin levels can differentiate among these conditions.

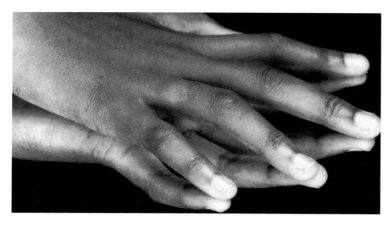

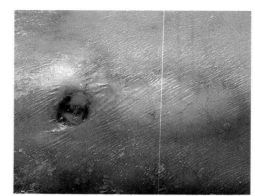

FIG. 9.31 Necrobiosis lipoidica diabeticorum is characterized by the presence of yellow waxy skin lesions that exhibit reddened components. Small areas of ulceration also may be seen. (Courtesy of Dr. B. Cohen)

FIG. 9.30 Diabetic sclerdactyly is seen in this patient's inability to flatten the palms and fingers as he presses both hands together. (Courtesy of Dr. A. Rosenbloom)

POSTPRANDIAL HYPOGLYCEMIA

Post gastric surgery
Diabetes mellitus
Galactosemia
Hereditary fructose intolerance
Reactive or functional hypoglycemia

FIG. 9.32

FASTING HYPOGLYCEMIA

Increased Substrate Utilization
    Hyperinsulinism—endogeneous
        Insulinoma
        Nesidioblastosis
        Autoimmune hypoglycemia
        Infants of diabetic mothers
        Beckwith-Wiedemann Syndrome
        Leprechaunism

Decreased Substrate Production
    Inborn errors of carbohydrate metabolism
        Defects of gluconeogenesis
        Glycogen storage diseases
    Inborn errors of protein metabolism
        Maple syrup urine disease
        Methylmalonic aciduria
    Inborn errors of fat metabolism
        Systemic carnitine deficiency
        Carnitine acetyltransferase deficiency
        Hydroxymethylglutaryl CoA lyase deficiency
        Acyl CoA dehydrogenase deficiency
    Counter regulatory hormone deficiency
        Cortisol
        Thyroid
        Glucagon
        Growth hormone
        Catecholamines
    Ketotic hypoglycemia
    Hepatic and renal disease
    Extra pancreatic neoplasms
    Reye's syndrome

FIG. 9.33

INSULIN-DEPENDENT DISEASES
Diabetes Mellitus

Diabetes mellitus represents one of the most common of the chronic diseases seen by the endocrinologist. Prior to the institution of aggressive insulin therapy, children with diabetes mellitus and short stature were seen frequently in endocrine clinics and represented instances of the Mauriac syndrome. This syndrome is characterized by poorly controlled diabetes, short stature, hepatomegaly, and sexual infantilism. This is now a very rare occurrence. In a carefully treated child with type I or insulin-dependent diabetes mellitus, growth rate should be indistinguishable from that of a normal child. However, one physical finding still frequently seen in diabetic patients is that of limited joint mobility. Figure 9.30 shows the inability of a diabetic child to flatten the palms because of waxy thickened skin in the areas of the proximal and distal interphalangeal joints. Although this phenomenon is not as yet completely understood, it has been associated with poor diabetic control. The development of specific skin lesions such as necrobiosis lipoidica diabeticorum also may be associated with diabetes. Figure 9.31 shows such a lipid-filled skin lesion, which may occasionally be seen in a child with type I diabetes.

DRUG-INDUCED HYPOGLYCEMIA

Insulin
Oral hypoglycemic agents
Ethanol
Salicylates
Propanolol
Miscellaneous other drugs
Ackee fruit

FIG. 9.34

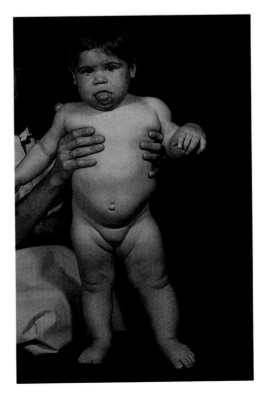

FIG. 9.35 Beckwith-Wiedimann syndrome. Note hemihypertropy on the left side, along with the prominence of the tongue. (Courtesy of Dr. D. Becker)

Hypoglycemia

The differential diagnosis of hypoglycemia is broad and involves many systems. A useful classification divides hypoglycemic states into those associated with the postprandial period (Fig. 9.32), those which occur during a fasting or catabolic stress (Fig. 9.33), and iatrogenic or drug-induced hypoglycemias (Fig. 9.34). Specific syndromes associated with hypoglycemia may be diagnosed at first glance during the patient's examination. The most striking of these is Beckwith-Wiedemann syndrome (Fig. 9.35), associated with macrosomia, macroglossia, omphaloceles, hemihypertrophy, and embryonal tumors. The hypoglycemia has been attributed to hyperinsulinism. These individuals may require aggressive treatment with diazoxide or in fact may come to partial or complete pancreatectomy because of the severity of the hypoglycemia.

Another rare cause of hypoglycemia, which may be quickly diagnosed, is leprechaunism. A small wizened infant presenting with severe recurrent hypoglycemia can readily be diagnosed as having leprechaunism. The etiology of the hypoglycemia seems to be that of hyperinsulinism and an abnormal cellular responsiveness to insulin's action. In this case, however, the hyperinsulinism seems to be a state associated with an unusual response to insulin with hypoglycemia, as opposed to simple hyperinsulinism.

SUMMARY

As seen in the above illustrations, endocrine imbalances may result in dramatic alterations in a child's phenotype. These alterations should be readily recognized, and thus direct the diagnostic approach. Careful attention to the appearance of children requiring evaluation by a physician should allow early diagnosis of endocrine disorders, resulting in prompt therapeutic intervention and in restoration of the child's appearance and overall state of well-being.

BIBLIOGRAPHY

Bacon GE, Spencer ML, Hopwood NJ, Kelch RP: *A Practical Approach to Pediatric Endocrinology*, ed 2. Chicago, Year Book, 1982.

Frasier SD: *Pediatric Endocrinology*. Orlando, Florida, Grune & Stratton, 1980.

Hung W, August GP, Glasgow AM: *Pediatric Endocrinology*. Hyde Park, New York, Medical Examination, 1983.

Kaplan SA: *Clinical Pediatric and Adolescent Endocrinology*. Philadelphia, WB Saunders, 1990.

Williams RH: *Textbook of Endocrinology*, ed 7. Philadelphia, WB Saunders, 1985.

PEDIATRIC NUTRITION AND GASTROENTEROLOGY

J. Carlton Gartner Jr., M.D.

NUTRITIONAL REQUIREMENTS		
Age	Calories (kcal/kg/day)	Protein (gm/kg/day)
0–12 months	100	2.5–3
1–7 years	75–90	1.5–2.5
7–12 years	60–75	1.5–2.5
12+ years	30–60	1.0–1.5

FIG. 10.1

ADVANTAGES OF BREAST FEEDING
Convenience
No sterilization required
Maternal-infant bonding
Less frequent hospitalizations
Possible increase in IQ
Optimal absorption of nutrients, vitamins, and trace elements
Possible protection from allergen exposure
Less obesity

FIG. 10.2

Nutrition and gastroenterology are areas closely related to the daily activities of most pediatricians. As a world health problem, the cycle of diarrhea, poor nutrition, and consequent absorptive disorders causes untold harm. This chapter will initially deal with nutritional assessment and malnutrition in children and then with some rarer nutritional deficiencies that may be diagnosed by careful examination and limited laboratory testing. This will supplement material already available in standard textbooks. The gastroenterology section will feature the conditions that may be diagnosed on clinical grounds, including cystic fibrosis, and will include several hepatic disorders based on our extensive experience as a transplant center.

NUTRITION

Normal Nutrition

Any discussion of nutrition in infancy must begin with the normal requirements (Fig. 10.1). Fortunately, human milk, the perfect infant feeding, exists worldwide. Breast milk has many advantages beyond the issues of maternal and infant bonding (Fig. 10.2). The only supplements required by nursing infants are fluoride, and vitamin D in dark-skinned infants in a "sunlight-deprived" environment. An iron source may be required in exclusively breast-fed babies in the latter part of the first year. As a general rule, content and absorption of nutrients from human milk are ideal for all infants with the possible exception of the infant with very low birth weight, who may have higher electrolyte, calcium, phosphorus, and vitamin requirements. Figure 10.3 shows the major components of formula and cow's milk compared with human milk.

Nutritional awareness is mandatory for child health workers, given the importance of growth and development during infancy and childhood. Each pediatric visit, whether for routine care or serious illness, should include at least a basic nutritional assessment. This may include dietary, clinical, anthropometric, and detailed laboratory data. In a healthy child this process involves only a brief dietary history (adequate formula in sufficient quantity) and a plot of height, weight, and head circumference on standard curves. The ill child may require more careful assessment to clarify acute and/or chronic malnutrition in order to plan effective therapy.

Clinical Observations of Malnutrition

The clinical signs of chronic malnutrition are relatively easy to recognize. However, a cycle of recurrent gastrointestinal disturbances is the most common prodrome to undernutrition.

COMPARISON OF MILKS—SELECTED COMPONENTS

	Human Milk	Formula	Whole Cow's Milk
Component			
Protein (g/dl)	1.2	1.5	3.3
Source	Human	Skim milk	Whey/casein
% calories	7	9	20
Fat (g/dl)	4	3.8	3.7
Source	Human	Soy/coconut	Butter fat
% calories	54	50	50
Carbohydrate (g/dl)	6.8	6..9	4.9
Source	Lactose	Lactose	Lactose
% calories	40	41	30
Osmolality (mEq/liter)	300	290	288
Renal solute load (mEq/liter)	87	90	226
Na^+ (mEq/liter)	7	9	24
K^+ (mEq/liter)	13	18	35
Ca^{++} (mg/liter)	340	440	1,150
P (mg/liter)	140	300	920
Ca/P ratio	2.2	1.5	1.3
Iron (mg/liter)	0.5	0 or 12	1
Vitamin D (IU)	22	420	444
Fluoride (mg/liter)	0.01	0*	0.02

Unless water added to concentrate.

FIG. 10.3

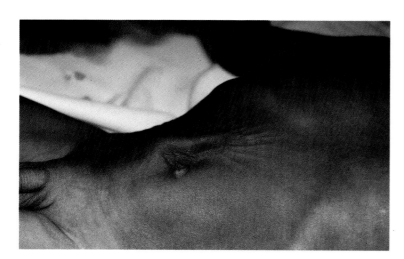

FIG. 10.4 Dehydration. Poor skin turgor is indicative of decreased extracellular volume. In this patient with severe dehydration, skin remains tented after release and retracts quite slowly.

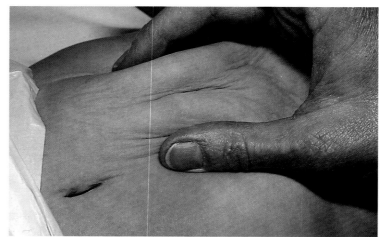

FIG. 10.5 Hypernatremic dehydration. The skin often has a "doughy" texture when the dehydration is associated with elevation of serum sodium.

Dehydration must be recognized early (dry mucous membranes, oliguria) before more serious complications ensue (depressed fontanelle, sunken eyes, diminished skin turgor) (Figs. 10.4, 10.5). Rapid treatment and follow-up of nutritional depletion may interrupt the vicious cycle of malnutrition.

Perhaps the major advance in world health in recent years is the use of oral rehydration solutions (ORS) to effectively treat gastroenteritis. Numerous studies have shown the advantages of this inexpensive, readily available mixture, which does require potable water and appropriate dilution.

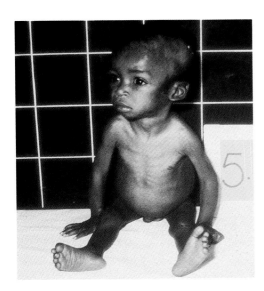

FIG. 10.6
Marasmus. Note profound wasting and sparse hair, producing a characteristic simian appearance.

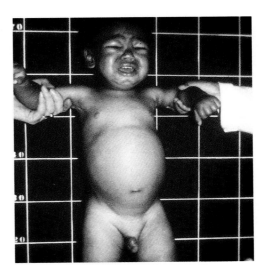

FIG. 10.7
Kwashiorkor. This patient has a typical "sugar baby" appearance with generalized edema. Note the periorbital and limb edema.

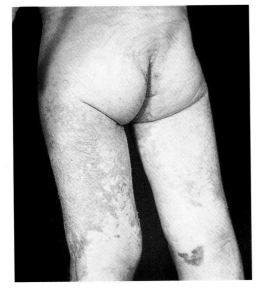

FIG. 10.8 The rash of kwashiorkor is scaly, erythematous, and may weep, especially in edematous areas.

Clinical descriptions of malnutrition differentiate between marasmus (caloric deficiency with wasting of tissue) and kwashiorkor (protein deficiency with edema). More recently it has become evident that these conditions often overlap and have a similar pathogenesis. For both conditions, physical signs and descriptions are helpful in patient evaluation and treatment. Malnourished children are often apathetic and have decreased physical activity. Marasmus is characterized by a marked weight-for-height reduction with emaciation, loss of subcutaneous fat, lusterless and sparse hair, and poor nail growth, producing a rather simian appearance (Fig. 10.6).

A classic kwashiorkor patient looks well-nourished ("sugar babies") without wasting. The initial "moon face" of kwashiorkor is often mistaken for good nutrition. In fact the child is often edematous, which becomes striking after nutritional repletion (Fig. 10.7). These children usually suffer acute protein deficiency in addition to preexisting caloric deprivation. Skin changes in kwashiorkor include hyper- and hypopigmentation with a scaly, weeping dermatitis that may ulcerate and desquamate (Fig. 10.8). The rash is often more prominent in skin areas that are chronically irritated (groin in infants and areas of peripheral edema). It resembles pellagra but is seen in areas other than those exposed to sunlight.

FAILURE TO THRIVE

In many areas of the world, the gap between the well- nourished and the severely malnourished infant or child is filled by the problem commonly known as failure to thrive. Definitions of this condition are often vague, but failure to grow at an appropriate *rate* is a reasonable description. Generally weight is affected first, with height and head circumference decrements occurring later. Although organic disorders are possible, in industrialized countries most of these children are categorized as having ``nonorganic'' problems related to the environment or to parenting. A careful history and physical examination with very selected laboratory tests usually can exclude true disease states. The most important factor is a careful dietary history that includes volumes, formula dilution, amount of emesis, etc. Growth curves are most helpful and often can prevent overinvestigation of children with normal variations in growth (Fig. 10.9A,B).

Anthropometric Measurements and Laboratory Tests

After the initial clinical exam of the malnourished patient is completed, anthropometric measurements should be made. These enable large groups of children to be followed sequentially, and aid in distinguishing between acute and chronic malnutrition and assessing the effects of protein or total calories. Using standard curves such as 1976 National Center for Health Statistics charts, height-for-age deficit (actual height divided by expected height-for-age [50th percentile] x 100) and weight-for-height deficit (actual weight divided by expected weight-for-height [50th percentile] x 100) may be calculated.

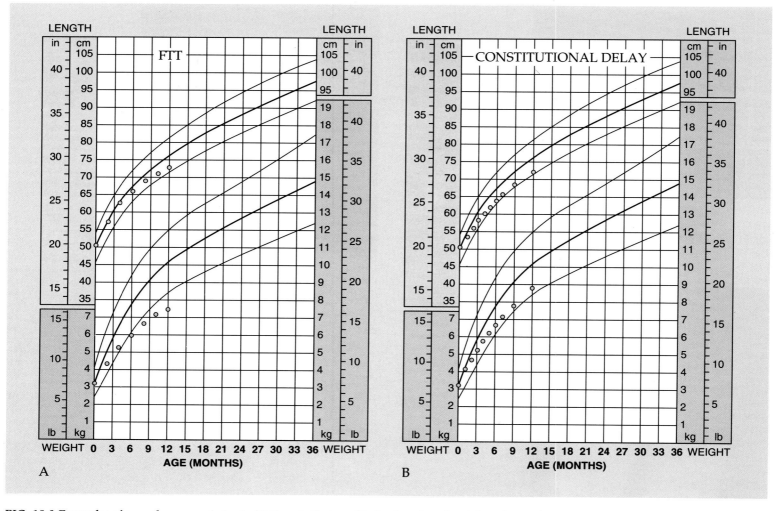

FIG. 10.9 Examples of growth curves. A, typical failure to thrive with deceleration of weight gain. B, slow growth but at a normal rate consistent with constitutional delay.

Diminished height for age most commonly reflects chronic undernutrition, while low weight for height may indicate more acute malnutrition. Grading of nutritional status is done using these two parameters (Fig. 10.10). In addition, measurements of triceps skinfold thickness and midarm muscle circumference aid in further delineating protein and calorie deficits (Fig. 10.11). The measurements must be done carefully (Figs. 10.12, 10.13). After these are completed, comparison is made with standards (see Bibliography, Walker and Hendricks, pp 17–23) and the predominant deficiencies can be defined.

Laboratory testing can be helpful in some malnourished children. Not only is the degree of chronicity of the insult confirmed, but certain specific deficiencies may be uncovered. Unfortunately, an inexpensive laboratory test for early malnutrition is not yet available. Amino acid nomograms may aid early diagnosis but are expensive and require a sophisticated laboratory. Decreases in body proteins are helpful but reflect the time for normal body catabolism. Consequently, retinol binding protein ($t_{1/2}$ 12 hours) and transferrin ($t_{1/2}$ 9 days) indicate more current nutritional status than the standard albumin ($t_{1/2}$ 20–24 days). An additional aid in assessing lean body mass is a comparison of 24-hour creatinine excretion to standard norms for height (creatinine height index).

As infection is a major cause of morbidity and mortality in the malnourished patient, a basic immunologic assessment is indicated. Total lymphocyte counts and skin tests are a minimal baseline, as the major effects are in the T-lymphocyte system.

Therapy

After clinical, anthropometric, and laboratory assessments are completed, decisions about aggressive nutritional repletion or mere maintenance therapy can be made. Obviously patients with hypoproteinemia and major changes in weight for height will need more vigorous therapy. Parenteral nutrition should be considered for patients with profound injury to the gastrointestinal tract (Fig. 10.14). This major advance in nutrition-

GRADING OF NUTRITIONAL STATUS

Grade	Height for Age	Weight for Height
I	<95%	<90%
II	<90%	<80%
III	<85%	<70%

FIG. 10.10

ANTHROPOMETRIC ASSESSMENT OF NUTRITIONAL STATUS

Measurement	Deficiency	Indicated Deficiency
Weight for age	<90% of standard	Protein-Calorie
Height for age	<95%	Protein-Calorie
Weight for height	<90%	Protein-Calorie
Triceps skinfold	<5%	Calorie
Midarm muscle	<5%	Protein

FIG. 10.11

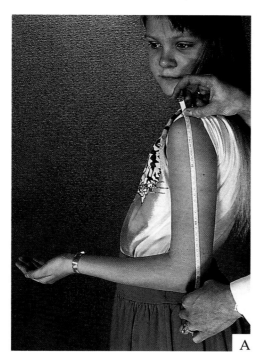
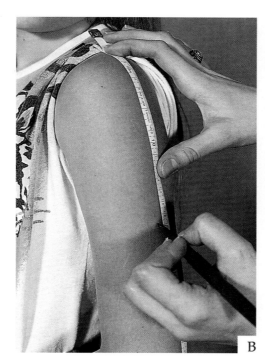
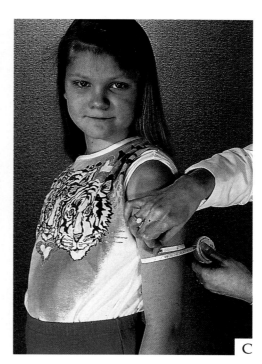

FIG. 10.12 *Midarm circumference.* **A,** *locate the midpoint of the arm with arm bent at 90° angle, tape at acromion and olecranon processes.* **B,** *mark at midpoint.* **C,** *make measurement at midpoint with arm hanging loosely.*

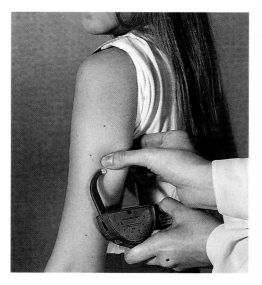

FIG. 10.13 *Triceps fatfold. Grasp a vertical pinch of skin and subcutaneous fat. The caliper jaw is placed over the skinfold at the midpoint mark while maintaining grasp of skinfold. Make reading to nearest 1 mm without excessive pressure. Average three readings for the final result.*

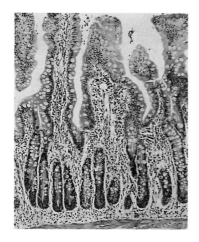
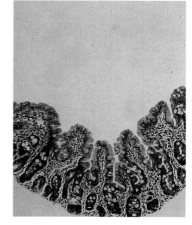

FIG. 10.14 *Normal jejunal mucosa with tall villi and deep crypts* (left) *complicating chronic diarrhea and malnutrition* (right).

NUTRITIONAL DEFICIENCIES WITH CHARACTERISTIC PHYSICAL SIGNS

Vitamin/Mineral	Signs/Symptom
Calcium, phosphorus, vitamin D	Rickets/osteomalacia
Vitamin A	Night blindness, xerophthalmia, Bitot's spots, follicular hyperkeratosis
Vitamin C	Scurvy: bone lesions, bleeding
Vitamin E	Hemolytic anemia, peripheral neuropathy
Vitamin K	Petechiae, ecchymoses
Thiamine B$_1$	Beriberi: heart failure, increased intracranial pressure
Niacin	Pellagra: dermatitis (sun-exposed areas)
Riboflavin B$_2$	Angular stomatitis, cheilosis
B$_6$	Anemia, dermatitis, neuropathy
B$_{12}$	Anemia, neuropathy
Folate	Anemia
Iron	Anemia, koilonychia
Biotin	Rash, hair loss
Essential fatty acids	Rash, coagulopathy
Zinc	Rash (acrodermatitis), growth failure, delayed sexual development, ageusia
Copper	Bone changes, hypopigmentation, anemia, neutropenia
Selenium	Heart failure

FIG. 10.15

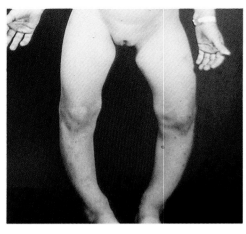

FIG. 10.16 Hypophosphatemic ricket marked by the obvious bowing.

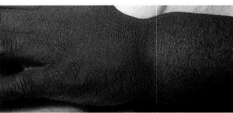

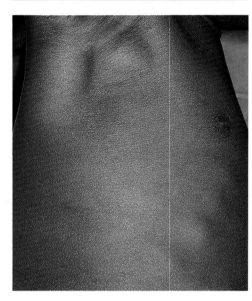

FIG. 10.17 Infantile rickets marked by widened wrists (top) and enlargement of the costochondral junction ("beading") (bottom). The latter occurred as the result of a rapid growth spurt following liver transplantation.

al therapy continues to be perfected by better mixtures, less cumbersome and better tolerated catheters, and home TPN using advanced programmable pumps. Recovery from intestinal injury is enhanced by intraluminal nutrition (which should be initiated as soon as possible). The industrialized countries fortunately have many modified and elemental formulas for children with acute or chronic digestive disturbances. As malnutrition has profound effects on intestinal absorption, several of these formulas may be invaluable. It is important to know the specific content of each product used. High osmolar formulas are often not tolerated, especially by the compromised small-bowel mucosa.

Prior to initiating nutritional therapy (or after a period of hyperalimentation) it is helpful to look for specific vitamin, mineral, and trace element deficiencies. The more common and previously well-described deficiencies are listed in Figure 10.15. It is often difficult to assign individual findings, such as angular stomatitis, to specific deficiencies in a child with chronic, severe malnutrition. Several deficiencies, often seen in a hospital population, will be discussed below.

Rickets (or osteomalacia in nongrowing bone) from vitamin D deficiency remains a world health problem. However, the increased survival of tiny premature infants has led to biochemical rickets from calcium or phosphorus deficiency.

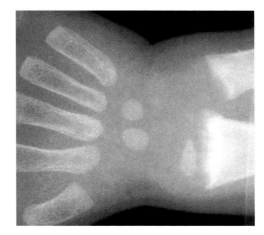
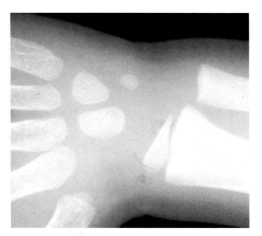

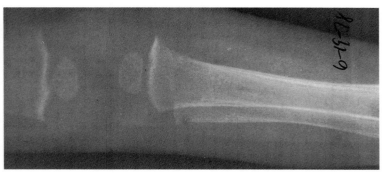

FIG. 10.18 Radiograph of the wrist in a patient with rickets (left) shows irregularity and widening of the epiphyses in the distal radius and ulna. With appropriate therapy (right), remineralization and healing occurs.

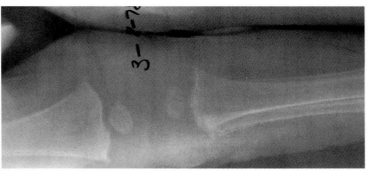
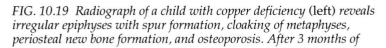

FIG. 10.19 Radiograph of a child with copper deficiency (left) reveals irregular epiphyses with spur formation, cloaking of metaphyses, periosteal new bone formation, and osteoporosis. After 3 months of intravenous copper (right), the child demonstrates healing of the metaphyses.

Increased supplements of both of these minerals leads to reversal of the changes. The resurgence of breast feeding, especially in dark-skinned or vegetarian populations, has produced clinical rickets. It should be noted that disorders of two other organ systems—liver and kidney—may produce clinical or biochemical osteomalacia. Poor bile flow and consequent malabsorption is the primary etiology in hepatobiliary disorders. Additionally, end-stage renal disease with failure of renal hydroxylation of vitamin D_3 or renal tubular wasting of phosphorus may cause poor bone matrix formation.

In all of the above conditions that cause osteomalacia, the physical changes are similar: poor growth, curvature of weight-bearing bones (Fig. 10.16), widening of epiphyses, and costochondral beading (Fig. 10.17). Softening of the skull (craniotabes) is seen in infants. With appropriate vitamin and mineral supplementation, radiographic healing occurs followed by bony remodeling (Fig. 10.18).

Deficiencies of other fat-soluble vitamins (E, K, A) may occur as well. Clinical vitamin E deficiency can progress from absence of peripheral deep-tendon reflexes to marked ataxia. Vitamin K deficiency, seen in patients with long-standing steatorrhea or liver disease, causes prolongation of the prothrombin time and can be associated clinically with easy bleeding and bruising. Vitamin A deficiency causes follicular hyperkeratosis, xerophthalmia, night blindness, and unusual shiny gray, triangular lesions on the conjunctivae (Bitot's spots).

Parenteral nutrition has been lifesaving, especially for neonates with major intestinal disorders complicated by malnutrition. Unfortunately, as trial-and-error methods were used in early hyperalimentation, numerous deficiencies were uncovered during prolonged periods of alimentation. Examples of this include fatty acid deficiency with the typical scaly dermatitis, and zinc deficiency with alopecia, diarrhea, and acrodermatitis; these conditions are now rare. Prior to reformulation of our own hyperalimentation mixture several years ago, other unusual problems were uncovered. A child on hyperalimentation for 6 months developed irritability, bone pain, and decreased hair pigmentation. Anemia and progressive neutropenia ensued, and a skeletal survey as well as copper and ceruloplasmin determinations confirmed copper deficiency. Bone changes included osteoporosis, metaphyseal spurs, and periosteal new bone formation. Hematologic and then bone changes reversed with copper administration (Fig. 10.19). Another patient with short-gut syndrome on home hyperali-

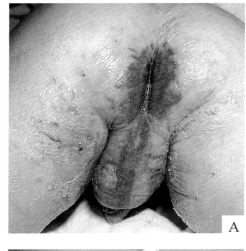

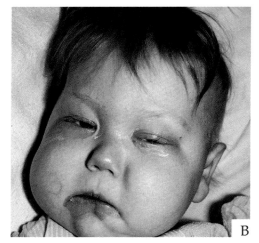

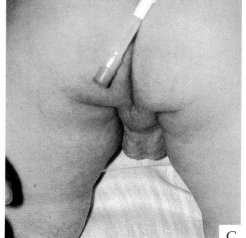

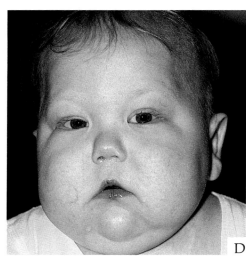

FIG. 10.20 Biotin deficiency. *A* and *B*, this child on chronic hyperalimentation developed dermatitis in perianal, perioral, and lid areas along with some thinning of hair. *C* and *D*, the rash has cleared dramatically after 4 days of biotin.

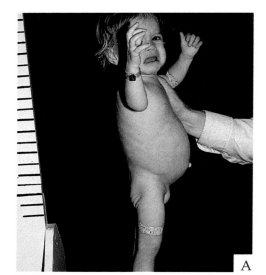

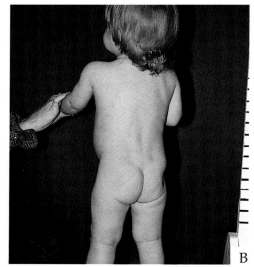

FIG. 10.21 Celiac disease. *A*, this child had a potbelly, vomiting, and weight loss as her major symptoms and was originally thought to have psychosocial failure to thrive. When celiac disease was suspected, the child was placed on a gluten-free diet. Note the protruding abdomen and wasted buttocks. *B*, after 10 weeks on the diet the improvement is obvious.

mentation developed a peculiar weeping dermatitis in the perioral, perianal, and lid areas along with lethargy and malaise. Changes reversed in only 4 days when intravenous biotin was added (Fig. 10.20).

Conclusion

Careful nutritional assessment followed by detailed clinical examination can uncover specific nutritional deficiencies as well as delineate the severity and chronicity of malnutrition.

These facts will then allow a more specific plan of nutritional repletion to be formulated using a combination of parenteral and enteral routes.

GASTROENTEROLOGY

Disturbances of gastrointestinal function are common in pediatric practice, perhaps second only to respiratory symptoms as a reason for office visits. However, clues to specific disorders are uncommon. This section will emphasize the major symp-

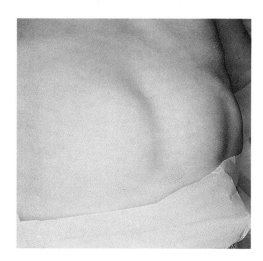

FIG. 10.22 Pyloric stenosis. The giant gastric waves are best seen just after a feeding.

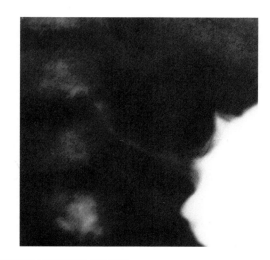

FIG. 10.23 This typical barium study in a patient with pyloric stenosis demonstrates a "stringlike" pyloric channel.

FIG. 10.24

PRESENTATIONS OF GASTROESOPHAGEAL REFLUX

Regurgitation
  "Spitting," rumination
  Emesis
  Failure to thrive

Esophagitis
  Irritability
  Colic
  Hiccups
  Anemia
  Hematemesis
  Stricture
  Protein-losing
    enteropathy
  Melena, occult blood loss

Behavioral
  Dystonic posturing
  Sandifer syndrome

Respiratory
  Wheezing, asthma
  Recurrent pneumonia
  Aspiration
  Laryngospasm
  Apnea

Neurologic
  Seizure-like episodes

Other
  Clubbing of digits
  Sudden infant death
    syndrome or apparent
    life-threatening event

toms which bring patients with GI disease to medical attention and define entities that may be diagnosed by examination. Later in this section we will also discuss cystic fibrosis and liver disorders.

Malabsorption

Malabsorption syndromes in pediatrics range from single sugars (lactase deficiency) to more complex multinutrient problems such as those associated with the short-bowel syndrome. The physical signs usually are those of malnutrition. Most clinicians, however, suspect celiac disease when they see a child with "potbelly" and wasted extremities and buttocks. A gluten-free diet is prescribed, and the results are quite rapid and dramatic (Fig. 10.21). As this is a lifelong condition, careful confirmation by repeated small intestinal biopsies is indicated.

Vomiting

Recurrent vomiting is a frequent symptom in childhood, most commonly associated with diarrhea (gastroenteritis).

PYLORIC STENOSIS

Early onset, a forceful projectile quality, continued hunger, and associated constipation are characteristic of hypertrophic pyloric stenosis. Giant gastric peristaltic waves and the typical firm pyloric olive are noted on examination (Fig. 10.22). In questionable cases, radiographs may be confirmatory by demonstrating a stringlike pyloric channel (Fig. 10.23). Abdominal ultrasonography can also demonstrate the pyloric tumor.

REFLUX

Gastroesophageal reflux is a common and usually self-limited condition beginning in early infancy. Many of these children have emesis even in the newborn nursery. Very characteristic are frequent episodes of emesis beginning immediately after feeding and continuing for several hours. Presentations of this disorder are multiple and include neurologic and/or behavioral abnormalities (Sandifer syndrome) characterized mainly by peculiar extension movements of the head and neck (Fig. 10.24). The problem usually lessens and gradually disappears by 1 year of age. Complicated reflux—failure to grow, aspiration, esophagitis, hemorrhage, apnea—is less frequent. Clinical

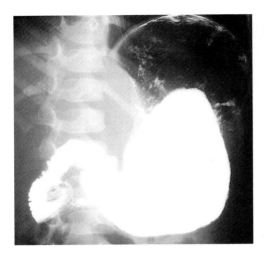

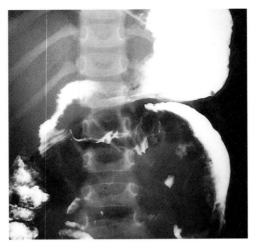

FIG. 10.25 Upper GI series demonstrates poor flow through the duodenum (left) and mass effect of the hematoma displacing other loops of bowel (right).

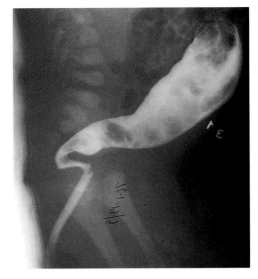

FIG. 10.26 The tapered transition zone to a normal-caliber colon is characteristic of Hirschsprung's disease.

diagnosis is sufficient in mild cases, but more persistent or difficult problems may require further diagnostic testing. Barium swallow is helpful but diagnostic of abnormality in only 50 percent of the cases. Twenty-four hour (or shorter) esophageal pH-probe measurements, esophagoscopy and/or biopsy, aspiration nuclear scans, and esophageal manometric studies may all be necessary before arriving at a final assessment. Additionally, psychophysiologic factors may predominate in the rumination syndrome. In late stages these children regurgitate constantly and swallow in a self-stimulating fashion.

Therapy in mild cases includes frequent small feedings and maintenance of an upright position. This is usually accomplished by elevating the head of the crib and keeping the infant in a prone position. By increasing intra-abdominal pressure, the "infant seat" actually worsens reflux. The value of thickened feedings (rice cereal added to formula) is still debated, although infants seem to cry less on this regimen. Variable results have been obtained with drug therapy using bethanechol or metoclopramide. Persistent, complicated reflux requires surgery—usually a Nissen-type fundoplication.

TRAUMA

No discussion of pediatric differential diagnosis is complete without a mention of trauma or child abuse. The GI tract may figure in subtle forms of abuse: chronic diarrhea from laxative abuse and feigned bleeding episodes are reported (Münchausen syndrome by proxy). Likewise, vomiting may be induced by occult trauma or abuse. Blunt injury to the abdomen, such as that from a bicycle handlebar, may produce an intramural duodenal hematoma with partial or complete obstruction and a fullness or mass on radiographic abdominal examination (Fig. 10.25). Resolution usually takes place slowly, and parenteral nutrition may be required for a period of time. As with other suspicious injuries, skeletal survey and detailed family evaluation are mandatory if the trauma is not explained by an obvious accident.

Constipation

Chronic constipation is usually seen on a functional basis and is often related historically to problems at the time of toilet training. Overflow incontinence (encopresis) may result and is usually manageable by a period of catharsis and bowel "retraining'" in preschool or younger school-age children. Occasionally, major psychopathology is uncovered, especially in the older child, and appropriate intervention is necessary. Bladder dysfunction with recurrent urinary tract infections may be associated with major long-standing constipation.

Examination of the child with constipation usually reveals palpable stool in the descending colon and rectum. If the history dates to early infancy and obstipation is present as well, one should consider Hirschsprung's disease. Barium enema radiographic studies are usually diagnostic (Fig. 10.26), though rectal biopsy for ganglion cells and special stains are necessary for confirmation. In older children, rectal manometric studies may be helpful in separating organic from functional disorders.

Abdominal Pain

Recurrent abdominal pain (RAP), often vague and nonspecific, is found in as many as 25 percent of school-age children. Typically, the pain is episodic, unrelated to meals, and centrally located in the abdomen; in addition, the child may appear pale. The definition includes the "rule of 3," i.e., patient older than 3 years, with more than three episodes over at least 3 months. Despite careful evaluation, a precise etiology is seldom determined. In one long-term followup study at the Mayo Clinic, the only condition which appeared to be missed, though rarely, was regional enteritis. Unfortunately, 20 percent of children with recurrent abdominal pain are subjected to laparotomy. Less than 5 percent of these children will have an organic disorder. The history and examination clues that warrant further investigation are listed in Figure 10.27.

CLUES TO ORGANIC DISEASE IN RECURRENT ABDOMINAL PAIN

Weight loss
Nocturnal pain
Recurrent emesis
Regular school attendance
Easygoing personality
Stable home environment
Heme-positive stools
Abnormal physical exam findings—clubbing, perianal skin tags, abdominal mass
Abnormal screening lab test results—decreased albumin, increased ESR, anemia, increased lipase/amylase

FIG. 10.27

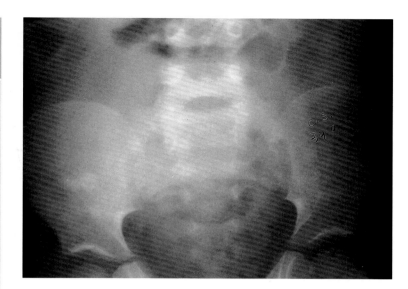

FIG. 10.28 An appendiceal fecalith can be seen in the right lower quadrant in this child with surgically proven acute appendicitis.

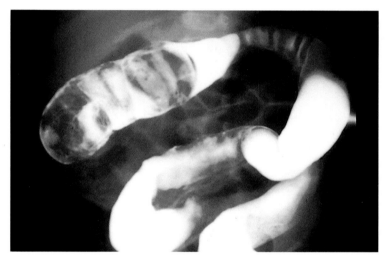

FIG. 10.29 Intussusception. Barium outlines the intussuscepted segment. Unfortunately, this lesion required laparotomy, as reduction did not occur during the barium enema.

GI HEMORRHAGE—CHILDREN OLDER THAN 1 YEAR

Upper	Lower
Esophageal varices	Colonic polyps
Gastric ulcers	Anal fissure
Gastritis	Intussusception
Duodenal ulcer	Meckel's diverticulum
	Ulcerative colitis
	Regional enteritis
	Hemorrhoids

FIG. 10.30

Acute appendicitis may not have the classic sequence in pediatric patients, and suspicion must be high in any acute illness. All too often perforation has occurred prior to the diagnosis, and an appendiceal fecalith may be a good though infrequent clue (Fig. 10.28).

Less than one-third of patients with intussusception will have the classic triad: colicky pain, currant jelly stools, and an abdominal mass (Fig. 10.29). Neurologic symptoms such as lethargy or seizure are occasional clues to the diagnosis. Reduction by barium enema simplifies management of this disorder in most instances.

bright blood per return indicates loss from the lower gastrointestinal tract. Portal hypertension, often of extrahepatic origin, is suggested by splenomegaly which may only become evident when volume status has been normalized after a recent hemorrhage. Other clues of chronic liver disease or colitis may be helpful. Perioral melanotic spots (Peutz-Jeghers syndrome,) and other manifestations of intestinal polyposis syndromes (such as Gardner syndrome) can be detected by examination. The common disorders causing gastrointestinal hemorrhage are listed in Figure 10.30 (see also Chapter 17, Pediatric Surgery).

Hemorrhage

The etiology of GI hemorrhage usually requires detailed endoscopic and x-ray examination. In younger infants, particularly neonates, the diagnosis may remain unclear in over 50 percent with a benign outlook. Generally, melanotic stools or frank hematemesis indicate upper gastrointestinal bleeding, whereas

Diarrhea

Major clues to the etiology of diarrhea can be found when the stool is carefully examined. Small bowel diarrhea is usually watery and free of mucus. Unabsorbed sugar is easily detected by the Clinitest® tablet, although heating and acidification are necessary if sucrose is present.

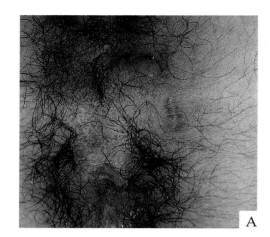

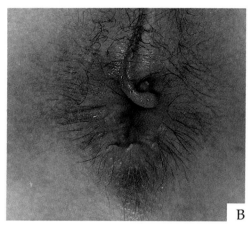

FIG. 10.31 *A, in this patient with Crohn's disease, the slightly raised, erythematous lesion eventually drained and represented a fistulous opening. B, note a scar from previous incision and drainage. Perianal skintags are common in Crohn's disease and a good clue to diagnosis.*

A

B

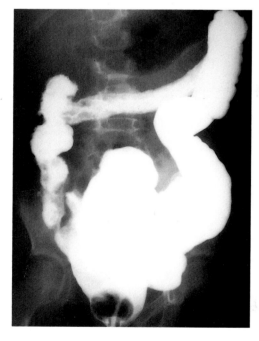

FIG. 10.32 *Crohn's disease. This growth curve demonstrates a falloff prior to onset of disease symptoms and continued poor growth through many exacerbations requiring steroid therapy. Home hyperalimentation has maintained weight gain.*

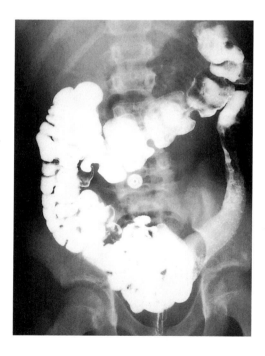

FIG. 10.33 *X-ray findings in Crohn's disease. Segmental narrowing of the left colon.*

FIG. 10.34 *X-ray findings in ulcerative colitis. There is narrowing and loss of haustral markings, especially in the transverse colon. Mucosal irregularities are prominent in the right colon.*

Stool pH also may be low (<5) in the presence of undigested carbohydrate. Excessive neutral fat (triglyceride) or split fat (fatty acid) supports the presence of malabsorption and can be easily detected. Neutral fat can be seen if several drops of water are added to the specimen. If 2 drops of 95% alcohol and 2 drops of stain (oil red-Sudan III) are added, smaller and more definite globules may be seen. Heating with acetic acid may be necessary to see split fat clearly under the microscope.

Infectious diarrhea often produces stools with blood or mucus. Stool leukocytes, another possible clue, can be seen more easily when 2 drops of water and 1 drop of methylene blue are added to a fresh stool smear before microscopic examination (see Sondheimer reference). Whereas chronic diarrhea

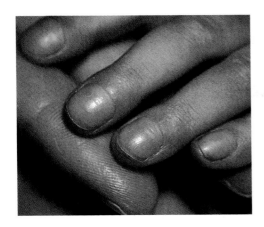

FIG. 10.35 *Osteoarthropathy (clubbing). Note thickening and loss of the angle at the nail bed.*

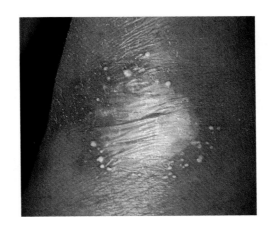

FIG. 10.36 *Pyoderma gangrenosum associated with inflammatory bowel disease. Initial papulopustules coalesce to form a deep necrotic lesion.*

may be caused by malabsorption, chronic nonspecific or toddler's diarrhea is common and self-limited unless severe dietary restrictions are initiated. Stools are loose and often contain undigested fibers, but no carbohydrate or fat. Occasionally, these children do better when placed on a diet containing unrestricted fat. The health beliefs of some parents, such as the benefits of low fat, low cholesterol foods, may contribute to the problem. Again, stool exam is helpful, especially a search for *Giardia lamblia* in children who are not thriving.

INFLAMMATORY BOWEL DISEASE

Crampy abdominal pain with mucus and blood suggests large-bowel involvement, and numerous clues may suggest chronic inflammatory bowel diseases such as Crohn's disease or ulcerative colitis. While clinical distinctions are at times blurred in these latter disorders, severe perianal disease with fistulas and fissures along with perianal skintags is more common in Crohn's disease (Fig. 10.31). Additionally, poor growth prior to major GI symptoms is often a clue to Crohn's disease (Fig. 10.32). Rectal disease is characteristic of ulcerative colitis, whereas perianal disease is less common. Histologically, Crohn's disease is characterized by transmural inflammation with granuloma formation and skip areas. This deep inflammatory process accounts for the tendency to form fistulas and abscesses. Crypt abscesses are often seen in ulcerative colitis and help distinguish this disorder from many other causes of acute colitis. Radiographically, Crohn's disease may involve the entire bowel, with segmental narrowing, skip areas, and fistula formation (Fig. 10.33). Ulcerative colitis is a mucosal inflammation confined only to the large bowel (Fig. 10.34).

Osteoarthropathy, or clubbing in its mildest form, is seen not only in many conditions in which there is overt cardiopulmonary disease such as cyanotic heart disease or lung disease but also in gastrointestinal diseases (especially Crohn's) and liver disorders. Pathogenetic mechanisms are not clear, but shunting from right to left via pulmonary or abdominal vessels is a possibility. Earliest signs of osteoarthropathy are softening and loss of a normal angle at the base of the nail (Fig. 10.35).

Many rashes accompany inflammatory bowel disease, including erythema nodosum, erythema multiforme, papulonecrotic lesions, and ulcerative erythematous plaques. Perhaps the most characteristic rash is pyoderma gangrenosum. Initial lesions are papular, then become bullous, and finally deeply ulcerated and necrotic. The most frequent locations are the cheeks, thighs, feet, hands, legs, and inguinal regions (Fig. 10.36).

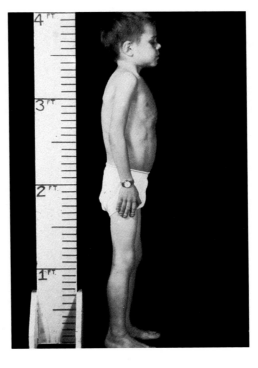

FIG. 10.37 *Cystic fibrosis. This child presented with chronic cough. Note an increased AP chest diameter and overall poor nutrition as well as clubbing.*

Cystic Fibrosis

Cystic fibrosis is the most common inherited lethal disorder in whites, with predominantly pulmonary and GI manifestations. Clues to the diagnosis of cystic fibrosis are myriad and involve multiple systems. Few clinicians would fail to think of the diagnosis with meconium ileus, chronic cough, failure to thrive, and malabsorptive stools, so a few less common presentations were selected for discussion here.

Edema in an infant who is breast-fed or on soy formula and consuming adequate calories should strongly suggest cystic fibrosis. As noted in the section on kwashiorkor, these infants often appear well-fed but quite thin after fluid is diuresed. The older child with asthma or recurrent bronchitis should be examined closely for signs of chronic lung disease. Subtle increases in AP chest diameter, clubbing, and rather poor general nutrition make a sweat test mandatory (Fig. 10.37) (see Pediatric Pulmonary Disorders chapter).

FIG. 10.38

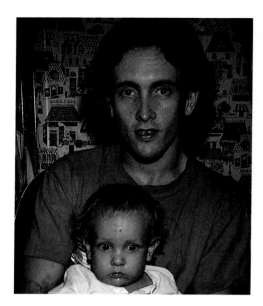

FIG. 10.39 Alagille syndrome. The child has intrahepatic biliary hypoplasia, butterfly vertebrae, and mild pulmonic stenosis. The father does not have liver disease, but he does have moderate pulmonic stenosis and poor growth. Note the narrow, thin face and pointed chin of both father and child.

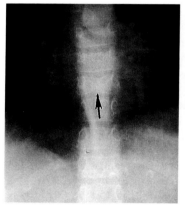
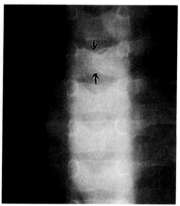

FIG. 10.40 These x-rays illustrate defects in the vertebral arches which lead to the "butterfly" appearance.

CHRONIC LIVER DISEASE

Infancy

Obstructive jaundice is the major clue to most hepatobiliary disorders in early infancy. Exceptions to this rule are metabolic or storage diseases (glycogen storage, Gaucher's disease, etc.) in which organomegaly is the prominent finding. Neonatal obstructive jaundice has a large group of diagnostic possibilities—extra-hepatic biliary atresia and neonatal "giant cell" hepatitis being the most common (Fig. 10.38). Although not specific, acholic stools are a sensitive marker of complete obstruction. Clues to individual disorders occasionally are present. Intrahepatic biliary atresia (biliary hypoplasia, paucity of bile ducts) is seen either in syndromic (Alagille syndrome) or nonsyndromic form. Peculiar facies (deeply set eyes, narrow chin), persistent posterior embryotoxon, pulmonary artery abnormalities, and butterfly vertebrae are characteristic of Alagille syndrome or arteriohepatic dysplasia (Figs. 10.39 and 40). This condition has been localized to chromosome 20. Many individuals have only a few features of the disorder; prognosis is variable. These patients often suffer from xanthoma formation and severe pruritus which may occasionally be features of other chronic liver diseases (Fig. 10.41). The choledochal cyst is a surgically correctable cause of jaundice and may be palpable (Fig. 10.42).

Extrahepatic biliary atresia (EBA), with an incidence of 0.65/10,000 live births, is the most common cause of end-stage pediatric liver disease. Approximately 350 children are born with this condition in the United States every year. EBA may be associated with abnormalities of other organ systems, situs inversus viscerum, and polysplenia with or without congenital heart disease. Additionally, GI tract anomalies such as malrotation (Fig. 10.43) and vascular anomalies (Fig. 10.44) may rarely complicate initial surgery and later liver transplantation.

Childhood

Children with chronic liver disease and cirrhosis have many clinical features in common. The liver is usually firm, often irregular and enlarged, though in late stages it may decrease in size. Splenomegaly follows portal hypertension. Portosystemic venous anastomoses lead to the development of dilated vessels in the abdominal wall (caput medusae) and gastrointestinal tract (varices, hemorrhoids) (Fig. 10.45). Ascitic fluid may form and, when in sufficient quantity, flank dullness and fluid wave may be elicited. Ultrasonography may detect even smaller amounts of free fluid. Spider nevi, dilated vascular channels which disappear with pressure, are seen in normal adolescents but should suggest chronic liver disease if other historical or examination clues are present (Fig. 10.46).

Wilson's disease is one of the chronic liver disorders that can be reversed with therapy. Presentations include hepatitis,

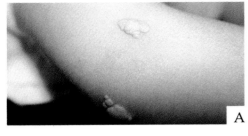

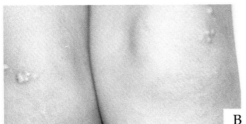

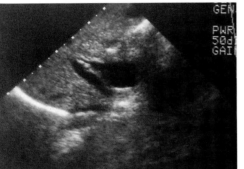

A

B

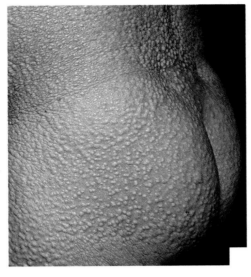

FIG. 10.41 *Xanthomas in chronic liver disease. Characteristic areas in the early stages of disease are "pressure points" such as elbows* **(A)** *and knee* **(B)***; later, xanthomas may become generalized* **(C)***.*

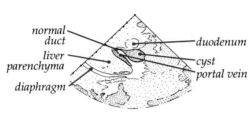

normal duct
liver parenchyma
diaphragm
duodenum
cyst
portal vein

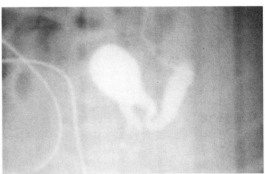

FIG. 10.42 *Ultrasound of infant with obstructive jaundice demonstrates cystic structure below the liver (left). Intraoperative cholan-* *giogram in same patient defines cyst and gallbladder along with hepatic and cystic ducts (right).*

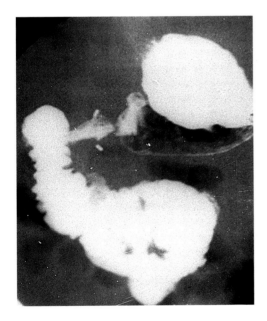

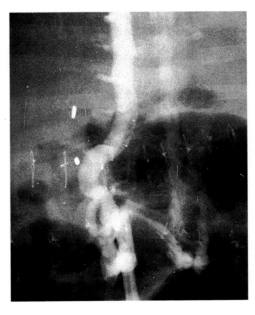

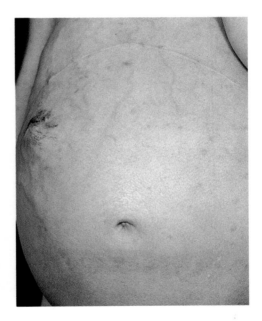

FIG. 10.43 *Malrotation in biliary atresia. The duodenal "C" loop is not closed and is displaced to the right.*

FIG. 10.44 *Vascular anomaly in biliary atresia. The inferior vena cava is interrupted and continues as an azygous vein.*

FIG. 10.45 *Chronic liver disease/portal hypertension. This child had biliary atresia with good bile flow following a portoenterostomy procedure. Cirrhosis developed late, with physical signs of prominent abdominal veins and ascites.*

neuropsychiatric disturbances, hemolytic anemia, and cirrhosis. The clinician must establish a diagnosis in any child older than 4 years with persistent transaminase elevation. Serum ceruloplasmin is usually reduced and 24-hour copper excretion elevated. However, measurement of hepatic copper may be necessary in some patients. Kayser-Fleischer rings occasionally are visible without the use of a slit lamp (Fig. 10.47). Therapy with copper-chelating agents such as penicillamine must be initiated before irreversible cirrhosis develops. Both the chronic liver failure and the neurologic disorder may be effectively treated by transplantation.

Finally, one chronic hepatic disorder can usually be recognized by examination alone. The healthy-appearing child with massive splenomegaly and a large, firm left lobe of the liver with no stigmata of chronic liver disease except GI hemorrhage almost certainly has congenital hepatic fibrosis (Fig. 10.48). It should be remembered that these children may be part of the spectrum of polycystic kidney disease in childhood, and renal function studies are warranted (Fig. 10.49). Therapy for this condition may include shunting procedures for portal hypertension, as liver function may remain normal indefinitely.

BIBLIOGRAPHY

Ament M: Inflammatory disease of the colon: ulcerative colitis and Crohn's colitis. *J Pediatr* 1975;86:322–334.

Balistreri WF: Neonatal cholestasis. *J Pediatr* 1985;106:171–184.

Barness L, et al: *Pediatric Nutrition Handbook*. Evanston, Illinois, American Academy of Pediatrics, 1979, 1985.

Berman WF, Holtzapple PG: Gastrointestinal hemorrhage. *Pediatr Clin North Am* 1975;23:885–895.

Berwick D: Nonorganic failure to thrive. *Pediatr Rev* 180;1:265–270.

Cox K., Ament MA: Upper gastrointestinal bleeding in children and adolescents. *Pediatrics* 1979;63:408–413.

Fitzgerald JF: Constipation in children. *Pediatr Rev* 1987;8:299–302.

Gartner JC: Recurrent abdominal pain—who needs a workup? *Contemp Pediatr* 1989;6:62–82.

Herbst JJ: Gastroesophageal reflux. *J Pediatr* 1981;98:859–870.

Orenstein S, Orenstein D: Gastroesophageal reflux and respiratory disease in children. *J Pediatr* 1988;112:847–858.

Scheinberg IH, Sternlieb I: *Wilson's Disease*. Philadelphia, WB Saunders, 1984.

Sondheimer JM: Office stool examination: a practical guide. *Contemp Pediatr* 1990;7:63–82.

Suskind RM (ed.): *Textbook of Pediatric Nutrition*. New York, Raven Press, 1981.

Suskind RM, Varma RN: Assessment of nutritional status of children. *Pediatr Rev* 1984;5:195–202.

Walker WA: Benign chronic diarrhea of infancy. *Pediatr Rev* 1981;3:153–158.

Walker WA, Hendricks KM: *Manual of Pediatric Nutrition*. Philadelphia, WB Saunders, 1985.

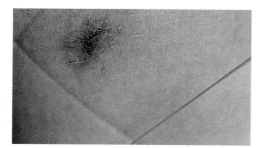

FIG. 10.46 Spider nevus. The vascular lesion blanches with compression by a glass slide, but it reappears when pressure is released.

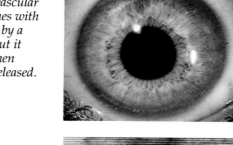

FIG. 10.47 Kayser-Fleischer ring appears as brownish discoloration in the posterior part of the cornea, as defined by slit lamp examination. Early KF rings may be seen only by slit lamp and begin at the superior and inferior poles.

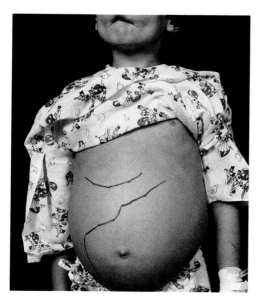

FIG. 10.48 Congenital hepatic fibrosis. This clinically well child had hematemesis and hypersplenism with normal liver function studies. Note massive splenic size and large left lobe of liver. Portosystemic shunting was effective therapy.

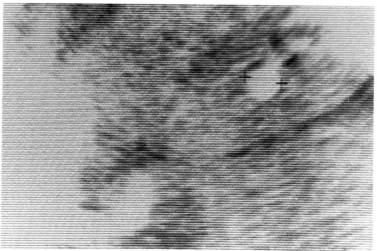

FIG. 10.49 Ultrasonogram of the kidney in a patient with congenital hepatic fibrosis reveals a cystic structure.

PEDIATRIC HEMATOLOGY AND ONCOLOGY

J. Malatack, M.D. ◆ Julie Blatt, M.D. ◆ Lila Penchansky, M.D.

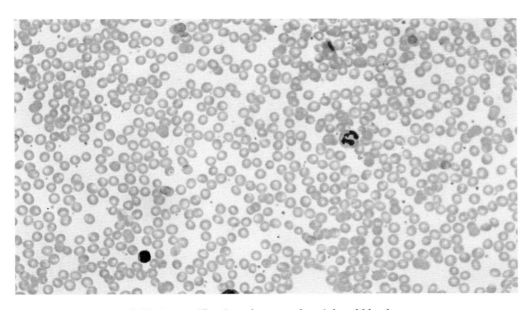

FIG. 11.1 *Low power (100x) magnification of a normal peripheral blood smear.*

HEMATOLOGY

The tools of the clinical pediatric hematologist have evolved over recent years, as techniques previously limited to research and laboratory settings have moved into the realm of normal investigation and therapeutics. Despite such advances, however, the core of hematologic diagnosis resides in a thorough medical history, physical examination, evaluation of the patient's peripheral blood, complete blood and reticulocyte counts and, occasionally, bone marrow examination. In contrast to much of pediatric diagnosis, laboratory results carry a disproportionate weight in the evaluation of the patient with hematologic problems.

We will first highlight common hematologic conditions as well as selected rarer entities. In this context, peripheral blood smear and basic diagnostic tests are used to evaluate nonmalignant hematologic disease including signs and symptoms of clotting abnormalities. Then, attention will be given to hematologic findings in leukemia and solid tumors.

The Peripheral Blood Smear

The peripheral blood smear serves two major functions: first, it provides confirmation of the values given on the standard Coulter counter printout, which may falsely report elevated white blood cell (WBC) counts due to the presence of nucleated red blood cells (RBCs). In addition, the presence of red cell fragments may result in falsely elevated platelet counts. Second, review of the peripheral smear allows the diagnostician to perform the differential WBC count at the same time as examination of red cell, white cell, and platelet morphology.

A systematic approach to the evaluation of the smear can maximize the amount of information extracted. First, the slide is scanned under low power, and an area is chosen in which the red cells are just barely touching (Fig. 11.1). Areas in which the red cells are too dense or too sparse are fraught with artifact. Under low power, both mononuclear and polymorphonuclear cells are visible. By using the high-dry or oil lens, the examiner can observe normal red cell morphology. The normal

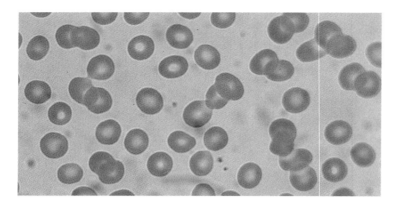

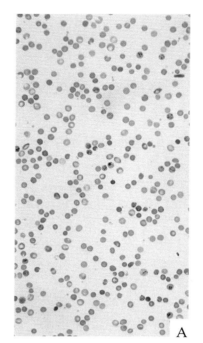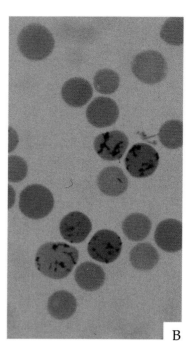

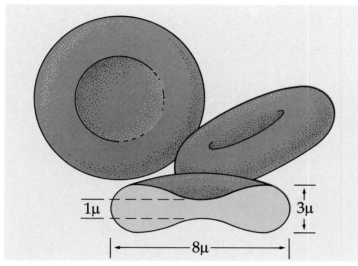

FIG. 11.2 High-power (400x) magnification of a normal peripheral blood smear (top). Schematic drawing of a red blood cell (RBC) in two views demonstrates features of the normal biconcave disc (bottom).

FIG. 11.3 **A**, reticulocyte-stained peripheral blood smear in a patient with high (18 percent) reticulocyte count. The more darkly stained cells are reticulocytes. The patient had hemolytic anemia. **B**, oil immersion view of reticulocyte-stained peripheral blood from the same patient. Higher power reveals reticulin staining of the red cells.

RBC appears as a biconcave disc with an area of central pallor surrounded by an otherwise homogeneous red circle (Fig. 11.2). Beyond the newborn period, during which time it is larger, the RBC is about the size of the nucleus of the small lymphocyte.

Following an evaluation of red cell morphology, a white cell differential count can be performed and the morphology of the cells assessed. A blood smear made from anticoagulated blood may have artifacts such as vacuolation of the WBCs. Finally, platelets should be scrutinized for number (each platelet found on a high-dry field represents approximately 10,000 to 15,000 platelets per mm^3).

The Red Blood Cell

The RBC is the most ubiquitous of the blood's cellular components. Its primary function is to mediate the exchange of respiratory gases (oxygen and carbon dioxide) between the lungs and body tissues. This is accomplished by the critical biochemical features of its oxygen-carrying intracellular component, hemoglobin (Hgb). Hemoglobin's oxygen-binding sites are completely saturated by passage of the RBC through the lungs. As the cells circulate through the systemic capillaries,

the hemoglobin releases 25 percent of its bound oxygen to the tissues. However, the amount of oxygen released in the tissue may be significantly increased under certain conditions (fever, acidosis, level of 2 to 3 DPG), allowing some compensation for a decrease in hemoglobin. Nonetheless, a decrease in hemoglobin eventually leads to tissue hypoxia, which triggers a release of erythropoietin. This induces an increase in red cell production, which brings the critical red cell mass back toward normal values.

Red Cell Production

Red cell production usually occurs in the bone marrow, but under conditions of disease, it also can occur in extramedullary locations such as the spleen. For the first 48 hours after it has joined the peripheral circulation, a newly formed red cell or reticulocyte, can be stained by a supravital dye for easy identification. Generally, the reticulocyte count is a reflection of the replacement of senescent red cells. Since the red cell life span is approximately 120 days, 0.83 percent of the red cell mass must be replaced by reticulocytes every day. Since reticulocytes maintain their staining characteristics for approximately 48 hours, the normal reticulocyte count (percentage of peripheral red cells that are reticulocytes) is approximately 1.66 percent, ranging from 0.83 to 2.49 percent. This figure is 1 to 2 percent higher in menstruating females. Increased reticulocyte counts are also a reflection of increased red cell loss through either hemolysis or hemorrhage. Decreased reticulocyte counts are indicative of decreased red cell production (Fig. 11.3).

HEMOGLOBIN (HGB) AND MEAN CORPUSCULAR VOLUME (MCV) VALUES AT VARIOUS AGES

Age	Hemoglobin (g/dl)	MCV (fl)
Birth (cord blood)	16.5	108
1 to 3 days (capillary)	18.5	108
1 week	17.5	107
2 weeks	16.5	105
1 month	14.0	104
2 months	11.5	96
3 to 6 months	11.5	91
0.5 to 2 years	12.0	78
2 to 6 years	12.5	81
6 to 12 years	13.5	86
12 to 18 years—female	14.0	90
male	14.5	88
18 to 49 years—female	14.0	90
male	15.5	90

FIG. 11.4 (Adapted from Dallman PR, in Rudolph A (ed): Pediatrics, ed 16. New York, Appleton-Century-Crofts, 1977, 1111)

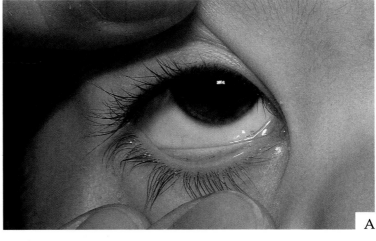

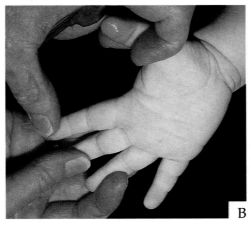

FIG. 11.5 **A**, pale conjunctivae in a patient with severe anemia. **B**, pale palmar creases in a child with a hemoglobin level of 4 g/dl.

Anemia

Increased red cell loss or decreased red cell production can both result in an overall decrease in RBC mass below a critical level, leading to anemia. This is the most common abnormality of red cells, and it is identified as decreased hemoglobin and hematocrit. Recognition that a child's hemoglobin is too low requires knowledge of age, sex, and race-related normal values. At any given age, anemia is defined as a value greater than 2 standard deviations below the mean (Fig. 11.4). For children 6 months of age until puberty, a hemoglobin level of less than 11 g/dl is a useful definition of anemia and an indication for evaluation. Alternatively, an inappropriate drop in hemoglobin may also be significant: the 5-year-old child who has a hemoglobin level of 11.5 g/dl but who, 1 month earlier, had a level of 13 g/dl, may require evaluation.

Severe anemia from any cause may elicit symptoms of fatigue, decreased appetite, and in extreme cases, shock, congestive heart failure, or even stroke. Physical examination of the anemic child may reveal pallor, although in the fair-skinned or very dark-skinned child this may be easily missed, even given an extremely low level of hemoglobin, unless palmar creases or conjunctivae are also examined for pallor (Fig. 11.5). Vital signs may be normal, but with severe anemia, heart rate increases.

Prior to embarking on a workup in a child with low hemoglobin, it is worth considering whether the reported blood value is accurate. Reasons for inaccuracy include poor quality control in the use of the Coulter counter, dilution of blood drawn from venous lines, falsely elevated values—particularly in neonates when the CBC is obtained by heel or fin-

ger stick. Anemia, when it does occur, may be an isolated finding or it may be part of the spectrum of pancytopenia in which WBCs and platelets also are decreased.

Conceptionally, anemia occurs as a result of one of the following:

1. decreased bone marrow production of RBCs.
2. increased destruction, of either mature red cells peripherally, or of their precursors while they are still in the bone marrow (ineffective erythropoiesis).
3. hemorrhage.
4. combinations of the above.

Anemias due to decreased red cell production include microcytic anemia, pure red cell aplasia, and megaloblastic anemia. Hemolytic anemias, characterized by increased RBC destruction without evidence of blood loss or ineffective erythropoiesis, include red cell membrane defects, intracellular RBC defects, and extra RBC factors causing hemolysis.

Anemias Due to Decreased Red Cell Production

Red cell morphology generally categorizes the type of anemia that may be present in a patient, and may suggest certain pathogenic mechanisms.

HYPOCHROMIC/MICROCYTIC ANEMIAS
Hypochromic/microcytic anemias represent the most common type of isolated failure of RBC production. Microcytosis exists when the mean corpuscular volume (MCV = hematocrit x 10/red cell number in millions per mm³) is low, or when the

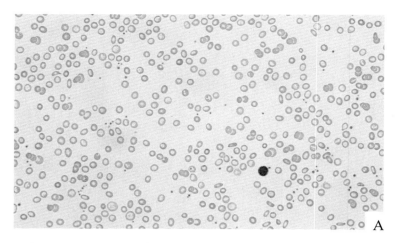

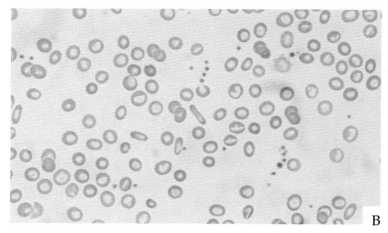

FIG. 11.6 *A, microcytic, hypochromic anemia of iron deficiency anemia. This 16-month-old patient has a history of excessive milk intake. Note the marked central pallor of the RBC with a small rim of hemoglobin, as well as its small size in comparison to that of the adja-* *cent small lymphocyte nucleus. B, peripheral blood smear of patient with iron deficiency. Frequent "cigar cells" can be seen in addition to the microcytic, hypochromic red cells.*

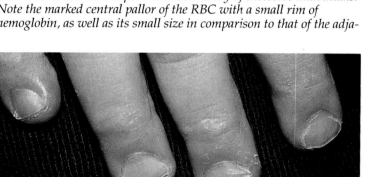

FIG. 11.7 *Spooning of fingernails in child with iron deficiency anemia.*

red cells themselves are smaller than the nuclei of the small lymphocytes. Hypochromia, a decrease in the concentration of intracellular content, is recognized when the mean corpuscular hemoglobin concentration (MCHC = hemoglobin in g/dl x 10/hematocrit) is decreased, or when the hemoglobinized rim of the red cell is less than two-thirds the diameter of the entire cell. Normally, the ratio of red cell volume to the intracellular RBC content is homeostatically maintained. As the concentration of intracellular content decreases for any reason, the volume of the cell also decreases.

The differential diagnosis of hypochromic/microcytic anemias includes iron deficiency, lead poisoning, thalassemia minor (both alpha and beta types), thalassemia major (Cooley's anemia), chronic infection, chronic inflammatory states, and sideroblastic anemia.

Iron Deficiency Anemia

Iron deficiency anemia is the most common of the pediatric hypochromic/microcytic anemias. Iron deficiency is only a laboratory finding, not a diagnosis. The causes of iron deficiency must be elucidated through a careful history and physical examination. While poor nutrition is the most common cause of iron deficiency, other causes such as hemorrhage or malabsorption also must be considered. Iron deficiency anemia occurs in infants whose rapidly increasing red cell mass outstrips the dietary iron intake. This lack of iron leads to failure of hemoglobin production and the formation of hypochromic, microcytic cells. Since the normal full-term infant has adequate iron reserve to accommodate the increas-

ing red cell mass through the first 5 months of life, iron deficiency is usually not seen until the second half of the first year of life. It is detected most often in the 10- to 18-month-old child.

The typical clinical history is that of an infant fed noniron-containing whole cow's milk who, from early infancy, takes large volumes of milk and little else. These children often are large, but their pallor will belie their apparent robust size. Whole cow's milk is not only deficient in dietary iron, but it often leads to enteropathy with gastrointestinal blood loss, exacerbating the child's iron-deficient status.

Figure 11.6A shows the peripheral blood smear of a 16-month-old child who had been fed large amounts of whole milk from 3 months of age. The RBCs are microcytic and hypochromic. The platelets are characteristically increased (particularly when the enteropathy is present), although they may be normal or even decreased. In severe iron deficiency anemia, anisocytosis (varied size of RBCs) and poikilocytosis (varied RBC shape) may be prominent. Nonspecific abnormalities of RBC morphology may also occur, such as the presence of microovalocytes (cigar cells) (Fig. 11.6B) or basophilic stippling (see Fig. 11.11).

The child with iron deficiency may be asymptomatic despite a significant degree of anemia. However, when symptoms are present, irritability is the prominent finding. Children have also been shown to demonstrate decreases in Bayley I.Q. scores, as well as occasional peculiar physical findings such as "spooning" of the finger and toenails (koilonychia) (Fig. 11.7) and glossitis.

Iron deficiency must be differentiated from thalassemia and lead poisoning. While patient history will generally suggest the appropriate diagnosis, the distinction can be made, for the most part, on the basis of a few laboratory tests. Review of the peripheral smear (see Fig. 11.6A) should first confirm the presence of microcytosis and/or hypochromia, which, like the measurements of hemoglobin, are susceptible to technical errors. In thalassemia minor, the hemoglobin is generally not less than 9 g/dl; moreover, for a given degree of anemia, the MCV tends to be lower in the child with thalassemia than in the child with iron deficiency. These trends may be reflected in the Mentzer Index, which mathematically relates the MCV to the red cell number (Mentzer Index = MCV/number of

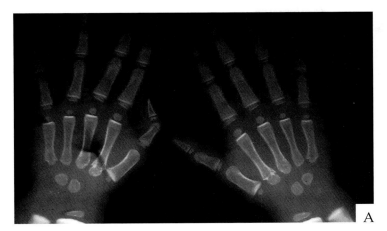

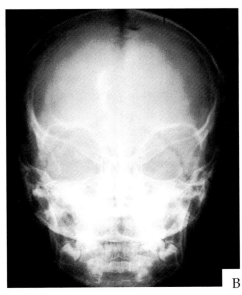

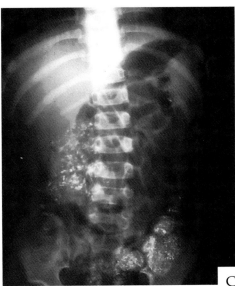

FIG. 11.8 A, hand radiograph of child with lead intoxication reveals marked linear increases in the density of the metaphyses. These should not be confused with the growth arrest lines seen following a variety of illnesses. B, skull film of patient with lead intoxication, with encephalopathy. Note the split sutures indicative of increased intracranial pressure. C, abdominal radiograph of a child with a history of pica and lead intoxication reveals radio-dense lead-containing paint chips scattered throughout the colon.

RBC/10⁶). Mentzer indices greater than 13.5 suggest iron deficiency while values less than 11.5 indicate thalassemia minor. In practice, we have not found the index to be helpful, since most children with mild anemias may have intermediate index values. Other helpful clues to the diagnosis can come directly from the RBC number. RBC numbers can be helpful since children with iron deficiency usually have a low RBC number whereas thalassemia tends to produce RBC numbers greater than $5 \times 10^6/mm^3$. The red cell distribution width ($SD_{RBC\ vol}/MCV \times 100$) is a reflection of the degree of anisocytosis and is significantly larger in iron deficiency than in thalassemia trait.

The clinical history, along with the results of the CBC, differential, platelet and reticulocyte counts, and review of the peripheral smear will be sufficient for diagnosis in most instances of microcytic hypochromic anemia. Occasionally, other more specific laboratory tests may be needed. If the evaluation prior to obtaining a specific test strongly suggests the presence of iron deficiency, a therapeutic trial of oral iron may be a reasonable approach. However, the physician is obliged to follow the patient until the blood count has returned to normal; improvement is not enough. The coexistence of lead poisoning and iron deficiency is well documented. Hence, partial response to iron therapy does not eliminate lead poisoning from diagnostic consideration.

Choosing between specific studies such as serum iron and total iron binding capacity (used together to calculate iron saturation) or ferritin and free erythrocyte protoporphyrin (FEP) is often a matter of personal preference. In addition, when the degree of anemia is mild, the results of any combination of tests may be equivocal. FEP has the advantage of screening for lead poisoning or porphyria. Ferritin is an acute phase reactant, and may be elevated into the low normal range in a child with a concurrent inflammatory process. Iron saturation and ferritin levels both have age-related normal values. Children up to age 15 have serum ferritin levels less than 10 µg/mg, indicating iron deficiency. Transferrin saturation confirms iron deficiency if it is under 12 percent for children 5 to 10 years old, and under 16 percent for older children. Free erythrocyte protoporphyrin levels indicate iron deficiency if they are over 90 µg/dl RBC for infants and preschoolers up to age 4 years, and over 70 µg/dl RBC for older children.

Lead Poisoning

Lead intoxication leads to a microcytic anemia. However, nonhematologic manifestations of lead intoxication, particularly neurologic complications, often dominate the picture. The spectrum of clinical presentations of lead intoxication ranges from vague symptoms of abdominal pain, vomiting, malaise, and behavioral changes to acute encephalopathy, with rapid progression to coma and death. Late physical findings may include papilledema. Significant radiographic changes also are seen in lead intoxication (Fig. 11.8A-C).

Lead intoxication occurs as a result of excessive environmental lead intake. Both aerosolized and oral lead-containing, environmental contaminants are major sources of lead intoxi-

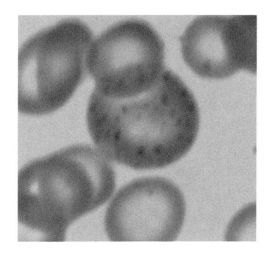

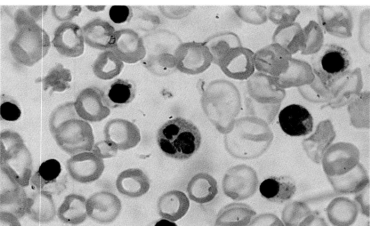

FIG. 11.10 Peripheral blood smear of child with thalassemia major. Note the microcytic hypochromic anemia and prominent nucleated red cells surrounding the polymorphonuclear cells and lymphocytes.

FIG. 11.9 Microcytic hypochromic anemia due to lead intoxication. Note prominent basophilic stippling. This finding is not specific for lead intoxication and may be seen in thalassemia and, though rarely, in iron deficiency.

cation. While clearly a common mechanism in lead poisoning, pica, associated with flaking lead paint, represents neither the only, nor the prevailing, cause of lead intoxication. The finger-sucking behavior of children in homes where lead paint has become an intimate part of house dust is perhaps a more important factor.

Hematologic abnormalities of lead intoxication are a direct result of the effect of lead on several cellular enzymes involved in heme production. Lead inhibits these enzyme systems, impairing iron utilization as well as globin synthesis. Thus, despite normal intracellular levels, iron is unable to be incorporated into heme, and hemoglobin production fails. Reduced hemoglobin production leads directly to the microcytic hypochromic anemia. Basophilic stippling is a secondary and inconsistent hematologic manifestation of lead intoxication, that occurs as a result of inhibition of yet another RBC enzyme, 5-pyrimidine nucleotidase. This enzyme normally removes nucleotide chains from the RBC after its nucleus has been extruded. In lead poisoning, these chains persist, and the nucleotide remnants stain blue on a normal Wright's stain, causing a stippling of the red cell (Fig. 11.9). While basophilic stippling is more prominent in lead intoxication, it is also present in thalassemia and iron deficiency. Its presence on the peripheral smear is nonspecific.

Differentiating lead intoxication from iron deficiency can, at times, be difficult. Also, lead intoxication and iron deficiency may coexist, further confusing the diagnosis. Both lead poisoning and iron deficiency cause erythrocyte protoporphyrin to accumulate in blood. The FEP is elevated in both conditions, although extremely high levels are seen more commonly in lead intoxication. Further testing, such as determination of blood lead level, is necessary to determine the cause of elevated FEP. When suspicion of lead intoxication exists, a lead level should be obtained. Recent information incriminating even low-level lead intoxication as a cause of disturbed cognitive function, underscores the necessity for clinicians to consider this diagnosis. Silent lead intoxication with blood levels of 15 μg/dl remains a significant pediatric health problem, and may not be associated with the signs of chronic, high level lead poisoning described above.

Thalassemia

Thalassemia is a term applied to a group of genetic disturbances decreasing hemoglobin production and leading to anemia and/or altered levels of the various hemoglobins in the blood.

Thalassemia trait is also responsible for hypochromic/microcytic anemia. In patients with beta thalassemia trait, hemoglobin electrophoresis usually reveals an increasein Hgb A_2 and Hgb F, whereas in patients with alpha thalassemia trait the findings may be normal. This costly test probably is overused in the evaluation of hypochromic/microcytic anemia. Hemograms on parents may be helpful is they show a micro-cytosis in at least one parent, further suggesting a diagnosis of thalassemia trait. Should a diagnosis of thalassemiabe suggested by any of the studies already discussed, both parents should have hemograms performed. While the index child may suffer from thalassemia trait, it is conceivable

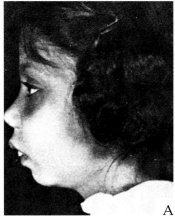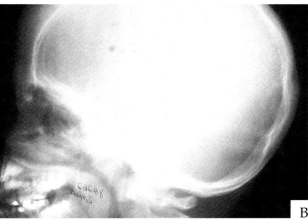

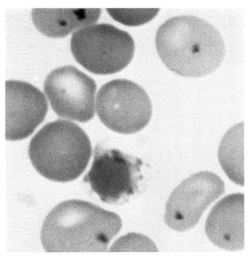

FIG. 11.11 **A,** *maxillary hyperplasia due to increased marrow space in child with thalassemia major.* **B,** *skull radiograph of the* *same patient demonstrates an increased marrow cavity of the skull and facial bones.*

FIG. 11.12 *Ringed sideroblast (iron-containing normoblast) on iron stain of the bone marrow. They are present in patients with sideroblastic anemia.*

that both parents may also have thalassemia trait, and a subsequent child may be born with thalassemia major, a disease with serious implications regarding both morbidity and mortality. Appropriate genetic counseling would be indicated.

Thalassemia major (Cooley's anemia) causes hypo-chromic/microcytic anemia which results from ineffective erythropoiesis due to an imbalance between alpha and beta globin chain synthesis. The peripheral blood smear shows hypochromia, microcytosis, target cells, basophilic stippling and often, large numbers of nucleated RBCs (Fig. 11.10A,B). Beta/thalassemia major is associated with increased marrow activity which is ineffectively attempting to correct the degree of anemia. The increased marrow activity expands the marrow cavity, producing a characteristic bony hyperplasia evidenced by physical and radiographic findings (Fig. 11.11). Untreated patients with Cooley's anemia have chronic, severe anemia, marked hepatosplenomegaly, scleral icterus, listlessness, and may have high output cardiac failure secondary to severe anemia. In addition, malocclusion may occur due to malar hypertrophy. This picture should not be confused with thalassemia trait, iron deficiency, or lead poisoning. Thalassemia major generally presents after the first 6 months of life at a time when beta chain synthesis increases. Hydrops fetalis may be due to alpha thalassemia major. Ethnicity may be an important clue in the history: beta thalassemia trait tends to occur in patients of African or Mediterranean extraction, whereas alpha thalassemia trait tends to occur in blacks or Orientals. Thalassemia major is largely restricted to people of Mediterranean or Middle Eastern heritage.

Chronic Inflammatory States

Chronic inflammatory states, such as chronic infection or collagen vascular diseases (particularly juvenile rheumatoid arthritis), may lead to microcytic hypochromic anemia. While the symptoms of the child's primary illness usually clarify the diagnosis, there are, occasionally, cases in which a chronic subclinical infection (particularly of the urinary tract) may go undiagnosed. Differentiating a chronic inflammatory state from other causes of hypochromic/microcytic anemia is usually more easily done on clinical than laboratory grounds. One laboratory study that may be of value is the serum ferritin determination. The ferritin is decreased in iron deficiency, whereas in chronic inflammatory states it is usually elevated.

Sideroblastic and Other Anemias

The sideroblastic anemias are characterized by the presence of a population of hypochromic microcytic cells in the peripheral blood, as well as sideroblasts in the bone marrow (Fig. 11.12). The sideroblastic anemias, very rare in pediatrics, can either be hereditary or acquired. The hereditary anemia is caused by a deficiency of an enzyme or enzyme activity required for hemoglobin production. The acquired form may arise secondary to drug or toxin (lead being the most important of those in childhood) reactions, malignancy, inflammatory endocrine disease, or may be idiopathic.

Copper deficiency and chronic disease, although generally resulting in normocytic anemia, may occasionally cause a microcytic picture.

MACROCYTIC ANEMIA

Macrocytic anemia (MCV >100 fl on the Coulter indices) may be associated with decreased RBC production. Some causes of macrocytosis may be associated with hemorrhage or hemolysis, and a brisk reticulocytosis which accounts for the large red cells on the peripheral smear. Such causes of macrocytic anemia usually are easily recognized and differentiated from macrocytic anemias based on bone marrow failure.

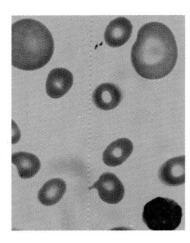

FIG. 11.13 Peripheral blood smear of patient with megaloblastic anemia. Note the enlarged red cell (macrocyte) at the upper left. It is much larger than the normal small lymphocyte in the same field.

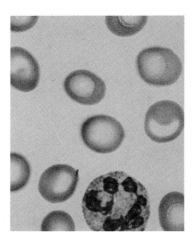

FIG. 11.14 A hypersegmented polymorphonuclear leukocyte in patient with phenytoin-induced folate deficiency.

Macrocytosis is relatively uncommon in pediatric patients outside the neonatal period (see Fig. 11.4). The differential diagnosis of macrocytosis includes reticulocytosis, Down syndrome, pure red cell aplasia (which also may be normocytic), hypothyroidism, liver disease, and megaloblastic anemia.

Megaloblastic Anemias

These anemias constitute another group of conditions characterized by failure of adequate red cell production. Although the etiology of the megaloblastic anemias may vary, common morphologic abnormalities of the erythropoietic cells exist. The hallmark is the megaloblast, a nucleated marrow red cell with a lacy chromatin pattern and a dyssynchrony of maturation between cytoplasm and nucleus. The morphologic alterations are a direct result of decreased nucleoprotein (DNA) synthesis compared with cytoplasmic protein synthesis, which stems from a relative decrease in the factors needed in DNA replication, namely folate or cobalamin (vitamin B_{12}). From a morphologic standpoint red cells are the primary cells affected by megaloblastic changes.

On the peripheral blood smear, the red cells are large in size (macrocytes), and they display a great deal of variation in their shapes (Fig. 11.13). These macrocytic cells are generally normochromic.

While red cells are primarily affected in megaloblastic anemia, all of the actively dividing marrow cells fail to have normal DNA duplication and will become involved in the pathologic process. Neutrophils are the second most likely cells to display morphologic abnormalities. These cells, like the RBCs, are large, and hypersegmentation of the nucleus is a pathognomonic finding (Fig. 11.14). Neutropenia is common. The more severe and prolonged megaloblastic anemias may lead ultimately to thrombocytopenia, with large bizarre platelets on the peripheral blood smear. Megaloblastic changes in each cell line are summarized in Figure 11.15.

Laboratory diagnosis requires measurement of folate and B_{12} levels in the serum and RBCs. Since a typical Western world diet is very unlikely to lead to either folate or B_{12} deficiency, a low level of either should raise questions of altered bioavailability or peculiar diet. Goat's milk is folate deficient (though in recent years many canned goat's milk products are folate-supplemented), and an infant on a goat's milk diet may become folate-depleted over time. Fad diets are often not structured thoughtfully, and may lead to folate deficiency. When the diet is not peculiar, various drugs which either decrease folate absorption (phenytoin) or interfere with folate metabolism (methotrexate) may lead to megaloblastic changes. Gastrointestinal tract pathology may be the primary disease causing malabsorption of folate or B_{12} and secondary megaloblastic changes. Pernicious anemia is a specific cause of failure of B_{12} absorption because of the absence or deficiency of intrinsic factor required for B_{12} absorption. Glossitis (see Fig. 11.8) or angular stomatitis seen in B_{12} deficiency can be a helpful physical finding in differential diagnoses.

NORMOCYTIC, NORMOCHROMIC ANEMIA

The third morphologic subgroup of anemia includes those with normochromic and normocytic red cells. These anemias are most easily analyzed on the basis of an algorithm beginning with a reticulocyte count. These normocytic, normochromic anemias with low reticulocyte counts develop because of failed RBC production. The differential diagnosis of this group includes pure red cell aplasia, dyserythropoietic anemia, renal disease, infection, and drug-induced aplasia. When low-reticulocyte, normocytic, normochromic anemia occurs in the presence of a decrease in WBCs and platelets, the diagnosis is much more ominous and includes leukemia, aplastic anemia, and tumor infiltration of the marrow.

Pure Red Cell Aplasia

Pure red cell aplasia can be either acquired or congenital. The congenital form (referred to variously as congenital hypoplastic anemia, chronic idiopathic erythroblastopenia, chronic congenital aregenerative anemia, erythropoiesis imperfecta or Blackfan-Diamond syndrome) is characterized by onset of anemia by 6 months of age with a low absolute reticulocyte count. Approximately 25 percent of patients with Blackfan-Diamond have minor congenital anomalies including thumb anomalies and/or a Turner (see Genetics, Chapter 1) phenotype. Some of the patients go into spontaneous remission; others may remit years after onset of signs of the disease; still others respond to corticosteroid therapy. A final subgroup does not improve,

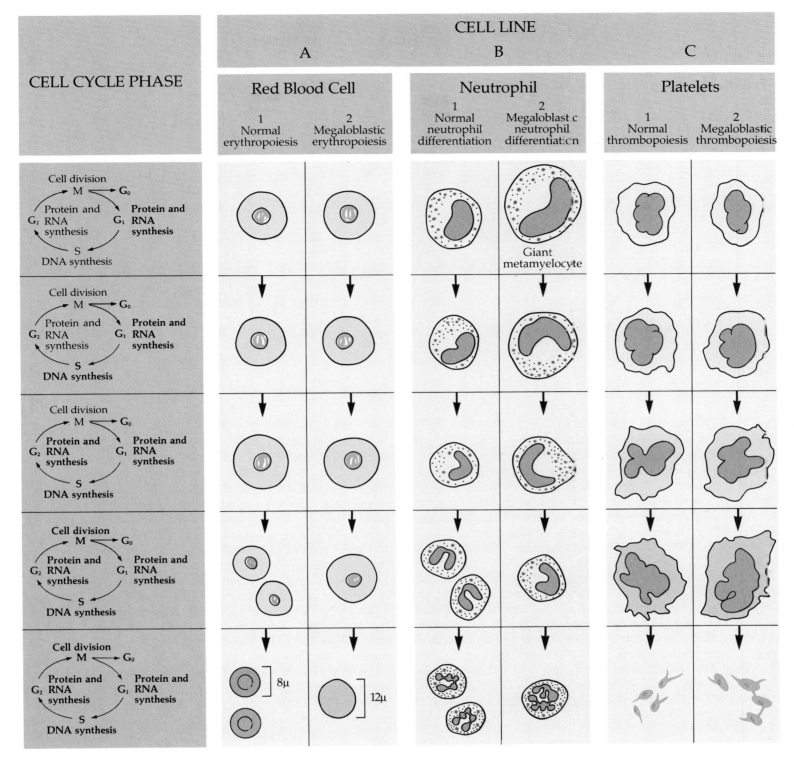

CELL CYCLE PHASE	CELL LINE					
	A		B		C	
	Red Blood Cell		Neutrophil		Platelets	
	1 Normal erythropoiesis	2 Megaloblastic erythropoiesis	1 Normal neutrophil differentiation	2 Megaloblastic neutrophil differentiation	1 Normal thrombopoiesis	2 Megaloblastic thrombopoiesis

FIG. 11.15 Schematic comparison of normal cellular maturation and megaloblastic differentiation of three cell lines. The cell cycle phase is identified to the left of the figure. Note that megaloblastic cells fail to undergo DNA replication and cellular division at S and M phases, respectively, leading to large red cells, hypersegmented polys, and large bizarrely shaped platelets.

and remains transfusion-dependent for the rest of their lives. Blackfan-Diamond red cell aplasia has an associated macrocytosis on the peripheral blood smear. However, we have included it in the discussion of normocytic normochromic anemias, because it must be distinguished from the most frequently acquired pure red cell aplasia, transient erythroblastopenia of childhood (TEC), which is normocytic and normochromic.

TEC occurs in 1- to 4-year-old children and appears 2 weeks to 2 months following a respiratory or gastrointestinal illness. Differentiating TEC from Blackfan-Diamond is important because TEC is transient and self-limited, while Blackfan-Diamond is chronic. Blackfan-Diamond may be most responsive to steroids when therapy is begun early in the course of the disease. Fortunately, it has been noted that Blackfan-

RBC Characteristic	**FEATURES DIFFERENTIATING CONGENITAL HYPOPLASTIC ANEMIA FROM TRANSIENT ERYTHROBLASTOPENIA OF CHILDHOOD**	
	Disease	
	Congenital Hypoplastic Anemia	Transient Erythroblastopenia of Childhood
Hemoglobin (Hgb)	Increased fetal Hgb	Normal fetal Hgb
Cellular antigen	i	I
MCV	Increased	Normal
RBC enzyme activity	Normal or high	Low

FIG. 11.16

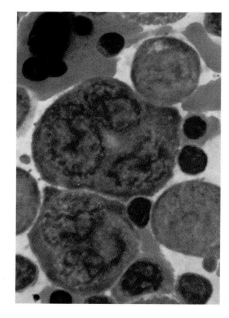

FIG. 11.17 Congenital dyserythropoietic anemia type III. Note the centrally located gigantoblast.

Diamond red cells have fetal characteristics, while TEC has age-appropriate red cell characteristics (Fig. 11.16).

Non-TEC acquired pure red cell aplasia is rare in pediatrics. In adults, pure red cell aplasia is sometimes suspected on an autoimmune basis and is frequently associated with thymoma. Autoimmunity rarely is the etiology in children, and thymoma is extremely rare. Drugs, particularly chloramphenicol, have been responsible for a significant percentage of pure red cell aplasias.

While the peripheral blood smear from a patient with RBC aplasia is often nonspecific (although it may show atypical lymphocytes as vestiges of a residual viral infection), the bone marrow aspirate may rarely be more specific. It may demonstrate the vacuolated erythroblasts of the chloramphenicol effect, or the multinucleated giant cells indicative of the rare congenital dyserythropoietic anemia (Fig. 11.17). Low reticulocyte, normocytic, normochromic anemia with depressed WBCs and platelets is discussed in the pancytopenia section of this chapter.

The Hemolytic Anemias

Normocytic, normochromic anemias with increased reticulocyte counts but without evidence of blood loss are most likely due to hemolytic processes. However, the reticulocyte count may not be elevated if measured within a few days of onset of the hemolysis. Patients with hemolytic anemia can suffer from any of the symptoms common to all anemias; however, in addition, they will develop an indirect hyperbilirubinemia with or without clinical icterus. Other laboratory evidence of hemolysis is present, including increased carboxyhemoglobin, increased LDH and SGOT, and decreased haptoglobin.

Differential diagnosis of hemolytic anemia rests largely in the recognition of specific morphologic abnormalities on the peripheral blood smear (Fig. 11.18) followed by appropriate specific laboratory tests.

NORMOCYTIC, NORMOCHROMIC ANEMIA WITH ELEVATED RETICULOCYTE AND SPHEROCYTE LEVELS
Coombs-Positive Hemolytic Anemia

Direct and indirect Coombs tests, which evaluate the patient's blood for the presence of anti-RBC antibody and complement on red cells or in the serum, respectively, will identify the immunohemolytic anemias. The antibody- and complement-mediated red cell destruction will produce spherocytes on the peripheral blood smear (Fig. 11.19). Coombs-positive hemolytic anemia in the newborn period most often represents an isoimmune hemolytic anemia. This is caused by a maternal antibody which has crossed the placenta into the neonate, hemolyzing the newborn red cells (i.e., maternal antibodies form to fetal red cell antigens when fetal blood gains entry into maternal circulation via a break in placental integrity. Maternal antibodies cross the placenta and cause fetal red cell hemolysis. In the majority of cases of isoimmune hemolytic anemia, the maternal antibody is directed at ABO or Rh red cell antigens. When Rh antigen is the antibody target, the blood smear will not show spherocytes.

Hereditary Spherocytosis

Coombs-negative hemolytic anemia with spherocytes most often represents hereditary spherocytosis (HS) which is the most common cause of genetically determined hemolytic anemia in the Caucasian population. HS is transmitted most frequently as an autosomal dominant trait, and it is named for the peculiar appearance of the RBCs on the peripheral blood smear. The red cell membrane defect, which appears to be due to inherent membrane instability, leads to loss of membrane. Membrane repair occurs, which decreases the normal RBC surface-to-volume ratio, causing the normal, bioconcave-disc configuration to assume a more geometrically efficient spherical shape (Fig. 11.20). The direct consequence of this new morphology is a less pliable cell. The inability of this new cell to deform during transit through the splenic microcirculation

CLASSIFICATION OF COMMON RED CELL HEMOLYTIC DISORDERS BY PREDOMINANT MORPHOLOGY*

Spherocytes
  Hereditary spherocytosis
  ABO incompatibility in neonates[†]
  Immunohemolytic anemias with IgG- or C3-coated red cells[†]
  Hemolytic transfusion reactions[†]
  Severe burns, other red cell thermal injuries

Bizarre Poikilocytes
  Red cell fragmentation syndromes (microangiopathic and macroangiopathic hemolytic anemias)
  Hereditary elliptocytosis in neonates

Elliptocytes
  Hereditary elliptocytosis
  Thalassemias
  (Other hypochromic-microcytic anemias)
  (Megaloblastic anemias)

Spiculated or Crenated Red Cells
  Acute hepatic necrosis (spur cell anemia)
  Uremia
  Abetalipoproteinemia

Prominent Basophilic Stippling
  Thalassemias
  Unstable hemoglobins
  Lead poisoning[‡]

Irreversibly Sickled Cells
  Sickle cell anemia
  Symptomatic sickle syndromes

Intraerythrocytic Parasites
  Malaria
  Babesiosis
  Bartonellosis

Target Cells
  Hemoglobins S, C, D, and E
  Hereditary xerocytosis
  Thalassemias
  (Other hypochromic-microcytic anemias)
  (Obstructive liver disease)
  (Postsplenectomy)

Nonspecific or Normal Morphology
  Embden-Meyerhof pathway defects
  HMP shunt defects
  Adenosine deaminase hyperactivity with low red cell ATP
  Unstable hemoglobins
  Paroxysmal nocturnal hemoglobinuria
  Dyserythropoietic anemias
  Copper toxicity (Wilson's disease)
  Erythropoietic porphyria
  Vitamin E deficiency
  Hypersplenism

*Nonhemolytic disorders of similar morphology are enclosed in parentheses for reference.
[†]Usually associated with positive Coombs test.
[‡]Disease sometimes associated with this morphology.

FIG. 11.18 (Adapted by permission from Nathan DG, Oski FA (eds): Hematology of Infancy and Childhood, ed 2. 1981, WB Saunders, Philadelphia, 483)

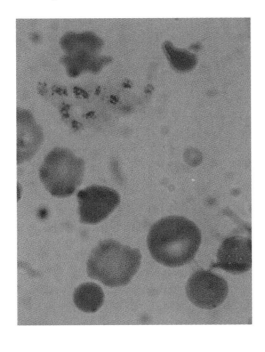

FIG. 11.19 Coombs-positive hemolytic anemia. Note spherocytes and a large RBC with polychromasia indicating the presence of regenerative anemia.

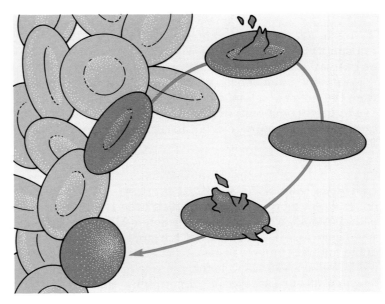

FIG. 11.20 Schematic drawing shows a developing spherocyte due to the process of repeated membrane fragmentation, loss, and repair.

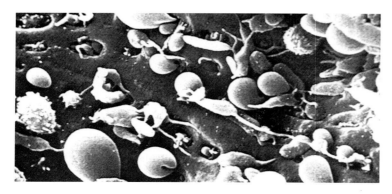

FIG. 11.21 RBCs being deformed as they traverse the microcirculation of the splenic sinusoids. (Reproduced by permission from Zucker-Franklin D, Greanes MF, Grossi CE, Marmont AM: Atlas of Blood Cells, Milan, Italy, Ermes, 1981)

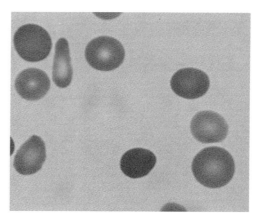

FIG. 11.22 Peripheral blood smear of patient who underwent splenectomy for hereditary spherocytosis (HS). Note the presence of small perfectly round cells without an area of central pallor. The MCHC may be normal but often is increased in patients with HS. Reticulocytosis also may be prominent.

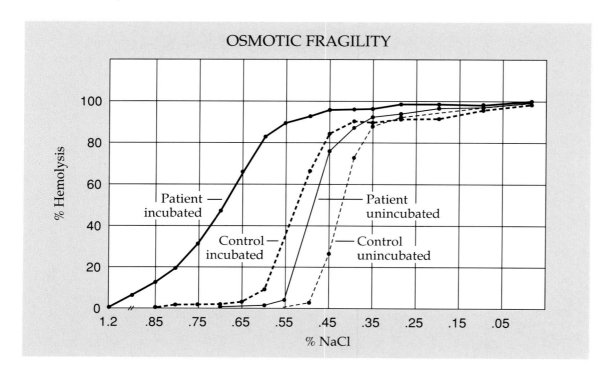

FIG. 11.23 Osmotic fragility of unincubated and incubated RBCs from a normal individual and from a patient with hereditary spherocytosis. The striking increase in fragility produced by incubation of hereditary spherocytosis RBCs is obvious.

leads to RBC destruction (Fig. 11.21). The characteristic smear of HS may show increased numbers of spherocytes following splenectomy when spherocytes are less likely to be removed from the circulation (Fig. 11.22). Osmotic fragility testing (Fig. 11.23), used commonly in patients with suspected HS, is an excellent confirmatory test, but is not pathognomonic for the diagnosis.

Elliptocytosis

Hereditary elliptocytosis (HE) (Fig. 11.24) is another membrane defect morphologically distinct from HS. However, the pathophysiology of red cell destruction in HE is similar to HS. Also, like HS, HE appears to be transmitted as an autosomal dominant trait. In most instances, hereditary elliptocytosis is a mild, well-compensated hemolytic anemia that is clinically insignificant unless splenic hypertrophy develops due to another disease process. The elliptocyte form bears only a superficial similarity to that of the "cigar cell" of iron deficiency anemia (see Fig. 11.6). Unlike the cigar cells, the elliptocytes of HE have normal size, a normal MCV, and are true elliptocytes. Elliptocytes also may be found in the peripheral blood smear of thalassemia or in megaloblastic anemia.

Hereditary stomatocytosis leads to still another morphologic defect. Its infrequency precludes a more lengthy discussion, but it is included here for completeness.

Acanthocytic/Echinocytic Anemias

A number of hemolytic anemias are characterized by spiculated red cells referred to as acanthocytes or echinocytes (Fig. 11.25). Abetalipoproteinemia, which generally presents as a neurologic disorder with progressive ataxia, is also characterized by retinitis pigmentosa, fat malabsorption, and the absence of chylomicrons, VLDLs and LDLs. Roughly 50 to 90 percent of the red cells on peripheral smear are acanthocytes, which develop as a direct result of the alterations of the serum lipids. Altered membrane lipid composition changes the fluidity of the RBC, which leads to the acanthocytic form. Malabsorption of fat-soluble vitamins in abetaliproproteine-

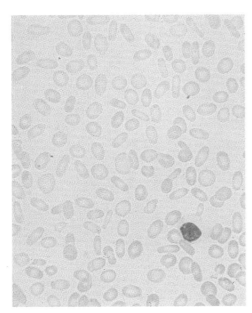

FIG. 11.24 Peripheral blood obtained incidentally from a 3-year-old child with elliptocytosis. Over 90 percent of the cells are elliptocytes. The child had a history of neonatal jaundice, but had been well before and has been well since.

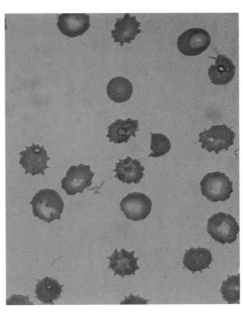

FIG. 11.25 Spiculated cells seen in a patient suffering from acute hepatic necrosis. The associated hemolytic anemia—spur cell anemia—was severe.

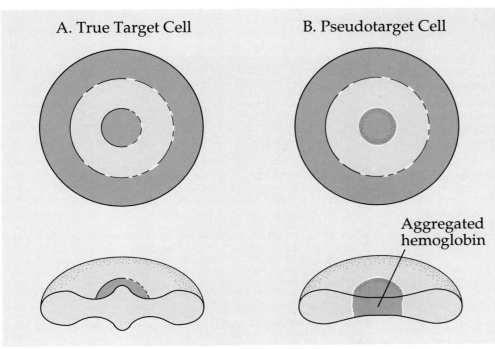

FIG. 11.26 Schematic depiction of the morphology of the true target cell **A** as compared with that of a pseudotarget cell **B**.

mia results in vitamin E deficiency, leaving the red cells subject to oxidative injury. However, despite altered membrane fluidity and vitamin E deficiency, hemolysis in abetalipoproteinemia is mild.

Spur cell anemia is another disorder characterized by acanthocytes. The hemolysis in this disorder, in contrast to abetalipoproteinemia, is brisk. Spur cell anemia develops in the setting of sudden and massive liver injury arising from any cause, e.g., hepatitis with acute yellow atrophy, shock liver, hepatic infarction. The hepatic decompensation leads to increased serum lipid and cholesterol, which lead, in turn, to increased RBC membrane cholesterol content, thus altering RBC membrane fluidity. Spiculated cells in lesser number can also be seen in uremia and anorexia nervosa as well as severe malnutrition. Probably the most frequent cause of spiculated RBCs on the peripheral blood smear is inadequate slide preparation. Thus, when confronted with such a slide, review of repeated peripheral blood smears is prudent.

Target Cells

Target cells draw their name from their target-like appearance on peripheral blood smear. They are most often seen as a secondary response to a process which either increases red cell membrane or decreases red cell content, leading to increase in the surface area-to-volume ratio of the red cells (Fig. 11.26A). In a dried smear, the excess surface accumulates and bulges outward in the area that is normally the red cell's central pallor, producing the characteristic target cell morphology. Liver diseases of any type (particularly obstructive hepatopathy), with their secondary alteration of serum lipids leading to membrane lipid loading, are well-known causes of target cell formation. Splenectomy decreases reticuloendothelial remodeling of reticulocytes, removes lipid-loaded RBC membranes and leads to targeted RBCs. Mechanisms previously discussed, which decrease red cell intracellular content (the microcytic hypochromic anemias), also induce target formation. Finally, a rare autosomal recessive condition, familial

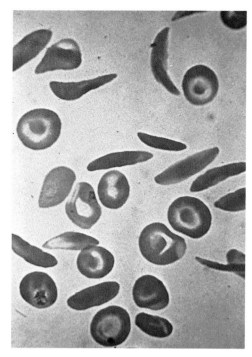

FIG. 11.27 Peripheral blood smear of a black child with HgbSS disease. Note the prominent targets and sickle cells, and the Howell-Jolly body.

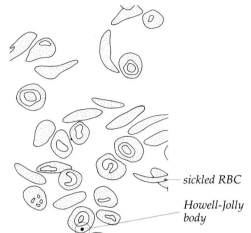

sickled RBC

Howell-Jolly body

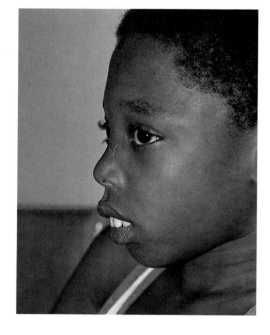

FIG. 11.28 Peripheral smear of SC disease with target cells. Sickled cells are less frequent in this disease than in SS disease.

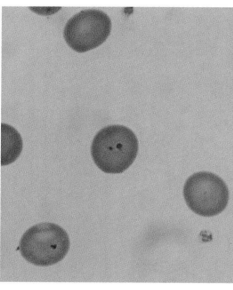

FIG. 11.29 "Heinz body prep" of 2-week-old infant with brisk hemolytic anemia. Note the dark-staining material in two of the red cells.

FIG. 11.30 Maxillary hyperplasia in a child with sickle cell anemia.

lecithin-cholesterol acyltransferase (LCAT) deficiency, characterized by anemia, corneal opacities, hyperlipidemia, proteinuria, chronic nephritis, and premature atherosclerosis, have prominent target cells on peripheral blood smear.

Additionally, targets (or, more accurately, pseudotargets) occur with various hemoglobinopathies. This happens more often in hemoglobin C, but also in hemoglobin S, D, and E (Figs. 11.27, 11.28) due to aggregation of hemoglobin in the central region of the red cell (see Fig. 11.26B).

Intracellular Red Cell Defects

HEMOGLOBINOPATHIES

The hemoglobinopathies often result in a characteristic and even diagnostic peripheral blood smear. They can be responsible for hemolysis due to unstable hemoglobin variants or to altered (decreased) hemoglobin solubility.

Unstable Hemoglobin Variants

Unstable hemoglobin variants, unlike most hemolytic hemoglobinopathies, rarely have a characteristic morphology—although basophilic stippling and Heinz bodies may be noted on special staining of the peripheral blood (Fig. 11.29). The Heinz bodies represent globin aggregates that have precipitated intracellularly. Red cells in Heinz body anemias usually are normocytic, but may be hypochromic as a result of red cell splenic "pitting" of precipitated hemoglobin. Because the precipitated hemoglobin may be mistaken for reticulum, reticulocyte counts may be spuriously high. Methylene blue staining of red cells after they have incubated for a few hours can demonstrate the Heinz bodies. Hemolysis may be mild (Hgb Köln) or brisk (Hgb Bristol), or it may be induced by drugs such as sulfonamides (Hgb Zurich).

Unstable hemoglobinopathies have an autosomal dominant pattern of inheritance, and affected individuals are heterozy-

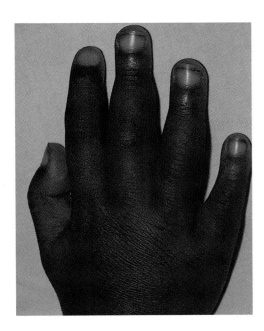

FIG. 11.31 Dactylitis (hand-foot syndrome) in a 3-year-old girl with sickle cell disease. This syndrome, which primarily affects toddlers, is seen less frequently in older children after the bone marrow of the small bones of the hands loses hematopoietic activity.

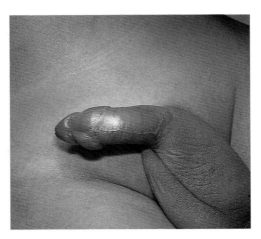

FIG. 11.32 Priapism in an adolescent. Erection had persisted for 12 hours, and had become extremely painful for the patient.

gotes. A homozygous state would, in most cases, be incompatible with life. Congenital Heinz body hemolytic anemia (CHBA) is an important cause of congenital hemolytic anemia. CHBA, though frequently a persistent process in the older infant, has been observed to resolve. At least some of these self-limited cases may represent the presence of unstable gamma hemoglobin which normally disappears as the infant ages. The precipitate-unstable hemoglobin secondarily increases membrane fragility, leading to the hemolysis seen in this disorder.

Sickle Cell Disease

Of the hemoglobinopathies that have altered hemoglobin solubility, none are as well known or as ubiquitous as sickle cell anemia. Substitution of valine for glutamic acid at position six in the beta chain of the hemoglobin molecule leads to the cross-linking of one beta chain to a second beta chain when the hemoglobin is in its deoxygenated state. This cross-linkage tips the solubility balance, leading to the sickling of the red cell (see Fig. 11.27). While sickle cell disease is seen predominantly in black patients, it is by no means exclusive to blacks, with Mediterranean and Middle Eastern peoples also being affected.

The clinical signs and symptoms of sickle cell anemia are due to decreased survival and altered rheology of the sickled red cell. As with any chronic hemolytic state, marrow cavity enlargement occurs, leading to maxillary hyperplasia and the so-called sickle cell facies (Fig. 11.30). Altered rheology, which occurs because sickle cells lose the ability to deform in the microcirculation (see Fig. 11.21) leads to a log-jam phenomenon, causing various tissue infarctions and painful crises. This same log-jamming, when occurring in certain locations, gives rise to clinical manifestations such as dactylitis (Fig. 11.31) in the toddler, priapism (Fig. 11.32), splenic sequestration, and skin ulceration.

It also may lead to the two most life-threatening complications of sickle cell disease: overwhelming infection with encapsulated organisms (most often pneumococcus), and stroke. The increased infectious risk in the sickle cell patient has multiple mechanisms, but by far, the most important are splenic dysfunction due to congested blood flow and then, ultimately,

splenic infarction. Stroke appears to occur only after larger cerebral arteries are damaged due to the effect of altered rheology and sickling in the vasa vasorum and on the nutrient layer of blood flow through these large cerebral vessels.

The sickle cell patient's peripheral smear is diagnostic of a sickling disorder (see Fig. 11.27).

Sickle cell disease is an autosomal recessive disorder with the heterozygote having a significant but less than 50 percent proportion of hemoglobin of the sickle cell type. Heterozygous carriers of the sickle cell gene, while suffering a number of difficulties, (e.g., poor urine-concentrating ability, occasional episodes of renal papillary necrosis with hematuria), have normal life expectancies and are virtually free of any significant consequences of their heterozygote state.

An effective screening test—the Sickle-Dex® or Sickle-Quick®—is widely available. It identifies the child with at least 20 percent hemoglobin S. It is not useful for distinguishing sickle cell disease from the heterozygous sickle cell trait. Additionally, it may fail to detect a hemoglobinopathy on the basis of a non-S hemoglobin and it may also fail to detect a neonate who has not yet started to synthesize significant amounts of S hemoglobin.

Hemoglobin C Disease

Though less common than sickle cell disease, disease associated with hemoglobin C is not rare in the black population. As in sickle cell disease, hemoglobin C disease (Hgb C) occurs due to one amino acid change. The change, again like hemoglobin S, is at the sixth position of the beta chain, but is a lysine rather than a valine replacement. In its homozygous form, Hgb C is a mild disorder characterized by hemolytic anemia and splenomegaly. The tendency of Hgb C to aggregate into precipitates is responsible for the characteristic target (actually a pseudotarget, see Fig. 11.26B) morphology of the Hgb C homozygous and Hgb C trait (heterozygous) cells on the peripheral blood smear (see Fig. 11.28). Vaso-occlusive phenomena are not associated with this disease, though target cells are formed on the dried peripheral blood smear. However, Hgb C, when paired in a double heterozygous state with Hgb S, is associated with vaso-occlusive phenomena, though less severely than Hgb SS.

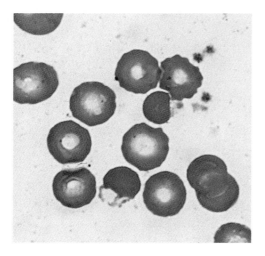

FIG. 11.33 Peripheral smear of patient with G_6PD deficiency in the midst of a hemolytic episode. Note blister cells with hemoglobin condensed in the remaining (nonblistered) portion of the cell.

LIST OF DRUGS USUALLY ASSOCIATED WITH CLINICALLY SIGNIFICANT HEMOLYSIS IN G_6PD DEFICIENCY

Antimalarials	Sulfa Drugs	Miscellaneous
Pamaquine	Salicylazosulfapyridine	Fava beans
Pentaquine	N-Acetylsulfanilamide	Nalidixic acid
Primaquine	Sulfapyridine	Naphthalene
Quinocide	Sulfamethoxypyridazie	Phenylhydrazine
	Thiazolsulfone	Toluidine blue
Antipyretics/Analgesics		Acetylphenylhy-drazine
Acetanilid		
Aminopyrine		
Antipyrine		

FIG. 11.34

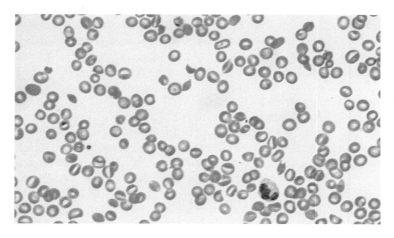

FIG. 11.35 Peripheral blood smear of a child with disseminated intravascular coagulation (DIC) secondary to meningococcemia. Note RBC fragments and decreased platelets.

Red Blood Cell Enzyme Abnormalities

Abnormalities of the RBC enzymes also may lead to hemolysis. While almost any of the RBC enzymes involved in red cell glycolysis or free radical detoxification via the Pentose shunt may be responsible for hemolysis, glucose-6-phosphate-dehydrogenase (G_6PD) deficiency is, by far, the most frequent. A second enzyme, pyruvate kinase, when deficient, also leads to a hemolytic state. Pyruvate kinase deficiency, though far less frequently seen than G_6PD deficiency, is prevalent enough to deserve attention in this discussion. The blood smears of patients with RBC enzyme deficiency-induced hemolysis often are normal though occasionally, with G_6PD deficiency, a suspicious morphology may be present (Fig. 11.33).

Over 75 variants of G_6PD have been identified for which enzyme activity may be elevated or severely deficient. Clinical syndromes may vary as well, with the degree of hemolysis paralleling inversely the level of G_6PD activity. In all instances, the hemolysis is due to the intracellular generation of free radicals and peroxides which fail to be detoxified by the G_6PD-deficient patient.

Chronic hemolysis is extremely mild and only subclinical in the common types. Hemolysis associated with $Gd^{Mediterranean}$ is severe and abrupt and parallels inversely the severe enzyme deficiency. In contrast, hemolysis with Gd^{A-} may be severe but self-limited when the enzyme deficiency is mild. In addition, some agents that trigger hemolysis with $Gd^{Mediterranean}$ may be tolerated by patients with Gd^{A-}. A list of some of the drugs associated with clinically significant hemolysis in G_6PD deficiency is provided (Fig. 11.34).

Pyruvate kinase (PK) deficiency is the second most prevalent enzyme abnormality of the red cell that leads to hemolysis; however, it is a far second, indeed, with one case of pyruvate kinase deficiency occurring worldwide for 500,000 cases of G_6PD deficiency. Like G_6PD deficiency, wide clinical variability exists with PK deficiency. Mild, fully compensated hemolytic anemia may occur, as well as severe neonatal hemolysis and hyperbilirubinemia. Hemoglobins range from 6 to 10 g/dl with normochromic anemia with normocytic or macrocytic indices, depending on the degree of reticulocytosis. The reticulocyte count can range from 5 percent to as high as

CLINICAL EQUIVALENT OF VERIFIED EXPERIMENTAL DIC-TRIGGERING AGENTS

Gram-negative septicemia

Necrotizing enterocolitis

Shock due to any cause

Endothelial damage (virus, bacteria, rickettsia, heat stroke)

Trauma/burns

Ascitic fluid (LaVeen shunt)

Hypoxia-acidosis, severe hyaline membrane disease

Malignancies (acute leukemia, neuroblastoma, rhabdomyosarcoma)

Dead fetal twin

Hemolysis tranfusion reaction

Small for gestational age (placental infarct)

Purpura fulminans

Localized giant hemangioma

FIG. 11.36 (Modified from Corrigan JJ: Disseminated intravascular coagulopathy. Pediatr Rev 1979, 1(2):39)

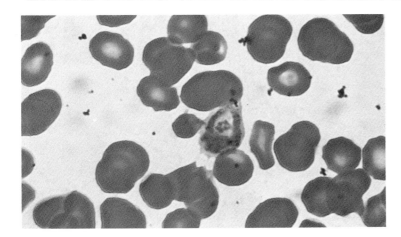

FIG. 11.37 A peripheral blood smear prepared by the so-called "thick prep" method. Plasmodia vivax malaria are seen intracellularly in the RBC in the center of the smear.

90 percent in the splenectomized patient. For the subgroup of patients with severe, transfusion-dependent disease, splenectomy may ameliorate or eliminate the need for transfusions.

HEMOLYSIS CAUSED BY EXTRA RED BLOOD CELL FACTORS
Microangiopathic Hemolysis

Hemolysis of red cells can occur not only due to intrinsic abnormalities of the red cell but also as a result of alterations in the red cell environment. Disseminated intravascular coagulation (DIC), which may be triggered by many differing pathologies, has, as its common manifestation, the hemolysis of RBCs and utilization of platelets and clotting factors. Regardless of the trigger, production of fibrin in the microcirculation and fibrin deposition in capillaries causes shearing of the red cells as they cross these capillary beds (Fig. 11.35). The clinical presentation of DIC is dominated by the clinical presentation of the original disease. In pediatrics, infection with shock is, by far, the most frequent cause of DIC. Patients may manifest petechiae, purpura, and persistent bleeding from

venipunctures. A list of diseases known to trigger DIC is listed in Fig. 11.36.

Localized microangiopathic changes of the peripheral blood smear also may be seen without fully developed DIC. In these instances, the fragmentation of the red cells occurs during transit through the involved organ or tissue (e.g., kidney in hemolytic uremic syndrome, and hemangioma in Kasabach-Merritt syndrome).

Malaria

Malaria is the most frequent cause of hemolysis on a worldwide scale. The patient who contracts the disease after being fed upon by the tropical Anopheles mosquito, is parasitized within the red cells with organisms at the merozoite stage (Fig. 11.37). The parasitization causes a clinical picture of intermittent fever, chills, and jaundice, and may lead to encephalopathy, massive hemolysis with hemoglobinuria (black water fever), and death. The cause of the hemolysis has been attributed to multiple mechanisms, including altered red cell osmotic fragility, membrane loss of negative surface charge,

NORMAL LEUKOCYTE AND DIFFERENTIAL COUNTS*

	12 months	4 years	10 years	21 years
Leukocytes, Total	11.4(6.0-17.5)	9.1(5.5-15.5)	8.1(4.5-13.5)	7.4(4.5-11.0)
Neutrophils, Total	3.5(1.5-8.5) (31%)	3.8(1.5-8.5) (42%)	4.4(1.8-8.0) (54%)	4.4(1.8-7.7) (59%)
Neutrophils, Band Forms	0.35 (3.1%)	0.27(0-1.0) (3.0%)	0.24(0-1.0) (3.0%)	0.22(0-0.7) (3.0%)
Neutrophils, Segmented	3.2 (28%)	3.5(1.5-7.5) (39%)	4.2(1.8-7.0) (51%)	4.2(1.8-7.0) (56%)
Eosinophils	0.30(0.05-0.70) (2.6%)	0.25(0.02-0.65) (2.8%)	0.20(0-0.60) (2.4%)	0.20(0-0.45) (2.7%)
Basophils	0.05(0-10) (0.4%)	0.05(0-0.20) (0.6%)	0.04(0-0.20) (0.5%)	0.04(0-0.20) (0.5%)
Lymphocyte	7.0(4.0-10.5) (61%)	4.5(2.0-8.0) (50%)	3.1(1.5-6.5) (38%)	2.5(1.0-4.8) (34%)
Monocytes	0.55(0.05-1.1) (4.8%)	0.45(0-0.8) (5.0%)	0.35(0-0.8) (4.3%)	0.30(0-0.8) (4.0%)

Values are expressed as cells x 10³/µl. Means values are given; ranges are in parentheses. Percent is for mean values.

FIG. 11.38 (Reproduced by permission from Altman PL, Dittmer DS (eds): Blood and Other Body Fluids, Washington, DC, Federation of American Societies for Experimental Biology, 1961)

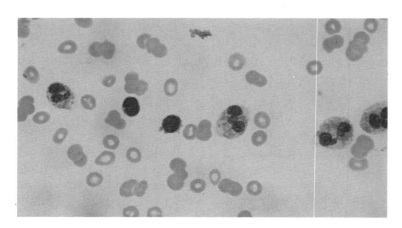

FIG. 11.39 Peripheral blood smear showing neutrophilia and increased band forms (shift to the left) in a child with pneumococcal sepsis.

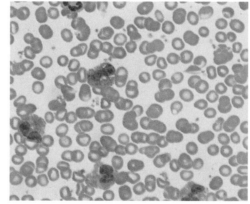

FIG. 11.40 Eosinophilia with an increase in white blood cell count. This patient suffered from a parasitic infection that triggered the increase in eosinophils.

direct injury by the parasite, autoimmunity, splenic pitting, and hypersplenism.

White Blood Cells

Normal values for total white blood cell (WBC) number and differential counts are age-related (Fig. 11.38). Black patients may have lower granulocyte counts than Caucasians of the same age. Both leukocytosis and leukopenia are common pediatric problems. Generally, these are due to increases or decreases in specific types of WBC. Few of the most common causes of neutrophilia (Fig. 11.39), neutropenia, eosinophilia (Fig. 11.40), lymphocytosis (Fig. 11.41), lymphopenia, or monocytosis (Fig. 11.42) are primary hematologic disorders. It will usually be obvious from the clinical context which type of disease is operative in a given case. The pertinent history and

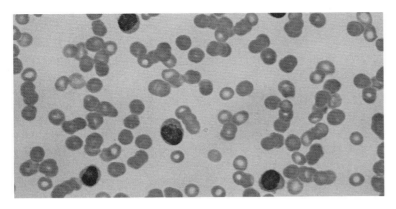

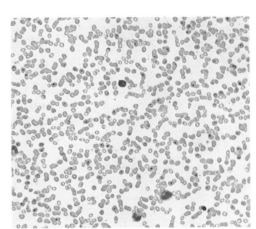

FIG. 11.42 Monocytosis in a child recovering from chemotherapy-related neutropenia.

FIG. 11.41 Lymphocytosis seen in a peripheral blood smear from a child with pertussis.

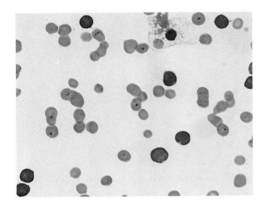

FIG. 11.43 Peripheral blood smear of a child with acute lymphocytic leukemia (ALL). Note the decreased platelets on the smear and the absence of normal WBCs.

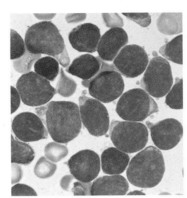

FIG. 11.44 Bone marrow aspirate from the child with ALL whose peripheral blood is shown in Figure 11.45. Note the monotonous pattern of the blastic cells (L1).

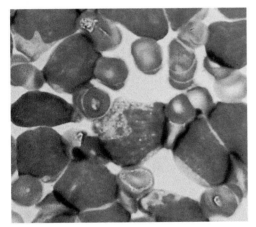

FIG. 11.45 Bone marrow aspirate shows L2 lymphoblasts in another patient with ALL. These lymphoblasts are larger and more heterogeneous in appearance than the L1 lymphoblasts and the nuclear to cytoplasm ratio is lower than that for L1 lymphoblasts. The nucleoli are prominent.

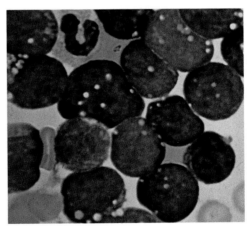

FIG. 11.46 L3 lymphoblasts represent the third morphologic presentation of ALL in this bone marrow aspirate. These lymphoblasts are large deeply staining cells that often are vacuolated.

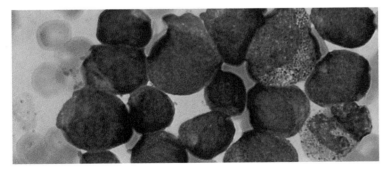

FIG. 11.47 Peripheral blood smear shows an Auer rod (red barlike figure in the cytoplasm) in a myeloblast of a patient with acute non-lymphocytic leukemia (ANLL).

physical findings related to increases or decreases in WBC numbers are outlined throughout this atlas.

LEUKEMIA AND LEUKEMOID REACTIONS

In some cases, a leukocytosis may result from an increase in the number of immature rather than mature WBCs of any given cell line (a so-called "shift to the left"). Leukemia (Fig. 11.43) is the prototype, and Figures 11.44–47 illustrate the varied appearances of blast cells. Figure 11.48 shows a leukemoid reaction, which is characterized by a high white count (usually greater than 50,000/mm³) with an increase in the number of immature myeloid cells.

There are many etiologies for leukemoid reactions, including Down syndrome and sepsis. Leukemoid reactions must be

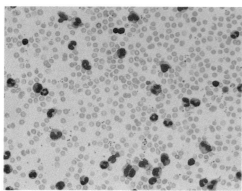

FIG. 11.48
Leukemoid reaction
in a patient with
pneumococcal sepsis.
A higher magnifica-
tion would reveal
toxic granulations
and Döhle bodies (see
Fig. 11.54) in the
polymorphonuclear
leukocytes.

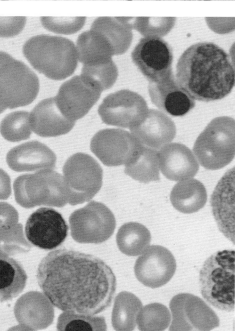

FIG. 11.49
Leukoerythroblastosis
seen on a peripheral
blood smear.

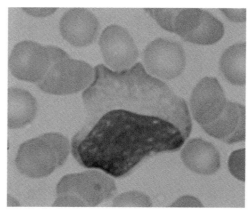

FIG. 11.50 An atypi-
cal lymphocyte from
patient with infec-
tious mononucleosis.
The nucleus is large
and the cytoplasm is
abundant. Note that
where the lymphocyte
cytoplasm abuts a red
cell, the lymphocyte
deforms around it.

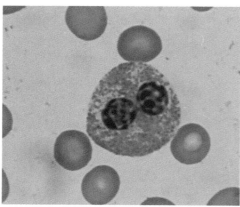

FIG. 11.51 Pelger-
Huët anomaly. Note
the uniform bilobed
nucleus of the
granulocyte.

distinguished from leukemia, and while this is definitively accomplished on the basis of a bone marrow aspirate, peripheral blood studies can facilitate a diagnosis. The leukocyte alkaline phosphatase (LAP) level is increased in leukemoid reaction and decreased in chronic myelogenous leukemia. Another differential diagnostic consideration is that of leukoerythroblastosis (Fig. 11.49) in which increased numbers of immature granulocytes are accompanied on smear by nucleated red cells and red cell fragments, teardrops, target cells, and large platelets. This morphologic picture, in turn, has a long list of causes that includes the spectrum of myeloproliferative disorders ranging from myelofibrosis to chronic myelogenous leukemia, polycythemia vera, or essential thrombopenia.

MORPHOLOGIC ABNORMALITIES

With or without an absolute increase in numbers of specific WBC subsets, there may be morphologic abnormalities in the white blood cell. Increased numbers of young lymphocytes that are not lymphoblasts often are accompanied by morphologic abnormalities, the most common of which is the atypical lymphocyte (Fig. 11.50). This is a large cell with an irregular plasma membrane which often "hugs" adjacent red cells. Its nucleus also is large, and nucleoli may be visible. The abundant cytoplasm is typically basophilic, and may contain vacuoles and azurophilic granules. Morphologic subtypes of atypical lymphocytes may occur, but clinically, their recogni-

tion is of little use. Although infectious mononucleosis comes to mind when atypical lymphocytes are seen, these lymphocytes are not specific, and may be present in many other situations, especially viral illnesses.

Morphologic abnormalities of the granulocytic series, while less common, may provide clues to diagnosis. The hypersegmented neutrophil, which may be an early clue to vitamin B_{12} deficiency, has been noted above (see Fig. 11.14). This needs to be distinguished from familial hypersegmentation by looking at the peripheral smears of family members.

Neutrophil Abnormalities

Occasionally, mature neutrophils may be abnormally large in members of a given family—the so-called hereditary giant neutrophils. The Pelger-Huët anomaly (Fig. 11.51) is sometimes acquired as an adult and generally spurs a search for occult malignancy. However, it carries no such connotation in children. Increased numbers of nuclear appendages also may be seen in the neutrophils of patients with trisomy 13-15 (Fig. 11.52). These, however, may be difficult to distinguish from normal neutrophil "drumsticks," which are nuclear appendages that occur in 2 to 10 percent of neutrophils of normal females.

Vacuoles can occur in any white cell for a variety of reasons, including artifact from anticoagulant, infections, or storage diseases. Certain types of inclusions, such as those seen in

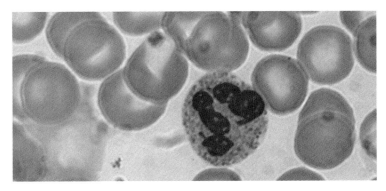

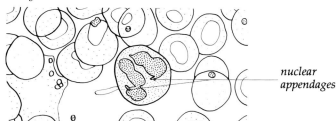

FIG. 11.52 Nuclear appendages, which can be seen normally in female polymorphonuclear leukocytes. An increase in appendages is seen in trisomy 13–15.

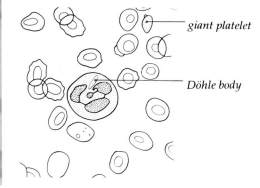

nuclear appendages

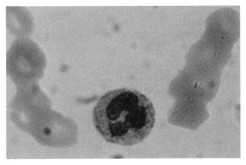

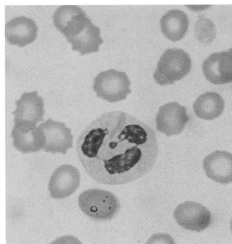

FIG. 11.53 Toxic granulations and a Döhle body are found in child with sepsis. The Döhle body appears as a gray-blue staining area, which in this cell is located at the inferior border of the cell.

FIG. 11.54 The May-Hegglin anomaly showing a Döhle body in the white cell, and giant platelets that may be decreased in number.

giant platelet

Döhle body

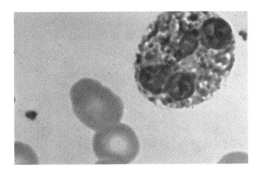

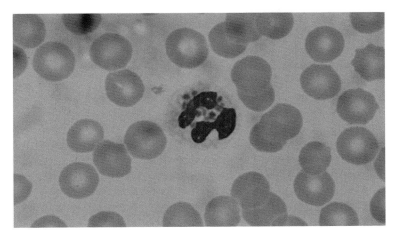

FIG. 11.55 Polymorphonuclear leukocytes with prominent granules characterize Alder-Reilly bodies as seen in Hurler's disease.

FIG. 11.56 Peripheral blood smear of a child with Chédiak-Higashi syndrome. (Courtesy of Dr. William Zinkham)

Gaucher's disease, are limited to bone marrow histiocytes and are not detected on examination of the peripheral smear.

Toxic granulations, which are prominent azurophilic granules, are another common type of white cell inclusion. They are nonspecific, but can be seen in both viral and bacterial infections (Fig. 11.53). Toxic granulations are to be distinguished from the hereditary dense granulation that may occasionally be present in the neutrophils of normal individuals. Döhle bodies, pale blue inclusions that usually are located peripherally in the cytoplasm of neutrophils, may coexist with toxic granulations. Together with giant platelets, Döhle bodies are seen in patients with the dominantly inherited May-Hegglin anomaly (Fig. 11.54).

Alder-Reilly bodies, or Reilly bodies, are metachromatic prominent granules when stained with toluidine blue. When present in any white cells, they are virtually pathognomonic of Hurler's disease (Fig. 11.55). Coarse azurophilic neutrophilic granules that resemble Alder-Reilly bodies but are nonmetachromatic have been reported in Batten disease. Likewise, large greenish-brown neutrophil inclusions are characteristic of the rare patient with Chediak-Higashi syndrome (Fig. 11.56). Such granules may appear in eosinophils and basophils as well.

White cells also may acquire inclusions by engulfing particles from their surroundings. Erythrophagocytosis (Fig. 11.57) is a nonspecific finding that is presumably immune-mediated

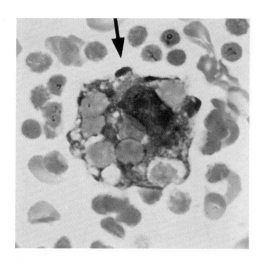

FIG. 11.57 Prominent erythrophagocytosis in which numerous RBCs are engulfed by white cell cytoplasm.

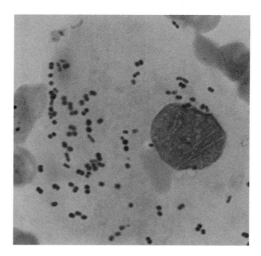

FIG. 11.58 Intracellular bacteria on Wright's stain of a buffy coat smear from a neutropenic patient. Note the numerous darkly stained bacteria in the cytoplasm.

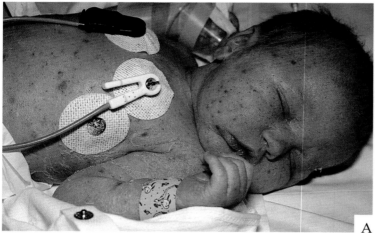

A

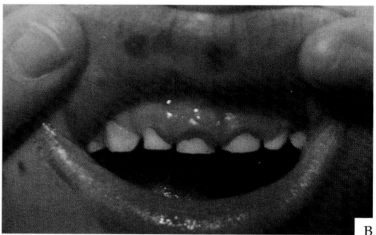

B

FIG. 11.59 **A**, tiny petechiae and larger ecchymosis in an infant with severe immune thrombocytopenia. **B**, purpura occurring on the oral mucosa or retina is called "wet purpura," and may suggest an increased tendency for major bleeding in the thrombopenic patient.

and seen in viral infections and primary diseases of the reticuloendothelial system. LE cells of systemic lupus erythematosus are a diagnostically useful example of cellular phagocytosis, although in general, they are not seen on routine peripheral blood smears. Figure 11.58 shows a buffy coat preparation from a patient with suspected sepsis, demonstrating intracellular bacteria. In most of these white cell anomalies, the clinical diagnosis will often be suspected on the basis of presenting signs and symptoms even before the hematologic abnormality is identified. One exception to this rule is the toddler with moderate to severe neutropenia which may be chronic yet benign. Many of these children will be entirely asymptomatic, and the neutropenia is an incidental finding. However, chronic benign neutropenia is a diagnosis of exclusion. The differential diagnosis is reviewed elsewhere.

Bleeding Disorders

Excessive bleeding or bruising is a common complaint during childhood. The hematologic causes (to be distinguished from child abuse, trauma, vascular anomalies, etc.) fall into two categories: disorders of platelets and coagulopathies. The child with mucocutaneous bleeding or purpura (petechiae or ecchymoses [Fig. 11.59A,B]) is most likely to fall into the first; bleeding into deep tissue or joints is most likely to be a reflection of the second. Patients with either of these problems may have

bleeding precipitated by trauma or surgery, and may develop hematuria, guaiac-positive stools, menorrhagia, or CNS bleeding. Frequent epistaxis, while possibly related to bleeding disorders, is more likely to have a nonhematologic cause such as nose picking, dry mucous membranes, or rarely, hypertension. Nonetheless, documentation of these problems or a positive family history will usually call for laboratory evaluation, which will likely include a CBC, differential, and platelet count, and a basic coagulation workup consisting of measurements of prothrombin time (PT) and partial thromboplastin time (PTT). It should be noted that not all children with purpura are thrombocytopenic.

PLATELET DISORDERS

A CBC and peripheral blood smear will reveal a platelet count which, if normal, is in the 150,000/mm^3 to 450,000/mm^3 range. The smear will not give information regarding the less often seen diseases of platelet function, but it will confirm quantitative abnormalities. Clinically, thrombocytopenia may be inapparent until counts are significantly depressed below normal, and frank purpura is infrequently seen with counts greater than 20,000/mm^3. It is important to ascertain that the decreased platelet number is not a spurious finding by repeating the test and reviewing the blood smear. The child whose peripheral blood smear is shown in Figure 11.54, unfortunately underwent a splenectomy for presumed idiopathic throm-

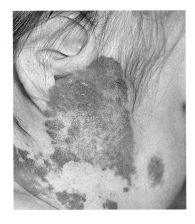

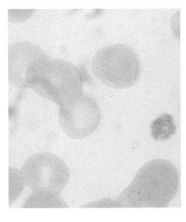

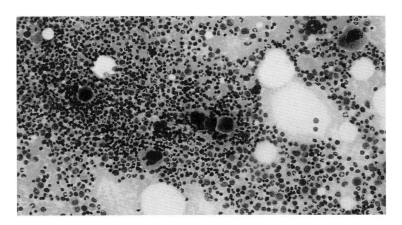

FIG. 11.60 Hemangioma of child with Kasabach-Merritt sydrome.

FIG. 11.61 Megathrombocyte in the peripheral blood of a patient with idiopathic thrombocytopenic purpura (ITP).

FIG. 11.62 Bone marrow aspirate in ITP, with prominent megakaryocytes. In children with thrombocytopenia—on the basis of decreased platelet production—megakaryocytes will be decreased in number.

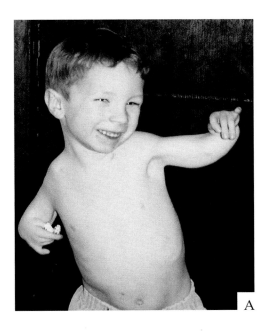

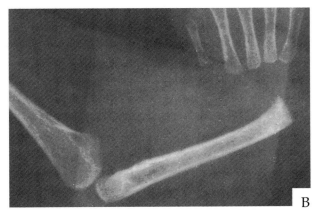

A

B

FIG. 11.63 A, child with TAR syndrome. B, radiograph of the same patient. Note the absence of radii.

bocytopenic purpura (ITP). However, the platelet count persistently was reported as less than 20,000/mm³, while the manually performed platelet count number was considerably higher. The Coulter counter had ignored these large platelets and incorrectly counted them as WBCs.

Isolated thrombocytopenia may result either from decreased production or from increased destruction. The etiologies for the latter are numerous, and include the idiopathic or immune thrombocytopenias, hypersplenism, DIC, consumption related to intracardiac defect or bypass surgery, washout from exchange transfusion, local microangiopathic disease (hemolytic uremic syndrome), or local thrombosis (renal vein thrombosis).

DIC has already been discussed as a cause of hemolysis and occurs most often in the pediatric age range as a secondary phenomenon due to shock in bacterial, or less frequently, viral sepsis (see Fig. 11.40). DIC also is seen in Kasabach-Merritt syndrome when platelet consumption occurs within the endothelial maze of massive strawberry and cavernous hemangiomas (Fig. 11.60).

The clinical setting often helps in distinguishing when thrombocytopenia is due to destruction as opposed to reduced

production, and in identifying the more immediate reason for the pathophysiology. Some combination of peripheral blood smear, bone marrow aspirate, antiplatelet antibody testing, and/or therapeutic trial of intravenous high dose gammaglobulin may define the diagnosis. The peripheral smear may reveal large platelets (megathrombocytes) (Fig. 11.61). The bone marrow may show abundant megakaryocytes (Fig. 11.62) and no infiltrative process. Antiplatelet antibodies may be present, and the patient may respond quickly to the gammaglobulin. All this may suggest ITP. Isoimmune thrombocytopenia seen in the newborn period occurs when fetal platelets cross the placenta into the maternal circulation and may, dependent on the platelet antigens, trigger a maternal production of IgG aimed at the foreign fetal platelet antigen. These antiplatelet antibodies can now cross the placenta and lead to infant thrombocytopenia.

Patients with isolated thrombocytopenia on the basis of failure of production will have decreased or absent megakaryocyte precursors. Differentiation of the various causes of decreased production, such as thrombocytopenia-absent radius (TAR) syndrome (Fig. 11.63) and amegakaryocytic thrombocytopenia, may rest on clinical findings. Patients with

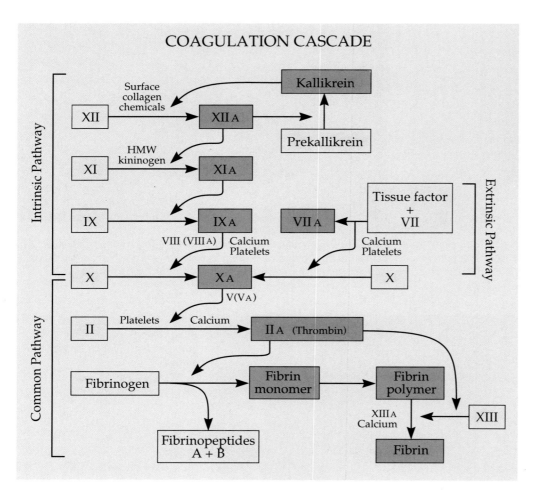

COAGULATION CASCADE

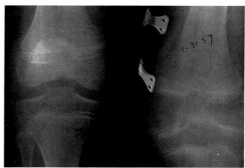

FIG. 11.65 Hemophiliac arthritis following recurrent hemarthroses. Note the widened joint space on the left knee as compared to that of the normal right knee.

FIG. 11.64 The prothrombin time (PT) measures the extrinsic/common pathway, while the partial thromboplastin time (PTT) measures the intrinsic/common pathway.

TAR syndrome may have a number of other congenital problems such as leukemoid reactions, congenital heart disease, and failure to thrive. Their thrombocytopenia will frequently resolve as they grow older. Rarely, thrombocytopenia may be due to a combination of decreased production and increased destruction. This can be seen in sepsis, collagen diseases, and Wiskott-Aldrich syndrome.

Qualitative or functional platelet defects may also lead to a bleeding diathesis. In the setting of normal platelet number and normal clotting studies, the possibility of poorly functioning platelets needs to be considered. The bleeding time in the child with a platelet count greater than 100,000/mm³ is probably the simplest and best test of platelet function, although it can also be abnormal in diseases of connective tissue (e.g., Ehlers-Danlos). The highly specialized tests necessary to confirm a diagnosis of platelet dysfunction are available in most large centers. Information in addition to that mentioned above, which may point to a reason for platelet dysfunction, includes a history of drug exposure either by direct ingestion by the patient or, in some cases, via breast feeding (aspirin alone or as a component of another medication is the best known, and will affect platelet studies for the 7- to 10-day life of the platelet), history of uremia, hypothyroidism, hyperbilirubinemia, and inflammatory bowel disease. Von Willebrand's disease (VWD) is a relatively common disorder in which the bleeding time is generally increased with or without an increase in the PTT. VWD usually is inherited in an autosomal dominant fashion, although it may also occur sporadically. It is not strictly a disorder of platelet function; rather, the disease is caused by an abnormality of the factor VIII molecule which binds platelets to the endothelium. The tendency to bleed may vary from patient to patient and from time to time in any given patient. Patients frequently are asymptomatic, being detected when an abnormal bleeding time or PTT is noted as part of a preoperative screen or when mucosal bleeding such as menorrhagia is demonstrated. Hemarthroses are not generally seen in children with von Willebrand's disease, even when the PTT is prolonged.

COAGULOPATHIES

Coagulopathies occur when the circulating factors necessary for normal coagulation are deficient from either lack of production of excessive consumption. Coagulopathies can occur either as genetic defects, as in the decreased production of normal procoagulants (hemophilia) or as acquired conditions resulting in depressed factor production (vitamin K deficiency, liver disease) or over-utilization of factors (DIC).

Whatever the cause of coagulopathy, the measurement of the partial thromboplastin time (PTT) and prothrombin time (PT) are the first steps in clarifying the diagnosis. The clotting system is shown in Figure 11.64. The PTT evaluates the intrinsic and common pathway while the PT evaluates the extrinsic

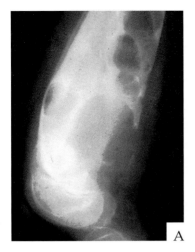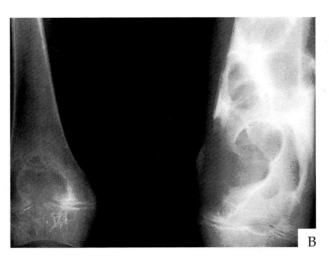

FIG. 11.66 **A**, pseudotumor of the femur due to recurrent hemarthroses with subsequent bony destruction of the knee and adjacent bony structure. **B**, note that the opposite knee also demonstrates early destructive changes in the distal femur and joint.

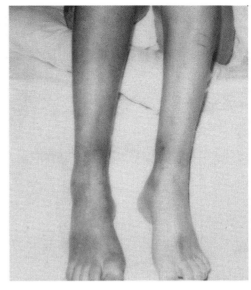

FIG. 11.67 Swollen, discolored leg in a child with deep venous thrombosis due to protein C deficiency. (Courtesy of Dr. R. Kellogg)

and common pathway. Values for these screening tests are age-related so that normal newborns, especially premature infants, have prolonged PTs and PTTs compared with older children. These screening tests, while sensitive enough to detect the mild, moderate, or severe deficiencies of hemophilia, will be normal in carriers with approximately 50 percent factor levels.

Hemophilia A and B

While deficiencies have been reported for every procoagulant, factor VIII deficiency (hemophilia A) and factor IX deficiency (hemophilia B) make up the vast majority of hemophilias. Because both hemophilia A and B are transmitted in an X-linked recessive inheritance pattern, hemophilia is found nearly always in males. Hemophiliacs may have variable degrees of factor deficiency and commensurate levels of clinical disease. Patients with mild hemophilia have factor activity between 5 and 30 percent, and in general, only suffer from bleeding if they undergo surgery or suffer major trauma. Patients with moderate hemophilia have a factor activity of 1 to 5 percent, and suffer localized hemorrhage in response to trauma. Finally, patients with less than 1 percent factor activity (the most frequent genotype) have spontaneous soft tissue hemorrhage or bleeding associated with only minor trauma.

Patients with hemophilia often present in the newborn period at the time of circumcision. Those infants who escape clinical problems at that time generally do not present until 12 to 18 months of age—when they have become more mobile and minor trauma from falls precipitates bleeding. Although the clinical manifestations of hemophilia can affect any organ, the musculoskeletal, CNS, and urinary systems predominate. The most common of the clinical manifestations include hemarthroses and soft-tissue bleeding with intramuscular hematomas. Secondary hemophiliac arthropathy also may occur, with knees, elbows, and ankles being the most commonly involved joints. Recurrent, untreated hemorrhages may lead to contractures (Fig. 11.65) and painful arthritis (Fig. 11.66). Finally, intramuscular bleeding can cause compartment syndromes with secondary peripheral nerve palsies.

Decreases in clotting factor production may be acquired as well as inherited. Hepatic synthesis of clotting factors may be depressed in the vitamin K-deficient patients. Vitamin K deficiency in the newborn may be suggested by cephalohematomas, bleeding from scalp or mouth sites, or intracranial hemorrhage, particularly if there has been inadvertent omission of prophylactic vitamin K administration, breast feeding, antibiotics, or maternal ingestion of vitamin K inhibitors in the last trimester.

The PT, PTT, or both tests, may be prolonged for a variety of reasons other than hemophilia or depressed factor production. The presence of acquired inhibitors of coagulation (lupus-like anticoagulants), which most often are defined in a coagulation laboratory by "mixing" studies, is one such reason. Children who have received antibiotics, especially the penicillins, may develop inhibitors which may persist for even months after discontinuation of medication. Although lupus anticoagulants have been associated with thrombotic and bleeding events, the lupus-like anticoagulants in otherwise well children have been associated with neither. DIC with consumption of clotting factors, as well as platelets, will also prolong the PTT and PT (see Fig. 11.35).

Far less common than bleeding, thrombotic events may also occur. Once again, either inherited deficiency of anticoagulants (protein C and S, antithrombin III) (Fig. 11.67) or acquired alteration in normal coagulation balance (paroxysmal nocturnal hemoglobinuria, tumors, nephrotic syndrome, deep catheter, dehydration, and medications) are possible.

Pancytopenia

Pancytopenia refers to a reduction in all three formed elements of the blood. In an analogous manner to anemia, pancytopenia is not a single disease entity but rather may result from a number of disease processes. Pancytopenia may occur due to bone marrow failure or to extramedullary cellular destruction (as seen in autoimmune disease, particularly SLE), or as a combination of depressed marrow function and increased cellular

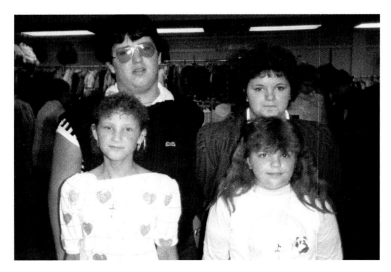

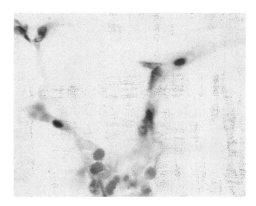

FIG. 11.69 Bone marrow biopsy of patient with acquired aplastic anemia. Stromal marrow cells are present with virtually no hematopoietic cells.

FIG. 11.68 A patient with Fanconi's anemia (shortly after bone marrow transplantation) and her three siblings. The patient (front left) presented with a hemoglobin of 3.5 g/dl, short stature, and increased skin pigmentation. Note the patient's diminutive size with respect to her more robust siblings.

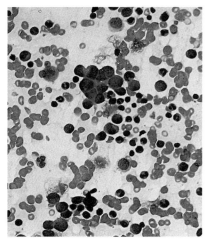

FIG. 11.70 Pseudorosettes (clumps of tumor cells) are particularly characteristic of a neuroblastoma metastasized to the bone marrow.

destruction. When pancytopenia is due to destruction of the formed elements of the blood, invariably there is another underlying disease. On the other hand, the pancytopenia due to bone marrow failure can be divided into genetically predisposed (constitutional) marrow failure syndromes, acquired marrow failure syndromes, and marrow replacement.

The most frequent of the constitutional marrow failure syndromes is Fanconi's anemia. Fanconi's anemia is a familial disorder marked by the association of pancytopenia and marrow hypoplasia with a variable constellation of congenital anomalies of the skin, skeleton, central nervous system, and genitourinary tract (Fig. 11.68). Fragility of the chromosomes further characterizes this syndrome, and it occurs even in the absence of physical anomalies. Patients can present with anemia very early in life but generally develop signs of marrow failure in mid childhood. The abnormal chromosomes are the most characteristic laboratory finding and chromosome breaks, gaps, and rearrangements are common.

Acquired marrow failure syndromes (aplastic anemia) occur as a result of an insult to the bone marrow from a variety of sources including drugs, toxins, solvents and radiation, as well as autoimmune and postinfectious disorders. Nevertheless a full 50 percent of aplastic anemia cases have no apparent insulting agent and are idiopathic in origin.

The clinical course of aplastic anemia from any of these causes is that of inexorable bone marrow failure with anemia, thrombocytopenia and leukopenia, leading ultimately to death from bleeding or infection if spontaneous recovery or successful intervention fails to occur.

While the peripheral smear will reveal a paucity of platelets and WBCs with a low reticulocyte count and normochromic normocytic anemia, a marrow biopsy generally is needed to clarify the diagnosis (Fig. 11.69).

Marrow replacement, another cause of pancytopenia, occurs either with a hematopoietic malignancy such as leukemia (see Fig. 11.44) or from solid tumors invading the marrow (Fig. 11.70). Both a direct "crowding out" phenomenon and an alteration of the marrow "milieu" appear to contribute to marrow failure.

ONCOLOGY
Cancer in Children

Almost 7,000 new cases of cancer in children less than 15 years of age are reported in the United States each year, reflecting an annual incidence of approximately 10/100,000. Whereas mortality was once the rule, it is now less than 40 percent. Thus, the majority of children with cancer have a curable illness.

The job of recognizing the signs and symptoms of malignancy usually falls to the pediatrician or family practitioner. In this section, we will highlight most of the common and some of the exotic presentations which should raise suspicion that a child may have cancer, with a view toward facilitating prompt referral to a pediatric oncologist. For details about specific cancers and their management we recommend more comprehensive texts.

Signs and Symptoms

Red flags which signal malignancy—both leukemias and solid tumors—may be detected in the course of history taking, physical examination, or review of a few basic laboratory tests. These may be direct effects of tumor (mass effects) or secondary to "humors" produced by cancerous or reactive cells (so-called paraneoplastic syndromes). The child with cancer may be entirely asymptomatic when routine physical exam suggests an abnormality. However, frequent nonspecific systemic complaints include fatigue, weight loss, fever (which may or may not have a discernable pattern or an infectious source), and night sweats (most commonly but not exclusively associated with Hodgkin's disease). Less common systemic complaints include diarrhea, failure to thrive, and pruritus

GROUPS AT HIGH RISK OF CANCER*

Hereditary cutaneous syndromes (xeroderma pigmentosum)

Neurocutaneous syndromes (neurofibromatosis)

Chromosomal abnormalities (Down syndrome, Bloom syndrome)

Hereditary or acquired immunodeficiency (ataxia-telangiectasia)

Autoimmune diseases

Congenital malformations or syndromes (hemihypertrophy, Beckwith-Weidemann syndrome)

Sibling with cancer

History of prior cancer

Intrauterine (diethylstilbestrol) or postnatal (chemotherapy immunosuppression), irradiation

Metabolic diseases (alpha$_1$ antitrypsin deficiency)

*Disease category followed by example

FIG. 11.71

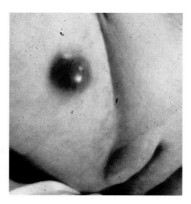

FIG. 11.72 Subcutaneous nodule in child with neuroblastoma. Lesions, which occasionally may be seen with leukemia or other solid tumors, may be dark ("blueberry muffin") or skin-colored. (From Pearson H: Tumors of the sympathetic nervous system, in Altman AJ, Schwartz AD (eds): Malignant Diseases of Infancy, Childhood, and Adolescence, ed 2. WB Saunders, Philadelphia, 1983, 368–388)

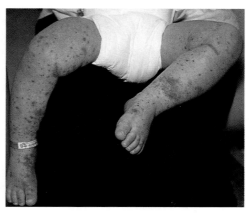

FIG. 11.73 Purpuric lesions in a child with neuroblastoma and tumor-related coagulopathy. Similar lesions may be due to isolated thrombocytopenia.

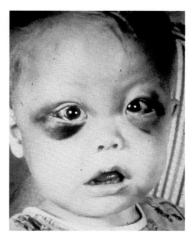

FIG. 11.74 Raccoon eyes, indicative of retroorbital tumor (usually neuroblastoma), may involve supra- or infraorbital areas. "Shiners" due to trauma or abuse may be part of differential diagnosis. (Courtesy of H. Pearson, Yale-New Haven Hospital)

(again, associated with Hodgkin's disease). Among the more localizing complaints are headaches and vomiting which are often but not always most prominent in the morning (brain tumors), constipation or voiding difficulty (pelvic tumors), hypertension (renal tumors, neuroblastoma, or pheochromocytoma), bone pain and/or limp (due to cortical lesions of primary bone or metastatic tumors, or to extensive intramedullary disease as in leukemia).

All of these complaints are more likely to have an etiology which is not malignant. However, persistence (2 weeks is a reasonable though not absolute guideline) or undue severity may give these red flags increased significance. Similarly, in the context of a number of predisposing, underlying diseases (Fig. 11.71), malignancy should be considered earlier. Certainly, children with a history of one cancer, by virtue of genetics or as a "late effect" of anticancer therapy, are at greater risk of a second cancer. Cancer in a parent or sibling, while heightening anxiety about the possibility of cancer in a child, is rarely, by itself, a major predisposing factor. The notable exception is the infant or toddler who has an identical twin with leukemia. In this child, the risk may be as high as 25 percent.

Specific physical findings may be sought when a particular diagnosis is suspected. For example, subcutaneous nodules should be looked for in infants with neuroblastoma (Fig. 11.72). However, even without knowledge about particular tumors, careful physical examination will disclose signs of malignancy in addition to those mentioned above. What follows is a listing of such signs by organ system.

SKIN

Examination of the skin should be complete, to look for cancerous lesions and cutaneous manifestations of extracutaneous cancers, as well as to pick up signs of a variety of precancerous or cancer-associated diagnoses (Fig. 11.71). Even in Caucasian children, skin color may be deceptive. Thus, pallor, a result of anemia, may be most readily appreciated by examination of subconjunctival or palmar creases (see Hematology section). Purpura, small petechiae or large ecchymoses, (see Hematology Section) are most common on the lower extremities or at sites of trauma, but they should be sought elsewhere on the body including on the retina or oral mucosa ("wet purpura"). Easy bruisability usually is due to thrombocytopenia, although patients with platelet counts greater than 20,000/mm^3 may well have no spontaneous bleeding tendency. Infrequently, purpura may be due to coagulopathy without thrombocytopenia (Fig. 11.73). Bleeding at a particular location may suggest a more specific diagnosis. For example, racoon eyes (Fig. 11.74) are periorbital ecchymoses attributable to

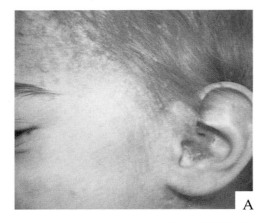

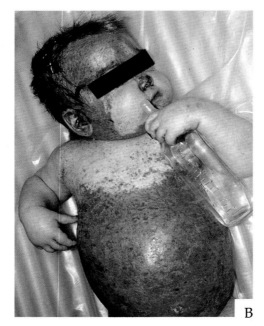

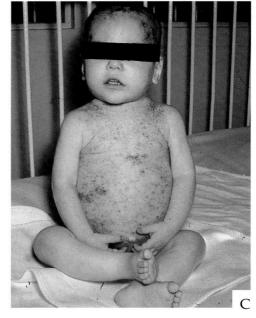

FIG. 11.75 **A**, seborrhea in infant with histiocytosis X. **B**, hemorrhagic or **C**, papular rashes also are seen in some children with this group of diseases. (Courtesy of Dr.P.Gaffney, Children's Hospital of Pittsburgh)

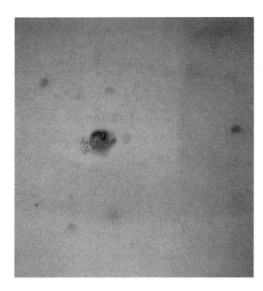

FIG. 11.76 Melanoma. In addition to location (see text), suspicious signs are red-brown-black color that tends to be diffuse at the periphery, crusting, bleeding, pain, or itcing.

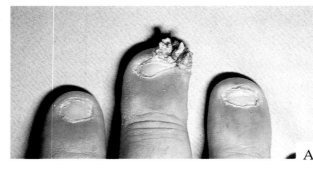

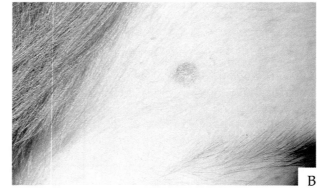

FIG. 11.77 **A**, squamous cell carcinoma. **B**, basal cell carcinoma on forehead of a seven-year-old boy who had received prophylactic cranial radiation as part of his treatment for acute lymphoblastic leukemia 5 years before he developed a second cancer. (**A**, courtesy of Dr. J. Zitelli, University of Pittsburgh School of Medicine. **B**, reproduced by permission from Pratt CB, Douglass EC: Management of the uncommon cancer of childhood, in Pizzo PA, Poplack DG (eds): **Principles and Practice of Pediatric Oncology.** Philadelphia, JB Lippincott, 1988, 759–182)

retroorbital tumor, notably neuroblastoma; isolated vaginal bleeding may be seen with rhabdomyosarcoma or yolk sac tumors arising in the vagina; gross or microscopic hematuria is sometimes seen in children with Wilms' tumor.

Seborrhea, which is usually a benign finding, may be one of the cutaneous manifestations of histiocytosis X (Fig. 11.75A-C; see Chapter 8, Dermatology), in which disease it can be more or less severe. Melanoma (Fig. 11.76), though extremely rare in childhood, is most likely to result from transformation of pigmented or junctional nevi. These precancerous lesions should be removed prophylactically when they occur on the palms, soles, genitalia, anorectal mucosa, nail beds, or lower extremities. Squamous and basal cell carcinomas (Fig. 11.77A,B) arise most often in the setting of heritable diseases such as xeroder-

ma pigmentosum or basal cell nevus syndrome. Although Kaposi's sarcoma has been described in only 1 percent of pediatric AIDS patients (predominantly in the adenopathic form), the increasing incidence of AIDS makes recognition of the cutaneous manifestations (see Chapter 4, Allergy and Immunology) important.

HEAD AND NECK

Findings on head, eyes, ears, nose, and throat (HEENT) exam may include macrocephaly, bulging fontanelle, and/or superficial venous distension due to increased intracranial pressure and hydrocephalus from primary or metastatic tumor involving the brain (Fig. 11.78). Chronic draining ears (Fig. 11.79A,B) and inappropriate loosening of teeth are seen with histiocyto-

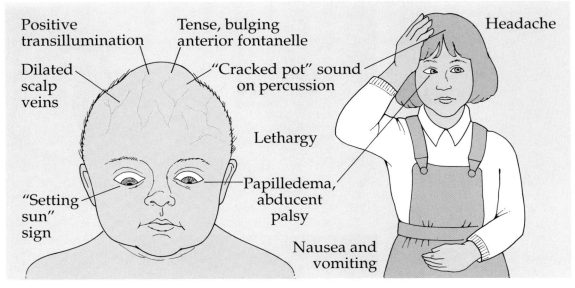

Positive transillumination

Dilated scalp veins

"Setting sun" sign

Tense, bulging anterior fontanelle

"Cracked pot" sound on percussion

Lethargy

Papilledema, abducent palsy

Nausea and vomiting

Headache

FIG. 11.78 Macrocephaly and superficial venous distension secondary to increased intracranial pressure in an infant with a CNS glioma. The older child may, instead, show changes in mental status, vomiting, or focal neurologic signs. (Reproduced by permission from Resident and Staff Physician, November 1980, by Romaine Pierson Publishers, Inc.)

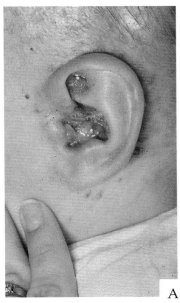

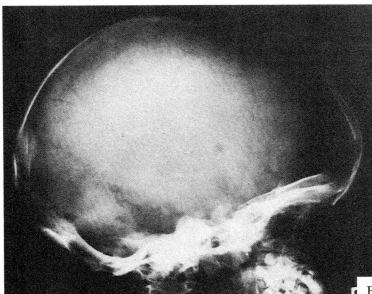

A

B

FIG. 11.79 **A**, otorrhea in child with histiocytosis. **B**, x-ray shows destruction of mastoid bone in same child. (**A**, courtesy of Dr. P. Gaffney, Children's Hospital of Pittsburgh)

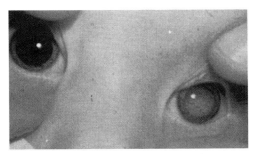

FIG. 11.80 Cat's eye reflex or leukocoria in child with retinoblastoma. (Reproduced by permission from Abramson D: Retinoblastoma. CA 1982; 32:133)

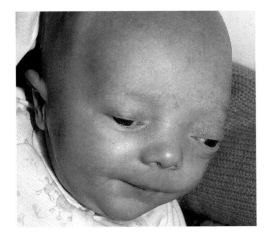

FIG. 11.81 Proptosis in child with retroorbital rhabdosarcoma. Note also, large head secondary to increased intracranial pressure. (Courtesy of Dr. V. Albo, Children's Hospital of Pittsburgh)

sis. Otorrhea also may be seen with other head and neck tumors such as rhabdomyosarcoma.

Ocular Findings

Cat's eye reflex or leukocoria with an absent red reflex are characteristic of retinoblastoma (see Chapter 19, Ophthalmology) and should be sought as part of the routine physical in the neonate and young child. This is often best appreciated from a frontal photograph of the child (Fig. 11.80), and therefore may be brought to the attention of a physician by a parent. Strabismus (see Chapter 19, Ophthalmology), particularly when first seen after infancy, may be a sign of an orbital tumor or intracranial pathology, and even if intermittent, merits attention. Similarly, proptosis (Fig. 11.81), characteristic of orbital rhabdomyosarcoma or histiocytosis, also deserves attention.

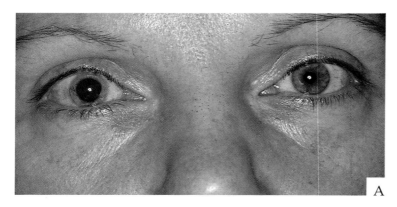
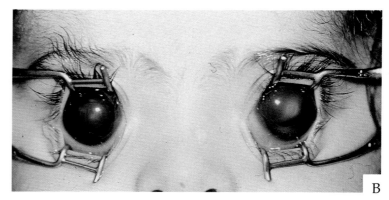

FIG. 11.82 **A**, heterochromia iridis in adult who had had Wilms' tumor as a child. **B**, aniridia. (**A**, courtesy of Dr. J. Roen)

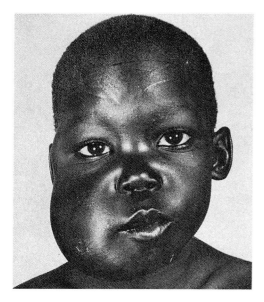

FIG. 11.83 Burkitt's lymphoma of the jaw in African child. (Courtesy of Dr. I. Magrath, National Cancer Institute)

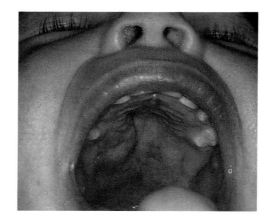

FIG. 11.84 Intraoral extension of intracranial rhabdomyosarcoma. The lesion was first detected by the child's dentist, and biopsied by an ENT specialist who did not suspect malignancy.

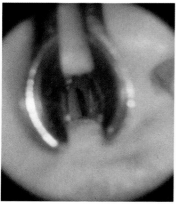
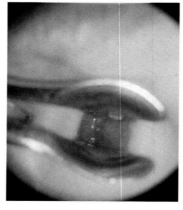

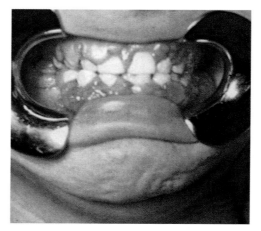

FIG. 11.86 Gingival hypertrophy due to leukemic invasion of gums. (Reproduced by permission from Bluefarb, SM: Dermatology. Kalamazoo, MI, Upjohn, 1984)

FIG. 11.85 Intranasal glioma occluding right nostril. The normal left nostril is also shown. (Courtesy of Dr. S. Stool, Children's Hospital of Pittsburgh)

Heterochromia (Fig. 11.82A), usually a benign oddity, may be associated with Wilms' tumor or with cervicothoracic neuroblastoma (pre- or postoperatively, where it occurs alone or as part of Horner's syndrome). Aniridia (Fig. 11.82B), when it occurs sporadically and not as an autosomal dominant trait, also has been associated with Wilms' tumor.

Orofacial Findings

Although masses such as the jaw lesion shown in Figure 11.83 will likely be referred early to an oncologist, intraoral (Fig. 11.84) or intranasal (Fig. 11.85) masses are more likely to masquerade as nonmalignant lesions, which may forestall correct diagnosis. These may be entirely asymptomatic or they may cause local bleeding or difficulty in swallowing or breathing. Gingival hyperplasia can be seen in children with leukemia, especially the acute myelomonocytic kind (Fig. 11.86).

While most physicians look for cervical adenopathy, it is important to remember the other lymph node groups which may be involved by focal or generalized adenopathy in leukemias, lymphomas, or solid tumors. A schematic diagram

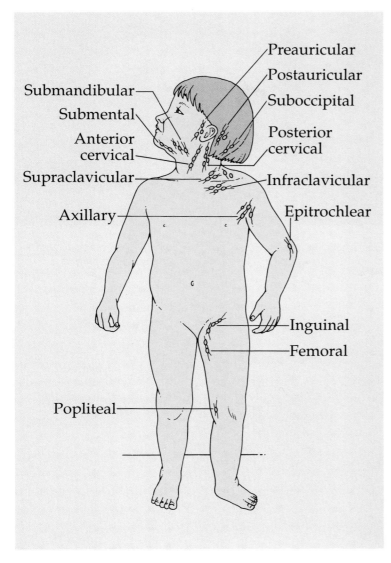

FIG. 11.87 Lymph node regions palpable on physical exam. Rarely, retroperitoneal nodes may become so enlarged as to be palpable.

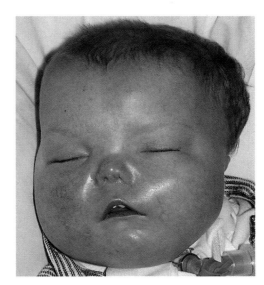

FIG. 11.88 Superior vena cava syndrome. Discoloration of the face and neck with venous distention. The mediastinal masses which produce these findings may pose considerable anesthetic risk.

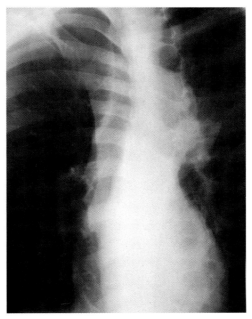

FIG. 11.89 Paravertebral mass and associated scoliosis.

depicting the major lymph node regions is presented in Figure 11.87. Although large, rock-hard nodes that are fixed to the subcutaneous tissue are most convincing for malignancy, texture and size can be misleading. Because Hodgkin's disease and non-Hodgkin's lymphoma can both occur concurrently with or following infectious mononucleosis, a positive mono spot test may be a false reassurance. Therefore, persistent adenopathy, even in that setting, should be followed closely. The algorithms for workup of adenopathy and indications for biopsy are reviewed in Chapter 12, Infectious Diseases.

In addition to the lymph nodes, examination of the neck may disclose jugular venous distension which may be subtle or fulminant, and associated with varying degrees of facial fullness, plethora, and respiratory distress (Fig. 11.88). The superior vena cava syndrome is an oncologic emergency which may be caused by any mediastinal mass, but in pediatrics, the most common etiology is lymphoma (Hodgkin's disease or non-Hodgkin's lymphoma). Goiters or nodular thyroids with or without bruits may be seen in patients with thyroid carcinoma.

CHEST

External examination of the chest may disclose obvious skeletal or other chest wall masses which may be asymptomatic or associated with localizing or pleuritic pain. Scoliosis has been associated with paravertebral tumors (Fig. 11.89). Respiratory distress may be due to an intrathoracic process or abdominal distension from a mass or ascites. Wheezing or cough commonly are due to airway compression by a mediastinal mass (see below). However, such tumors are most likely to be asymptomatic. They are detected on chest x-ray performed for some other reason, or as part of a staging workup in a child in whom cancer is suspected or diagnosed on the basis of some other findings.

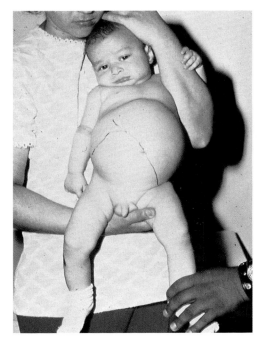

FIG. 11.90
Abdominal swelling with hepatospleno-megaly in child with neuroblastoma. (Reproduced by per-mission from Pearson H: Malignant Diseases of Adolescents in Childhood. *Philadelphia, WB Saunders)*

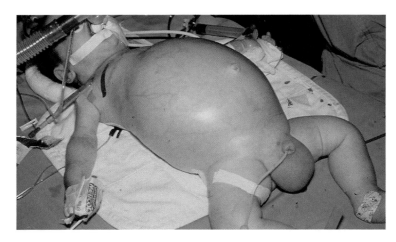

FIG. 11.91 *Superficial venous distension in child with intraabdominal tumor. (Courtesy of Dr. D. Nakayama, Children's Hospital of Pittsburgh)*

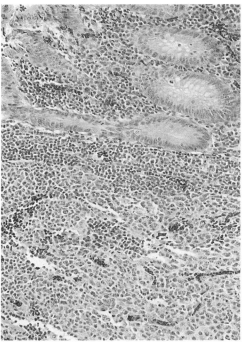

FIG. 11.92
Microscopic picture of the appendix, showing involvement with non-Hodgkin's lymphoma. Malignant cells, pre-dominating in the lower half of the slide, are large, with clear cytoplasm, and irreg-ularly shaped nuclei.

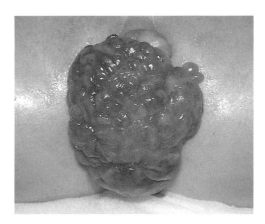

FIG. 11.93 *Sarcoma botryoides in child with multiple con-genital anomalies. Note grape-like appearance of lesion.*

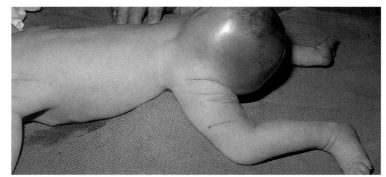

FIG. 11.94 *Sacrococcygeal teratoma.*

ABDOMEN

An observant parent may be the first person to detect abdomi-nal swelling or mass (see Chapter 17, Surgery) which may be due to hepato- and/or splenomegaly (Fig. 11.90), the flank mass of Wilms' tumor, the often more centrally located retroperitoneal neuroblastoma, other intraabdominal tumors, or ascites. Superficial venous distension (Fig. 11.91) may signal deep venous obstruction related to intraabdominal tumor. These findings, even when obvious, may be asymptomatic or associated with vomiting, diarrhea, constipation, respiratory embarrassment, or decreased urine output. Primary intestinal tumors, notably non-Hodgkin's lymphoma, may masquerade as an acute abdomen such as appendicitis (Fig. 11.92), or pro-vide a lead point for intussusception. The pediatric surgeon, recognizing these possibilities, will need to send specimens for careful pathologic review.

UROGENITAL TRACT

Involvement of the genitourinary system or perianal area by tumor may be reflected in the obstructive symptoms already described. Sarcoma botryoides (Fig. 11.93) is a subtype of rhabdomyosarcoma named for its grapelike appearance. Classically, it involves the vagina, but may also involve the mucosal surfaces of other hollow organs such as the bladder or larynx. This tumor and sacrococcygeal teratoma (Fig. 11.94) usually are grossly apparent. However, both may present as intraabdominal or pelvic masses. The latter may need to be distinguished from a meningomyelocele and other spinal

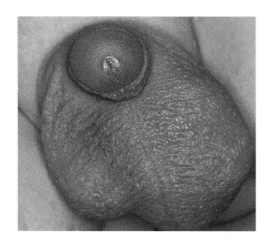

FIG. 11.95 Unilateral scrotal swelling in infant with left testicular mass.

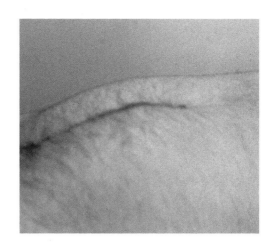

FIG. 11.96 Abdominal distension and hirsutism in a young girl with adrenocortical carcinoma. (Courtesy of Dr. P. Lee, Children's Hospital of Pittsburgh)

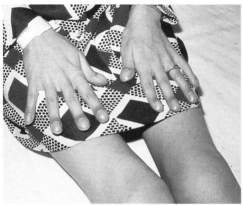

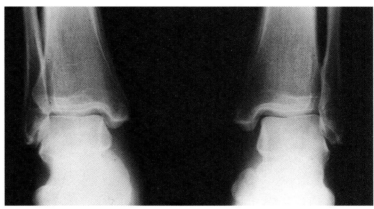

FIG. 11.97 Clubbing (left) and bone lesions (right) in child with hypertrophic osteoarthropathy secondary to hepatocellular carcinoma not involving the lung. (Courtesy of Dr. K.S. Oh, Children's Hospital of Pittsburgh)

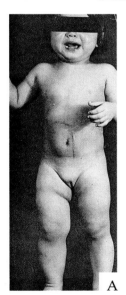

A

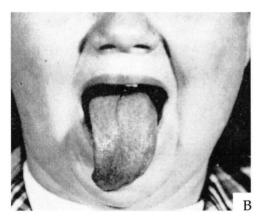

B

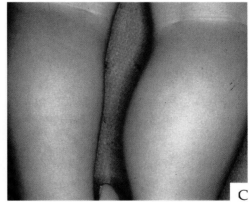

C

FIG. 11.98 A and B, hemihypertrophy. C, asymmetry due to soft tissue sarcoma of left calf. (A and B, reproduced by permission from Fraumeni JF, Geiser CF, Manning MD: Wilms' tumor and congenital hemihypertrophy report of five new cases and review of literature. Pediatrics 1967;40:886–899. C, courtesy of Dr. D. Nakayama, Children's Hospital of Pittsburgh)

tumors, but, as with these other diagnoses, it may cause peripheral neurologic abnormalities.

Testicular enlargement (Fig. 11.95; see Chapter 17, Surgery) may be secondary to involvement by metastatic leukemia or lymphoma (in which case bilateral swelling may be seen), or to primary testicular tumors. Priapism (see Fig. 11.32) is a rare concomitant of chronic myelogenous leukemia. Isosexual precocity, particularly in a boy, may be caused by a tumor of the CNS, gonads (ovaries or testes), or adrenal gland. Other endocrinopathies such as Cushing's syndrome, diabetes insipidus, and hypoglycemia also have been described as presenting manifestations of pediatric cancer. Particularly in the case of adrenal tumors (Fig. 11.96), early diagnosis contributes to curability.

MUSCULOSKELETAL SYSTEM

Bone and joint manifestations of pediatric cancer are relatively common. Arthralgia, or full-blown arthritis, is a well-described (so-called JRA-like) presentation of acute lymphocytic leukemia (ALL). Findings may be migratory, and typically involve knees, wrists, and fingers. Bone pain, as discussed above, also is common. Hypertrophic osteoarthropathy, probably one of the paraneoplastic syndromes, has been described in children with hepatomas, not all of whom have advanced disease at the time of presentation (Fig. 11.97). Hemihypertrophy (Fig. 11.98; see Chapter 9, Endocrinology) or relative enlargement of one or more parts (usually legs or feet) of one side of the body, has been associated with the subsequent development of a number of solid tumors as well as

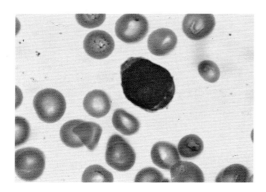

FIG. 11.99 Blasts in peripheral blood of a baby who also had hepatosplenomegaly and thrombocytopenia, but who turned out to have a viral illness instead of leukemia.

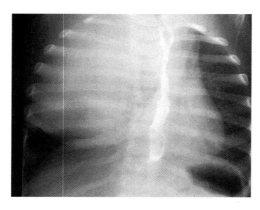

FIG. 11.100 Posterior mediastinal mass in child with neuroblastoma. Calcification, not present in this film, may be seen in 50 percent

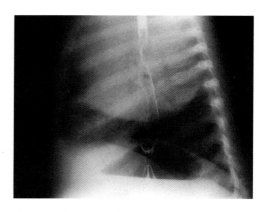

of cases. (Courtesy of Dr. J. Medina, Children's Hospital of Pittsburgh)

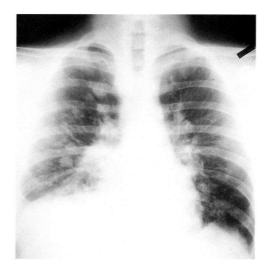

FIG. 11.101 Pulmonary nodules in an adolescent with metastatic sarcoma.

with leukemia, and should be distinguished from hemiatrophy, which is not a predisposing condition. A mass involving one extremity (Fig. 11.98C) is not usually confused with hemihypertrophy. Deep vein thromboses may be due to vessel compression by tumor or to a paraneoplastic effect.

NERVOUS SYSTEM

Neurologic symptoms of pediatric cancer include headaches and vomiting as noted above. In addition, seizures or changes in mental status may be due to primary or metastatic intracranial tumors, or to metabolic abnormalities. Cranial nerve palsies (see Fig. 11.78) may be localizing or false-localizing signs. Opsoclonus-myoclonus (dancing eyes, dancing feet) is a much talked about, infrequently seen, and poorly understood syndrome most closely associated with neuroblastoma. Spinal cord tumors or tumors that press on the cord may present with bowel-bladder dysfunction, paresthesias, and changes in gait. Pain on percussion over the vertebral column may be an early sign of cord compression, and should be actively sought in the child with suspected cancer in whom it may be another of the oncologic emergencies.

Laboratory Aids to Diagnosis

EVALUATION OF BLOOD AND BONE MARROW SPECIMENS

In the case of leukemias, or occasionally solid tumors, a complete blood count (CBC) ordered with a differential and platelet count may provide the first suggestion of malignancy, particularly in the child with persistent but minimal and nonlocalizing symptoms. Careful attention should be paid to abnormalities in the white blood cell count (which may be increased or decreased), hemoglobin, and platelet count. Although thrombocytopenia is commonly associated with leukemia, thrombocytosis can rarely be seen in that disease; it is characteristic of neuroblastoma or hepatic cancers, even when the bone marrow is not involved. While blasts are not specific for leukemia (Fig. 11.99), their presence should hasten

further workup. However, blasts in the peripheral blood never preclude the need to examine the bone marrow. Conversely, the absence of blasts does not rule out a diagnosis of leukemia, and a child who is subsequently found to have leukemia may have a CBC which is entirely normal at the time of presentation. Because multiple special studies including flow cytometry and chromosomal analysis are needed for evaluation of bone marrow specimens, it is our strong belief that a child who warrants a bone marrow workup should be referred to a pediatric oncologist.

EVALUATION OF METABOLIC ABNORMALITIES

Metabolic abnormalities may be a reason for morbidity and mortality. Therefore, a battery of "tumor" chemistries also should be ordered in the child with a suspicion of cancer. These would include electrolytes, blood urea nitrogen, creatinine, uric acid, lactate dehydrogenase, calcium, and phosphorus, the results of which should be checked "stat," and liver function tests. Even in children with primary or metastatic disease involving the liver, SGOT, SGPT, bilirubin, and alkaline phosphatase levels may all be normal. Although 24-hour urine collections can be used to measure the catecholamine metabolites HVA and VMA in children with sus-

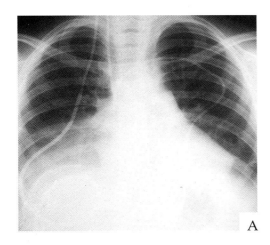

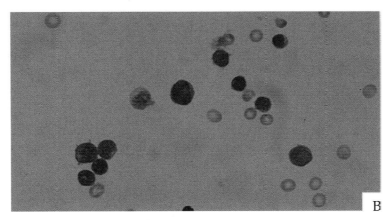

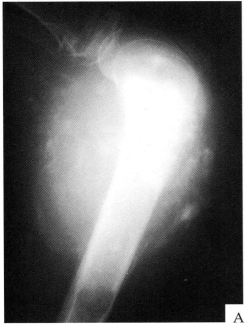

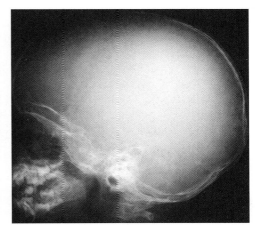

FIG. 11.104 Lytic lesions in child with leukemia. Similar lesions may be due to metastatic solid tumors.

FIG. 11.103 *A*, x-ray of child with osteosarcoma shows soft tissue swelling, calcification, cortical bone destruction with increased osteodensity, and new bone formation (Codman's triangle). *B*, Ewing's sarcoma shows cortical destruction and soft tissue swelling of diaphysis of femur. (Courtesy of J. Medina, Children's Hospital of Pittsburgh)

pected neuroblastoma, in many hospitals, random urine samples can be tested with similar accuracy and much greater ease. Because it may take a prolonged period of time to get these results back, further evaluation may need to be done without waiting.

MEDIASTINAL MASSES

The likely etiology of mediastinal masses (see Chapter 17, Surgery) depends to a certain extent on location. Tumors of the posterior mediastinum (especially when calcified on x-ray) are commonly neurogenic (e.g., neuroblastoma or its benign counterpart ganglioneuroma (Fig. 11.100) or lymphomas. Tumors of the anterior mediastinum are thymomas, teratomas, or lymphomas. Middle mediastinal masses or hilar adenopathy are most likely to be leukemic or lymphomatous. Parenchymal pulmonary nodules, when tumor-related, are likely to be asymptomatic and are most commonly due to metastatic sarcoma or Wilms' tumor (Fig. 11.101). Neuroblastoma classically avoids the lung parenchyma until late in a patient's course. It is important to be aware that pleural effusions, though relatively rare in pediatric cancers, may be malignant, and cytologies should be considered if a diagnostic thoracentesis is done (Fig. 11.102).

EVALUATION OF BONE PAIN

In evaluating bone pain (see above), plain radiographs often are ordered by the primary pediatrician. Frequent findings include the destructive lesions of primary bone tumors. Osteosarcoma most frequently occurs in the metaphysis of a long bone of the lower extremity while Ewing's sarcoma is more commonly a diaphyseal lesion (Fig. 11.103). Lytic or blastic lesions may be seen in patients with leukemia, lymphoma, and metastatic tumors (Fig. 11.104); metaphyseal lucencies and growth arrest lines are nonspecific findings of chronic disease but are most commonly associated with ALL (Fig. 11.105). Diffuse osteopenia (Fig. 11.106) is, presumably, an effect of tumor-produced bone resorbing factors. However, a normal plain film should never exclude the possibility of malignancy as a cause of bone symptoms. A bone scan or repeat plain film may be indicated after an arbitrary interval.

SPECIALIZED TECHNIQUES

The reasons for obtaining a chest x-ray are discussed above. Whether more specialized radiographic studies such as intravenous pyelograms, sonograms, CT scans (always with and without contrast), and magnetic resonance imaging scans are ordered by the generalist or are not done until referral to a specialist is a decision which should depend on:

1. How sick the child is, and whether the studies can be obtained in a timely fashion.

2. Knowledge of how reliable the diagnostic radiology services are at a particular hospital.

3. The ability to get good copies of the studies sent with the patient when he is ultimately transferred.

Whether the child with suspected malignancy should have a tissue biopsy (other than a bone marrow) at the referring institution is also controversial. Under optimal circumstances, the surgeon should be familiar with the requirements of cancer operations, and adequate fresh tissue should be available with which to confirm a specific tumor diagnosis. It is often most convenient for the biopsy to be done at the institution where the oncologist is located.

Bibliography

Lanzkowsky P (ed): *Pediatric Oncology: a Treatise for the Clinician*, New York, McGraw Hill, 1983.

Miller DR, Pearson HA, Baehner RL, McMillan LW: *Smith's Blood Diseases of Infancy and Childhood*, ed 4. St. Louis, CV Mosby, 1978.

Nathan DG, Oski FA: *Hematology of Infancy and Childhood*, ed 2. Philadelphia, WB Saunders, 1981.

Oski FA, Naiman JL: *Hematologic Problems of the Newborn*, ed 3. Philadelphia, WB Saunders, 1982.

Pizzo PA, Poplack DG (eds): *Principles and Practice of Pediatric Oncology*. Philadelphia, JB Lippincott, 1989.

Wintrobe MM, et al: *Clinical Hematology*, ed 8. Philadelphia, Lea & Febiger, 1981.

Zucker-Franklin D, Greanes MF, Grossi CE, Marmont AM: *Atlas of Blood Cells*. Milan, Italy, Ermes, 1981.

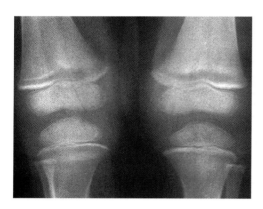
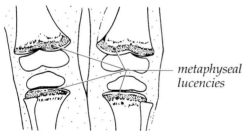
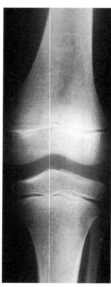
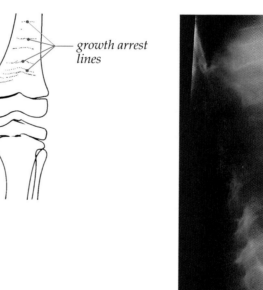
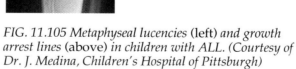
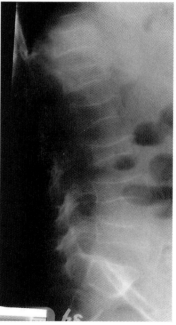

FIG. 11.105 Metaphyseal lucencies (left) and growth arrest lines (above) in children with ALL. (Courtesy of Dr. J. Medina, Children's Hospital of Pittsburgh)

FIG. 11.106 Diffuse osteopenia in ALL. This child was followed for many months by an orthopedist before an abnormal hemogram prompted referral to a hematologist.

PEDIATRIC INFECTIOUS DISEASE

Holly W. Davis, M.D. ◆ Raymond B. Karasic, M.D.

In selecting infectious diseases for presentation in an atlas format, we have chosen to emphasize common and serious disorders in which visual findings tend to be prominent. Modes of presentation, patterns of clinical evolution, and spectrum of severity will be stressed. The following topics will be covered: infectious exanthems, mumps, bacterial skin and soft-tissue infections, infectious lymphadenitis, bacterial bone and joint infections, and congenital and perinatal infections.

INFECTIOUS EXANTHEMS

Exanthematous disorders are numerous, commonly encountered and, having many similarities, often are a source of clinical confusion. In establishing a diagnosis the clinician should attend not only to the basic character of the exanthem but also to its mode of spread, its distribution, the evolution of lesions, and the constellation of associated symptoms. In some of these illnesses, the presence of a characteristic oral enanthema can be helpful in establishing the diagnosis.

Viral Exanthems

Along with mumps, three exanthems—measles or rubeola, rubella, and varicella—continue to be referred to as the usual childhood diseases. Although immunization has markedly decreased the incidence of measles, mumps, and rubella compared with the pre-vaccine era, there has been a major resurgence of measles and a less dramatic increase in cases of mumps over the past decade. Varicella remains as common as ever, although a new varicella vaccine is awaiting licensure.

RUBEOLA (NINE-DAY OR RED MEASLES)
Measles is a highly contagious, moderate to severe acute illness with a typical prodrome and mode of evolution. Prodromal symptoms consist of fever, malaise, dry cough, coryza, and conjunctivitis with clear discharge and marked photophobia (Fig. 12.1A). One to two days after onset, a pathognomonic enanthem (Koplik's spots) appears on the buccal mucosa (Fig. 12.1B). Lesions consist of tiny bluish white dots surrounded by red halos, which increase in number and then fade over a 2- to 3-day period. The exanthem is seen first on day 3 or 4, as prodromal symptoms and fever peak in severity. It is a blotchy, erythematous blanching maculopapular eruption that appears at the hairline and spreads cephalocaudally over 3 days, ultimately involving the palms and soles (Fig. 12.1C,D). Once generalized, the rash becomes confluent over proximal areas but remains discrete distally. Older lesions tend to develop a rusty hue as a result of capillary leak and cease to blanch with pressure. Fading commences after 3 days with clearing 2 to 3 days later. Fine branny desquamation of the most severely involved areas may ensue. Generalized adenopathy may be present in moderate to severe cases.

During the acute phase of this illness, most patients are quite ill systemically. They are lethargic, have moderate to severe malaise and anorexia, and prefer to be left alone to sleep in a darkened room.

The incubation period for measles is 9 to 10 days, and patients are contagious from approximately 4 days before the appearance of rash until about 4 days after. The attack rate in exposed susceptible individuals is greater than 90 percent. Morbidity is rather high and mortality not uncommon, especially in third world countries. The peak season for measles is late winter through early spring. Potential complications (resulting either from extension of the primary infection or from secondary invasion by bacterial pathogens) include otitis media, pneumonia, obstructive laryngotracheitis, and acute encephalitis.

RUBELLA (GERMAN MEASLES)
While rubella has little or no prodrome in children, adolescents, like adults, may experience 1 to 5 days of low-grade fever, mild malaise, adenopathy, headache, sore throat, and coryza. Fever, if present at all in young children, is low-grade and rarely lasts more than a day. The exanthem is a discrete pinkish-red fine maculopapular eruption which, like measles, typically begins on the face and spreads cephalocaudally (Fig. 12.2A). The rash becomes generalized within 24 hours, then begins to fade, clearing completely by 72 hours. Forscheimer spots, an enanthem consisting of small reddish spots on the soft palate, are seen in some patients on day 1 of the rash and

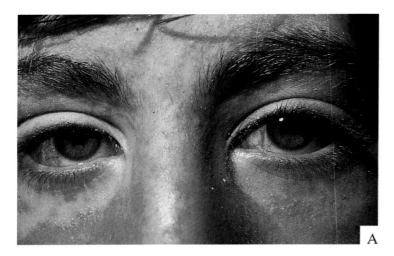

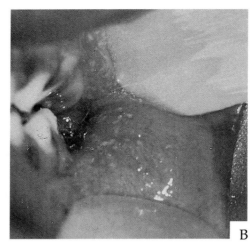

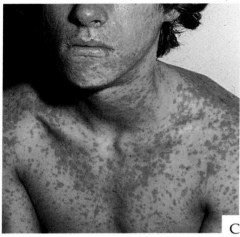

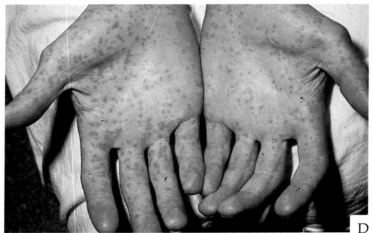

FIG. 12.1
Rubeola/measles.
A, during and after the prodromal period, the conjuctivae are injected and produce a clear discharge. This is associated with marked photophobia.
B, Koplik's spots, bluish-white dots surrounded by red halos, appear on the buccal and labial mucosa a day or two before the exanthem and begin to fade with onset of the rash. **C ,** the measles exanthem is a blotchy erythematous blanching maculopapular eruption that appears at the hairline and spreads cephalocaudally over 3 days **(D)** ultimately involving the palms and soles. With evolution lesions become confluent at proximal sites. (**A, C** and **D,** courtesy of Dr. Michael Sherlock)

can be helpful in differential diagnosis (Fig. 12.2B). Adenopathy, often generalized, is a common but not invariable feature. Occipital, posterior cervical, and postauricular nodes tend to be those most prominently enlarged. Arthritis and arthralgias are frequent in adolescent and adult females, beginning on day 2 to 3 and typically lasting 5 to 10 days. Large or small joints may be affected.

Many patients infected with rubella do not manifest this typical picture. Up to 25 percent of infected individuals are asymptomatic yet are capable of transmitting the virus to others. In some, the rash may last only 1 day and it may involve only the trunk; in others, the exanthem is absent and the patient will appear to have pharyngitis or an upper respiratory tract infection. Since a number of other viruses, including adenoviruses, coxsackie viruses and echoviruses, can produce a rubella-like picture, exact diagnosis requires serologic testing. Such testing is important if the patient is pregnant or has been in contact with a pregnant woman, or if arthritis is a prominent feature simulating the picture of acute rheumatic fever or rheumatoid arthritis.

Peak incidence occurs in late winter and early spring, and patients are contagious from a few days prior to a few days after appearance of the exanthem. The incubation period ranges from 14 to 21 days. Complications are rare in childhood and include arthritis, purpura with or without thrombocytopenia, and mild encephalitis. The major complication results from spread of the virus to susceptible pregnant women and their fetuses, resulting in congenital rubella syndrome (see section on congenital infections). When such an exposure is thought to have occurred, acute and convalescent titers should be obtained

from the index patient, and the pregnant woman should be tested for hemagglutination inhibition antibody. If this is positive, immunity can be assumed; if it is negative, she should be retested in 2 weeks. If antibody is detected in the second specimen, infection has occurred and the fetus is at risk.

VARICELLA (CHICKENPOX)

Varicella in the normal host is a relatively benign albeit highly contagious illness caused by the varicella-zoster virus. A brief prodrome of low-grade fever, upper respiratory tract symptoms, and mild malaise may occur, followed rapidly by the appearance of a pruritic exanthem. Lesions appear in crops and evolve rapidly over several hours. Most patients will have three crops although some may have only one and others may have as many as five. Initial crops involve the trunk and scalp, while subsequent crops are distributed more peripherally; thus, the mode of spread is centrifugal. The presence of scalp lesions with the initial crop often is helpful in diagnosing the patient who presents early in the course of the disease. Lesions begin as tiny erythematous papules that rapidly enlarge to form thin-walled superficial central vesicles surrounded by red halos. Vesicular fluid changes promptly from clear to cloudy; then drying begins, resulting in an umbilicated appearance. As surrounding erythema fades, a central crust or scab is formed, which sloughs after several days. A hallmark of this exanthem is the finding of lesions in all stages of evolution within a relatively small geographic area of skin (Fig. 12.3A). Generally, all scabs have sloughed by 10 to 14 days. Scarring usually does not occur unless lesions become secondarily infected. It is important to recognize that the lesions of varicel-

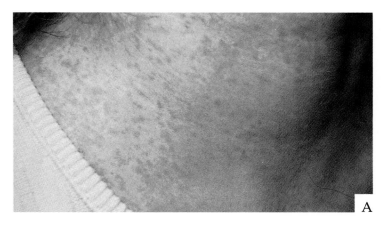
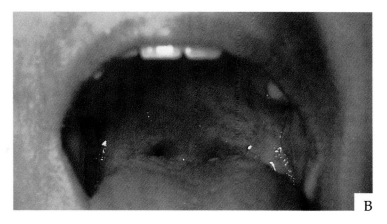

FIG. 12.2 Rubella/german measles. **A,** the exanthem of rubella usually consists of a fine pinkish-red maculopapular eruption that appears first at the hairline and rapidly spreads cephalocaudally. Lesions tend to remain discrete. **B,** the presence of red palatal lesions (Forscheimer spots), seen in some patients on day 1 of the rash, and occipital and posterior cervical adenopathy are suggestive findings of rubella. (Courtesy of Dr. Michael Sherlock)

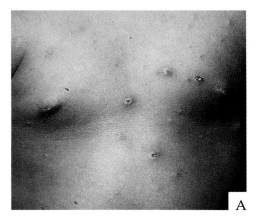
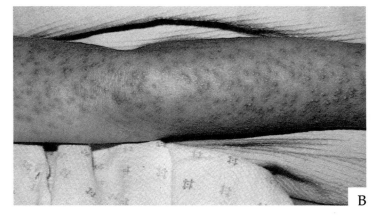
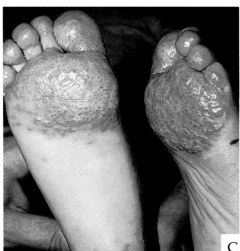
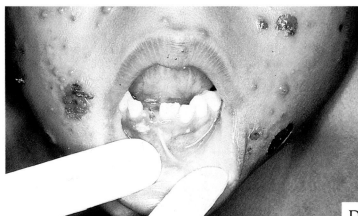

FIG. 12.3 Varicella/chickenpox. **A,** the characteristic finding of lesions in all stages of evolution is seen on the trunk of this child. Note the presence of papules, vesicles, and umbilicated and scabbed lesions, all within a small geographic area. **B** and **C** in this child with underlying eczema, the first crop of vesicles appeared in clusters at sites previously affected by eczema. The flexor surface of his arm is covered with numerous discrete lesions, and, vesicles are confluent over the plantar surface of his toes and on the balls of his feet. **D,** on mucosal surfaces, thin-walled vesicles may form, which rapidly rupture, forming painful shallow ulcers. (**B** and **C,** courtesy of Dr. Michael Sherlock; **D,** courtesy of Dr. Ellen Wald)

la, like other viral exanthems, tend to appear first and cluster most heavily at sites of prior skin irritation, such as the diaper area or sites of eczematous dermatitis (Fig. 12.3B,C).

An enanthem is commonly seen and consists of thin-walled vesicles that rapidly rupture to form shallow ulcers (Fig. 12.3D). Other mucosal surfaces may be affected as well. While skin lesions are pruritic, those present on oral, rectal, or vaginal mucosa or those involving the external auditory canal or tympanic membrane can be very painful necessitating analgesia. Systemic symptoms generally are mild, although low-grade to moderate fever may be present during the first few days. In most cases pruritus is the child's major complaint. In adolescents, however, as in adults, the illness is more likely to be severe with prominent systemic symptoms and with more extensive exanthematous involvement.

Varicella occurs year round, with peak periods in late autumn and late winter through early spring. The period of communicability begins 1 to 2 days before the appearance of lesions and lasts until all lesions have crusted over. The incubation period ranges from 10 to 20 days, with high secondary attack rates in susceptible individuals. The most common complication in normal hosts is secondary bacterial infection of excoriated skin lesions. Such infection can range from impetigo to cellulitis. Other complications, though rare, include pneumo-

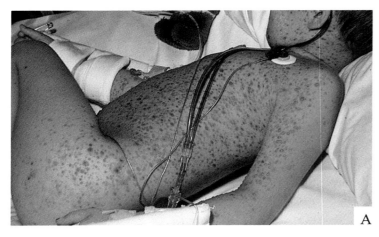

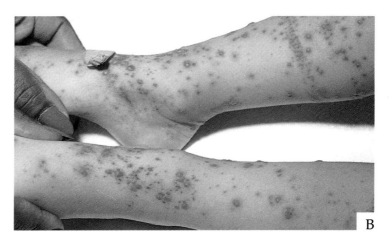

FIG. 12.4 Disseminated hemorrhagic varicella. **A,** in the immunocompromised child skin lesions tend to be hemorrhagic and nearly conflu-

ent. **B,** lesions also evolve more slowly than usual, remaining vesicular for a prolonged period.

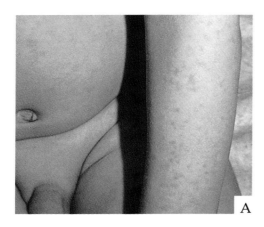

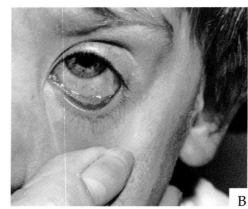

FIG. 12.5 Adenovirus. **A,** this discrete erythematous blanching maculopapular rash was generalized when first noted, and occurred in association with pharyngitis and **(B)** nonpurulent conjunctivitis. (Courtesy of Dr. Michael Sherlock)

nia, hepatitis, and encephalitis. The onset of these complications typically is heralded by a secondary fever spike concurrent with an increase in general systemic symptoms. With encephalitis, an altered level of consciousness occurs along with other signs of neurologic dysfunction. Reye's syndrome, an encephalopathy of unclear etiology, is a well-recognized but fortunately rare complication that can occur as a child is recovering from acute varicella. Repetitive pernicious vomiting is followed by an altered level of consciousness in which periods of lethargy alternate with periods of delirium or combativeness.

In the immunocompromised host with deficient cellular immunity, varicella is a severe and often fatal disease with CNS, pulmonary, and generalized visceral involvement. Skin lesions often are hemorrhagic and tend to remain vesicular for a prolonged period of time (Fig. 12.4). In the potentially compromised host who has not had varicella previously (including those on short-course high-dose steroids), parents must be forewarned of these dangers and instructed to notify their physician immediately of any possible exposure. This enables the administration of varicella-zoster immune globulin within 96 hours of exposure, thus reducing the severity of illness.

ADENOVIRUS INFECTIONS

There are approximately 30 distinct types of adenoviruses capable of producing a variety of clinical illnesses including conjunctivitis, upper respiratory tract infections and pharyngitis, croup, bronchitis, bronchiolitis and pneumonia (occasionally fulminant), gastroenteritis, myocarditis, nephritis, cystitis, and encephalitis. An exanthem occasionally accompanies other symptoms, and a variety of rashes have been described. The

eruption may consist of discrete nonspecific blanching maculopapular lesions or it may be morbilliform, rubelliform or, on occasion, petechial. Typically the rash is generalized when first noted. The most readily identifiable clinical constellation consists of conjunctivitis, rhinitis, pharyngitis and a discrete blanching maculopapular rash (Fig. 12.5). Anterior cervical and preauricular lymphadenopathy, low-grade fever, and malaise are common associated findings. The peak season for adenovirus infections in temperate climates is late winter through early summer, and patients are maximally contagious during the first few days of illness. The incubation period ranges from 6 to 9 days.

COXSACKIE HAND-FOOT-AND-MOUTH DISEASE

Of the enteroviruses, coxsackie group A16 produces the most distinctive exanthem, known as "hand-foot-and-mouth disease." Patients may have a brief prodrome consisting of low-grade fever, malaise, sore mouth, and anorexia, during which time lesions are absent. Within 1 to 2 days oral lesions and, soon thereafter, skin lesions appear. The former consist of shallow, yellow ulcers surrounded by red halos. They are found most frequently on the labial and buccal mucosal surfaces but also may affect the tongue, soft palate, uvula, and anterior tonsillar pillars (Fig. 12.6A,B). These enanthematous lesions usually are only mildly painful. Early in the illness, small vesicles may be seen on the palate or mucosal surfaces. The cutaneous lesions begin as erythematous macules on the palmar aspect of the hands and fingers, the plantar surface of the feet and toes, and the interdigital surfaces. Occasionally, the buttocks may be involved as well. They evolve rapidly to form small thick-

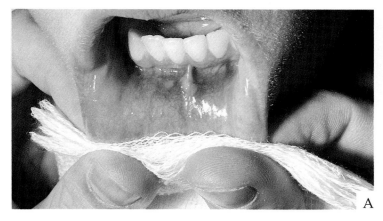

A

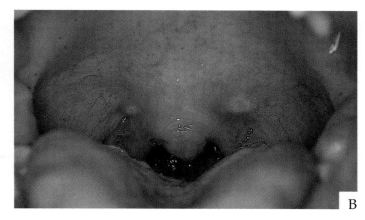

B

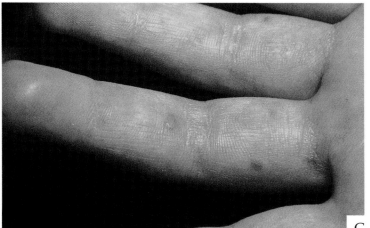

C

FIG. 12.6 Coxsackie hand-foot-and-mouth disease. The exanthem of this disorder is characterized by mildly painful, shallow yellow ulcers surrounded by red halos. These may be found on (A) the labial or buccal mucosa, the tongue, (B) soft palate, uvula, and anterior tonsillar pillars. When oral lesions occur in the absence of the exanthem, the disorder is called herpangina. C, the exanthem of coxsackie hand-foot-and-mouth disease involves the palmar, plantar and interdigital surfaces of the hands and feet, and consists of thick-walled gray vesicles on an erythematous base. (C, courtesy of Dr. Michael Sherlock)

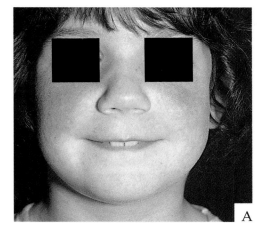

A

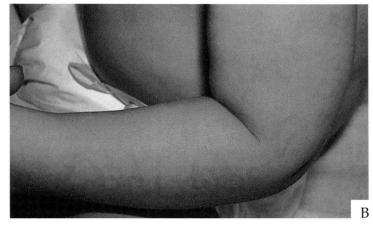

B

FIG. 12.7 Erythema infectiosum (fifth disease). A, on day 1, warm erythematous nontender circumscribed patches appear over the cheeks. These fade on the following day as (B) an erythematous lacy rash develops on the extensor surfaces of the extremities. (Courtesy of Dr. Michael Sherlock)

walled gray vesicles on an erythematous base (Fig. 12.6C), which may feel like slivers, be pruritic, or be asymptomatic. Over 90 percent of patients with disease caused by coxsackie A16 have oral lesions and about two-thirds have the exanthem. In those cases where cutaneous manifestations are absent, the process is called herpangina (caused by coxsackie and other enteroviruses) and may resemble early herpes gingivostomatitis. However, coxsackie ulcers are less painful, are less likely to involve gingival surfaces, and are not associated with the high fever and intense gingival erythema, edema, and bleeding typical of herpes (see Fig. 12.10).

Coxsackie hand-foot-and-mouth disease is highly contagious with an incubation period of approximately 2 to 6 days. The duration of symptoms ranges from 2 days to 1 week. The peak season is late summer through early fall.

Other enteroviral syndromes produced by the coxsackie group and by echoviruses include a mild, nonspecific febrile illness with myalgias, headache, and abdominal pain; generalized exanthems that may be maculopapular, vesicular, or urticarial; encephalitis, acute cerebellar ataxia, and myelitis; pleurodynia; myocarditis; hemorrhagic conjunctivitis; and gastroenteritis.

ERYTHEMA INFECTIOSUM (FIFTH DISEASE)

Erythema infectiosum is a mildly contagious illness, caused by parvovirus B19, that principally affects preschool and young school-age children. It occurs year round with a peak incidence in late winter and early spring. The disorder is characterized primarily by its exanthem, as fever and constitutional symptoms are unusual. Occasionally, headache, nausea, myalgias, and peripheral polyarthralgias are reported. The rash begins on the face, with large, bright red erythematous patches appearing over both cheeks (Fig. 12.7A). These patches are warm but nontender, and have circumscribed borders that usually are macu-

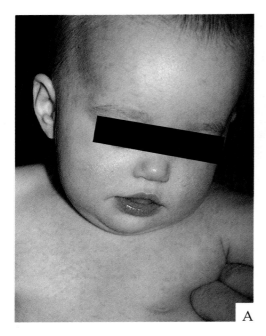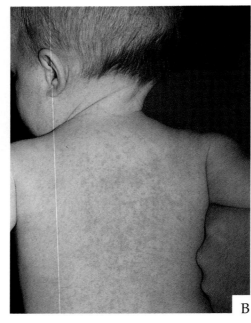

*FIG. 12.8 Roseola infantum/exanthem subitum. **A** and **B**, the exanthem of this disorder usually appears abruptly after 3 days of high fever and irritability. It is morbilliform in appearance and is characterized by discrete rose-pink macules. It may be generalized when first noted or may start centrally and spread centrifugally. Scalp involvement is prominent.*

A

B

lar but may be slightly raised. They are easily distinguished from those of cellulitis and erysipelas (see Figs. 12.35 and 12.36) by their symmetry and lack of tenderness, and by the absence of high fever and toxicity. On the following day the facial lesions begin to fade and a symmetric, macular or slightly raised, lacy erythematous rash appears on the extensor surfaces of the extremities (Fig. 12.7B). The rash may spread over the next day or so to the flexor surfaces, buttocks, and trunk. Resolution occurs within 3 to 7 days of onset.

Recent studies have found that the virus is transmitted primarily by respiratory secretions and—following transmission—replicates in red cell precursors in the bone marrow. It then may cause a biphasic illness with fever and nonspecific symptoms accompanied by red cell suppression occurring approximately a week later, followed by the appearance of the exanthem characteristic of fifth disease 1 to 2 weeks hence. Viral shedding ceases prior to this latter phase. Although red cell suppression due to parvovirus does not result in anemia in normal individuals, it can cause aplastic crisis in patients with sickle cell disease, other hemoglobinopathies, and other forms of hemolytic anemia.

ROSEOLA INFANTUM (EXANTHEM SUBITUM)

Roseola infantum is a febrile illness that primarily affects young children between the ages of 6 and 36 months. Recent studies have confirmed the long-held belief that roseola is a viral illness; the causative agent is now known to be human herpesvirus 6. The clinical course begins abruptly with rapid temperature elevation, which occasionally precipitates a febrile seizure. Anorexia and irritability are the major associated symptoms. Examination reveals no source for the fever, which usually is higher than 39°C. Administration of an antipyretic produces only a transient decrease in temperature, which then rises rapidly to its former height. While most patients do not look toxic, many undergo a sepsis workup and lumbar puncture because of the combination of unexplained high fever and marked irritability. Fever persists for approximately 72 hours, whereupon the patient abruptly defervesces. In most cases an erythematous morbilliform exanthem appears simultaneously with defervescence, but in a small percentage of patients it develops 1 day before or after fever lysis. Lesions are discrete

rose-pink macules or maculopapules that begin first on the trunk and then spread rapidly to the extremities, neck, face, and scalp (Fig. 12.8). They may last from several hours to a day or two before resolution.

While cases occur year round, roseola appears to be more common in late fall and early spring. Secondary cases are uncommon except in institutional settings. The duration of communicability is unclear, but the incubation period is thought to be 10 to 15 days.

INFECTIOUS MONONUCLEOSIS

Infectious mononucleosis is an acute, usually self-limited illness of children and young adults caused by the Epstein-Barr (EB) virus. Transmission of EB virus can occur by intimate oral contact (i.e., kissing), via shared eating utensils, or by transfusion. The incubation period usually ranges from 30 to 50 days, although it is shorter (14 to 20 days) with transfusion-acquired infection.

In its most typical form, infectious mononucleosis is characterized by fever, fatigue, pharyngitis, lymphadenopathy, splenomegaly, atypical lymphocytosis, and a positive heterophil antibody response. Nevertheless, most young children with EB virus infection do not have classic mononucleosis; instead, they tend to have either a nonspecific illness, which is clinically indistinguishable from other common viral diseases, or—less frequently—subclinical infection.

Clinical Features of Mononucleosis

The illness often begins with a prodrome, which lasts from 3 to 5 days, consisting of fatigue, malaise, and anorexia, often in association with headache, sweats, and chills. Photophobia and edema of the eyelids and periorbital tissues may be noted in some patients. The acute phase usually is heralded by a fever which may show wide daily fluctuations. Pharyngitis and cervical node enlargement then become apparent. The sore throat tends to increase in severity over several days before abating and may be associated with significant dysphagia. Tonsillar and adenoidal enlargement can range from mild to marked, and the tonsillar surface may vary in appearance from one of mild erythema to one of severe exudative inflammation with palatal and uvular edema (Fig. 12.9A). Halitosis

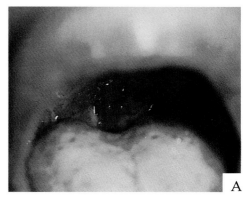

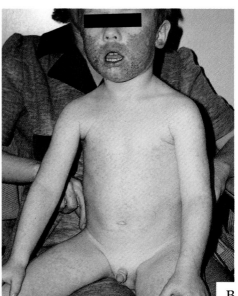

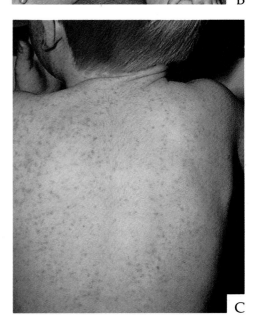

A

B

C

FIG. 12.9 EB virus mononucleosis. **A,** severe pharyngotonsillitis is seen in this child whose tonsils are markedly enlarged and covered with a gray exudate. The uvula is erythematous and edematous. **B and C,** in this child with EB virus mononucleosis, a diffuse erythematous maculopapular rash was part of the clinical picture. Lesions on his face are hemorrhagic and confluent as a result of prior irritation. (He had practiced shaving 2 days before.) Note also the swelling in the region of the tonsillar node and the fact that the child is mouth breathing as a result of adenoidal hypertrophy. (**B and C,** courtesy of Dr. Michael Sherlock)

An exanthem is seen in 5 to 10 percent of patients with mononucleosis, although this percentage is greatly increased in those treated with ampicillin for pharyngeal or respiratory symptoms. Usually an erythematous maculopapular rubelliform rash, the exanthem can be morbilliform, scarlatiniform, urticarial, hemorrhagic, or even nodular in character (Fig. 12.9B,C).

Less common manifestations or complications of mononucleosis include pneumonitis with a pattern of a diffuse atypical pneumonia; hematologic abnormalities such as direct Coombs-positive hemolytic anemia and thrombocytopenia; icteric hepatitis; neurologic disorders such as acute cerebellar ataxia, encephalitis, aseptic meningitis, myelitis and Guillain-Barré syndrome; and, rarely, myocarditis and pericarditis. Neurologic and hepatic involvement occasionally can be fulminant, resulting in death. Other major complications include acute upper airway obstruction due to tonsillar and adenoidal hypertrophy, and splenic rupture, which may occur spontaneously or as a result of minor trauma, repeated palpation, or the increase in intra-abdominal pressure associated with defecation. While younger patients are somewhat less subject to the less usual manifestations and complications of mononucleosis, they are more vulnerable to acute upper airway obstruction as a result of tonsillar and adenoidal hypertrophy. Moreover, children under 5 years of age who develop significant tonsillar and adenoidal enlargement during the course of EB virus infection are more likely to have secondary otitis media, and may, subsequent to resolution of the acute process, become subject to recurrent bouts of otitis media, tonsillitis, and sinusitis as a result of persistent tonsillar and adenoidal hypertrophy.

Diagnostic Methods

A number of laboratory studies may be helpful in suggesting or confirming the diagnosis of infectious mononucleosis. A classic finding is that of lymphocytosis of 50 percent or more, with at least 10 percent atypical lymphocytes. These atypical lymphocytes will vary in appearance in contrast to the monotonous forms seen with leukemia. There is considerable variability, however, in the degree of lymphocytosis and in its timing. Eighty percent or more of patients will have mild elevations in liver enzymes early in the course of their disease. Most commonly the diagnosis is confirmed by finding heterophil antibodies in the serum toward the end of the first week or at the beginning of the second week of illness. Currently rapid slide tests, of which the Monospot is best known, are the most prevalent method of detecting heterophil antibodies. Although the presence of heterophil antibodies is highly specific for infectious mononucleosis, the sensitivity of the test is limited in that only about 85 percent of adolescents (and a smaller percentage of younger children) with mononucleosis ever develop measurable heterophil antibodies. Although EB virus infection can be confirmed by measuring specific EB virus antibody titers, such studies are usually reserved for severe, prolonged, or atypical heterophil-negative cases of suspected EB virus infection.

Differential Diagnosis of Mononucleosis

In view of the multiple modes of presentation and the wide variability in severity of illness, clinical manifestations, and clinical course, there exists a broad range of differential diagnostic possibilities. In patients presenting with fever and exudative tonsillitis, the principal diagnostic considerations include group A streptococcal pharyngitis, diphtheria, and

and palatal petechiae are common. Approximately one-third of patients develop severe pharyngeal manifestations. The anterior cervical lymph nodes are routinely enlarged, and posterior cervical adenopathy is characteristic. In classic cases the adenopathy becomes generalized toward the end of the first week. Involved nodes are firm, discrete, and mildly to moderately tender. Approximately 50 percent of patients develop splenomegaly in the second to third week of illness, and about 10 percent have associated hepatic enlargement.

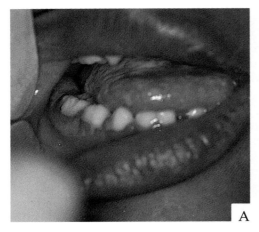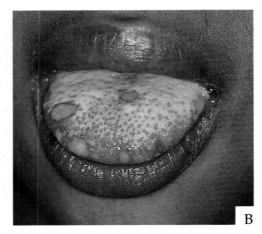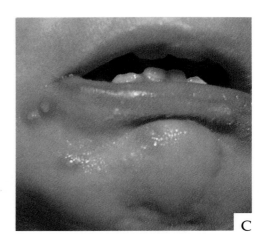

FIG. 12.10 Herpes simplex infections. **A,** herpetic gingivostomatitis is characterized by discrete mucosal ulcerations and by gingival erythema, edema and friability in association with fever, dysphagia and cervical adenopathy. **B,** numerous yellow ulcerations with thin red halos are seen on the patient's tongue as well. **C,** these thick-walled vesicles on erythematous bases were noted in this child who had early findings of intraoral involvement, as well. (**C,** courtesy of Dr. Michael Sherlock)

other viral causes of pharyngitis. When lymphadenopathy and splenomegaly are the predominant features, the differential diagnosis includes cytomegalovirus infection, toxoplasmosis, malignancy, and drug-induced mononucleosis (caused by phenytoin, para-aminosalicylic acid, and diaminodiphenylsulfone). In patients with severe hepatic involvement, EB virus infection can simulate other forms of viral hepatitis as well as leptospirosis. While the history and some aspects of the clinical picture may help in distinguishing one disease entity from another, specific serologic tests often are required.

HERPES SIMPLEX INFECTIONS

The herpes simplex viruses produce infections that primarily involve the skin and mucous membranes, although in neonates, in the immunocompromised host, or, rarely, in a normal host, infection can result in disseminated disease and central nervous system involvement. Like other herpesviruses, herpes simplex virus—after producing initial (primary) infection—often enters a latent or dormant stage within local sensory ganglia; once latent, the virus can be reactivated at any time, causing recurrent infection. There are two distinct serotypes of herpes simplex virus, types 1 and 2. Herpes simplex type 1 is the more common pathogen and can produce a variety of clinical syndromes. In contrast, herpes simplex type 2 virus usually is a genital pathogen (see Chapter 18, Gynecology), although occasionally it is the source of oral lesions and is the usual agent associated with neonatal herpes (see section on congenital infections).

Diagnosis of symptomatic herpes simplex infections often can be made on clinical grounds alone, particularly in cases of primary infection. When the diagnosis is in question, a Giemsa-stained (Tzanck) smear of scrapings obtained from the base of a vesicle (see Chapter 18) usually will demonstrate ballooned epithelial cells with intranuclear inclusions and multinucleated giant cells when the lesion is herpetic. Viral cultures yield results in 24 to 72 hours. Acute and convalescent titers are less useful and are of no help during recurrences.

Primary Herpes Simplex Infections

Over 90 percent of primary infections due to herpes simplex type 1 are subclinical; nevertheless, because the virus is ubiquitous, symptomatic primary infections are common. One of the most prevalent forms of primary infection is *herpetic gingivostomatitis*. Patients with this condition typically have high fever, irritability, anorexia, and mouth pain; infants and toddlers often drool copiously. The gingivae become intensely erythematous, edematous, and friable and tend to bleed easily. Small yellow ulcerations with red halos are seen routinely on the buccal and labial mucosae, on the gingivae and tongue, and often on the palate and tonsillar pillars, as well (Fig. 12.10A,B). Within a short time yellowish-white debris builds up on mucosal surfaces and halitosis becomes prominent. Thick-walled vesiculopustular lesions also may develop on the perioral skin (Fig. 12.10C). The anterior cervical and tonsillar nodes are enlarged and tender. Symptoms range in duration from 5 to 14 days, but the virus may be shed for weeks following resolution. The severity of illness can vary from mild to marked. Young children with prolonged high fever and intense pain may become dehydrated and ketotic and should be followed closely and hydrated as needed. The diffuseness of the ulcerations and mucosal inflammation and the intense gingivitis help to distinguish this disorder from herpangina (see Fig. 12.6) and exudative tonsillitis, as well as from other forms of gingivitis.

Primary herpetic infections involving the skin typically present with fever, malaise, localized lesions, and regional adenopathy. The skin lesions generally result from direct inoculation of previously traumatized skin, for example, at the site of an abrasion, burn, or small cut. The lesions consist of deep, thick-walled painful vesicles on an erythematous base; they usually are grouped but may occur singly. As they evolve over several days, the vesicles become pustular, coalesce, ulcerate, and then crust over. As a result, the lesions may simulate those of bacterial infection, but the presence of grouped vesicles and the relative sparseness of bacteria on Gram stain support the clinical diagnosis of herpes, which can be confirmed by positive findings on Giemsa-stained scrapings from the base of the lesion.

While the virus can infect any area of the skin, the lips and fingers or thumbs (as in *herpetic whitlow*) are the most common sites of involvement (see Figs. 12.10 and 12.11). Occasionally the eyelids and periorbital tissues are affected (Fig. 12.12); this can lead to keratoconjunctivitis, which is diagnosed by the presence of characteristic dendritic ulcera-

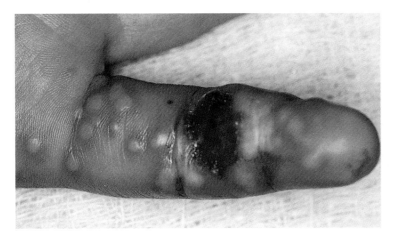

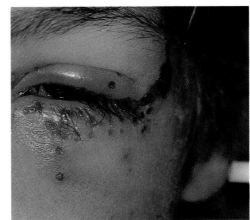

FIG. 12.12 Ocular herpes may be limited to involvement of the lids and periorbital skin but can spread to involve the conjunctiva, cornea, and deeper structures with devastating results.

FIG. 12.11 Herpetic whitlow. Grouped thick-walled vesicles on an erythematous base that are painful and tend to coalesce, ulcerate, and then crust are the characteristic findings of herpetic whitlow.

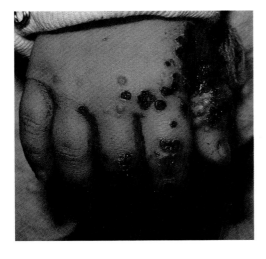

FIG. 12.13 Eczema herpeticum (Kaposi's varicelliform eruption). Primary herpes simplex infection in a child with underlying eczema produced crops of hemorrhagic vesiculopostular lesions limited to areas of preexisting dermatitis, which then ruptured and crusted. (Courtesy of Dr. Michael Sherlock)

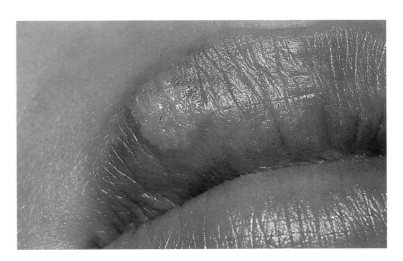

FIG. 12.14 Recurrent herpes labialis (cold sore). Following a brief prodrome of burning, these grouped vesicles filled with yellow fluid erupted on this child's upper lip.

tions visible on slit-lamp examination (see Chapter 19, Ophthalmology). Because this complication carries a risk of permanent visual impairment, urgent ophthalmologic consultation is indicated whenever there is any suspicion of ocular herpetic infection.

Eczema Herpeticum (Kaposi's Varicelliform Eruption)
Patients with atopic eczema and other forms of chronic dermatitis are at risk for a particularly severe form of primary herpes simplex infection and thus should avoid contact with people with active herpetic infections. The illness is heralded by the onset of high fever, irritability, and discomfort. Lesions appear in crops and primarily involve areas of previously affected skin. Typically they evolve to form pustules, which rupture and form crusts over the course of a few days. Occasionally these lesions become hemorrhagic (Fig. 12.13). Multiple crops can appear over 7 to 10 days, simulating varicella. However, the slower evolution of lesions, the tendency of such lesions to become hemorrhagic, their concentration in eczematous areas, and the persistence of fever and systemic symptoms for as long as 1 week help to distinguish this disorder from varicella. Severity ranges from mild to fulminant and is dependent in part on the extensiveness of the preceding der-

matitis. When the area of involvement is large, fluid losses can be severe. There also is a significant risk of secondary bacterial infection. Up to 40 percent of cases are fatal.

Recurrent Herpes Simplex Infection
As mentioned earlier, following primary infection the herpes simplex virus becomes latent within the ganglia that lie in the region of initial involvement; reactivation of the latent virus results in localized recurrences at or near the site of previous infection. Fever, sunlight, local trauma, menses, and emotional stress are recognized triggers and, since the mouth is the major site of primary infection, labial and perioral lesions (cold sores) are seen most commonly. Many patients report a prodrome of localized burning along with stinging or itching prior to the eruption of grouped vesicles. These vesicles contain yellow serous fluid, and they often appear smaller and less thick-walled than primary lesions (Fig. 12.14). After 2 to 3 days, the vesicular fluid becomes cloudy, and then crusts form. Although fever and systemic symptoms are absent, regional nodes may be enlarged and tender. The localization of the lesions to a small area helps to distinguish them from those of herpes zoster. Prodromal symptoms and discomfort help to distinguish recurrent herpes simplex from impetigo and from contact dermatitis.

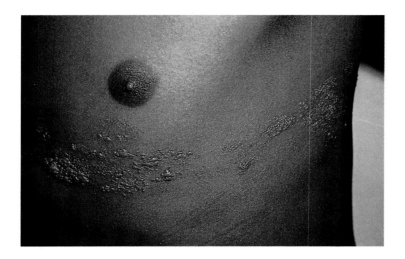

FIG. 12.15 Herpes zoster. The dermatomal distribution of these grouped vesicles is a hallmark of herpes zoster. The vesicles are rather thin-walled and coalescent, and they lie on an erythematous base. (Courtesy of Dr. Michael Sherlock)

HERPES ZOSTER (SHINGLES)

The varicella-zoster virus, like other herpesviruses, takes up permanent, albeit generally quiescent, residence in its host following initial infection, i.e., varicella. Generally the virus lies dormant in the genome of sensory nerve root cells, but it can reactivate as does herpes simplex. Mechanical and thermal trauma, infection, and debilitation all have been postulated as triggers. In the reactivated form, herpes zoster, lesions consist of grouped thin-walled vesicles on an erythematous base, which are distributed along the course of a spinal or cranial sensory nerve root (Fig. 12.15). They evolve from macule to papule to vesicle and then to a crusted stage over a few days. Hyperesthesia or nerve root pain may precede, accompany, or follow the eruption, and has no correlation with severity of the rash. Pain, if present at all in pediatric patients, rarely is severe and generally is short lived, unless a cranial nerve dermatome is involved. Fever and constitutional symptoms may or may not be part of the picture, but regional adenopathy is common.

Thoracic dermatomes are involved in the majority of cases, and are followed in frequency by cervical, trigeminal, lumbar, and facial nerve regions. Cranial nerve involvement may produce a puzzling prodrome consisting of severe headache, facial pain, or auricular pain with no evident cause, lasting up to several days prior to appearance of the eruption. Lesions appear unilaterally on the tonsillar pillars and uvula with involvement of the maxillary branch of the trigeminal nerve on the buccal mucosa and palate with involvement of the mandibular division and on the face, cornea, and tip of the nose with involvement of the ophthalmic branch (see Chapter 20, Oral Disorders). When the geniculate ganglion is affected, vesicles are seen in the external auditory canal in concert with facial paralysis. Although varicella can be transmitted by patients with herpes zoster, contagion generally is less of a problem since most have lesions on areas that are covered by clothing and most do not have involvement of the oropharynx.

Bacterial Exanthems

STREPTOCOCCAL SCARLET FEVER

While most commonly associated with pharyngitis and impetigo, the group A ß-hemolytic streptococci are frequently the cause of an illness associated with a generalized exanthem known as scarlet fever, or scarlatina. The exanthem is produced by an erythrogenic toxin excreted by the streptococcus. Streptococcal infections occur year round, although pharyngi-tis and scarlet fever have a peak incidence in winter and spring. Transmission requires close contact to permit the direct spread of large droplets, and those with nasal infection are particularly effective sources. Anal carriers as well as contaminated food sources also have been responsible for outbreaks. The incubation period for scarlet fever ranges from 12 hours to approximately 7 days. Patients are contagious during the period of the acute illness and may transmit the organism during active subclinical infection as well. An average of 50 percent of family members living with an index case will become secondarily infected, and up to half of these individuals will have subclinical disease.

Once a severe illness with high morbidity and mortality, scarlet fever has become modified over the past several decades to a much milder illness. In the classic case, which is seen less than 10 percent of the time, the patient experiences an abrupt onset of fever, chills, malaise, headache, sore throat, and vomiting; abdominal pain also may be a prominent complaint. Within 12 to 48 hours the exanthem appears and rapidly generalizes, usually beginning on the trunk and spreading peripherally, but sometimes spreading cephalocaudally. The face is flushed with perioral pallor. The remaining skin becomes diffusely erythematous and is covered by tiny pinhead-sized papules, giving the appearance of a sunburn with goose bumps. The texture is sandpapery on palpation and the erythema blanches with pressure (Fig. 12.16A,B). The skin may be pruritic, but it is not tender. Many patients also will have urticaria and dermatographism. In severe cases vesiculation may occur. Following generalization the rash becomes accentuated in skin folds or creases, and 1 to 3 days after its appearance petechiae may appear in a linear distribution along the creases, forming "Pastia's lines" (Fig. 12.16C). Examination of the oropharynx in the "textbook" case discloses large, very erythematous and edematous tonsils that often are covered by exudate, along with palatal erythema and petechiae (see Chapter 22, Otolaryngology). The uvula may be erythematous and edematous as well. The tongue also shows characteristic findings. During the first two days it has a white coating through which erythematous papillae project, resulting in a "white strawberry tongue." Subsequently the white coat peels leaving a glistening red surface with prominent papillae, which is referred to as a "red strawberry tongue" (Fig. 12.16D). Tender cervical adenopathy is seen in 30 to 60 percent of cases. Without benefit of treatment the rash, fever, and pharyngitis resolve within 1 week; with treatment improvement is relatively rapid. Desquamation occurs regardless of treatment,

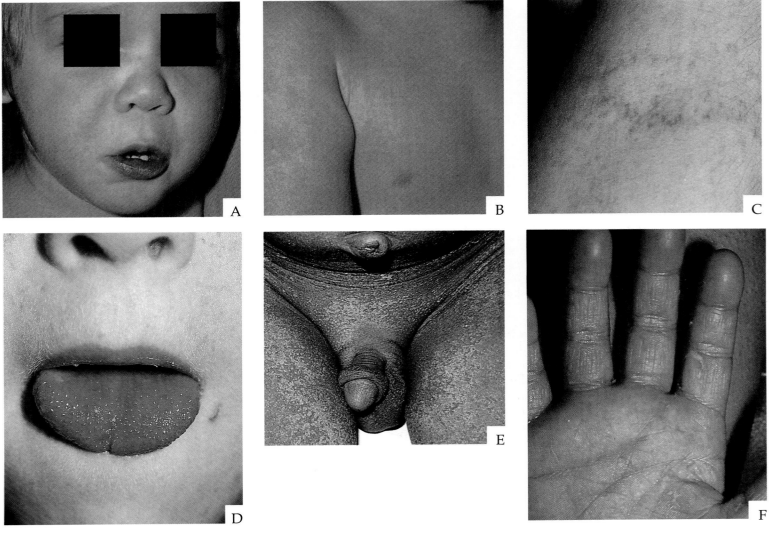

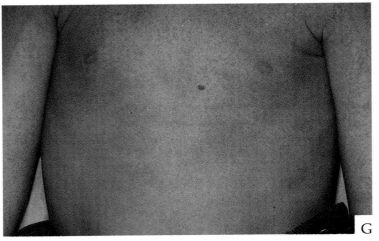

FIG. 12.16 Streptococcal scarlet fever. **A** and **B**, in the classic case of this disease the exanthem is characterized by a flushed face, perioral pallor and a diffuse blanching erythematous rash that has a sandpapery consistency on palpation. **C**, within 1 to 3 days of onset, Pastia's lines may be noted. **D**, the characteristic red strawberry tongue with glistening surface and prominent papillae is seen a few days after onset. **E** and **F**, desquamation occurs in fine thin flakes as the acute phase of the illness resolves, and is proportional to the intensity of the exanthem. **G**, there is a wide spectrum in severity and manifestations. In this child with streptococcal scarlet fever, the rash has a patchy distribution with accentuation in the axillae and other skin creases. (**A**, **B**, and **E** courtesy of Dr. Michael Sherlock)

and begins several days after onset, occurring in a cephalocaudal distribution (Fig. 12.16E,F). The skin is shed in fine thin flakes (in contrast to the thick flakes that characterize desquamation following staphylococcal exanthems [see Figs. 12.17 and 12.19]), and the extent of this process is directly proportional to the intensity of the exanthem.

Diagnosis is easy in the classic case, but the wide spectrum in severity of disease and in its manifestations can occasionally cause confusion. Fever may be absent or low grade, and malaise may be minimal. Pharyngitis may be mild (without exudate, petechiae, or marked erythema) or absent, even when the throat is the site of infection. In such cases tongue findings may be absent as well. When streptococcal skin or wound infections are the primary site of infection, the oropharynx is normal. The appearance of the exanthem may vary also. In some children it is patchy but continues to be most prominent near skin folds (Fig. 12.16G). An occasional child may have diffuse petechiae. Still others may present with fever and/or nasopharyngitis and urticaria as their initial manifestations. In dark-skinned children, erythema and perioral pallor may be difficult to appreciate and the papules may be larger, thus producing a texture less like sandpaper.

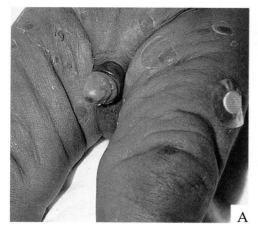 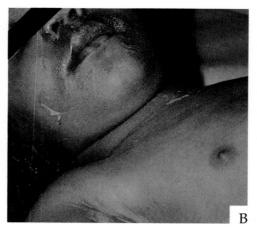 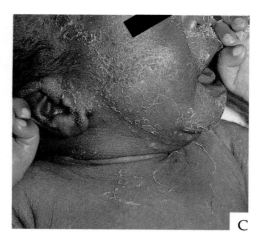

FIG. 12.17 *Staphylococcal scalded skin syndrome.* **A,** *this infant shows evidence of epidermal separation and has numerous ruptured bullae over the inguinal region and thighs.* **B,** *in this older child, symptoms were mild and only the skin of the face, axillae, and perineum showed signs of epidermal separation. Note the evidence of a positive* Nikolsky's sign on her upper lip and cheek, which resulted when she wiped her nose. **C,** a denuded area is evident on the upper chest and thick flakes have begun to form on the face. Culture of the purulent nasal discharge was positive for Staphylococcus aureus. (Courtesy of Dr. Michael Sherlock)

Recognition of scarlet fever followed by treatment with a 10-day course of penicillin or erythromycin is important not only to shorten the course of the illness but also to prevent rheumatic fever and pyogenic complications, the most common of which include adenitis, otitis, sinusitis, and peritonsillar and retropharyngeal abscesses. Therefore, in patients with fever or nasopharyngitis and urticaria and in children with scarlatiniform eruptions, a screening throat culture for group A streptococci should be obtained regardless of presence or absence of other symptoms. Poststreptococcal nephritis, however, is not prevented by antimicrobial therapy.

STAPHYLOCOCCAL EXANTHEMS

Coagulase-positive staphylococci are ubiquitous organisms that are carried at any given time by approximately one-third of the population. While the hallmark of staphylococcal infection is the abscess, numerous forms of infection are seen, and at least three distinct generalized exanthematous disorders have now been identified: staphylococcal scalded skin syndrome; staphylococcal scarlet fever; and toxic shock syndrome. In each case the organisms at the primary site of infection release exotoxins, which then produce the characteristic rash. Transmission may occur via direct contact with persons who are infected or who are carriers. Sites of carriage include the nose, skin, axilla, perineum, hair, and nails. Spread of infection also may occur via airborne particles or through contact with contaminated objects or food. Draining skin lesions, nasal discharge, and contaminated hands constitute particularly important sources of transmission. Traumatic or surgical wounds, burns, insect bites, areas of preexisting dermatitis, viral skin lesions, and prior viral respiratory tract infection all serve as major predisposing conditions.

Staphylococcal Scalded Skin Syndrome

A disorder seen most commonly in infants and young children, staphylococcal scalded skin syndrome is caused by phage group II coagulase-positive staphylococci. The primary infection usually is mild, with purulent nasopharyngitis, conjunctivitis, impetigo, and infections of the umbilicus and circumcision sites seen most commonly. Rarely, sepsis, pneumonia, or other severe invasive staphylococcal infections may precede the onset of the exanthem.

The infecting organisms produce an epidermolytic exotoxin, which is spread hematogenously and which causes cleavage of the skin between the epidermis and the dermis. This process may begin within hours or days of the appearance of signs of the primary infection, and typically its onset is heralded by prodromal symptoms of fever and irritability, often accompanied by vomiting. These symptoms are followed by the development of a diffuse erythroderma that spreads rapidly from head to toe and simulates the appearance of a sunburn. In contrast to streptococcal scarlet fever, the involved skin is tender, even to light touch. Within 1 to 3 days, thin-walled, flaccid bullous lesions appear, which rupture soon after formation (Fig. 12.17A). Simultaneously larger portions of the epidermis begin to separate in sheets, and during this phase the placement of light lateral traction on the skin will cause the epidermis to pull away from the dermis leaving a raw weeping surface; this separation of the skin in response to stroking is called Nikolsky's sign (Fig. 12.17B). Following exfoliation the surface gradually dries, forming large, thick flakes (Fig. 12.17C).

There is a broad spectrum of severity for this syndrome. In severe cases the patient appears toxic and in considerable pain. The patient may shed large portions of skin, resulting in significant fluid losses that may be accompanied by difficulties with temperature regulation. In mild cases (see Fig. 12.17B) toxicity is absent and only localized areas of skin are denuded, with the face and perineum constituting the primary sites of shedding. The causative organism can be isolated from the site of primary infection, but it is absent—at least initially—from the bullae and from sites of skin separation.

Staphylococcal Scarlet Fever

Staphylococcal infection can result in an exanthem that initially is indistinguishable in appearance from that produced by group A ß-hemolytic streptococci. The illness is characterized by fever, irritability, and moderate malaise, followed by the abrupt onset of a generalized erythematous rash, often of sandpapery consistency, with accentuation in the skin creases. In contrast to the exanthem seen in streptococcal scarlet fever, the involved skin usually is tender, the tongue is normal, and there is no palatal enanthem. Evolution of lesions also differs, as within 2 to 5 days the skin begins to crack and fissure, espe-

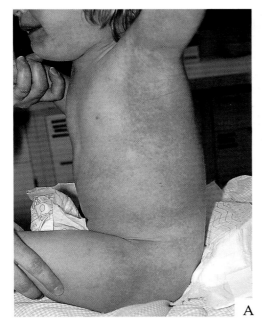

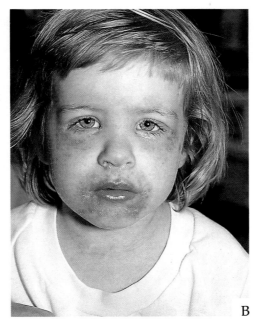

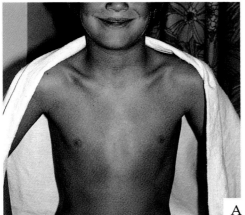

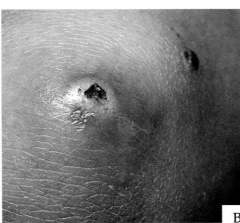

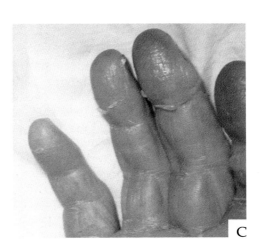

FIG. 12.18 Staphylococcal scarlet fever. *A,* in this patient, nasopharyngitis and purulent conjunctivitis antedated the development of a generalized sandpaper-like rash which was tender to the touch. *B,* the skin in the periorbital and perioral areas has begun to crack, fissure, and weep serous fluid.

FIG. 12.19 Toxic shock syndrome. *A,* this young boy presented with diffuse erythroderma fever, chills, myalgias, headache, vomiting, and orthostatic dizziness with mild widening of his pulse pressure. *B,* examination disclosed an infected knee abrasion, which grew S. aureus. *Though his illness was relatively mild, the association of gas-*trointestinal symptoms and orthostatic changes suggested TSS, which was confirmed by laboratory studies and by *(C)* subsequent desquamation. This begins periungually and the skin is shed in thick casts. *(C,* courtesy of Dr. George Pazin, Presbyterian University Hospital of Pittsburgh)

cially in the perioral and periorbital areas and in the skin creases (Fig. 12.18). It is then shed in large, thick flakes over 3 to 5 days. Local skin and wound infections are common antecedents and their presence often enables presumptive identification of staphylococci as causative agents early in the course of the disease. However, when nasopharyngitis is the source of primary infection, the picture can be very difficult to distinguish from that of variants of streptococcal infection, in which the strawberry tongue and palatal petechiae often are absent. The same may be true when a local infection with lymphangitis is the source. In such cases the tendency for the staphylococcal rash to be tender may be the major clinical distinction, pending Gram stain and/or culture results. Unless the primary infection is severe enough to warrant parenteral treatment, oral antimicrobial therapy is sufficient.

Toxic Shock Syndrome

Toxic shock syndrome (TSS) is the third syndrome of staphylococcal origin to be characterized by a generalized exanthem. It is seen in children and adults who have localized infections caused by coagulase-positive staphylococci of phage groups I or III, and in menstruating women and girls whose vaginas are colonized with these organisms. In the latter subgroup of patients (who may not have a history of prior vaginal discharge), there is a strong correlation with tampon use, suggesting that the impedence of normal menstrual flow and/or the presence of secondary abrasions may contribute to development of this syndrome. Patients with nonmenstrually associated TSS often have an obvious primary focus of infection in the form of a skin lesion, an abscess, or purulent conjunctivitis (see Fig. 12.19B).

In its full-blown form, TSS begins with a prodrome consisting of low-grade fever, malaise, myalgias, and vomiting. This is followed by an abrupt increase in fever with chills, worsening myalgias, repetitive vomiting, abdominal pain, orthostatic dizziness, and weakness. Soon thereafter, patients develop diffuse erythroderma, mimicking a sunburn (Fig. 12.19A). Conjunctivitis with photophobia, oropharyngeal erythema, and a strawberry tongue are common features. Subsequently, severe watery diarrhea, hypotension, and oliguria may become prominent, accompanied by alterations in level of consciousness. This often necessitates massive volume replacement and

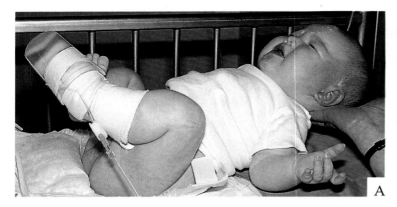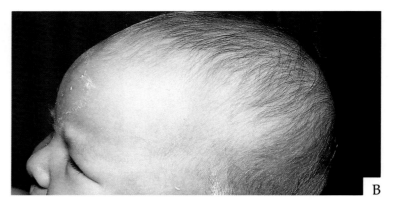

FIG. 12.20 Meningitis. **A,** *nuchal rigidity and a positive Brudzinski's sign are demonstrated. On attempted passive flexion of the neck, the infant grimaces with pain, neck stiffness limits flexion, and the knees* and hips are flexed to reduce traction on the meninges. **B,** *this infant also was found to have a bulging anterior fontanelle when sitting quietly, reflecting increased intracranial pressure.*

vasopressor therapy. In severe cases, adult respiratory distress syndrome may develop. Many patients have muscle tenderness and weakness as well as diffuse abdominal tenderness without peritoneal signs. A small proportion develop nonpitting edema of the face, hands, and feet. Over the ensuing days, petechiae and a secondary maculopapular rash may be noted along with oral ulcerations. Desquamation is routine, usually beginning a week after onset of the rash. It is most prominent over the palms and soles and in the periungual areas, and the skin is shed in thick casts (Fig. 12.19C). Parenteral antimicrobial therapy directed against *Staphylococcus aureus* is designed to eradicate any focus of infection and reduce the risk of recurrence.

Clinical and laboratory findings in severe cases suggest a process in which there is diffuse vascular leakage with third-spacing of fluids, electrolytes, and serum proteins. Secondary hypotension and hypoperfusion result in azotemia. Toxin-related hepatic changes may also be noted. As recognition of TSS has increased, the existence of a wide spectrum of severity has become apparent. Mild cases mimic the picture of staphylococcal scarlet fever. Such patients tend to have smaller gastrointestinal losses and less difficulty with fluid shifts and attendant complications.

MENINGOCOCCAL EXANTHEMS

Neisseria meningitidis is capable of producing a number of clinical illnesses, two of which—acute meningococcemia, and meningococcosis or chronic meningococcemia—are characterized in part by a generalized exanthem. The organism is carried in the upper respiratory tract of humans who, though usually asymptomatic, nevertheless may transmit the organism via droplet spread of respiratory secretions. The majority of persons so exposed become carriers and produce antibodies but do not develop clinical disease. Clinical illness is most common in children under 5 years of age, with a peak incidence between 6 and 12 months of age. A secondary peak of lesser magnitude is seen in adolescence. Susceptibility to disease appears to be related to a lack of bactericidal antibody or to a failure to produce antibody in response to infection. It is still unclear as to whether or not antecedent viral respiratory infection is a predisposing factor.

While meningococcal infection occurs year round, the peak season for these illnesses is late winter and early spring. Invasive disease occurs both endemically and epidemically. Persons who have intimate contact with infected patients, e.g.,

other members of the same household or persons in "closed communities" such as military barracks, dormitories, or daycare centers, are at highest risk of becoming secondarily infected. The incubation period following exposure ranges from 1 to 10 days, with most clinical cases developing in less than 4 days. Secondary attack rates range from 0.3 to 10 percent and are highest during epidemic outbreaks. Any mucosal surface is subject to infection, which may remain localized or may serve as the source of invasive disease.

Acute Meningococcemia

The two major invasive forms of meningococcal disease are meningitis and septicemia, which may occur singly or in combination. Patients usually experience a prodromal period ranging in length from a few hours to 5 days. During this phase, symptoms of upper respiratory tract infection or nasopharyngitis in association with fever are typical. Patients also may have lethargy, headache, myalgias, arthralgias, and vomiting. Following this, an abrupt change occurs, characterized by increased fever with chills (or occasionally hypothermia), worsening malaise, and progressive lethargy. In the 90 percent in whom meningitis is the primary manifestation, vomiting, irritability (often with a high-pitched cry in infants), and nuchal rigidity are prominent (Fig. 12.20A). Infants may also have a bulging fontanelle (Fig. 12.20B). Delirium, combativeness, stupor, and seizures also may develop. While some of these patients also have meningococcemia, they are less likely to develop cutaneous manifestations than are those without meningitis. Endotoxic shock and disseminated intravascular coagulation (DIC) also are unusual, and mortality is relatively low.

In contrast, approximately 10 percent of patients develop a picture of overwhelming sepsis with little or no evidence of meningitis. In these patients the abrupt change in clinical picture described above typically heralds the development of a rash in association with manifestations of shock, including mottling, distal coolness with decreased capillary refill or cyanosis, and either widened pulse pressure or frank hypotension. Up to 85 percent of these patients will have cutaneous lesions involving the trunk and extremities. Such lesions may consist of tender pink macules; petechiae, which often are palpably raised; and purpura, which when present is most prominent on the extremities and may progress to form areas of frank necrosis (Fig. 12.21). The combination of purpura and shock is termed the "Waterhouse-Friderichsen" syndrome and

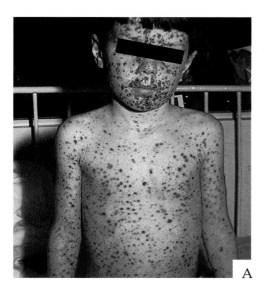

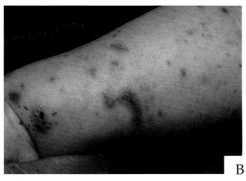

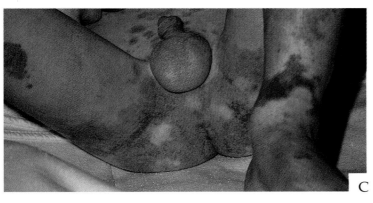

FIG. 12.21
Meningococcemia.
A, *this youngster manifests the generalized purpuric and petechial rash characteristic of acute meningococcemia.* **B,** *petechiae are more apparent in this close-up of an infant. Gram stain of petechial scrapings may reveal organisms.* **C,** *purpura may progress to form areas of frank cutaneous necrosis, especially in cases with DIC.*

gram-negative diplococci. Cultures of blood, CSF, and petechial lesions should be performed unless the severity of illness precludes lumbar puncture. Counter-immunoelectrophoresis of urine, CSF, or blood may provide rapid confirmation. Because of the potential for deterioration, aggressive empiric antimicrobial therapy and vigorous supportive measures should be instituted promptly whenever meningococcemia is suspected.

There are a number of differential diagnostic possibilities, which include other forms of bacterial sepsis, bacterial endocarditis, Rocky Mountain spotted fever, and various other disorders characterized by thrombocytopenia. Some forms of septicemia due to gram-negative bacilli may be clinically indistinguishable from meningococcal septicemia initially. Similarly *Haemophilus influenzae* type b septicemia as well as pneumococcal septicemia may be associated with the development of petechiae, though in these cases they are not palpable. The purpuric lesions of staphylococcal sepsis tend to become pustular early on, and the site of primary infection also helps distinguish this organism. Adenoviral and streptococcal infections may produce petechial rashes but usually do not cause a septic picture. Other clinical characteristics help to distinguish patients with thrombocytopenia due to immune thrombocytopenic purpura, acute leukemia and mononucleosis, while the centripetal mode of spread of the petechial rash of Rocky Mountain spotted fever, and the initial distribution and subsequent mode of spread of the lesions of Henoch-Schönlein purpura, help to distinguish these illnesses. Differentiation can be particularly difficult in the case of a child presenting with high fever with no source other than that of an upper respiratory tract infection and a petechial rash. These findings may represent early nonfulminant meningococcemia, but they also can be part of the picture of viral illness or another bacterial process; in such cases observation and/or presumptive therapy may be necessary.

Meningococcosis (Chronic Meningococcemia)
Meningococcosis, a disorder more indolent than acute meningococcemia, is defined as meningococcal sepsis with a fever of greater than 1 week's duration, without meningitis. The average length of symptoms prior to diagnosis is 6 to 8 weeks. In most cases symptoms are intermittent, and in all cases they consist of fever and chills (without rigor), associated with an exanthem in nearly 95 percent of cases. The rash waxes and wanes, often in association with the fever. Lesions may consist of tender erythematous subcutaneous nodules, erythematous macules and papules, or petechiae, occurring singly or in combination. Urticarial lesions are seen occasionally. The feet, legs, upper arms, and trunk are the sites most commonly involved. Mild malaise and myalgias tend to accompany the fever, and headache and arthralgias also are common. In childhood cases swelling of hands, feet, knees, and ankles may occur intermittently, without evidence of warmth or erythema; however, when the legs are involved, the child may refuse to walk.

The diagnosis of meningococcosis can be difficult, since early blood cultures often are negative (although children are more likely than adults to have positive cultures), and skin lesions generally are negative for organisms, both on smear and culture. Throat culture usually is negative, as well. Leukocytosis is seen with the fever. The sedimentation rate may be normal or elevated. Thrombocytopenia is seen occasionally. Close followup and monitoring of the clinical course, combined with repeated blood cultures, is the best way to con-

has been associated in some but not all instances with adrenal hemorrhage and secondary adrenal insufficiency. Evolution may be fulminant, resulting in prostration within a few hours, or it may be slower, occurring over a period lasting up to 24 hours. Patients with a short prodrome, fulminant progression, and early appearance of purpuric lesions have a particularly poor prognosis. Over 60 percent of such patients have clinical evidence of hypotension and DIC on presentation, and approximately 50 percent have no leukocytosis, suggesting that their immune system has been overwhelmed. Only about 20 percent of these patients have meningitis. Mortality in such cases approaches 40 percent, while only 3 percent of those with slower progression succumb. Most deaths occur within 24 hours of presentation and are the result of a combination of circulatory collapse and congestive heart failure due to endotoxic shock and myocarditis.

In many cases the diagnosis can be suspected clinically and is confirmed by laboratory findings. Gram-stained smears of petechial lesions and buffy coat preparations often will reveal

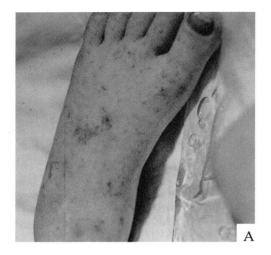 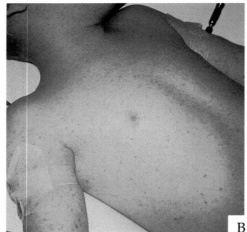

*FIG. 12.22 Rocky Mountain spotted fever. **A,** the exanthem characteristic of this disease first appears distally on wrists, ankles, palms, and soles. It may be petechial from the outset, or it may start as an erythematous, blanching macular or maculopapular eruption, which then becomes petechial as it spreads centripetally. **B,** in this child the rash has become generalized. Both petechial and blanching erythematous lesions are present. (**A,** courtesy of Dr. Ellen Wald, Children's Hospital of Pittsburgh; **B,** courtesy of Dr. T. F. Sellers, Jr.)*

firm the diagnosis. Of the patients not diagnosed and treated, approximately one-third ultimately will develop severe localized infection (after an average of 10 weeks of illness) with meningitis, carditis, nephritis, and ocular infection occurring most commonly.

Rocky Mountain Spotted Fever

Rocky Mountain spotted fever is an acute potentially severe exanthematous disease caused by the organism *Rickettsia rickettsii*. These obligate intracellular parasites usually are transmitted to man via the bite of an infected tick, which injects organisms while it feeds on the host. Once injected, the organisms multiply in the endothelium of small blood vessels and are spread hematogenously, resulting in a widespread vasculitis characterized by focal inflammation and thrombosis with secondary vascular leakage. Because ticks are active during warm months, the peak seasons for this disorder are spring and summer. The incubation period ranges from 2 to 14 days with an average of 4 to 8 days. Two-thirds of cases occur in children under 15 years of age. Yearly outbreaks tend to occur in circumscribed geographic areas. Mortality is as high as 5 to 7 percent and often is due to failure to diagnose and treat the condition in its early phase.

Onset may be acute or gradual and is characterized by fever and headache. The headache, which may be frontal or generalized, typically is severe, unremitting, and unresponsive to analgesia. Headache may not be a major complaint in very young children, however. Other less constant symptoms include chills, anorexia, nausea and vomiting, sore throat, abdominal pain, diarrhea, arthralgias, and myalgias. Respiratory symptoms are uncommon. The spleen is enlarged in 30 to 50 percent of cases, but adenopathy is not prominent. The exanthem usually is noted on or about the third day of illness, but it may appear as late as the beginning of the second week.

In the majority of patients, the characteristic appearance and mode of spread of the exanthem is the most helpful clue to clinical diagnosis. The rash begins on wrists, ankles, palms, and soles, usually appearing as an erythematous, blanching, fine macular or maculopapular eruption. It then spreads centripetally and becomes petechial (Fig. 12.22) although occasionally lesions are petechial from the outset. In some cases, the eruption is not prominent and may even be transient, making diagnosis difficult. Conjunctival injection, with photophobia and petechial hemorrhages, often develops simultaneously with the rash. Firm, nonpitting, nondependent edema, beginning in the periorbital region and then generalizing, tends to occur a few days after the onset of symptoms. In severe cases CNS symptoms develop with disease progression and range in severity from restlessness, irritability, and anxiety to confusion, delirium, and coma with or without seizures and focal neurologic signs. Myocarditis, DIC, renal failure, and cardiovascular collapse are features of advanced disease.

White blood cell counts are normal or low in the first few days and then tend to rise. Thrombocytopenia is common. Other laboratory abnormalities include hyponatremia due to fluid shifts and renal losses; hypoproteinemia due to vascular and renal losses, and hepatic dysfunction; abnormal liver function tests; and hyperkalemia with increasing cell death.

Because there is no diagnostic test capable of providing prompt definitive results, and because the early institution of antimicrobial treatment is crucial to a favorable outcome, the diagnosis of Rocky Mountain spotted fever must be made on clinical grounds and as early as possible. The diagnosis should be suspected in any child with fever, headache, toxicity, and a centripetally spreading petechial rash, especially when the patient's history suggests or confirms an exposure to ticks. The *R. rickettsii* organisms are sensitive to both chloramphenicol and tetracyclines, and recovery is the rule if therapy is begun during the first week of illness. If treatment is delayed beyond the first week, however, the outcome may be unfavorable despite antimicrobial therapy and vigorous supportive measures. Subsequent serologic confirmation may be made using complement fixation tests or a variety of other assays. Immunofluorescent examination of skin biopsy specimens obtained 4 to 8 days from onset can provide earlier confirmation, but often this test is not readily available.

MUMPS (EPIDEMIC PAROTITIS)

Mumps is an acute viral illness that preferentially involves glandular and neural tissues. While salivary glands, especially the parotid glands, are the most common sites of clinical involvement, the CNS may be affected as well as other glandular tissues. In as many as one-third of cases, infection is subclinical. Peak incidence is in late winter and spring. The incubation period is 16 to 18 days, with patients being contagious from 1 to 7 days prior to onset of clinical symptoms and for 5 to 9 days thereafter. Asymptomatic individuals also can transmit the virus.

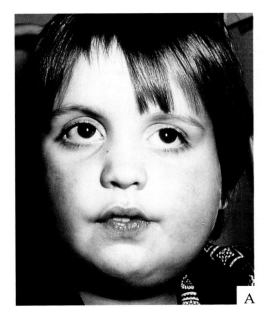 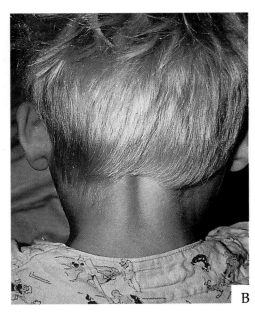 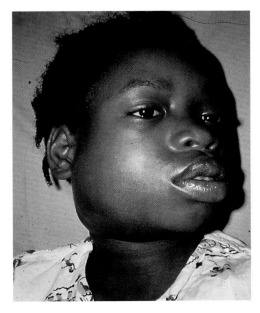

FIG. 12.23 Mumps. **A,** this young boy presented with unilateral parotid swelling, which was indurated and moderately tender. Visually it was appreciated best in this view, which reveals swelling anterior and inferior to his left ear. **B,** bilateral postauricular

swelling (right greater than left) can be appreciated when the patient is viewed from behind. Secondary displacement of the auricle is evident on the left. (**A,** courtesy of Dr. G. D. W. McKendrik. **B,** courtesy of Dr. Michael Sherlock)

FIG. 12.24 Suppurative parotitis. This patient presented with high fever, chills and marked enlargement of the right parotid gland which was severely painful and exquisitely tender. The overlying skin is erythematous, and purulent material was seen draining from Stenson's duct. (Courtesy of Dr. Sylvan Stool, Children's Hospital of Pittsburgh)

Prodromal symptoms consist of fever, headache, malaise, and anorexia. In the typical case these symptoms are followed within 24 hours by the onset of an earache or face pain, which older children often can localize to the region of the pinna. Pain is aggravated by chewing and by stimulation of salivation (in particular, by sour foods). Parotid swelling generally becomes noticeable within the next 24 hours, increases gradually over the next few days, and then abates over a similar period of time. Fever may persist for the duration of swelling but can disappear early in the course. On examination, an area of tender indurated swelling, extending from the preauricular area through the subauricular space to the postauricular region, can be palpated (Fig. 12.23A). With pronounced enlargement the pinna is pushed up and out (Fig. 12.23B). The gland is mildly to moderately tender to palpation. The color of the overlying skin is normal. Intraoral examination may reveal erythema and edema of Stensen's duct. Bilateral involvement is usual, although one gland will tend to enlarge before the other, and up to 25 percent of symptomatic patients will have unilateral inflammation.

This "typical picture" is but one of many possible variants of clinical mumps. In some cases the parotid gland is spared and the submaxillary or sublingual salivary glands may be the primary site of involvement. In the former instance, indurated swelling is found below the mid-portion of the mandible; in the latter case bilateral submental swelling is seen externally with sublingual swelling noted intraorally.

Preauricular swelling and induration, the Stensen's duct abnormality, and the absence of prominent overlying erythema help to distinguish parotid swelling from cervical adenitis involving the tonsillar node. In confusing cases and in cases where submaxillary or sublingual salivary glands are involved, closely simulating adenopathy, the patient can be

given lemon juice to sip or a lemon wedge to suck. In patients with mumps, this will result in a prompt increase in the size of the affected gland and in pain as salivation is stimulated, whereas no such change will be seen in patients with adenopathy. In cases of bacterial parotitis, the patient is likely to have high fever and to show signs of toxicity. The overlying skin is erythematous, with exquisite tenderness found on palpation (Fig. 12.24). Inspection of Stensen's duct while the gland is massaged usually will show purulent drainage.

While it has been estimated that up to 75 percent of mumps patients may have CSF pleocytosis, symptomatic meningoencephalitis is seen only in about 10 percent of patients. CNS symptoms usually follow parotitis, but can develop prior to or even in the absence of salivary gland involvement. There is a wide spectrum in severity of these symptoms, ranging from isolated headache and malaise with fever to frank nuchal rigidity with nausea, vomiting, and severe alterations in sensorium. Fortunately, permanent sequelae are rare, although children recovering from severe mumps meningoencephalitis may not return to normal levels of school performance for up to 6 months or a year.

Mumps orchitis is much less common in boys than in men, who have a 20 to 30 percent incidence. Orchitis usually follows salivary gland enlargement but may occur in its absence. Fever, chills, headache, nausea, vomiting, and lower abdominal pain are prominent and develop with the onset of painful, generally unilateral testicular swelling. Epididymitis is an invariable accompaniment. Duration of this process ranges from 3 to 7 days. Oophoritis, seen in an occasional female patient, presents with a secondary temperature spike, nausea, vomiting, and severe lower abdominal pain and tenderness. Involvement may be unilateral or bilateral, and when unilateral and on the right side, it may be indistinguishable from

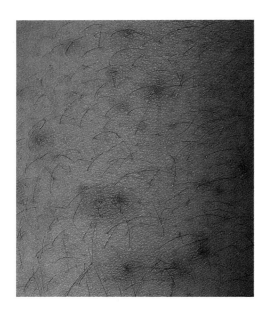

FIG. 12.25
Folliculitis. The extensor surfaces of the extremities and other hair-bearing areas are the most common sites of this superficial infection of hair follicles. Lesions begin as erythematous nodules at the base of a hair shaft and then evolve to form a central pustule with a thin red rim.

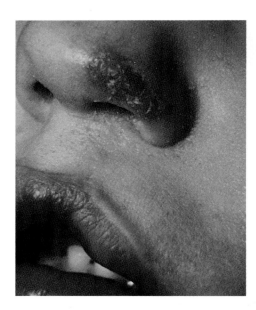

FIG. 12.26
Streptococcal impetigo. This impetiginous lesion has evolved from a papule to a vesicle that ruptured, producing this characteristic honey-colored crust. (Courtesy of Dr. Michael Sherlock)

appendicitis. Pancreatitis is an uncommon though potentially severe manifestation. Patients tend to have sudden onset of excruciating epigastric pain in association with fever, chills, repetitive vomiting, weakness, and prostration. This, too, tends to last for 3 to 7 days. Thyroiditis, mastitis, bartholinitis, and dacryocystitis have been reported in isolated cases as well.

BACTERIAL SKIN AND SOFT-TISSUE INFECTIONS

Superficial bacterial skin infections occur with a relatively high frequency in childhood. In the majority of cases, the causative organisms are inoculated through a small wound such as a superficial cut, an abrasion, an insect bite, or a burn. Infection may occur at the time of the injury if the pathogen has colonized the site previously, or it may occur subsequently via scratching, touching, or contamination with dirt. In some cases a preexisting dermatitis, by breaking down the skin barrier, sets the stage for secondary infection. The ever-present risk of infection in patients with preexisting dermatitis must be kept in mind, especially when steroids are being prescribed.

While most superficial infections are relatively minor in severity, diagnosis and proper treatment are important to reduce further spread of infection and to prevent its transmission to others. Deeper skin and soft-tissue infections, while less common, have the potential for causing greater morbidity and even mortality. As with superficial lesions, inoculation from without is the most common mode of acquisition. In a number of instances, however, these infections represent metastatic foci of bacteremic spread.

Group A ß-hemolytic streptococci and coagulase-positive staphylococci are the organisms most commonly responsible for skin and soft-tissue infections. Both organisms commonly reside in the nasopharynx, and staphylococci routinely colonize the skin, a phenomenon that is less likely, though still possible, with streptococci. Both organisms are transmitted readily by carriers or persons with active nasopharyngeal or skin infections. The fact that each pathogen produces relatively characteristic clinical features can help, to some extent, in making clinical diagnoses. Staphylococci, for example, are somewhat more likely to remain localized, stimulating suppuration and tissue necrosis, whereas streptococcal infection tends to spread along tissue planes and through lymphatics and thus is more commonly associated with secondary cellulitis, lymphangitis, and regional adenopathy.

FOLLICULITIS

Folliculitis refers to superficial infection and/or irritation of hair follicles. The scalp, face, extensor surfaces of the extremities, and buttocks are the most common sites of involvement. Patients with dry, atopic skin and keratosis pilaris (a condition in which follicles become blocked by keratin plugs) are particularly prone to this problem (see Chapter 8, Dermatology). Additional predisposing factors include seborrhea, excessive sweating, poor hygiene, and topical application of or contact with oils, tars, and adhesives. In each of these situations, obstruction of follicles occurs, setting the stage for inflammation and secondary infection. Following occlusion, a superficial erythematous nodule develops around the hair. The lesion then evolves to form a thin-walled central pustule with a narrow red rim (Fig. 12.25). The lesions may itch or burn and subsequently may drain and crust. While healing of a given lesion occurs in 7 to 10 days without treatment, multiple crops may occur. With scratching the infection may be spread to other areas, and secondary impetiginous lesions may develop. Coagulase-positive staphylococci are the pathogens usually identified, although other skin colonizers may participate. Oral antimicrobial therapy directed at the staphylococcus and treatment or avoidance of the predisposing condition are the measures indicated to clear the process.

On occasion the early lesions found in some forms of tinea capitis and tinea corporis may mimic folliculitis, although itching usually is more prominent in fungal infections and the surrounding rim of erythema tends to be wider. Tinea should be suspected especially when folliculitis is localized to the hairline of the scalp (see Chapter 8). Older lesions, when present, may help in distinguishing between fungal and bacterial infections. Gram stains, KOH preparations, and cultures can be useful in evaluating questionable cases.

IMPETIGO

Impetigo is a superficial infection of the epidermis caused by streptococci, staphylococci, or both. Exposed portions of the body including the face, extremities, hands, and neck are the most common sites of involvement. Lesions teem with organ-

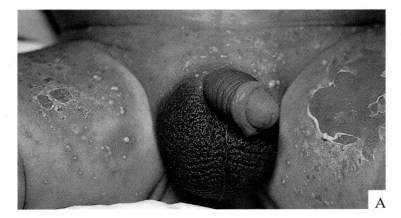

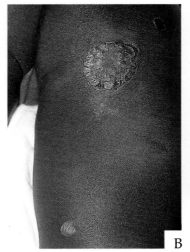

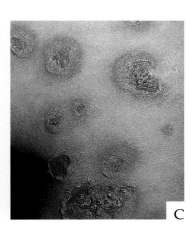

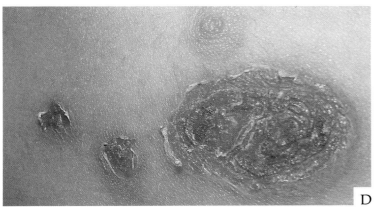

FIG. 12.27 *Staphylococcal impetigo.* **A,** *this infant with staphylococcal diaper dermatitis has multiple small thin-walled pustules that rupture rapidly and coalesce, leaving a shallow base and a superficial peeling rim.* **B,** *the various stages of bullous impetigo are evident in this child. An unruptured flaccid bulla is seen near an older lesion that has spread outward and crusted peripherally, and another that has just ruptured.* **C,** *in this child with staphylococcal impetigo older lesions have central crusts with bullous rims that are spreading outward.* **D,** *the findings of long-standing impetigo are seen in this youngster whose lesions are crusted in rings. Note also the smaller satellites surrounding the larger primary lesion.*

isms and serve as a potential source of transmission to others. In temperate climates the disorder has a peak incidence in summer and early fall because of increased exposure of the body surface to insect bites, injury, and colonization by pathogenic organisms. In warm climates impetigo is prevalent year round. Although impetigo has traditionally been considered a streptococcal disease, recent evidence suggests that *Staphylococcus aureus* has eclipsed the group A streptococcus as the predominant cause of impetigo.

In patients without preexisting dermatitis, lesions tend to be localized, but when the child has an antecedent condition such as eczema, the infection can spread rapidly to involve extensive areas.

In cases due to group A streptococci alone, the lesion begins as a papule and evolves rapidly to form a small thin-walled vesicle with an erythematous halo. The initially serous vesicular fluid becomes cloudy and the vesicle ruptures, forming a superficial honey-colored crust (Fig. 12.26). If the crust is lifted, a shallow, smooth, weeping, erythematous base is revealed. Secondary enlargement and tenderness of the regional lymph nodes is common.

The initial macules of primary staphylococcal impetigo may evolve rapidly to form small thin-walled pustules (Fig. 12.27A) or the larger flaccid bullae of bullous impetigo. The latter contain slightly cloudy fluid and often are a centimeter or more in diameter. In either case the pustules or bullae rupture rapidly leaving a shallow erythematous base surrounded by a superficial peeling rim (Fig. 12.27B). In cases of more long-standing or combined infection, lesions may crust centrally and enlarge centrifugally. This may result in the formation of a superficial central scab surrounded by a bullous rim or a dried lesion with multiple concentric rings (Fig. 12.27C,D). Lesions may coalesce over time and satellite lesions may form around larger primary lesions. Regardless

of type, impetigo frequently is pruritic and the patient is stimulated to scratch, thereby spreading the infection to other sites or even inoculating the offending bacteria deeper into the skin.

The possible source of the causative organisms may be the patient's own skin or nasopharynx or those of another infected person. In patients with facial and perinasal lesions, the nose is the most likely site of origin. Oral antimicrobial therapy is preferred for eradication and is particularly important when the source of infection is the nasopharynx or when lesions are extensive, although topical antibacterial therapy with mupirocin is effective for small numbers of lesions on the extremities and may reduce the spread of infection to others. If the patient has a predisposing dermatosis, this too must be treated.

On occasion, infection with other organisms can simulate the picture of impetiginous lesions. One form of tinea capitis produces lesions identical to those of streptococcal impetigo (see Chapter 8). Hence, when small pustules and golden-crusted lesions are seen on the scalp or at the hairline, Gram stain and KOH preparation are indicated to ensure correct diagnosis. *Candida* can produce tiny pustules, which rupture and have a superficial peeling rim, at times simulating staphylococcal infection in the diaper area. However, with candidal diaper dermatitis, lesions are smaller (pinpoint in size), pustules are more evanescent, the inflammation is more diffuse and the erythema more intense than with staphylococcal impetigo (see Chapter 8). In confusing cases a KOH preparation and/or Gram stain can be used to clarify the etiology.

ECTHYMA

Ecthyma is an ulcerative skin infection that penetrates more deeply than impetigo to involve the dermis. The disorder is most prevalent in tropical climates. Poor hygiene, insect bites, and trauma are the major predisposing factors, accounting for the fact that the lower extremities and the buttocks are the

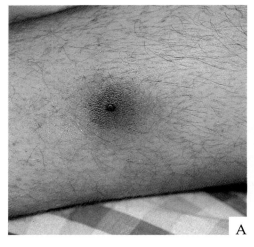

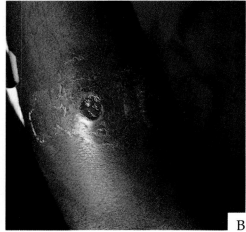

FIG. 12.28 Ecthyma. **A,** in focal ecthyma due to inoculation of group A streptococci, the lesion initially consists of a central vesicle or pustule (that rapidly crusts over) on a painful indurated erythematous base. **B,** with progression a deep widening ulcer forms, as seen in this child following removal of the overlying crust. (Courtesy of Dr. Ellen Wald, Children's Hospital of Pittsburgh)

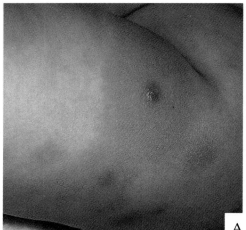

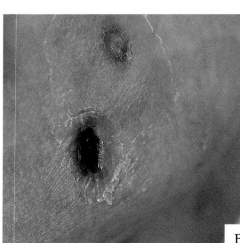

FIG. 12.29 Metastatic ecthyma. Pseudomonas septicemia may result in metastatic ecthymatous lesions that begin as pink macules, become hemorrhagic **(A)** and ultimately necrose centrally to form a black eschar **(B).** (Courtesy of Dr. Ellen Wald, Children's Hospital of Pittsburgh))

usual sites of involvement. Initially, lesions may resemble impetigo, consisting of a vesicle or a pustule on an erythematous base, which then ruptures and crusts over. In ecthyma, however, the lesions are painful, and the crusts harder, thicker and more adherent than in impetigo, and the surrounding area of erythema is indurated. The ulcerative base beneath the crust gradually deepens and enlarges. Unroofing the crust uncovers a round, deep, punched-out ulcer with raised borders (Fig. 12.28). The size of the lesions ranges from 1/2 to 3 cm. Without treatment these lesions take weeks to heal, leaving a circumscribed scar.

In most cases ecthyma is the result of direct inoculation of organisms through the skin, with group A ß-hemolytic streptococcus being the usual pathogen. On occasion staphylococci or pseudomonas may be causative; the latter organism, when infecting a small wound, is more likely to produce a central abscess that exudes a greenish or bluish purulent exudate when its crust is lifted. Pseudomonas septicemia also may result in metastatic ecthymatous lesions, which begin as pink macules, evolve to hemorrhagic papules, and then necrose centrally to leave a dark eschar on an erythematous base (Fig. 12.29). Subsequently, ulceration occurs, associated with deep necrosis. This metastatic form of ecthyma is distinguished easily from primary cases by virtue of the formation of multiple lesions and the presence of systemic signs of sepsis.

Abscesses of the Skin and Soft Tissues

Abscesses are localized collections of purulent material, which are buried in a tissue, an organ, or in a confined space. They result from the deep seeding of pyogenic organisms, which, in

the case of abscesses involving the skin and its appendages, usually are coagulase-positive staphylococci. As the area of inflammation expands outward, central necrosis occurs and the process tends to produce an increase in pressure with resultant pointing toward the surface or spread along tissue planes, and further local tissue destruction. Drainage is essential for healing, as the abscess contents provoke a continuing inflammatory response, and antimicrobials are generally unable to penetrate to the necrotic center of the lesion. Abscesses of the skin and soft tissues are categorized in part according to the site of involvement and in part according to the structure involved. The types most commonly encountered in childhood will be discussed below.

PARONYCHIA (PERIUNGUAL ABSCESS)

A paronychia is a relatively superficial abscess that develops under the cuticle or along the nail fold of a finger or a toe. Staphylococci and occasionally streptococci gain access through a traumatized hangnail or through lesions created by clipping a cuticle or by chewing on the fingers. Occasionally an ingrown toe nail is the predisposing condition, and in such cases the nail, which usually was cut improperly, grows laterally into the nail fold, lacerating the soft tissue and setting the stage for infection. In typical cases, erythema, pain, and tenderness develop at the site of injury, and are followed rapidly by suppuration (Fig. 12.30). The infection then advances from the portal of entry around the nail fold and, if treatment is delayed, it can burrow beneath the base of the nail creating a subungual abscess (onychia). Occasionally secondary lymphangitis may develop. Drainage is accomplished readily by

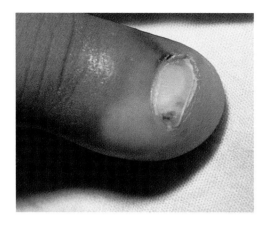

FIG. 12.30 Paronychia. Chewing on a hangnail predisposed this child to the development
of a paronychia. Initially, erythema developed
near the hangnail, and was followed rapidly
by suppuration.

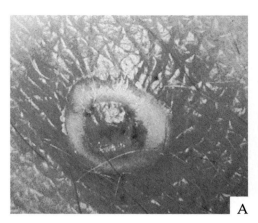

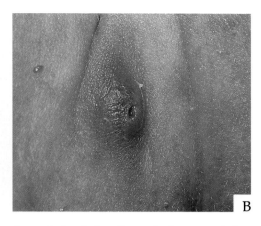

FIG. 12.31 Furuncle. **A,** in this well-developed furuncle, the abscess has burrowed to
the surface and the skin has thinned centrally
and begun to necrose. There is a wide surrounding rim of erythema and induration. **B,**
furuncle located on the neck of a young infant
had spontaneously ruptured and drained,
earlier in the day, but was beginning to
enlarge again. (**A,** courtesy of Dr. Bernard
Cohen, Children's Hospital of Pittsburgh)

undermining the involved portion of the cuticle and nail fold
with a scalpel blade. Unless secondary complications have
developed, subsequent soaking usually is sufficient for healing,
although oral antistaphylococcal agents hasten the process.

ABSCESSES OF SKIN APPENDAGES
Furuncle

A furuncle, or boil, is a perifollicular dermal abscess that is
usually caused by coagulase-positive staphylococci, perhaps
in concert with other skin flora. It may be the result of extension of a superficial folliculitis or of direct inoculation via
minor trauma. Hairy areas subject to friction and/or maceration are particularly vulnerable. Skin contact with occlusive
agents such as oils, tars, and adhesives is another common
predisposing factor. Older children and adolescents have a
much higher incidence than do younger children.

The lesion begins as a small dermal nodule around a hair follicle, which initially may produce a sensation of mild discomfort
and itching. As it gradually increases in size, pain worsens and
is aggravated by touching and motion of the involved area.
With expansion, the overlying skin becomes reddened, central
necrosis begins to occur, and with increased inflammation and
pressure the infection begins to seek egress. In the case of most
furuncles, the abscess burrows toward the surface of the skin,
which becomes thinned and shiny as the abscess becomes fluctuant (Fig. 12.31). Application of warm compresses can hasten
this process. At this point incision and drainage are indicated.
Without intervention, spontaneous drainage of bloody purulent
material ultimately occurs in most cases, and the patient experiences prompt relief of pain. In areas such as the nape of the neck
or the upper back, where the overlying skin is thick enough to
resist external pointing, the process may take a path of lesser
resistance, burrowing outward from the center through the subcutaneous tissues and along fascial planes. If this process is not
interrupted by early surgical intervention, the result is the gradual formation of a *carbuncle* which consists of an extremely
painful, exquisitely tender, multilocular mass of interconnected
dermal and subcutaneous abscesses, with multiple points of
partial drainage at the skin surface. Carbuncle formation often
is accompanied by fever, chills, and increasing malaise, and
there is a significant risk of secondary bacteremia. Even with
treatment, sloughing and extensive scarring tend to result.

Hidradenitis Suppurativa

In hidradenitis suppurativa, an apocrine gland is the site of
infection and abscess formation. Hence, localization in these
cases is limited to the axillae, perineum, and areolae, and the
disorder is not seen until the onset of puberty. Occlusion, maceration, and poor hygiene are major predisposing factors, fos-
tering inflammation of the gland with resultant obstruction
and providing a favorable environment for multiplication of
staphylococci and anaerobic bacteria. As the inflammatory
process expands, the gland ultimately ruptures and an abscess
forms. In contrast to the perifollicular furuncle, this infection is
deeper and slower to localize and suppurate. It begins as a
firm, mildly tender nodule that enlarges very gradually,
becoming increasingly uncomfortable and tender to the touch.
Recurrences are considerably more common with this disorder
than with furuncles.

ABSCESSES OF SPECIAL SITES

The breasts, scalp, and perianal areas are three specific sites of
abscess formation of particular importance in pediatrics.
Breast and scalp abscesses are discussed below. Perirectal
abscesses are described in Chapter 17, Surgery.

Breast Abscess

Breast abscesses occur with a small but significant frequency
in pediatric patients with incidence peaks in the neonatal and
pubertal age groups. Newborns greater than 31 weeks gestation at delivery have the highest incidence, due in part to
physiologic hypertrophy of breast tissue as a result of stimulation by maternal hormones. Colonization of the skin
and/or the nasopharynx with potentially virulent organisms
(*S. aureus* or coliforms) during delivery or in the nursery is
another important predisposing factor. Up to 25 percent of
affected infants have overt staphylococcal diaper dermatitis
at the time of presentation. Minor local trauma also is
thought to be a predisposing factor. The majority of cases
occur during the second or third week following delivery,
but infection may occur as late as 8 weeks of age. The problem first manifests as swelling and tenderness of the affected
breast. Unilateral involvement is the rule. With time local
warmth and overlying erythema become evident, and it may
be possible to express a purulent discharge from the nipple

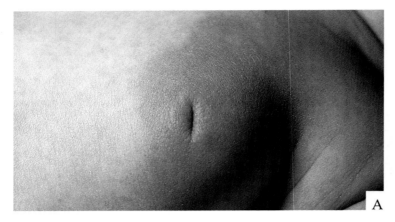

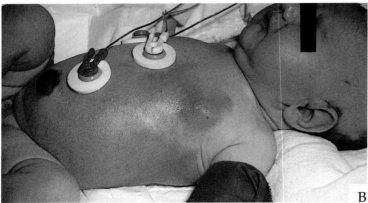

FIG. 12.32 Breast abscess. **A,** the typical manifestations of a breast abcess were seen in this neonate—swelling, induration, tenderness, warmth, and erythema. With compression, pus could be expressed from the nipple. **B,** this infant was not brought to the hospital until subcutaneous rupture and extensive cellulitic spread had occurred. She was febrile, toxic, irritable, and listless on presentation.

(Fig. 12.32A). Axillary adenopathy may be present as well. Only 25 percent of infants have low-grade fever, and other systemic symptoms are uncommon unless treatment is delayed. Depending on the time of presentation, a firm tender nonfluctuant nodule may be found on palpation, or the mass clearly may be fluctuant, indicating suppuration and necrosis. In the former instance parenteral antibiotic therapy and close monitoring for progression are indicated. In the latter instance prompt surgical incision and drainage are required. Broad-spectrum antimicrobial coverage should be provided pending culture results. Commonly recovered organisms include *S. aureus, Escherichia coli, Salmonella* species, *Streptococcus agalactiae, Proteus mirabilis,* and mixed flora. Delay in diagnosis and institution of treatment can result in subcutaneous rupture and cellulitic spread with secondary bacteremia (Fig. 12.32B). Delay in surgical drainage of fluctuant lesions also can result in permanent loss of breast tissue, which in females can produce a cosmetically deforming breast asymmetry that is first noted at puberty.

Breast abscesses may be seen again following puberty. Minor trauma, cutaneous infections, epidermal cysts, and duct blockages appear to be the common antecedent conditions. The clinical picture is similar to that seen in infants. Coagulase-positive staphylococci are the usual offending organisms.

Scalp Abscess

As is the case with breast abscesses, pyogenic infections of the scalp are particularly common in the neonatal period. Trauma

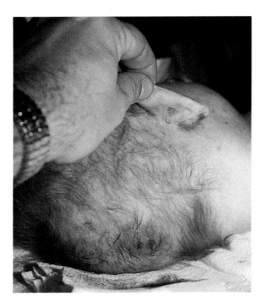

FIG. 12.33 Scalp abscess. Several days after discharge from the newborn nursery this infant presented with two scalp abcesses and an impetiginous lesion behind the right ear. The surface of the larger abscess is marked by two puncture wounds, which were the site of placement of monitor leads during labor. (Courtesy of Dr. Basil Zitelli, Children's Hospital of Pittsburgh)

is the predominant predisposing factor, and in neonates these abscesses commonly develop at the site of insertion of scalp leads for fetal monitoring during labor. Affected infants occasionally are found to have staphylococcal diaper dermatitis, as well. In the majority of cases, the infection is localized and consists of a tender nodule with overlying erythema (Fig. 12.33). The nodule commonly is fluctuant at the time of presentation, enabling prompt incision and drainage. Staphylococci and coliforms are the major pathogens recovered. Because of the neonate's immunologic immaturity, antimicrobial therapy also is recommended and in most cases can be administered orally. On rare occasions infection is extensive and takes the form of a necrotizing fasciitis (see below). In these patients and in the rare infant with a localized abscess and systemic symptoms, parenteral broad-spectrum antibiotic treatment (pending culture results) is indicated in addition to incision, drainage, and debridement.

When scalp abscesses are encountered in older children, care should be taken to determine the responsible pathogen. While staphylococci may be the source, invasive fungi are more likely to be the responsible organisms. These fungi produce a thick-walled boggy multilocular abscess termed a "kerion" (see Chapter 8). Gram stain and KOH preparations of purulent contents and of pulled hairs are important, for while incision and drainage is the treatment of choice for abscesses of bacterial origin, oral antifungal and steroid therapy are indicated for the kerion.

Lymphangitis

Inflammation of lymphatic channels is actually a secondary manifestation of infection at a distal site. The phenomenon is the result of invasion of lymphatic vessels by pathogenic organisms, which then spread along these channels toward regional lymph nodes. Group A ß-hemolytic streptococci, by virtue of elaborating fibrinolysins and hyaluronidases, are the most common source of lymphangitis, although wounds infected by staphylococci and *Pseudomonas* also may result in overt lymphangitis. Clinically, erythematous irregular linear streaks (which may be tender) are seen extending from the primary site toward the draining regional nodes (Fig. 12.34). The primary site may be an infected wound or an area of cellulitis.

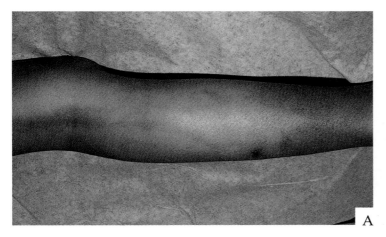

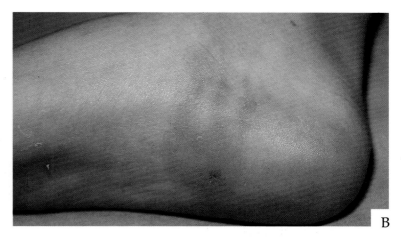

FIG. 12.34 Lymphangitis. **A,** an insect bite was the source of inoculation of group A streptococci in this child who subsequently developed secondary cellulitis and lymphangitis. The erythematous streaks coursing up the leg were tender and slightly indurated. **B,**

three distinct lymphangitic streaks are seen coursing up the instep from an area of cellulitis surrounding a puncture wound. Pseudomonas was the causative organism.

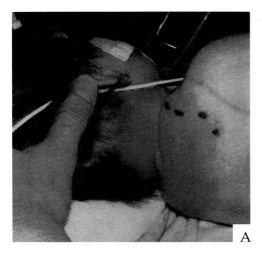

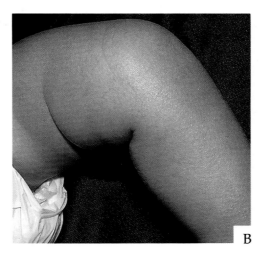

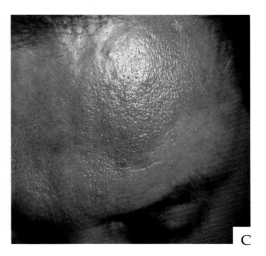

FIG. 12.35 Erysipelas. **A,** this 6-week-old infant presented with fever, lethargy, irritability, and hypotension in association with erysipelas. The purplish-red lesion was raised, indurated, and tender. The border, though irregular, was sharply demarcated from the adjacent skin. Cultures of blood and tissue aspirate grew group A streptococci. **B,** the

sharply circumscribed area of erysipelas on this toddler's leg was pink. On close inspection, one can see that the skin has a peau d'orange quality. **C,** this is seen more clearly in a close-up of an adolescent's forehead. (**C,** courtesy of Dr. James Ferante, St. Margaret Memorial Hospital, Pittsburgh, PA)

Systemic symptoms consisting of fever, chills, and malaise are often, but not invariably, present. Without appropriate antimicrobial therapy, cellulitis may develop or extend, and necrosis and ulceration may occur with attendant risk of bacteremia. Culture and Gram stain of material from the primary site will aid in selection of antimicrobials; however, presumptive initial therapy is necessary pending culture results.

Erysipelas

Group A ß-hemolytic streptococci are the source of this unusual distinctive infection involving a localized area of the dermis and superficial lymphatics. The causative organisms usually are found in the upper respiratory tracts of afflicted patients and are inoculated through a break in the skin that may elude detection on presentation. Hematogenous seeding has been postulated in some cases. Systemic symptoms are prominent and precede appearance of the characteristic skin lesion. The onset is abrupt and is heralded by fever and chills often in association with nausea, vomiting, and headache. This pro-

drome is followed by the appearance of an intensely painful skin lesion that consists of a circumscribed raised plaque that is usually a deep purplish-red in color but which may be red or even pink (Fig. 12.35A,B). The raised border, although irregular, is well demarcated and spreads centrifugally. Red lymphatic streaks may advance ahead of it toward the regional nodes. On close inspection the skin is seen to be edematous and may have a thickened "peau d'orange" character (see Fig. 12.35C). On palpation it is indurated, hot, and exquisitely tender. With evolution, small surface blebs containing yellow fluid may form. The face is the site most commonly involved, with the trunk, neck, and extremities being less frequent areas of localization. Patients may become bacteremic, developing metastatic foci of infection. Infants are at particular risk for systemic spread. The clinical picture of erysipelas is so characteristic that streptococcal infection can be presumed and parenteral antimicrobial treatment initiated. Cultures of tissue aspirate from the advancing border of the lesion and cultures of the nose and throat typically are positive for group A streptococci, as are blood cultures in septic patients.

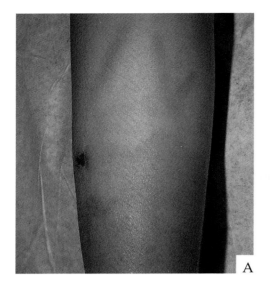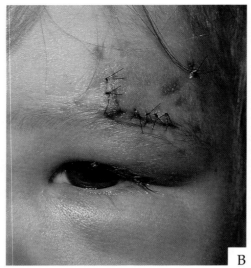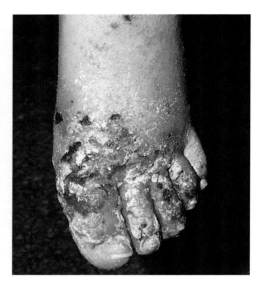

FIG. 12.36 Wound-related cellulitis. **A,** the infected mosquito bite that served as the source of cellulitis in this child can be seen on the left. The area of erythema was indurated and exquisitely tender. Note that the skin is smooth and the borders fade gradually into

the adjacent normal skin. **B,** mild erythema and edema are evident in the periorbital area of an infant whose laceration from a dog bite had been sutured 48 hours earlier. The edematous areas were indurated and tender.

FIG. 12.37 This patient with cellulitis of the foot had been on topical steroid therapy for contact dermatitis for about 48 hours when he experienced explosive onset of swelling, redness, and pain. Impetiginous changes are apparent, as well. (Courtesy of Dr. Michael Sherlock)

Cellulitis

Cellulitis is an infection of bacterial origin in which subcutaneous loose connective tissue is the primary site of inflammation. With progression, the process extends centrifugally through the subcutaneous tissue and also may ascend to involve the lower dermis. Although cellulitis may develop anywhere on the body, it occurs most commonly on the extremities and face. There are three major modes of origin:

1. Extension from a wound.
2. Hematogenous seeding.
3. Extension from a deeper infection.

Clinically, cellulitis is characterized by painful, tender, indurated subcutaneous swelling. The overlying skin is smooth, warm, often shiny, and usually erythematous (see Fig. 12.36). Occasionally it is pink or has a violaceous hue. In contrast to erysipelas, the margins or borders of both the edema and erythema are indistinct, fading imperceptibly into the surrounding tissues. Prior to therapy, rapid extension is the rule. Systemic symptoms are common, particularly when infection is due to hematogenous spread or to extension from deeper sites. In such cases fever, chills, malaise, and headache are typical. When hematogenous seeding is the source, toxicity may be marked.

WOUND-RELATED CELLULITIS

Extension of infection from an external wound such as a puncture, laceration, abrasion, or insect bite is perhaps the most common source of cellulitis, particularly in school-age children and in adolescents. Mild local erythema immediately surrounding a wound, an impetiginous lesion, or a pustule may have been noted prior to the abrupt onset of increased pain and the rapid evolution of subcutaneous inflammation that herald the development of cellulitis. In the majority of cases, the primary lesion is readily identifiable at the time of presentation (Fig. 12.36), but in some instances it may no longer be detectable. Occasionally, secondary infection of a preexisting dermatitis may result in a cellulitis that spreads with frightening speed (Fig. 12.37). Group A streptococci and coagulase-positive staphylococci are the organisms recovered most commonly in these circumstances. *Pseudomonas* and mixed flora may be responsible for cellulitis occurring secondary to puncture wounds of the foot (see Fig. 12.34B). While rapid peripheral spread, overt lymphangitis, and regional adenitis are regarded as highly characteristic of streptococcal infection, this same picture may be seen with cellulitis due to any of these wound-related pathogens. Fever and other systemic symptoms may be present with this form of cellulitis, but they are more likely to occur with cellulitis due to hematogenous seeding or to extension of inflammation from deeper structures.

Hands, feet, and extremities are the most common sites of wound-related cellulitis. This necessitates close assessment and monitoring for further spread and for secondary neurovascular compromise. Inward spread to tendon sheaths of a hand or a foot can have disastrous consequences; hence, cellulitis involving these structures must be treated aggressively, and clinical status must be monitored very closely. When an extremity is encircled by cellulitis, swelling and increased pressure can result in extensive damage distally if the area is not surgically decompressed.

Gram stain and culture of material obtained from the primary wound and/or from tissue aspirate from the center and margin of the inflamed area may be helpful in identifying the specific pathogen. Successful aspiration necessitates the use of a large syringe to provide high-pressure suction and may require prior injection of nonbacteriostatic saline. Blood cultures should be obtained in all patients with systemic symptoms. Prompt treatment is essential to prevent further spread and complications. Antimicrobial therapy often has to be selected empirically, pending culture results. Coverage for penicillinase-producing staphylococci is essential.

Major differential diagnostic considerations include angioedema due to insect bites and delayed hypersensitivity reactions to hymenoptera stings. The former is pruritic, nontender, and often has an identifiable central punctum, while the latter

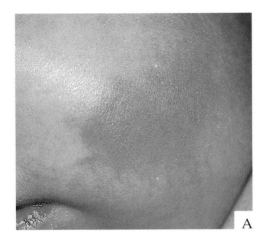

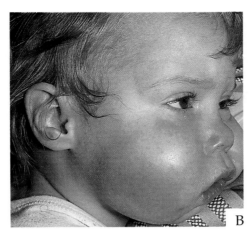

FIG. 12.38 Hematogenous cellulitis. **A,** this small erythematous patch with indistinct borders appeared on this infant's cheek shortly after the onset of fever, irritability, and anorexia. On palpation it was found to be indurated and tender. Blood culture was positive for H. influenzae type b. **B,** in this toddler, the evolution of buccal cellulitis due to H. influenzae was fulminant, resulting in unusually dramatic swelling.

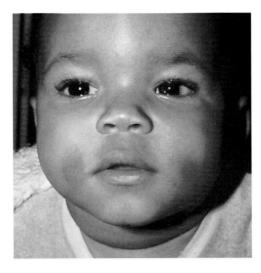

FIG. 12.39 Popsicle panniculitis. This older infant who had become fond of popsicles presented with bilateral areas of purplish swelling just lateral to the corners of his mouth. He was otherwise well. On palpation, mildly tender discrete indurated disc-shaped masses could be appreciated. These were localized areas of fat necrosis due to cold injury. (Courtesy of Dr. Michael Sherlock)

is pruritic, and mildly painful and tender (see Chapter 8). Both are unassociated with systemic symptoms or with adenopathy or lymphangitis. The history, lack of erythema, presence of ecchymotic discoloration, and absence of systemic symptoms all help to distinguish swelling due to trauma.

HEMATOGENOUS CELLULITIS

Hematogenous seeding is another common source of cellulitis, particularly in infants and young children. While young infants may present with sudden onset of sepsis followed soon thereafter by the appearance of cellulitis, older infants, toddlers, and preschool-age children commonly have antecedent upper respiratory tract symptoms. This prodrome is followed by the sudden development of a high fever that begins nearly simultaneously with the appearance of a nondescript area of swelling. Often this swelling is localized in the periorbital region (see Chapter 22), but at times may be located over a cheek, the neck, or an extremity. The overlying skin rapidly becomes pink, red, or violaceous as the area of edema spreads in extent and becomes indurated. Irritability, anorexia, and signs of toxicity become increasingly marked, in most cases prompting presentation for medical care within 24 hours. *H. influenzae* type b is a particularly likely source of this picture, but it is by no means the only organism to produce cellulitis in this age group or in these anatomical regions. *Streptococcus pneumoniae,* as well as group B streptococci (in infants under 3 months of age), can produce an identical picture.

Haemophilus influenzae type b does appear to be the sole pathogen responsible for cellulitis of the cheek, also termed "buccal cellulitis." In this form of cellulitis, a type limited exclusively to infants, the swelling and erythema are located over the midcheek near the mandibular ramus (Fig. 12.38). Localized erythema of the underlying buccal mucosa is a common associated finding. The systemic symptomatology and exquisite tenderness help to distinguish it from "popsicle panniculitis," which results from cold injury. The latter is characterized by formation of a mildly tender, discrete indurated disc-shaped subcutaneous mass located at the angle of the mouth, with reddish-purple discoloration of the overlying skin (Fig. 12.39). Systemic symptoms, induration, and tenderness also help to distinguish hematogenous cellulitis at other sites from sympathetic swelling and from angioedema due to insect bites (see Chapter 8).

The severity of illness with buccal cellulitis and the inevitability of bacteremia with its attendant risks warrant expeditious evaluation and treatment. Blood cultures are positive in a very high percentage of patients and may be supplemented by culture of tissue aspirates from the area of cellulitis. Counter-immunoelectrophoresis also may be helpful. High-dose antimicrobial therapy should be administered parenterally, and selected to ensure coverage for ß-lactamase-producing *Haemophilus.*

CELLULITIS DUE TO EXPANSION OF INFECTION FROM DEEPER STRUCTURES

Though less common than the other forms, cellulitis may result from extension of infection and inflammation from deeper structures. This possibility necessitates paying close attention to examination of underlying structures in evaluating any patient with evidence of cellulitis. Dental abscesses (see Chapter 20) and acute sinusitis (see Chapter 22) may underlie facial cellulitis. Osteomyelitis may produce secondary cellulitic changes of overlying soft tissues, especially following subperiosteal extension (see below). Suppurative lymphadenitis and subcutaneous rupture of skin, scalp, and breast abscesses are other common sources (see Fig. 12.32B). Fever, toxicity, and other systemic symptoms are not unusual with this form of cellulitis. Antecedent history along with findings on careful examination usually will result in identification of this type of cellulitis and in recognition of the primary source.

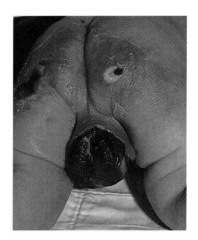

FIG. 12.40 Necrotizing fasciitis. The extent of cellulitis and tissue necrosis are visibly evident in this child who is recovering from necrotizing fasciitis due to group A streptococci. On presentation he was thought to have cellulitis but was more ill systemically and appeared much more uncomfortable than would be expected. Furthermore, on presentation the area of induration extended well beyond the overlying erythema. (Courtesy of Dr. Michael Sherlock)

Necrotizing Fasciitis

Variously termed necrotizing fasciitis or cellulitis, synergistic cellulitis or gangrene, necrotizing erysipelas and streptococcal gangrene, this dreaded disorder is a severe, deep, necrotizing soft-tissue infection, which at a minimum involves subcutaneous tissues and fascial sheaths and often extends to underlying muscle. This process spreads relentlessly along fascial planes producing edema, vascular thrombosis, and ever-widening necrosis, resulting in extensive soft-tissue destruction. Deep surgical and traumatic wounds are major predisposing factors, although injection sites, cutaneous ulcers, and abscesses may serve as the initiating condition. Diabetics with vascular disease have an especially increased risk. The extremities, perineum, buttocks, trunk, and abdominal wall are the most common sites of involvement. Causative organisms include group A ß-hemolytic streptococci, *S. aureus*, *Pseudomonas aeruginosa*, *E. coli*, and mixtures of aerobes, anaerobes, and facultative gram-negative rods.

Moderate to severe systemic symptoms are prominent clinically, and along with fever usually precede the appearance of cellulitic changes. The local area of inflammation initially may resemble ordinary cellulitis with nonraised, indistinct margins, and localized subcutaneous edema with overlying erythema. However, on careful palpation, it often is possible to appreciate that the edema and induration are deeper and far more extensive than the overlying erythema. Pain is remarkably severe early on and the lesion is exquisitely tender. With progression, the overlying skin itself may become edematous, simulating erysipelas. Later its color changes from red or purple to a patchy gray-blue and surface bullae, often filled with hemorrhagic fluid, may appear. At this point numbness and decreased sensitivity to pain may be noted centrally. With further evolution central necrosis or cutaneous gangrene supervenes (Fig. 12.40). When anaerobes are involved, crepitance may become evident clinically or subcutaneous emphysema may be visible on radiography.

As the localized process evolves, systemic symptoms increase. Signs of poor perfusion, pallor, and mottling often are accompanied by grunting respirations and by alterations in level of consciousness including disorientation, obtundation, and seizures. This picture may culminate in frank prostration, often in association with generalized edema. Common laboratory findings in advanced cases include anemia due to hemolysis and marrow suppression, proteinuria, hypoproteinemia, hypocalcemia due to saponification of necrotic fat, and hyponatremia. Blood and wound cultures are routinely positive.

Mortality ranges from 8 to 70 percent, depending on the series, and morbidity and disfigurement are common in survivors. Delays in diagnosis and inadequate surgical debridement are major factors in cases with poor outcome.

Early recognition is crucial to ensure appropriate intervention and improve prognosis. This can be particularly difficult in cases resembling ordinary cellulitis that initially improve on antimicrobial therapy before worsening. Necrotizing fasciitis should be suspected in any patient with cellulitis (particularly around a deep wound) who has unusually severe pain and systemic symptoms that are out of proportion to local findings. This can enable exploration before advanced skin changes and loss of sensation appear, signaling that necrosis already is extensive. If such changes are present, this process must be presumed. In early cases examination of frozen sections of biopsy material may confirm the diagnosis. Incision and passage of a probe also can be helpful. If the probe passes easily along fascial planes, the diagnosis is confirmed. Control necessitates wide excision with extensive exposure and debridement of all necrotic tissues, in combination with broad-spectrum antimicrobial therapy (guided in part by Gram' stain results). Aggressive supportive measures are important, as well.

INFECTIOUS LYMPHADENITIS

Lymph nodes respond to both systemic and local infections with increased cellular multiplication and activity, clinically manifest as enlargement and tenderness. When enlargement and degree of inflammation are mild, this often is called "reactive adenopathy." Nodes usually are 2 cm or less in diameter, and they are discrete, slightly firm or rubbery in consistency, and mobile. Discomfort and tenderness are mild. However, when enlargement is marked and inflammation is pronounced, the phenomenon is termed "adenitis." In this condition, the lymph node itself is infected. Nodes usually exceed 2 to 3 cm in diameter, and overlying soft tissues may become edematous, making it difficult to distinguish exact margins. With progression, the overlying skin often becomes erythematous and may become adherent, reducing mobility. Discomfort and tenderness are usually, but not always, marked. Depending on the causative organism, suppuration may occur.

Adenopathy may be generalized or regional, but adenitis tends to be localized to a single node. Whereas adenitis is invariably of infectious etiology, adenopathy also may be a feature of collagen vascular disease, or it may be of neoplastic origin. Malignant nodes usually are very firm or hard, but occasionally they are rubbery in consistency. They also may be discrete but, not infrequently, they are matted and often appear fixed or poorly mobile. Tenderness is unusual. Depending on the type of malignancy, the adenopathy may be isolated to one region, or it may be generalized and associated with hepatosplenomegaly and with such systemic symptoms as anorexia, fatigue, weight loss, night sweats, and bone pain. Many of the infectious diseases associated with generalized or cervical adenopathy have been discussed earlier in this chapter. Figure 12.41 presents in tabular form some of the distinguishing features of the adenopathy characteristic of these disorders. Neoplastic diseases are discussed in Chapter 11.

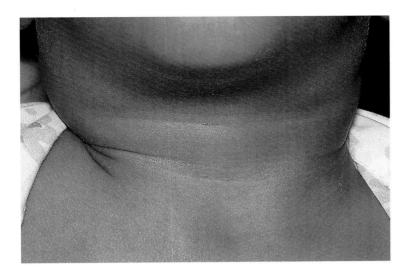

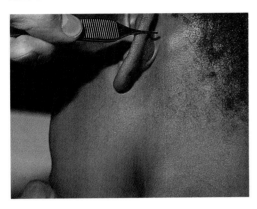

FIG. 12.43 Cervical adenopathy. Bilateral enlargement of the tonsillar nodes in this child was associated with viral pharyngitis.

FIG. 12.44 Acute postauricular lymphadenitis. This child presented with folliculitic and crusted scalp lesions and a tender 1.5-cm postauricular node with overlying erythema. The initial suspicion of bacterial infection was not confirmed. KOH preparation and fungal culture identified tinea capitis as the primary process.

with secondary infection of seborrhea, impetigo, wound infections, tinea capitis, or head lice infestation (Fig. 12.44). Conjunctival infections may result in adenitis of the preauricular node. The teeth, gingivae, and tongue are drained by lymphatics coursing to the submental and submandibular nodes, which can be secondarily involved in cases of dental abscess, gingivitis, and stomatitis. Infections of the external auditory canal and the auricle may drain to the preauricular or postauricular nodes, while those involving the neck may affect the anterior or posterior cervical chain.

While the number of potential causative organisms is high, an individual pathogen often can be implicated by careful history-taking and physical examination. Differentiation also must be made from other masses that may be present in the cervical region, many of which are congenital and subject to secondary infection, simulating adenitis. A number of these and their clinical characteristics are enumerated in Fig 12.45.

THE AXILLARY AND EPITROCHLEAR LYMPH NODES

Over a dozen nodes occupy the axilla. Those in the anterior pectoral portion drain the breast and chest wall, those in the lateral or mid-portion receive drainage from the hand and arm (see Fig. 12.50B), and those in the posterior subscapular region drain portions of the back. The epitrochlear node receives lymphatic vessels from the fingers, hand, and skin of the forearm, but it is a much less common site of adenitis than are the axillary nodes. Wound and skin infections, cellulitis, and herpes zoster are major sources of axillary adenitis in childhood.

THE INGUINAL LYMPH NODES

The inguinal nodes are divided into two groups by Poupart's ligament, with those above the ligament being termed inguinal nodes and those below it termed femoral (Fig. 12.46 and see Fig. 12.48). The inguinal group receives lymphatics from the external genitalia, anus, umbilicus, lower abdomen and back, buttocks and upper thigh, and also may drain the lower leg. Thus, in addition to wound and skin infections, perianal, intra-abdominal, and genital infections may serve as sources of inguinal adenitis. The femoral nodes primarily drain the foot and lower leg. The popliteal nodes receive drainage from the foot and lower leg, but like the epitrochlear nodes, they are unusual sites of adenitis.

Having contrasted the general features of acute lymphadenitis with those of adenopathy, as well as having discussed the regions of involvement and their likely sources, we now can look at the characteristics of adenitis produced by the various causative organisms.

Acute Suppurative Lymphadenitis

Group A ß-hemolytic streptococci and coagulase-positive staphylococci are responsible for the majority of cases of acute lymphadenitis, regardless of anatomical region. Together they account for up to 80 percent of cases of cervical adenitis alone. In recent years staphylococcal infections have surpassed in frequency those due to streptococci. Other than culture of a specimen obtained by needle aspirate, there is no way to distin-

DIFFERENTIAL DIAGNOSIS OF CERVICAL ADENOPATHY/ADENITIS

Type of Mass	Usual Site	Character	Time of Appearance
Lymphangioma	Preauricular, submental, submandibular, supraclavicular	Soft, compressible; transilluminates; margins often indistinct; may increase in size with crying or straining; nontender unless infected	Birth to 2 years
Hemangioma	Preauricular, postauricular, may occur along or under sternocleidomastoid	Soft, compressible; margins often indistinct; increases in size with crying, straining, and dependency; nontender unless infected	Birth to 1 year; gradually enlarges during first year, then regresses
Branchial cleft cyst	Preauricular, at mandibular angle, along anterior border of sterno-cleidomastoid, suprasternal	Discrete; usually has overlying or nearby pore or fistula, which may retract with swallowing; nontender unless infected	Present at birth; often not noticed until infection produces enlargement, pain, and overlying ery-thema with or without drainage
Thyroglossal duct cyst	Midline, often at level of hyoid or just below	Discrete; usually has overlying pore or fistula; moves with tongue movement	Present at birth; often not noticed until infection produces enlargement, pain, and overlying erythema with or without drainage
Dermoid cyst	Midline, often submental or suprasternal	Discrete, smooth; doughy or rubbery; nontender; does not retract with swallowing	Infancy/childhood
Laryngocele	Just lateral to midline along anterior border of sternocleidomastoid	Soft, compressible, may gurgle on compression; increases in size with straining or crying; nontender unless infected; may have associated stridor or hoarseness; may have air-fluid level on x-ray	Infancy/childhood
Esophageal diverticulum	Paratracheal, usually on the left	Soft, compressible; increases in size with crying or straining; nontender; may have history of dysphagia and/or aspiration	Infancy/childhood
Sialadenitis	Preauricular, extending under and behind ear, submandibular, submental	Firm; mildly tender when viral; exquisitely tender when suppurative, with pus exuding from orifice; pain increased with eating, especially lemons; elevated serum or urine amylase	Any age
Teratoma	Midline or paramedian	Solitary; firm with irregular border; rapid increase in size; may have calcifications on x-ray	Infancy/childhood

FIG. 12.45

Type of Mass	Usual Site	Character	Time of Appearance
Thyroid goiter	Isthmus (midline), and lobes (paratracheal)	Diffuse enlargement; usually smooth contour and soft consistency, occasionally nodular; moves with swallowing	Occasionally neonatal (with maternal ingestion of iodides); childhood in endemic areas (iodine-deficient water); childhood/adolescence in familial cases
Graves' disease	Isthmus (midline), and lobes (paratracheal)	Diffuse enlargement; smooth contour and soft consistency; moves with swallowing; associated signs of thyrotoxicosis and exophthalmos	Childhood/adolescence
Hashimoto's thyroiditis	Isthmus (midline), and lobes (paratracheal)	Diffuse enlargement; distinct contours; firm or rubbery; surface may be irregular; may have neck soreness and dysphagia; may have symptoms of mild hyperthyroidism	Childhood/adolescence
Thyroid carcinoma	Usually in lateral lobe or at junction of isthmus and lobe	Solitary mass; firm or hard and differs in consistency from rest of gland; may have associated adenopathy; may have past history of irradiation	Childhood/adolescence
Leukemia	Any cervical node or nodes	Firm to hard; often enlarges rapidly; may be fixed or matted; nontender; often other regions involved; often hepatosplenomegaly; may have fever, anorexia, weight loss, bone pain, pallor, petechiae	Any age
Non-Hodgkin's lymphoma	Spinal accessory, supraclavicular	Firm to hard; enlarges rapidly; may be fixed or matted; nontender; often other regions are involved; may have fever, anorexia, weight loss, bone and joint pain	5-15 years
Hodgkin's disease	Anterior or posterior cervical, preauricular, supraclavicular	Firm, occasionally rubbery; slow growing; may be mobile, fixed or matted; nontender; often otherwise asymptomatic; may have fever, malaise, weight loss, night sweats hepatosplenomegaly	Usually >5 years
Rhabdomyo-sarcoma	Nasopharyngeal, parotid, anterior or posterior cervical	Primary nasopharyngeal: symptoms of enlarged adenoids; later serosan-.guineous nasal discharge, weight loss, cranial nerve deficits, and secondary node enlargement Primary parotid or cervical: hard, painless, nontender mass	Any age, but more common in early childhood

FIG. 12.45

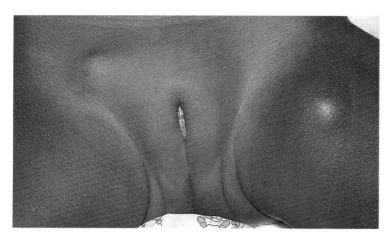

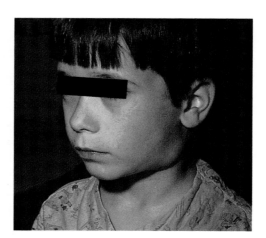

FIG. 12.47 Acute suppurative lymphadenitis. This youngster was seen within 24 hours of onset of painful enlargement of the left tonsillar node. There was mild overlying edema and the node was markedly tender. (Courtesy of Dr. Michael Sherlock)

FIG. 12.46 Subacute lymphadenitis of a right inguinal and left femoral node resulted in dramatic swelling in this toddler. Atypical mycobacteria were found to be causative.

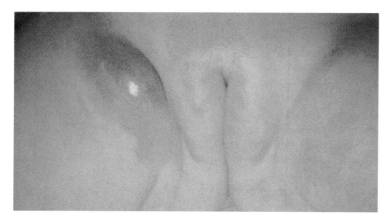

FIG. 12.48 Acute suppurative lymphadenitis. Increased pain and erythema, thinning of the overlying skin, and fluctuance on palpation signal that central necrosis has occurred. (Courtesy of Dr. Michael Sherlock)

guish between the two clinically, as the clinical picture for both consists of sudden, painful, and rapid enlargement, usually of a single node. The involved node is firm and exquisitely tender, and may range in diameter from 2 to 6 cm (Fig. 12.47). Within 24 to 72 hours the overlying soft tissue becomes edematous and the skin erythematous. As many as 50 percent of patients may be febrile and some appear toxic; bacteremia develops in a small percentage. Left untreated, suppuration occurs during the next several days and is detectable as central fluctuance. Simultaneously, thinning of the overlying skin may be noted as the process points to the surface (Fig. 12.48). Occasionally the abscess may point inward rupturing into the soft tissues and dissecting along tissue planes with potentially catastrophic effects. Prompt institution of antimicrobial therapy can significantly alter this course. When high-dose oral therapy is started prior to development of overlying cellulitic changes, such changes may be prevented and enlargement halted, followed by regression. Even cases with swelling and erythema at the start of therapy may not progress to suppuration. Patients with high fever and toxicity require parenteral treatment, as do children who fail to improve on oral medication. Suppuration necessitates incision and drainage.

Cervical nodes, especially the tonsillar and anterior cervical,

are the most common sites of adenitis due to streptococci or staphylococci. Patients usually are young children with a peak incidence between 1 and 4 years. Many have a history of antecedent rhinitis, often associated with impetiginization of the anterior nares and anterior cervical adenopathy. Cough, anorexia, vomiting, and fever also may be present. These findings may persist or they may clear prior to the onset of adenitis. In older children, a recent episode of pharyngitis may be reported, and in a small percentage, adenitis develops in association with a peritonsillar abscess (see Chapter 22). Secondarily infected dermatitis, insect bites, impetigo, and wound infections may precede the onset of adenitis in other patients, in which case the node affected depends on the primary site. These infections, as well as cellulitis, are common antecedents of axillary and inguinal adenitis due to streptococci and staphylococci. Primary sources may be evident at the time adenitis develops, but often they have healed. It is also important to remember that invasive forms of tinea capitis may closely mimic streptococcal and staphylococcal infection, both in the appearance of the primary lesion and in the character of the secondary adenitis, although progression to suppuration is unusual.

Although streptococci and staphylococci are the predominant pathogens causing acute lymphadenitis, occasionally anaerobic bacteria—including Actinomyces—are responsible. The vast majority of cases caused by anaerobes are secondary to dental disease, including dental abscesses, gingivitis, and stomatitis; as a result, the submental or submandibular nodes are more likely to be affected. On occasion the adenitis appears simultaneously with facial cellulitis stemming from a dental abscess (see Chapter 20).

Actinomycotic adenitis, though unusual, has a distinctive clinical course. Enlargement of the affected node is gradual, and on palpation it is firm and lumpy, has an irregular border, and is mildly to moderately tender. Over time the center blackens and necroses, and a chronic draining sinus may form. Microscopic examination of the discharge discloses characteristic sulfur granules.

Mycobacterial Lymphadenitis

Although the incidence of tuberculosis has decreased markedly in developed countries, Mycobacterium tuberculosis and non-

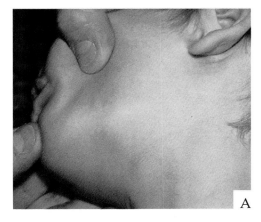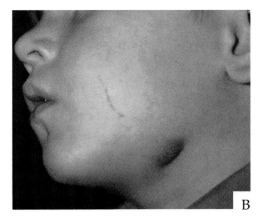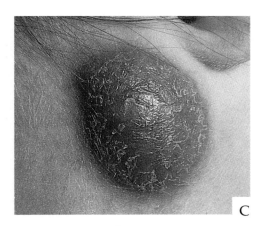

FIG. 12.49 Mycobacterial adenitis. **A,** early in the course of adenitis due to M. tuberculosis *or atypical mycobacteria, enlargement of the node is gradual, tenderness is mild, and there is little or no sign of warmth or overlying inflammation.* **B,** *after a few to several weeks the* overlying skin becomes thickened, tense, discolored, and adherent to the node. **C,** *this node was fluctuant, indicating suppuration.* (Courtesy of Dr. Michael Sherlock)

tuberculous or atypical mycobacteria (especially *Mycobacterium avium-intracellulare*) continue to be important causes of lymphadenitis. Recognition of mycobacterial lymphadenitis is important, as its management is considerably different from that caused by other bacteria. Both groups of mycobacteria cause similar clinical findings. Nodal enlargement is gradual and persistent. The node is slightly to mildly tender and initially there is little or no sign of warmth or overlying inflammation (Fig. 12.49A and see Fig. 12.46). After a few to several weeks the node becomes adherent to the overlying skin, which in turn becomes thickened and tense, with overlying reddish or reddish-purple discoloration (Figs. 12.49B, C). Suppuration may occur several weeks to months after onset, and this may result in rupture through the overlying skin with formation of a chronically draining sinus. The risk of chronic drainage may be increased if aspiration or incision and drainage are attempted. While local clinical findings are similar, there are historical and other differences that can help to distinguish tuberculous adenitis from atypical mycobacterial adenitis.

TUBERCULOUS LYMPHADENITIS
Children with tuberculosis may be of any age and frequently have a positive history of exposure to an infected adult. Posterior cervical and supraclavicular nodes are the most common sites involved, and in a small percentage of cases adenitis is bilateral. Generalized adenopathy may be noted in as many as 20 percent of patients. Up to 50 percent have systemic symptoms that may include fever, cough, night sweats, anorexia, and malaise. Chest radiographs reveal findings suggestive of tuberculosis in 75 percent of cases; the sedimentation rate exceeds 30 in up to 80 percent; and the PPD is positive with more than 10 mm of induration. Treatment of tuberculous adenitis is pharmacologic, with excision reserved for cases with chronic drainage.

ADENITIS DUE TO ATYPICAL MYCOBACTERIA
Patients with atypical mycobacterial adenitis usually are under 4 years of age and are unlikely to have a history of exposure to tuberculosis. A submandibular, preauricular, anterior cervical, inguinal, or epitrochlear node may be the site of involvement. Bilateral adenitis and generalized adenopathy do not occur and systemic symptoms are rare. Chest radio-

graphs rarely are abnormal; only one third have elevated sedimentation rates; and the PPD is intermediate or positive with induration ranging from 5 to 10 mm. Atypical mycobacteria invariably are resistant to multiple drugs, hence excisional biopsy generally is the treatment of choice. Spontaneous regression can occur, however, making observation a reasonable course if suppuration and/or drainage have not occurred.

Adenitis Associated with Animal or Vector Contact

In a number of children, acute local lymphadenitis is the result of inoculation of a pathogen via an animal scratch or bite, from the bite of an insect vector transmitting a pathogen from an animal host, or by contact with a contaminated animal carcass. In some of these disorders, systemic symptoms are prominent; in others the local adenitis is the primary manifestation.

PASTEURELLA MULTOCIDA ADENITIS
Suppurative adenitis due to *P. multocida* may occur in patients who develop local infection at the site of a scratch or bite inflicted by a dog or cat. Soon after the manifestations of local infection appear at the primary site, a regional node enlarges and becomes tender. Overlying swelling and redness are common and suppuration may occur early. This picture is clinically indistinguishable from adenitis due to streptococci or staphylococci, but often *P. multocida* infection can be suspected by history. Axillary and inguinal nodes are the most common sites of involvement. Systemic symptoms are unusual.

CAT SCRATCH DISEASE
Adenitis is a primary feature of cat scratch disease, which is due to an as yet unidentified pleomorphic bacillus that is seen in Warthin-Starry silver-stained sections of biopsied nodes. Low-grade fever may occur in about 25 percent of affected patients. Ninety percent have a history of either an antecedent cat scratch or of contact with cats or kittens. While inoculation via a cat scratch is the most common means of infection, splinters, puncture wounds, and dog scratches also have been implicated. Incidence is highest in fall and winter in temperate climates, with cases occurring with equal frequency year-round in tropical areas. Most patients are in the 5- to 14-year

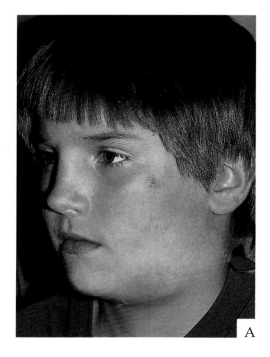

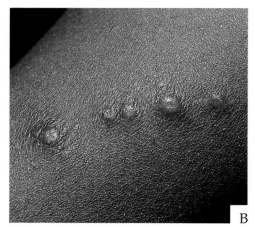

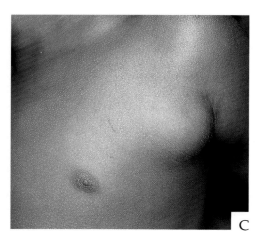

FIG. 12.50 Cat scratch disease. **A,** this boy presented with mildly painful "swollen glands." The left preauricular and tonsillar nodes were enlarged, firm and mildly tender. An ulcerated papule, evident on his left cheek, was the site of a scratch by one of his kittens 2 weeks before. **B,** a line of papules is seen on the forearm of a 3-year-old at the site of a scratch by his new kitten 3 weeks prior to presentation. **C,** marked enlargement of an ipsilateral axillary node had prompted his visit. The node was firm and only mildly tender. (**A,** courtesy of Dr. Kenneth Schuit)

age range, but family clusters that include younger children and adults have been reported.

Onset of symptoms begins 3 to 30 days following inoculation, with 7 to 12 days being the most common time. A red papule or series of papules is commonly noted at the site of inoculation. Shortly thereafter, one or more regional nodes enlarge, becoming mildly painful and tender (Fig. 12.50). Involved nodes are firm, and overlying warmth and mild redness may develop within a few days of enlargement. In order of frequency, axillary, cervical, submandibular, preauricular, epitrochlear, and inguinal nodes have been reported as sites of involvement. In cases involving a preauricular node, associated conjunctivitis is common and suggests conjunctival inoculation as the source. Discomfort generally subsides in 4 to 6 weeks, but the node may remain enlarged or may fluctuate in size for months. Suppuration occurs in about one third of patients.

As skin-test materials generally are unavailable and because methods of culturing the organism are still in the process of being developed, diagnosis is made primarily on the basis of history, clinical picture and course, and/or pathologic findings on excisional biopsy. When infection is suspected, expectant followup is recommended. If suppuration occurs, aspiration is believed by most authorities to be preferable to incision and drainage because of concerns that the latter procedure may lead to prolonged drainage and scarring. In protracted or atypical cases excisional biopsy is suggested.

TULAREMIA

Francisella tularensis may produce an illness in which adenitis is prominent in concert with systemic symptoms. Rabbits, hares, muskrats, and voles serve as endemic sources of this pathogen. Children may acquire the glandular or ulceroglandular form of the disease by handling or skinning dead animals, following an animal bite (especially that of a cat who hunts rabbits), or occasionally from the bite of an insect vector. The incubation period ranges from 1 to 21 days. Onset is abrupt and characterized by fever, chills, headache, myalgias, vomiting, and possibly photophobia. Within 2 days, axillary, epitrochlear or inguinal adenitis is noted, and soon thereafter a painful papule appears distal to the involved node at the site of inoculation. This ruptures within 1 to 2 days, forming a central ulcer with a raised edge. The involved node is firm and tender and may be associated with overlying erythema. Generalized adenopathy and hepatosplenomegaly may be noted in some cases, and in the second week of illness a blotchy erythematous maculopapular rash (or occasionally a vesicular, pustular or nodose exanthem) may appear. Without treatment fever may persist for 2 to 3 weeks, and the ulcer may take as long as a month to heal. The diagnosis is suggested by history, clinical picture and course, and is confirmed by serologic tests. Streptomycin is the treatment of choice.

BUBONIC PLAGUE

Now rare in developed countries, this infection continues to appear sporadically in people who live or hunt in areas in which infection is endemic in the wild rodent population. Its usual means of transmission is via flea bite, but on occasion inoculation occurs through a break in the skin as a result of handling an infected carcass. Thus inguinal and axillary nodes are the most common sites of bubo formation. The incubation period ranges from several hours to 10 days and is terminated by the abrupt onset of high fever, chills, malaise, weakness, and headache. Pain in the area of a regional node precedes rapid nodal enlargement. The node is fixed, firm, and exquisitely tender with overlying edema. Purplish discoloration is common. The inoculation site may appear normal, or it may be manifest as a skin abscess. Rapid progression of systemic symptoms occurs, with the patient appearing toxic and apprehensive, and often manifesting delirium and signs of neurologic dysfunction. DIC and septic shock may supervene if treatment is not instituted promptly. When infection is suspected the node should be aspirated for culture, blood cultures should be obtained, and broad-spectrum parenteral therapy instituted.

General Approach to Diagnosis of Lymphadenitis

Because of the wide range of pathogens that can produce lymphadenitis, meticulous care must be taken in the process of clinical assessment. The history should include questions concerning antecedent and current signs and symptoms, which may include prior wounds such as cuts, bites, punctures, splinters, or scratches distal to the inflamed node. Exposure to other ill persons or to animals, as well as recent travel, should be determined. Questions also must be asked about the presence or absence of systemic symptoms and about the rapidity of evolution of the adenitis itself. A history of past problems and medication intake is important as well. Physical examination must include precise measurement of size of the inflamed node, in addition to inspection of overlying soft tissue and palpation to determine contour, consistency, and degree of tenderness. The region drained by the involved node must be inspected for clues as to the probable primary source of infection. Finally, close attention should be paid to the child's general status and to other portions of the reticuloendothelial system, e.g., to other nodal regions as well as to the liver and spleen.

With the above information the specific pathogen may be evident on clinical grounds alone or the differential diagnostic possibilities may be considerably narrowed, permitting confirmation by a minimum of laboratory tests. Close follow-up is important for all children treated as outpatients, to monitor their clinical course and response to therapy.

BACTERIAL BONE AND JOINT INFECTIONS

Osteomyelitis

The anatomy and physiology of growing bone place children at particular risk for bacterial infection, and in fact 85 percent of cases of osteomyelitis occur in children under 16 years of age. The highest incidence occurs in infancy with a secondary peak between 8 to 12 years, in most series. During infancy males and females are affected with equal frequency but, thereafter, males predominate in a ratio of 2–3 to 1. The advent of antimicrobial therapy and advances in diagnostic techniques have significantly altered the course and outcome. Mortality has fallen from 25 percent in the pre-antibiotic era, to 1 to 2 percent; morbidity has dropped from 50 percent to less than 15 percent.

S. aureus and ß-hemolytic streptococci are the most commonly identified pathogens in all age groups. *H. influenzae* type b is a major cause of septic arthritis in toddlers, but is an infrequent pathogen in osteomyelitis. Gram-negative organisms account for a small percentage of cases. Salmonella is of particular importance in children with sickle hemoglobinopathies, and pseudomonas often is isolated in cases resulting from puncture wounds of the foot. In 15 to 20 percent of cases no causative organism is identified, often as a result of suppression by prior antibiotic therapy. Once bacteria become established within bone, they stimulate an inflammatory response with formation of exudate. As this collects, local pressure increases, promoting extension outward and causing further vascular stasis and thrombophlebitis. The resultant ischemia causes local bone necrosis. With further progression dead bone can form a sequestrum surrounded by purulent material, which becomes inaccessible to antimicrobial penetration.

An appreciation of the anatomic and physiologic features of bone in general and of growing bone in particular is essential to an understanding of the pathophysiology of osteomyelitis in childhood. Nutrient vessels enter the diaphysis from the periosteum and extend to the metaphysis (or, in flat and irregular bones, to the area adjacent to the epiphysis) where terminal arterioles form loops and empty into larger sinusoidal veins. This area is one of sluggish, somewhat turbulent blood flow, which is prone to thrombosis and which serves as an ideal site for bacterial deposition in the face of bacteremia. Because they are devoid of phagocytic macrophages, the sinusoidal veins lack a major line of defense against bacteria.

In infants under 8 to 12 months of age, a number of additional factors facilitate the extension of infection, once it is present. As the epiphyseal plate has not fully formed, the nutrient arterioles penetrate into the epiphysis; hence rupture of infection into the adjacent joint is common. The cortex of the infant's metaphysis is thin and the trabeculae are fewer in number, facilitating penetration outward to a more loosely attached periosteum, as well as extension toward the diaphysis. Thus infants are far more likely to have extensive involvement, even with early diagnosis. Once the epiphyseal growth plate has formed, it serves as a relatively effective barrier to joint extension, substantially reducing the frequency of secondary septic arthritis, although sympathetic joint effusions are not uncommon. Exceptions to this are cases of hematogenous osteomyelitis involving the proximal metaphysis of the humerus or femur and of the distal fibula, where the synovium of the adjacent joint inserts so as to include the metaphysis within the joint.

There are two major mechanisms through which bones become infected. Hematogenous spread accounts for over 50 percent of cases in childhood. Areas of rich blood supply and sluggish flow are most vulnerable to bacterial seeding; hence the metaphyseal portions of long bones and the subepiphyseal portions of flat and irregular bones are the usual sites of involvement in this category. Trauma may be a predisposing factor, perhaps by virtue of producing local small-vessel occlusion with secondary stasis, anoxia, and necrosis. Children with sickle hemoglobinopathies are particularly susceptible to hematogenous osteomyelitis as a result of their vulnerability to bacteremia and sepsis, and because their bones are predisposed to sludging and infarction.

Spread from a contiguous focus of infection accounts for most of the remaining cases of osteomyelitis in childhood. Infections of fracture sites, surgical wounds, and puncture wounds, or extension of infection from an adjacent cellulitis or abscess serve as the predisposing conditions, with localization dependent on the original site of injury or infection.

While important in adults, peripheral vascular disease is rarely a predisposing condition in childhood. When such cases are seen, the patient usually is an adolescent with long-standing diabetes mellitus, and the small bones of the hands or feet are the most common sites of involvement.

In addition to categorization by mode of spread or acquisition, osteomyelitis is further subdivided into acute, subacute, and chronic forms according to duration of symptoms. Of these, the acute form is by far the most common. The major clinical finding in each form is localized bone pain, which typically is constant, severe, and exacerbated by movement. The overlying soft tissues may be warm, swollen, and occasionally erythematous, but in contrast to the findings in cellulitis, they generally are not indurated. Spasm of overlying muscles is

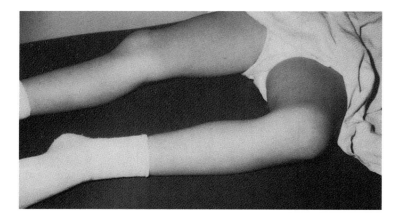

FIG. 12.51 Acute osteomyelitis. Fever, hip and thigh pain, and refusal to walk were the chief complaints of this 5-year-old child with osteomyelitis of the proximal femur. On inspection she lay still, holding the left leg externally rotated and flexed at the hip and knee. This same position also is adopted by children with acute arthritis of the hip.

often intense, adding to discomfort, and the adjacent joint may be held in flexion. Beyond these common features there is a wide range of clinical expression. Appreciation of this spectrum is important to ensure early diagnosis, thus resulting in a more favorable outcome.

ACUTE OSTEOMYELITIS
Acute Hematogenous Osteomyelitis

In the acute hematogenous form of osteomyelitis, the mode of presentation and clinical findings are age dependent, although most patients present within 1 week of onset of symptoms.

Infants under 6 months of age often have no systemic signs of infection. However, a small percentage have low-grade fever, and a few may present with a frankly septic picture. Early on, irritability and anorexia are the major manifestations. Within a few days evidence of pain on movement and/or of decreased use of a limb may be noted (pseudoparalysis). At this time or soon after, localized soft-tissue swelling develops. This often extends rapidly to involve the entire extremity, reflecting rapid spread of infection in the underlying bone. For the same reason tenderness also is diffuse. Furthermore multiple bones may be involved. Careful attention must be given to joint examination because of the high risk of early joint extension and secondary septic arthritis.

In children 8 months to 2 years of age, fever and signs of toxicity are common although not universal. History and/or persistent signs of antecedent upper respiratory tract or skin infection are present in over 50 percent of cases. In many cases systemic symptoms consist primarily of fever and irritability in association with refusal to walk, a limp, or decreased use of an extremity. A small percentage present with more severe systemic symptoms, including chills, lethargy, irritability, anorexia, vomiting, and dehydration. At this age children often are unable or unwilling to point to the site of discomfort, but on observation may be found to avoid moving the involved extremity or to hold a particular joint in flexion *consistently*. Soft-tissue swelling and warmth may be noted overlying a metaphysis, but this often is subtle or absent in early cases, and it is undetectable in cases where the proximal femur is involved. Comparative circumferential measurements of suspected areas and painstaking care in first eliciting the child's cooperation, and then in palpating for evidence of muscle spasm and/or point tenderness, are well worth the effort when osteomyelitis is suspected. Even then, focal tenderness may be difficult to detect early in the course.

Children over 2 years of age with acute osteomyelitis are usually febrile but rarely toxic. They are more likely to complain of and point to a specific site of pain, and point tenderness generally is easy to elicit unless presentation is very early. Older patients describe the pain as deep, intense, and constant. Signs of adjacent joint flexion and of nearby muscle spasm are common (Fig. 12.51) but, again, overlying soft-tissue swelling may be subtle. Unless a sympathetic effusion has developed, the adjacent joint may be passively moved through its full range of motion, although this will exacerbate the pain.

When bones other than the long bones of the extremities are the site of infection, the clinical picture can be especially confusing. Osteomyelitis of the pelvic bones can mimic numerous other conditions. While fever and an abnormal gait are the most common presenting complaints, lower abdominal and groin pain, hip and/or buttock pain, sciatica, and thigh pain (with swelling) each can be prominent early complaints in individual patients. Often the initial clinical picture is more suggestive of appendicitis, pelvic abscess, or infection of the hip or femur than of pelvic osteomyelitis. Diagnosis necessitates a high level of suspicion and great care in examination. In patients presenting with abdominal complaints, the lack of rebound tenderness, lesser prominence of gastrointestinal symptoms, onset of pain in the lower abdomen rather than in the periumbilical region, and normal findings on rectal examination can help to distinguish the process from that of acute appendicitis. Furthermore, while the majority of patients have pain on hip motion in one or more planes, range of motion either is normal or only slightly limited, and with careful examination point tenderness usually can be detected.

Acute Osteomyelitis Due to Contiguous Spread

Acute osteomyelitis as a result of contiguous spread of infection must be suspected in patients with prior puncture wounds, deep lacerations, surgical incisions, open fractures, abscesses, or cellulitis who experience a sudden onset of increased pain at the wound site. This pain is perceived as deep, severe and constant, and is aggravated by movement. In these cases soft-tissue cellulitis is a common associated finding and fever is usual. Often, when extension of primary soft-tissue infection is the source, the patient may have worsened clinically after a period of improvement on antimicrobial therapy or may have failed to show the expected response to therapy.

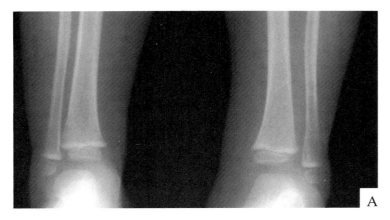

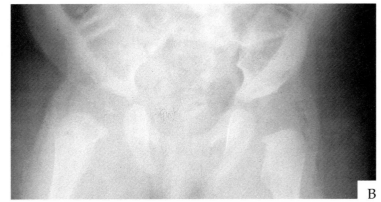

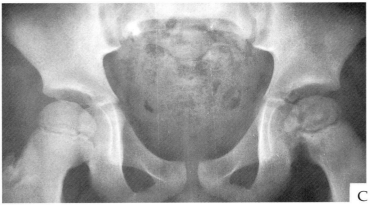

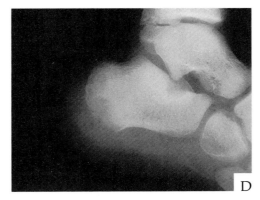

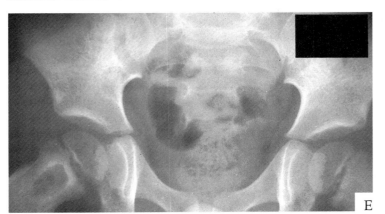

FIG. 12.52 Acute osteomyelitis. Radiographic changes lag behind the clinical in osteomyelitis. **A,** the first noticeable change, about 3 days after onset, is deep soft-tissue swelling, seen here adjacent to the metaphysis of the distal tibia on the left. **B,** in this neonate a radiolucency is evident in the proximal metaphysis of the right femur, which also is displaced upward and laterally. On aspiration of the hip, purulent fluid was obtained confirming the suspicion of rupture of the infection into the hip and of secondary septic arthritis. **C,** the epiphysis and proximal metaphysis of the left femur have a moth-eaten appearance in this older child. **D,** deep and superficial soft-tissue swelling overlie the radiolucent lesion of the calcaneus in this boy who developed pseudomonas osteomyelitis following a puncture wound of the heel. **E,** the late changes of a lytic lesion with sclerotic margins are seen in the right femoral metaphysis of this child who was completing his course of therapy. (**A,** courtesy of Dr. Jocelyn Ledesma-Medina; **B, C,** and **E,** courtesy of Dr. Roderigo Dominguez; **D,** courtesy of Dr. Ellen Wald)

Diagnostic Methods in Acute Osteomyelitis

Standard radiographic and laboratory studies are of somewhat limited use in the diagnosis of acute osteomyelitis. The sedimentation rate is elevated in the vast majority of cases and exceeds 40 in about 80 percent. This finding is helpful primarily in confirming that an inflammatory process is the source of symptoms. White blood cell counts, while sometimes elevated with a left shift in differential, may be normal in as many as 50 percent of cases and thus are less useful.

Radiographic changes lag behind the clinical process and can be subtle. The first noticeable change, seen about 3 days after onset of symptoms, is the presence of deep soft-tissue swelling displacing fat lines adjacent to a metaphysis (Fig. 12.52A). In ensuing days the swelling increases to obliterate fascial planes, and then extends to involve subcutaneous tissues. These soft-tissue changes can be very difficult to appreciate when osteomyelitis involves bones of the trunk or pelvis; however, in cases of pelvic osteomyelitis, clouding of the obturator foramen, distortion of the fascial planes around the adjacent hip, or even displacement of the bladder may be detectable. When a sympathetic joint effusion is present or when rupture into the adjacent joint has resulted in secondary septic arthritis, joint-space widening and/or bony displacement may be evident (Fig. 12.52B). Bony changes are not visible radiographically until 7 to 10 days after onset in untreated patients. These changes consist of periosteal elevation followed by focal evidence of bony lysis, and subsequently, by sclerosis or new bone formation at the margins of the lytic lesion (Fig. 12.52C–E). Early diagnosis and treatment may completely prevent development of bony radiographic changes.

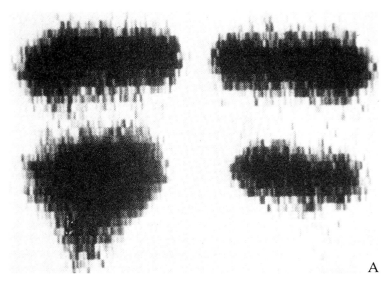

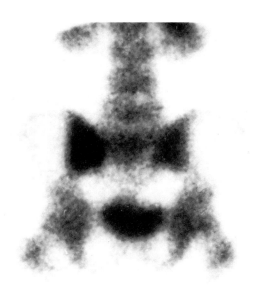

A

B

FIG. 12.53 Technetium scan findings in acute osteomyelitis. **A,** in this radionuclide scan, selectively increased uptake is seen in the proximal right tibial metaphysis. The uptake in the epiphyses is normal reflecting active bone growth. **B,** this youngster presented with a puzzling picture of abdominal pain suggestive of an acute abdomen. A bone scan was obtained after other studies were unrevealing. The increased uptake in the right sacroiliac area helped to identify osteomyelitis as the source of symptoms. (Courtesy of Dr. Ellen Wald, Children's Hospital of Pittsburgh)

Technetium scanning has provided a better means of early identification and localization of sites of acute osteomyelitis. It can be positive as early as 24 to 48 hours after onset of symptoms, revealing discrete areas of increased uptake (Fig. 12.53A). The procedure has been particularly useful as a diagnostic adjunct in cases of pelvic and vertebral osteomyelitis in which the mode of presentation has simulated the clinical picture of another condition (Fig. 12.53B, and see Fig. 12.56C). It also can be helpful in distinguishing osteomyelitis from cellulitis, septic arthritis, and acute bony infarcts. With cellulitis, intense deep soft-tissue uptake is seen with faint diffuse uptake in underlying bone; in septic arthritis the scan may be normal, or when accompanied by overlying cellulitis, it may show increased periarticular soft-tissue uptake; in early infarcts, uptake is decreased. Scans also are helpful in delineating additional areas of involvement in the small percentage of cases with multiple sites. Standard radiographs remain important, however, in identifying fractures and malignancies, which may simulate the appearance of osteomyelitis on bone scan. Bone scans have the additional limitation of an occasional false-negative reading, possibly due to local ischemia. When clinical suspicion remains high, a repeat technetium scan or a gallium scan (which identifies purulent exudate) should be considered or aspiration should be performed.

Vigorous attempts must be made to isolate the causative organism in order to optimize therapy on the basis of known sensitivities and a determination of bactericidal levels. Aspiration of the site of maximal tenderness or maximal uptake as revealed by bone scan can be very useful in that it provides material for Gram stain and culture. In cases where purulent material is obtained, operative drainage should be considered strongly. Even in the absence of exudate, flushing the aspirating needle with culture media often will enable isolation of the causative organism. Blood cultures are positive in over 50 percent of cases of acute hematogenous osteomyelitis and should be drawn in all suspected cases.

Complications of osteomyelitis include secondary septic arthritis with resultant joint damage, epiphyseal injury with long-term morbidity from impaired bone growth, progression to chronic osteomyelitis (now seen in less than 4 percent of cases), and rarely pathologic fractures. The rate of complications is highest in young infants who often have extensive bony involvement and secondary septic arthritis by the time the diagnosis is made. Care in clinical assessment and aggressive attempts to confirm the diagnosis of acute osteomyelitis as early as possible are as important in ensuring good outcome and minimizing complications as are adequate antimicrobial therapy and recognition of the need for surgical intervention where appropriate. Close collaboration between pediatrician and orthopedic surgeon is essential to optimize decisions regarding the route and duration of pharmacotherapy, and the need for and timing of surgical intervention when indicated.

SUBACUTE OSTEOMYELITIS

Approximately 10 percent of cases of hematogenous osteomyelitis have an insidious onset and a subacute course, often characterized by mild to moderate local pain in an extremity, with or without swelling. Fever is unusual and other systemic symptoms are absent. Typically the patient has had symptoms for a few to several weeks prior to presentation. In some instances this subacute course appears to be related to partial suppression of the infection by antibiotics that have been administered for infection at another site (such as for otitis media, tonsillitis, or impetigo). In these patients pain may improve during the period of antimicrobial therapy only to worsen once they stop taking the medication. In other cases in which antibiotics have not been prescribed, reduced bacterial virulence is postulated. On examination local tenderness is evident and overlying soft-tissue swelling may be noted. By the time diagnosis is made, multiple sites are involved in as many as 20 percent of patients. However, secondary sites may not be symptomatic.

While white blood cell counts usually are normal, the sedimentation rate is elevated in most (but not all) patients. Blood cultures rarely are positive. Radiographs may show one of

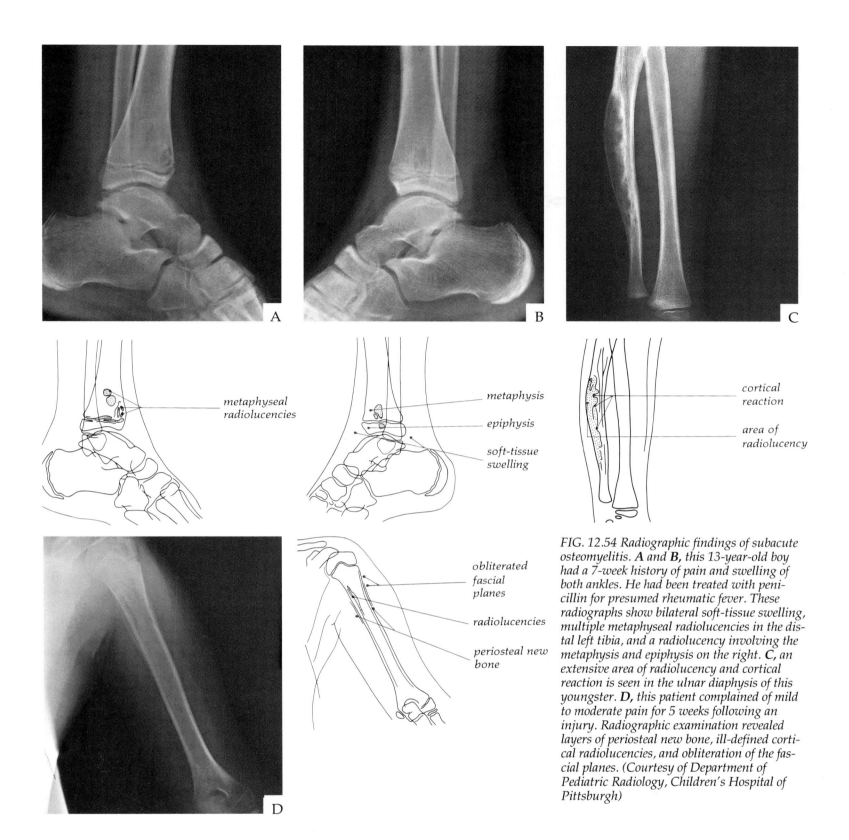

FIG. 12.54 Radiographic findings of subacute osteomyelitis. **A** and **B,** this 13-year-old boy had a 7-week history of pain and swelling of both ankles. He had been treated with penicillin for presumed rheumatic fever. These radiographs show bilateral soft-tissue swelling, multiple metaphyseal radiolucencies in the distal left tibia, and a radiolucency involving the metaphysis and epiphysis on the right. **C,** an extensive area of radiolucency and cortical reaction is seen in the ulnar diaphysis of this youngster. **D,** this patient complained of mild to moderate pain for 5 weeks following an injury. Radiographic examination revealed layers of periosteal new bone, ill-defined cortical radiolucencies, and obliteration of the fascial planes. (Courtesy of Department of Pediatric Radiology, Children's Hospital of Pittsburgh)

several possible findings. In children presenting within a few weeks of onset who have taken antibiotics, radiographic findings may simulate the deep soft-tissue swelling characteristic of early acute osteomyelitis. Other configurations include an isolated metaphyseal radiolucency surrounded by reactive bone (Brodie's abscess); a metaphyseal radiolucency with loss or disruption of cortical bone simulating a tumor; excessive cortical reaction in the diaphysis simulating an osteoid osteoma; or multiple layers of subperiosteal new bone overlying the diaphysis, at times mimicking the appearance of Ewing's sar-

coma (Fig. 12.54). While a bone scan is not of great use in distinguishing subacute osteomyelitis from a primary bone tumor, it can be very helpful in revealing other sites of involvement. Because the long course, clinical picture and radiographic findings of this infection often are indistinguishable from those of a neoplastic process, biopsy generally is required to establish the diagnosis and to isolate the causative organism. In the vast majority of cases, a coagulase-positive staphylococcus is found. Surgical curettage, immobilization, and antimicrobials are the mainstays of treatment.

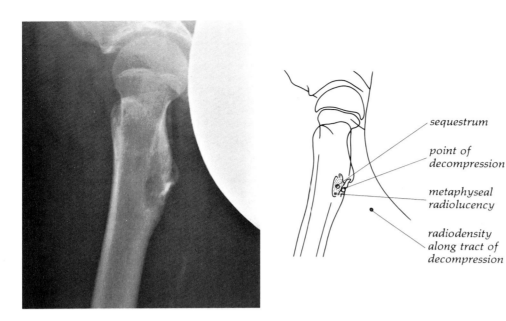

sequestrum

point of decompression

metaphyseal radiolucency

radiodensity along tract of decompression

CHRONIC OSTEOMYELITIS

With the advent of antimicrobial therapy and improvements in diagnostic techniques, chronic osteomyelitis has become a relatively rare entity in countries where there is ready access to medical care. Delay in diagnosis, inadequate antimicrobial and/or surgical therapy, and unusually resistant organisms are the major factors associated with this outcome. Pathophysiologically, extensive necrosis, sequestrum formation as a result of bone death, and decompression via fistulization through the overlying soft tissues are characteristic (Fig. 12.55). Patients continue to be troubled by local pain of varying severity and by chronic draining sinuses. Aggressive surgical curettage and long-term antimicrobial therapy are required to achieve resolution but, despite this, permanent functional disability and deformity are not uncommon once osteomyelitis has progressed to a chronic phase.

JUVENILE DISCITIS AND VERTEBRAL OSTEOMYELITIS

Inflammation of an intervertebral disc space in childhood is a puzzling disorder, both in terms of the elucidation of its exact pathophysiology and its mode of presentation. Prior to the third decade of life, vascular channels penetrate through the vertebral end plates and communicate with the intervertebral disc. Thus it is thought that hematogenously spread organisms are more likely to alight in the disc space of children and adolescents, whereas thereafter they may lodge in vascular arcades adjacent to the subchondral plate of the vertebra itself. This factor has been used to explain the higher frequency of discitis in childhood and the relative infrequency of acute vertebral osteomyelitis prior to adulthood. However, differences in clinical picture, the lower frequency of isolation of pathogens, and evidence that immobilization alone is effective in treating discitis—while antimicrobial therapy is required in vertebral osteomyelitis—have led to speculation that disc-space inflammation may be due to a low-grade viral or bacterial infection.

Known predisposing conditions in adults include urinary tract infections, pelvic inflammatory disease and bowel and urinary tract surgery, while in children they include upper respiratory tract infection, gastroenteritis, and genitourinary infection. The importance of antecedent trauma is unclear. Hematogenous spread may occur through the valveless veins of Batson's plexus or via the vertebral branches of the posterior spinal arteries. In both discitis and vertebral osteomyelitis, coagulase-positive staphylococci are the organisms most commonly isolated, followed by streptococci, gram-negative enteric pathogens, and corynebacteria. The lumbar spine and the lower thoracic spine are the most common sites of involvement for both entities.

The clinical picture of discitis, which is seen predominantly in children under age 4, is dominated by pain and progressive limp. Often the pain is perceived as focal back pain of progressively worsening severity. In a few instances it may be perceived as primarily worse in the flank, abdomen, or hip. It is constant, may be aggravated by sitting, standing, or movement, and typically is worse at night. Children who are too young to describe their pain may present with a picture of irritability and refusal to walk or even sit. In some cases increased irritability has been noted during diaper changes. Adoption of an abnormal posture is a frequent finding. Most commonly this posture is one of exaggerated lumbar lordosis, but in some cases the lumbar spine may be held stiff and straight. Toddlers may assume a knee-chest position. Fever often is present during the first week or two of symptoms, but it may be absent and often is low grade. Other systemic symptoms are unusual. Occasionally abdominal distension is prominent, raising suspicion of intra-abdominal pathology.

Failure to remember that vertebrospinal pathology may result in a limp or refusal to walk, and thus failure to examine carefully the backs of such patients, often results in long delays in diagnosis. Such examination may reveal paravertebral muscle spasm with guarding and exquisite focal tenderness, although in some cases tenderness may be vague or absent. Resistance to flexion and extension of the spine is common, and in the young may simulate meningeal signs. Pain on straight-leg raising and hip motion also may be encountered.

The sedimentation rate is elevated unless symptoms have been present for many, months, but white blood cell counts are

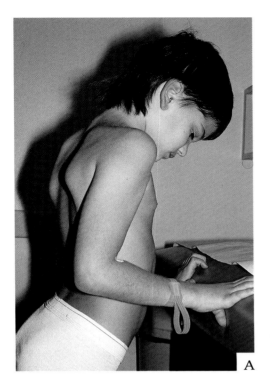

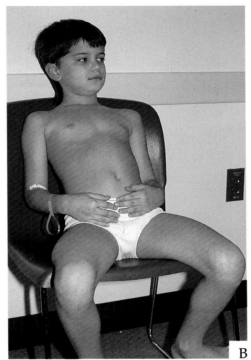

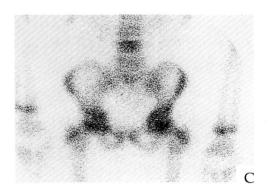

FIG. 12.56 Vertebral osteomyelitis. This 10-year-old boy presented with a 2-week history of intermittent fever, malaise, and steadily worsening lower back and left hip pain, exacerbated by movement. **A** and **B**, he had an exaggerated lumbar lordosis and extreme limitation of flexion both standing and sitting. The straight leg raising test also accentuated his pain. **C**, bone scan revealed selectively increased uptake in the L_4 vertebral body. (**C**, courtesy of the Department of Pediatric Radiology, Children's Hospital of Pittsburgh)

elevated only during the first few weeks. Specific radiographic changes do not appear until 2 to 6 weeks after onset, at which point disc-space narrowing becomes evident. In ensuing weeks irregularities of the adjacent vertebral end plates become apparent. The loss of normal lumbar lordosis or the presence of local scoliosis may be noted early on. A technetium scan can reveal focal increased uptake as early as 1 week after onset of symptoms. Culture of biopsy specimens of the disc space, when obtained early in the course, may yield an offending organism but commonly is negative after a few weeks of symptoms. Blood cultures rarely are positive. The majority of patients improve symptomatically with immobilization alone, and the process appears to resolve after several weeks of casting.

The clinical picture of vertebral osteomyelitis, seen in older children and adolescents, usually is one of insidious onset of gradually progressive back pain that is constant, aggravated by movement, and resistant to analgesics. Fever is absent or low grade. Occasionally the onset is acute with fever and generalized systemic symptoms accompanying the abrupt appearance of pain. In the rare cases reported in young children, onset usually has been acute and the clinical picture dominated by abdominal and/or flank pain, with associated tenderness and often guarding. In some patients paraspinous or spinous process tenderness, back stiffness, an exaggerated lumbar lordosis, and pain on leg motion or lower extremity weakness also may be noted (Fig. 12.56). Laboratory findings are similar to those of children with discitis, with the exception that blood cultures obtained in the acute phase generally are positive. Early radiographic findings also are similar, but following the appearance of disc-space narrowing, frank destructive lesions of the vertebral body are seen. Cultures of operative biopsy specimens usually are positive for *S. aureus.* Antimicrobial therapy is necessary to achieve clinical resolution, and surgical debridement is more likely to be required.

Septic Arthritis

Bacterial invasion of the synovial membrane with resultant septic arthritis is a condition with a high potential for long-term morbidity. Release of lysosomal enzymes by attracted leukocytes, abscess formation, development of granulation tissue, and ischemia resulting from increased intra-articular pressure act in concert to damage the articular surface and to promote synovial fibrosis and bony ankylosis. Early diagnosis and treatment are essential to prevent or at least to minimize the extent of irreversible damage. This, however, is hindered in many cases by overlap, in both clinical picture and laboratory findings, with viral and other forms of acute arthritis.

Septic arthritis is a disorder primarily of young children with two-thirds to three-fourths of cases occurring in patients under 5 years of age. Males are affected twice as often as females. Ninety percent of cases are the result of hematogenous seeding in the course of bacteremia, and while in most cases the affected joint becomes the primary site of localization, it is not uncommon for septic arthritis to develop in a child with bacterial meningitis or pneumonia, often becoming manifest early in the course of treatment. As many as 40 percent of patients have a history and/or signs of an antecedent upper respiratory tract infection at the time of diagnosis. This is especially common in cases caused by *H. influenzae* type b. Streptococcal skin and soft-tissue infections may antedate septic arthritis due to this pathogen. In older children or in adolescents, gonococcal urethritis, vaginitis, and/or cervicitis assume importance as antecedents to hematogenous seeding (see Chapter 18, Gynecology). Prior trauma also may predispose and is reported in a significant number of cases. In approximately 10 percent of patients, the septic arthritis is secondary to rupture of a primary osteomyelitis into the joint space. Direct penetrating injury accounts for a small percentage (see Chapter 21, Orthopedics).

FIG. 12.57

RELATIVE FREQUENCY OF PATHOGENS IN SEPTIC ARTHRITIS ACCORDING TO AGE			
Neonate	**1 Month–2 Years**	**2–5 Years**	**>5 Years**
S. aureus	H. influenzae type b	S. aureus	S. aureus
Group B streptococci	Group A streptococci	Group A streptococci	Group A streptococci
Gram-negative enteric pathogens	S. pneumoniae	H. influenzae type b	Neisseria gonorrhoeae
	N. meningitidis	N. meningitidis	P. aeruginosa
	P. aeruginosa	S. pneumoniae	
	Salmonella species		

Bacterial pathogens are isolated in 65 to 75 percent of cases, either from synovial fluid culture, blood culture, or both. The relative frequency of pathogens varies considerably with patient age, as shown in Figure 12.57. Children with sickle hemoglobinopathies occasionally develop salmonella septic arthritis. Failure to isolate an organism can be explained in some instances by suppression due to prior antibiotic administration.

The knee, hip, elbow, and ankle are the joints most commonly affected. The wrist and shoulder are involved less often, with other joints being rare sites of septic arthritis. In over 90 percent of cases, only a single joint is affected. *Neisseria gonorrhoeae* is the organism most commonly associated with multiple joint involvement, but other pathogens may be responsible, particularly coagulase-positive staphylococci and also *H. influenzae* type b. The hip and shoulder joints, when involved, are particularly prone to damage. Clinical signs may be subtle and thus diagnosis often is delayed. Further, as the synovium inserts distal to the epiphysis of the proximal humerus and femur, compromise of the blood supply to the epiphysis is more likely to occur as a result of increased intra-articular pressure.

The typical clinical picture of hematogenous septic arthritis is one of a young child who presents with moderate to high fever and signs of toxicity, in association with severe localized joint pain, overlying swelling, and marked limitation in range of motion. The fever may be quite acute in onset or it may have been present for a few days, but presentation tends to occur soon after the onset of joint symptoms. Variations in this picture depend in part on the age of the patient, the joint involved, the causative organism, and the duration of symptoms. Infants and toddlers cannot describe focal pain and thus they tend to present with fever and irritability, the latter aggravated by movement. Refusal to bear weight or decreased use of an extremity may or may not have been noted by the family. When a knee, ankle, wrist, or elbow is involved, local swelling and warmth usually are evident (Fig. 12.58). However, with early presentation swelling may be subtle and high fever may make differential warmth hard to distinguish. Surface erythema often is absent. When a hip is involved, swelling and warmth are not evident externally and pain may be referred to the knee or thigh. Often the position adopted by the patient is the best diagnostic clue. To minimize intra-articular pressure and pain, the child prefers to lie still with the knee and hip flexed and with the hip externally rotated (see Fig. 12.51). In cases of septic arthritis of the shoulder, subtle swelling may or may not be evident, but the shoulders may not be held at the same level and the arm on the involved side will be held against the chest to splint the joint.

Septic arthritis of the sacroiliac joint, which accounts for about 1 percent of cases, can present a particularly confusing picture, often mimicking hip or intra-abdominal disease. Only one-third of patients have an acute presentation, and the remainder have a subacute course. Buttock pain, limp, and fever are the most common presenting complaints. Unilateral radicular pain is described by as many as one-third of patients. Findings of lower abdominal and rectal tenderness in association with normal hip motion may fool the examiner who fails to recognize that leg and buttock pain necessitate meticulous examination of the lower back. Such an exam will reveal tenderness over the involved sacroiliac joint, and pelvic compression will replicate the pain as will hyperextension of the ipsilateral hip, with the patient supine and dangling his leg over the edge of the table.

Limitation of joint motion and evidence of pain on motion are perhaps the most valuable clinical clues to the diagnosis of septic arthritis. Limitation usually is severe unless presentation occurs very early, and motion provokes marked discomfort. In young patients with fever and decreased use of an extremity but without clear-cut swelling, localization often is possible if, after careful inspection and palpation for bony tenderness, each joint is gently moved while the examiner carefully guards the other joints, without touching them. Diagnosis can be particularly difficult in neonates and very young infants, who may be afebrile and often will have no systemic symptoms. In such cases decreased use of an extremity often is the earliest clue. Pain on motion usually is evident, however, even before the appearance of localized swelling.

When septic arthritis is the result of rupture of a focus of osteomyelitis into a joint, distinction between the two processes can be very difficult to establish clinically. Focal pain generally is of longer duration, but as most cases occur in infants under 8 months this clue often is unavailable. In older children the hip, shoulder, and ankle are the major sites of this secondary form of septic arthritis. These children usually will have a history of prolonged focal pain, antedating a brief period of respite, followed by the sudden return of pain that is markedly aggravated by joint motion. In the days following a penetrating joint injury, a sudden increase in pain and swelling should lead to immediate suspicion of secondary septic arthritis.

Because of the high cost of delays in diagnosis in terms of morbidity, any child with fever, acute onset of pain, and limit-

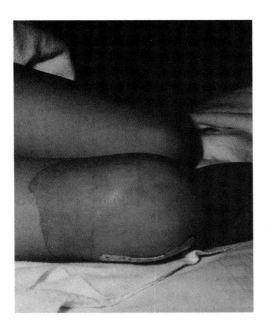

FIG. 12.58 Septic arthritis. This 8-year-old boy awoke suddenly at 3 AM with severe knee pain. By 8 AM he was febrile and had marked swelling and extreme limitation of movement. There was no overlying erythema. Examination of joint fluid revealed gram-positive cocci in chains, with a white blood cell count of 24,000. Cultures were positive for group A streptococci.

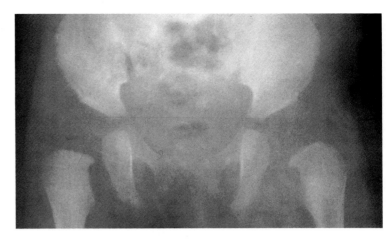

FIG. 12.59 Radiographic findings of septic arthritis. While radiographs may be normal early on, in most cases joint-space widening can be detected. In this infant who presented with fever, toxicity, and refusal to move the left leg, capsular swelling and displacement of the proximal femur are readily apparent. (Courtesy of Dr. Roderigo Dominguez, University of Texas)

ed motion of a joint should be presumed to have septic arthritis until proven otherwise. These findings should prompt expeditious diagnostic investigation. Plain radiographs with comparison views should be obtained without delay and inspected carefully for even subtle signs of joint-space widening or capsular distention, although in early cases findings may be normal. When the hip is the suspected site of pathology, lateral and upward displacement of the femoral head may be noted along with displacement of the gluteal fat lines (Fig. 12.59). A bone scan is perhaps the best method of evaluating the child with suspected septic arthritis of the sacroiliac joint and is also useful in identifying patients with underlying osteomyelitis.

Arthrocentesis should be considered early, as examination of joint fluid is the study most likely to yield definitive results. A heparinized syringe should be used to prevent spontaneous clotting. Positive findings on Gram stain are particularly helpful; cultures are positive in 60 percent or more of cases. Pleocytosis is common with two-thirds of patients having more than 50,000 white blood cells. It is crucial to remember, however, that there is considerable overlap with nonbacterial arthritis in cell counts, differential counts, and protein and glucose levels found on examination of synovial fluid. Thus septic arthritis cannot be ruled out when these values are within the normal range.

Peripheral white blood cell counts and sedimentation rate may add suggestive evidence, but again there is overlap with viral arthritis. As many as 20 percent of patients have white blood cell counts under 10,000, although most have a significant left shift. The sedimentation rate may be markedly elevated, but it is under 40 in as many as 45 percent of cases. Blood cultures are positive in up to 40 percent of patients. Counter-immunoelectrophoresis studies may be helpful in identifying the responsible pathogen before culture results are available and in cases where cultures prove negative.

Diagnosis thus is dependent on assessment of the assembled data including clinical course, physical findings, and results of multiple laboratory studies. Even with a negative Gram stain, empiric antimicrobial therapy selected to cover the most likely pathogens (see Fig. 12.57) should be started, pending culture results, for cases in which septic arthritis is deemed likely on

the basis of the available findings. As is true of osteomyelitis, collaboration between pediatric and orthopedic colleagues is essential, for drainage of infected material is essential to good outcome.

Any disorder associated with acute arthritis must be considered as part of the differential diagnosis. In some instances the clinical picture of an obvious viral or vasculitic syndrome enables differentiation. The polymigratory picture of acute rheumatic fever and the much less acute onset of juvenile rheumatoid arthritis help to distinguish these conditions. Adenopathy, visceromegaly, anemia, and radiographic changes help distinguish malignant joint infiltration.

CONGENITAL AND PERINATAL INFECTIONS

A number of pathogens that produce relatively mild or even subclinical disease in children and adults can cause severe disease with devastating sequelae when infection is acquired prenatally or perinatally. Toxoplasmosis, rubella, cytomegalic inclusion disease, herpes simplex infection (the TORCH diseases), and congenital syphilis are well-known sources of pathology. In addition sepsis, meningitis, pneumonia, and other infections due to numerous perinatally acquired bacterial pathogens are the cause of significant neonatal morbidity and mortality, especially in infants born prematurely. Because of the breadth of this subject and because of limitations of space, we have elected to limit discussion to three disorders that tend to produce distinctive physical findings.

Congenital Toxoplasmosis

Toxoplasma gondii is an intracellular protozoan that is acquired primarily from consumption of infected raw or undercooked meat, or via ingestion or inhalation of oocysts excreted in cat feces. Occasionally transmission occurs via transfusion or organ transplantation. While most cases of postnatal infection are thought to be subclinical, a mononucleosis-like syndrome and cervical adenopathy have been identified as clinical features, and it may well be that in many cases the clinical picture simulates a viral illness and thus the true cause goes unrecognized.

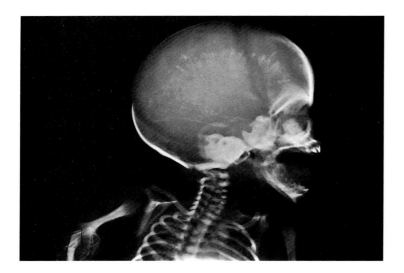

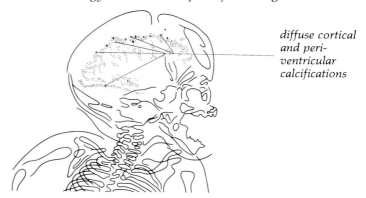

FIG. 12.60 Congenital toxoplasmosis. Microcephaly, ventricular dilatation, and cerebral calcifications were prominent findings in this infant with severe congenital toxoplasmosis. (Courtesy of Department of Pediatric Radiology, Children's Hospital of Pittsburgh)

diffuse cortical and peri-ventricular calcifications

Prenatally acquired infection has the potential for serious harm to the developing fetus. It is estimated that in the United States 1-2 per 1000 live-born infants have congenitally acquired toxoplasmosis. Maternal infection during pregnancy results in fetal infection less than 50 percent of the time, however. Risk of transmission to the fetus increases as gestation advances, but the severity of fetal injury is greater the earlier the infection occurs during pregnancy. Major sites of involvement are the CNS, retina, choroid, and muscles. As a result of these factors, 70 percent of congenitally infected infants appear normal at birth, about 10 to 20 percent are overtly symptomatic, and approximately 10 percent have detectable chorioretinitis without other abnormalities (see Chapter 19, Ophthalmology). Infected infants without signs of disease and those with mild chorioretinitis alone are at risk for progressive ocular and, on occasion, CNS involvement if not diagnosed and treated. In many instances, however, the diagnosis is not suspected until signs of visual impairment, strabismus, or developmental delay prompt careful ophthalmologic and neurologic assessment.

In severely affected infants, the clinical picture may closely simulate that of other congenital infections, especially cytomegalovirus. These infants tend to be small for gestational age, may be microcephalic or hydrocephalic, develop early onset jaundice, have hepatosplenomegaly and diffuse adenopathy, and often are covered with petechial and purpuric lesions or with a generalized maculopapular rash. Seizures are common in these infants as is a CSF pleocytosis with increased protein and xanthochromia. Skull radiographs may reveal diffuse cortical calcifications in contrast to the periventricular pattern seen with cytomegalic inclusion disease (Fig. 12.60). Interstitial pneumonitis and myocarditis may be prominent features as well. These infants have a high risk of severe neurodevelopmental sequelae, if they survive. Other infants may appear normal initially but may rapidly develop signs of neonatal myocarditis with minimal CNS manifestations, although they too may have cerebral calcifications, as do many infants with apparently isolated chorioretinitis.

Diagnosis is best confirmed by IgM fluorescent antibody testing or, in cases presenting with ocular findings later in infancy, by the Sabin-Feldman dye test. Treatment with pyrimethamine and triple sulfa or sulfadiazine for a 4-week course appears to interrupt the infection and prevent the progression of ocular and CNS injury.

Congenital Rubella

Despite its usually mild manifestations when acquired postnatally, prenatal infection with rubella virus is a far from benign process. Intrauterine death, variable constellations of congenital anomalies, and severe perinatal illness may result. The mother may or may not have symptomatic illness. In the viremic phase the virus is transmitted to the placenta, and then in most instances to the fetus. If the fetus becomes infected, mitotic activity is reduced and focal cytolysis and vascular injury occur, resulting in congenital malformations. The earlier in gestation the infection occurs, the greater the potential for injury. Of fetuses infected during the first 8 weeks, 39 percent will spontaneously abort or be stillborn, 25 percent will have gross anomalies noted at birth, and 36 percent will appear normal. Ultimately 85 percent of all liveborn infants infected during the first 8 weeks will be found to have sequelae. Infections in the ensuing 12 weeks pose a gradually decreasing risk of anomalies, and those occurring thereafter do not cause defects. The most commonly encountered anomalies are central diffuse cataracts, congenital heart disease (patent ductus arteriosus, pulmonary artery stenosis, pulmonary valvular stenosis), and sensorineural deafness (usually bilateral, occasionally unilateral), seen singly or in combination.

There is thus a wide range of clinical manifestations. Some infants at risk are normal. Some appear normal at birth but later are found to have hearing loss. A number are small for gestational age and at birth have evidence of congenital heart disease and ocular anomalies including microphthalmia, glaucoma, cataracts that may be central or diffuse, and pigmented retinopathy (see Chapter 19). While usually present at birth, ocular findings may be missed unless careful ophthalmologic examination is performed. Many of these infants develop jaundice within 24 hours of delivery and have hepatosplenomegaly and diffuse adenopathy as well.

Ten to twenty percent of liveborn infants with congenital rubella manifest signs of severe disseminated infection at or shortly after delivery. In addition to early jaundice, hepatosplenomegaly and adenopathy, they often have signs of myocarditis with ischemic changes on electrocardiography, interstitial pneumonitis, thrombocytopenia with petechiae and purpura, and signs of CNS dysfunction that may range from lethargy and hypotonia to frank meningoencephalitis. Radiographs may reveal bony abnormalities consisting of metaphy-

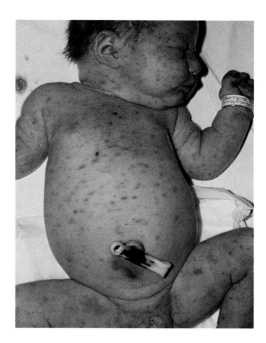

FIG. 12.61 Congenital rubella. This newborn had the full-blown picture of the "expanded rubella syndrome," including a generalized blueberry muffin rash, diffuse petechiae, hepatosplenomegaly, early onset of jaundice and neurologic depression. (Courtesy of Dr. Michael Sherlock)

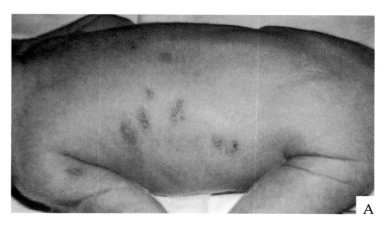

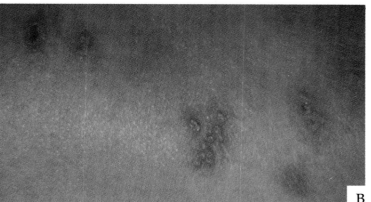

FIG. 12.62 Neonatal herpes simplex type 2 infection. **A** and **B**, although normal at birth, this infant developed sudden onset of fever, lethargy, and decreased feeding at 6 days of age. On examination multiple grouped vesicular lesions were noted on the trunk and scalp. The liver and spleen were markedly enlarged and very firm. He had a fulminant course resembling that of septic shock, and died within 24 hours. (Courtesy of Dr. Michael Sherlock)

seal lucencies and irregular epiphyseal mineralization. In some cases a rubelliform rash may be noted, or a characteristic raised bluish papular eruption, termed a "blueberry muffin rash," may be evident due to dermal erythropoiesis (Fig. 12.61). Most of these severely affected infants are microcephalic in addition to being small for gestational age. Survivors of this "expanded rubella syndrome" have a high likelihood of deafness and significant psychomotor retardation.

In a small percentage of cases of congenital rubella, delayed manifestations may surface. These include anemia toward the end of the first month, and at 3 to 4 months of age the insidious onset of interstitial pneumonitis and the appearance of a chronic generalized rubelliform exanthem. Still later immunodeficiency may be detected. Feeding difficulties, chronic diarrhea, and failure to thrive are common.

Infants with congenital rubella are chronically and persistently infected, and tend to shed live virus in urine, stools, and respiratory secretions for up to a year. Hence, they should be isolated in hospitals and kept away from susceptible pregnant women when sent home. Diagnosis can be confirmed by viral culture and specific IgM titers.

Neonatal Herpes Simplex Infection

Infants born vaginally to mothers with genital herpes simplex type 2 are at significant risk for acquisition of infection. Typically the mother is asymptomatic and the infant appears totally normal at birth. Signs of infection may develop any time within the first 4 weeks, but usually they appear 4 to 8 days postpartum. Infection may be localized to the skin, eye, mouth, or central nervous system, or it may be systemic. In the latter instance, onset begins with fever or subnormal temperature in association with lethargy, poor feeding, vomiting and jaundice. The liver and spleen are enlarged and often are remarkably firm. Respiratory distress supervenes, followed by a picture that is indistinguishable from that of septic shock with DIC. Approximately three-fourths of affected infants have typical herpetic skin or mucosal lesions (Fig. 12.62). The scalp and face are the sites most commonly involved. Occasionally lesions are limited to the conjunctiva or to the

oral mucosa. In the absence of these lesions, accurate diagnosis is extremely difficult. Mortality is high, exceeding 50 percent, but has been reduced by early recognition and systemic antiviral therapy. Nevertheless, morbidity remains high in survivors. Infants with localized skin, eye, and/or oral involvement have a relatively good prognosis. Those with localized CNS disease have a better survival rate than those with systemic infection but they share severe morbidity.

Less frequently infections may occur prenatally as a result of ascent from the lower genital tract through ruptured membranes, or as a result of maternal viremia. With prenatal acquisition, the infant may die in utero or may be born with jaundice, skin lesions, and signs of systemic infection.

BIBLIOGRAPHY

Barton LL, Feigin RD: Childhood cervical lymphadenitis: a reappraisal. *J Pediatr* 1974;84:846–852.

Barton LL, Friedman AD: Impetigo: a reassessment of etiology and therapy. *Pediatr Derm* 1987;4:185–188.

Cherry JD: Newer viral exanthems. *Adv Pediatr* 1969; 16:233–286.

Chesney PJ, Davis JP, Purdy WK, et al: Clinical manifestations of toxic shock syndrome. *JAMA* 1981;246: 741–748.

Clain A: *Demonstrations of Physical Signs in Clinical Surgery*, ed 16. Littleton, Mass, John Wright-PSG, 1980.

Committee on Infectious Diseases, American Academy of Pediatrics: *Report of the Committee on Infectious Diseases—the 1988 ed Book,* ed 21. Evanston, Illinois, Am Acad Pediatr, 1988.

Dich VQ, Nelson JD, Haltalin KC: Osteomyelitis in infants and children. *Am J Dis Child* 1975;129:1273–1278.

Feigin RD, Cherry JD: *Textbook of Pediatric Infectious Disease,* ed 2. Philadelphia, WB Saunders, 1987.

Fleisher G, Ludwig S, Campos J: Cellulitis: bacterial etiology, clinical features and laboratory findings. *J Pediatr* 1980; 97:591–593.

Hanshaw JB, Dudgeon JA: *Viral Diseases of the Fetus and Newborn.* Philadelphia, WB Saunders, 1978.

Krugman S, Katz SL, Gershon AA, Wilfert CM: *Infectious Diseases of Children,* ed 8. St. Louis, CV Mosby, 1985.

Lascari AD, Bapat VR: Syndrome of infectious mononucleosis. *Clin Pediatr* 1970;9:300–304.

Leibel RL, Fangman JJ, Ostrovsky MC: Chronic meningococcemia in childhood. *Am J Dis Child* 1974;127:94–98.

Mandell GL, Douglas RG Jr, Bennet JE: *Principles and Practice of Infectious Diseases,* ed 3. New York, Churchill Livingstone, 1990.

May M: Neck masses in children: diagnosis and treatment. *Pediatr Ann* 1976;5:517–535.

Morrey BF, Bianco AJ, Rhodes KH: Septic arthritis in children, *Pediatr Clin North Am* 1975;6:923–934.

Nixon GW: Acute hematogenous osteomyelitis. *Pediatr Ann* 1976;5:65–81.

Rapkin RH, Bautista G: *Haemophilus influenzae* cellulitis. *Am J Dis Child* 1972;124:540–542.

Season EH, Miller PR: Primary subacute pyogenic osteomyelitis in long bones of children. *J Pediatr Surg* 1976;11:347–353.

Toews WH, Bass JW: Skin manifestations of meningococcal infection. *Am J Dis Child* 1974;127:173–176.

Tofte RW, Williams DN: Toxic shock syndrome: evidence of a broad clinical spectrum. *JAMA* 1981;246:2163–2167.

Wannamaker LW, Ferrieri P: Streptococcal infections–updated. *DM* Oct 1975;1–40.

Wilson HD, Haltalin KC: Acute necrotizing fasciitis in childhood. *Am J Dis Child* 1973;125:591–595.

13

NEPHROLOGY

Demetrius Ellis, M.D.

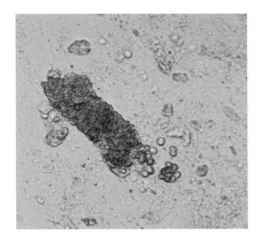

FIG. 13.1 Red blood cell cast from a patient with post-streptococcal glomerulonephritis. These casts are almost always associated with glomeru-lonephritis or vas-culitis, and virtually exclude extrarenal disorders of bleeding.

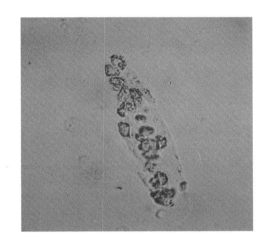

FIG. 13.2 White blood cell cast from a patient with chronic glomeru-lonephritis.

The manifestations of renal and genitourinary disorders range from readily apparent, gross structural abnormalities to subtle abnormalities of the urinary sediment. In this chapter, examples of physical findings, as well as characteristic urinary findings and radiographs will be utilized, to demonstrate the broad spectrum of these disorders in the pediatric population.

GLOMERULAR DISORDERS
Nephritis and Nephrosis

In children suspected of having a glomerular disease, the urinary sediment can provide important clues that may expedite the diagnosis and help formulate therapeutic plans. A classic example of nephritic syndrome is that of acute poststreptococcal glomerulonephritis, in which the urinalysis reveals variable levels of proteinuria, and granular, red (Fig. 13.1) and, less frequently, white blood cell casts (Fig. 13.2). On the other hand, the urine of children with classical nephrotic syndrome, such as minimal change disease, shows heavy proteinuria (>40 mg/m^2/hr), free fat droplets and oval fat bodies, and little or no hematuria or other sediment abnormalities.

Unlike patients with nephrotic syndrome, those with acute nephritic syndromes are usually hypertensive, have very darkly-colored urine, and tend to have a depressed glomerular filtration rate. Several disorders exhibit features of both nephritis and nephrosis. The nephrotic syndrome in childhood is generally due to one of 5 major disorders: minimal change disease, mesangial proliferative glomerulonephritis, focal glomerulosclerosis, membranous nephropathy, and membranoproliferative glomerulonephritis. Minimal change is the most common, comprising over 70 percent of all cases of nephrosis in children. It is so named because of its virtually normal light microscopic histology, negative immunofluorescence, and fusion of epithelial cell foot processes on electron microscopy. Laboratory features include selective proteinuria, normal complement levels, and decreased IgG levels while IgM levels are increased. Minimal change nephrotic syndrome usually is benign, with more than 95 percent of patients maintaining adequate renal function.

Mesangial proliferative nephrosis exhibits diffuse proliferative changes with negative or variable deposition of mesangial IgG, IgM, and C^3. It represents 15 to 20 percent of nephrosis in childhood. Serum complement levels are normal, but hematuria is common.

Focal glomerulosclerosis accounts for approximately 10 percent of nephrotic syndrome in childhood. It demonstrates focal and segmental sclerosis, with IgM and C^3 deposition within affected glomeruli. Hematuria, pyuria, poorly selective proteinuria but normal C^3 levels are characteristic of laboratory features. The majority of children with mesangial proliferation or focal glomerulosclerosis will progress to renal failure about 6 years after the onset of the disease.

Membranous glomerulopathy is an unusual cause of nephrotic syndrome in children, but has unique histopathologic changes seen by microscopy. Capillary walls appear

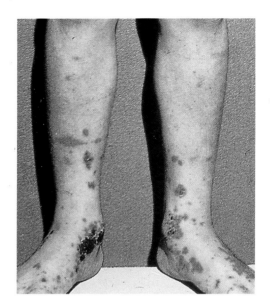

FIG. 13.3 Older child with severe Henoch-Schönlein purpura vasculitis resulting in cutaneous necrosis just below and anterior to the right malleolus.

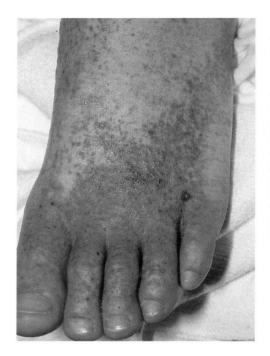

FIG. 13.4 The typical vasculitic rash of Henoch-Schönlein purpura is evident in the dorsum of the foot of this 15-year-old youngster. He went on to develop rapidly progressive glomerulonephritis and pulmonary hemorrhage which were managed by pulse methylprednisolone.

thickened, and the basement membrane has argyrophilic spikes on special staining. Immunoglobulin G deposits can be seen within the capillary walls, and electron microscopy shows subepithelial deposits. Protein excretion is variably selective, serum C^3 is normal, and patients are prone to renal vein thrombosis. Ultimate renal function is maintained in 50 to 70 percent of children with this disorder.

Membranoproliferative glomerulonephritis is subdivided into two types: Type I has lobular changes along with the mesangial proliferative changes and subendothelial deposits seen on electron microscopy. Hematuria is common, and serum C^3 is intermittently low. Over half of patients will avoid chronic dialysis. Type II disease has C^3 capillary and mesangial immune deposits. Hematuria, persistently reduced serum C^3, and the presence of C^3 nephritic factors are laboratory features of Type II. The disorder is also known as dense deposit disease because of enhanced osmiophilic staining observed by electron microscopy. Unlike Type I, almost all patients with Type II disease will progress to end-stage renal disease.

ACUTE GLOMERULONEPHRITIS

The most common causes of acute glomerulonephritis in children include poststreptococcal or postpneumococcal glomerulonephritis, IgA nephritis, Henoch-Schönlein purpura, and hemolytic uremic syndrome. In some instances, these disorders may have an aggressive clinical course characterized by oliguria, hypertension, and rapid reduction in glomerular filtration rate, in which case the designation of rapidly progressive glomerulonephritis (RPGN) is given. The renal biopsy in such patients often demonstrates cellular or acellular crescents and inflammatory infiltrates. Several other chronic glomerulonephritides such as membranoproliferative glomerulonephritis and membranous glomerulopathy may also evolve into RPGN.

In addition to the clinical symptoms, the antinuclear antibody titer, streptococcal titers, quantitative serum immunoglobulin concentrations, and C^3 and C^4 levels often are helpful

in differentiating several of the glomerulonephritides. Serum complement levels are particularly helpful since only a few of these conditions are associated with depressed complement levels. In poststreptococcal glomerulonephritis, the complement levels are only transiently reduced and return to normal concentrations within 8 weeks following the onset of the renal symptoms.

A typical situation is that of a child 3 to 10 years of age, who presents with mild periorbital edema, headache, and decreasing urine output during the preceding few days. The urine is described as being smoky or tea-colored. Medical history reveals that 2 weeks earlier, the patient experienced a febrile illness with painful pharyngitis for which he received no medical attention. Clinical examination reveals a blood pressure of 140/105 mm Hg, mild periorbital edema, and tenderness on palpation of the kidneys. A urinalysis shows 2+ protein, 3+ blood, and a SG of 1.020. Red blood cell casts (see Fig. 13.1) are seen on urinalysis. Laboratory studies are consistent with mild renal insufficiency. Also found are a protein excretion of 1.1 g/24 hours, a low plasma C^3 level, and elevated streptozyme and anti-DNAase B-titers, evidence which strongly implicates a streptococcal infection in the pathogenesis of the glomerulonephritis. Generally, complete, spontaneous recovery of all renal abnormalities occurs within 5 weeks with conservative management, although hematuria may persist for about 1 year or longer.

CHRONIC GLOMERULONEPHRITIS

White blood cell casts may be seen in the urine sediment of patients with acute or chronic glomerulonephritis and vasculitis, as well as pyelonephritis and other disorders resulting in tubulointerstitial nephritis. The cast shown in Figure 13.2 occurred in a child with systemic lupus erythematosus whose only presenting symptom was mild back pain. Urinalysis demonstrated 2+ protein, microhematuria, pyuria without bacteria, and red and white blood cell casts. Diagnosis was confirmed by immunologic findings including low serum C^3

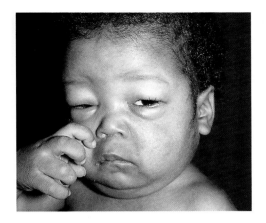

FIG. 13.5 Marked eyelid edema in a 2-year-old boy with minimal change nephrotic syndrome. Eyelid edema in any child should prompt the performance of urinalysis rather than the presumption of allergy.

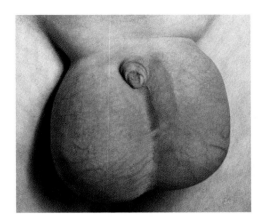

FIG. 13.6 Severe scrotal edema in a 6-year-old boy with nephrotic syndrome.

and C^4 levels, a positive fluorescent antinuclear antibody titer, and antibodies against double-stranded DNA. Renal biopsy revealed diffuse proliferative lupus nephritis. Note that formation of tubular casts is aided by diminished urine flow, high urinary solute concentration, and the hyaline matrix of plasma- and tubule-derived protein in which cells become embedded. Several acute glomerular syndromes may progress to chronic glomerulonephritis. In the final stages, many such patients develop hypertension and severe renal failure (uremia). On renal ultrasonography, the kidneys appear small and fibrosed.

HENOCH-SCHÖNLEIN PURPURA

Three weeks after a respiratory infection, a 2-year-old boy presented with generalized malaise, abdominal pain, periorbital edema, and difficulty walking "as if his legs were hurting." One day later he developed an ecchymotic, purpuric rash, the characteristic clinical manifestation of Henoch-Schönlein purpura. The rash was distributed over the extensor surfaces of the extremities and on the buttocks, but spared the trunk. Individual lesions faded over 1 week, but new lesions appeared or recurred over several weeks. Other cutaneous manifestations of the vasculitic lesions in this disorder are shown in Figures 13.3 and 13.4.

Some patients initially develop an urticarial-type eruption which subsequently becomes macular or maculopapular. Occasionally, younger patients develop an angioneurotic-like edema of the scalp, face, or the dorsum of hands or feet. Ninety percent of children with Henoch-Schönlein purpura have a prodrome consisting of an upper respiratory infection 1 to 3 weeks prior to the onset of symptoms, and 80 percent have melena, hematemesis and/or arthritis mostly involving the ankles and knees. About half of the patients have renal involvement ranging from simple microhematuria and a variable degree of proteinuria to oliguria and renal failure. In contrast to adults, use of multiple medications is rarely related to the onset of this condition in children.

There are no distinct biochemical features of this condition. Some patients have leukocytosis and an elevated serum IgA level. In the absence of severe proteinuria, hypoalbuminemia and edema are often due to protein-losing enteropathy. Platelet counts and coagulation studies are normal. The skin rash is essential for the diagnosis of Henoch-Schönlein purpura since the renal abnormalities may otherwise closely resemble a similar disorder known as IgA nephropathy (Berger's disease).

NEPHROTIC SYNDROME

Children with nephrotic syndrome rarely have an underlying systemic illness or a history of drug intake, and hence are designated as having primary or idiopathic nephrotic syndrome. Patients with poststreptococcal glomerulonephritis, Henoch-Schönlein purpura, IgA nephritis, or systemic lupus erythematosus, as well as rare patients treated with nonsteroidal and inflammatory agents, lithium, colchicine, and other drugs, may also be associated with nephrotic range proteinuria, i.e., ≥ 40 mg/m^2/hr.

Minimal change disease is the single most common cause of idiopathic nephrotic syndrome in childhood. Generalized edema and rapid weight gain are characteristic features of this condition, with the former showing a predilection for the eyelids, pleural spaces, abdomen, scrotum, and lower extremities (Figs. 13.5, 13.6). Although edema per se usually provokes few complaints from most patients, at times it may be disfiguring, and it may produce skin induration and breakdown or interference with respiratory, genitourinary, or gastrointestinal function. Symptoms may occasionally be confused with allergic edema. However, the findings of severe proteinuria, hypoalbuminemia, and hypercholesterolemia usually lead to correct diagnostic and treatment measures.

Of special interest is nephrotic syndrome presenting in the newborn period or in the first 2 to 3 months of life. Acquired immunodeficiency syndrome (AIDS) has recently been added to the list of systemic diseases underlying infantile nephrotic syndrome, and is increasingly recognized as a cause of this disorder in infants and young children. Focal glomerulosclerosis is the most common underlying histopathologic lesion.

HEMATURIA

Isolated gross or microscopic hematuria is probably the most common symptom prompting nephrologic assessment in children. Many such children have symptomless microscopic hematuria often detected as part of routine office visits or physical examinations prior to participation in sport activities. Because of the large number of conditions associated with per-

ALGORITHM FOR DIAGNOSIS OF HEMATURIA

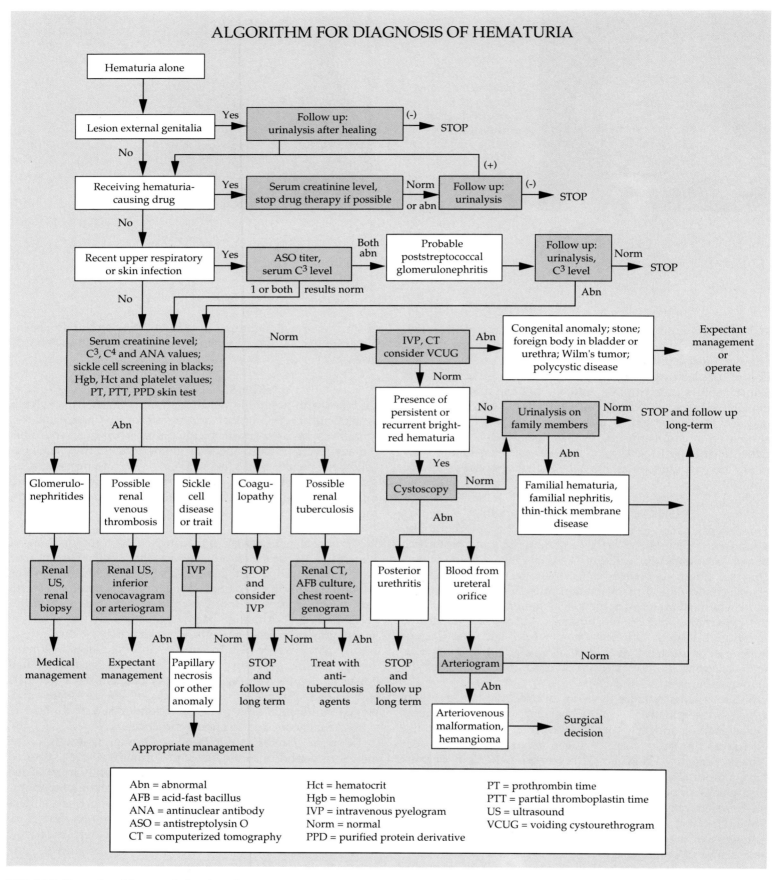

FIG. 13.7 (Reproduced by permission from Brewer ED, Benson GS: Hematuria: algorithms for diagnosis. JAMA 1981; 246:877. Copyright 1981, American Medical Association)

Clinical history

Family history of nephrolithiasis
Immobilization or other protracted illness or stress
High dietary purine intake
Excessive salt and/or calcium ingestion
Large and infrequent meals
Excessive intake of vitamins or over-the-counter medications
Symptoms of urinary tract infection or history of pyelonephritis
Source and calcium content of drinking water
Polyuria-polydypsia

Physical diagnosis

Band keratopathy and other signs of hyperparathyroidism
Elfin facies and other features of William's syndrome

Radiologic studies

Ultrasound—especially sensitive in identifying renal calculi and nephrocalcinosis
KUB—for the identification of ureteral stones; radiopaque stones include calcium oxalate, cystine
Intravenous urography—identifies urological abnormalities and confirms obstruction. Especially helpful in detecting radiolucent calculi such as uric acid, urates, matrix, and xanthine
^{125}I–hippurate scan—may provide differential renal function or suggest obstruction in children in whom an intravenous pyelogram poses high risk.

Urinary studies

Urinalysis—may reveal pyuria or bacteriuria, inability to lower urinary pH or to concentrate the urine, flat hexagonal crystals pathognomonic of cystinosis
Urine culture
Screening with cyanide—nitroprusside (cystinosis)
Timed urine collections on two or more occasions for determination of creatinine, sodium, potassium, calcium, phosphorus, magnesium, oxalate, citrate, cystine and uric acid

Biochemical studies

Creatinine, BUN, electrolytes, total CO_2, albumin, calcium, phosphorus, magnesium, and uric acid; plasma parathyroid hormone levels if indicated
Chemical analysis of gravel or stones

FIG. 13.8

sistent hematuria in children, several algorithms have been devised to aid in the systematic evaluation of this condition (Fig. 13.7).

History and clinical symptoms may point toward trauma, viral cystitis, drug-induced hematuria or cystitis, etc. Detection of the most common causes of hematuria, including glomerulonephritis or urinary tract infection, can be readily achieved by the finding of cellular casts in a carefully performed examination of the urinary sediment or by appropriate bacterial cultures. Moreover, the absence of red blood cells in a child with positive orthotolidine reagent color change on the dipstick may lead to the correct diagnosis of conditions associated with rhabdomyolysis or hemolysis. Once these simple measures are undertaken, one relies on biochemical techniques to investigate renal function, hyperexcretion of metabolites resulting in nephrolithiasis (see below), hemoglobinopathies, bleeding diathesis, or immunologic assessment of an underlying glomerulonephritis. Measurement of calcium and creatinine concentrations in a single voided urine sample also should be included in the minimal initial assessment of asymptomatic hematuria, since hypercalciuria is found in a large proportion of such children. Identification of possible disorders by such methods may help determine the need for further assessment. Thus, the finding of a nephritic sediment obviates the need for any radiologic procedures, while the presence of a single well-documented urinary tract infection in a child under 8 years of age may require cystographic and ultrasonographic evaluation. In the absence of any physical signs such as an abdominal mass to suggest Wilm's tumor or neuroblastoma, malignancies of the kidney or urinary tract rarely present with isolated gross or microscopic hematuria. Renal ultrasonography coupled with Doppler evaluation of the renal vessels is useful in screening for the presence of tumor, polycystic kidney disease, or renal venous thrombosis in newborns and young infants. Computed tomography scanning or nuclear magnetic resonance techniques may provide fine anatomic resolution of such masses.

Invasive cystography or arteriography are rarely indicated in the evaluation of structural lesions underlying isolated hematuria in children. A ^{99m}technetium dimercaptosuccinic acid (DMSA) renal scan may disclose renal scars suggestive of chronic pyelonephritis in children with or without vesicoureteral reflux. Finally, a renal biopsy may be helpful in making a definitive diagnosis in cases of suspected renal parenchymal disease manifested by hematuria.

Pediatric Nephrolithiasis

The diagnosis of nephrolithiasis should be entertained in any child presenting with acute onset of flank or abdominal colicky pain. In children, renal colic is poorly localized and is often described as diffuse abdominal pain. Small stones may produce no pain at all, and are detected only after an episode of gross hematuria, pyuria, or urinary tract infection. Thus, a strong index of suspicion is required on the part of the clinician so that appropriate diagnostic studies may be undertaken. Relatively few children pass gravel or stones and the kind of crystals found in the urine are rarely of diagnostic value. While dietary phytate is a more common cause of endemic stones in the Far East, and urinary tract infection is more common in Europe, metabolic disorders predominate in children with nephrolithiasis in the United States. The clinical history and laboratory evaluation often reveal the cause of the stones. Biochemical analysis of the calculus is, therefore, of little diagnostic importance. One diagnostic approach to pediatric nephrolithiasis is shown in Figure 13.8.

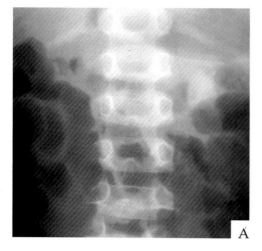

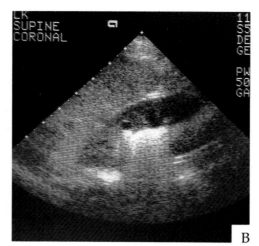

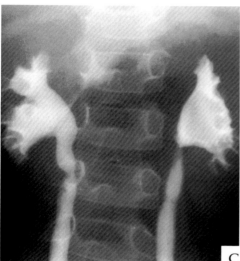

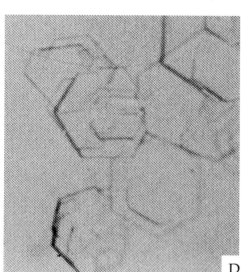

FIG. 13.9 Six-year-old boy, born of a consanguineous marriage, presented with diffuse abdominal pain, oliguria, and mild renal failure. **A**, plain film of the abdomen showed a slight opacity in the area of the left kidney. **B**, renal ultrasound demonstrated a distinct shadow produced by the calculus. **C**, an intravenous pyelogram showed the relatively radiolucent stone within the left renal pelvis. Multiple small calculi produced the dilatation and partial obstruction of both ureters. **D**, the pathognomic flat hexagonal crystals found in the urine aided the diagnosis of cystinuria.

The most common calculus in childhood consists of calcium oxalate. Such calculi frequently occur in children with idiopathic hypercalciuria, which may be silent or may be manifested by painless microscopic or recurrent gross hematuria for many years before frank nephrolithiasis occurs. Hypercalciuria is found in 35 percent of all children evaluated for hematuria. Screening for hypercalciuria may be done utilizing a single voided urine specimen; a calcium to creatinine ratio exceeding 0.2 is highly suggestive of this condition, which may then be confirmed by a 24-hour urine collection having a calcium content ≥4 mg/kg body weight. The nonabsorptive form of hypercalciuria appears to have an autosomal dominant inheritance underlying a renal tubular defect and net loss of calcium independent of the amount of dietary calcium ingested. The absorptive form may be associated with increased serum concentrations of calcitriol resulting in increased fractional absorption of calcium at the intestinal level. Premature infants in whom high dosages of furosemide have been given to control fluid retention associated with bronchopulmonary dysplasia may develop hypercalciuria, nephrolithiasis, and nephrocalcinosis. Other disorders predisposing to nephrolithiasis include hyperparathyroidism, cystinuria (Figure 13.9A–D), hyperoxaluria, defects of purine

metabolism and distal (type I) renal tubular acidosis (Fig. 13.10A-C). Urinary tract infections and/or obstructive uropathy are also important. Laboratory studies and the radiologic location and appearance of the stone often provide clues as to the cause and treatment of the nephrolithiasis.

Apart from available medical therapies and traditional surgical techniques, specific conditions may be treated by newer modalities, such as extracorporeal shock-wave lithotripsy and stone fragmentation through pulse laser energy.

Renal Venous Thrombosis

Volume depletion secondary to diarrhea or vomiting (Fig. 13.11), hypotension due to any etiology, hypercoagulable or hyperviscocity states (hematocrit more than 65 percent) or indwelling catheters in the vicinity of the renal veins especially predispose infants to renal vein or intrarenal venous thrombosis. Older children with severe nephrotic syndrome are also prone to this disorder. Among children, 75 percent of all cases of renal venous thrombosis occur in the first month of life, and 50 percent of all cases are bilateral. The typical clinical features of renal vein thrombosis are a palpable renal mass in 60 percent of infants; hematuria and thrombocytopenia occur in

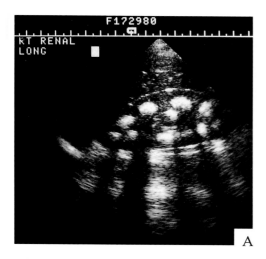

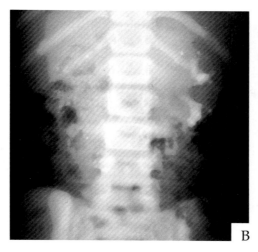

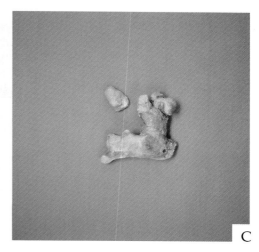

FIG. 13.10 *A, renal ultrasound demonstrates severe nephrocalcinosis in an 8-year-old girl who failed to thrive and showed familial type I renal tubular acidosis. Notice the multiple echogenic shadows produced by the calcium deposits within the renal parenchyma. B, a* staghorn calculus in the left renal pelvis of another child with renal tubular acidosis. *C, appearance of calculus removed at operation. The shape of the calculus generally conforms to the pelvocaliceal system.*

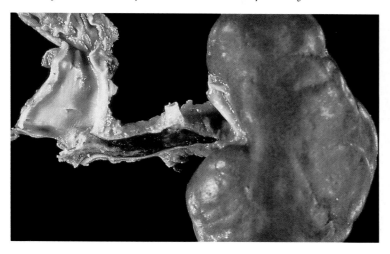

FIG. 13.11 *Twelve-year-old boy with ulcerative colitis, who died following a bout of severe diarrhea and dehydration. Apart from dural sinus thrombosis, the left renal vein contained this partially organized clot.*

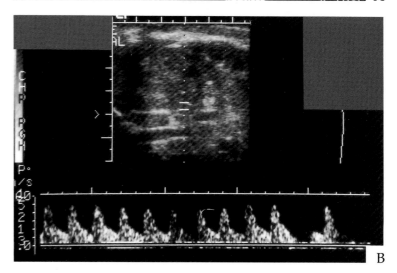

excess of 90 percent of the patients. Renal function may be normal, particularly in unilateral renal vein thrombosis or in bilateral disease that does not result in oliguria. The renal ultrasound is the diagnostic procedure of choice, particularly when coupled with Doppler examination of the renal and adjacent major vessels (Fig. 13.12).

VESICOURETERAL REFLUX

Vesicoureteral reflux is a congenital condition in which the normal valve mechanism of the ureterovesicular junction is impaired, leading to reflux of bladder urine into the ureter and/or kidneys. In a young child with urinary tract infection, such reflux of infected urine is a major risk factor for the development of pyelonephritis, renal scarring, and chronic renal damage.

The severity of vesicoureteral reflux is assessed by the findings on voiding cystourethrograms, and classified according

FIG. 13.12 *Renal venous thrombosis. A plethoric 2-day-old infant of a diabetic mother (hematocrit 75 percent) was found to have an abdominal mass in the right abdomen on routine physical examination. Laboratory evaluation disclosed hematuria and thrombocytopenia without elevation in BUN or serum creatinine concentrations. A, notice the absence of venous pulsations in the lower panel on the Doppler study of the right renal vein while arterial pulsations remained intact. B, subsequent serial renal ultrasound studies showed a progressive reduction in the size of the right kidney despite recanalization of the venous thromboses.*

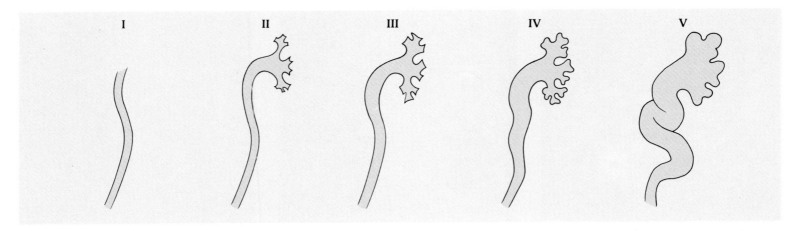

FIG. 13.13 *Grades of vesicoureteral reflux, schematically presented.*

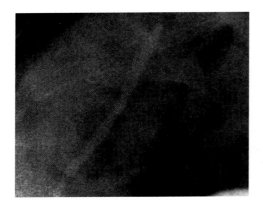

FIG. 13.14 *Grade I reflux: cystourethrogram shows reflux only into the ureter.*

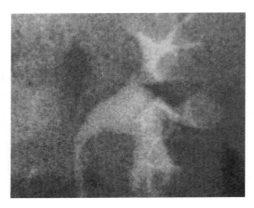

FIG. 13.15 *Grade II reflux: cystourethrogram shows complete reflux into the ureter, pelvis, and calyces; no dilatation.*

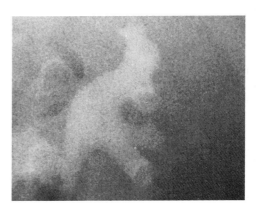

FIG. 13.16 *Grade III reflux: cystourethrogram shows complete reflux with mild dilatation of the ureter and renal pelvis, but only slight blunting of the calyces.*

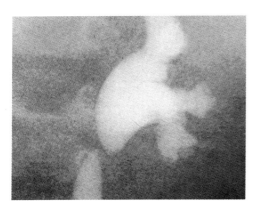

FIG. 13.17 *Grade IV reflux: cystourethrogram shows complete reflux with moderate dilatation of the ureter, pelvis, and calyces; complete obliteration of sharp angle of fornices.*

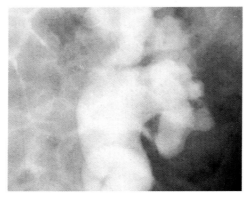

FIG. 13.18 *Grade V reflux: cystourethrogram shows gross dilatation of the ureter, pelvis, and calyces; obliteration of the papillary impressions of the calyces.*

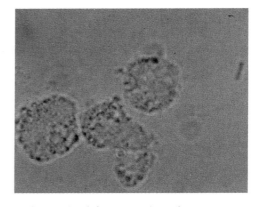

FIG. 13.19 *High-power view of unspun urine shows several white blood cells and a rod-shaped organism, suggestive of bacterial cystitis.*

to the following international grading system (Fig. 13.13):

Grade I—reflux into the ureter only (Fig. 13.14).

Grade II—complete reflux into the ureter, pelvis, and calyces without any dilation of the structures (Fig. 13.15).

Grade III—complete reflux with mild dilatation and/or tortuosity of the ureter, and mild dilatation of the renal pelvis but only slight blunting of the calyceal fornices (Fig. 13.16).

Grade IV—complete reflux with moderate dilatation of the ureter, renal pelvis, and calyces; complete obliteration of the sharp angle of the fornices with maintenance of the papillary impressions of the calyces (Fig. 13.17).

Grade V—gross dilatation and tortuosity of the ureter with gross dilatation of the renal pelvis and calyces; obliteration of the papillary impressions of the calyces (Fig. 13.18).

Grades I through III have a high rate of spontaneous resolution, and patients with such findings should be placed on sup-

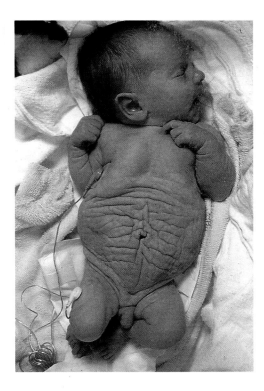

FIG. 13.20 Newborn with prune-belly syndrome shows the characteristic wrinkled and redundant skin covering the abdominal wall. On palpation, no abdominal muscular tissue or muscular tone could be detected.

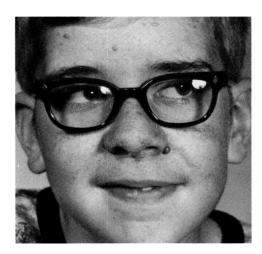

FIG. 13.21 This 6-year-old patient with tuberous sclerosis demonstrates characteristic papules distributed across the bridge of the nose and the nasolabial folds. He was originally diagnosed as having polycystic kidney disease because of abdominal distention and bilateral renal enlargement prior to the onset of any skin lesions.

pressive antibiotic regimens to ensure maintenance of sterile bladder urine. Grades IV and V are generally associated with significant anatomic abnormalities of the ureteral orifice, and often require surgical correction.

Bacterial Cystitis

Young children presenting with an acute onset of fever, emesis, dysuria, suprapubic pain, and a urinary sediment such as that shown in Figure 13.19 should be suspected of having bacterial cystitis. Many more cells and bacteria may be seen when urine is examined after centrifuging at 3,000 rpm for 5 minutes. By far, the most common organism cultured from patients with acute or chronic urinary tract infections is *Escherichia coli,* with pseudomonas or proteus species occasionally found, particularly in patients with abnormal genitourinary anatomy.

While the diagnosis of urinary tract infection is established by appropriate urine cultures, the site of infection may not be apparent when one considers the presenting symptoms or urinalysis findings alone. Evaluation with pyelography and micturition cystourethrography should be performed in all children under the age of 8 years following documentation of their first urinary tract infection. Such studies will usually define structural abnormalities leading to obstructive nephropathy or vesicoureteral reflux, and are essential in planning medical and surgical management of these patients.

DEVELOPMENTAL/HEREDITARY DISORDERS

Developmental Abnormalities

The number of congenital malformations associated with renal abnormalities is too large to discuss individually in this chapter. Renal abnormalities should be suspected in any child with one or more congenital abnormalities. In this chapter, only a selected number of syndromes will be considered in which

renal abnormalities are serious, relatively common, and the physical findings may serve to facilitate the diagnosis.

PRUNE-BELLY SYNDROME (EAGLE-BARRETT SYNDROME)

This syndrome usually consists of the absence of abdominal musculature, renal and urinary tract abnormalities, and cryptorchidism (Fig. 13.20). Males are affected more severely and 20 times more frequently than females. Although there is generally no ureteral obstruction, the ureters are dilated and tortuous, and 75 percent exhibit reflux. The bladder is enlarged despite low renal pelvic and intravesical pressures. Infection is quite common because of urinary stasis.

The major determinant of prognosis in these patients is the degree of associated cystic renal dysplasia. Intestinal malrotation is a common associated abnormality; anomalies of the limbs and heart may occur, but these are uncommon. Infertility in males is universal even when it is possible to surgically place the testes into their normal intrascrotal position. Libido and orgasm, however, remain normal. Early orchiopexy may well improve the chances for fertility and prevent testicular neoplasia.

TUBEROUS SCLEROSIS

Tuberous sclerosis is a neurocutaneous syndrome inherited as an autosomal-dominant trait with marked variability of expression. The full syndrome is characterized by myoclonic seizures, mental deficiency, foci of intracranial calcifications, depigmented "ash leaf" cutaneous patches, and pathognomonic skin lesions which are fibroangiomatous nevi (adenoma sebaceum). The latter may be present during the first year of life, but may not be noted until the age of 4 to 7 years, when they take the form of discrete yellowish papules distributed along the bridge of the nose and the nasolabial folds (Fig. 13.21). Patients with tuberous sclerosis may have hamartomas in many organs and tissues. Renal angiomyolipoma causing genitourinary symptomatology may suggest the diagnosis of polycystic kidney disease in patients with minimal skin or cen-

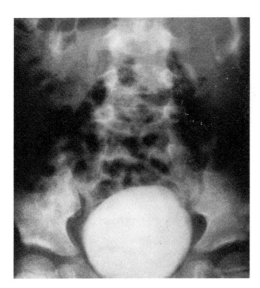

FIG. 13.22 Intravenous pyelogram of the patient in Figure 13.21 shows enlarged kidneys with the collecting system stretched and distorted by multiple soft-tissue masses, later found to be renal angiomyolipoma.

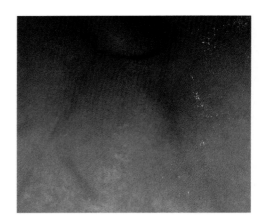

FIG. 13.23 Imperforate anus. This male newborn has an absent median raphe and anal atresia. On further study he was found to have agenesis of the right kidney, severe dysplasia in the left kidney, and a communication of the blind-ended rectal pouch and the prostatic urethra.

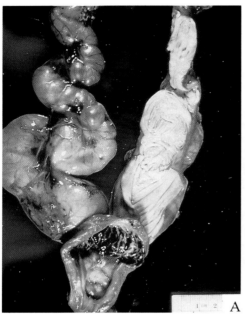

A

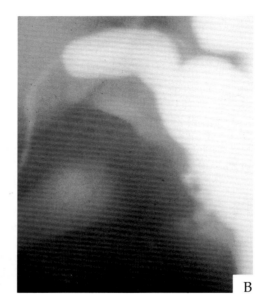

B

FIG. 13.24 **A**, autopsy findings of a newborn with posterior urethral valves. Notice the marked enlargement and tortuosity of the ureters and the small, thick-walled, muscular bladder. **B**, an antemortem voiding cystourethrogram shows the markedly dilated proximal urethra typical of this condition.

tral nervous system involvement (Fig. 13.22). Although small asymptomatic cysts are common in autopsy cases of tuberous sclerosis, large renal cysts may be discovered early in infancy and suggest the diagnosis of autosomal dominant PKD. Hypertension and renal insufficiency may further confuse the diagnosis. In such instances, the diagnosis of tuberous sclerosis is confirmed by family history and the development of other features of the syndrome.

IMPERFORATE ANUS

Because of common embryologic origins and the anatomic proximity of the genitourinary and lower gastrointestinal tracts, children with imperforate anus have a high incidence of genitourinary and lower spinal abnormalities. A high imperforate anus (at or above the supralevator muscle) (Fig. 13.23) is associated with a 50 percent incidence of genitourinary anomalies, mainly unilateral renal agenesis, neurogenic bladder, or vesicoureteral reflux. In males, one usually finds a fistulous communication between the blind end of the rectal pouch and the prostatic urethra. In females, the rectum often communicates with the vagina or posterior fourchette. All children with imperforate anus should undergo evaluation of the genitouri-

nary tract with renal ultrasound and voiding cystourethrography, and must be monitored for urinary tract infection.

POSTERIOR URETHRAL VALVES

The most common obstructive lesions of the lower urinary tract in infants are posterior urethral valves. Such folds traverse the urethra from a point just distal to the verumontanum to the proximal limit of the membranous urethra, and cause obstruction to urinary flow with consequent enlargement of the prostatic urethra, hypertrophy of the bladder neck, trabeculation of the bladder, and significant dilatation of the upper urinary tract. Children with posterior urethral valves may present as infants with renal failure and profound electrolyte imbalance. Older children may present with abdominal masses, voiding disturbances, or infection. Diagnosis is made radiologically by voiding cystourethrography (Fig. 13.24), and confirmed endoscopically. Although urinary diversion is frequently required, some patients can be treated directly with transurethral valve ablation. Surgery is usually successful in achieving urinary drainage, but in many cases, associated renal dysplasia may lead to chronic renal failure during infancy or childhood.

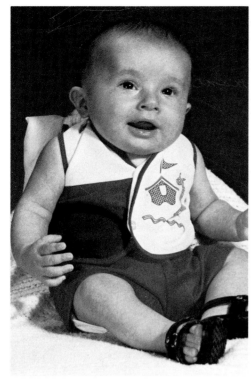

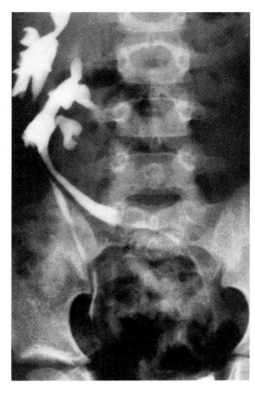

FIG. 13.25 An infant with Klippel-Feil syndrome (**left**) demonstrates a short neck (fused cervical vertebrae) and nonfunctioning right thumb due to lack of tendons to this digit. Intravenous pyelogram (**right**) reveals crossed renal ectopia of the left kidney, while the ureter from the left kidney crosses the midline and inserts into the left side of the trigone.

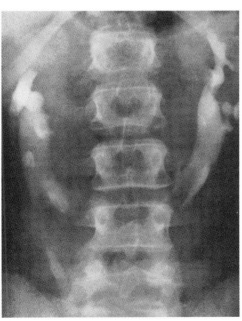

FIG. 13.26 Horseshoe kidney. This excretory urogram was performed as part of the evaluation for gross hematuria following abdominal injury in the child. Notice the unusual and oblong configuration of the collecting system resulting from fusion of the lower renal poles.

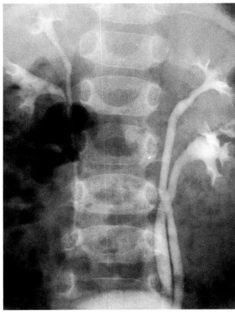

FIG. 13.27 Excretory urogram shows bilateral duplication of the urinary collecting system. This child has recurrent urinary tract infections due to vesicoureteral reflux in the ureter from the left lower pole. Ureteral duplication is incomplete on the right side (Y-type).

CROSSED RENAL ECTOPIA

Children with this developmental anomaly generally present with an abdominal mass or with hematuria following minor trauma. Obstruction at the ureteropelvic junction is quite common. The location of the ectopic kidney may be cryptic, as in the pelvic region, and can be best demonstrated by a renal radionuclide scan. Crossed renal ectopia, renal agenesis, and/or duplication of the collecting system are often found in association with Klippel-Feil syndrome (Fig. 13.25), but has also been associated with cervicothoracic vertebral anomalies, and with Müllerian duct aplasia in females.

HORSESHOE KIDNEY

This condition results from fusion of the lower renal poles during development (Fig. 13.26). Although generally asymp-

tomatic, patients with horseshoe kidney may present with (1) hematuria after trauma to the pelvic area; (2) a midline abdominal mass; or (3) a ureteropelvic junction obstruction, a common associated finding in this condition.

DUPLICATION OF THE URINARY COLLECTING SYSTEM

This is one of the most common of all genitourinary abnormalities. It is sometimes familial, and more common in females than in males. About 30 percent of the duplications are bilateral (Fig. 13.27), but with much variation in the extent of duplication. This condition occurs when the kidney is penetrated by two separate ureteral buds during nephrogenesis. When present, vesicoureteral reflux usually occurs in the ureter from the lower pole, while ureteral obstruction occurs almost exclusive-

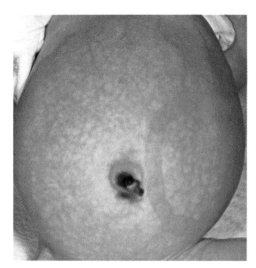

FIG. 13.28 This infant with infantile polycystic kidney disease shows marked abdominal distention and bilaterally enlarged kidneys, as indicated by the outlined area.

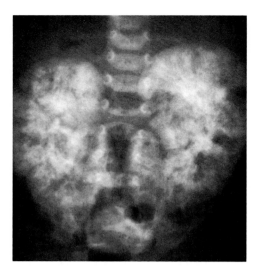

FIG. 13.29 Intravenous pyelogram of the patient in Figure 13.28 shows the characteristic mottled nephrogram, with brushlike medullary opacification secondary to retention of contrast material in dilated cortical and medullary collecting ducts.

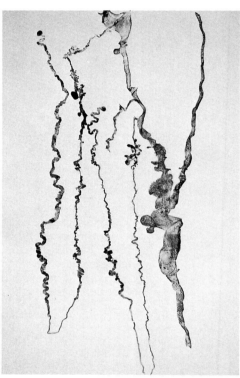

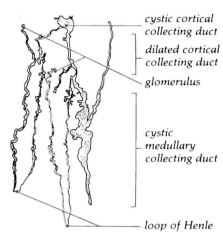

cystic cortical collecting duct

dilated cortical collecting duct

glomerulus

cystic medullary collecting duct

loop of Henle

FIG. 13.30 The cystic areas are apparent in the microdissected nephron tree shown in this photograph. (Courtesy of Dr. G. Fetterman)

ly in the ureter from the upper renal segment. Reflux into a duplicated system is unlikely to resolve spontaneously. These associated problems may predispose patients to recurrent infection or hydronephrosis necessitating surgical correction.

Hereditary and Metabolic Disorders

POLYCYSTIC KIDNEY DISORDERS (PKD)

These disorders have been recently reviewed by K. Zerres et al. Three major forms of cystic kidney diseases may present in childhood. Although autosomal dominant PKD and cystic renal dysplasia are far more common (1/1,000), the autosomal recessive PKD (1/40,000) is a much more serious disorder during childhood. Cystic renal dysplasia has no defined inheritance pattern, and is often associated with other syndromes. Only a few of the better known causes of PKD will be presented here.

Autosomal Recessive (Infantile) PKD

With the exception of the most severe manifestations of the disease, prenatal diagnosis by renal ultrasonography is not usually reliable until the second half of pregnancy. This disorder has variable expression, so that the severity of the cystic malformation often determines the age and mode of presentation. About 85 percent of cases begin during infancy. Oligohydramnios and associated pulmonary hypoplasia may result in life-threatening respiratory difficulties and talipes in the neonate, while abdominal masses and hypertension are common presenting signs in later infancy; hepatic enlargement, portal hypertension, growth failure, and progressive renal insufficiency occur more commonly in the school-age child. Pancreatic cysts are rare, and usually do not produce digestive difficulties. Hyponatremia often occurs in infancy and may relate to nonosmotic release of vasopressin particularly in the setting of pulmonary disease, excessive renal salt

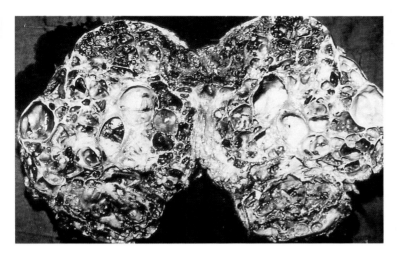

FIG. 13.31 *Autosomal dominant (adult type) polycystic kidney disease. Notice replacement of normal renal parenchyma by fluid-filled cysts.*

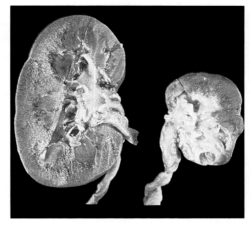

FIG. 13.32 *Unilateral renal hypoplasia/dysplasia. In contrast to the normal right kidney, the left is markedly small. The parenchyma in the upper pole is normal, but microscopic examination of the lower pole showed several morphologic features of dysplasia.*

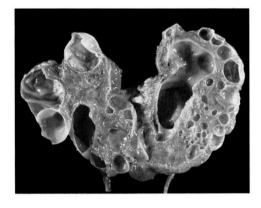

FIG. 13.33 *Bilateral cystic renal dysplasia. Multiple cysts of variable size are seen throughout the cortex and medullary regions.*

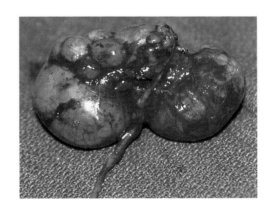

FIG. 13.34 *A less severe form of multicystic renal dysplasia involving mainly the midportion of the kidney.*

wasting, extracellular volume contraction, and inadequate dietary salt replacement.

Congenital hepatic fibrosis is always present in this condition, and may predominate over kidney involvement in some of the patients. Hypersplenism and hematemesis are frequent in such patients. Liver pathology may be similar in other autosomal recessive syndromes associated with PKD.

Infantile PKD, with diffuse cystic involvement of both kidneys, is transmitted by autosomal-recessive inheritance. One fourth of siblings have PKD, but parental involvement is rare. The cysts are initially small, but can enlarge with age to produce palpable flank or abdominal masses (Fig. 13.28). The condition may be differentiated from bilateral hydronephrosis of any etiology by thorough radiologic evaluation which may include sonography, cystography, and intravenous pyelography. The intravenous pyelogram in Figure 13.29 shows a characteristic mottled nephrogram, with the retention of contrast material in dilated medullary and cortical collecting ducts producing brushlike medullary opacification with streaks radiating to the outer portion of the kidney. This correlates well with the pathologic findings in such kidneys of cystic dilation localized to the medullary and cortical collecting ducts. This localization is best demonstrated by isolated nephron microdissection (Fig. 13.30).

Autosomal Dominant (Adult-Type) PKD

This is one of the most common inherited disorders, and accounts for 10 percent of all patients with end-stage renal disease in the United States. Renal cysts are usually demonstrated in one of the parents and in 50 percent of the siblings of affected individuals. Although clinical manifestations such as pain from enlarging, bleeding or infected cysts, nephrolithiasis, hypertension, and renal insufficiency generally occur in the third to fifth decades of life, symptoms of nephromegaly, abdominal distention, and hypertension may occur during infancy. One third of patients have berry aneurysms that may produce fatal central nervous system hemorrhage. Cysts in the liver are rare in children, but occur in about one third of adults with this disorder.

The early renal radiographic appearance may be indistinguishable from that of autosomal recessive PKD. However, the cystic changes may not become apparent until the second decade of life, after which time they are unlikely to occur. Thus, exclusion of this disorder may require periodic monitoring by renal ultrasound during the first two decades of life. Pathologically, the cysts evolve to become very large and asymmetrical, and involve all parts of the nephron (Fig. 13.31). New techniques in genetic linkage analysis provide a prenatal diagnosis for this condition that is reliable in up to 95 percent of the cases.

Cystic Renal Dysplasia

Pathologically, abnormal renal morphogenesis includes processes leading to both deficient parenchyma (hypoplasia) (Fig. 13.32) and abnormally differentiated parenchyma (dysplasia) (Figs. 13.33, 13.34). These conditions often coexist, and, despite the presence of cysts, the kidneys may be too small to appreci-

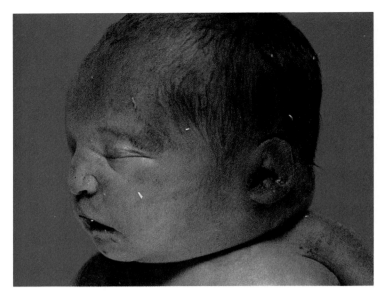

FIG. 13.35 Potter facies. This infant with bilateral multicystic dysplasia died 12 hours of age with pulmonary insufficiency. The altered facies produced by the fetal compression syndrome of oligohydramnios includes small, posteriorly rotated ears, micrognathia, a beaked nose, and wide-set eyes. (Courtesy of Dr. MacPherson, Magee-Women's Hospital, Pittsburgh)

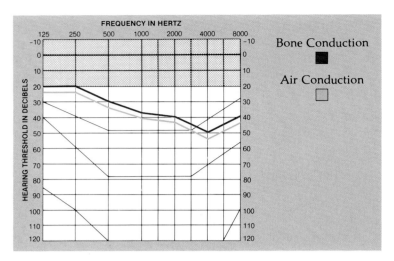

FIG. 13.36 In Alport syndrome, a loss of high-frequency auditory perception may be found in 40 percent of patients. Since the hearing deficit may be most marked at frequencies between 4,000 and 8,000 Hz, it may be initially detected only by audiometric testing.

ate by bimanual examination (i.e., bracing the flank and back with the fingers of one hand while gradually producing deep abdominal compression with the other hand). When bilateral, these renal disorders are frequently detected during the first few weeks of life. The infant usually demonstrates poor weight gain, pallor, emesis, and tachypnea. Many of the early symptoms are secondary to metabolic acidosis resulting from renal insufficiency. The amount of urine output bears little relationship to the degree of renal failure as reflected by the serum creatinine and blood urea nitrogen concentrations. Collectively, these conditions constitute the most common cause of chronic renal failure in children.

Patients with renal *hypoplasia* often have gastrointestinal, central nervous system, cardiac, and pulmonary abnormalities, but other abnormalities of the genitourinary tract are rarely present. Obstruction of the gastrointestinal or genitourinary tracts is commonly found in patients with dysplasia, while less common anomalies may include Down syndrome, as well as tracheoesophageal fistula, ventriculoseptal defect, and lumbosacral dystrophies which together make up the VATER association.

It should be emphasized that cystic dysplasia may be a major component of several syndromes with distinct additional malformations. Many of these syndromes have defined inheritance patterns. The overall risk for siblings of children with isolated forms of dysplasia/hypoplasia is usually less than 10 percent, but may be higher if one of the parents has renal agenesis or a kidney that is affected by the same process. Pediatricians should be aware of several of the more common syndromes described below.

Multicystic dysplasia is the most common cause of abdominal masses in newborns. There is usually complete loss of the renal architecture and, microscopically, there are primitive ducts, fibrosis, and islands of cartilage representing the distinctive features of dysplasia. This condition is more often unilateral than bilateral, may be discovered by prenatal sonography or it is often diagnosed during the neonatal period after palpation of a "lumpy" intra-abdominal mass of variable size which often transilluminates. Because atresia of the ureter is usually present, urine output and renal function will depend on the presence of bilateral involvement as well as the degree of associated renal dysplasia. Very large multicystic kidneys can interfere with respiration or produce mechanical intestinal compression. Radionuclide scanning, renal ultrasonography, and retrograde urography are usually sufficient to establish the diagnosis. Because a large percentage of multicystic kidneys spontaneously involute, the prevailing opinion, although somewhat controversial, is that unilateral and asymptomatic multicystic kidneys do not need to be removed. However, correction of any associated obstructive abnormalities that may be present in the contralateral kidney is of vital importance.

POTTER'S SEQUENCE

Potter's sequence can occur in any cystic disorder severe enough to produce oligohydramnios or anhydramnios. Oligohydramnios from any cause leads to a complex syndrome of fetal compression. Although chronic leakage of amniotic fluid may be responsible for oligohydramnios, it most commonly occurs secondary to decreased fetal urine formation because of renal agenesis or severe underlying renal structural disorders. The relative lack of amniotic fluid during fetal life leads to pulmonary hypoplasia and fetal compression, which consequently results in abnormal positioning of the hands, talipes, and altered facies characterized by abnormally small pos-

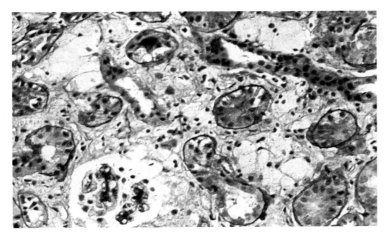

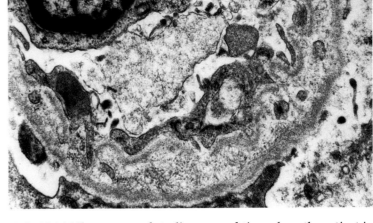

FIG. 13.37 *Renal biopsy of a 6-year-old male with high-frequency hearing loss and persistent hematuria and proteinuria reveals multiple aggregations of foam cells and areas of glomerular sclerosis.*

FIG. 13.38 *Ultrastructural studies on renal tissue from the patient in Figure 13.37 reveal the characteristic lamellation and irregularities of the glomerular basement membrane, diagnostic of Alport syndrome.*

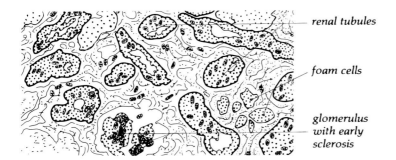

renal tubules

foam cells

glomerulus with early sclerosis

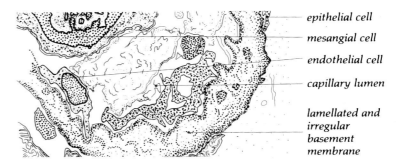

epithelial cell

mesangial cell

endothelial cell

capillary lumen

lamellated and irregular basement membrane

teriorly rotated ears, a small chin, a beaked nose, and unusual facial creases (Fig. 13.35). Infants with Potter's syndrome die of respiratory insufficiency secondary to the severe associated abnormalities of pulmonary development.

ALPORT SYNDROME

Alport syndrome, or hereditary progressive nephritis, is characterized by recurrent hematuria, progressive renal failure, and neurosensory deafness. It is transmitted by autosomal-dominant inheritance with variable penetrance. The most common clinical feature is persistent or recurrent hematuria which may be recognized early in childhood. Proteinuria is absent or mild in the early stages of the disease, but increases as it progresses. The course is commonly one of slowly progressive renal failure, often accompanied by hypertension which is more severe in males than in females. The majority of patients with Alport syndrome have neither deafness nor ocular defects, but loss of high-frequency auditory perception occurs in as many as 40 percent of patients, and thus, may be used as a clinical marker in family studies (Fig. 13.36).

Alport syndrome must be differentiated from the many benign forms of childhood hematuria as well as from other progressive glomerular disorders. Diagnosis relies on careful family history, audiologic or ocular abnormalities, and renal histopathologic features such as the presence of foam cells and glomerular sclerosis on light microscopy (Fig. 13.37), and

ultrastructural alterations of the glomerular capillary basement membrane (Fig. 13.38). There is no specific treatment for this disorder, and progressive end-stage renal disease is supported with dialysis or renal transplantation.

HYPOPHOSPHATEMIC RICKETS

Rickets is a disturbance of growing bone in which defective mineralization of the matrix leads to an abnormal accumulation of uncalcified cartilage and osteoid. Hypophosphatemic vitamin D–resistant rickets is an X-linked inherited disorder which presents clinically during the first year of life with hypophosphatemia, short stature, and rickets. Normal muscle tone and strength, the absence of tetany or convulsions, and the predominance of rachitic changes in the lower extremities aid the clinical differentiation of this specific disorder from other forms of childhood rickets. Biochemical differentiaton consists of low plasma phosphorus, normal or borderline low plasma calcium, a normal parathyroid hormone level, the absence of aminoaciduria, a normal 25-hydroxyvitamin D level, and a 1,25-dihydroxyvitamin D level which is low for the level of hypophosphatemia. The pathogenesis of the disorder is believed to involve a renal tubular phosphate leak which is accompanied by an inappropriately low 1,25-dihydroxyvitamin D synthesis by renal tubular cells. The characteristic radiologic features of hypophosphatemic rickets, as in all forms of childhood rickets, include early widening of the

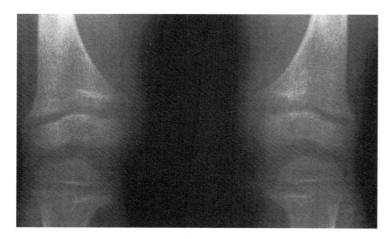

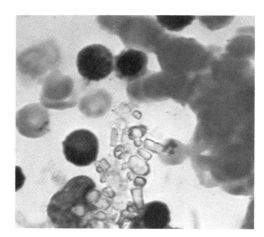

FIG. 13.40 Diagnosis of cystinosis is often confirmed by the finding of cystine crystals in bone marrow aspirate from affected individuals, as seen here.

FIG. 13.39 Hypophosphatemic rickets. Radiograph of the knees of a 2-year-old female who presented with bow legs. Note the widened space between the metaphyses and epiphyseal ossification center, cupping and splaying of the metaphyses of the femur and tibia, and an overall decreased density of bone. (Courtesy of Dr. M. Goodman, Children's Hospital of Pittsburgh)

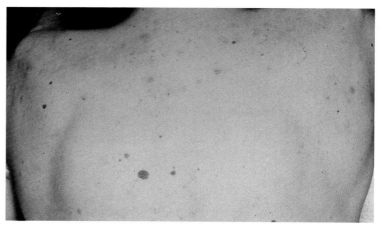

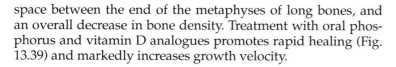

FIG. 13.41 Fabry's Disease. The small, red-purple papules are angiokeratomata. This young man had hematuria and minimal proteinuria, but no renal insufficiency.

space between the end of the metaphyses of long bones, and an overall decrease in bone density. Treatment with oral phosphorus and vitamin D analogues promotes rapid healing (Fig. 13.39) and markedly increases growth velocity.

CYSTINOSIS

Cystinosis is an autosomal-recessive metabolic disorder which is characterized by the intralysosomal accumulation of cystine in most body tissues. After degrading intracellular protein, the cystinotic lysosomes are unable to transport cystine into the cytoplasm due to a recently discovered defect in the specific lysosomal transport system for this amino acid. In its nephropathic form, the disease presents with global proximal tubular dysfunction (Fanconi syndrome) and progressive glomerular damage. The clinical manifestations of this renal tubular dysfunction include failure to thrive, renal tubular acidosis, and rickets which results from persistent urinary losses of bicarbonate and phosphorus. Also associated with this disorder are low molecular weight proteinuria and glycosuria.

Cystinotic children show a number of clinical features not obviously related to the renal abnormalities. The majority have blonde hair and a fair complexion; this, in association with growth failure and rickets, results in strikingly similar appearance between unrelated patients. Clinical diagnosis is established by ophthalmologic examination, which detects a characteristic peripheral retinopathy, and by slit-lamp examination, which detects the deposition of crystalline material in the conjunctiva and cornea. Diagnosis is confirmed by the finding of cystine crystals in the bone marrow of affected patients (Fig. 13.40), and by the presence of elevated levels of cystine in fibroblasts or peripheral leukocytes.

Treatment of nephropathic cystinosis consists of correction of the metabolic abnormalities induced by the tubular dysfunction. Patients thus receive alkali, phosphorus, potassium supplements, and often, vitamin D analogues. Despite such therapy, renal function progressively deteriorates, and most patients require end-stage renal disease therapy in the first

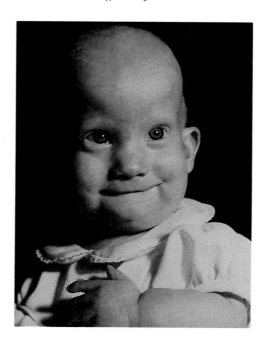

FIG. 13.42 Brachycephaly, short stubby fingers, alopecia and short stature in a 2-year-old girl with Jeune's syndrome and moderate renal failure.

decade of life. There is no specific treatment available for this metabolic disorder. Treatment with cysteamine delays, but does not prevent multiorgan injury. Patients with this condition may benefit from synthetic growth hormones, since growth failure may persist despite successful kidney or kidney/liver transplantation.

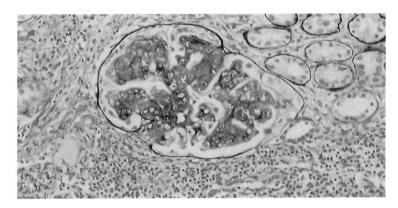

FIG. 13.43 Distinctive glomerular lesion of diffuse mesangial sclerosis in Drash syndrome. Notice the spongy and "solid" appearance of the mesangium without proliferative changes, and the obliteration of the capillary lumina. Interstitial inflammation and dilated tubules also are apparent.

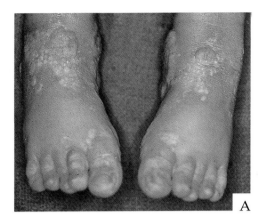

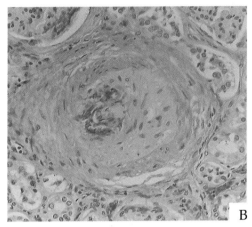

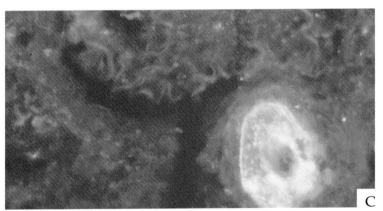

FIG. 13.44 *A*, *large xanthomatous subcutaneous deposits of cholesterol in the dorsal aspect of the feet of a 5-year-old boy with Alagille syndrome. B, renal failure occurred secondary to diffuse renal arteriolar occlusion in lipid-laden endothelial cells and macrophages. C, striking autofluorescence of the lipids is seen within such occluded vessels.*

ANGIOKERATOMA CORPORIS DIFFUSUM (FABRY'S DISEASE)

The diagnosis of Fabry's disease is usually made in childhood by recognition of its characteristic dermal telangiectasias, especially over the trunk (Fig. 13.41). This is one of the renal X-linked disorders for which prenatal diagnosis is possible through measurement of α-galactosidase (ceramide trihexodase A) in amnionic fluid cells or chorionic villi, or by gene analysis. The absence of this enzyme leads to lysosomal accumulation of an abnormal neutral glycosphingolipid in the vascular smooth muscle of the glomeruli, heart, sympathetic ganglia, and skin. Peripheral nerve involvement results in limb paresthesias and pain. Thrombosis and hemorrhage in these vessels may result in myocardial or cerebrovascular ischemia while progressive renal failure is usually preceded by hypertension, proteinuria, and hematuria.

JEUNE'S SYNDROME

Because many of the children born with Jeune's syndrome have severe and, usually, lethal pulmonary agenesis, the condition is also known as asphyxiating thoracic dystrophy. However, many children overcome the early respiratory difficulties, and may present with small thoracic cage, brachycephaly, short limbs, abnormal radiologic features of the pelvic bones, and a variety of renal manifestations ranging from mild to moderate glomerular and/or tubular changes to microcystic renal dysplasia (Fig. 13.42). We have successfully transplanted four uremic children with Jeune's syndrome and have noticed marked improvement in their growth and bone disease, as well as excellent neurologic and intellectual development.

DRASH SYNDROME

This condition is characterized by Wilm's tumor, male pseudohermaphrodism, and nephropathy. Although most children present with an abdominal mass, there may be a history or clinical evidence of edema, reflecting the severe proteinuria. Because 70 percent of such children have nephrotic syndrome in the first month of life, they are often mistaken as having congenital or Finnish-type nephrotic syndrome. However, instead of the typically microcystic proximal tubule, and Bowman's space and mesangial proliferation found in the latter disorder, the characteristic lesion is that of diffuse mesangial sclerosis (Fig. 13.43). This progressive disorder leads to

hypertension, hyperkalemia that is disproportional to the reduction in glomerular filtration rate (hyporeninemic hypoaldosteronism), and progression to renal failure at 1 to 4 years of life. Despite the absence of ambiguous genitalia, the phenotypically female youngster whose biopsy is shown in Figure 13.43 had an XY karyotype and absence of testes, ovaries, fallopian tubes, and uterus on abdominal laparotomy performed at the time of renal transplantation.

ALAGILLE SYNDROME

The main components of this disorder, which is also known as arteriohepatic dysplasia, are absence of intrahepatic bile ducts leading to cholestatic jaundice, unusual facies, posterior embryotoxon, vertebral defects, and pulmonary artery hypoplasia. Children with this condition have high circulating concentrations of total cholesterol, phospholipids, triglycerides, pre-ß and ß lipoproteins, and elevated apolipoproteins. Thus, large lipid accumulations in the skin and other tissues are common (Fig. 13.44A). Various renal abnormalities have

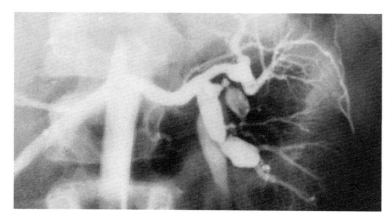

FIG. 13.45 *Arteriogram of a 12-year-old patient who presented with malignant hypertension shows multiple areas of stenosis alternating with aneurysmal dilatation in the distal segment of the renal artery, characteristic of fibromuscular dysplasia.*

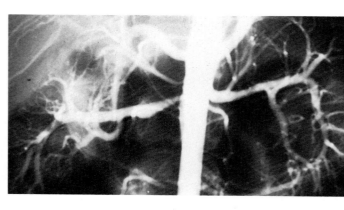

FIG. 13.46 *Arteriogram of a 13-year-old patient with neurofibromatosis who presented with mild mental retardation and a blood pressure of 140/100 shows narrowing of the renal artery close to its origin from the aorta, in contrast to the distal involvement of fibromuscular dysplasia.*

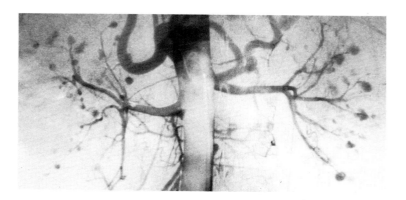

FIG. 13.47 *This arteriogram is from a 12-year-old girl who presented with weight loss, fever, abdominal pain, and malignant hypertension. Note the diagnostic features of renal involvement with polyarteritis nodosa, characterized by multiple thrombi and aneurysms.*

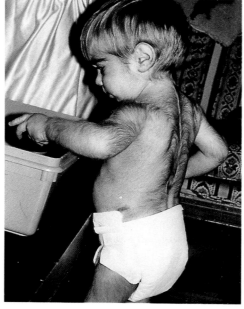

FIG. 13.48 *Two-year-old boy with generalized hirsutism secondary to treatment with cyclosporine.*

been increasingly appreciated in association with Alagille syndrome. In one recent report, 18 of 26 such patients had glomerular lesions characterized by mesangial lipidosis. Although severe renal dysfunction is uncommon, children surviving advanced stages of liver failure may also develop severe renal failure. The latter may occur in association with liver failure ("hepatorenal syndrome"), or may result from marked occlusion of renal arteries by lipid-laden or foam cells as in the case shown in Figure 13.44B,C.

RENOVASCULAR HYPERTENSION
Renal Artery Stenosis

Although only 5 percent of pediatric hypertension is caused by renal artery stenosis, detection of this abnormality is particularly important since a cure usually can be achieved. The basic pathophysiology of all renovascular hypertension involves activation of the renin-angiotensin-aldosterone system. If a lesion in the minor or major branches of the renal artery significantly decreases renal perfusion pressure, it causes an increased renin release from the affected kidney. The high plasma renin activity leads to increases in angiotensin II levels with subsequent increases in total peripheral vascular resistance. This also leads to increased adrenal aldosterone production with resultant renal sodium and water retention and expansion in extracellular fluid volume.

Renovascular hypertension should be suspected in any hypertensive child with the physical finding of high-pitched bruits heard in the flank or abdominal areas, or when stigmata of syndromes associated with arterial abnormalities are present (e.g., homocystinuria, Marfan syndrome, and the phakomatoses). Patients with renovascular hypertension may show abnormalities on intravenous urography (delayed appearance of contrast in the affected kidney, difference in renal length, ureteric notching), abnormalities on radionuclide renal scans, or elevated plasma renin activity. Renal arteriography together with selective renal vein renin sampling is the definitive diagnostic procedure for all pediatric patients with suspected renovascular hypertension.

Intrinsic diseases of the renal artery include fibromuscular dysplasia, thrombotic and embolic lesions, aneurysms, arteritis, and arteriosclerosis. The lesions of fibromuscular dysplasia involve multiple areas of stenosis alternating with aneurysmal

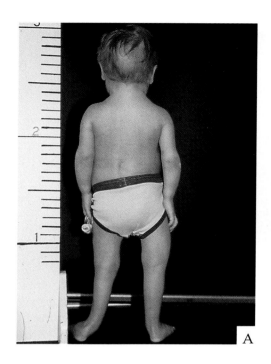

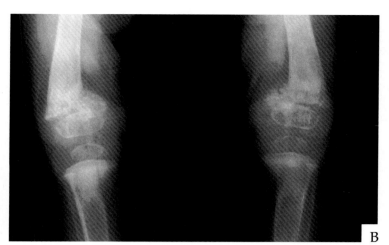

FIG. 13.49
Autonomous hyperparathyroidism and severe renal osteodystrophy in a 6-year-old boy with renal failure due to posterior urethral valves. A, bossing of the occiput. B, radiograph shows distal femoral and proximal tibial areas, as well as subperiosteal erosion of the cortical bone and active rickets in the epiphyseal ossification centers.

dilatation in the distal two-thirds of the main renal artery (Fig. 13.45). Pheochromocytoma and neurofibromatosis may also be associated with renal artery disease. Although difficult to differentiate from fibromuscular dysplasia histologically, the narrowing of the renal artery associated with neurofibromatosis generally begins within 1 cm of the origin from the aorta, distinguishing it from distal involvement of fibromuscular dysplasia (Fig. 13.46). The majority of pediatric patients with polyarteritis nodosa have renal involvement with hypertension, which leads to arterial lesions characterized by multiple thrombi and aneurysms (Fig. 13.47). Such arteriographic findings are diagnostic in the child with hypertension accompanied by weight loss, fever, and systemic manifestations of diffuse arteritis.

Correction of renovascular hypertension due to intrinsic disease of the renal artery include surgical revascularization of the kidneys or dilatation of discrete stenoses by transluminal angioplasty. Diffuse arteritis, which may cause renovascular hypertension in children with underlying systemic diseases, is treated medically with corticosteroids, immunosuppressives, or anticoagulants depending on the nature of the primary disease process. Young children with bilateral renal artery stenosis together with coarctation of the abdominal aorta represent a most challenging management problem. The small caliber vessels, and possible scarring in the vessel walls render bypass or reconstructive surgery a most difficult task. Transluminal angioplasty is also ineffective in most cases. At our center, we have successfully managed this problem by staged bypass of the coarctation and autotransplantation of one kidney, followed by autotransplantation of the remaining kidney at a later time.

Hirsutism

Although there are many endocrinologic causes of hirsutism, a number of drugs used in children with renal disorders are capable of producing this condition. Marked hirsutism gener-

ally accompanies the use of minoxidil or diazoxide, which are potent antihypertensive agents causing direct relaxation of arteriolar smooth muscle. Cyclosporine, the immunosuppressive agent used to combat tissue allograft rejection after organ transplantation has a dose-dependent effect on hair growth (Fig. 13.48). Hirsutism and alteration in body image may be a major determinant of drug compliance, particularly in adolescent girls undergoing organ transplantation.

CHRONIC RENAL FAILURE
Renal Osteodystrophy

Renal osteodystrophy, or "renal rickets," is the osseous manifestation of chronic renal failure, and results primarily from two major pathologic processes: (1) relative deficiency of 1,25-dihydroxyvitamin D, which leads to impaired mineralization of cartilage and bone, resulting in rickets and osteomalacia; and (2) an excess of parathyroid hormone, which leads to osteitis fibrosa cystica, the classic bone disease of primary hyperparathyroidism. In any given patient, each of these pathologic processes may occur with varying severity, giving a wide range of clinical and radiologic presentations. In children, renal osteodystrophy is clinically characterized by growth retardation, bone pain, and deformity of long bones. The radiologic features in children include increased thickness and fraying of the radiolucent zone in the region of growth plates, subperiosteal erosion of the cortices of long bones and phalanges, and changes in bone density including osteoporosis, osteosclerosis, or coarsening of the trabecular pattern of long bones (Figs. 13.49, 13.50).

Prevention or treatment of this disorder consists of hormone replacement and aggressive medical control of the mineral imbalance, metabolic acidosis, and malnutrition. When the glomerular filtration rate decreases below 50 ml/min/1.73 m², these children are begun on commercially available 1,25-dihydroxyvitamin D_3, which is normally synthesized by healthy

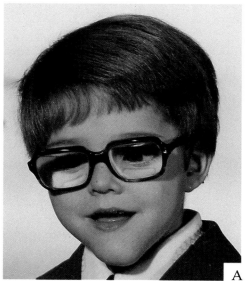

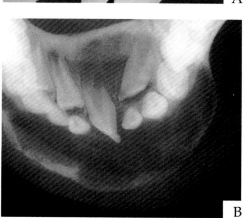

FIG. 13.50 **A**, this 5-year-old boy with moderate renal failure secondary to obstructive uropathy, was admitted for evaluation of loose teeth, marked protrusion of the mandible, and exploration of a radiolucent mandibular tumor. **B**, surgery was canceled after biochemical evaluation was consistent with renal osteodystrophy. Biopsy revealed a brown tumor resulting from intense osteoclastic activity and bone resorption. Medical treatment resulted in regression of the tumor and the prognathia, bone remineralization, strengthening of the dental ridge, and dental preservation.

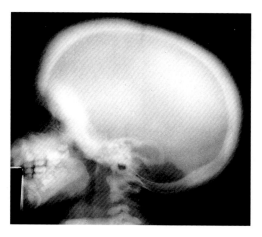

FIG. 13.51 Facial and radiologic features of the anemia of renal failure and extramedullary erythropoiesis in the same child shown in Figure 13.49. Notice the thickened cranial table with the brush-like projections.

kidneys. Calcium carbonate preparations also are given to reduce intestinal absorption of dietary phosphate while simultaneously providing calcium supplementation and intestinal acid-neutralizing capacity which helps to control the metabolic acidosis and hydrogen deposition in bone.

Anemia of Renal Failure

Severe anemia in chronic renal failure is due to the inability of the damaged kidneys to secrete sufficient amounts of erythropoietin. In untreated children with end-stage renal failure, the hemoglobin levels are often lower than in adults (5 to 7 g/dl), and severely limit the tolerance to physical activity. Good overall nutrition and replacement of folic acid and other erythroactive water-soluble vitamins lost through dialysis treatments only partially obviate the need for blood transfusions. Thus, many patients develop the facial features and radiographic appearance of Cooley's anemia (Fig. 13.51). The recent availability of recombinant erythropoietin may help improve the quality of life and prevent hemosiderosis, allergic reactions, infections, and other risks associated with frequent blood transfusions.

Growth Failure

Growth failure remains a major problem for children receiving dialysis, and may persist following successful renal transplantation. Recombinant human growth hormone has shown great promise in clinical trials of selected children with growth fail-

ure before or following renal transplantation. This agent may be effective even in children with normal concentrations of endogenous growth hormone.

BIBLIOGRAPHY

Alagille D, Estrada A, Hadchouel M, et al: Syndromatic paucity of interlobular bile ducts (Alagille syndrome or arteriohepatic dysplasia): review of 80 cases. *J Pediatr* 1987; 110:195.

Brewer ED, Benson GS: Hematuria: algorithms for diagnosis. *JAMA* 1981; 246:877–880.

Gilli G, Berry AC, Chantler C: Syndromes with a renal component, in Holliday MA, Barratt TM, Vernier RL (eds): *Pediatric Nephrology*, ed 2. Baltimore, Williams & Wilkins, 1987.

Grupe WE: Relapsing nephrotic syndrome in childhood. *Kidney Int* 1979; 16:75–85.

Habib R, Dommergues J-P, Gubler M-C, et al: Glomerular mesangiolipidosis in Alagille syndrome (arteriohepatic dysplasia). *Pediatr Nephrol* 1987; 1:455–464.

Harms E: Prenatal diagnosis of inborn errors of metabolism with renal manifestations. *Pediatr Nephrol* 1987; 1:540–545.

Jensen JC, Ehrlich RM, Hanna MK, et al: A report of four patients with the Drash syndrome and a review of the literature. *J Urol* 1989; 141:1174–1176.

Kaplan BS, Kaplan P, Rosenberg HK, et al: Polycystic kidney disease in childhood. *J Pediatr* 1989; 22:867–880.

Kaplan MR: Hematuria in childhood. *Pediatr Rev* 1983; 5:99.

Laufer J, Boichis H: Urolithiasis in children: current medical management. *Pediatr Nephrol* 1989; 3:317–31.

McCrory WW: Glomerulonephritis. *Pediatr Rev* 1983; 5:19–25.

Sibley RK, Mohan J, Mauer SM, Vernier RL: A clinicopathologic study of forty-eight infants with nephrotic syndrome. *Kidney Int* 1985; 27:544–552.

Stapleton FB: Idiopathic hypercalciuria: association with isolated hematuria and risk for urolithiasis in children. *Kidney Int* 1990; 37:807–811.

Strauss J, Abitbol C, Zilleruelo G, et al: Renal disease in children with the acquired immunodeficiency syndrome. *N Engl J Med* 1989; 321:625–630.

West CD, McAdams AJ: The chronic glomerulonephritides of childhood. Parts I and II. *J Pediatr* 1978; 93:1–12, 167–176.

Zerres K: Genetics of cystic kidney diseases. *Pediatr Nephrol* 1987; 1:397–404.

Zerres K, Volpel MC, Weib H: Cystic kidneys: genetics, pathologic anatomy, clinical picture, and prenatal diagnosis. *Hum Genet* 1984; 68:104–135.

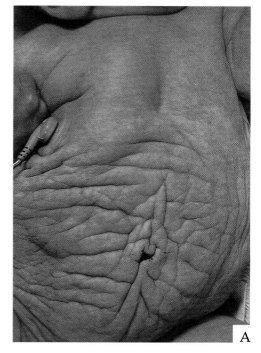

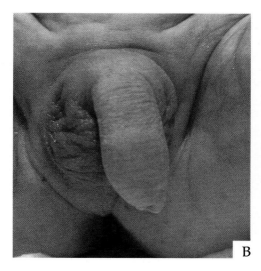

FIG. 14.4 **A,** classic appearance of prune-belly syndrome in a neonate. **B,** empty scrotum of the same infant.

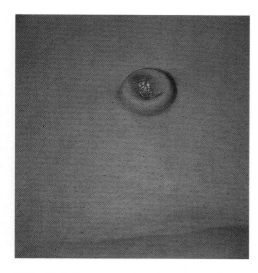

FIG. 14.5 Patent urachus in a girl with recurrent umbilical drainage and inflammation.

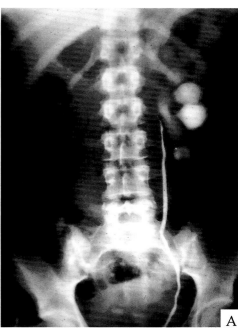

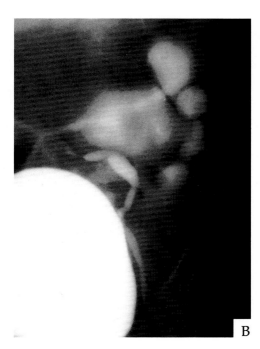

FIG. 14.6 **A,** retrograde ureterogram defines of obstruction at the ureteropelvic junction. B, the coexistence of vesicoureteric reflux and UPJ obstruction is seen in this voiding cystourethrogram.

Several lesions may result from persistence of the urachus: patent urachus, vesicourachal diverticulum, urachal cyst, and alternating urachal sinus. *Patent urachus* results when the urachal lumen fails to obliterate, and the bladder communicates with the umbilicus (Fig. 14.5). Umbilical drainage, inflammation, or infection may result. The differential diagnosis includes persistent omphalomesenteric duct. Voiding cystourethrography is important in making this diagnosis and excluding infravesical obstruction. *Urachal cysts* may become infected and present in infancy through adulthood with suprapubic or infraumbilical pain, tenderness, a palpable mass, or inflammation. Urinary tract infection with irritative voiding symptoms may result. Sonography or computerized tomography are diagnostic. *Urachal diverticula* usually are inconsequential.

HYDRONEPHROSIS
Ureteropelvic Junction Obstruction

Lesions of the ureteropelvic junction (UPJ) are a common cause of hydronephrosis. UPJ obstruction may present as prenatal hydronephrosis, neonatal flank mass, urinary tract infection, or recurrent abdominal pain in the older child and adolescent. In many cases of significant obstruction, the kidney may not be palpably enlarged. UPJ obstruction may be documented by sonography or intravenous pyelography and confirmed by retrograde pyelography (Fig. 14.6A). Voiding cystourethrography is important, particularly in infants in whom vesicoureteric reflux may coexist. In some cases, reflux is the primary lesion, with the UPJ kink as a secondary lesion

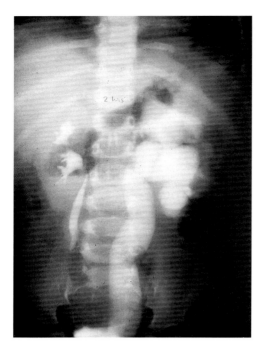

FIG. 14.7 Left megaureter with hydronephrosis.

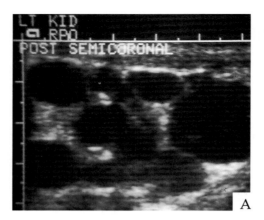

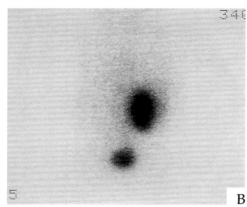

FIG. 14.8 **A**, ultrasound examination of a multicystic kidney. **B**, nuclear medicine scan of a nonfunctional left multicystic dysplastic kidney (posterior view). The top blot represents the right kidney and the lower one is the bladder.

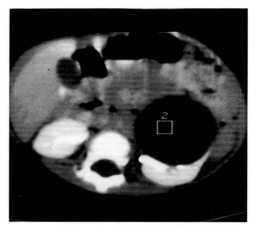

FIG. 14.9 Computed tomogram of a huge left renal cyst which presented as a left upper quadrant abdominal mass.

(Fig. 14.6B). Not all hydronephrotic kidneys are truly obstructed and, in borderline cases, diuresis renography (nuclear medicine) or percutaneous antegrade pressure perfusion studies (Whitaker test) may be necessary to determine whether surgical intervention is warranted. Some dilated but nonobstructed infant kidneys spontaneously return to a normal or near-normal appearance with time (see previous discussion).

Megaureter

The term megaureter is descriptive of a large ureter, with or without hydronephrosis (Fig. 14.7). Megaureter may be the result of massive vesicoureteric reflux, obstruction at the ureterovesical junction, or it may be nonobstructive. In fact, experience with neonatal megaureter has shown that a great many of these lesions, if studied by diuresis renography or Whitaker protocols, are proven to be nonobstructive and will resolve spontaneously. True obstructive megaureters require excision of the abnormal distal ureter and tapered reimplantation. A nonrefluxing megaureter is thought to be due to either local neurologic or, more likely, muscular abnormalities of the distal ureter that interfere with normal peristalsis.

A megaureter usually is discovered on prenatal sonography or presents as a urinary tract infection. Calculi may form in them.

MULTICYSTIC RENAL DYSPLASIA

Multicystic renal displasia (see Chapter 13, Pediatric Nephrology) is the second most common cause of renal enlargement in the neonate, and may be discovered by prenatal sonography, serendipitously, or during the evaluation of an abdominal mass. Multicystic renal dysplasia must be differentiated from hydronephrosis, and the combination of sonography and radionuclide scan is diagnostic (Fig. 14.8). Since contralateral vesicoureteric reflux is not uncommon, voiding cystourethrography should be performed in all patients to detect reflux into the solitary functioning kidney. A percentage of multicystic kidneys (at least 15 percent but perhaps much higher) spontaneously involute as determined by followup sonography, and there is still debate about the indications for nephrectomy. The Urology Section of the American Academy of Pediatrics has instituted a registry for longitudinal followup of these patients.

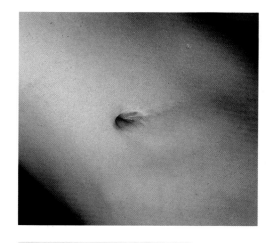

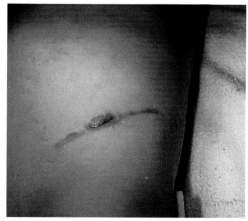

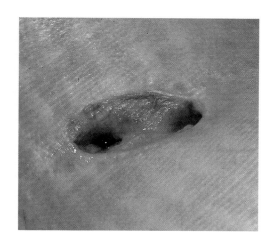

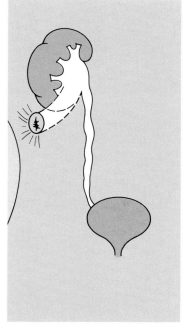

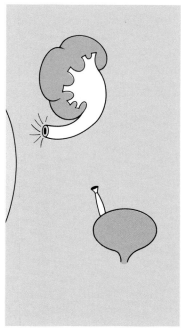

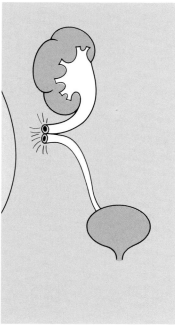

FIG. 14.10 Cutaneous pyelostomy.

FIG. 14.11 End ureterostomy.

FIG. 14.12 Loop ureterostomy. Note double-barrelled stoma.

SIMPLE RENAL CYSTS

Simple cysts were thought to be rare in children until the advent of high-resolution ultrasound technology. They are now frequently detected, albeit much less commonly than in adults, in whom the incidence increases with age. As a result, the traditional admonition to surgically explore all cysts in children has been replaced with the policy of radiographic evaluation similar to that in adults. Simple cysts should be treated as benign. Most cysts are discovered serendipitously while evaluating the urinary tract for infection-related symptoms, but large cysts occasionally present as abdominal masses. Radiologic evaluation usually includes sonography, but computed tomography (Fig. 14.9) and even cyst puncture for aspiration and contrast studies may be used to confirm the nature of the cyst. The differential diagnosis includes cystic Wilms' tumor, multilocular cystic dysplasia, duplication anomaly with hydronephrosis, and adult polycystic disease.

CUTANEOUS URINARY DIVERSION

Although permanent urinary diversion in children is rarely performed in this age of intermittent catheterization and urinary tract reconstruction, temporary diversion still has an important role in difficult situations. Understanding the anatomic relationships of urinary stomas is an integral part of caring for children with diversions.

Cutaneous Pyelostomy
The renal pelvis is marsupialized to the skin (Fig. 14.10). This is an uncommon diversion except in small infants with severe hydronephrosis and compromised renal function.

End Ureterostomy
A single stoma is created, which usually requires using the distal ureter (Fig. 14.11).

Loop Ureterostomy
A double-barrelled stoma is created, allowing access to both the proximal and distal ureter (Fig. 14.12).

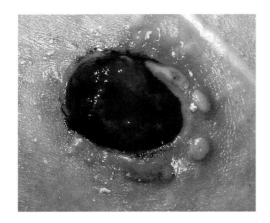

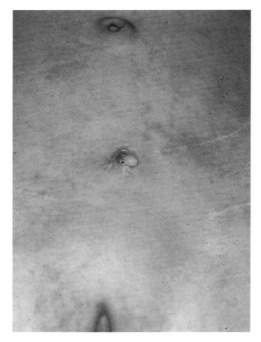

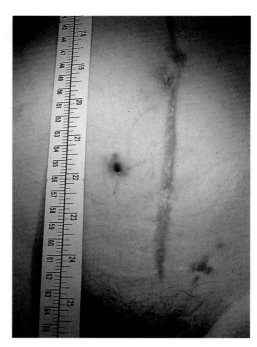

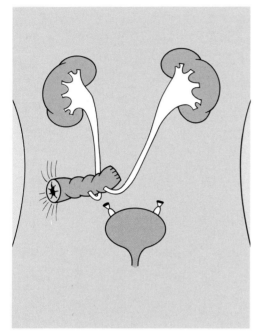

FIG. 14.13 Ileal conduit.

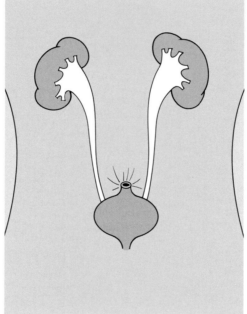

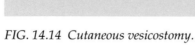

FIG. 14.14 Cutaneous vesicostomy.

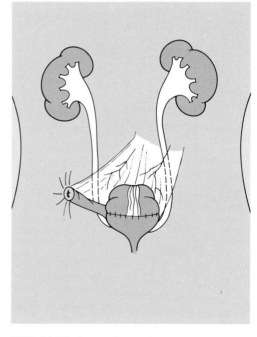

FIG. 14.15 Appendicovesicostomy.

Intestinal Diversion

An isolated segment of bowel is interposed between the skin and ureters. The normal continuity of the intestinal tract is restored (Fig. 14.13).

Cutaneous Vesicostomy

This is probably the most commonly created temporary diversion in children, usually done in cases of urethral valves, neuropathic bladder, prune belly syndrome, and occasionally severe vesicoureteric reflux. It is basically a vesicocutaneous fistula, and in the small infant it is simply covered with a diaper (Fig. 14.14).

Appendicovesicostomy

A continent diversion intended to allow intermittent catheterization of the bladder when urethral access is difficult (Fig. 14.15).

Nephrostomy

This percutaneous or operatively placed catheter is a temporary urinary diversion or upper tract access for contrast or manometric evaluations (Fig. 14.16).

EXSTROPHIC ANOMALIES

Classic Exstrophy

Bladder exstrophy occurs in approximately 1 of every 40,000 live births. It predominates in males, and is thought to result from premature rupture of the cloacal membrane. The infant usually is otherwise healthy. Examination reveals a red mucosal surface of varying size on the suprapubic abdominal wall,

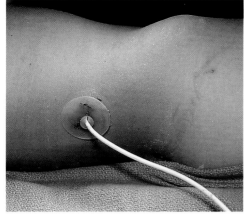

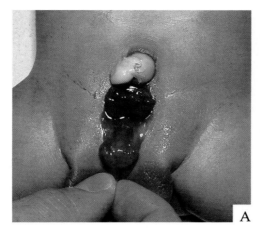

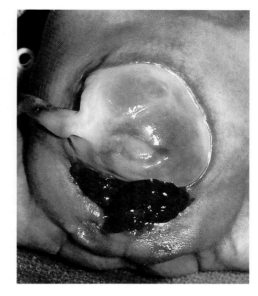

FIG. 14.18 Cloacal exstrophy.

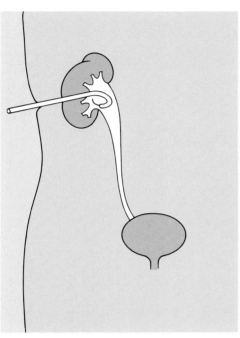

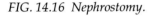

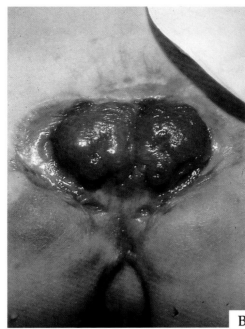

FIG. 14.16 Nephrostomy.

FIG. 14.17 **A**, classic bladder exstrophy in a male infant with a small bladder. **B**, bladder exstrophy in a female. Note the separated openings to each hemivagina.

which is the entire bladder opened as a book. On the inferior bladder surface, the trigone and ureteral orifices are visible, freely effluxing urine. The penis is epispadiac and lies dorsally tethered against the bladder. When the penis is retracted downward, the entire mucosal surface of the urethra is seen to be splayed open (Fig. 14.17A). In severe cases, the penis may be bifid or rudimentary, and sex assignment may be questionable. The scrotum may be normal or bifid, and testes may be undescended. Inguinal hernias are common. The pubic symphysis is widespread. In the female, a hemiclitoris and duplicate vagina are common (Fig. 14.17B). The delicate bladder surface should be kept moist until urologic consultation is obtained. Prompt upper tract evaluation and neonatal closure are routine. Pelvic osteotomy may be necessary to achieve successful closure.

Cloacal Exstrophy

Cloacal exstrophy is a rare anomaly (1 in 200,000 births). It represents an embryological mishap similar to that resulting in classic exstrophy, except that rupture of the cloacal membrane

occurs before the urorectal septum has completed its descent to separate the hindgut from the bladder. The resulting constellation is severe, with long-term survival little better than 50 percent in most cases. Most children have a large omphalocele, and a majority have meningomyelocele and hydrocephalus. Examination of the exstrophic mucosa reveals that the bladder is divided into two widely separated halves, with a strip of bowel mucosa in the middle. This strip is the ileocecal segment, usually accompanied by a long, prolapsed tubular structure which is the terminal ileum (Fig. 14.18). Separate orifices enter the appendix and a short, blind colon. The anus is imperforate. The genitalia are usually hypoplastic, widely separate, and sex assignment is almost universally female. A multi-specialty approach should be taken to the infant with cloacal exstrophy.

Epispadias

Epispadias represents the opposite end of the spectrum of exstrophic anomalies. Approximately 55 percent of patients are males with penopubic epispadias and incontinence. These boys have a radiographically widened pubic symphysis, and a

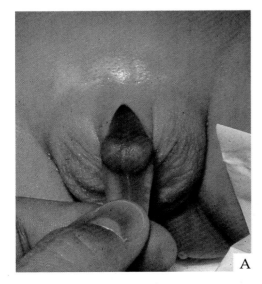

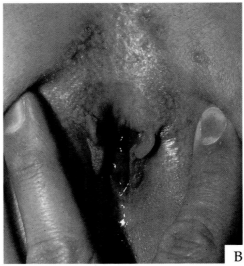

FIG. 14.19 **A,** penopubic epispadias with incontinence in a male infant. **B,** female epispadias reveals a patulous urethra and widespread hemiclitoris.

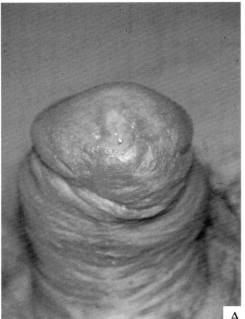

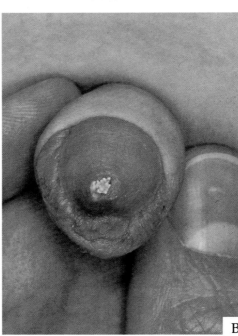

FIG. 14.20 **A,** urinary retention secondary to severe chronic balanitis (balanitis xerotica obliterans). **B,** urinary retention secondary to an impacted urethral calculus.

broad spade-like penis with the urethra opened fully on its dorsal surface. The penis usually is tethered dorsally, and the patient is usually incontinent (Fig. 14.19A). A small percent of boys demonstrate continence and penile or balanitic epispadias. In girls, incontinence usually is accompanied by a very wide urethra and a bifid clitoris (Fig. 14.19B). The cosmetic appearance of the genitalia in both sexes can be improved by genitoplasty, but the larger problem is incontinence, which is accentuated by small bladder capacity. Staged surgical correction is the rule. Sonography and voiding cystourethrography should be performed in all cases.

URINARY RETENTION

Acute urinary retention in infants and children is usually voluntary, and associated with severe acute cystitis, urethritis, meatitis (in the male), or vaginitis. In the male, urethral valves (anterior, posterior), urethral stricture (congenital, traumatic),

and meatal stenosis with meatitis (Fig. 14.20A) should be considered. Retention in the female may be caused by severe labial adhesions or uncommon lesions such as a prolapsed ureterocele. Bladder or urethral calculus (Fig. 14.20B) can be ruled out by a plain abdominal film and ultrasound examination. Severe constipation may be coincident with retention, as may acute neurologic changes associated with spinal cord injury or transverse myelitis. Intermittent catheterization is extremely valuable in managing the bladder until diagnostic evaluations can be completed.

NEUROVESICAL DYSFUNCTION

Neurovesical dysfunction in childhood may be either congenital (meningocele, myelomeningocele, intradural lipoma, diastematomyelia, sacral agenesis) or acquired (trauma, transverse myelitis, spinal cord tumor). Independent of etiology, the evaluation and management of the child with neurovesical

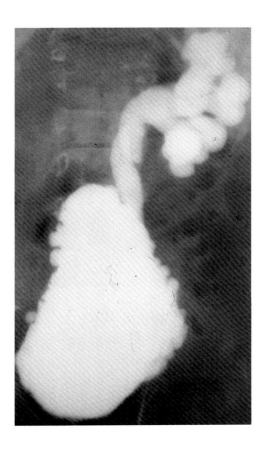

FIG. 14.21 Severe bladder trabeculation and vesicoureteric reflux in a child with myelomeningocele.

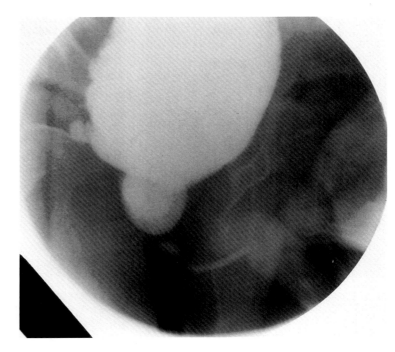

FIG. 14.22 Voiding cystourethrogram of a boy with Hinman-Allen syndrome shows severe dilation of the prostatic urethra thought to represent urethral valves. Severe bilateral hydronephrosis resulted from vesicoureteric reflux.

dysfunction is extremely important in order to preserve renal function, prevent renal damage from infection, and provide social continence. The pediatrician caring for an infant with neurovesical dysfunction should ensure that periodic evaluation of the child's urinary tract is carried out. This evaluation may include radiographic and/or urodynamic studies, and should be repeated several times during the first year of life or after injury, and at least yearly thereafter. Danger signs may include infection, fevers, or a change in a normal pattern of bladder or bowel continence (Fig. 14.21).

Uninhibited bladder contractions and discoordinated voiding are seen in various other neurologic conditions, and may also result in bladder dysfunction severe enough to cause not only incontinence or retention of urine, but also upper tract deterioration. Multiple sclerosis and other demyelinating diseases are examples. Severe cerebral palsy is frequently associated with incontinence, and when bladder dysfunction is severe, upper tract deterioration may result.

NON-NEUROGENIC VESICAL DYSFUNCTION

The "non-neurogenic neurogenic bladder," or what is termed the Hinman-Allen syndrome, is a little known but very important entity that may result in incontinence and renal failure. This syndrome represents a learned disorder of micturition, and usually presents as day and night incontinence, fecal soiling, and urinary tract infection. Many children display behavioral problems. The syndrome seems to be at the far end of the spectrum of the frequency/urgency syndrome commonly seen in childhood. Most children have urinary urgency to the point

of incontinence, although overflow incontinence from a full bladder may also occur (the lazy bladder syndrome). On occasion, the child has disordered micturition without symptoms of incontinence, and may present with urinary tract infection or renal failure. The diagnosis of dysfunctional voiding is one of exclusion, made after ruling out occult neuropathy, since the uroradiographic findings often mimic neurovesical dysfunction (Fig. 14.22). If child and family are cooperative, bladder retraining using a timed, double voiding regimen may be effective, frequently augmented with biofeedback. In severe cases, intermittent catheterization may be necessary to reverse hydronephrosis. When renal function is in jeopardy and patient cooperation is minimal, temporary urinary diversion may be appropriate. Many children with this disorder require behavioral or psychologic therapy in combination with thoughtful urologic management.

ANOMALIES OF THE MALE GENITALIA
Hypospadias

Hypospadias is a common anomaly which occurs in approximately 1 in 150 male births. The configuration of the urethra varies from mild glanular hypospadias to a severe perineal hypospadias with chordee. In describing the appearance of the hypospadiac penis, it is important to refrain from nonspecific terms such as "first degree" and "minimal." Proper definition of the anomaly should give an accurate description of the location of the meatus (glanular, coronal, subcoronal, distal shaft, midshaft, proximal shaft, penoscrotal, scrotal, perineal), and the presence or absence of chordee (Fig. 14.23A–F). If hypospa-

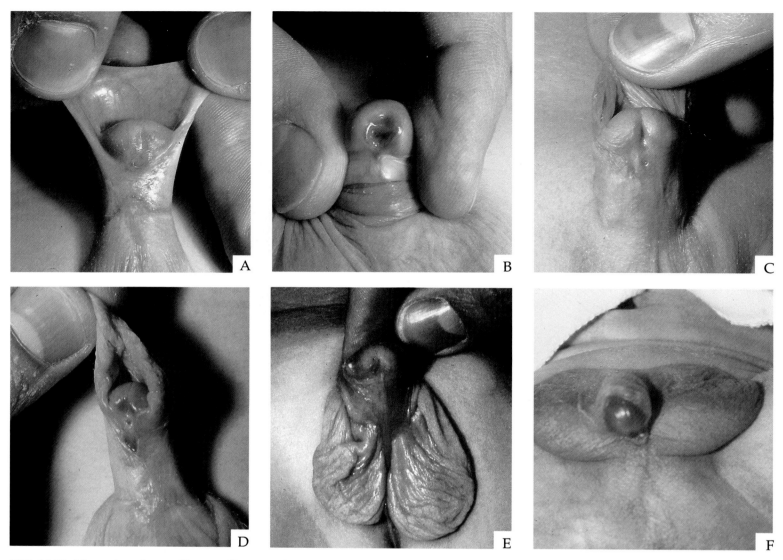

FIG. 14.23 *The various forms of hypospadias, revealing location of the meatus. **A**, the typical appearance of the "dorsal hood" prepuce seen in association with hypospadias. **B**, glandular hypospadias. **C**, subcoronal hypospadias. **D**, midshaft hypospadias. **E**, scrotal hypospadias with bifid scrotum but without chordee. **F**, perineal hypospadias with chordee.*

dias is associated with cryptorchidism, the karyotype should be determined. Voiding cystourethrography is not indicated in hypospadias except in severe lesions or in boys with a history of urinary tract infection. Renal sonography is likely to be abnormal in boys with proximal hypospadias. Infants with hypospadias should not be circumcised, because the dorsal preputial skin may be necessary for penile reconstruction. Repair is usually undertaken at 1 year of age.

Chordee

Chordee without hypospadias occurs much less frequently than chordee with hypospadias. Chordee may be a minor problem related to skin tethering, or it may be due to a congenitally short urethra, in which case surgical correction requires division of the urethra and interposition of a skin tube. If chordee is suspected in the neonate, circumcision should be delayed until examination under anesthesia and artificial erection can determine whether either circumcision or repair is appropriate (Fig. 14.24).

Penile Torsion

Torsion of the penis may be congenital or acquired. Congenital torsion may be severe and related to anomalous development of the corporal bodies, but most commonly, it is mild and related to dysgenetic subcutaneous fascia (Fig. 14.25). Acquired torsion may occur after circumcision.

Webbed Penis

This minor anomaly is easily corrected with a V-Y scrotoplasty (Fig. 14.26). Webbing is caused by the transposition of scrotal skin onto the ventral penile shaft at the penoscrotal junction. The ill effects are purely cosmetic in nature.

Buried Penis

Buried penis may occur as a primary finding in the neonate, but it is most common after circumcision (Fig. 14.27). Buried penis is usually the result of a thick suprapubic fat pad, and

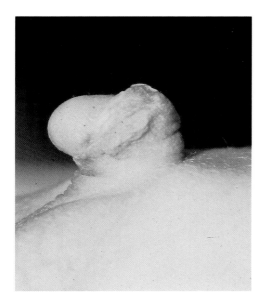

FIG. 14.24 *Chordee not associated with hypospadias.*

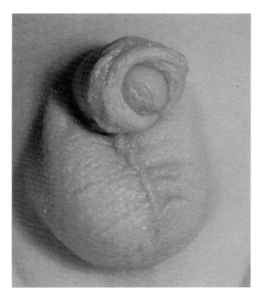

FIG. 14.25 *Mild counterclockwise penile torsion.*

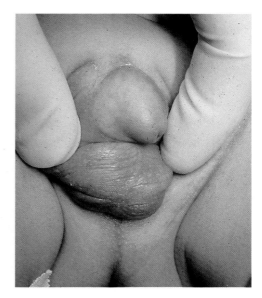

FIG. 14.26 *Webbed penis.*

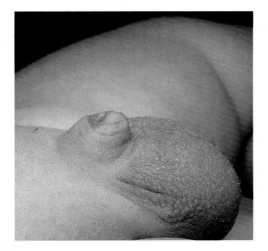

FIG. 14.27 *Buried penis after circumcision.*

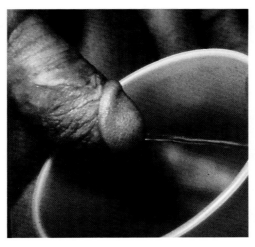

FIG. 14.28 *Observation of the urinary stream in suspected meatal stenosis reveals a full stream.*

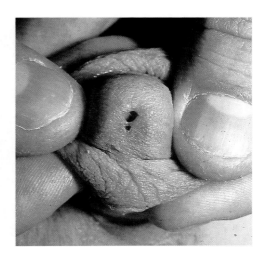

FIG. 14.29 *Meatal bridge.*

resolves with normal development. In severe cases, dysgenetic subcutaneous fascial bands bind the penis down. In general, penile stretch length should be measured and confirmed to be normal. The child should then be observed. Buried penis after circumcision may be similar to congenital buried penis, and observation may be the rule. In this situation, removal of more skin might leave the penile shaft skin deficient. If caused by a severe phimosis that covers the glans completely, surgical intervention may be necessary to open the phimotic ring and remodel the shaft skin.

Postcircumcision Lesions

MEATAL STENOSIS

Relative meatal stenosis is common after circumcision, secondary to mild recurrent meatitis. Mild to moderate stenosis usually is asymptomatic, but dysuria, strangury, or deflection of the urinary stream may bring the child to a physician's office.

Mere examination of the meatus is insufficient to document stenosis, and the urinary stream should be observed for a thin or upward stream, or for bulging of the meatus (Fig. 14.28). Meatotomy in the office under local anesthesia is curative.

MEATAL BRIDGES

These unusual lesions appear to result from meatal stenosis in which the ventral aspect of the meatus recanalizes, leaving a bridge of skin that may cause dysuria or deflection and spraying of the urinary stream (Fig. 14.29).

PREPUTIAL ADHESIONS

Fibrinous adhesions are a result of incomplete retraction of the prepuce during normal development or after circumcision. These adhesions will resolve spontaneously with normal hy-giene and development. Fibrous adhesions after circumcision result when the free edge of the circumcision adheres to the glans penis and, not properly cared for, grows onto the

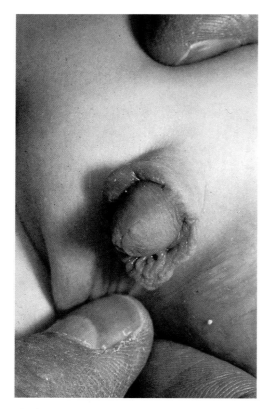

FIG. 14.30 *Preputial adhesions after circumcision.*

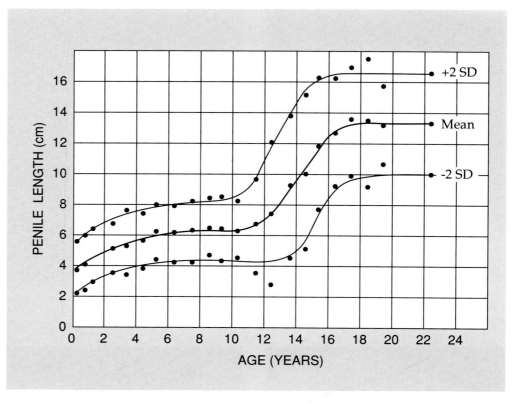

FIG. 14.31 *Cumulative frequency curves of penile length for age. (Reproduced from Lee PA, Mazur T, Danish R, et al: Micropenis I, criteria, etiologies, and classification.* Johns Hopkins Med J *1980;146:156)*

glans. The resulting bridge of skin may cause penile torsion or trap smegma, causing recurrent inflammation or infection (Fig. 14.30).

Microphallus

Microphallus (micropenis) is a small, normally formed penis less than 2 standard deviations below the mean (Fig. 14.31), which is thought to result from a disorder in the synthesis, metabolism, or utilization of testosterone. It is important to obtain an accurate penile stretch length and corporal shaft diameter. Karyotype, FSH, LH, and testosterone levels should be measured in addition to a diagnostic HCG stimulation test. Although a great deal of controversy exists about the long-term outlook for penile growth at puberty and about the appropriateness of female gender reassignment in infancy, most authors suggest a diagnostic trial of testosterone for 3 months before making a final decision about sex of rearing.

Diphallus

Diphallus is a rare entity usually associated with severe deformities of the lower urinary tract and genitalia. Complete evaluation of the upper and lower urinary tract is mandatory. In most cases of diphallus, one penis is dominant in erectile and urethral function, but in some, the bladder is septate or duplicate, and each phallus plays a significant role (Fig. 14.32).

Priapism

Priapism is a persistent painful erection in which the corporal bodies are firmly erect but the glans is soft (Fig. 14.33). The shaft and preputial skin may become very edematous, and the pain of priapism usually is severe. Priapism in children usually is related to an underlying disease state as opposed to the more common idiopathic variety seen in adults. It is most frequently associated with sickle cell disease, but may be seen in relation to pelvic malignancy, leukemia, blunt perineal trauma, or secondary to acute spinal cord injury. Sickle cell-related priapism should initially be treated as any other sickle cell crisis, with oxygenation, exchange transfusion, and alkalinization. Surgical therapy may be necessary in order to irrigate the corpora cavernosa or perform vascular bypass.

Lesions of the Scrotal Contents

The testis is an ovoid structure lying in a vertical plane in the scrotum in which it is quite mobile, moving up and down with cremasteric contraction and relaxation. Posterior and slightly lateral to the testis lies the epididymis, which may be closely applied to the body of the testis or attached by a somewhat longer mesoepididymis. The appendix testis and appendix epididymis are small embryological remnants attached to the upper anterior testis or head of the epididymis. These structures are not palpable in the normal state and are not constant findings in all males.

The Acute Scrotum

The acute scrotum is a urologic surgical emergency until proven otherwise. It is most imperative to rule out torsion of the spermatic cord. The most important aspects of evaluating the patient with an acute scrotum are history and physical examination. The nature of the onset of pain and swelling are

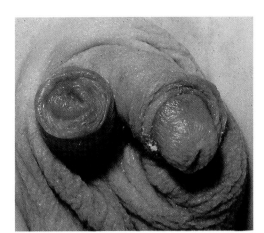

FIG. 14.32 Diphallus.

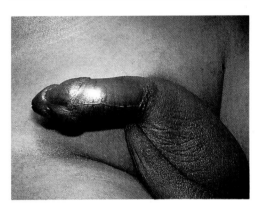

FIG. 14.33 Priapism.

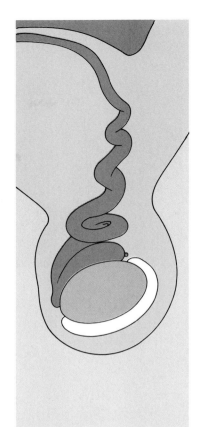

FIG. 14.34 Torsion of the spermatic cord.

important, as is a history of dysuria, fever, hematuria, previous urinary tract infection, urethral instrumentation, or perineal trauma. Examination of the scrotum starts with the normal testis, while observing the involved testis for its size, location, and anatomic orientation. The skin and wall of the scrotum are examined for edema, inflammation, and fluctuance. Mobility of the testis should be assessed, as should the presence or absence of a cremasteric reflux ipsilateral to the involved testis. Laboratory evaluation includes urinalysis, white blood count, and testicular flow scan if appropriate. The bottom line is expeditious evaluation with a liberal approach to exploration if the diagnosis is uncertain.

Torsion of the Spermatic Cord

Torsion of the spermatic cord is the most significant condition that must be excluded in cases of scrotal pain and swelling (Fig. 14.34). Since the testis deprived of its normal blood supply has, at most, a few hours before irreverisble injury destroys spermatogenic potential, acute swelling of the scrotum is a diagnostic and surgical emergency until torsion has been adequately excluded as an etiology. Torsion may occur at any age.

Prenatal torsion is thought, in most cases, to represent extravaginal torsion, or torsion of the entire scrotal contents including the covering tunics. It occurs during descent of the testis, and usually presents at birth as a firm, nontender mass high in the scrotum or at the scrotal inlet. Frequently there is fixation to the overlying skin as a part of the inflammatory response. Although a point of current controversy, the classic teaching has been that these testes are not salvageable, being more important for the contralateral testis to have normal scrotal fixation and not be prone to asynchronous torsion. Although

"salvage" of a testis after prenatal torsion is unlikely, acute torsion can occur during delivery and may be a reversible situation. A scrotal mass at birth should thus be considered a surgical emergency until proven otherwise. If observation is chosen because the involved testis appears unsalvageable, most pediatric urologists now feel that delayed exploration of the contralateral testis should be undertaken to insure that a "bell-and-clapper" deformity does not predispose the solitary testis to later torsion.

Intravaginal torsion (within the tunica vaginalis) may occur at any age. Most patients present with acute, painful swelling of the scrotum, many with lower abdominal pain, nausea, and vomiting. It is not unusual for a boy to awaken from sleep with pain, but torsion also can occur after scrotal trauma or during almost any activity. On occasion, torsion presents a much more insidious onset as a dull scrotal pain of subacute nature. Dysuria is usually absent, and urinalysis is normal, but leukocytosis may develop rapidly. Examination may vary depending on the time elapsed after the acute episode. Most patients are very uncomfortable. The scrotum is reddened and swollen, with the testis elevated due to foreshortening of the spermatic cord. The contralateral testis may have a more transverse orientation than normal. In the acute stage, a hydrocele may develop. The testis may have an abnormal orientation, with the epididymis located in an abnormal position. The cremasteric reflex usually is absent, and elevating the testis to the pubic symphysis increases pain (negative Prehn's sign). When inflammation has progressed, the scrotum becomes a firm, homogeneous mass in which all anatomic landmarks are lost.

If torsion is suspected, attempting to detorse the cord by gentle twisting in either direction may allow the cord to untwist, at least partially. If detorsion occurs, relief of pain is

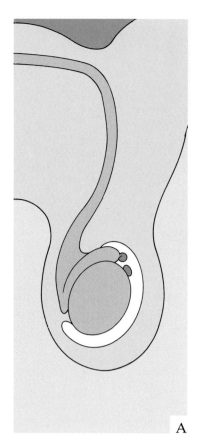

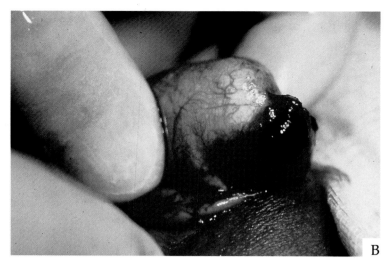

FIG. 14.35 **A**, *torsion of appendix testis/epididymus.* **B**, *operative findings after torsion of an appendix epididymis.*

instantaneous. Nuclear blood flow scanning, if immediately available, may be helpful in many instances. Ultrasound examination and Doppler flow studies have a high incidence of misleading findings.

Torsion of Testicular Appendages

The appendix testis and appendix epididymis are embryological remnants that are normally undetectable on routine examination. Torsion of an appendix, which can occur in the early pubertal age group, may be difficult to differentiate from torsion of the spermatic cord. Early after the onset of acute scrotal pain, a small tender mass may be palpable on the upper anterior surface of the testis or epididymis (Fig. 14.35A). In light-skinned children, the swollen, dark, infarcted appendage may be visible through the scrotal skin (the "blue dot" sign of Dresner) (Fig. 14.35B). In later presentations, the entire testis and scrotum may become inflamed and indistinguishable from torsion of the spermatic cord.

Epididymitis

Epididymitis may be secondary to bacterial infection, reflux of sterile urine into the ejaculatory ducts, or to ectopic insertion of a ureter into the seminal vesicle or vas deferens. The clinical presentation of epididymitis may be indolent or acute, as seen with torsion. Fever often accompanies epididymitis, and the urinary sediment may reflect infection. Examination of the scrotum in early stages demonstrates a tender, slightly swollen epididymis (Fig. 14.36), but later the entire scrotal contents are replaced by an inflammatory mass. The cremasteric reflex is present, and elevation of the testis on the pubis may relieve pain (Prehn's sign). A radionuclide scan will demonstrate increased blood flow. If torsion of the spermatic cord cannot

be excluded, surgical exploration must be carried out promptly. All children with epididymitis should undergo complete upper and lower urinary tract radiographic evaluation after resolution of the acute process.

Chronic Scrotal Swelling

VARICOCELE

A varicocele consists of dilated veins of the pampiniform plexus of the spermatic cord (Fig. 14.37). Varicoceles occur primarily on the left side and rarely before puberty. They may be bilateral. The postulated causes of varicocele vary from hormonal to hydrostatic. The postulated etiology of testicular injury from varicocele varies from hormonal deficiencies to temperature effects. Most varicoceles decompress in the supine position. Those that do not decompress, or present with acute onset on either side may lead to concern about lesions in the kidney or retroperitoneum causing obstruction to venous outflow. Most varicoceles are asymptomatic and are noted by the child incidentally, or discovered on routine examination. Pain secondary to varicocele is uncommon.

Infertility is found in approximately 33 percent of adults with varicoceles, and because semen analyses are not generally available in children, controversy has arisen over the proper management of adolescents. It is common practice to ablate varicoceles in patients with testicular atrophy or bilateral varicocele. In patients with minimal or no testicular atropy, an LHRH stimulation test may demonstrate hormonal deficiencies, giving reason for correction.

SPERMATOCELE

Spermatoceles are common in adults, and they are recognized frequently in adolescents as well. They are painless cystic masses located in the epididymis or testicular adenexa sepa-

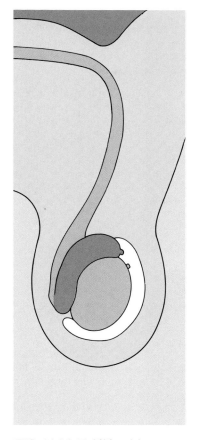

FIG. 14.36 Epididymitis.

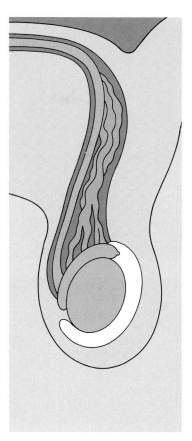

FIG. 14.37 Varicocele.

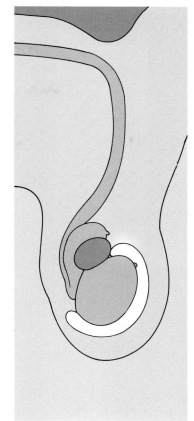

FIG. 14.38 Spermatocele.

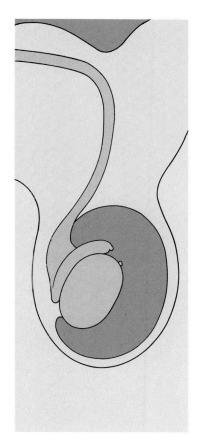

FIG. 14.39 Hydrocele.

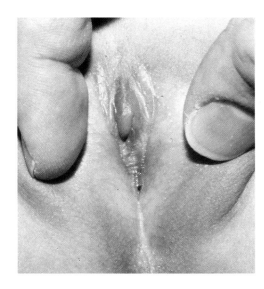

FIG. 14.40 Labial adhesions. Only a small opening remains anteriorly.

rate from the testis (Fig. 14.38). They vary in size, but are usually less than 1 cm in diameter. They are mobile, transilluminate, and do not change in size. Spermatoceles contain sperm and are retention cysts of the epidymis or tubules of the rete testis. Excision is not recommended in routine cases because of the potential for scarring of epididymal tubules and subsequent infertility.

HYDROCELE

Hydroceles are fluid accumulations within the tunica vaginalis or processus vaginalis (Fig. 14.39). They may be small or large, are usually painless even if they are large, and may be tense enough to obscure palpation of the testis. They transillumi-

nate. Simple scrotal hydroceles are common in neonates, and usually resolve spontaneously over several months. If the processus vaginalis remains patent, a communicating hydrocele results, and may present with periodic increase and decrease in scrotal size. If a segment of processus vaginalis fails to obliterate, a hydrocele of the cord may result. This cystic, nontender mass in the groin may need to be differentiated from a sarcoma of the spermatic cord by exploration.

LESIONS OF THE FEMALE GENITALIA

Labial adhesions are common in the prepubertal age group. They represent fusion of the labia minora, postulated to be caused by inflammation of the thin vaginal mucosa which simply adheres in the midline. Fusion begins posteriorly, and may progress until almost complete fusion results (Fig. 14.40). On inspection, the vaginal introitus may be closed with the exception of a small anterior opening. Severe fusion may be associated with dysuria, postvoid dribbling as the urine voided into the vagina drains out, or urinary tract infection. Although most adhesions will lyse spontaneously as puberty approaches and the vaginal epithelium cornifies, problems of hygiene and discomfort bring many girls to the physician for evaluation and treatment.

Labial fusion must be separated mechanically. This is usually performed easily in the office, after application of a lidocaine ointment to the introitus. Lysis should be followed by the application of estrogen cream to the area for several days, to thicken the vaginal mucosa. Unfortunately, many physicians think that mere application of estrogen will cure the problem. This is untrue. After lysis, simple hygiene should prevent recurrence.

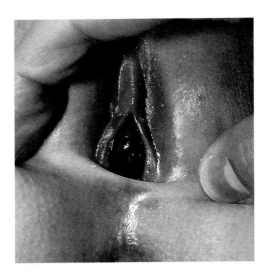

FIG. 14.41 Urethral prolapse. This is a chronic case in which the initial hemorrhagic nature of the acute prolapse has resolved with observation, leaving a protuberant, edematous urethra.

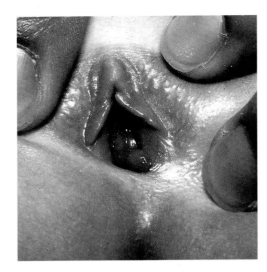

FIG. 14.42 A small polyp of the posterior vaginal fourchette.

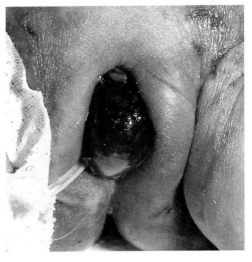

FIG. 14.43 Prolapsed ureterocele. The catheter enters the urethra.

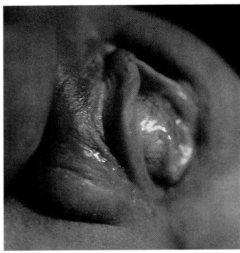

FIG. 14.44 Paraurethral cyst.

Urethral Prolapse

Prolapse of the urethra occurs almost exclusively in black girls. Its cause is unknown. The presentation is usually bloody spotting, with occasional mild dysuria. Examination reveals a reddened or dark circumferential prolapse of the urethra with an otherwise normal introitus (Fig. 14.41).

Urethral Polyps

Small polyps may originate from the urethral meatus or hymenal ring (Fig. 14.42). These usually are thin mucosal tags that cause no symptoms and require no specific treatment. Fleshy polyps or multiple polyps should be examined closely and biopsied to exclude malignancy such as sarcoma botryoides (see Chapter 11, Pediatric Hematology/Oncology).

Prolapsed Ureterocele

Prolapse of a large ureterocele through the urethral orifice should be considered in the differential diagnosis of all interlabial masses in infants and children (Fig. 14.43). Ureteroceles are cystic dilations of the distal ureter, which are located in the bladder or urethra and may prolapse through the urethral meatus as reddened or even necrotic mucosal surfaces. A prolapsed ureterocele, unlike urethral prolapse, will not present a symmetric orifice but rather, an asymmetrical protrusion through the urethra. Catheterization alongside the prolapse may locate the lumen of the urethra. Prolapse of a ureterocele may be associated with a palpable distended bladder or flank mass (hydronephrosis). Ultrasound examination of the bladder and kidneys will demonstrate unilateral or bilateral hydronephrosis, or hydronephrosis of a segment of a complete ureteral duplication, usually the upper pole of an obstructed renal unit. Voiding cystourethrography with intravenous urography or radionuclide studies and, occasionally, direct puncture of the ureterocele with contrast injection, may be appropriate to define the anatomy of the malformation.

Paraurethral Cysts

Cystic lesions of the paraurethral or vaginal mucosa may be found on routine examination, and are usually asymptomatic. They rarely cause voiding symptoms, and occasionally present, in older girls, as palpable interlabial masses. Normal mucosa overlies the cyst, which usually displaces the urethral meatus slightly from the midline. Most cysts rupture spontaneously, but aspiration or marsupialization may be necessary (Fig. 14.44).

Congenital Obstruction of the Vagina

Vaginal obstruction may occur as a result of an imperforate hymen, vaginal atresia or septa, or urogenital sinus malformation. Fusion anomalies of the müllerian structures may result

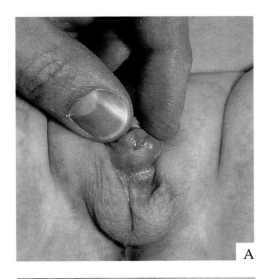
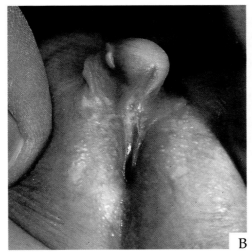
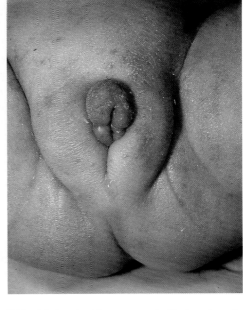

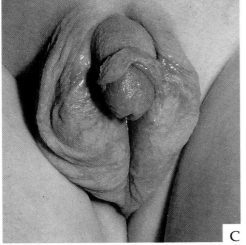
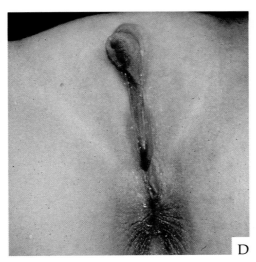

FIG. 14.46 *Ambiguous genitalia in a female with a high imperforate anus.*

FIG. 14.45 *Examples of conditions manifesting as ambiguous genitalia.* **A,** *congenital adrenal hyperplasia.* **B,** *mixed gonadal* *dysgenesis.* **C,** *true hermaphrodism.* **D,** *posteriorly displaced urogenital sinus.*

in a septate vagina or bicornuate uterus with one obstructed segment. Neonates or infants may present with abdominal masses or urinary retention, while girls with didelphia or bicornuate uterus may present with pelvic pain or menstrual irregularities at puberty. Examination of the infant may reveal a distended vagina with a bulging hymenal membrane. If a vaginal septum or atresia is the cause of the obstruction, external genital examination may be normal, and a complete pelvic examination with vaginoscopy may be necessary. Ultrasound examination of the pelvis may be helpful. All girls with uterine or vaginal anomalies should undergo sonographic or intravenous pyelographic evaluation of the upper urinary tract given the high incidence of upper tract anomalies in this group. This is particularly important in girls with unilateral renal agenesis.

AMBIGUOUS GENITALIA

The human genitalia begin as undifferentiated structures which, early in gestation, are identical in both genetic sexes. The combined effect of genetic, hormonal, and local influences modify the structure and function of the genitalia, to produce genital structures appropriate to the genetic sex of the individ-

ual (see Chapter 9, Pediatric Endocrinology). When abnormal development takes place, genitalia of indeterminate nature may result. The recognition of abnormal genitalia is the first step in the evaluation of intersex. It must be kept in mind that the combination of hypospadias and unilateral cryptorchidism should be considered as representative of intersex until proven otherwise. Examination of the genitalia in suspected intersex cases should include assessment of phallic length and diameter, presence or absence of gonads and their size, assessment of labioscrotal and perineal anatomy, rectal examination, ultrasound examination of the pelvis, and flush genitogram (urethrogram) to delineate urethral/vaginal structures. A full genetic and endocrine evaluation should be carried out as well (Fig. 14.45).

Genital Ambiguity Associated with Imperforate Anus

The embryological deformity that produces a high imperforate anus in the female occasionally also influences the formation of the external genitalia by presumed local factors. The end result may be genitalia that appear to be masculinized (Fig. 14.46).

GENITAL TRAUMA

Injury to the genitalia may be the result of minimal trauma or may be a part of multiple trauma. Although genital trauma may not be life-threatening, proper management may be very important to the later well-being and psychosocial development of the patient. This is particularly important in children. Trauma to the penis or scrotum should always raise the question of urethral injury. This is easily ruled out in the emergency room or x-ray department by injecting contrast (intravenous contrast in case of extravasation into vascular structures) through the urethral meatus, using a blunt-tipped syringe or a small catheter. Once urethral injury has been excluded, urethral catheterization can be performed safely. Scrotal trauma mandates close evaluation of the testes, and if injury is discovered, examination and repair should be performed in the operating room (Fig. 14.47). Scrotal and testicular trauma is not uncommon in breech delivery, when the scrotum is the presenting part. Prompt urologic assessment should be sought.

Ultrasound examination of the testes may be helpful if massive edema or hematoma preclude thorough examination. If injury is suspected, surgical exploration is the most conservative approach.

BIBLIOGRAPHY

Belman AB, Kaplan GW: *Genitourinary Problems in Pediatrics.* Philadelphia, WB Saunders, 1981.

Gillenwater JY, Grayhack JT, Howards SS, Duckett JW (eds): *Adult and Pediatric Urology.* Chicago, Year Book, 1987.

Kelalis PP, King LR, Belman AB (eds): *Clinical Pediatric Urology.* Philadelphia, WB Saunders, 1985.

Lee PA, Mazur T, Danish R, et al: Micropenis I, criteria, etiologies, and classification. *Johns Hopkins Med J* 1980;146: 156–163.

Williams DI, Johnston JH (eds): *Paediatric Urology.* London, Butterworth, 1982.

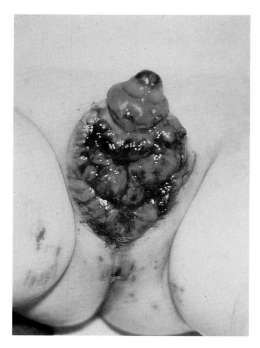

FIG. 14.47 *Perineal trauma. The testes were injured, but the urethra was intact.*

15

PEDIATRIC NEUROLOGY

Henry B. Wessel, M.D.

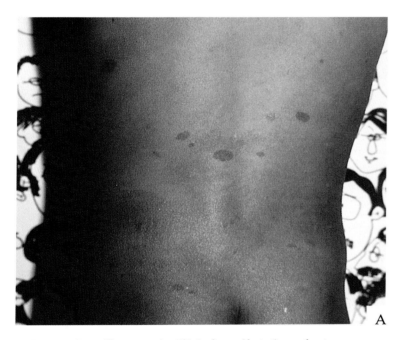

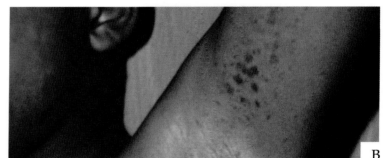

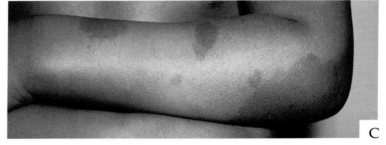

FIG. 15.1 Neurofibromatosis. Clinical manifestations of cutaneous pigmentary abnormalities. **A,** most common are multiple café-au-lait spots over the trunk. **B** and **C,** also seen are axillary freckling or extensive areas of hyperpigmentation. (Courtesy of Dr. Michael Sherlock)

The primary objective of the traditional systematic neurologic examination is to determine the functional integrity of the central and peripheral nervous systems. This cornerstone of neurologic physical diagnosis permits detection and localization of neurologic dysfunction, the first step in neurologic differential diagnosis. Neurologic evaluation also includes careful inspection for skin lesions, abnormalities of head shape and volume, disturbances of gait and posture, and abnormalities of muscle bulk, findings which may provide important additional diagnostic clues. This chapter will concentrate on selected neurologic disorders which are accompanied by physical signs that can be detected on visual inspection.

NEUROCUTANEOUS SYNDROMES

The neurocutaneous syndromes or phakomatoses are congenital, often inherited disorders with prominent cutaneous and neurologic manifestations. The simultaneous involvement of skin and nervous system, both derivatives of embryonic ectoderm, suggests that these disorders may be caused by an unknown abnormality of the embryonic epiblast. Although the clinical and pathologic features of the phakomatoses are diverse, these syndromes share a propensity for malformations and hamartomatous tumors of multiple organs. Among the more frequently encountered phakomatoses are neurofibromatosis, tuberous sclerosis, Sturge-Weber syndrome, ataxia telangiectasia, and linear sebaceous nevus.

Neurofibromatosis 1

Neurofibromatosis 1 or NF-1 (previously known as von Recklinghausen's neurofibromatosis) is the most common of the neurocutaneous syndromes. Inherited as an autosomal-dominant disorder, NF-1 affects about 1 in 4,000 individuals. The

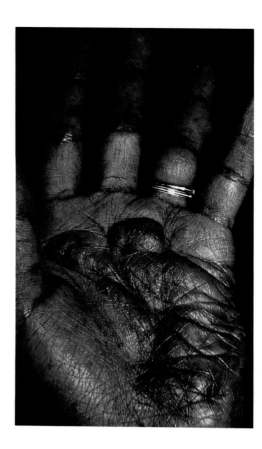

FIG. 15.2
Neurofibromatosis.
Extensive plexiform
neurofibroma of the
palm. (Courtesy
of Dr. Michael
Sherlock)

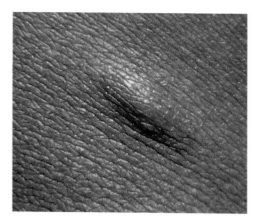

FIG. 15.3
Neurofibromatosis.
Subcutaneous neu-
rofibroma along the
course of a nerve
trunk. (Courtesy of
Dr. Michael Sherlock)

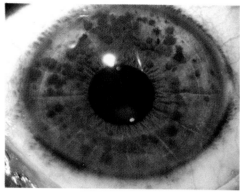

FIG. 15.4
Neurofibromatosis.
Pigmented hamar-
tomas of the iris
(Lisch nodules).

NF-1 gene has been localized to chromosome 17. Characteristic clinical manifestations include multiple hyperpigmented skin macules (café-au-lait spots), intertriginous freckling, multiple skin neurofibromas, and iris hamartomas (Lisch nodules). Associated abnormalities may include optic gliomas, other central nervous system tumors of glial or meningeal origin, neurofibromas of spinal or peripheral nerves, pheochromocytoma, macrocephaly, cognitive impairment or bony abnormalities.

Diagnostic criteria for neurofibromatosis 1 are met if two or more of the following are found:

1. Six or more café-au-lait macules over 5 mm in greatest diameter in prepubertal children and over 15 mm in greatest diameter in postpubertal individuals.
2. Two or more neurofibromas of any type or one plexiform neurofibroma.
3. Axillary or inguinal freckling.
4. Optic glioma.
5. Two or more Lisch nodules (iris hamartomas).
6. A distinctive osseous lesion such as sphenoid dysplasia or thinning of long bone cortex with or without pseudarthrosis.
7. A first-degree relative (parent, sibling, or child) with NF-1 by above criteria.

Multiple café-au-lait spots, the most frequently encountered cutaneous abnormality, are brown hyperpigmented macules, usually most numerous over the trunk (Fig. 15.1A). Although solitary café-au-lait spots may be seen in normal individuals, the occurrence of four or more such lesions is uncommon. Other abnormalities of cutaneous pigmentation may include axillary or inguinal freckling or extensive areas of hyperpigmentation (Fig. 15.1B,C). Hyperpigmented skin lesions almost always precede neurologic symptoms. However, they are not necessarily present at birth and may be inconspicuous in early childhood, becoming more prominent at puberty.

Additional cutaneous manifestations of neurofibromatosis may include extensive plexiform neuromas at the terminal distribution of nerve fibers (Fig. 15.2) or small subcutaneous nodules—neurofibromas—scattered along the course of nerve trunks (Fig. 15.3).

Pigmented hamartomas of the iris, termed Lisch nodules, are found in over 90 percent of patients with NF-1 who are 6 years of age or older, and occur in nearly one third of younger patients (Fig. 15.4). They do not occur in normal individuals. These hamartomas are asymptomatic, and do not correlate with the extent or severity of other manifestations. However, they are helpful in establishing diagnosis.

Skeletal abnormalities are found in 51 percent of affected individuals. The characteristic findings (Fig. 15.5) include :

1. Severe angular scoliosis with dysplasia of vertebral bodies.
2. Defects of the posterior-superior wall of the orbit.
3. Congenital bowing and pseudarthrosis of the tibia, fibula, femur, or clavicle.
4. Disorders of bone growth associated with elephantoid hypertrophy of overlying soft tissue.
5. Erosive bony defects produced by contiguous neurogenic tumors.
6. Scalloping of the posterior margins of the vertebral bodies corresponding to saccular areas of dilatation of the spinal meninges.

Magnetic resonance imaging frequently shows areas of increased signal intensity on T2-weighted images of the globus pallidus, brain stem, or cerebellar white matter (Fig. 15.6). Believed to represent hamartomas, these regions of abnormal signal intensity do not appear to correlate with neurologic dysfunction. However, their presence does help confirm the diagnosis of neurofibromatosis. Computed tomography (CT) seldom demonstrates corresponding abnormalities.

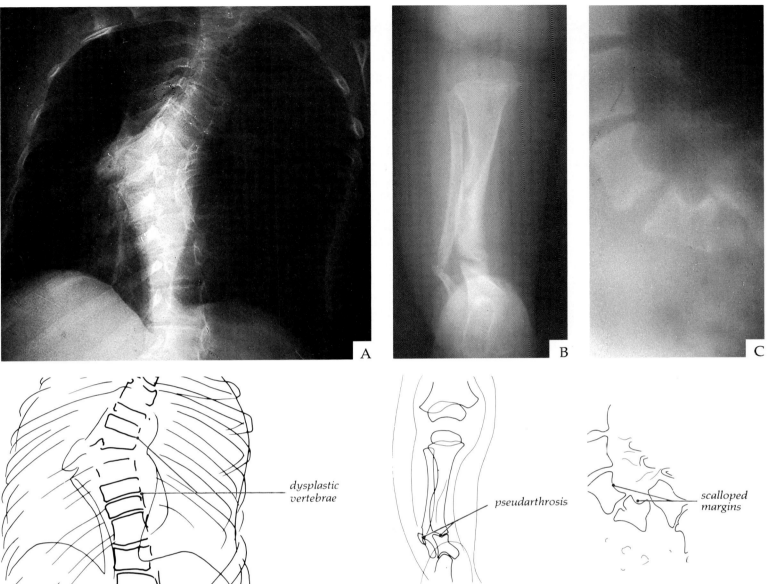

FIG. 15.5 Neurofibromatosis 1. Radiographic manifestations of skeletal abnormalities. **A,** severe angular scoliosis and vertebral dysplasia. **B,** congenital bowing and pseudarthrosis of the tibia and fibula. **C,** scalloping of posterior margins of the vertebral bodies was due to dural ectasia. (Courtesy of Department of Radiology, Children's Hospital of Pittsburgh)

Neurofibromatosis 2

Neurofibromatosis 2 or NF-2 (also known as bilateral acoustic neurofibromatosis) is a distinct genetic disorder characterized by autosomal dominant inheritance of bilateral acoustic neuromas with a penetrance of over 95 percent. The NF-2 gene is probably located on chromosome 22. Symptoms usually first appear in the teens or early twenties, when pressure on the vestibulocochlear or facial nerve complex results in impaired auditory discrimination, hearing loss, tinnitus, unsteadiness, or facial weakness. Presenile lens opacities are found in half the patients examined, and may precede the onset of symptoms referable to acoustic neuroma. Other Schwann-cell tumors of cranial nerves, spinal roots, or spinal cord, as well as multiple central nervous system tumors of meningeal or glial origin may develop. Cutaneous manifestations such as café-au-lait spots, cutaneous neurofibromas, and intertriginous freckling are less common in NF-2 than in NF-1.

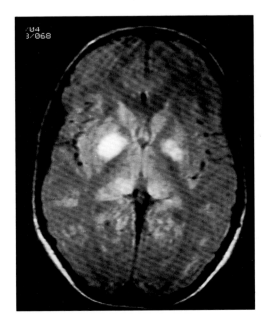

FIG. 15.6
Neurofibromatosis 1:
MRI T2-weighted
image demonstrates
high signal areas in
the region of the
globus pallidus bilaterally. (Courtesy of
Division of
Neuroradiology,
University Health
Center of Pittsburgh)

DIAGNOSTIC FEATURES OF TUBEROUS SCLEROSIS

**Primary Features
(only one required for definitive purposes)**

Shagreen patches
Ungual fibroma
Retinal hamartoma
Facial angiofibroma (adenoma secaceum)
Subependymal glial nodules (by CT or MRI)
Renal angiomyolipomata

**Secondary Features
(two required for presumptive diagnosis)**

Hypopigmented macules (ash-leaf spots)
Gingival fibromas
Bilateral polycystic kidneys
Cardiac rhabdomyomata
Cortical tubers (by MRI)
Radiographic "honeycomb" lungs
Infantile spasms
Myoclonic, tonic, or atonic seizures
First-degree relative with tuberous sclerosis
Giant cell astrocytoma

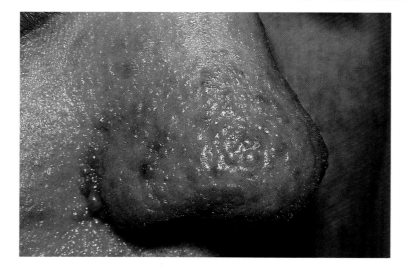

FIG. 15.8 Tuberous sclerosis: adenoma sebaceum. This adolescent boy had adenoma sebaceum in a characteristic malar distribution. Lesions were especially prominent over his nose.

Diagnostic criteria for neurofibromatosis 2 are met by an individual with:

1. Bilateral eighth-nerve masses seen on CT or MRI, or
2. A first-degree relative with NF-2 and either
   a. A unilateral eighth-nerve mass, or
   b. Two of the following:
      Neurofibroma
      Meningioma
      Glioma
      Schwannoma
      Juvenile posterior subcapsular lenticular opacity.

Tuberous Sclerosis

Tuberous sclerosis is an autosomal-dominant neurocutaneous disorder in which the more prominent features include seizures (96 percent), mental retardation (60 percent), intracranial calcification (49 percent), tumors of various organs including the brain, heart, liver and kidneys, and cutaneous lesions. The abnormal gene is located near the ABO locus on the long arm of chromosome 9. Seizures are the most frequent presenting complaint. The reported prevalence of the disorder is 1 in 150,000, though this may be an underestimate since manifestations can be inconspicuous. Diagnostic features are summarized in Fig. 15.7.

The characteristic skin lesion of tuberous sclerosis is the angiofibroma (adenoma sebaceum). These are seen as erythematous papules distributed over the nose and malar region (Fig. 15.8). Approximately 40 percent of children with tuberous sclerosis demonstrate these lesions by 3 years of age.

Ovoid depigmented nevi with irregular borders, termed "ash-leaf" spots, are another common cutaneous manifestation (Fig. 15.9). These generally appear earlier than adenoma sebaceum and may be present at birth. They are detectable by 2 years of age in over half of affected children. While resembling vitiligo, they differ in that they are not completely devoid of melanin. In fair-skinned infants, these nevi may be demonstrable only under Wood's light.

Another valuable cutaneous marker is the shagreen patch, a plaque of thickened skin with a cobblestone or orange peel texture (Fig. 15.10). Histologically, the shagreen patch is a connective tissue nevus.

Additional dermatologic manifestations of tuberous sclerosis include periungual and dental fibromas and macular areas of hyperpigmentation. Recognition of the cutaneous features can suggest an etiologic diagnosis in some patients presenting with mental retardation or seizures.

In patients with tuberous sclerosis, CT often demonstrates intracranial calcifications that appear as multiple scattered areas of increased density adjacent to the walls of the lateral

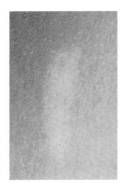

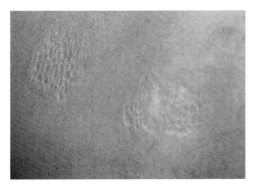

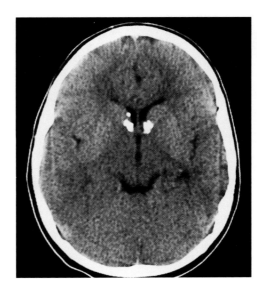

FIG. 15.9 Tuberous sclerosis. Ash-leaf spot, an oval depigmented nevus with irregular borders. (Courtesy of Dr. Michael Sherlock)

FIG. 15.10 Tuberous sclerosis. Shagreen patch. This plaque of thickened skin with a cobblestone texture is distinctive, but is one of the less common cutaneous manifestations of tuberous sclerosis. (Courtesy of Dr. Michael Sherlock)

FIG. 15.11 Tuberous sclerosis. This CT scan through the foramina of Monro shows the multiple periventricular calcific deposits characteristic of this disorder. (Courtesy of Division of Neuroradiology, University Health Center of Pittsburgh)

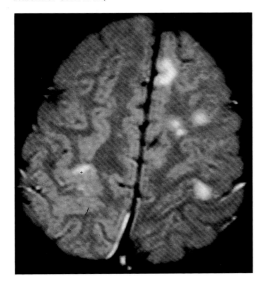

FIG. 15.12 Tuberous sclerosis. MRI demonstrates multiple cortical tubers which appear as areas of increased signal intensity in this T2-weighted image. The signal abnormalities actually arise predominantly within the white matter subjacent to the tuber. (Courtesy of Division of Neuroradiology, University Health Center of Pittsburgh)

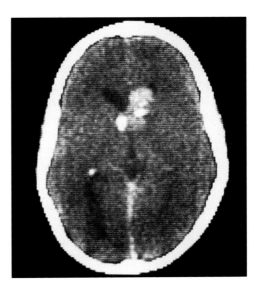

FIG. 15.13 Tuberous sclerosis. CT scan demonstrates a large subependymal astrocytoma which intermittently obstructed the ventricular system, producing episodic symptoms of increased intracranial pressure. (Courtesy of Division of Neuroradiology, University Health Center of Pittsburgh)

and third ventricles (Fig. 15.11). CT is superior to MRI for demonstration of small calcifications. No relationship has been established between the extent of periventicular calcification and clinical severity as judged by developmental function or seizure frequency. CT may also demonstrate typical intracranial calcifications in asymptomatic individuals who lack external manifestations of the disorder. This can help identify subclinical cases and improve accuracy of genetic counseling in affected families.

The characteristic gross abnormality of the brain is the presence of multiple gliotic nodules (hamartomas) of varying size, which constitute the tubers for which this disorder is named. These are located over the convolutions of the cerebral hemispheres and beneath the ependymal lining of the lateral and third ventricles. Heterotopic nodules of identical structure may be found in the cerebral white matter as well. While cortical tubers are rarely apparent on CT, they are readily identified by MRI (Fig. 15.12). More severely affected patients have a greater number of cerebral cortical lesions detected by MRI, suggesting that MRI may be useful in predicting eventual clinical severity in young children with newly diagnosed tuberous sclerosis.

Tumors may arise from either the cortical or the subependymal tubers, complicating the course of the disease by producing increased intracranial pressure and other symptoms associated with intracranial mass lesions (Fig. 15.13).

Visceral lesions associated with tuberous sclerosis include cardiac rhabdomyomas, renal hamartomas and mixed embryonal tumors, and hepatic hamartomas. The cardiac rhabdomyomas are usually asymptomatic, but occasionally an affected newborn may present with obstructive congestive heart failure. Renal lesions are often unimportant functionally, but can produce albuminuria or hematuria. Chronic renal failure and malignant transformation of renal tumors are quite rare. Hepatic hamartomas are clinically insignificant.

Sturge-Weber Syndrome

The cardinal manifestations of Sturge-Weber syndrome are:

1. A vascular nevus or "port wine" stain over the face, involving the cutaneous distribution of the ophthalmic division of the trigeminal nerve.
2. Ipsilateral leptomeningeal angiomatosis with associated intracranial calcifications.
3. A high incidence of mental retardation and ipsilateral ocular complications.

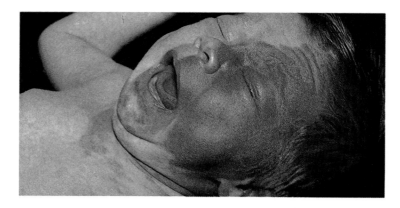

FIG. 15.14 *Sturge-Weber syndrome. Nonelevated purple cutaneous hemangioma in a trigeminal distribution, including the ophthalmic division.*

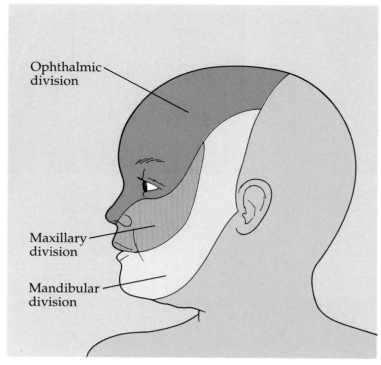

FIG. 15.15 *Sturge-Weber syndrome. Cutaneous distribution of division of the trigeminal nerve. Only patients with facial vascular nevi (port wine stains) which involve the ophthalmic division are at risk for associated neuro-ocular symptoms.*

The vascular nevus (Fig. 15.14) is usually present at birth and consists of a pink-to-purple macular cutaneous hemangioma. Only patients with lesions involving the cutaneous distribution of the ophthalmic division of the trigeminal nerve (i.e., forehead and upper eyelid) are at risk for associated neuro-ocular complications (Fig. 15.15). Repeated ophthalmologic examination and CT are indicated only in this high-risk group.

The coincidence of seizures and facial vascular nevus should suggest the diagnosis of Sturge-Weber syndrome, which can be confirmed by CT scan (Fig. 15.16). These scans may be normal at birth, but subsequently show areas of gyriform contrast enhancement corresponding to the leptomeningeal angiomatosis. Serial examinations often demonstrate progressive ipsilateral cerebral atrophy. Additional findings may include serpiginous calcifications of brain parenchyma underlying vascular malformations of the pia. These intracranial calcifications are first seen on CT scan but become evident on plain skull films by the end of the second decade.

Associated ocular abnormalities are often encountered. Buphthalmos or coloboma may be present at birth, and glaucoma frequently develops in infancy or later childhood (Fig. 15.17). Dilated vessels in the sclera, conjunctiva, and retina are common, while angiomatous malformations of the choroid occasionally occur.

The estimated incidence of facial cutaneous angioma is 1 in 5,000, and the estimated frequency of the complete syndrome is 1 in 30,000. Among patients with the complete syndrome, seizures occur in 90 percent and contralateral hemiparesis eventually develops in one third. While most cases are sporadic, genetic determination has not been ruled out. There are, however, no reported cases of direct transmission from parent to child.

Ataxia Telangiectasia

Ataxia telangiectasia is a multisystem, autosomal-recessive degenerative disorder characterized by ataxia, oculocutaneous telangiectasia, immunodeficiency, and a high incidence of neoplasia. The nature of the basic underlying defect is unknown.

Ataxia is the usual presenting feature, and the course of the neurologic disturbance is rather stereotypic. Tremors of the head may be seen before 1 year of age, and unsteadiness of gait is evident when the child first walks. Progressive global ataxia and slurred, scanning, dysarthric speech are typical during the early school-age years. Loss of deep-tendon reflexes and impairment of position and vibratory sensation are evident by the end of the first decade. Adolescence is marked by choreoathetosis, dystonic posturing, gaze apraxia, and progressive dementia.

The characteristic cutaneous manifestations of this disorder appear by 6 years of age. Telangiectases first appear on the bulbar conjunctivae (Fig. 15.18), and develop later over the malar regions, ears, antecubital fossae, neck, and upper chest.

Neuropathologic changes are widespread, with the cerebellum being the site of maximal degeneration. Loss of Purkinje and basket cells, thinning of the granular cell layer, and mild changes in the molecular layer are characteristic findings.

Systemic manifestations include major defects in both cellular and humoral immunity. Deficiencies of IgA and IgM are characteristic, and together with impaired cellular immunity, contribute to susceptibility to the recurrent respiratory infections which mark this disorder (see Chapter 4, Allergy and Immunology).

Linear Sebaceous Nevus

The sebaceous nevus of Jadassohn is usually present at birth, presenting as a yellow-tan, waxy linear lesion (Fig. 15.19) which contains a papillomatous excess of sebaceous glands. This nevus may be found on the scalp, face, neck, trunk, or

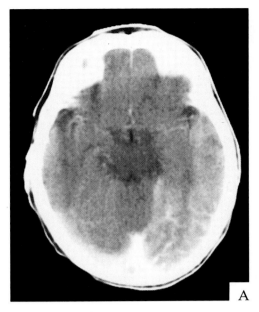

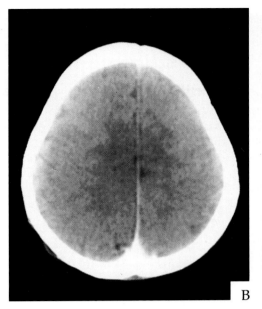

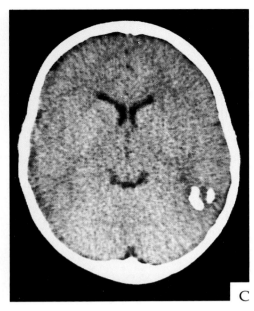

FIG. 15.16 Sturge-Weber syndrome. Although the CT scan is usually normal at birth, findings such as gyriform contrast enhancement, seen here in the left occipital, temporal, and parietal lobes *A,* and associated hemispheric atrophy *B,* may be observed by age 4 months. *C,* serpigi-

nous parenchymal calcifications may be observed in the older child. (Courtesy of Division of Neuroradiology, University Health Center of Pittsburgh)

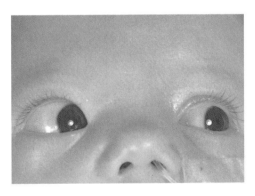

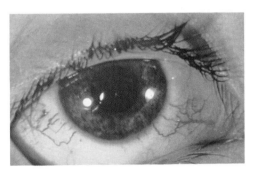

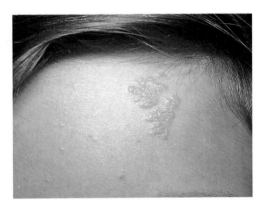

FIG. 15.17 Buphthalmos. Enlargement of the cornea of right eye is evident. This is one of the associated ocular findings in Sturge-Weber syndrome. (From Booth IW, Wozniak ER: Pediatrics. Baltimore, Williams & Wilkins, 1984, 32)

FIG. 15.18 Ataxia telangiectasia. Such telangiectases in the bulbar conjunctiva usually develop between 3 months and 6 years of age.

FIG. 15.19 Linear sebaceous nevus of Jadassohn. This yellow-tan, waxy-appearing lesion became elevated at puberty and was associated with seizures and mental retardation.

extremities. With time, the lesion becomes unsightly. This phenomenon as well as a 15 to 20 percent risk of malignant degeneration has led practitioners to recommend early surgical excision. While this lesion usually occurs as an isolated abnormality in otherwise normal individuals, an association with seizures and mental retardation has been reported. The risk of associated neurologic abnormalities is greatest when the cutaneous lesion is located in the midfacial area.

CENTRAL NERVOUS SYSTEM MALFORMATIONS

Malformations of the central nervous system are a leading cause of neurologic and developmental disability in infants and children. Although CNS malformations are not necessarily accompanied by external dysmorphic features, distur-

bances of cranial volume, abnormalities of head shape, and skin lesions overlying the dorsal midline should alert the physician to the possibility of associated CNS dysmorphogenesis.

Macrocephaly

Macrocephaly is defined as a head circumference greater than two standard deviations above the mean for age, sex, and gestation. It is a phenomenon which can be caused by a myriad of conditions (Fig. 15.20), including excessive accumulation of cerebrospinal fluid (hydrocephalus); intracranial mass lesions (tumors, subdural effusions); thickening or enlargement of the skull (primary skeletal dysplasias); or a true increase in brain substance (megalencephaly) such as is seen in Soto syndrome, achondroplasia, the neurocutaneous syndromes, and certain

Early Infantile (Birth to 6 Months)

Hydrocephalus (progressive or arresting)
    Induction disorders (congenital malformations)
        Spina bifida cystica, cranium bifidum, Chiari
        malformations (types I, II, and III), aqueductal
        stenosis, holoprosencephaly
    Mass lesions
        Neoplasms, A-V malformations, congenital cysts
    Intrauterine infections
        Toxoplasmosis, cytomegalic inclusion disease,
        syphilis, rubella

Peri- or postnatal infections
    Bacterial, granulomatous, parasitic
Peri- or postnatal hemorrhage
    Hypoxia, vascular malformation, trauma
Hydranencephaly
Subdural effusion
    Hemorrhagic, infectious, cystic hygroma
Normal variant (often familial)

Late Infantile (6 Months to 2 Years)

Hydrocephalus (progressive or arresting)
    Space occupying lesions
        Tumors, cysts, abscesses
    Postbacterial or granulomatous meningitis
    Dysraphism
        Dandy-Walker syndrome, Chiari Type I
        malformation
    Posthemorrhagic
        Trauma or vascular malformation
Subdural effusion
Increased intracranial pressure syndrome
    Pseudotumor cerebri
        Lead, tetracycline, hypoparathyroidism,
        steroids, excess or deficiency of vitamin A,
        cyanotic congenital heart disease
Primary skeletal cranial dysplasia (thickened or
    enlarged skull), osteogenesis imperfecta,
    hyperphosphatemia, osteopetrosis, rickets

Megalencephaly (increase in brain substance)
    Metabolic CNS diseases: Leukodystrophies (e.g.,
        Canavan, Alexander), lipidoses (Tay-Sachs),
        histiocytosis, mucopolysaccharidoses
    Proliferative neurocutaneous syndromes
        von Recklinghausen, tuberous sclerosis,
        hemangiomatosis, Sturge-Weber
    Cerebral gigantism
        Soto syndrome
    Achondroplasia
    Primary megalencephaly
        May be familial, and unassociated or associated
        with abnormalities of cellular architecture

Early to Late Childhood (After 2 Years)

Hydrocephalus (arrested or progressive)
    Space-occupying lesions
    Preexisting induction disorder
        Aqueductal stenosis, Chiari Type I malformation
    Postinfectious
    Hemorrhagic

Megalencephaly
    Proliferative neurocutaneous syndromes
    Familial
Pseudotumor cerebri
Normal variant

(From Gabriel RS: Malformations of the central nervous system, in Menkes JH (ed): Textbook of Child Neurology, ed 2. Philadelphia, Lea & Febiger, 1980)

FIG. 15.20

lipidoses, leukodystrophies, and mucopolysaccharidoses. Primary megalencephaly may occur as a benign familial trait.

Evaluation of the child with a head which is abnormally large or which appears to be growing at an excessive rate should include:

1. Evaluation of serial measurements of head circumference.
2. Measurement of the parents' head circumferences and exploration of family history for evidence of macrocephaly or neurologic and cutaneous abnormalities.
3. Developmental history.
4. Careful examination for evidence of increased intracranial pressure, developmental delay, skeletal dysplasia, abnormal transillumination, cranial bruits, ocular abnormalities, or organomegaly.

Plain skull x-rays may provide evidence of increased intracranial pressure (see Fig. 15.34), identify intracranial calcification (Fig. 15.21), or detect primary skeletal dysplasias (Fig. 15.22). CT or MRI allow assessment of ventricular size

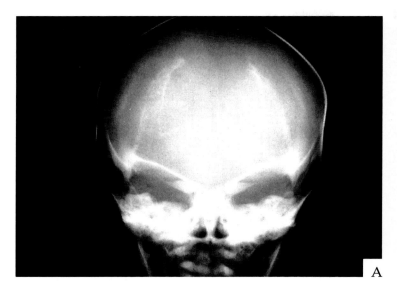

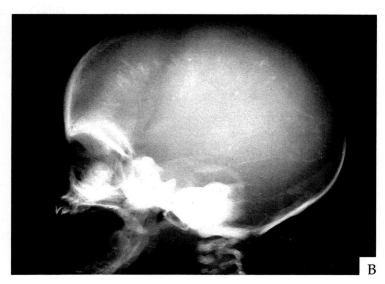

A

B

FIG. 15.21 Macrocephaly. **A,** frontal and **B,** lateral radiographs reveal bilaterally symmetrical, paraventricular cerebral calcifications in asso-

ciation with cranial enlargement. (Courtesy of Department of Radiology, Children's Hospital of Pittsburgh)

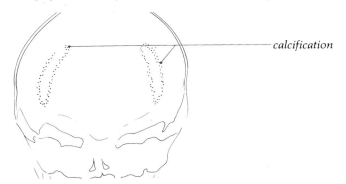

calcification

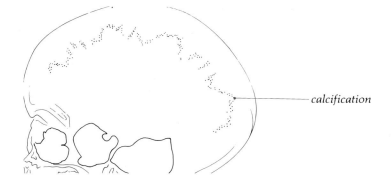

calcification

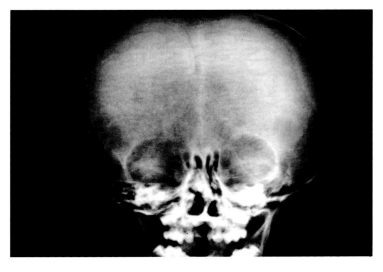

FIG. 15.22 Macrocephaly. Plain skull radiographs allow detection of primary skeletal dysplasias. In this case note the mosaic rarification of the cranial vault and multiple wormian bones characteristic of osteogenesis imperfecta. (Courtesy of Department of Radiology, Children's Hospital of Pittsburgh)

and permit detection of intracranial mass lesions and chronic subdural effusions. CT is the method of choice for demonstration of intracranial calcification and detection of fresh blood.

HYDROCEPHALUS

Hydrocephalus is an imbalance between cerebrospinal fluid (CSF) production and resorption of sufficient magnitude to result in a net accumulation of fluid within the ventricular system. Impaired CSF resorption may occur secondary to obstruction of CSF pathways within the ventricular system (noncommunicating hydrocephalus) or as a result of obstruction of the subarachnoid space (communicating hydrocephalus). Hydrocephalus secondary to CSF overproduction is rare, but does occur in some cases of choroid plexus papilloma (see Fig. 15.38). Noncommunicating hydrocephalus is often due to aqueductal stenosis or congenital malformations of the fourth ventricle, and accompanies tumors or vascular malformations of the posterior fossa which compress the cerebral aqueduct or obstruct outflow from the fourth ventricle. Causes of communicating hydrocephalus include intracranial hemorrhage, meningitis, cerebral venous or dural sinus thrombosis, and diffuse infiltration of the meninges by malignant cells.

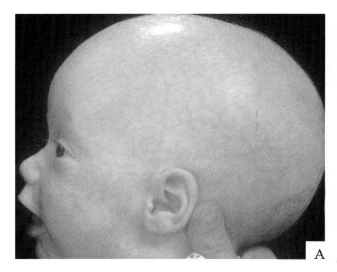
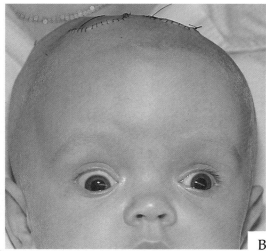

FIG. 15.23 Infantile hydrocephalus. **A,** characteristic enlarged head, thinning of the scalp, distended scalp veins, and a full fontanelle. **B,** paresis of upward gaze is seen in an infant with hydrocephalus due to aqueductal stenosis. It appears more apparent on the right. This phenomenon is often termed the "sunsetting" sign. (**A,** from Booth IW, Wozniak ER: Pediatrics. Williams & Wilkins, Baltimore, 1984, 108. **B,** courtesy of Dr. Albert Biglan, Children's Hospital of Pittsburgh)

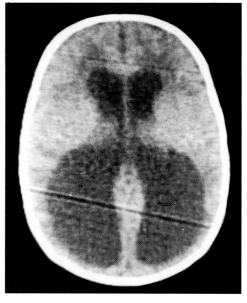

FIG. 15.24 Infantile hydrocephalus. CT scan demonstrates a dilated ventricular system and thinning of the cortical mantle. (Courtesy of Division of Neuroradiology, University Health Center of Pittsburgh)

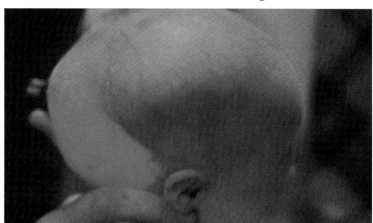

FIG. 15.25 Dandy-Walker malformation. Transillumination demonstrates a posterior fossa cyst. Note also the bulging occiput, prominent scalp veins, and enlargement of the head. (Courtesy of Dr. Michael J. Painter)

The clinical manifestations of hydrocephalus in infancy are stereotypic. The head is either excessively large at birth or grows at an abnormally rapid rate, becoming macrocephalic over the first few months. The forehead is disproportionally large, and the face appears small in relation to the calvarium. The scalp is thin and glistening; its veins are distended, often becoming strikingly dilated when the infant cries. The anterior fontanelle is large, tense, and nonpulsatile, and the sutures are excessively wide (Fig. 15.23). Divergent strabismus, abducens nerve paresis, and impaired upgaze are important ocular findings. With severe hydrocephalus there may be involuntary, forced, conjugate, downward deviation of the eyes so that the inferior half of the iris is hidden by the lower eyelid, producing the "sunsetting" sign(Fig. 15.23B). Neurologic abnormalities include developmental delay, persistence of early infantile automatisms, and spasticity and hyperreflexia of the lower extremities.

CT or MRI will demonstrate enlargement of the ventricular system and thinning of the cortical mantle, and may provide additional anatomic information concerning etiology (Fig. 15.24).

Infantile hydrocephalus must be distinguished from other causes of macrocephaly in infancy such as chronic subdural hematoma, expanding porencephalic cyst, and certain degenerative disorders which may produce abnormal enlargement of the head (see Fig. 15.20). In premature infants with suspected hydrocephalus, the normally rapid postnatal head growth must be taken into account.

DANDY-WALKER MALFORMATION

Dandy-Walker malformation is a primary developmental abnormality characterized by progressive cystic enlargement of the fourth ventricle beginning early in fetal life. This is accompanied by enlargement of the posterior fossa and upward displacement of the tentorium, torcula, and transverse sinuses. Associated hydrocephalus is almost universal, and may be present at birth or develop later during infancy or childhood. Of affected individuals, 60 percent show signs of hydrocephalus and increased intracranial pressure by 2 years of age.

Clinical manifestations of Dandy-Walker malformation are variable, and depend upon the severity and rate of progression of the associated hydrocephalus. Symptomatic children often have an unusually prominent bulging occiput in addition to the usual findings of hydrocephalus. In children under 1 year of age, transillumination of the skull effectively demonstrates

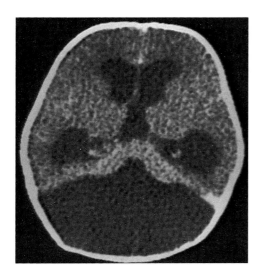

FIG. 15.26 Dandy-Walker malformation. CT scan shows a posterior fossa cyst, a small cerebellar remnant, and associated hydrocephalus.

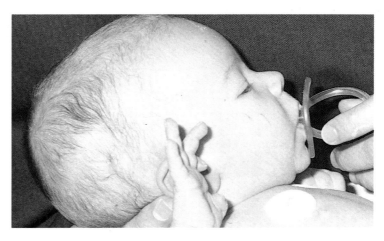

FIG. 15.27 Hydranencephaly. Patient, age 3 weeks, has a deceptively normal appearance with little to suggest a severe brain abnormality.

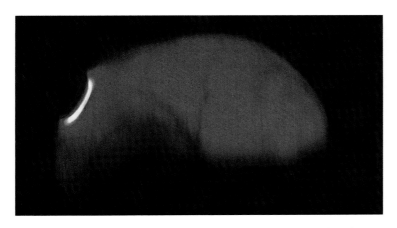

FIG. 15.28 Hydranencephaly. Transillumination of the skull lights up the calvarium, suggesting the diagnosis.

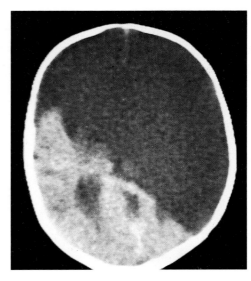

FIG. 15.29 Hydranencephaly. CT scan demonstrates replacement of the cerebral hemispheres by a large water-dense cavity with residual islands of brain tissue in regions of the occipital poles and right inferior temporal lobe. (Courtesy of Division of Neuroradiology, University Health Center of Pittsburgh)

the posterior fossa cyst (Fig. 15.25). Ataxia, nystagmus, and cranial nerve deficits may also be prominent.

Plain skull x-rays demonstrate posteroinferior enlargement of the cranial vault, thinning and ballooning of the occipital squama, and upward displacement of the torcula. CT or MRI will confirm the presence of a large posterior fossa cyst along with a small cerebellar remnant and associated hydrocephalus (Fig. 15.26).

Hydranencephaly

Hydranencephaly is a severe anomaly of the brain characterized by the absence of the cerebral hemispheres despite intact meninges and a normal skull. Affected children often appear deceptively normal at birth, with little to suggest the presence of a severe brain abnormality (Fig. 15.27). Since newborn infants function at a subcortical reflex level, even complete absence of the cerebral hemispheres may not interfere with normal reflexes. However, within the first few weeks of life, developmental arrest, decerebration, hypertonia, and hyperreflexia become apparent in the hydranencephalic infant. Most do not live beyond 6 to 12 months, although survival for several years is occasionally reported. Seizures are common, and progressive enlargement of the head may complicate nursing care.

Diagnosis may be suggested if, on transillumination of the skull, the entire calvarium is lit up (Fig. 15.28). It must be noted, however, that severe hydrocephalus and bilateral subdural hygromas may present a similar appearance.

CT scan demonstrates a large water-dense cavity replacing the cerebral hemispheres with islands of residual brain tissue at the base (Fig. 15.29). To distinguish this disorder from massive bilateral subdural hygromas, cerebral angiography is required to confirm absence of the cerebrum.

Microcephaly

Microcephaly is defined as a head circumference which is more than two standard deviations below the mean for age, sex, and gestation. Apart from cases due to premature closure of the sutures (generalized craniosynostosis), microcephaly reflects an abnormally small brain, and can be a symptom of any disorder which impairs brain growth (Fig. 15.30). The neurologic manifestations range from minor (poor fine motor

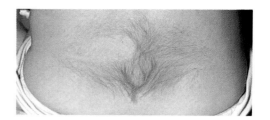

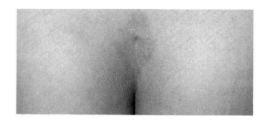

CAUSES OF MICROCEPHALY

Genetic defects
  Autosomal-recessive
  Autosomal-dominant

Disorders of karyotype
  Trisomies
  Deletions
  Translocations

Intrauterine infections
  Rubella
  Cytomegalic inclusion disease
  Toxoplasmosis
  Congenital syphilis
  Herpes virus

Prenatal irradiation

Exposure to drugs and chemicals during gestation
  Ethyl alcohol (fetal alcohol syndrome)
  Phenytoin
  Trimethadione
  Methyl mercury

Maternal phenylketonuria

Perinatal insults
  Traumatic
  Anoxic
  Metabolic
  Infectious

FIG. 15.30

FIG. 15.31 Occult spinal dysraphism. Note hairy patch over lumbar region, here associated with diastematomyelia. (Courtesy of Dr. Michael J. Painter)

FIG. 15.32 Occult spinal dysraphism. Sacral sinus tract associated with intraspinal dermoid tumor. (Courtesy of Dr. Michael J. Painter)

FIG. 15.33 Occult spinal dysraphism. CT scan demonstrates an intraspinal lipoma in a child who presented with a subcutaneous lipoma over the lumbar spine.

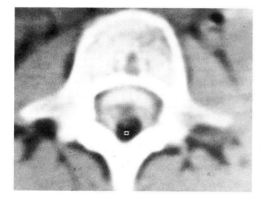

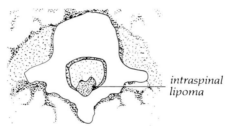

intraspinal lipoma

skills, mild intellectual impairment) to profound (decerebration, chronic vegetative state). Diagnostic evaluation should include family history, prenatal history, search for associated congenital anomalies, karyotyping, amino acid screening, and serologic studies for intrauterine infection. Plain skull x-rays can detect craniosynostosis, while CT scan is most useful in identifying intracranial calcifications. MRI is preferred for delineation of recognizable patterns of central nervous system dysmorphogenesis.

Occult Spinal Dysraphism

Development of the human nervous system begins early in the third week of gestation with proliferation of ectodermal cells in the dorsal midline to form the neural plate. By the end of the fourth week, the neural plate has invaginated and then fused in the midline to form the neural tube. The cerebrum, diencephalon, midbrain, and brainstem will develop from the rostral portion of the neural tube. The caudal portion separates from the overlying ectoderm forming the precursor of the spinal cord and becomes surrounded by mesodermal elements destined to form the vertebral bodies and supporting soft-tissue structures. Midline spinal cord/vertebral skeletal defects,

termed "spinal dysraphism," result from defective closure of the caudal neural tube. Abnormal neural tube closure beginning early in the embryologic sequence produces dysraphic states which involve both neural and skeletal elements (myelomeningocele), while later-occurring closure defects produce congenital anomalies restricted to the posterior elements of the vertebrae (spina bifida occulta).

Occult spinal dysraphism is a defect of intermediate severity in which vertebral anomalies are associated with underlying intraspinal tumors or developmental abnormalities. Its presence is often betrayed by cutaneous abnormalities such as a hairy patch (Fig. 15.31), skin tag, port wine stain, hemangioma, subcutaneous lipoma, or sinus tract (Fig. 15.32). Patients found to have such skin lesions overlying the lumbosacral spine should have spinal radiographs taken. If these reveal underlying vertebral abnormalities, neuroradiologic investigations are indicated, as early surgical intervention can prevent the development of progressive neurologic deficits. Common intraspinal lesions include dermoid tumors, intraspinal lipomas (Fig. 15.33), and diastematomyelia.

While some patients with occult spinal dysraphism may show signs of neurologic dysfunction and talipes equinovarus from birth, most develop symptoms insidiously after a symp-

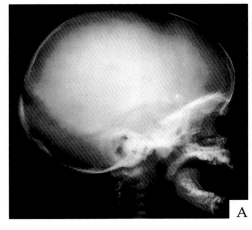 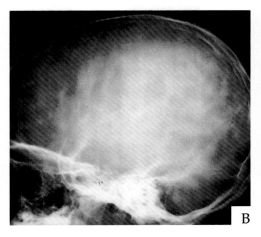 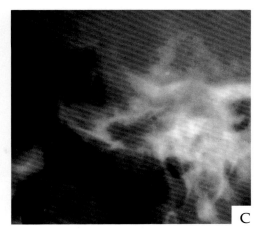

FIG. 15.34 Findings of increased intracranial pressure that may be seen on standard skull radiographs. **A**, widening of the cranial structures. **B**, prominent convolutional markings on the inner table of the skull (beaten silver skull). **C**, erosion of the sella turcica, in this case due to a craniopharyngioma. (**A**, Courtesy of Department of Neuroradiology, University Health Center of Pittsburgh. **B** and **C**, courtesy of Dr. Jocelyn Medina, Children's Hospital of Pittsburgh)

from birth, most develop symptoms insidiously after a symptom-free interval. Dysfunction usually begins at around 3 years of age, but many do not develop problems until school age or adolescence. Presenting complaints may include back or leg stiffness, clumsiness, mild weakness or numbness of the lower extremities, or problems with bladder dysfunction. Objective findings may consist of decreased tone and deep-tendon reflexes in the lower extremities; patchy decreases in sensation; and foot deformities consisting of broadening and shortening, deepening of the arch, and contractures of the toes. Patients with associated tethering of the spinal cord tend to present during a period of rapid growth with back, leg, or buttock pain; signs of lower limb spasticity; and, on occasion, bowel and bladder dysfunction.

Objective findings may consist of decreased tone and deep-tendon reflexes in the lower extremities; patchy decreases in sensation; and foot deformities consisting of broadening and shortening, deepening of the arch, and contractures of the toes. Patients with associated tethering of the spinal cord tend to present during a period of rapid growth with back, leg, or buttock pain; signs of lower limb spasticity; and, on occasion, bowel and bladder dysfunction.

INCREASED INTRACRANIAL PRESSURE

The cranial cavity is occupied by brain, blood, and cerebrospinal fluid. An increase in the volume of any of these compartments, unless accompanied by a concomitant decrease in one or both of the other compartments, results in increased intracranial pressure. Increased intracranial pressure can result from a wide variety of disorders and is itself hazardous. Recognition of associated signs and symptoms permits early diagnosis and prompt intervention to forestall progressive brain injury or catastrophic neurologic deterioration.

Primary Signs and Symptoms

The clinical manifestations of increased intracranial pressure vary with age. In infants, examination of the anterior fontanelle allows reliable assessment of intracranial pressure. In the normal quiet infant, held in upright or sitting posture, the anterior

fontanelle is either flat or slightly concave. Under these conditions, an anterior fontanelle which bulges above the contour of the calvarium and which is excessively firm on palpation is always abnormal. Because the cranial sutures are not fused in infants and young children, increased intracranial pressure rapidly produces separation of the bony plates of the skull. In infants, this can be detected by palpation; in older children, x-rays of the skull may be needed to identify widened cranial sutures (Fig. 15.34A). Prominent convolutional markings on the inner table of the skull (Fig. 15.34B) are a less useful radiographic sign, as they are frequently seen on skull x-rays of normal children. However, when secondary to increased intracranial pressure, they are preceded by suture diastasis and changes in the sella turcica (Fig. 15.34C). An excessive rate of head growth is a prominent feature of chronically increased intracranial pressure in infants and children up to 3 years of age. Associated findings may include frontal prominence and distended scalp veins. If the ability to accommodate for increased intracranial pressure by expansion of the calvarium is exceeded, other symptoms appear. These may include listlessness, irritability, poor feeding, vomiting, failure to thrive, paresis of upward gaze, increased tone, hyperactive stretch reflexes, and high-pitched cry. Papilledema is uncommon.

In older children and adults, the most consistent clinical features of increased intracranial pressure include headache, vomiting, visual disturbances, and papilledema. Headaches are of variable severity. They may be constant or intermittent and either generalized or localized to frontal, temporal, or occipital head regions. In some cases, they recur on early arising or awakening and are accompanied by vomiting. The headaches may be exacerbated by sneezing, coughing, or straining. Vomiting due to increased intracranial pressure is no different than vomiting from other causes. It is seldom projectile and is not necessarily accompanied by headache.

Horizontal diplopia (double vision) secondary to paralysis of one or both abducens nerves is the most common visual disturbance. Initially double vision may occur only on lateral gaze toward the side of the paretic lateral rectus. This may be intermittent and may not be accompanied by limitation of ocular motility sufficient to be seen by the examiner. With progression, diplopia becomes constant and is present even with the eyes in the primary position and an internal strabismus results

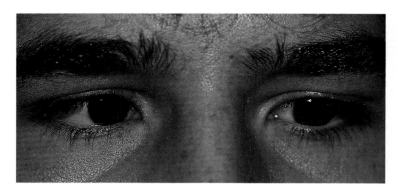

FIG. 15.35 Left abducens (sixth cranial nerve) palsy. This boy presented with headaches and diplopia and was found to have papilledema and a left abducens palsy. Note that his left eye cannot move past the midline on left lateral gaze. (Courtesy of Dr. Kenneth Cheng, Children's Hospital Pittsburgh)

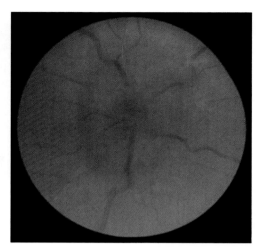

FIG. 15.36 Papilledema. Fundus photograph shows blurring of the optic disk margin, elevation and hyperemia of the optic nerve head, and distention of the retinal blood vessels. (Courtesy of Dr. Kenneth Cheng, Children's Hospital of Pittsburgh)

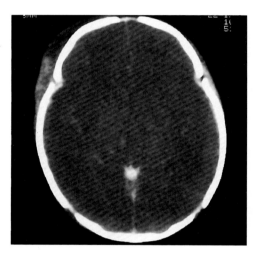

FIG. 15.37 Cerebral edema. CT performed 24 hours after severe hypoxic-ischemic injury. Note obliteration of the cerebral ventricles, loss of gray-white differentiation, and homogeneous "ground-glass" appearance. (Courtesy of Department of Neuroradiology, University Health Center of Pittsburgh)

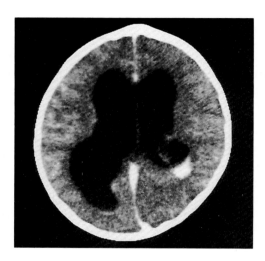

FIG. 15.38 Choroid plexus papilloma. CT of an infant who presented with excessively rapid head growth. There is an enhancing mass within the body of the left lateral ventricle and associated ventricular enlargement (hydrocephalus) secondary to excessive secretion of cerebrospinal fluid by the tumor. (Courtesy of Dr. Michael Painter, Children's Hospital of Pittsburgh)

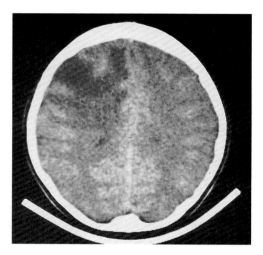

FIG. 15.39 Hemispheric oligodendroglioma. CT scan of patient presenting with seizures demonstrates a low-density mass lesion in the right frontal lobe. (Courtesy of Dr. Michael Painter, Children's Hospital of Pittsburgh)

(Fig. 15.35). Selective vulnerability of the sixth cranial nerve to increased intracranial pressure may be explained by its long intracranial course and proximity to rigid structures. Other visual disturbances may include transient obscurations, visual field deficits, and impaired upgaze.

Sustained intracranial hypertension produces papilledema, a passive swelling of the optic disk (Fig. 15.36). The observation of papilledema in a child with headache, vomiting, or visual disturbances confirms the presence of increased intracranial pressure. Absence of venous pulsations or the presence of associated flame-shaped hemorrhages can help distinguish papilledema from other causes of blurred optic disk margins.

Increased intracranial pressure may be accompanied by changes in personality and behavior, deteriorating school performance, decreased appetite and activity, and alterations in level of consciousness.

Causes of Increased Intracranial Pressure

Causes of increased intracranial pressure include cerebral edema, mass lesions, trauma, CNS infections, pseudotumor cerebri, and hydrocephalus.

Cerebral edema (Fig. 15.37), an expansion of brain volume due to an increase in brain content of water and salt, is a response of brain tissue to a variety of insults. Vasogenic cerebral edema results from the alterations in vascular permiability produced by brain tumor, trauma, abscess, and hemorrhage. Cytotoxic cerebral edema, caused by swelling of brain cells (neurons and glia) is usually caused by infection, hypoxia, ischemia, or toxins.

Intracranial mass lesions (tumor, hemorrhage, abscess, vascular malformations) produce increased intracranial pressure by (1) occupying space; (2) causing cerebral edema; (3) obstructing cerebrospinal fluid pathways; and (4) altering

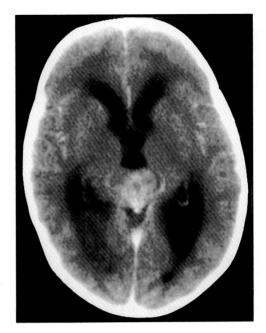

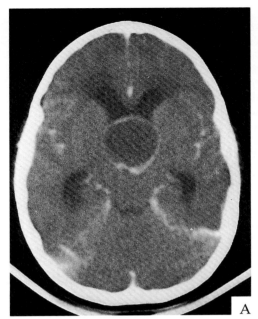

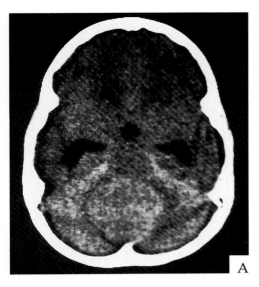

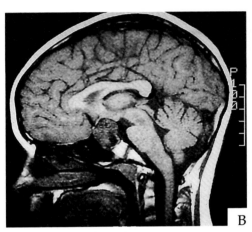

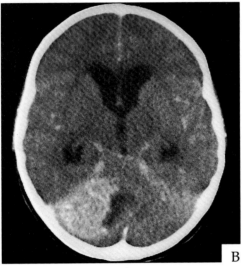

FIG. 15.40 Pineal region tumor. CT scan of a patient who presented with headache, lethargy, and vomiting and paresis of upward gaze shows an enhancing mass in the pineal region and severe obstructive hydrocephalus (Courtesy of Department of Neuroradiology, University Health Center of Pittsburgh)

FIG. 15.41 Craniopharyngiom. **A,** CT scan shows a large spherical suprasellar mass, obliteration of the third ventricle, and associated hydrocephalus. **B,** MRI provides superior visualization of the anatomic relations of this tumor to the optic chiasm and hypothalamus. (Courtesy of Department of Neuroradiology, University Health Center of Pittsburgh)

FIG. 15.42 Cerebellar neoplasms. **A,** midline ependymoma filling the fourth ventricle and invading the cerebellar vermis. **B,** glioblastoma of the right cerebellar hemisphere. (**A,** courtesy of Dr. Michael Painter, Children's Hospital of Pittsburgh, **B,** courtesy of Department of Neuroradiology, University of Health Center of Pittsburgh)

blood flow. Choroid plexus papillomas, by virtue of secreting a large excess of cerebrospinal fluid, cause communicating hydrocephalus (Fig. 15.38). Although astrocytomas of the cerebral hemispheres (Fig. 15.39) most often present with seizures or contralateral motor difficulties, symptoms of increased intracranial pressure are the initial manifestations in 37 percent of cases and are present at the time of diagnosis in 80 percent. Pineal region tumors (Fig. 15.40) frequently obstruct the third ventricle or cerebral aqueduct, producing signs and symptoms of increased intracranial pressure accompanied by *Parinaud's syndrome* (impairment of upgaze with preservation of downgaze and retraction-convergence nystagmus with attempted upgaze) due to compression of the periaqueductal grey (see Fig. 15.23B). Hypothalamic region tumors such as

craniopharyngioma (Fig. 15.41) present with growth retardation or failure of sexual maturation accompanied by visual field defects due to compression of the optic chiasm. Hydrocephalus occurs in 25 percent.

Headache and vomiting accompanied by disturbances of gait and coordination are frequent presenting manifestations of posterior fossa tumors such as cerebellar astrocytoma, medulloblastoma, and ependymoma. Midline tumors involving the cerebellar vermis can produce truncal ataxia (Fig. 15.42A), whereas mass lesions of the cerebellar hemispheres often cause unilateral limb ataxia and horizontal nystagmus (Fig. 15.42B). The cardinal manifestations of brainstem glioma are cranial nerve palsies associated with contralateral hemiplegia and ataxia. Increased intracranial pressure is not an early feature.

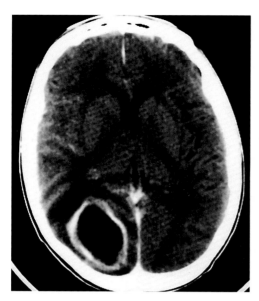

FIG. 15.43 Brain abscess. CT scan demonstrates a low-density mass lesion with an enhancing rim and surrounding edema in an immuno-suppressed patient with an Aspergillus abscess. Bacterial abscesses and neoplasms can present a similar CT appearance. (Courtesy of Department of Neuroradiology, University Health Center of Pittsburgh)

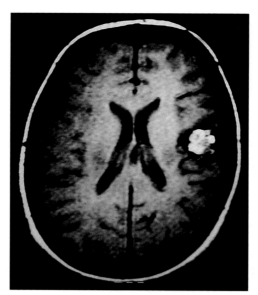

FIG. 15.44 Intracranial hemorrhage. Enhanced MRI demonstrating a cerebral hemangioma with associated old hemorrhage. (Courtesy of Dr. Michael Painter, Children's Hospital of Pittsburgh)

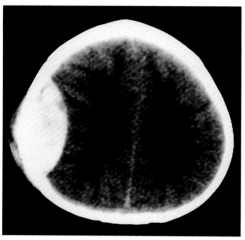

FIG. 15.45 Epidural hematoma. Blunt head trauma followed by vomiting, progressive obtundation, and decreased movement of the left arm and leg. CT scan shows a large lens-shaped epidural hematoma over the right hemisphere. (Courtesy of Department of Neuroradiology, University Health Center of Pittsburgh.

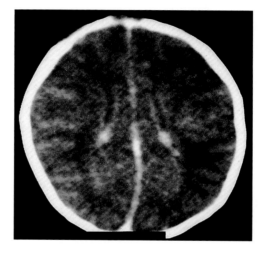

FIG. 15.46 Bacterial meningitis. Infant with fever, lethargy, nuchal rigidity, and tense distended fontanelle. CT scan shows contrast enhancement of the cortical gyri and ependyma of the lateral ventricles. (Courtesy of Department of Neuroradiology, University Health Center of Pittsburgh)

Brain abscesses (Fig. 15.43) are uncommon in the absence of predisposing factors such as chronic otitis or sinusitus, chronic pulmonary infection, dental abscesses, cyanotic congenital heart disease, or immunosuppression. Unless accompanied by prodromal symptoms of fever, headache, lethargy, and malaise, brain abscesses may be impossible to distinguish from other intracranial mass lesions on clinical grounds.

Spontaneous intracranial hemorrhage (Fig. 15.44) secondary to rupture of a vascular malformation or arterial aneurysm is rare in the pediatric population. Leakage of small amounts of blood into the subarachnoid space produces symptoms (fever, hesdache, stiff neck) that mimic bacterial meningitis. In such cases, the correct diagnosis may be first suspected when lumber puncture yields grossly bloody fluid. The presentation of large subarachnoid hemorrhages is catastrophic, with sudden onset of excruciating headache followed by collapse and evidence of increased intracranial pressure.

Head trauma results in increased intracranial pressure by provoking cerebral edema or causing intracranial hemorrhage. The modes of presentation of cerebral contusion, subdural hematoma, and post-traumatic cerebral edema are discussed in Chapter 6. Features of epidural hematoma (Fig. 15.45) in childhood which differ from those encountered in adults bear emphasis here. Infants and young children with epidural hematoma frequently will not have suffered immediate loss of consciousness following the traumatic event. Associated linear skull fractures are less common than in adults, and the source of bleeding into the epidural space is generally ruptured

epidural veins rather than lacerations of the middle meningeal artery. Often, persistent lethargy and intermittent vomiting are the only initial signs. Headache, papilledema, and localizing signs may not emerge for several hours to several days. Once neurologic signs and symptoms do appear they may progress rapidly to coma and death or evolve slowly over several days before producing brainstem compression.

Bacterial meningitis (Fig. 15.46) produces increased intracranial pressure by causing cerebral edema and impairing reabsorption of cerebrospinal fluid. Signs and symptoms are discussed in Chapter 12, Infectious Diseases. While cerebral edema and intracranial hypertension may complicate the course of viral encephalitis, the usual presentation is with seizures, behavioral change, and altered level of consciousness.

Pseudotumor cerebri is a syndrome of increased intracranial pressure which occurs in the absence of hydrocephalus or an intracranial mass. Pseudotumor cerebri is associated with the use of certain drugs (steroids, tetracycline, vitamin A, oral contraceptives), occurs as a complication of otitis media or sinusitis, and can be caused by a variety of endocrine and metabolic disturbances. However, in many instances it is idiopathic. The presenting symptom is headache. Papilledema is the rule and abducens nerve palsy is not uncommon (see Figures 15.35 and 15.36). There may be associated nausea and vomiting, but most children do not appear acutely ill. Progressive papilledema may lead to optic atrophy and treatment is essential to prevent loss of vision. Pseudotumor cerebri is a diagnosis of

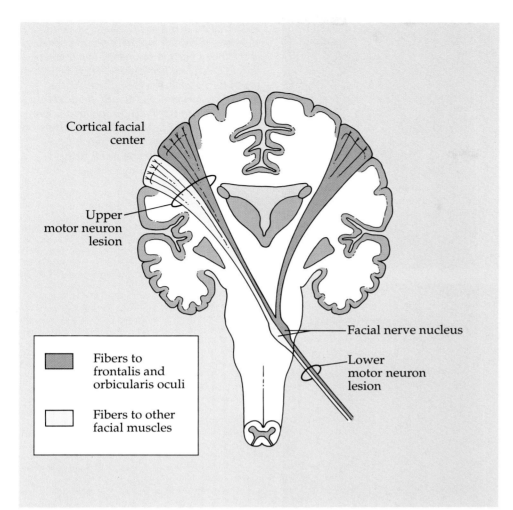

FIG. 15.47 Central motor control of facial muscles. The portion of the facial nerve nucleus which supplies the lower half of the face receives predominantly crossed fibers originating from the opposite cerebral hemisphere; that portion which innervates the upper half receives fibers from both cerebral hemispheres. (Modified by permission from Haymaker W: Bing's Local Diagnosis in Neurological Diseases, ed 15. St. Louis, CV Mosby, 1969)

Cortical facial center

Upper motor neuron lesion

Facial nerve nucleus

Lower motor neuron lesion

Fibers to frontalis and orbicularis oculi

Fibers to other facial muscles

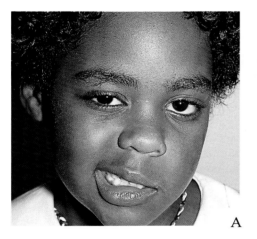
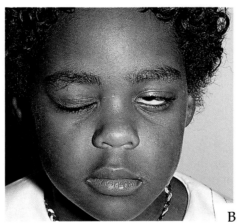

A B

FIG. 15.48 Peripheral facial weakness. Flaccid weakness of entire left face due to a lesion of the left facial nerve. A, flattening of nasolabial fold and inability to retract the corner of the mouth. B, inability to fully close the eye.

exclusion. CT scan or MRI must be done to rule out hydrocephalus or a mass lesion. Examination of the cerebrospinal fluid is unremarkable apart from increased opening pressure.

FACIAL WEAKNESS

The cortical motor center controlling muscles of facial expression is located in the lower third of the precentral gyrus (Fig. 15.47). Motor fibers arising in the cerebral cortex travel through the corona radiata, internal capsule, and cerebral peduncle into the pons, where the majority decussate to supply the facial (VIIth) nerve nucleus on the opposite side. Some fibers, destined to terminate in that portion of the facial nerve nucleus which innervates muscles in the upper half of the face,

do not decussate. Thus, while the portion of the facial nerve nucleus which supplies the lower half of the face receives predominantly crossed fibers originating from the opposite cerebral hemisphere, that portion which innervates the frontalis and the orbicularis oculi has bilateral supranuclear control.

Peripheral Facial Weakness

A lesion of the VIIth nerve nucleus or emergent facial nerve results in flaccid weakness of the entire face on the same side. On the affected side the face is smooth with flattening of the nasolabial fold, drooping of the corner of the mouth, and inability to smile, frown, retract the corner of the mouth, wrinkle the forehead, or close the eye (Fig. 15.48). Causes of periph-

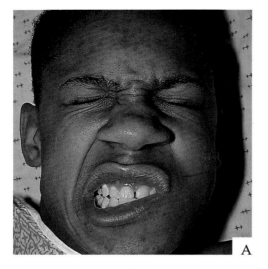

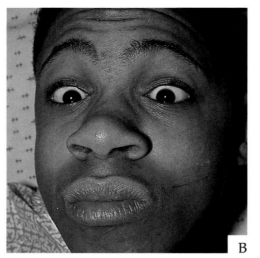

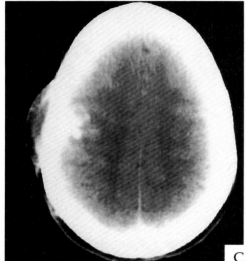

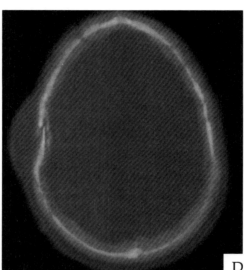

FIG. 15.49 *Central facial weakness.* **A** and **B**, *weakness of the left face with relative sparing of the upper portion secondary to a lesion of the right cerebral hemisphere. There is flattening of the nasolabial fold and inability to retract the corner of the mouth, while ability to close the eye and wrinkle the forehead is preserved.* **C** *and* **D** *CT scans shows the depressed fracture of the temporal bone which was responsible for this central facial palsy.*

eral facial weakness include infection, trauma, hypertension, cerebellopontine angle mass, tumors of the pons, and acute idiopathic paralysis (Bell's palsy).

Central Facial Weakness

With a lesion above the level of the facial nerve nucleus (i.e. an upper motor neuron lesion), there is weakness of the lower part of the face on the opposite side, but relative sparing of the upper portion of the face so that the ability to wrinkle the forehead (frontalis muscle) and to voluntarily close the eyes (orbicularis oculi) is preserved (Fig. 15.49).

NEUROMUSCULAR DISORDERS

Weakness is the most common presenting symptom of neuromuscular disease. If time is taken to determine the ways in which the weakness interferes with normal activities and uncover the types of tasks that the patient finds difficult, the distribution and severity of muscle weakness can be predicted from the clinical history. Determining the mode of onset and pattern of progression of the symptoms is essential in differential diagnosis and selection of diagnostic studies. Since many neuromuscular disorders are genetically determined, a complete family history must be obtained.

Essential components of the physical examination of patients with neuromuscular disease include inspection, palpation, percussion, evaluation of the deep-tendon reflexes, and assessment of muscle strength. Inspection can reveal muscle wasting and atrophy, abnormal spontaneous activity, and abnormal resting postures. Palpation permits assessment of muscle consistency, determination of muscle tone, and detection of muscle tenderness. Percussion is useful in detecting myotonia. Assessment of muscle strength includes both individual muscle testing and functional evaluation. The strength of individual muscles is recorded using a standardized system:

0–no contraction.
1–flicker or trace contraction.
2–active movement with gravity eliminated.
3–active movement against gravity.
4–active movement against gravity and resistance.
5–normal power.

Functional evaluation of muscle strength is accomplished by observing the patient rising from the floor, rising from a chair, stepping onto a stool, climbing stairs, walking on heels, hopping on toes, and raising the arms above the head. This permits rapid detection of proximal weakness of the hips and shoulders, and distal weakness of the legs.

Duchenne Muscular Dystrophy

The muscular dystrophies are genetically determined disorders characterized by progressive degeneration of skeletal muscle, usually following a latency period of seemingly normal devel-

CLINICAL FEATURES OF THE MUSCULAR DYSTROPHIES

	Duchenne	Becker	Fascioscapulo-humeral	Limb-Girdle	Myotonic
Inheritance	X-linked recessive	X-linked recessive	Autosomal-dominant	Autosomal-recessive	Autosomal-dominant
Age of onset	Early childhood	Late childhood, adolescence	Variable, childhood through early adult life	Childhood to early adult	Highly variable
Pattern of weakness	Pelvic girdle, shoulder girdle	Pelvic girdle, shoulder girdle	Face, shoulder girdle	Pelvic girdle, shoulder girdle	Face, distal limbs
Rate of progression	Rapid	Slow	Very slow	Variable	Variable
Associated features	Pseudohyper-trophy of calves	Pseudohyper-trophy of calves	None	Pseudohyper-trophy rare	Myotonia
Systemic features	Mental retardation, abnormal ECG, cardio-myopathy	Occasional mental retardation	None	None	Frequent mental retardation, heart block, cataracts, premature balding, testicular tubular atrophy, diabetes

FIG. 15.50

opment and function. The various clinical types of muscular dystrophy are traditionally classified on the basis of patterns of inheritance, distribution of initial weakness, age of onset of clinical manifestations, and rate of progression (Fig. 15.50).

Duchenne muscular dystrophy, affecting 1 in 3,500 male births, is characterized by X-linked recessive inheritance: early onset; symmetrical and initially selective involvement of pelvic and pectoral girdles; pseudohypertrophy of the calves; very high levels of activity of certain serum enzymes, notably creatine kinase; and relentless progression leading to wheelchair confinement by adolescence and death owing to cardiorespiratory insufficiency by age 20 years.

Duchenne muscular dystrophy is caused by a deletion mutation affecting the Xp21 region on the short arm of the X-chromosome. Dystrophin, the large cytoskeletal protein normally encoded by this gene locus, is absent from the muscle fibers of patients with Duchenne dystrophy. The precise function of dystrophin in maintaining the integrity of muscle and the mechanism by which dystrophin deficiency produces progressive muscle destruction remain to be determined. Becker muscular dystrophy, an allelic disorder affecting 1 in 30,000 male births, is distinguished clinically by later age of onset, slower rate of progression, and longer survival, and biochemically by the presence of dystrophin of abnormal molecular weight.

Clinical manifestations of Duchenne muscular dystrophy do not usually appear until the second year of life. Early developmental milestones are normally attained, although the first

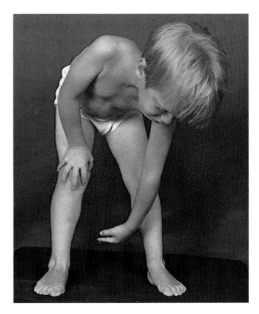

FIG. 15.51 Duchenne muscular dystrophy. This child, age 5, has difficulty rising. Unilateral hand support on the knee is required to get erect.

attempts at walking may be delayed. Gait is often clumsy and awkward from the start, and the ability to run is never normally attained. Difficulty in climbing stairs, frequent falls, and progressive difficulty in rising from the floor are early features. In order to rise from the floor, the child may, at first, need only to push with one hand on a knee (Fig. 15.51). However, as weak-

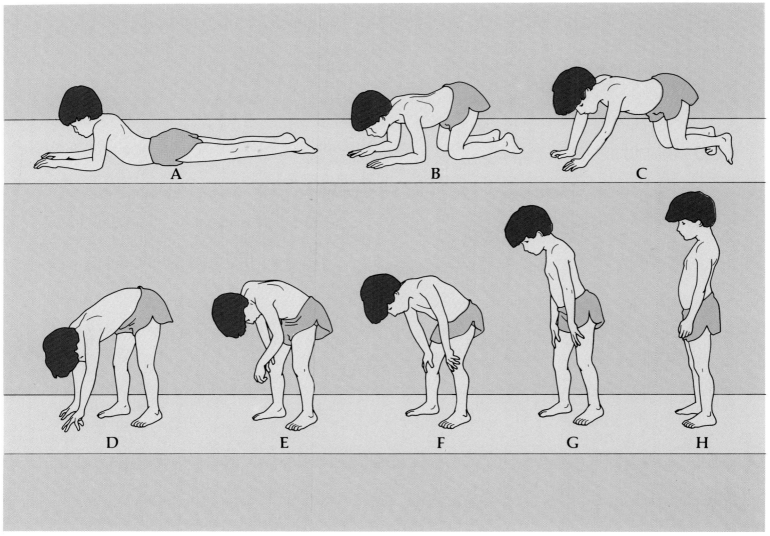

FIG. 15.52 The Gower maneuver. This series of diagrams illustrates the sequence of postures used in attaining the upright position. *A–C,* first the legs are pulled up under the body, and the weight is shifted to rest on the hands and feet. *D,* the hips are then thrust in the air as the knees are straightened and the hands are brought close to the legs. *E–G,* finally, the trunk is slowly extended by the hands walking up the thigh *H,* until the erect position is attained.

ness of the extensors of the hips becomes more pronounced, rising from the floor becomes increasingly difficult and requires the use of the hands to "climb up the legs" (the Gower maneuver) (Fig. 15.52).

Progressive gluteal weakness leads to the assumption of a compensatory posture characterized by a broadened base, accentuated lumbar lordosis, and forward thrusting of the abdomen (Fig. 15.53). Although weakness of the arms is not a common early symptom, proximal upper extremity weakness is easily detected on clinical examination when the child is lifted with the examiner's hands placed beneath the arms. There is marked laxity of the shoulder girdle musculature associated with upward displacement of the shoulders and abnormal rotation of the scapulae(Fig. 15.54A). In addition, spontaneous winging of the scapulae may be prominent (Fig. 15.54B).

Weakness of the neck flexors, as evidenced by marked head lag when pulled to sit from the supine position (Fig. 15.55), is an early finding. Enlargement of muscles, particularly in the calves (Fig. 15.56), is a common feature by 5 or 6 years of age. The abnormally enlarged muscles have an unusually firm rubbery consistency on palpation. Early in the clinical course this increase in muscle volume may be due to true hypertrophy, with muscle strength proportional to bulk. Later, infiltration by fat and connective tissue sometimes maintains this bulk in spite of loss of muscle fibers. This is called "pseudohypertrophy."

Charcot-Marie-Tooth Disease (Hereditary Motor-Sensory Neuropathy, Type I)

Charcot-Marie-Tooth disease is an autosomal-dominant demyelinating form of peroneal muscular atrophy. Onset of symptoms is usually in the second decade, the presenting complaints being foot deformities and gait abnormalities. Often, pes cavus or hammer-toe deformities develop in early childhood long before more overt symptoms appear. The clinical picture is quite variable, and as most affected persons do not consult a physician for their neurologic problems, the majority remain undiagnosed. The astute physician will consider the diagnosis when a patient who presents with unrelated symptoms is found to have pes cavus or hammer toes and symmetrical distal weakness.

Muscle weakness and atrophy begin insidiously in the foot and leg muscles. The intrinsic muscles of the foot are often affected first, followed by involvement of the peronei, anterior

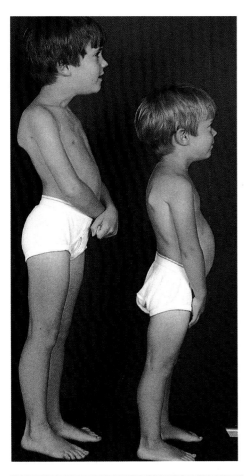

FIG. 15.53 Duchenne muscular dystrophy. These brothers, ages 5 and 8, show progressive compensatory postural adjustments, with broadening of stance, accentuated lumbar lordosis, and forward thrusting of the abdomen.

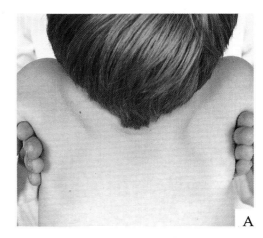

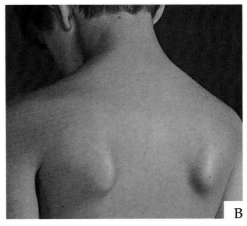

FIG. 15.54 **A,** duchenne muscular dystrophy. This child, age 5, demonstrates weakness and hypotonia of shoulder girdle musculature. Upward displacement of shoulders and abnormal rotation of scapulae are seen when the child is lifted with the examiner's hands under his arms. **B,** spontaneous winging of the scapulae can be noted in this 8-year-old.

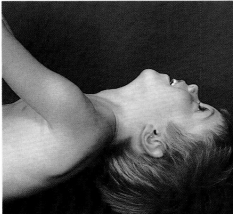

FIG. 15.55 Duchenne muscular dystrophy. This 5-year-old has neck flexor weakness. Note marked head lag when the patient is pulled to sit from the supine position.

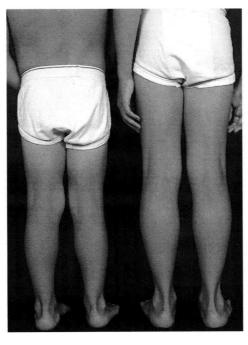

FIG. 15.56 Duchenne muscular dystrophy. Enlargement of calves in brothers ages 5 and 8.

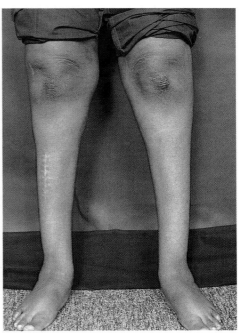

FIG. 15.57 Charcot-Marie-Tooth disease. Patient, age 15, with distal muscular atrophy of the lower extremities ("stork-leg" appearance).

tibial muscles, long toe extensors, intrinsic hand muscles, and gastrocnemius. Weakness and atrophy may spread to the more proximal muscles of the leg and forearm. The degree of muscle wasting is often mild; however, in some cases the loss of muscle mass in the distal lower extremities is severe, giving rise to a striking "stork-leg" appearance (Fig. 15.57). With involvement of the distal upper extremities there may be obvious wasting of the intrinsic hand muscles and development of secondary "claw deformities" (Fig. 15.58). Deep-tendon reflexes are first lost in the gastrocnemius and soleus, and subsequently in the quadriceps femoris and upper limbs. Sensation may be mildly impaired in the distal lower extremities.

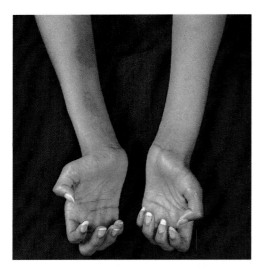

FIG. 15.58 Charcot-Marie-Tooth disease. This 15-year-old demonstrates atrophy of forearm and intrinsic hand muscles and "claw-hand" deformity.

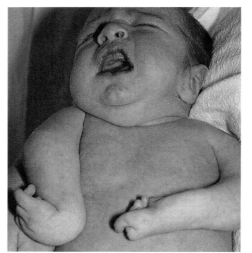

FIG. 15.59 Congenital cervical spinal atrophy. This 2-day-old infant has flaccid paresis limited to the upper extremities and associated congenital flexion contractures.

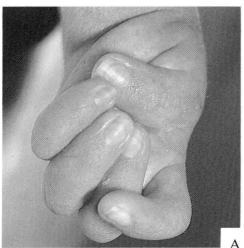

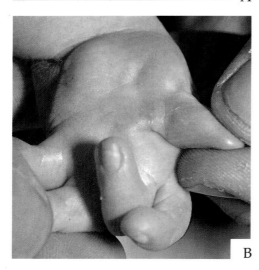

A

B

FIG. 15.60 Congenital cervical spinal atrophy. Wasting and atrophy of intrinsic hand muscles with flexion contractures of the fingers **A**, and poorly developed transverse palmar creases **B**, can be seen in this 2-day-old.

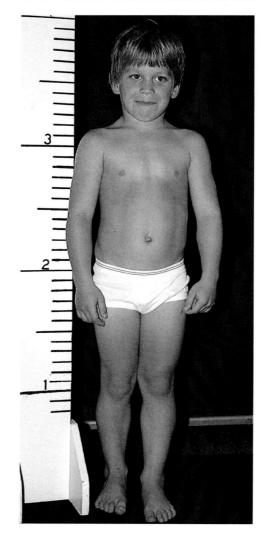

FIG. 15.61 Myotonia congenita. Patient, age 8, demonstrates generalized muscular hypertrophy, giving a well-developed athletic appearance.

Congenital Cervical Spinal Atrophy

This rare disorder presents at birth with dramatic flaccid paresis of the upper extremities (Fig. 15.59). The presence of congenital flexion contractures suggests chronic denervation which must have occurred in utero, and allows this syndrome to be distinguished from injury to the cervical spine or brachial plexuses during delivery (see Chapter 2). Abnormalities in the formation of the transverse palmar creases are present in all cases (Fig. 15.60), suggesting a prenatal insult during the first trimester. The disorder is nonprogressive.

Myotonia Congenita

Myotonia congenita is an inherited disorder of skeletal muscle in which muscle stiffness is the only complaint. Both autosomal-dominant and autosomal-recessive forms occur. The clinical symptoms are rather stereotypic. After a period of inactivity, the muscles stiffen and are difficult to maneuver; however, with continued activity, the stiffness diminishes and movement becomes almost normal. Typically, the child moves clumsily with a stiff awkward gait and falls often. However, as activity continues, he begins to walk freely, and with adequate "warm-up" is able to run without difficulty.

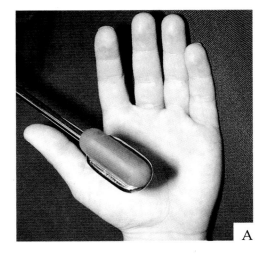
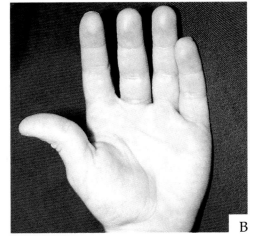

*FIG. 15.62 Myotonia congenita. **A,** percussion of the thenar eminence is followed by **B,** involuntary opposition of the thumb and visible contraction of the thenar muscles which lasts for several seconds.*

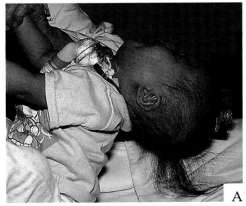
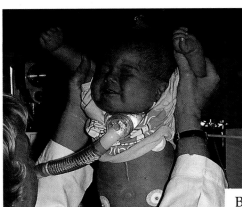

*Fig. 15.63 Hypotonic infant. **A,** abnormal traction response. Head falls into extreme extension. Limbs fail to flex to counter traction. **B,** when held under the arms, the infant tends to slip through the examiner's hands.*

Generalized muscular hypertrophy is a frequent finding on examination, with affected children often presenting an unusually well-developed athletic appearance (Fig. 15.61). This belies their sedentary habits and physical ineptitude due to muscle stiffness. Clinically, the myotonia may be demonstrated following sustained contraction of a group of muscles, as produced by clenching the hand or by percussion of the thenar eminence (Fig. 15.62).

THE HYPOTONIC INFANT

Since depression of postural tone is manifested by paucity of movement, unusual postures, diminished resistance to passive movement, and increased range of movement of joints, the hypotonic infant has been likened to a rag doll. The legs lie externally rotated and abducted, with their lateral surface in contact with the bed while the arms are either extended at the sides or flexed so that the hands lie beside the head. When the infant is pulled by the hands from supine (traction response), the head falls into extreme extension and the limbs fail to flex to counter the traction (Fig. 15.63A). In horizontal suspension, with the chest and abdomen supported by the examiner's hand, the hypotonic infant drapes limply like an inverted "U". When held under the arms, the hypotomic infant tends to slip through the examiner's hands (Fig. 15.63B). Because maintenance of normal postural tone requires functional integrity of both the central and peripheral nervous system, hypotonia is a common symptom of many disorders affecting the brain, spinal cord, peripheral nerve, and muscle (Fig. 15.64). Hypotonia also occurs as a nonspecific manifestation of systemic illness. The term "benign congenital hypotonia" is reserved for infants with isolated depression of postural tone which resolves with growth and maturation, usually by 1 year of age.

THE HYPOTONIC INFANT: DIFFERENTIAL DIAGNOSIS

Disorders of the Central Nervous System	Disorders of Peripheral Nervous System

Chromosome disorders
  Trisomy
  Prader-Willi
    syndrome
  Other
	Spinal muscular atrophies

	Congenital polyneuropathies
Other genetic defects	Transient neonatal myasthenia

Static Encephalopathies
  Congenital
    malformation
  Perinatal acquired
  Post- natal acquired
	Congenital myasthenic
	  syndromes

	Congenital muscular
	  dystrophy
	  Myotonic
	  Fukuyama type
	  Other

Inborn errors of
  metabolism
  Amino acid
  Organic acid
  Urea cycle
  Peroxisomal disorders
  Lysosomal disorders
	Congenital myopathies

	Metabolic myopathies
	Systemic illness

Neonatal spinal cord
  injury
	Benign congenial
	  hypotonia

FIG. 15.64

BIBLIOGRAPHY

Bell WE, McCormick WF: *Increased Intracranial Pressure in Children*, ed 2. Philadelphia, WB Saunders, 1978.

Brooke MH: *A Clinician's View of Neuromuscular Diseases*, ed 2. Baltimore, Williams & Wilkins. 1987.

Chao DH: Congenital neurocutaneous syndromes of childhood. III. Sturge-Weber disease. *J Pediatr* 1959;55:635–649.

Dubozitz V: *The Floppy Infant*, ed 2. Philadelphia, JB Lippincott,1980.

Emery AEH: *Duchenne Muscular Dystrophy.* Oxford, Oxford University Press, 1987.

Enjolras O, Riche MC, Merland JJ: Facial port-wine stains and Sturge-Weber syndrome. *Pediatrics* 1985;76:48–52.

Fenichel GM: *Clinical Pediatric Neurology: A Signs and Symptoms Approach.* Philadelphia, WB Saunders, 1988.

Goldstein SM, Curless RG, Post JD, Quencer RM: A new sign of neurofibromatosis on magnetic resonance imaging of children. *Arch Neurol* 1989:46:1222–1224.

Gomez MR (ed): *Tuberous Sclerosis,* New York. Raven Press, 1979.

Hoffman EP, Fishbeck KH, Brown RH, et al: Characterization of dystrophin in muscle-biopsy specimens from patients with Duchenne's or Becker's muscular dystrophy. *N Engl J Med* 1988; 318:1363–1368.

Martuza RL, Eldridge R: Neurofibromatosis 2. *N Engl J Med* 1988;318:684–688.

Menkes JH: *Textbook of Child Neurology,* ed 3. Philadelphia, Lea & Febiger, 1980.

Osborne JP: Diagnosis of tuberous sclerosis. *Arch Dis Child* 1988;63:1423–1425.

Paller AS: The Sturge-Weber syndrome. *Pediatr Dermatol,* 1987: 4:300–304.

Riccardi VM: Von Recklinghausen neurofibromatosis. *N Engl J Med* 1981;305:1617–1627.

Roach ES, William DP, Laster DW: Magnetic resonance imaging in tuberous sclerosis. *Arch Neurol* 1987:44:301–303.

Swaiman KF: *Pediatric Neurology; Principles and Practice.* St. Louis, CV Mosby, 1989.

Warkany J, Lemire RJ, Cohen MM: *Mental Retardation and Congenital Malformations of the Central Nervous System.* Chicago, Year Book, 1981.

PEDIATRIC PULMONARY DISORDERS

Blake E. Noyes, M.D. ◆ David M. Orenstein, M.D.

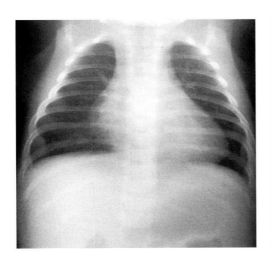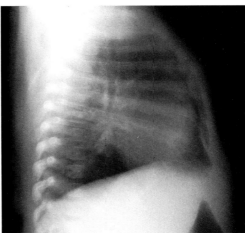

FIG. 16.1 Normal posteroanterior (left) and lateral (right) chest radiographs in a 2-month-old infant.

The chest radiograph in pediatric patients is unique in that normal findings may vary with age. In the chest x-ray of a normal infant (Fig. 16.1), the width of the chest on the lateral projection is about the same as the transverse dimension on a frontal projection and the lungs may appear relatively radiolucent. Further, in contrast to the older child (more than 2 years of age), the cardiothoracic ratio in the infant may be as high as 0.65. The width of the superior mediastinum at this age may also be striking because the thymic shadow is particularly prominent during the first few months of life before the normal process of involution occurs. The normal chest x-ray of an older child (Fig. 16.2) shows the diaphragm on an inspiratory film at the eighth or ninth rib posteriorly (sixth rib anteriorly), a cardiothoracic ratio of 0.5 and pulmonary vessels extending two thirds of the way to the periphery. In most situations, a lateral radiograph should accompany the posteroanterior (PA) view because some pathologic findings may be missed on a single projection. For example, a lateral x-ray yields the best information about the anterior mediastinum and the tracheal air column, and may also reveal a small pleural effusion that is unsuspected on the basis of a PA radiograph alone. In combination with the PA view, the lateral projection may help localize an abnormal finding to a particular lobe or segment.

COUGH

The youngster with persistent or chronic cough represents one of the most common and vexing problems in pediatrics. In most circumstances, the tracheobronchial tree is kept clean by airway macrophages and the mucociliary escalator, but cough becomes an important component of this defense system when excessive or abnormal materials are present, or when mucociliary clearance is reduced, as during a viral respiratory illness. A cough achieves clearance of airway secretions and inhaled particulate matter by a combination of the high airflow velocities generated during the expiratory phase of the cough, and by the compression of smaller airways which "milks" the secretions into larger bronchi where they can then be eliminated by a subsequent cough. Cough is generally produced by a reflex response arising from cough receptors located in ciliated epithelia in the lower respiratory tract, but can be suppressed or initiated at higher cortical centers.

One of the most common causes of cough in pediatric patients is the self-limited cough of an acute viral lower respiratory illness or bronchitis that lasts 1 to 2 weeks. The cough that persists longer than 2 weeks is potentially more worrisome. A diagnostic approach to chronic cough is best served by considering the age of the child (Fig. 16.3).

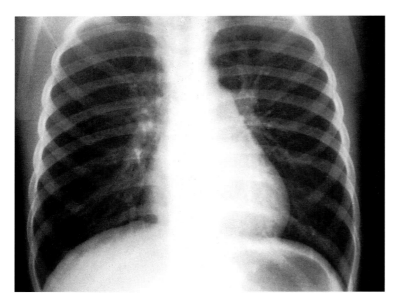

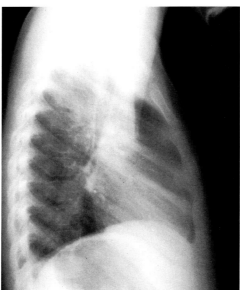

FIG. 16.2 Normal posteroanterior (top) and lateral (left) chest radiographs in a 6-year-old child.

CAUSES OF COUGH ACCORDING TO AGE

CAUSES OF COUGH ACCORDING TO AGE

Infancy (Under 1 Year)

Congenital and neonatal infections
    Chlamydia
    Viral (e.g., RSV, CMV, rubella)
    Bacterial (e.g., pertussis)
    Pneumocystis carinii
Congenital malformations
    Tracheoesophageal fistula
    Vascular ring
    Airway malformations (e.g., laryngeal cleft)
    Pulmonary sequestration
Cystic fibrosis
Reactive airway disease
Recurrent viral bronchitiolitis/bronchitis
Gastroesophageal reflux
Interstitial pneumonitides
    Lymphoid interstitial pneumonitis
    Diffuse interstitial pneumonitis

Preschool

Inhaled foreign body
Reactive airway disease
Suppurative lung disease
    Cystic fibrosis
    Bronchiectasis
Right middle lobe syndrome
Ciliary dyskinesia syndromes
Upper respiratory tract disease
Recurrent viral infection/bronchitis
Passive smoking
Gastroesophageal reflux
Interstitial pneumonitides
Pulmonary hemosiderosis

School Age to Adolescence

Reactive airway disease
Cystic fibrosis
Mycoplasma pneumoniae infection
Psychogenic or habit cough
Cigarette smoking
Pulmonary hemosiderosis
Interstitial pneumonitides
Ciliary dyskinesia syndromes

Common to All Ages

Recurrent viral illness
Asthma
Cystic fibrosis
Granulomatous lung disease
Foreign body aspiration
Pertussis infection

    However, there are several causes of persistent cough that are common to all pediatric age groups, such as recurrent viral bronchitis, hyperactive airways disease, cystic fibrosis, granulomatous lung disease (e.g., tuberculosis), foreign body aspiration, and pertussis.

Age and Cause of Chronic Cough

INFANCY (UNDER 1 YEAR)

Cough starting at birth or shortly afterwards may be a sign of serious respiratory disease and must be evaluated assiduously. Cough beginning at this time raises the possibility of congenital infections like cytomegalovirus (Fig. 16.4) or rubella, which are often associated with other findings such as hepatosplenomegaly, thrombocytopenia, or central nervous system involvement. Pneumonia due to *Chlamydia trachomatis* (Fig. 16.5) generally develops after the first month of life and presents as an afebrile pneumonitis with congestion, wheezing, fine diffuse rales, a paroxysmal cough, and, in approximately 50 percent of cases, a prior or concomitant inclusion conjunctivitis. Pneumonia due to *Bordetella pertussis* may be a life-threatening illness,

FIG. 16.3

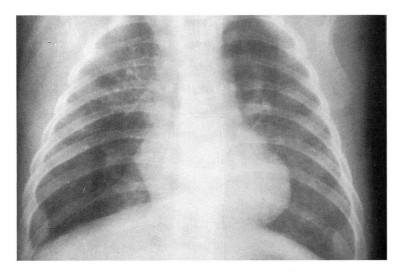

FIG. 16.4 *Pneumonia due to cytomegalovirus in an infant.*

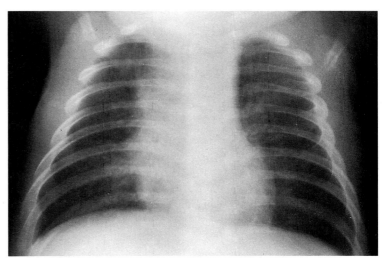

FIG. 16.5 *Pneumonia due to* Chlamydia trachomatis *in a 3-month-old infant with inclusion conjunctivitis.*

FIG. 16.6 *Fatal pertussis in a 6-week-old demonstrates the typical radiographic pattern of perihilar involvement.*

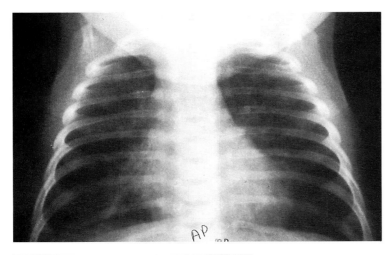

FIG. 16.7 *Tracheoesophageal fistula.* **A,** *frontal projection shows feeding tube passing no further than proximal esophagus.* **B,** *barium swallow in same infant reveals aspiration of barium into the tracheobronchial tree.*

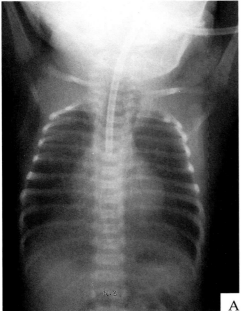

A

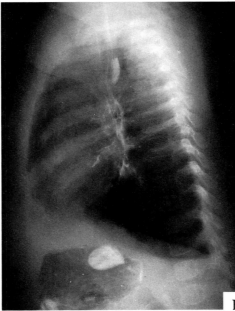

B

characterized by severe paroxysmal coughing episodes followed by cyanosis and apnea, and often associated with an inspiratory "whoop." The latter finding may be missing in very young infants or those weakened by the recurrent coughing spasms. The chest radiograph (Fig. 16.6) may show perihilar infiltrates, atelectasis, hyperinflation and, in some cases, intersti-

tial or subcutaneous emphysema. More recently, *Ureaplasma urealyticum* and *Pneumocystis carinii* have been recognized as causes of pneumonia and, hence, persistent cough, in this age group.

Congenital malformations such as tracheoesophageal fistula (Fig. 16.7) or laryngeal cleft or web can produce cough via chronic aspiration of gastric contents, milk, or saliva. Both of

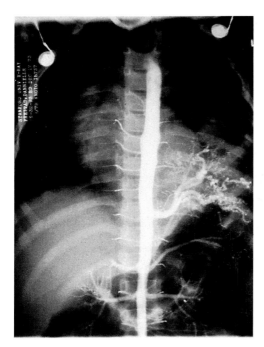

FIG. 16.8 Pulmonary sequestration. Aortic angiogram demonstrates anomalous origin of pulmonary blood supply from abdominal aorta to the left lower lobe in a 7-year-old girl with extralobar sequestration.

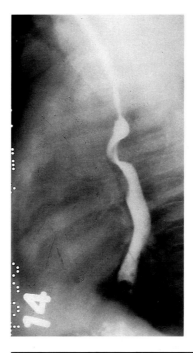

FIG. 16.9 Vascular ring. Barium swallow in a toddler with posterior compression of esophagus and trachea from a vascular ring. (Courtesy of Department of Radiology, Children's Hospital of Pittsburgh)

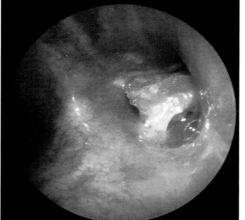

FIG. 16.11 Portion of a carrot lodged in the right mainstem bronchus, as seen through a rigid bronchoscope. (Courtesy of Dr. S. Stool, Children's Hospital of Pittsburgh)

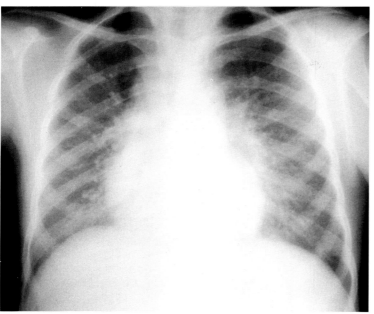

FIG. 16.10 Lymphocytic interstitial pneumonitis in a 10-year-old boy shows a diffuse increase in interstitial markings.

these anomalies are associated with feeding-related symptoms of coughing, choking, and occasionally cyanosis. Infants with neurologic disorders may have incoordination of swallowing and sucking reflexes that lead to inhalation of milk or gastric contents into the lung. Pulmonary sequestration (Fig. 16.8) and bronchogenic cysts are rare congenital anomalies that may compress the pulmonary tree or become infected, thereby producing a cough. The presence of aberrant major blood vessels generally causes inspiratory stridor and expiratory wheezing from tracheal compression (Fig. 16.9), but a brassy cough may also be observed, as may dysphagia from the associated esophageal constriction.

This triad of poor weight gain, steatorrhea, and chronic cough at this age makes cystic fibrosis a strong consideration and a sweat test is therefore mandatory. Reactive airway disease or bronchial hyperresponsiveness is a common and probably un-

derdiagnosed cause of cough in infancy. Either cough or persistent wheezing can be found in these infants, who may have a history of a previous viral lower respiratory illness or a positive family history of wheezing and/or asthma. Babies with gastroesophageal reflux may have a combination of wheezing and coughing and, in some cases, poor weight gain. The absence of a history of "spitting" does not eliminate gastroesophageal reflux as a diagnostic consideration in infants with persistent coughing, because occult reflux may stimulate bronchospasm via vagal reflexes.

Diffuse (DIP) and lymphocytic interstitial pneumonia (LIP) are rare causes of cough in children and are of unknown etiology. DIP presents with an insidious onset of cough, dyspnea, anorexia and weight loss, tachypnea, and scattered bibasilar crackles. Later, cyanosis and clubbing are noted on physical exam. LIP may present in a similar fashion but must also be

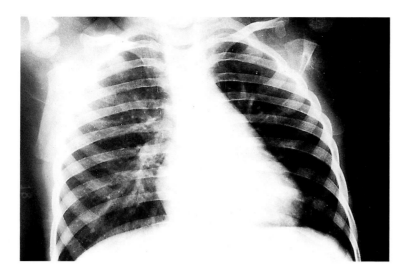

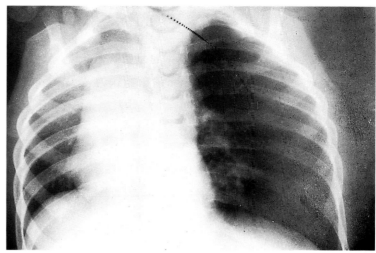

FIG. 16.12 *Inspiratory (left) and expiratory (right) radiograph in a child with an inhaled foreign body lodged in the left mainstem bronchus reveals hyperlucency of the left hemithorax and compensato-* ry shift of the mediastinal structures to the right, as the left lung does not empty in expiration.

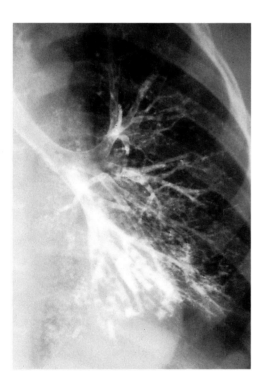

FIG. 16.13 *Bronchogram shows cylindrical bronchiectasis of the left lower lobe in a 5-year-old girl with recurrent pneumonias and chronic cough.*

suspected in those patients at risk for human immunodeficiency virus infection. The diagnosis of interstitial pneumonitis depends on tissue obtained at lung biopsy. An interstitial pattern on chest radiograph (Fig. 16.10) is seen with varying degrees of hyperinflation or patchy atelectasis.

PRESCHOOL

The two most common reasons for a persistent cough in this age group are recurrent viral infections with bronchitis and reactive airway disease. The child with reactive airway disease may not manifest the common finding of audible wheezing or dyspnea, but rather presents with cough during vigorous activity or exposure to noxious inhalants such as cigarette smoke.

Upper respiratory tract disease and sinusitis have been implicated in the pathogenesis of chronic cough, presumably through the stimulation of pharyngeal cough receptors by upper airway secretions. Parental smoking without evidence of reactive airways may be a cause of cough in a small population of preschool children. Gastroesophageal reflux more commonly causes cough at a younger age but may appear in preschool children as well. The interstitial pneumonitides may also produce a chronic cough in this age group.

An inhaled foreign body either in the esophagus or tracheobronchial tree is an important cause of chronic cough, especially in toddlers. A history of gagging or choking may be absent at this age, physical examination may be unrevealing, and the plain chest radiograph may be normal. Subtle differences in air entry into homologous lung segments detected by the differential (two-headed) stethoscope may be the only indication of a foreign body in the airway. Cough is present in over 90 percent of cases, but a quiescent period may occur after inhalation and cough may disappear as irritant receptors adjust to its presence. A mobile foreign body may result in the recurrence of cough as new receptors are stimulated by the object. Although inspiratory and expiratory radiography and fluoroscopy are essential in the evaluation of a child who may have inhaled a foreign body, they may be normal and a bronchoscopy may be necessary to confirm or disprove the presence of a foreign object (Fig. 16.11). Unilateral air trapping demonstrated by inspiratory and expiratory radiographs (Fig. 16.12) is strongly suggestive of an inhaled foreign body.

Suppurative lung diseases such as cystic fibrosis or bronchiectasis (Fig. 16.13) from any other causes (e.g., tuberculosis) characteristically result in a chronic cough producing purulent sputum. Right middle lobe syndrome, commonly associated with enlargement of lymph nodes surrounding the right middle lobe bronchus in tuberculosis, has also been described in asthma and a number of other illnesses and may cause chronic cough. Recurrent infection of the middle lobe can ultimately lead to the development of bronchiectasis or fibrosis.

Disorders of ciliary motility may produce insidious symptoms of productive cough, nasal drainage, recurrent middle ear infections, and fever. Clinical findings include basilar crackles and, later, radiographic changes of recurrent lower lobe infections and eventually bronchiectasis. Repetitive infections occur unless measures such as chest physical therapy, postural drainage, and liberal use of antibiotics are employed.

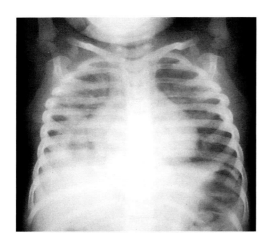

FIG. 16.14
Idiopathic pulmonary hemosiderosis in a youngster with hemoptysis and wheezing and mostly right-sided radiographic involvement.

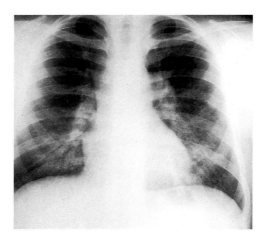

FIG. 16.15
Mycoplasma pneumonia in an adolescent shows typical lower-lobe involvement by chest x-ray. (Courtesy of Dr. A. Urbach, Children's Hospital of Pittsburgh)

It is now recognized that the classic triad described by Kartagener of situs inversus, sinusitis, and bronchiectasis fits only a limited number of patients because situs inversus occurs in only about half of all patients with immotile-cilia syndrome.

Pulmonary hemosiderosis is a potentially fatal disorder that has been described in association with cardiac or panorganic disease, glomerulonephritis (Goodpasture's syndrome), infantile hypersensitivity to cow's milk protein (Heiner's syndrome) and collagen-vascular diseases, and as an idiopathic form. Idiopathic pulmonary hemosiderosis (IPH) is a disease of unknown etiology characterized by episodes of dyspnea, cough and/or hemoptysis, wheezing, cyanosis, fever, and iron-deficiency anemia. Hematemesis or melena may be the only presenting complaints in some patients without symptoms referable to the respiratory tract. As a result of recurrent bleeding episodes, jaundice may be observed, and clubbing develops over time in some patients. Laboratory findings include iron-deficiency anemia and, in a small number of patients, peripheral eosinophilia. Radiographic findings (Fig. 16.14) are quite variable, with some patients demonstrating scant transient infiltrates and others showing widespread parenchymal infiltrates that resemble miliary tuberculosis. The finding of hemosiderin-laden macrophages obtained from sputum, gastric washings, or bronchoalveolar lavage is suggestive of the diagnosis, but a lung biopsy may be necessary. A percutaneous renal biopsy may be helpful in cases of hemosiderosis associated with Goodpasture's syndrome.

SCHOOL AGE TO ADOLESCENCE

Because in the first several years of school children are exposed to numerous respiratory viruses, recurrent viral bronchitis remains an important cause of chronic cough in this age group. Reactive airway disease continues to be a likely consideration in the patient presenting with a chronic cough. Patients in this age group are amenable to pulmonary function tests, including bronchodilator responsiveness or bronchial provocation studies as a means of confirming the diagnosis. Other disorders may present with chronic cough at this age, including cystic fibrosis, pulmonary hemosiderosis, interstitial pneumonitis, and ciliary dyskinesia syndromes.

Mycoplasma pneumoniae infection is an important cause of chronic cough among school age children. Although the lung is the primary site of infection, and cough is a striking feature of the disease, the gradual onset of extrapulmonary symptoms such as malaise, headache, fever, and sore throat may be the initial clues to the diagnosis. Cough is generally productive of

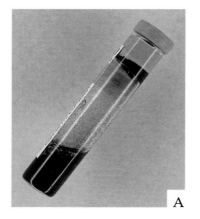 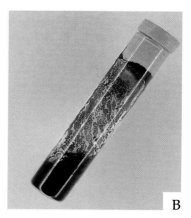

FIG. 16.16 Bedside cold agglutinins (see text for explanation of technique). **A,** purple-top tube before placing on ice. **B,** positive result shows agglutination of heparinized blood after exposure to cold. (Courtesy of Dr. H. Davis, Children's Hospital of Pittsburgh)

mucoid sputum, and hemoptysis may develop later in the course. The cough can persist for 3 to 4 months. Physical findings tend to be minimal, although crackles are generally the most common sign, with wheezing often noted in younger children. The chest radiograph is not diagnostic and the findings may be either interstitial or bronchopneumonic in character, with predilection for the lower lobes (Fig. 16.15). Bedside cold agglutinins are a simple means of confirming the suspected diagnosis and may be positive in about half of cases but are not specific. About 1 cc of blood is collected in an NaEDTA ("purple-top") tube and placed on ice for 30 to 60 seconds. By tilting the tube and examining whether there is blood agglutination that disappears upon rewarming to 37°C suggests a positive result (Fig. 16.16). A positive result correlates with a serum cold agglutinin titer of at least 1:64. During the acute stage of the illness the presence of specific IgM antibody to mycoplasma or a rise in the level of specific IgG antibody may confirm the diagnostic impression.

A psychogenic or habit cough may be observed following a lower respiratory illness. Habit cough may persist for weeks or months after the acute process has subsided. A psychogenic cough tends to be very loud and bizarre in nature and timing and is often described as "honking" or "barking." This type of

PEDIATRIC PULMONARY DISORDERS

FIG. 16.17

CHARACTERISTICS OF CHRONIC COUGHS AND ASSOCIATED CONDITIONS

Characteristic	Associated condition
Loose, productive	Cystic fibrosis, bronchiectasis, ciliary dyskinesia
Croupy	Laryngotracheobronchitis
Paroxysmal	Cystic fibrosis, pertussis syndromes, foreign body, *Mycoplasma, Chlamydia*
Brassy	Tracheitis, upper airway drainage, psychogenic cough tic
After feedings	Pharyngeal incoordination, pharyngeal mass, tracheoesophageal fistula, gastroesophageal reflux
Nocturnal	Upper respiratory tract disease, sinusitis, asthma, cystic fibrosis, gastroesophageal reflux
Most severe in morning	Cystic fibrosis, bronchiectasis
With exercise	Asthma (including exercise-induced), CF, bronchiectasis
Loud/honking/bizarre	Psychogenic cough
Disappears with sleep	Psychogenic cough

cough is short, nonproductive, and nonparoxysmal; it is quite disturbing to family members and classmates, to the point that the child may be excluded from school and other activities. It always disappears with sleep. The cough becomes more obvious with stressful situations or when parents (or physicians) express undue interest or anxiety regarding the cough. For this reason, extensive evaluations by medical personnel may merely exacerbate the problem when the diagnosis can be made on the basis of the characteristic quality of the cough.

Cigarette smoking in this group should also be a consideration and, unless the rapport between physician and adolescent is particularly strong, it is likely that the history will be unrevealing. Staining of the teeth or fingers or the presence of conjunctivitis may be indirect clues to the underlying cause of the cough.

Evaluation of Cough

Information obtained in the history may suggest the underlying cause of the cough (Fig. 16.17) and, perhaps more importantly, eliciting the cough during the physical exam can be very helpful. A loose or productive cough is suggestive of the presence of suppurative lung disease such as cystic fibrosis, other forms of bronchiectasis, or ciliary dyskinesia syndromes. The cough in these patients tends to be most severe in the morning as well, because inadequately cleared and excessive secretions pool in the tracheobronchial tree through the sleeping hours. A croupy sounding cough may be observed in patients with acute laryngotracheobronchitis and there may be associated wheezing. A dry or brassy cough generally is seen in patients with larger airway pathology, as in tracheitis or drainage from upper respiratory tract disease; a psychogenic cough may produce similar findings, but this type of cough may be distinguished from the others by its disappearance with sleep. As noted previously, a psychogenic cough

tends to be very loud, "honking," bizarre, and disruptive. A paroxysmal cough is seen in patients with pertussis syndrome, *Mycoplasma, Chlamydia,* foreign body inhalation, or cystic fibrosis. A coughing episode associated with feedings suggests the presence of pharyngeal incoordination or mass, tracheoesophageal fistula or gastroesophageal reflux. Nighttime coughing is noted in cystic fibrosis, asthma, gastroesophageal reflex and sinusitis, or upper respiratory tract disease. Cough occurring with or shortly after activities suggests asthma, cystic fibrosis or bronchiectasis.

Examination of the sputum also may be helpful in suggesting the diagnosis. Clear, mucoid sputum containing eosinophils is likely to represent asthma, whereas purulent green sputum is more suggestive of suppurative lung disease such as cystic fibrosis. A yellow color can be imparted to the sputum by breakdown products of white blood cells; therefore, yellow sputum can be seen with infection (polymorphonuclear leukocytes breaking down) or asthma (eosinophils breaking down). Bloody sputum can occur in cystic fibrosis, retained foreign body, idiopathic pulmonary hemosiderosis, tuberculosis, bronchiectasis or some infections. It is important to recognize that upper respiratory tract irritation may lead to the mistaken notion that hemoptysis is occurring. Hematemesis also may be mistaken for hemoptysis.

Clinical findings associated with a cough also may point to the correct nature of the problem. A cough occurring in the presence of poor weight gain and malabsorption makes cystic fibrosis a likely concern. A cough occurring with wheezing suggests asthma, and if evidence of rhinitis, conjunctivitis, or "allergic shiners" is present, allergic disease also may be a consideration (see Chapter 4, Pediatric Allergy and Immunology). A cough that is worse in spring and summer months, or only occurs after exercise, suggests asthma. A worsening of the cough in the winter is consistent with cold-induced bronchospasm or recurrent viral illnesses.

DIAGNOSTIC APPROACH TO COUGH

Complete history and physical examination
Chest and sinus radiographs
CBC with differential
Pulmonary function tests
   (including bronchoprovocation tests)
Sweat test (pilocarpine iontophoresis method)
Trial of bronchodilators
Sputum for Gram's stain, AFB, bacterial, viral,
   and fungal cultures
Quantitative immunoglobulins
Tuberculin skin test/anergy panel
Serology for *Mycoplasma pneumoniae*
Bronchoscopy
Barium swallow
pH probe/Bernstein test

FIG. 16.18

CAUSES OF RECURRENT OR CHRONIC STRIDOR

Croup
   Infectious
   Allergic/angioneurotic edema
Laryngomalacia
Tracheomalacia
Subglottic stenosis
Extrinsic airway compression
   Vascular ring
   Mediastinal mass
   Lobar emphysema
   Bronchogenic cyst
   Foreign body in esophagus
   Thyromegaly
Pharyngeal or laryngeal masses
   Papillomas
   Hemangiomas
   Laryngocele
   Webs
   Foreign body
Tracheoesophageal fistula
Vocal cord paralysis
Hysterical/psychogenic

FIG. 16.19

Diagnostic Approach to Cough

The approach to making a diagnosis in a patient presenting with persistent cough begins with a complete history in which some of the factors alluded to earlier (Fig. 16.18) are targeted. On physical examination, close attention to nutritional status, presence of associated upper respiratory tract disease, or clubbing of the digits is as important as the examination of the chest. Clubbing of the fingers raises the possibility of cystic fibrosis; any patient with this finding requires a sweat test performed by quantitative pilocarpine iontophoresis. On auscultation of the chest, a localized wheeze, particularly if associated with delayed air entry, is suggestive of a foreign body or focal airway lesion leading to narrowing. Inspiratory crackles may be noted in cystic fibrosis, bronchiectasis from other causes, interstitial lung disease, or pneumonias. Crackles also are present during one third to one half of untreated asthma attacks, even in the absence of infection.

Most patients with prolonged cough should have a chest x-ray and, if historical or physical findings are suggestive, sinus x-rays as well. Inspiratory and expiratory radiographs and fluoroscopy may be indicated if inhalation of a foreign body is suspected. A complete blood count with differential may suggest the diagnosis in some patients, with eosinophilia seen in allergic disease, lymphocytosis in pertussis and other viral diseases, and an increased proportion of neutrophils in bacterial infections. In a child old enough to cooperate, pulmonary function testing may detect lower airway obstruction and its reversibility with bronchodilator administration. Abnormalities of the shape of the inspiratory or expiratory loops during spirometry may suggest upper airway pathology (discussed below). In some cases, an outpatient trial of bronchodilators for

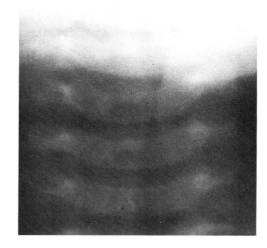

FIG. 16.20 The "steeple sign" shows subglottic narrowing of the trachea due to croup.

several weeks may serve to confirm the suspicion of cough-variant asthma. Failure to respond to this regimen suggests that asthma is not the problem, but also could be explained by noncompliance with the prescribed medications. Examination of sputum produced by the patient with Wright or Gram's stain or by cultures may lead to a diagnosis. The presence of eosinophils suggests allergic disease and polymorphonuclear leukocytes with organisms suggests a bacterial infection. Quantitative immunoglobulins and immunoglobulin subclasses may be helpful in detecting some immunodeficiencies, and an elevated IgE is suggestive of allergic disease. A PPD placed

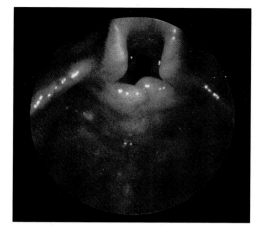 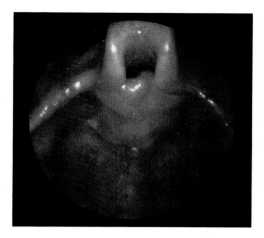 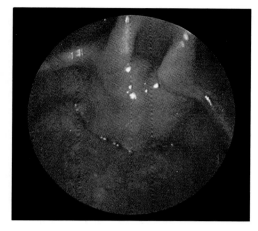

FIG. 16.21 *A sequence of photographs demonstrates the degree of air way compromise occurring during inspiration in laryngomalacia. The epiglottis is supported by a laryngoscope blade, but the progressive collapse of the other laryngeal structures during inspiration, especially* *the arytenoid cartilages, is shown clearly. (Reproduced by permission from Benjamin B:* Atlas of Pediatric Endoscopy. *London, Oxford University Press, 1981)*

in conjunction with other antigens of known immunogenicitiy (e.g., *Candida* or mumps) may be important in some patients. In the appropriate clinical setting, serologic studies for *Mycoplasma pneumoniae* are occasionally fruitful. A bronchoscopy may be extremely important to exclude the diagnosis of foreign body or airway malformation as the cause of chronic cough. If foreign body inhalation is likely (based on history and/or physical exam), bronchoscopy is essential and should be performed under general anesthesia with the rigid instrument, not with the flexible bronchoscope, in order to provide adequate airway control.

A bronchogram may confirm the diagnosis of bronchiectasis, and should be performed if surgical removal of the affected segment is contemplated. A barium swallow is useful in patients with suspected tracheoesophageal fistula or various pharyngeal disorders. Prolonged monitoring of the pH in the distal esophagus may confirm the suspicion of gastroesophageal reflux. The appearance of symptoms with acid infusion into the distal esophagus (Bernstein test) can confirm the causal relation between acid reflux and cough. Finally, on rare occasions, a nasal ciliary biopsy for examination by light and electron microscopy may be indicated in patients suspected of having ciliary dysmotility.

STRIDOR

There are a number of clinical entities that can produce persistent or recurrent stridor (Fig. 16.19) and some of these also may be associated with a chronic cough, as described earlier. Stridor is characteristically a harsh inspiratory noise created by obstruction of the larynx or the extrathoracic trachea. With a mild degree of airway narrowing, breath sounds may be normal when the infant or child is at rest, but with any activity that increases tidal breathing, e.g., crying, feeding, or agitation, inspiratory stridor may become noticeable.

The most common cause of inspiratory stridor in the pediatric population is infectious croup or acute laryngotracheobronchitis. The disease generally is due to a respiratory virus (parainfluenza, respiratory syncytial, influenza, or rhinovirus) and the patient typically has coryza for 24 to 48 hours before the appearance of croupy cough, hoarseness, and stridor. Occasionally the inflammatory process may spread to the smaller airways and produce wheezing in addition to these symptoms. The "steeple sign" is a characteristic radiographic sign on anteroposterior projections (Fig. 16.20) which may be accompanied by marked dilation of supraglottic structures, particularly on lateral films. In the majority of patients, serious airway obstruction does not occur and the disease is self-limited. Acute angioneurotic edema is a less common cause of stridor. In most cases it results from an allergic reaction and is potentially fatal.

Laryngomalacia and tracheomalacia may appear separately or together, and the stridor associated with laryngomalacia (Fig. 16.21) generally begins within the first month of life, varies with activity, may be expiratory, and is more noticeable in the supine position. Clinical symptoms may suggest the diagnosis, but bronchoscopic visualization of airway dynamics by flexible bronchoscopy is a safe and reliable method of confirming the suspicion of laryngomalacia. Tracheomalacia can produce stridor or wheezing as the compliant posterial tracheal wall collapses anteriorly with increased respiratory effort. Parents can be reassured that both of these entities are self-limited, become less marked after 6 to 10 months of age, and rarely cause significant problems.

Narrowing of the subglottic region can be congenital or acquired, as in subglottic stenosis associated with prolonged endotracheal intubation. Congenital subglottic stenosis improves as the child grows older, but that associated with tracheal intubation may require a tracheostomy, particularly if the infant remains dependent on ventilatory support.

Airway compression from extrinsic factors may produce stridor, depending on the site of obstruction. A vascular ring (see Fig. 16.9) can produce either inspiratory stridor or expiratory wheezing (see Chapter 5, Pediatric Cardiology). Diagnosis can be made by barium swallow, echocardiography, or bronchoscopy; the latter may demonstrate a pulsatile lesion com-

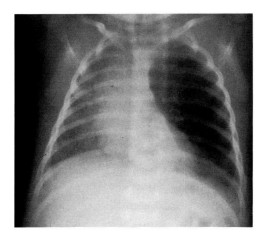

FIG. 16.22 *Congenital lobar emphysema of the left upper lobe shows hyperlucency of the affected globe, atelectasis of the lower lobe, and mediastinal shift.*

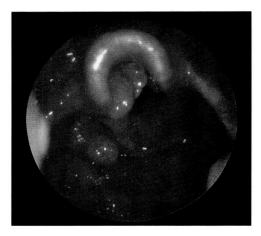

FIG. 16.23 *Multiple papillomas involving the larynx. (Reproduced by permission from Benjamin B: Atlas of Pediatric Endoscopy. London, Oxford University Press, 1981)*

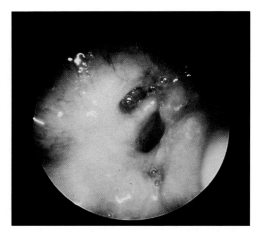

FIG. 16.24 *Expiratory view of a laryngeal web in an infant with inspiratory stridor that was exaggerated by crying noted at birth. The web is seen traversing the area of the glottis. Copyright: Boehringer Ingelheim International GmbH.*

pressing the trachea. Mediastinal masses or, occasionally, enlargement of the thyroid gland may produce tracheal compression and stridor. Congenital or acquired lobar emphysema usually produces tachypnea or some other respiratory symptoms such as cough, wheeze, or intermittent cyanosis, but stridor also may be noted. The chest radiograph in lobar emphysema (Fig. 16.22) demonstrates a large, hyperlucent area with few bronchovascular markings and usually compression atelectasis of adjacent lobes. Left upper lobe involvement is most common, but right middle lobe emphysema also is seen. For the infant who is growing well and in whom tachypnea is the primary manifestation, or in lobar emphysema associated with a mucous plug, conservative management is indicated.

A bronchogenic cyst in the newborn can cause stridor, as the cyst fills with air after birth and compresses large airways. It also can cause tachypnea, dyspnea, cyanosis, and diminished breath sounds on the affected side. Later, the cyst may become infected, leading to recurrent bouts of fever, cough, and hemoptysis. Finally, an esophageal foreign body may compress the compliant posterior wall of the trachea and produce stridor, cough, and dysphagia.

Congenital laryngeal or pharyngeal masses also can produce stridor by their obstruction to airflow. Laryngeal papillomatosis (Fig. 16.23) is a rare and life-threatening illness that generally presents in the first decade of life. Papillomas can involve the vocal cords as in the aforementioned figure, but there also may be widespread involvement of the remainder of the tracheobronchial tree. Although inspiratory stridor may be observed, hoarseness is a more common presenting feature. Hemangiomas of the larynx or trachea also may produce stridor or a brassy or dry cough. Cutaneous or mucosal hemangiomas noted during the physical exam may suggest the diagnosis. Laryngeal webs (Fig. 16.24), cysts, and laryngoceles are quite uncommon, are all accompanied by respiratory distress and stridor and, occasionally, by feeding difficulties and cyanosis. Diagnosis is made by bronchoscopy. A foreign body in the pharynx or larynx also may cause stridor.

CAUSES OF CHRONIC OR RECURRENT WHEEZING

Reactive airways disease
   Asthma
   Exercise-induced asthma
   Gastroesophageal reflux
   Hypersensitivity reactions (e.g., ABPA)
Cystic fibrosis
Aspiration
   Tracheoesophageal fistula
   Foreign body
   Gastroesophageal reflux
   Laryngeal cleft
   Pharyngeal dysmotility
Extrinsic masses
   Vascular ring
   Cystic adenomatoid malformation
   Lymph nodes
   Tumors
Ciliary dyskinesia syndromes
Tracheo- and/or bronchomalacia
Congestive heart failure
Bronchopulmonary dysplasia
Idiopathic pulmonary hemosiderosis/Heiner's syndrome
Endobronchial lesions, including localized stenosis
Interstitial pneumonitides
Bronchiolitis obliterans

FIG. 16.25

Vocal cord paralysis, either unilateral or bilateral, may present in the neonatal period, although in the case of unilateral paralysis several weeks may pass before the diagnosis is suspected. A weak or absent cry, hoarseness, inspiratory stridor

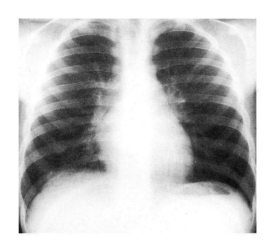

FIG. 16.26 The chest x-ray from an adolescent with asthma and allergic bronchopulmonary aspergillosis shows hyperinflation and patchy atelectasis.

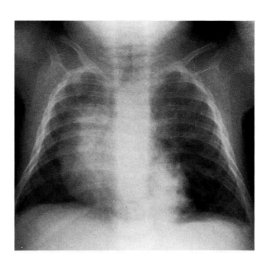

FIG. 16.27 Cystic areas in the left lower lobe caused by congenital cystadenomatoid malformation in an infant presenting with respiratory distress and wheezing.

with or without respiratory distress, and feeding difficulties are usual manifestations of vocal cord paralysis. Bilateral vocal cord paralysis may be seen with hydrocephalous, myelomeningocele, Arnold-Chiari malformation or other malformations of the brain. Both unilateral and bilateral cord paralyses are observed in patients with abnormalities of the cardiovascular system that are accompanied by cardiomegaly (ventricular septal defect or tetralogy of Fallot), or that cause abnormalities of the great vessels (e.g., vascular ring, transposition, patent ductus arteriosus). The diagnosis is best made by flexible bronchoscopy under minimal sedation so that vocal cord movement can be examined adequately.

The diagnosis of hysterical or psychogenic stridor is generally made during adolescence and is more common in girls. As in psychogenic cough, psychogenic stridor disappears with sleep and is more noticeable with anxiety or when excessive attention is drawn to the patient.

WHEEZING

Many of the diseases that produce chronic wheezing in pediatric patients (Fig. 16.25) overlap with entities that cause coughing or stridor. Wheezing usually is considered an expiratory sound from obstruction of airflow in intrathoracic airways, from the lower trachea "downstream" to the small bronchi and in the large bronchioles. Although most pediatricians recognize that not all wheezing results from bronchospasm, it *is* true that reactive airway disease is the most common cause of wheezing in pediatric patients. Reactive airway disease may take many different forms, including typical asthma, cough-variant asthma, exercise-induced asthma, and wheezing associated with gastroesophageal reflux. The development of increased wheezing in a previously well-controlled asthmatic patient should raise the possibility of allergic bronchopulmonary aspergillosis (ABPA). These patients often have an insidious onset of low-grade fever, fatigue, weight loss, and productive cough. Physical findings include expiratory wheezes and bibasilar crackles and, later in the course, clubbing of the digits. Radiographic features of ABPA (Fig. 16.26) include areas of consolidation, atelectasis, and evidence of

dilated bronchi radiating from the hila. Diagnosis can be made by positive skin test results with *Aspergillus fumigatus* antigens, elevated total serum IgE levels, elevation of specific IgE, presence of serum precipitins to *Aspergillus,* and isolation of *Aspergillus fumigatus* from the sputum culture. Pulmonary function studies may worsen considerably during episodes of ABPA with evidence of increased airway obstruction. There are a host of other hypersensitivity reactions producing extrinsic allergic alveolitis with wheezing and the reader is referred to any of the standard pulmonary texts listed in the bibliography for a further discussion of these entities.

Other disorders that have been discussed previously and can provoke wheezing include cystic fibrosis, aspiration events from any cause, and extrinsic masses that compress the airways. Among extrinsic masses that may cause wheezing, congenital cystic adenomatoid malformation is very rare. Symptoms generally begin at birth or shortly afterwards as normal lung is compressed by the lesion with the onset of tachypnea, respiratory distress, and cyanosis. Polyhydramnios at birth often is noted. Rarely, smaller cysts may be an incidental finding on chest x-ray or symptoms may develop after infection of the cysts occurs. The radiographic appearance (Fig. 16.27) is that of multiple cyst-like areas compressing normal lung with mediastinal displacement. It is usually confined to a single lobe and there is no apparent predilection for a particular lobe.

Bronchopulmonary dysplasia (BPD), one of the sequelae of hyaline membrane disease and its treatment, is associated with recurrent episodes of wheezing, respiratory distress, and tachypnea (see Chapter 2, Neonatology). Otherwise mild respiratory illnesses in these infants may progress to lower respiratory tract disease necessitating frequent hospitalizations. Patients with BPD may develop chronic respiratory insufficiency, pulmonary hypertension, and cor pulmonale. The frequency of wheezing episodes may diminish with age, although it appears that these patients continue to have airway hyperreactivity that is triggered by any number of different insults.

Miscellaneous causes of wheezing include idiopathic pulmonary hemosiderosis, endobronchial lesions associated with localized stenosis, interstitial lung disease, and bronchiolitis obliterans. The last has been described in an idiopathic form,

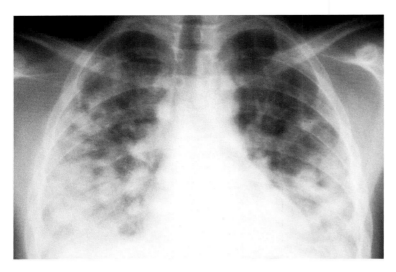

FIG. 16.28 *Bronchiolitis obliterans of unknown cause in a 12-year-old boy demonstrates extensive pulmonary involvement.*

following adenoviral infections or inhalation of toxic agents and in conjunction with other diseases (including rheumatoid arthritis) in adults. Patients may present initially with fever, cough, or tachypnea and subsequently develop dyspnea and wheezing. Physical findings include both wheezing and crackles. The radiographic pattern (Fig. 16.28) is that of diffusely increased interstitial markings with areas of atelectasis and consolidation. Complications of adenovirus-induced bronchiolitis obliterans include bronchiectasis, overinflation and recurrent atelectasis, and pneumonia. In many patients the prognosis is poor.

CYSTIC FIBROSIS

Cystic fibrosis (CF) is the most common fatal genetic disease among Caucasians in North America and afflicts 1 in 2,500 newborns in this group. The incidence in American blacks is about 1 in 17,000 and in people of Oriental background, 1 in 90,000. It is estimated that the carrier rate in Caucasians is 1 in 25. CF is a generalized exocrinopathy characterized by the inspissation of abnormally thick and tenacious secretions, principally involving the pancreas and lungs. In the lungs, the secretions cause obstruction of the airways resulting in recurrent infections and an inflammatory process that leads to bronchiolitis, bronchitis, bronchiectasis, and bronchiolectasis. Eventually, pulmonary function declines, and respiratory disease accounts for the vast majority of the deaths in CF. In the pancreas, ducts become obstructed by the abnormal secretions, preventing pancreatic enzymes from entering the duodenum and therefore preventing breakdown of dietary fat and protein. In 10 to 15 percent of patients with CF, pancreatic enzyme secretion is largely intact. This condition has recently been labeled "pancreatic sufficiency."

The disease is inherited as an autosomal recessive trait. Considerable excitement has been generated with the recent announcement of the isolation of the CF gene on the 7th chromosome. The basic defect appears to involve the inhibition of chloride transport across various epithelia resulting in abnormally viscid and poorly hydrated airway secretions. The prognosis for patients with CF has improved dramatically over the last several decades. In 1990, the median survival for patients rose to age 28 years.

PRESENTATIONS OF CYSTIC FIBROSIS

General
    Failure to thrive
    Salty taste to skin

GI/Nutritional
    Meconium ileus
    Foul-smelling stools, bloating, abdominal pain
    Rectal prolapse
    Intestinal impaction and obstruction
    Pancreatitis, acute and chronic
    Hypoproteinemia and edema
    Neonatal hyperbilirubinemia
    Cholelithiasis, cholecystitis
    Cirrhosis/portal hypertension
    Fat-soluble vitamin deficiency (A, D, E, K)

Metabolic
    Hyponatremic hypochloremic dehydration
    Heat stroke
    Metabolic alkalosis
    Diabetes mellitus

Respiratory
    Clubbing
    Asthma
    Chronic obstructive pulmonary disease
    Recurrent pulmonary infiltrates
    Chronic cough/sputum production
    Barrel chest
    Hemoptysis
    Pneumothorax
    Cor pulmonale
    Nasal polyps

Other
    Infertility (males)

FIG. 16.29

Presentations of Cystic Fibrosis

CF can present in any number of fashions (Fig. 16.29), but most symptoms are referable to respiratory or gastrointestinal involvement. The presenting sign in 5 to 10 percent of patients with CF will be meconium ileus, which is noted at or shortly after birth. Meconium ileus is a common cause of intestinal obstruction in the newborn period; these infants present with abdominal distention, bilious vomiting, and failure to pass meconium stools. Abdominal radiographs show dilated loops of small bowel and a ground-grass appearance in the cecal region, signifying pockets of air within the thick meconium. A barium or Gastrografin® contrast enema may show a very small distal colon (Fig. 16.30). In cases of meconium ileus associated with prenatal rupture and meconium peritonitis, abdominal calcification may be noted on plain radiographs, and at laparotomy thick, tar-like meconium is found in the terminal ileum (Fig. 16.31). Prolonged neonatal jaundice, generalized edema in a breast-fed or soy formula-fed infant, or hypoelectrolytemia with heat prostration are less common presentations of CF in early infancy.

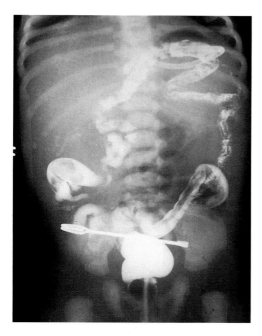

FIG. 16.30 Barium enema in a newborn with meconium peritonitis and evidence of a small, unused distal colon (note small extraluminal calcifications).

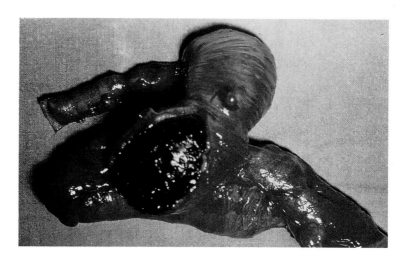

FIG. 16.31 Gross appearance of the thick, tar-like meconium found at laparotomy in meconium ileus.

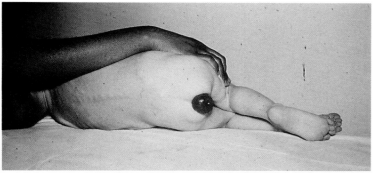

FIG. 16.32 Rectal prolapse in a toddler not previously recognized as having CF.

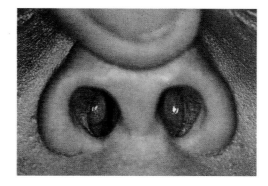

FIG. 16.33 Nasal polyps in a patient with CF.

A combination of poor weight gain, loose, foul-smelling, bulky stools and a voracious appetite are signs and symptoms that most clinicians associate with CF and rarely present a diagnostic problem. Rectal prolapse (Fig. 16.32) may be the presenting feature of CF in about 5 percent of cases, and may recur multiple times. Rarely, the patient may undergo a surgical procedure for the rectal prolapse before the underlying diagnosis is suspected. Rectal prolapse is thought to result from chronic malnutrition, reduced abdominal musculature, and voluminous stools. It does not generally pose problems once the diagnosis has been made and the patient started on supplemental pancreatic enzymes. Acute or chronic pancreatitis occurs occasionally, but only in patients with pancreatic sufficiency. These patients present with the acute onset of abdominal pain and vomiting, and may have recurrent bouts of pancreatitis before the pancreas "burns itself out." Laboratory evaluations that are diagnostic include elevations of serum lipase and amylase. The differential diagnosis in CF patients with acute abdominal pain and vomiting includes cholecystitis, appendicitis, and distal intestinal obstruction syndrome. The last is characterized by crampy abdominal pain, constipation, vomiting and, occasionally, a palpable mass in the right lower quadrant. There may be a history of missed pancreatic enzyme supplements, especially in adolescents. Other possible presenting manifestations in CF with respect to the gastrointestinal system include cirrhosis, portal hypertension, and esophageal varices, and clinical evidence of fat-soluble vitamin deficiency.

A chronic productive cough or wheezing in patients who have digital clubbing suggests the diagnosis of CF until proved otherwise. Patients may present with a history of recurrent pneumonia or a history of sinus disease; it is worth noting that the large majority of patients with CF demonstrate pansinusitis radiographically. Nasal polyps (Fig. 16.33) may be a presenting manifestation of CF and are seen in about 20 percent of patients sometime during the course of the disease. Other initial respiratory presentations are listed in Figure 16.29.

The clinical course and severity of the disease vary remarkably. For years many patients do not develop signs or symptoms of respiratory disease other than an intermittent, loose cough. Other patients have persistent symptoms from early infancy and are rarely without a cough. These patients tend to require frequent visits to the physician and frequent hospitalizations, and are more likely to have poor weight gain. Virtually all patients develop a loose, productive cough that may be blood-tinged during acute respiratory illnesses. Hemoptysis occurs in over half of adult patients with CF and a considerable proportion of adolescents as well. Tachypnea, dyspnea, diffuse crackles, and digital clubbing will develop in most patients. Later, diffuse bronchiectasis, hyperinflation, and a barrel chest deformity are noted. The usual cause of death in patients with CF is respiratory failure, often in conjunction with cor pulmonale.

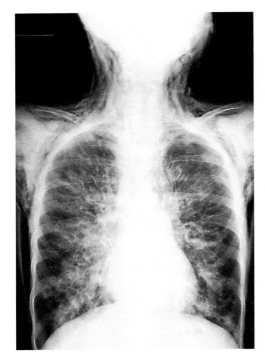

FIG. 16.34 A teenager with cystic fibrosis, severe respiratory disease, pneumomediastinum and massive subcutaneous emphysema.

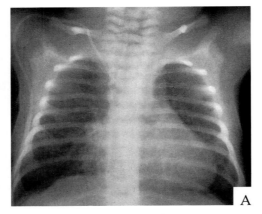

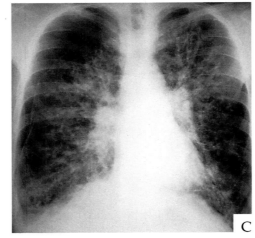

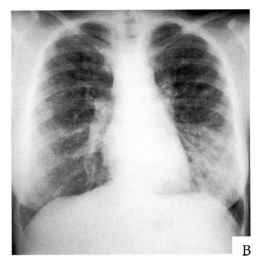

FIG. 16.35 Typical progression of radiographic changes in cystic fibrosis. **A,** 2-month-old child with hyperinflation and right middle lobe atelectasis. **B,** 15-year-old girl with peribronchial cuffing, hyperinflation, and bronchiectatic changes, particularly of the lower lobes. **C,** 21-year-old man with severe respiratory involvement and an unsuspected right pneumothorax.

Complications

The complications of CF include hemoptysis, pneumothorax, pneumomediastinum, hypertrophic pulmonary osteoarthropathy, distal intestinal obstructive syndrome (meconium ileus equivalent), liver disease, pancreatitis, and cor pulmonale. Among the respiratory complications, massive hemoptysis and pneumothorax with or without pneumomediastinum are potentially life-threatening. Blood streaking of sputum is not uncommon and massive hemoptysis from rupture of large blood vessels during chronic suppurative infections may occur in a small percentage of patients. Pneumothorax (see Fig. 16.35C) generally occurs from rupture of bullous lesions created from chronic airway obstruction and presents with acute onset of chest pain and shortness of breath with or without cyanosis. Pneumomediastinum and massive subcutaneous emphysema may result (Fig. 16.34). Hypertrophic pulmonary osteoarthropathy involving the knees and other major joints occurs in about 5 percent of patients with severe lung disease and is characterized by pain, swelling, and limitation of mobility of the affected joint. Right ventricular hypertrophy and cor pulmonale are findings in the terminal stages of many CF patients with severe pulmonary disease.

Radiographic Findings in Cystic Fibrosis

The radiographic findings in CF vary from early hyperinflation and patchy areas of atelectasis to a generalized increase in peribronchia markings with bronchiectasis, parenchymal densities, and large cystic areas noted in severe disease (Fig. 16.35A–C). The Brasfield scoring system is widely used as a means of classifying chest radiographs of these patients. It is based on a point system for findings such as hyperinflation, linear densities, cystic lesions, atelectasis, and right-sided cardiac enlargement or pneumothorax.

Diagnosis of Cystic Fibrosis

The recent identification and cloning of the CF gene may mean that DNA analysis will provide the diagnosis in the future. In the meantime, the sweat test performed by pilocarpine iontophoresis with quantitative analysis of chloride and/or sodium remains the laboratory evaluation of choice. The test must be performed in an experienced laboratory, such as those associated with one of the Cystic Fibrosis Foundation-approved CF centers. Both false negative and false positive results are alarmingly common in inexperienced hands. In the appropriate clinical setting of chronic lung disease, malabsorption or a family history of CF, a sweat chloride or sodium greater than 60 mEq/liter based on a collection of at least 100 mg of sweat is diagnostic of the disorder. Values below 40 mEq/liter are normal and those between 40 and 60 are suspicious for CF and should be repeated. In competent laboratories, false negative values are quite uncommon and the sweat test should be repeated in those cases where the suspicion is high. False positive values can occasionally occur, but disorders that cause this are readily distinguished clinically from CF. Other entities that elevate sweat chloride include adrenal insufficiency, ectodermal dysplasia, nephrogenic diabetes insipidus, hypothyroidism, mucopolysaccharidoses, glucose-6 phosphatase defi-

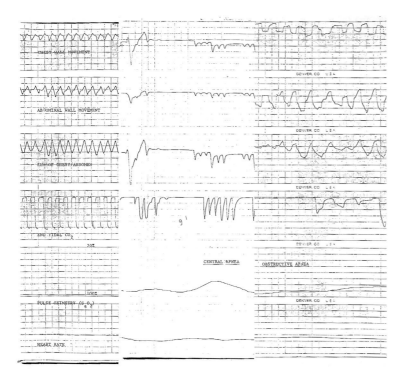

FIG. 16.36 *Representative set of tracings from a 6-channel sleep study recording. The first panel shows a normal tracing. In the center panel, the cessation of both respiratory efforts and airflow at the nose is shown in a patient with central apnea. The right panel depicts obstructive apnea with continued chest and abdominal wall motion despite a lack of airflow. The latter two tracings also demonstrate a significant fall in oxygen saturation during and after the apneic episode.*

ciency and hypoproteinemia, and anemia associated with malnutrition. Patients with CF who present with severe malnutrition and edema may have false negative values on initial sweat tests until their nutritional status improves. Newborn screening, recently adopted at many hospitals throughout the country, is based on the demonstration of elevated levels of immunoreactive serum trypsin by blood spot analysis. It is recommended that a single blood spot with elevation of serum immunoreactive trypsin (IRT) be repeated and, if this value remains high, a sweat chloride test should be performed. The false positive rate after two positive IRTs is quite high, at 20 percent, and the false negative rate may be as high as 10 percent.

APNEA AND SUDDEN INFANT DEATH SYNDROME

Sudden infant death syndrome (SIDS) is defined as the unexpected death of an infant who has been otherwise healthy and in whom there is no demonstrable pathologic basis for the death as determined by a thorough postmortem examination. The incidence of SIDS in the U.S. is reported to be 2 deaths per 1,000 live births, resulting in approximately 10,000 deaths annually. SIDS is the leading cause of death after the neonatal period, with a peak at 2 to 4 months postnatally and rarely occurring after 10 months of age. Most of these infants die soundlessly during sleep, without any obvious sign of agitation. Occasionally, a history of the recent onset of a viral illness may be elicited.

Clinically meaningful apnea can be defined as the absence of airflow for at least 20 seconds or apnea accompanied by cyanosis or bradycardia. Infants who experience these "apparent life-threatening events" are known to be at increased risk for SIDS, but the precise cause of SIDS remains elusive. Other infants at high risk for sudden death include those with a family history of SIDS (particularly in a sibling), premature infants with prolonged apnea and bradycardia, infants with significant illness such as bronchopulmonary dysplasia or congenital heart disease, infants with viral bronchiolitis (especially caused by respiratory syncytial virus), and infants born to mothers of lower socioeconomic class or whose mothers abused alcohol, drugs, or tobacco during pregnancy. Several different forms of apnea are recognized in pediatric patients: obstructive, central, and mixed (Fig. 16.36). Obstructive apnea is characterized by the lack of airflow at the nose or mouth despite continued respiratory efforts, whereas absence of airflow accompanied by the cessation of chest and abdominal wall movement distinguishes central apnea.

The number of hospital evaluations for infants with apneic episodes has undergone a dramatic increase in recent years, as has the number of infants who receive months of home apnea monitoring. There is no specific test or tests that can accurately predict the infant at risk for SIDS, and the assessment of an infant presenting with clinically significant apnea varies depending on findings uncovered during the initial history and physical examination. Factors that should be sought in an otherwise healthy infant include infection (sepsis, CNS infection, infantile botulism), cardiac disease (congenital or cardiac arrhythmias), metabolic disease (including electrolyte abnormalities), neurologic disease (seizures, intraventricular hemorrhage, increased intracranial pressure) and gastroesophageal reflux. Studies that may be helpful include a sleep study that measures respiratory and abdominal wall movement, airflow at the mouth or nose, pulse oximetry and heart rate and, in some cases, pH monitoring of the distal esophagus. Episodes of obstructive, mixed or central apnea, alone or together, may be observed during a sleep study evaluation (Fig. 16.36). Obstructive apnea can take place in the setting of extreme obesity, in infants with gastroesophageal reflux, severe laxity of the supraglottic structures, or in older patients with marked adenoidal or tonsillar enlargement. Central apnea may occur in infants with seizure disorders or central nervous system pathology such as intraventricular hemorrhage, in premature infants with immature respiratory control mechanisms, and in congenital central hypoventilation syndrome (Ondine's curse). Mixed apnea generally occurs when an obstructive apneic episode is followed by a central pattern of apnea.

Other studies that may be useful include ventilatory responses to hypercapnea or hypoxia, a chest x-ray, an electroencephalogram, Holter monitoring, and/or bronchoscopic evaluation of the airway, particularly in those patients with evidence of obstructive apnea. Laboratory evaluation may include any or all of the following: CBC, arterial or venous blood gases, chest radiography, electrocardiogram. Unfortunately, despite the battery of sophisticated tests available to the clinician, none is able to predict the subsequent risk for SIDS nor to determine which patients are appropriate candidates for home monitoring. As a result, a clinical judgment weighing the results of testing, the assessment of the home situation, and the seriousness of the original event is required for decisions regarding therapeutic intervention. Complicating this decision is the fact that there is no convincing evidence that home apnea monitoring will prevent SIDS.

DEGREES OF CLUBBING

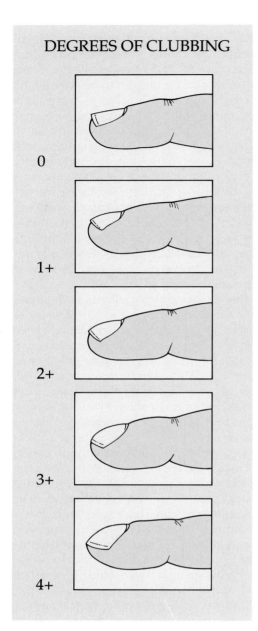

0

1+

2+

3+

4+

FIG. 16.37

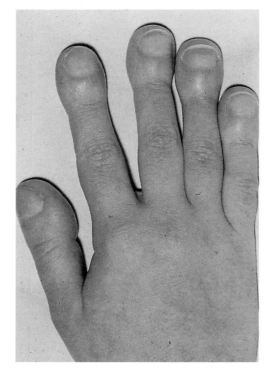

FIG. 16.38 Patient with cystic fibrosis and finger clubbing.

Pulmonary
    Cystic fibrosis
    Other bronchiectasis
    Pulmonary abscess
    Empyema
    Neoplasms
    Interstitial fibrosis
    Pulmonary alveolar
        proteinosis
    Interstitial pneumonitis
    Chronic pneumonia

Cardia
    Cyanotic congenital
        heart disease
    Subacute bacterial
        endocarditis

Gastrointestinal/hepatic
    Ulcerative colitis
    Crohn's disease
    Polyposis
    Biliary cirrhosis/biliary
        atresia

Familial
Thyrotoxicosis

FIG. 16.39

pulmonary function testing in children must take into account variability in performance by children and differences in age, height, weight, sex, and race. In children, PFTs may be useful in establishing the severity of respiratory disease, in guiding the choice of therapy and, in some cases, in measuring the response to a therapeutic regimen. In some diseases, such as cystic fibrosis or asthma, evidence of increasing airway obstruction may indicate the need for initiating or increasing the aggressiveness of therapeutic intervention.

The inspection of the shape of flow-volume curves generated during forced expiratory maneuvers is critical for the appropriate interpretation of PFT results (Fig. 16.41). The initial portion of the flow-volume curve is effort-dependent, but the terminal 75 percent of the expiratory maneuver is dependent on elastic recoil and airway resistance and is independent of patient effort. A normal-appearing flow-volume curve is shown in Fig. 16.41A. With increased airway resistance distal to the central, large airways, the curve becomes concave to the abscissa. This type of concavity, therefore, suggests obstruction to airflow (Fig. 16.41B). Patients with suspected reactive airways disease may develop this type of flow-volume curve following bronchoprovocation tests such as inhaled histamine, methacholine or cold air, or after exercise testing.

The restrictive pattern shown in Fig. 16.41C demonstrates preservation of expiratory flow function but a reduction in total lung volume. Neuromuscular disorders such as Duchenne's muscular dystrophy, or scoliosis, and interstitial lung disease are among the entities that typically produce this pattern on pulmonary function testing.

DIAGNOSTIC TECHNIQUES

The notion that "the examination of the lungs begins at the fingertips" is an important one, as digital clubbing may point to the presence of severe lung disease. Various stages of clubbing, from mild to severe, are depicted in Figures 16.37 and 16.38. Not all digital clubbing is associated with pulmonary disease (Fig. 16.39); nonpulmonary causes include cardiac, gastrointestinal, hepatic, and familial, as well as clubbing observed with thyrotoxicosis. Bronchiectasis from cystic fibrosis or from other infectious etiologies is the major cause of clubbing among all pulmonary diseases. Digital clubbing in any child with a chronic cough or wheezing warrants a thorough evaluation and investigation to determine the underlying disorder.

Diagnosis and treatment of children with respiratory complaints may be facilitated by the use of pulmonary function testing. With appropriate training, and with the technician's patience and encouragement, most children 5 years of age or older will cooperate with simple spirometry and measurements of lung volumes (Fig. 16.40). Interpretation of results of

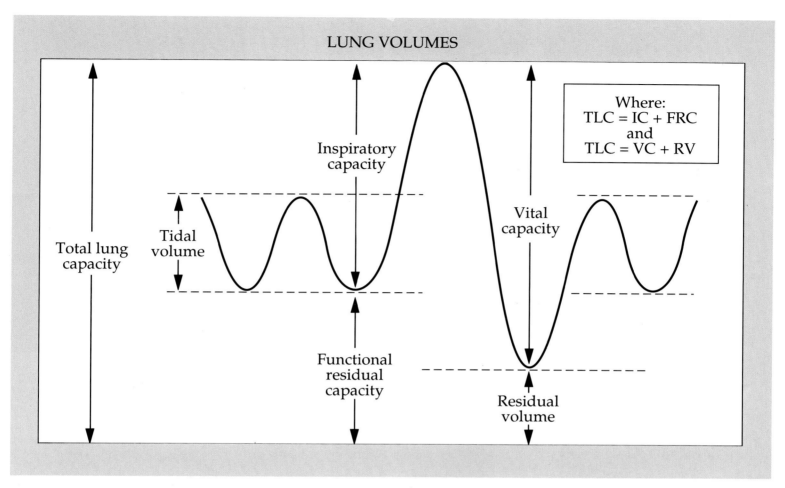

FIG. 16.40 Schematic representation of lung volumes.

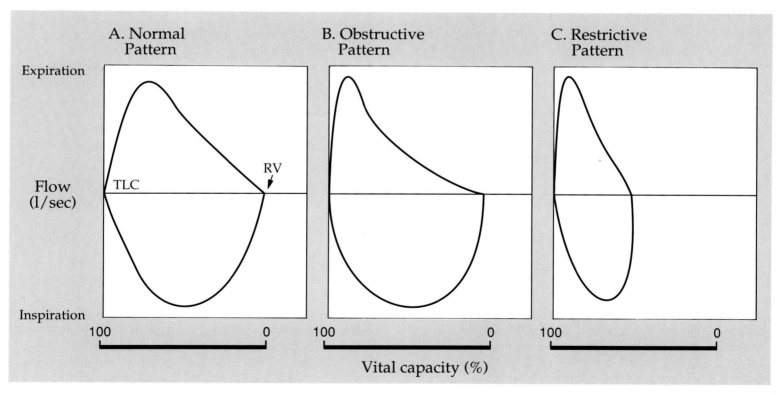

FIG. 16.41 Flow-volume curves obtained by spirometry. **A,** normal configuration of expiratory flow curve. **B,** reduced expiratory flow rates suggestive of obstructive airway disease. **C,** preservation of flow rates with a diminished vital capacity consistent with restrictive lung disease.

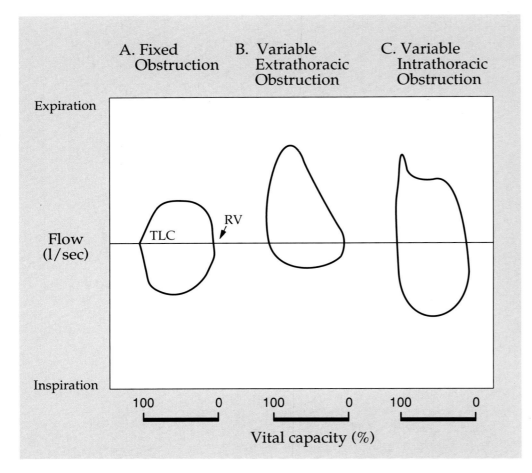

FIG. 16.42 **A,** *fixed obstruction of upper airways with reduction in inspiratory and expiratory flow loops.* **B,** *reduction in peak inspiratory flow observed in variable extrathoracic airway obstruction.* **C,** *reduction and flattening of the expiratory limb in variable intrathoracic obstruction.*

FIG. 16.43 *Flexible fiberoptic bronchoscope (Olympus BF3C10, 3.5-min OD) shown next to a 10-cent coin, for size comparison.*

The shape of the flow-volume curve may also be helpful in evaluating the presence of upper or central airway pathology (Fig. 16.42). Fixed obstruction of the upper airways, as in tracheal stenosis, produces a limitation and plateau of both the inspiratory and expiratory loops of the flow-volume curve. A reduced inspiratory flow and a plateau of the inspiratory loop are suggestive of variable extrathoracic obstruction seen in disorders such as laryngomalacia. Malacia of the intrathoracic trachea or major bronchi results in a picture of variable intrathoracic obstruction with reduction and flattening of the expiratory limb, since pleural pressures exceed pressure within the lumen.

Exercise testing can be a valuable tool to assess the cardiorespiratory fitness of a subject and may provide further information regarding a patient's respiratory reserve in addition to that found during routine pulmonary function tests. A progressive exercise study by bicycle ergometry can give important information regarding ventilatory effort, heart-rate responses, oxygen delivery and uptake, and carbon dioxide production. Evaluation of these parameters may provide information regarding exercise fitness and, if limited, identify whether the limiting factor is ventilatory or cardiac. Like PFTs, exercise testing can be utilized to assess the severity or progress of disease, evaluate effects of changes in treatment, and provide information about the safety or appropriateness of an exercise program in children with chronic lung disease.

Flexible fiberoptic bronchoscopy (Fig. 16.43) is a relatively new procedure available to the pediatric pulmonologist. It can

RANGE OF NORMAL ARTERIAL BLOOD GAS VALUES BY AGE

	pH	pCO_2	pO_2
Newborn	7.33-7.49	27-41	>60
Infant (<1 year)	7.34-7.46	26-41	>75
Older child	7.35-7.45	35-45	>75

FIG. 16.44

be extremely useful in the diagnosis of lesions of the pulmonary tree and in isolating organisms from patients with pneumonia. Compared with traditional open-tube ("rigid") bronchoscopy, flexible bronchoscopy offers the advantages of avoiding general anesthesia and allowing the study of airway dynamics during regular tidal breathing. Indications for pediatric flexible bronchoscopy include evaluation of stridor, unexplained or chronic cough or wheeze, suspected airway malformations or compression, atelectasis, or recurrent pneumonia. To obviate the need for open lung biopsy, flexible bronchoscopy and bronchoalveolar lavage may be particularly useful in immunosuppressed patients with unexplained pneumonia. Flexible bronchoscopy should not be attempted when there is a strong clinical or radiographic suggestion of inhaled foreign body. In these cases, rigid bronchoscopy is the procedure of choice to remove the object.

Arterial blood gas measurements are the standard for assessing gas exchange. Pulse oximetry and analysis of the CO_2 in exhaled air are useful noninvasive tools that have a place in a selected number of patients with respiratory embarrassment, but technical difficulties in interpretation and artifact can lead to serious errors in assessment. Venous or capillary blood gases can give accurate estimations of pH and PCO_2, but may significantly underestimate real PO_2. Normal arterial pH, PO_2, and PCO_2 values are provided in Figure 16.44.

ACKNOWLEDGMENT

The authors wish to thank Dr. Geoffrey Kurland for his assistance with photographs and clinical material.

BIBLIOGRAPHY

Benjamin B: *Atlas of Paediatric Endoscopy*. London, Oxford University Press, 1981.

Chernick V, Kendig EL: *Disorders of the Respiratory Tract in Children*, ed 5. Philadelphia, WB Saunders, 1990.

Eigen HE: The clinical evaluation of chronic cough. *Pediatr Clin North Am* 1982; 29:67–78.

Fishman AP: *Pulmonary Diseases and Disorders*, ed 2. New York, McGraw-Hill, 1988.

Lloyd-Still JD: *Textbook of Cystic Fibrosis*. Boston, John Wright, 1983.

Phelan PD, Landau LI, Olinsky A: *Respiratory Illness in Children*, ed 3. London, Blackwell Scientific Publications, 1990.

Singleton EB, Wagner MI, Dutton RV: *Radiologic Atlas of Pulmonary Abnormalities in Children*. Philadelphia, WB Saunders, 1988.

Taussig LM: *Cystic Fibrosis*. New York, Thieme-Stratton, 1984.

17
PEDIATRIC SURGERY

Don K. Nakayama, M.D.

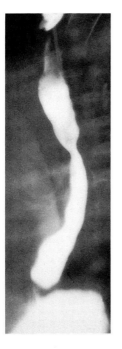

FIG. 17.1
Midthoracic compressions into the esophageal barium column identify the presence of vascular ring anomalies (in this case, pulmonary artery sling).

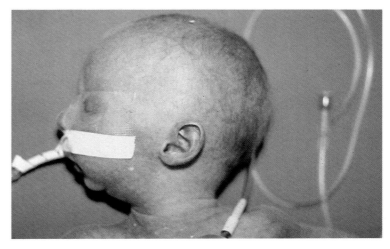

FIG. 17.2 In Pierre-Robin sequence, the hypoplastic mandible positions the tongue posteriorly, potentially obstructing the upper airway.

This chapter encompasses many common general pediatric surgical disorders, but is not intended to be an exhaustive survey. Emphasis is on surgical conditions likely to be encountered in general pediatric practice, amplified by the inclusion of some uncommon and rare disorders.

RESPIRATORY DISTRESS

Surgical causes of respiratory distress are uncommon, but demand immediate attention and should be considered in the evaluation of newborns and infants who demonstrate signs of dyspnea or stridor. Plain film evaluation should include both anteroposterior and lateral views of the chest, with special attention to the airway contour and lateral soft-tissue views of the upper airway. Examination under fluoroscopy gives valuable information of changes in airway contour and diaphragmatic motion during the respiratory cycle. Barium swallow helps to locate masses within the mediastinum and to establish the presence of a vascular ring anomaly (Fig. 17.1). Laryngoscopy and endoscopic examinations of the upper air-

way, the tracheobronchial tree, and esophagus become necessary when the procedures above fail to yield a clear-cut diagnosis. The different surgical causes of respiratory distress are grouped most conveniently by anatomic site: upper airway, thoracic, and extrathoracic.

Upper Airway

Newborn infants do not acquire the ability to breathe through the mouth until several days after birth. Thus an obstructive lesion of the upper airway must be considered in any infant who demonstrates cyclic dyspnea (recurring episodes of asphyxia followed by crying, mouth breathing, quiet, and then asphyxia again), or inability to nurse. An obstructive airway within the extrathoracic area forces the infant to gasp to breathe, because the upper airway tends to collapse onto the lesion at inspiration. The airway enlarges during expiration, which is relatively unlabored. The voice is normal unless the larynx itself is occluded. The differential diagnosis should include choanal atresia, tracheoesophageal fistula, esophageal

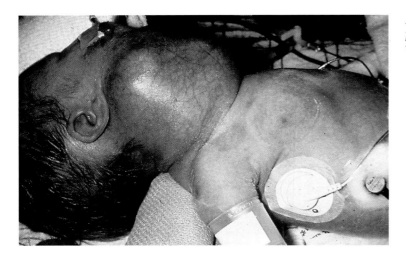

FIG. 17.3 *Cervical teratoma may compress the esophagus in utero, and produce polyhydramnios. After delivery, compression of the upper airway from the mass may create a surgical emergency.*

MEDIASTINAL MASSES IN CHILDHOOD

Anterior and Superior	Middle	Posterior
Teratoma, including dermoid cysts	Bronchogenic cysts	Neurogenic tumors
Normal thymus	Pericardial cyst	Enterogenous cysts
Lymphoma		Pulmonary sequestration
Vascular malformations		
Thymic cysts		
Cystic hygroma		
Intrathoracic goiter		

FIG. 17.4

atresia, vocal cord paralysis, foreign body, and tumors or other lesions in the naso- or oropharynx.

Passage of a nasogastric tube is a basic procedure during the initial evaluation of the newborn infant with possible airway obstruction. Inability to reach the pharynx suggests choanal atresia. The obstruction is bony in 90 percent, and membranous in 10 percent. About half of all cases are associated with other anomalies, including craniofacial, cardiovascular, and abdominal. Endoscopic examination or contrast roentgenography of the nasopharynx confirms the diagnosis. Maintenance of an oral airway and gavage feeding are necessary until transpalatal repair is performed.

Macroglossia may obstruct the oropharynx and cause respiratory distress. Diffuse enlargement of the tongue from lymphangioma is the most common cause. Hypertrophy of the tongue is characteristic of Beckwith-Wiedemann syndrome. In contrast, a hypoplastic and recessed mandible causes a normal-sized tongue to fall posteriorly and obstruct the airway in Pierre-Robin sequence (Fig. 17.2). Cleft palate and cardiac anomalies frequently complicate the latter condition. Placing the baby in the prone position may open the airway; this allows many infants to be managed without tracheostomy. The infant eventually learns to keep the tongue away from the larynx, and sufficient mandibular growth occurs. Some infants, however, still require tracheotomy.

Lesions of the larynx are characterized by a husky, hoarse, or whispered cry, or complete aphonia in association with dyspnea. Laryngeal atresia, webs, cysts, laryngomalacia, subglottic stenosis, and vocal cord paralysis are included in the differential diagnosis. The need for tracheotomy becomes urgent when a severe obstruction prevents placement of an orotracheal tube, as in cases of laryngeal atresia. Laryngeal cleft allows feedings in the pharynx to enter the airway directly through a defect between the arytenoids in the posterior larynx.

Cysts and other tumors that lie within the pharynx may cause upper airway obstruction. Examples include dermoids, branchial cleft remnants, lingual thyroid, intraoral thyroglossal duct cysts, hemangioma, duplications, and palatal teratoma (epulis). Large masses in the neck may compress the airway and cause dyspnea, such as cervical teratoma (Fig. 17.3).

Thoracic

MEDIASTINUM AND DIAPHRAGM

Mediastinal lesions cause respiratory distress through compression of the airway, and produce other clinical effects (dyspnea, plethora of the head and upper extremities) by compressing other structures nearby (esophagus, superior vena cava) (Fig. 17.4). Location of the mass within the mediastinum

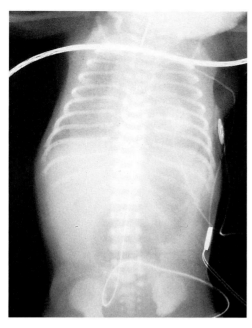

FIG. 17.5 The large thymus of the newborns and infants should not be confused with an upper mediastinal mass on chest film.

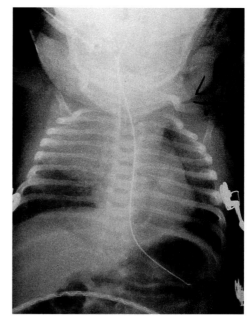

FIG. 17.6 Posterior mediastinal masses include esophageal duplication (illustrated here), neurenteric cysts, extralobar sequestration, anterior myelomeningocele, and neural tumors. Vertebral anomalies coexist frequently.

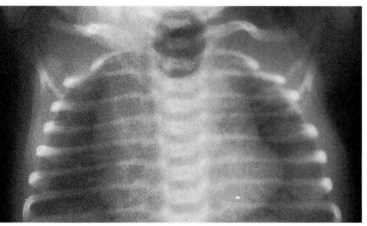

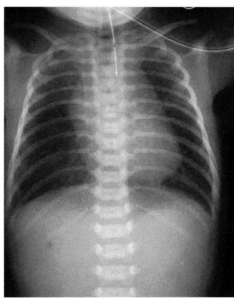

FIG. 17.7 A nasogastric tube lying in the upper mediastinum within a distended esophageal pouch identifies esophageal atresia; air within the gastrointestinal tract means that a distal tracheoesophageal fistula is also present.

FIG. 17.8 In contrast to Fig. 17.7, the absence of air in the abdomen means that no tracheoesophageal fistula is present, and the esophageal atresia (again identified by a coiled nasogastric tube in the upper mediastinum) is isolated.

and the age of the patient give the most important clues to the identity of mediastinal masses. Abnormalities of the superior and anterior mediastinum include cystic hygroma, lymphoma, teratoma, and dermoid cysts. Here the thymus is normally prominent in newborns and infants (Fig. 17.5). Pericardial and bronchogenic cysts arise in the middle mediastinum. Foregut duplications (Fig. 17.6), neurenteric cysts, extralobar sequestration, anterior myelomeningocele, and neurenteric tumors arise in the posterior mediastinum.

Inability to pass a nasogastric tube into the stomach (the same tube to exclude choanal atresia) makes the diagnosis of esophageal atresia. A fistula from the carina to the distal esophageal remnant (distal tracheoesophageal fistula) completes the most common combination of tracheoesophageal

anomalies (present in 85 percent of cases). The fistula allows air to fill the stomach, a feature on plain film that distinguishes cases of esophageal atresia associated with a distal tracheoesophageal fistula (Fig. 17.7) from those without a tracheoesophageal communication (pure esophageal atresia, Fig. 17.8). The third most common pattern of tracheoesophageal anomalies, tracheoesophageal fistula without esophageal atresia, has no esophageal obstruction, so a nasogastric tube passes freely into the stomach. The fistula arises from the trachea and passes distally into the esophagus, creating an "N" rather than a horizontal "H" shaped communication between the two structures. This angle may impede reflux of material from the esophagus into the trachea, including contrast. To keep the lungs free from foreign material, barium swallow to opacify

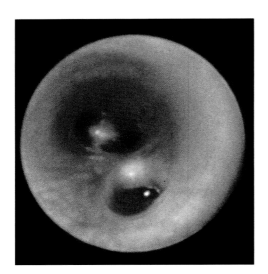

FIG. 17.9
Bronchoscopy visualizes tracheoesophageal fistula, seen as a posteriorly positioned orifice (bottom) in the upper trachea. The carina, seen toward the top of the picture, lies distally.

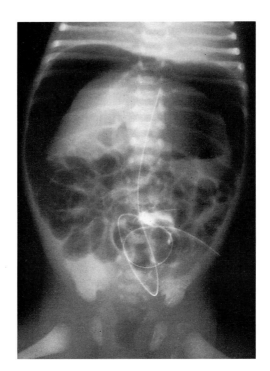

FIG. 17.10
Tracheoesophageal fistula allows air to be forced into the stomach during positive pressure ventilation either by bag and mask or through an endotracheal tube. The stomach may perforate or ventilation become suddenly ineffective if a gastrotomy is placed initially during surgical repair.

the fistula is not recommended. Its diagnosis requires confirmation by bronchoscopy (Fig. 17.9).

Respiratory distress results from the esophageal obstruction and the communication between the airway and esophagus. Babies with esophageal atresia salivate excessively and are unable to swallow feedings. The baby may aspirate formula and saliva pooled in the obstructed upper esophageal pouch. Gastric juice refluxes into the distal esophageal segment, and enters the tracheobronchial tree through the fistula. While awaiting surgical repair, the baby is kept in a flat, head-up position to minimize gastroesophageal reflux. An infant sump tube (Replogle tube) keeps the upper esophageal pouch decompressed. A problem arises when respiratory distress is severe, either from aspiration or from pulmonary immaturity. The gastrointestinal tract may offer less resistance to inflation than the lungs, so positive pressure ventilation by mask or endotracheal tube may force air into the stomach. Respiratory insufficiency may worsen and perforation of the stomach may occur (Fig. 17.10).

Congenital diaphragmatic hernia results from persistence of the foramen of Bochdalek (Fig. 17.11). Most (85%) are left-sided. Intestines enter the thorax during early gestation, inhibiting pulmonary development and leading to hypoplasia of the lung. Once placental circulation is interrupted at birth, respiratory distress develops rapidly. Because the intestines are in the chest, the abdomen appears scaphoid. The left hemithorax is dull to percussion, and breath sounds may be poor or absent. Heart sounds are best heard on the side opposite the hernia because of displacement of the mediastinum. Chest film reveals air-filled loops within the hemithorax that appear to push the mediastinum into the contralateral lung, which is collapsed. Cystic adenomatoid malformation may mimic the roentgenographic appearance of diaphragmatic hernia; the location of the stomach bubble is the abdomen in the former, and the chest in the latter. Respiratory insufficiency is severe, the result of pulmonary hypoplasia and pulmonary hypertension. Despite early operative repair and aggressive management with advance modalities of critical care, including extracorporeal membrane oxygenation, mortality remains high.

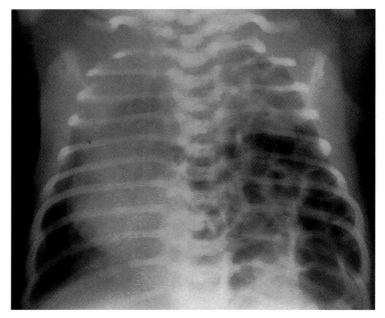

FIG. 17.11 Congenital diaphragmatic hernia allows intestines to enter chest in utero, and pushes the mediastinum to the contralateral side.

Persistence of the embryonic aortic arches creates complete vascular rings around the trachea and esophagus. Symptoms arise from compression of the trachea (dyspnea) and esophagus (dysphagia). Narrowing of the tracheal air contour within the mediastinum on chest film (Fig. 17.12) suggests the presence of vascular ring. Barium swallow shows compression on the esophagus (see Fig. 17.1) and confirms the diagnosis. Bronchoscopy (Fig. 17.13), a necessary part of the preoperative assessment, needs to be performed by the attending surgeon in the operating room, should the procedure induce closure of a critically narrowed airway. Aortography provides the necessary anatomic detail for surgery.

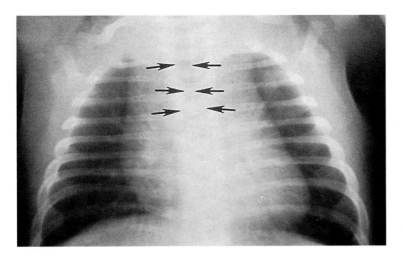

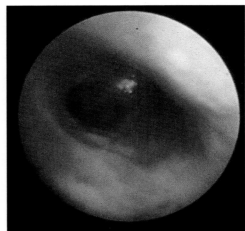

FIG. 17.13 Anterior compression of the trachea by an innominate artery with an anomalous leftward origin, as viewed at bronchoscopy.

FIG. 17.12 Narrowing (arrows) or disappearance of the tracheal air contour suggests the presence of tracheal compression by a vascular ring, an often subtle sign which should be followed by a barium swallow in the evaluation.

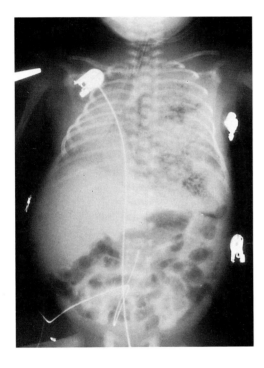

FIG. 17.14 Microcystic adenomatoid malformation of the left lung. Large cystic lesions can be mistaken for bowel loops herniating through a diaphragmatic hernia (Fig. 17.11).

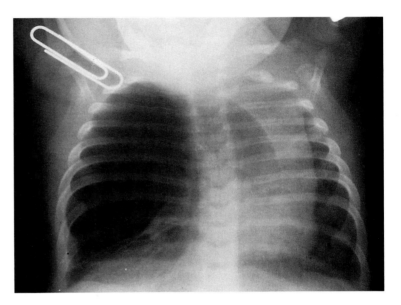

FIG. 17.15 Lobar emphysema, usually involving the upper lobes, may become hugely distended and may cause life-threatening respiratory distress.

Although an important cause of respiratory insufficiency, congenital heart disease is beyond the scope of this discussion (see Chapter 5).

LUNG

Anomalies of lung bud development lead to cystic diseases of the lung and pulmonary sequestration, the most common surgical causes of respiratory distress that arise within the lung itself. Growth of these lesions within the thorax compresses normal lung parenchyma, causing dyspnea early in life. Large or rapidly expanding lesions may require emergency surgical excision. Rupture of an expanding cyst is rare, except as a complication of diagnostic aspiration, which is not recommended except as a temporizing procedure before surgery in patients with severe symptoms. Some patients are relatively free from dyspnea and present later in infancy or childhood with cough, fever and recurrent pulmonary infections.

There are three varieties of cystic adenomatoid malformation of the lung, based upon the size of the cysts: large (1 to 4 cm, the type mistaken for diaphragmatic hernia on plain film), small (<1 cm, Fig. 17.14), and solid (noncystic). Like diaphragmatic hernia, cystic adenomatoid malformation can produce life-threatening symptoms soon after birth and may be complicated by pulmonary hypertension. Overexpansion of a segment or lobe of a lung leads to congenital lobar emphysema (Fig. 17.15). About half of all cases become symptomatic within the first week of life, but symptoms may not develop 1 to 4 or more months later. Chest films show a hyperlucent, overexpanded area of the lung, most frequently either upper lobes or

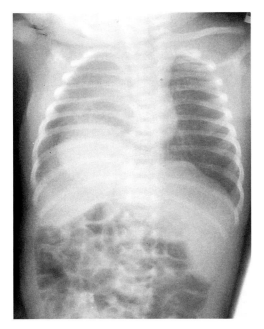

FIG. 17.16 Persistent infiltration of the lung parenchyma may indicate the presence of an intralobar sequestration, here involving the right lower lobe. Also seen is a right diaphragmatic hernia, a frequently associated malformation.

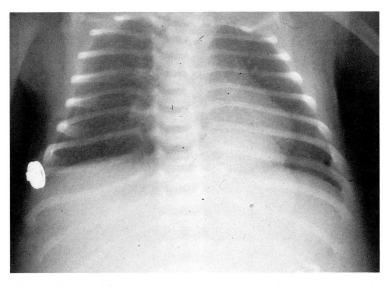

FIG. 17.17 Extralobar sequestration appears typically as a nonaerated intrathoracic mass in the lower posterior thorax, here on the left.

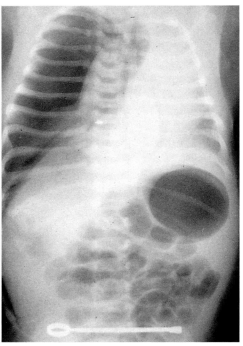

FIG. 17.18 This chest film shows typical radiologic signs of tension pneumothorax: mediastinal shift, flattening of the diaphragm and widening of the intercostal spaces.

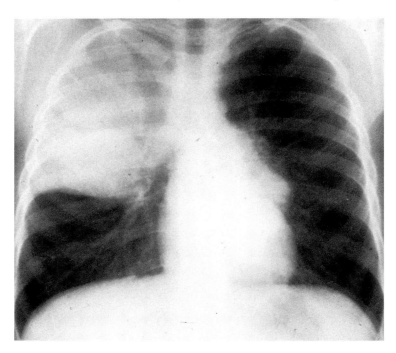

FIG. 17.19 Chest film in a child with allergic bronchopulmonary aspergillosis of the right upper lobe, which ultimately required resection.

the right middle lobe. Infants and children who develop dyspnea require resection. Asymptomatic lesions that do not cause significant compressive effects do not require removal. In patients with congenital lobar emphysema, positive pressure ventilation (upon anesthetic induction or during resuscitation) may cause acute cardiorespiratory decompensation by overdistending the affected lobe.

Pulmonary sequestrations are accessory lobes of lung tissue that reside separately from the architecture of the normal lung, either within a normal lobe (intralobar type, Fig. 17.16), or lying separately from the normal lobes of the lung, invested in its own pleura (extralobar type, Fig. 17.17). Most frequently found in the lower left posterior chest, many sequestrations

derive a systemic blood supply from the thoracic or abdominal aorta. A few cases retain a bronchial communication with the foregut. Most cases are asymptomatic and are found as an airless posterior mediastinal mass during repair of a diaphragmatic hernia or in a chest film taken for other indications. Recurring localized infection in a fluid-filled cyst is the most common presentation. Aortography or high-resolution Doppler ultrasound establishes the diagnosis by demonstration of a systemic arterial supply.

Pneumothorax may result from both blunt and penetrating trauma to the chest. It complicates positive pressure ventilation in critical care units and spontaneously breathing children with advanced cystic fibrosis. The ipsilateral thorax is expand-

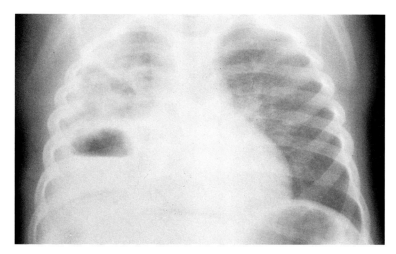

FIG. 17.20 Chest film in a child with a cavitary lung abscess.

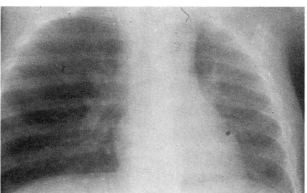 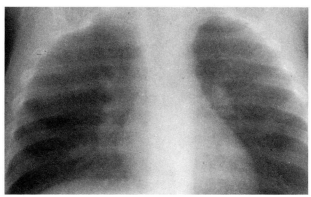

FIG. 17.21 Signs of a radiolucent foreign body are often subtle. Persistent overdistention of the right lung was due to right mainstem bronchial occlusion.

ed, is tympanic to percussion, and has decreased breath sounds. Breath sounds, however, may be transmitted from the opposite, unaffected side, particularly in infants. Tension pneumothorax causes the diaphragm to flatten and the mediastinum to shift to the opposite side (Fig. 17.18). The heart shifts as well, disturbing its relationship to systemic and pulmonary veins, thus embarrassing venous return. Hypotension results, and may preclude x-ray confirmation of the diagnosis. Needle decompression may be life-saving.

Resection may become necessary in pulmonary infections that persist despite antibiotic therapy or where the diagnosis remains in doubt. Failure of an infiltrate to resolve suggests the presence of a resistant organism (Fig. 17.19), development of a lung abscess, a diagnosis that becomes obvious when cavitation occurs (Fig. 17.20), or the presence of a pulmonary malignancy. A foreign body that occludes a bronchus (Fig. 17.21) may produce pulmonary consolidation.

Extrathoracic Causes

Abdominal distention of any cause elevates the diaphragm and decreases intrathoracic volume, and may lead to respiratory insufficiency. In newborns and infants, common causes include tumors, ascites, and intestinal obstruction. On pedi-

atric surgical services, the use of narcotics for postoperative pain control may lead to respiratory depression, apnea, and, on occasion, arrest.

VOMITING

The major surgical cause of vomiting is obstruction of the gastrointestinal tract. The clinical challenge is to distinguish the relatively few cases that require surgery from the many children with self-limited conditions and medical illnesses that cause vomiting but do not demand operation or even plain films, contrast studies, or medical and surgical consultation. Certain clinical signs direct attention to a surgical etiology. Bilious vomiting is a key finding in newborns and infants. When it occurs in an infant without abdominal distention, malrotation and volvulus becomes the paramount concern; when the abdomen is distended, distal small bowel obstruction must be considered. Blood in the stool may indicate the presence of intestinal ischemia, from, for example, intussusception or malrotation. Failure to pass meconium in the first day of life in term infants should increase suspicions that a congenital obstruction is present. Fever, abdominal pain, and tenderness upon palpation suggests peritonitis. An abdominal surgical scar identifies the child at risk for postoperative adhe-

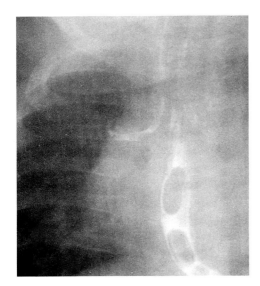

FIG. 17.22 Fluoroscopic examination of the infant during barium swallow must be of sufficient duration to allow the identification of episodes of reflux (here associated with aspiration into the tracheobronchial tree).

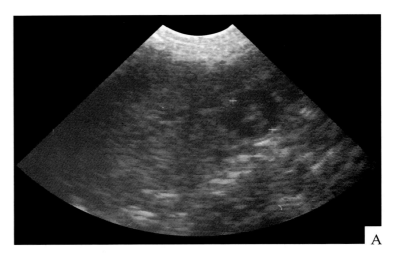

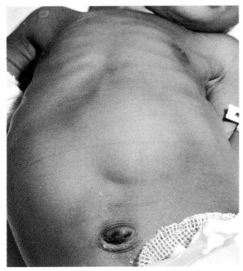

FIG. 17.23 Pyloric stenosis may cause epigastric distention by the obstructed stomach. This patient also demonstrates a visible wave of peristalsis, which moves from left to right.

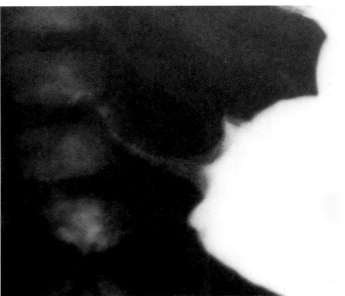

FIG. 17.24 Hypertrophic pyloric stenosis. *A*, ultrasonographic scan of the upper abdomen demonstrates the thickened pyloric muscle, indicated by the cursors. *B*, barium study of the stomach (bottom) shows thin streaks of barium in the pyloric canal. The hypertrophic pyloric muscle bulged into the gastric antrum produces a "reversed 3" configuration.

sion obstruction. A vomiting child must always be checked for a fixed, tender groin bulge.

Plain film evaluation should include both anterior-posterior and left lateral recumbent views (patient on his or her side, left side down, film taken "cross-table") of the abdomen. These views easily demonstrate air-fluid loops and free intra-abdominal air, if present.

Newborn infants have unique radiologic requirements. No radiographic contrast is needed to make the diagnosis of esophageal atresia and duodenal atresia. A small amount of air injected into the stomach through the gastric tube may help demonstrate the characteristic "double bubble" in the latter diagnosis. If air is present distal to the duodenal bulb, an upper gastrointestinal series is the examination of choice to establish the presence of normal intestinal rotation. Intra-abdominal calcification identifies perforation and meconium peritonitis. Digital rectal examination and the use of suppositories and enemas may decompress distended colon above the transitional aganglionic zone in Hirschsprung's disease, causing a valuable radiographic sign to disappear. Therefore, a contrast enema study of the distended infant with bilious vomiting should precede other manipulations of the anorectum. Barium provides excellent opacification of the transition zone, if present. If no transition zone can be demonstrated, water-soluble contrast is used. Encountering a microcolon sug-

gests meconium ileus, particularly if mucus cocretions ("rabbit pellets") are present, or small bowel atresia. A transition zone from a small left colon to a distended transverse colon identifies small left colon syndrome. Water-soluble contrast may relieve obstruction in both meconium ileus and small left colon syndrome. In cases where no radiographic diagnosis can be made, abdominal films obtained one to several days later may reveal delayed passage of administered contrast, a sign of Hirschsprung's disease.

The different surgical causes of vomiting are grouped most conveniently into two age groups: newborn infants and older infants and children.

Vomiting in Newborn Infants

A practical way to divide causes of vomiting in newborn infants distinguishes those cases associated with bilious versus nonbilious vomiting, and those cases that cause abdominal distention versus those that do not.

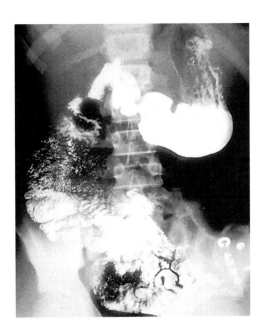

FIG. 17.25 The ligament of Treitz in malrotation is either absent or abnormally located, and the duodenum and small intestine lie on the right side of the abdomen. Duodenal obstruction may be partial (due to Ladd's bands, as seen here) or complete (due to volvulus).

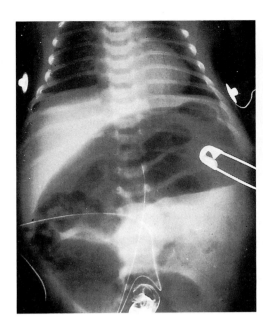

FIG. 17.26 Complete duodenal obstruction from midgut volvulus. Air in the distal gastrointestinal tract fails to rule out complete obstruction from volvulus, and distinguishes the diagnosis from duodenal atresia.

NONBILIOUS VOMITING

Nearly all infants have gastroesophageal reflux, the most common cause of nonbilious vomiting during the first year of life. The condition is self-limited, and three-fourths of infants are reflux-free by 9 months of age. The tendency toward vomiting is made worse by overfeeding, failure to burp the baby, and overstimulating the baby after feeding, so a careful feeding history may indicate the cause of vomiting.

A number of tests confirm the diagnosis and establish the need for surgery. In addition to demonstrating episodes of reflux, barium swallow (Fig. 17.22) rules out pyloric stenosis and malrotation and gives roentgenographic evidence of esophageal stricture and motility disturbances. Radionuclide milk scan detects episodes of reflux, quantifies esophageal and gastric clearance, and detects aspiration when radioactivity is present over lung fields. Placement of a pH probe into the distal esophagus gives the duration and number of reflux episodes, usually during an overnight period, and is the most sensitive test. The presence of esophagitis on biopsy of the distal esophageal mucosa confirms a complication of reflux that may require corrective surgery.

Even in severe cases, conservative management successfully controls vomiting. Surgical procedures to strengthen the lower esophageal antireflux mechanism (fundoplication procedures) are applied to those cases associated with complications: esophageal stricture, aspiration, failure to gain weight, and documentation of life-threatening episodes of apnea associated with reflux. Hiatal hernia is usually absent; in rare cases the stomach may slip through the hiatus into the chest, a situation that risks gastric volvulus. Reflux in children with neurologic handicaps are particularly severe and often require fundoplication. Fundoplication may render the child unable to vomit. Should adhesions from surgery form and obstruct the intestine distally, a closed loop obstruction results that may lead rapidly to intestinal ischemia. Immediate placement of a nasogastric tube is required in a child with a fundoplication who develops abdominal distention.

Pyloric stenosis is the most common surgical condition of the newborn period, present in 1 in 700 live births. Etiology is unknown, but heredity has some influence: it is more common in boys, it develops in 7 percent of children of affected parents, and is four times more likely to be present when the mother was affected. Vomiting begins at 1 to 6 weeks of age, generally about 3 weeks, and is frequently projectile. Peristalsis of a distended stomach may become visible (Fig. 17.23). The lesion itself is palpable in the epigastrium, between the midline and the right midclavicular line, having the consistency of a small, firm olive. The child must be relaxed and the stomach empty to allow adequate examination. Maneuvers that are sometimes helpful include raising the baby into a semirecumbent position to allow the pylorus to fall inferiorally and flexing the legs to relax abdominal muscles. When the mass is not palpable, the most productive alternative approach is a second physical examination in about an hour, when the child is sleeping and other examiners are long gone. An affected pylorus is palpable in 70 to 90 percent of cases. Once felt, no further tests are necessary before pyloromyotomy. If the diagnosis remains in doubt, an upper gastrointestinal series is preferred because other causes of vomiting can be diagnosed if pyloric stenosis is not present (Fig. 17.24). Ultrasound examination is a reliable alternative when an experienced sonographer is present.

BILIOUS VOMITING, NO ABDOMINAL DISTENTION

Malrotation is failure of the midgut (small intestine and right colon) to achieve its normal anatomic position during development. The cecum and colon lie in the left abdomen; the duodenum and small intestine lie on the right side. Retroperitoneal attachment is inadequate and the mesenteric pedicle is narrow, factors that easily lead to volvulus. Volvulus leads to high intestinal obstruction and vomiting (Figs. 17.25, 17.26). Twisting of the mesenteric vessels causes intestinal ischemia and midgut infarction (Fig. 17.27). Bloody stool or nasogastric drainage, the development of abdominal distention, guarding, abdominal wall erythema, and edema indicate

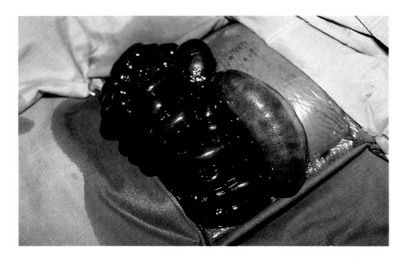

FIG. 17.27 Malrotation predisposes to volvulus and infarction of the entire midgut.

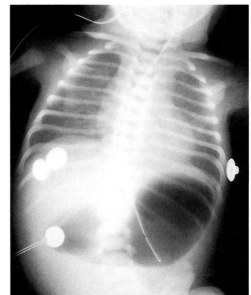

FIG. 17.28 Swallowed air distends the stomach and first portion of the duodenum in duodenal atresia, producing the characteristic "double bubble" on plain film and making other contrast studies unnecessary.

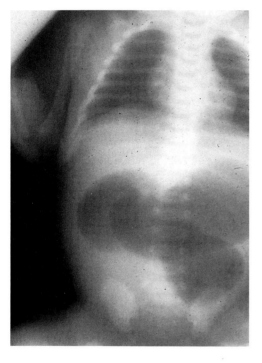

FIG. 17.29 Jejunal atresia distends only a few bowel loops proximally, distinguishing it from duodenal and ileal atresia.

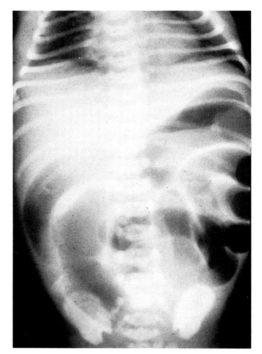

FIG. 17.30 Many intestinal loops become distended in patients with ileal atresia (pictured here), making the distinction between this diagnosis and other causes of distal bowel obstruction difficult. Other signs (such as intraperitoneal calcification indicating meconium peritonitis) and contrast enema become necessary to identify the cause of obstruction.

the development of intestinal gangrene. The result is death or extreme short gut syndrome if ischemia of the midgut is irreversible.

Although only a fraction of infants with bilious vomiting have malrotation, the consequences of missed cases are so grave that many surgeons recommend strongly that all newborn infants with bilious vomiting undergo urgent evaluation by upper gastrointestinal series. The key finding on contrast study is the location of the ligament of Treitz, which should be to the left of the vertebral column and behind the stomach bubble. An inadequately configured duodenal "C" loop that fails to cross to the left of midline and the proximal jejunal loops lying in the right side of the abdomen are diagnostic of malrotation (Fig. 17.25). The cecum on barium enema exami-

nation lies in the right upper quadrant or left side of the abdomen. Barium enema detects malrotation less reliably, because the cecum in the infant is mobile. The presence of a dilated duodenal loop (Fig. 17.26) suggests that obstruction has occurred, either from volvulus (Fig. 17.27) or by peritoneal bands overlying the duodenum (Ladd's bands). Plain films are not diagnostic. The obstructed midgut may fill with fluid and produce a "gasless" abdomen.

Duodenal atresia produces the characteristic "double bubble" on plain film (Fig. 17.28). Vomiting typically occurs soon after birth. Duodenal atresia frequently accompanies Down syndrome and congenital heart defects. Congenital stenosis of the duodenum, duodenal web, and annular pancreas cause partial duodenal obstruction, distinguished by the presence of

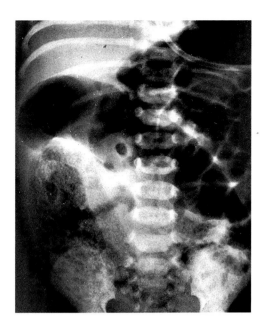

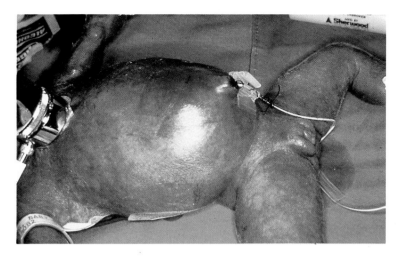

FIG. 17.31 This plain film shows two signs indicative of meconium ileus: a "soap bubble" mass in the right iliac fossa, produced by the impacted meconium and distended loops of different diameters, reflecting the gradual distention of the small bowel to the area of obstruction.

FIG. 17.32 Intense inflammation from free meconium in the peritoneal cavity (meconium peritonitis) may produce visible erythema and edema over the abdominal wall.

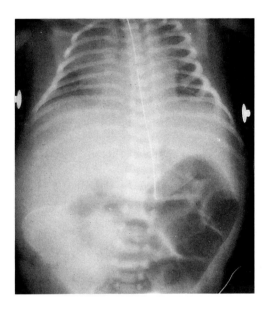

FIG. 17.33 Calcification in an area of meconium peritonitis in the right iliac fossa.

air distal to the dilated duodenal bubble. Because malrotation may also cause partial duodenal obstruction by Ladd's bands or volvulus, urgent contrast examination of the duodenal anatomy is required.

BILIOUS VOMITING, DISTENDED ABDOMEN

Small bowel atresias arise from intrauterine vascular insults. Their formation may occur relatively late in gestation, and meconium may have formed and passed distally by that time. Alone, passage of meconium after birth does not rule out the presence of an atresia. Proximal jejunal atresia results in upper abdominal distention, with only a few distended loops on abdominal plain film, which is diagnostic (Fig. 17.29). No contrast studies are needed. More generalized distention results from atresias located more distally, and contrast studies may be required to distinguish ileal atresia from other causes of distal bowel obstruction, such as Hirschsprung's disease and meconium ileus (Fig. 17.30). Distention develops 12 to 24 hours after birth. Distention present when the baby is born suggests meconium ileus or meconium peritonitis. Jejunoileal atresia may coexist with malrotation, meconium peritonitis, meconium ileus, and, rarely, Hirschsprung's disease. The different anatomic variants have been classified based upon whether the bowel and mesentery are intact. Two rare variants, "apple peel" atresia (the distal small bowel spirals around the ileocecal artery in a retrograde direction, a consequence of a major mesenteric arterial occlusion and multiple atresia ("string of sausages") are likely to leave the baby with short gut syndrome.

Meconium ileus is the first manifestation of cystic fibrosis in about 10 to 15 percent of affected children. A family history for cystic fibrosis is present in one-third of all cases. The meconium in cystic fibrosis is abnormally thick and tenacious, and impacts in the ileum, causing intestinal obstruction. Distally, the ileum and colon are tiny and contain concretions of mucus ("rabbit pellets"). The site of impact becomes hugely distended with meconium, seen as a "soap bubble" mass in the right iliac fossa on plain film (Fig. 17.31). No air-fluid levels are seen, because the meconium cannot easily form layers. The

gradual distention of small bowel along its length causes loops of bowel of different size to be seen on abdominal film. Contrast enema demonstrates the microcolon and "rabbit pellets" of inspissated mucus. Water-soluble contrast refluxed into the impacted ileum may result in passage of the meconium and relief of the obstruction in about half of patients with uncomplicated meconium ileus. Meconium ileus can be complicated by small bowel atresia, gangrene, volvulus of the impacted area, and perforation with meconium peritonitis. Presence of an atretic segment will, of course, prevent further passage of a contrast enema, a point that must be kept in mind during attempts at enema reduction of what is thought to be an uncomplicated case. Meconium peritonitis may cause an intense peritoneal reaction with erythema and edema of the abdominal wall (Fig. 17.32). Free meconium in the peritoneum calcifies, visible on plain film (Fig. 17.33).

In Hirschsprung's disease, intramural ganglion cells are absent in the distal rectum and for a variable distance proximally. No peristalsis occurs in the affected segment, causing a functional distal bowel obstruction. Symptoms in the newborn period are failure to pass meconium, abdominal distention,

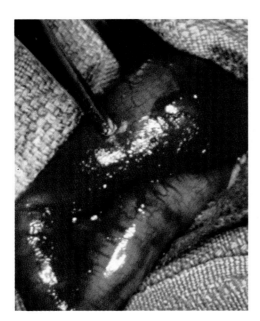

FIG. 17.34 Absence of intramural ganglion cells prevents intestinal peristalsis through segments affected by Hirschsprung's disease, causing a functional bowel obstruction. The involved segment appears narrow when compared with the distended, obstructed proximal bowel, which possesses normal ganglion cells.

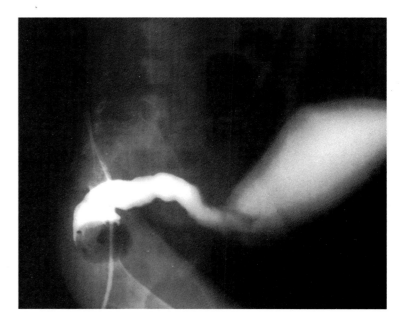

FIG. 17.35 Barium enema outlines the transition zone between the contracted (aganglionic) rectosigmoid lying distal to the obstructed, but normally innervated, colon. To demonstrate this sign, the examination must be conducted in an unprepped patient who has undergone neither enemas nor digital rectal examination.

and, later, bilious vomiting (Fig. 17.34). Gas-filled bowel loops fill the abdomen on plain film. Barium enema examination demonstrates the distended bowel (which has normal ganglion cells) tapering over a transition zone to the narrowed, aganglionic distal segment (Fig. 17.35). Barium enema should precede rectal examination or attempts at decompression. A suppository or saline enema may decompress the bowel proximal to the aganglionic zone, causing the diagnostic transition zone to disappear. The diagnosis is confirmed by suction rectal biopsy, a procedure that does not require anesthesia.

Symptoms from Hirschsprung's disease may not develop until later in infancy or childhood. Older children may have complaints of chronic constipation, abdominal distention, and failure to thrive. A potentially lethal complication of uncorrected Hirschsprung's disease is acute enterocolitis, which may be the presenting manifestation. The child has the acute onset of abdominal distention, fulminant diarrhea, and diarrhea. Urgent rectal biopsy to make the diagnosis and colostomy to decompress the bowel become necessary.

Vomiting in Older Infants and Children

Invagination of a portion of the intestine into itself, intussusception, causes both vomiting and abdominal pain (Fig. 17.36). Intussusception occurs most frequently between the ages of three and eighteen months; in this age group its etiology is usually not known. In contrast, the small number of cases occurring in older children have generally an anatomic abnormality that acts as a lead point for the intussusception. Examples include children with Meckel's diverticulum, intestinal lymphoma, polyps, cysts, areas of hemorrhage from Henoch-Schonlein purpura and hemophilia, and, for obscure reasons, children with cystic fibrosis and normal children who are recovering from operation (postoperative intussusception). Among cases of idiopathic intussusception, the great majority originate at or near the ileocecal valve. The classic clinical picture is of a well infant who suddenly appears to have violent abdominal pain and vomits. Soon thereafter he passes a normal stool and appears to recover, being relaxed, even playful and hungry. However, bouts of colic recur, causing the child to

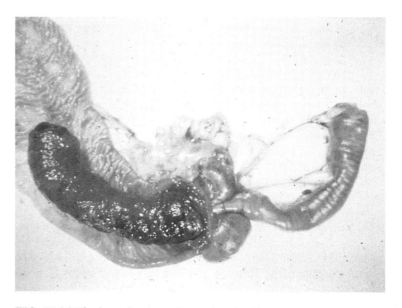

FIG. 17.36 The intestine invaginates into itself in intussusception. The ileum is pulled through the ileocecal valve into the colon, the most common pattern seen in infancy, pictured here.

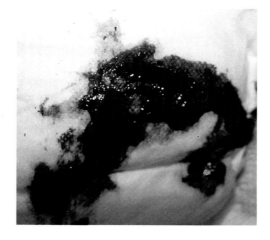

FIG. 17.37 The intussusceptum—the invaginated portion of bowel—becomes congested and ischemic, leading to the passage of bloody stool mixed with mucus.

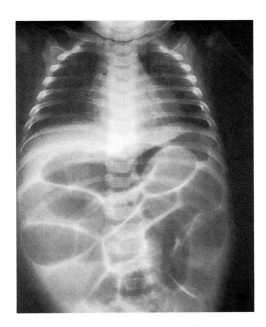

FIG. 17.38 Small bowel obstruction occurs late in intussusception.

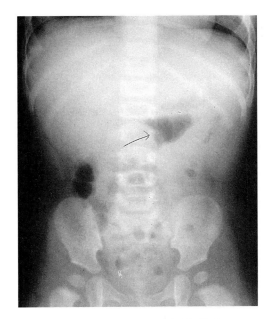

FIG. 17.39 In some cases the intussusceptum can be seen as a meniscus-shaped mass outlined by air in the colon.

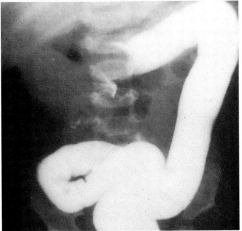

FIG. 17.40 Barium enema confirms the diagnosis by outlining the intussusceptum. The column of contrast can then be used to push the invaginated bowel proximally. Free reflux of contrast into the bowel proximally signals complete reduction of the intussusception.

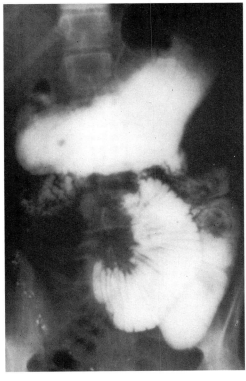

FIG. 17.41 Proximal small bowel intussusceptions require upper gastrointestinal series for diagnosis because enema studies cannot reliably reach the lesions. In contrast to those that occur after operations in infants and small children, those that occur de novo have a lead point, here a small bowel polyp in a patient with Peutz-Jegher's syndrome.

draw up his thighs and cry, or, alternatively, become pale, sweaty, and apathetic. Vomiting returns, and the baby begins to pass bloody stools. The vomiting at first is nonbilious, arising as a reflex response from traction on the involved mesentery. As obstruction becomes complete, vomiting later becomes bilious and the abdomen becomes distended. The intussusceptum (the segment of invaginated bowel) becomes engorged with blood and, with time, ischemic (Fig.17.37). "Currant jelly" describes the bloody mucus from the intussusceptum that appears in the diaper. On occasion the intussusceptum reaches the anus, where it can be felt on rectal examination. A sausage-shaped mass can be palpated in the majority of cases; because the process pulls the ileocecal area distally, the right iliac fossa may be scaphoid (Dance's sign).

Plain film of the abdomen may reveal obstruction (Fig. 17.38), an intussusceptum seen as a soft-tissue density meniscus outlined by air-filled distal colon (Fig. 17.39), or no abnormalities. Barium enema (Fig. 17.40) confirms the diagnosis and offers an opportunity to reduce the intussusception with a low rate of recurrence (less than 5 percent). Barium must be administered by gravity, without external manipulation of the bowel. Contrast must reflux freely into the small bowel to assure complete reduction and the absence of another intussusception in a more proximal location. A failed attempt requires immediate

operation, so a surgeon must be involved directly in the management of the child. Intussusception that recurs after barium enema reduction, or in older children, requires operative reduction and exploration for a possible lead point. Contrast enemas usually cannot reach intussusceptions that are restricted to the small bowel, so are useless in diagnosis and management. Upper gastrointestinal series with follow through into the small bowel may help diagnose small bowel intussusceptions (Fig. 17.41). Those that occur after operations cause small bowel obstruction and require reexploration, making contrast studies unnecessary. Small bowel intussusceptions require surgical reduction.

Volvulus around intraperitoneal bands and hernia can produce intestinal obstruction. Internal hernia from omphalomesenteric remnants may cause intestinal obstruction. Omphalomesenteric duct remnants may persist as a band that extends from the small bowel mesentery to the umbilicus. The

COMMON CAUSES OF GASTROINTESTINAL HEMORRHAGE

Upper		Lower	
Patients <1 year	**Patients >1 year**	**Patients <1 year**	**Patients >1 year**
Gastritis	Peptic ulcer	Anal fissure	Colonic polyps
Swallowed maternal blood	Varices	Intussusception	Intussusception
Peptic ulcer (duodenal and gastric)		Necrotizing enterocolitis	Meckel's diverticulum
Malrotation and volvulus		Meckel's diverticulum	Infectious diarrhea
		Malrotation and volvulus	Inflammatory bowel disease

FIG. 17.42

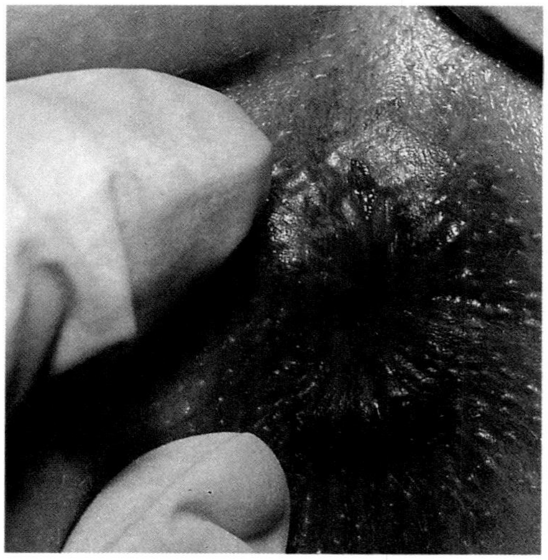

FIG. 17.43 Small tears in the anoderm may bleed, producing small amounts of blood on the stool of healthy infants.

omphalomesenteric artery originates the end artery of the superior mesenteric artery and extends to the tip of a Meckel's diverticulum, but remains suspended like a bowstring away from the mesentery and bowel. Inadequate retroperitoneal fixation of the bowel, considered a form of malrotation, leaves retroperitoneal pockets (paraduodenal hernia) into which small bowel can become entrapped. The most common source of intra-abdominal bands remains postoperative adhesions from prior surgery or abdominal trauma.

Incarcerated hernia, a common cause of intestinal obstruction, is discussed with inguinal-scrotal abnormalities below.

GASTROINTESTINAL BLEEDING

The evaluation of an infant or child bleeding from the gastrointestinal tract involves obtaining answers to a few basic questions. (1) Is it blood? Red dyes in sodas and food such as beets produce red stool, and ingested iron gives stool the appearance of melena. (2) In infants, is it maternal blood? The Apt test distinguishes maternal, adult hemoglobin from fetal hemoglobin, thus identifying blood in the newborn as swallowed during delivery or from the baby itself. (3) Does the bleeding come from an upper or lower source? Bilious fluid free of blood sampled from a gastric tube shows that the bleeding source is distal to the ligament of Treitz. Bright red blood passed from the rectum may be from an upper source with rapid transit to the rectum. A closely related question is whether the bleeding source is the gastrointestinal tract at all. Nosebleeds and hemoptysis may mimic upper tract bleeding; bleeding from the urinary tract or vagina may be interpreted as coming from the rectum. (4) Does the child have a coagulopathy? Gastrointestinal bleeding may be the initial manifestation of congenital or acquired coagulopathies, hematologic malignancy, and a complication of liver disease or medications. (5) How much has been lost? The volume of blood loss is often overestimated, but children in shock must be recognized

and treated aggressively. Postural vital signs, the appearance of the skin, and hematocrit reflect the amount of blood that has been lost. Bright red blood issuing in large amounts from the gastric tube or anus demands large-bore intravenous catheters and arrangements for prompt blood replacement to coincide with diagnostic workup.

The age of the patient, his or her appearance (how sick he or she appears), and the bleeding site (upper versus lower) give clues to the diagnosis. The discussion below will follow this format (Fig. 17.42).

Infants

The infant who has swallowed maternal blood looks well and has normal vital signs and hematocrit. The Apt test identifies the blood as having adult hemoglobin, establishing its source. (The mixture of one volume of the gastric aspirate and four parts of water is centrifuged. The supernatant is in turn mixed in a four-to-one ratio with 1 percent sodium hydroxide. If the liquid remains pink, the blood has fetal hemoglobin; if it turns

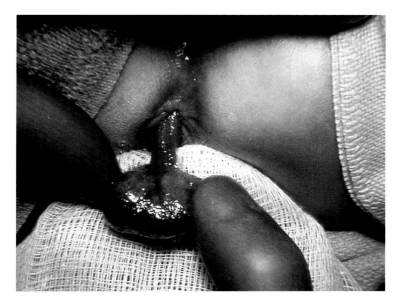

FIG. 17.50 Juvenile polyps are found most often in the rectosigmoid colon. On occasion they may prolapse through the anus.

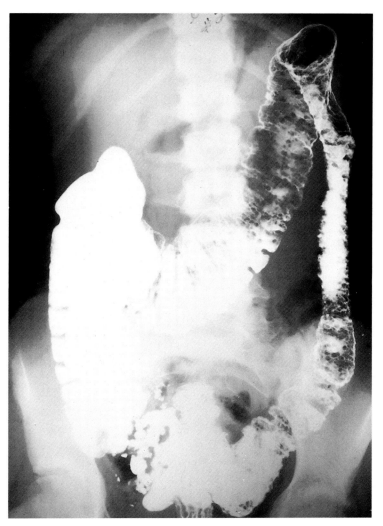

FIG. 17.51 Familial adenomatous polyposis. Barium enema study demonstrates multiple small polyps throughout the colon.

of vomiting, above), diverticulitis (clinically indistinguishable from appendicitis and rare), and persistent omphalomesenteric fistula.

Bleeding from esophageal varices arises from portal hypertension. Portal hypertension in childhood has two major causes: extrahepatic portal vein occlusion and cirrhosis. Omphalitis in the newborn, one of the complications of umbilical vessel catheterization, may cause thrombosis of the portal vein. Despite a successful portoenterostomy that clears jaundice, cirrhosis still may develop in cases of biliary atresia. Other causes of cirrhosis in childhood include congenital hepatic fibrosis, cystic fibrosis, alpha 1-anti trypsin deficiency, and end-stage liver disease following viral hepatitis. Endoscopy gives the most direct and reliable means of diagnosis of bleeding varices. Contrast opacification of the portal vein and its tributaries is necessary if surgical portal decompression becomes necessary (Fig. 17.49). However, most bleeding episodes are self-limited. Persistent bleeding is controlled effectively in nearly all cases by endoscopic injection of a sclerosant into the bleeding varix, and surgery is seldom necessary.

Vasculitis from Henoch-Schonlein purpura may cause lower tract bleeding in this age group. A viral or streptococcal infection may precede the development of arthralgias and confluent purpura primarily over the lower extremities. The diagnosis is made difficult when bleeding or abdominal pain precedes the appearance of the rash. Bloody diarrhea and abdominal pain may accompany hemolytic-uremic syndrome. Hemolytic anemia on blood count and smear, azotemia, and thrombocytopenia establish the diagnosis. Infectious diarrhea may produce bloody bowel motions. The diagnosis is suggested by fever and the presence of white cells in the stool, and is confirmed by culture.

Older Children

Juvenile polyps of the colon are benign hamartomas covered with flattened epithelium and granulation tissue (Fig. 17.50).

Children aged 2 to 8 years are affected most frequently. Most occur singly; when multiple, usually they number less than twelve. Two-thirds of symptomatic polyps occur in the rectum, and 90 percent occur distal to the sigmoid. Bleeding is painless, small in amount, and found on the surface of the stool. The polyp may prolapse out the anus. Surgical resection of those that prolapse out the anus, or endoscopic resection, is curative. Diffuse gastrointestinal juvenile polyposis is a rare entity that causes bleeding, diarrhea, rectal prolapse, intussusception, and protein-losing enteropathy. A life-threatening condition, diffuse juvenile polyposis requires total colectomy.

Adenomatous polyps are extremely rare as solitary colonic polyps in children. Children who are members of families with familial adenomatous polyposis usually develop symptoms at puberty or late adolescence. Innumerable adenomatous polyps carpet the colon, and cause bloody diarrhea, tenesmus, and abdominal pain (Fig. 17.51). Polyps associated with Peutz-Jegher's syndrome are also adenomatous, but are fewer in number and are located at all levels of the gastrointestinal tract from stomach to rectum. Mucocutaneous melanin spots are

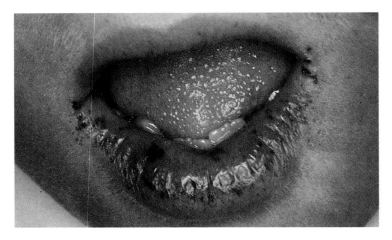

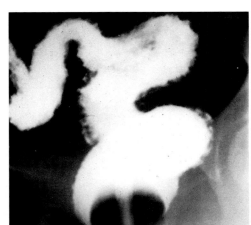

FIG. 17.53 Linear ulcerations and crypt abscesses fill and leave islands of mucosa, which appear as pseudopolyps on barium enema.

FIG. 17.52 The characteristic melanotic spots of Peutz-Jegher syndrome are seen on the lips, buccal mucosa, and anus.

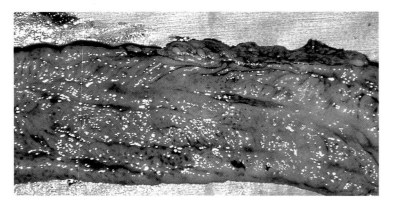

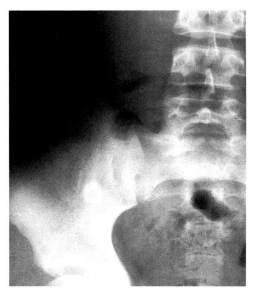

FIG. 17.55 A fecalith, the round calcification in the iliac fossa, obstructs the appendiceal lumen and initiates inflammatory processes that produce appendicitis.

FIG. 17.54 This opened colectomy specimen demonstrates the linear ulcerations in the mucosa of a patient with ulcerative colitis.

present on the lips and face, buccal mucosa, and fingers and may precede the development of abdominal symptoms by years (Fig. 17.52). Gastrointestinal bleeding is usually occult. Colic is the major abdominal symptom, caused by transient intussusception with a polyp as the lead point (Fig. 17.41).

The common causes of bleeding among children as they get older are those common among adults, such as peptic ulcer disease, gastritis, Mallory-Weiss tear, and inflammatory bowel disease (Figs. 17.53, 17.54). Endoscopy provides the most direct means to diagnosis.

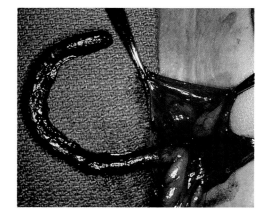

FIG. 17.56 The purple color of the appendix in this case of appendicitis contrasts with the pink color of the healthy serosa of the cecum at its base.

ABDOMINAL PAIN

Acute appendicitis is the most common surgical emergency of the abdomen in childhood and adolescence. Obstruction of the appendiceal lumen, commonly by a fecalith visible on abdominal plain film (Fig. 17.55), leads to appendiceal edema, ischemia, and ultimately necrosis and gangrene (Fig. 17.56). The classic progression of symptoms begins with vague periumbilical pain. Transmural inflammation follows, and produces fever and leukocytosis. As the appendix distends, the child loses his or her appetite and begins to vomit. When the inflamed appendix comes in contact with the abdominal wall, the child perceives the localization of pain in the right lower quadrant. Any sudden movement, such as coughing, walking,

jumping, or palpation by a physician causes pain at that point, so the child lies still on his or her side, legs drawn up at the hips, and resists examination. Involuntary guarding develops, detected on palpation as muscular spasm in the area where the child is most tender. Mild sedation, administered to facilitate examination, never masks true involuntary guarding. Tenderness may be mild in cases where a retrocecal appendix fails to impinge the anterior abdominal wall, but may produce

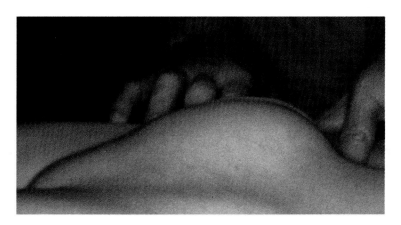

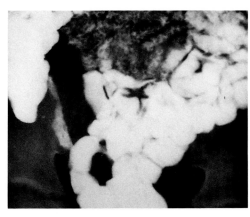

FIG. 17.58 Stricture of the terminal ileum, and segmental involvement of the small bowel and colon, are characteristic findings on barium enema examination of a child with Crohn's disease.

FIG. 17.57 A large ovarian cyst in a prepubertal girl can be demonstrated easily on abdominal exam.

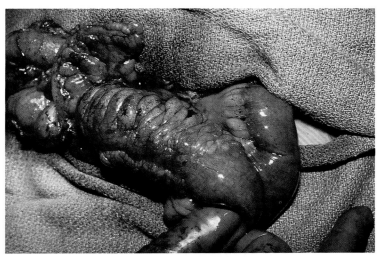

FIG. 17.59 Findings at laparotomy in Crohn's disease reveal petechiae over the serosa of thickened small bowel, which has mesenteric fat "creeping" over its surface.

instead a positive psoas or obturator sign. When the appendix perforates, pain at first decreases as the appendix decompresses. Perforation soils the peritoneum, and generalized peritonitis produces diffuse abdominal pain, distention, and rigidity. The omentum and adjacent loops of bowel may limit the perforation to the right lower quadrant, forming an abscess and creating a mass in the right lower quadrant.

Appendicitis occurring in children and adolescent boys seldom presents problems in diagnosis, and the rate of normal appendices removed (negative appendectomy) is less than 5 percent. The prevalence of acute salpingitis and other uterine tubo-ovarian pathology leads to a high negative appendectomy rate in adolescent girls. The fever and symptoms closely related to the onset of menses, tenderness on movement of the cervix, and absence of gastrointestinal complaints suggest acute salpingitis. A twisted ovarian cyst produces a mobile mass in the lower abdomen, and causes severe pain without gastrointestinal symptoms or abdominal tenderness (Fig. 17.57). Abdominal ultrasound helps to delineate the presence of ovarian cysts or tubo-ovarian abscess. Appendicitis in preschool children is difficult to diagnose at an early, nonperforated stage because of problems in obtaining precise details of clinical history and adequate physical examinations. Because diagnosis is often delayed, the rate of perforation among young children exceeds 50 percent. A number of extra-abdominal and systemic inflammatory conditions can cause abdominal pain, including otitis media, pneumonia, urinary infections, diabetes mellitus, Henoch-Schonlein purpura, rheumatic fever, and sickle cell disease. In all ages, other acute intestinal conditions can mimic closely acute appendicitis. Viral and bacterial enteritis is most common. Inflammatory bowel disease becomes more common in older children (Figs. 17.58, 17.59). Intussusception becomes more prevalent among the younger age group and should be considered, rather than appendicitis, in infants who exhibit abdominal pain and vomiting. Meckel's diverticulitis, clinically indistinguishable from acute appendicitis, results from peptic perforation of the diverticulum. It is the least common clinical manifestation of Meckel's diverticulum.

Other surgical causes of abdominal pain are uncommon in childhood. Right upper quadrant pain suggests a biliary tract

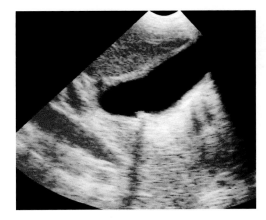

FIG. 17.60 Ultrasound examination of the right upper quadrant easily demonstrates stones within the gallbladder. An acoustic shadow extends beneath the stone.

pathology, particularly when jaundice coexists. Acute cholecystitis occurs in children with hemoglobinopathy or hematologic conditions that cause unusual degrees of hemolysis, and adolescent girls who develop "adult" cholesterol gallstones. Ultrasound examination reveals gallstones, distended gallbladder (Fig. 17.60), and biliary tract dilatation, if present. Right upper quadrant pain, jaundice, and mass represent the classic triad of choledochal cyst. Pancreatitis produces epigastric pain and the serum amylase becomes elevated. A child with pancreatitis who develops an epigastric mass requires an

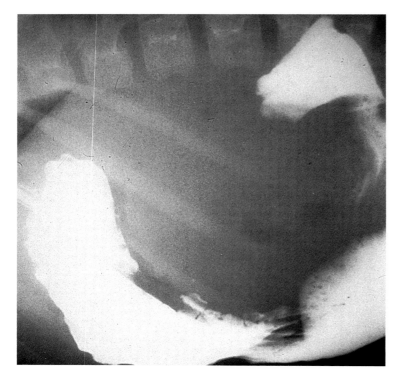

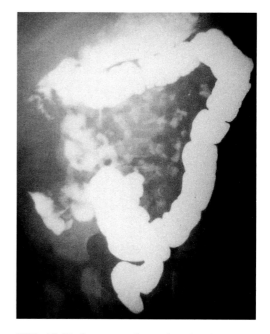

FIG. 17.61
Pancreatic pseudo-
cyst, a complication
of pancreatitis of any
cause, may grow
large enough to dis-
place the stomach
anteriorally.

FIG. 17.62 An omental cyst has displaced the
right colon.

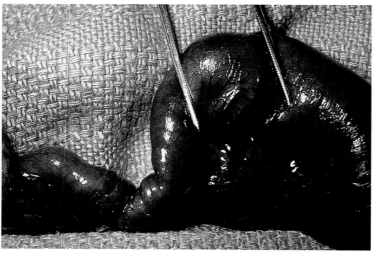

FIG. 17.63 Duplications typically lie within the mesentery and
involve the terminal ileum. They may be spherical (pictured here) or
tubular. An obstructed duplication may become palpable as an abdominal mass; one with ectopic gastric mucosa may produce gastrointestinal bleeding; one may act as a lead point for intussusception.

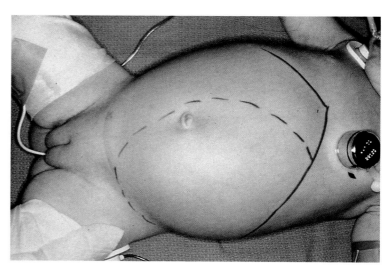

FIG. 17.64 The dashed line indicates the extent of a flank mass in an
infant with ureteropelvic junction obstruction.

ultrasound examination to rule out pancreatic pseudocyst (Fig. 17.61). Urinalysis and renal ultrasound identifies the urinary tract as the source of abdominal pain, usually located in the flank but sometimes the source of confusion when pain occurs more anteriorally.

ABDOMINAL MASSES

The etiology of abdominal masses includes congenital and neoplastic lesions, as well as complications of inflammatory conditions. Discovery of a mass requires early surgical consultation, as nearly half (45 percent) are surgical lesions. Of this group, neoplasm represents about 45 percent of lesions and

hydronephrosis causes about one-third (32 percent). Less common causes of abdominal masses include multicystic kidney, hydrocolpos, omental and mesenteric cysts (Fig. 17.62) and duplications (Fig. 17.63). A mass in a newborn infant is usually a benign obstructive renal lesion in 75 to 80 percent of cases. Unusual congenital intra-abdominal masses such as ovarian and omental cysts and duplications are frequently found during early infancy. In older age groups, the majority of masses are malignant tumors. Signs of inflammation, such as tenderness, fever, leukocytosis, and overlying tenderness suggest an inflammatory cause such as abscess from appendicitis, Crohn's disease, or an infected peritoneal cyst associated with a ventriculoperitoneal shunt.

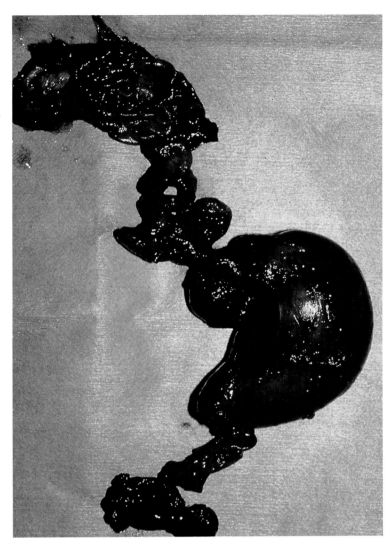

FIG. 17.65 *Irregular dilatations along the course of an obstructed duplicated ureter may become palpable as flank masses.*

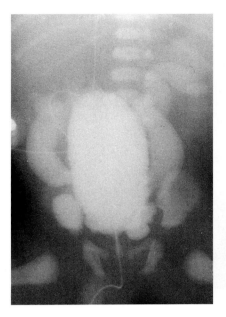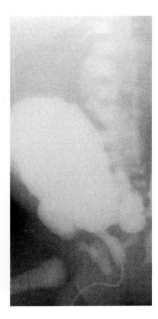

FIG. 17.66 *Posterior urethral valves cause dilatation of bladder and both upper tracts, seen here on a retrograde contrast study.*

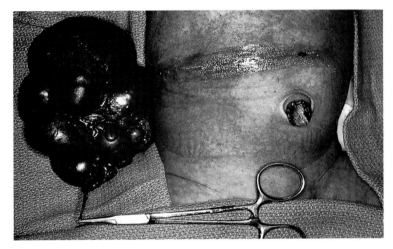

FIG. 17.67 *Multicystic kidney produces a knobby flank mass.*

Ultrasonography is useful early in the evaluation to distinguish between solid tumors from obstructive uropathy and other fluid-filled masses. Ultrasound identifies the lesion as arising from the kidney (such as Wilms' tumor) or outside the kidney (adrenal neuroblastoma). Intravenous pyelography locates the mass relative to the kidney and establishes whether both kidneys excrete dye and are thus functional, a point of obvious surgical importance should nephrectomy become necessary. Abdominal plain film, seldom diagnostic, may demonstrate calcifications from a neuroblastoma. Computed tomoraphy gives more precise anatomic information than ultrasonography, demonstrating enlarged lymph nodes and other masses within the chest or abdomen that might represent metastases. Contrast studies of the stomach and intestines are useful to identify inflammatory bowel disease or the relationship between masses and the gastrointestinal tract.

Genitourinary Obstructions

Hydronephrosis is the most common cause of abdominal mass in the newborn and is usually painless. In contrast, hydronephrosis in older children is rarely palpable and causes pain and urinary infection. Ureteropelvic junction obstruction results in a large, smooth flank mass that is treated by pyeloplasty (Fig. 17.64). Ureteral duplication causes ureteral dilatation, the upper pole ureter from obstruction, the lower pole ureter from reflux. The ureters may become palpable as a knobby flank mass (Fig. 17.65). Stasis within the ureters may cause urinary infection. Ureterocele associated with a duplicated system may obstruct the bladder. Posterior urethral valves are the most common cause of lower urinary obstruction in boys (Fig. 17.66). The distended bladder drains inadequately, and is palpable in the lower abdomen. Hydroureteronephrosis may be present and produce bilateral flank masses. Multicystic kidney produces a large, knobby mass in infants (Fig. 17.67), a diagnosis which is easily confirmed on ultrasonography.

An obstructed female genital tract may cause hydrometrocolpos in infancy, usually palpated as a smooth mass placed centrally in the lower abdomen, but occasionally as a huge mass that fills the abdomen. Symptoms may not arise until menarche, when the obstructed genital tract fills with blood,

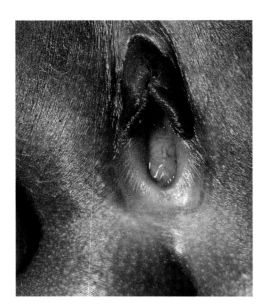

FIG. 17.68
Imperforate hymen. Accumulated secretions in the vagina and uterus caused bulging of the hymen and a pelvic mass in this newborn infant.

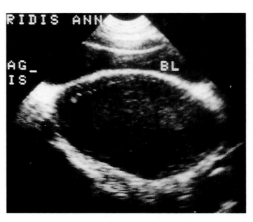

FIG. 17.69 *A pelvic mass arising at the expected time of menarche should suggest the presence of an obstructed uterine anomaly, here demonstrated by pelvic ultrasound as an oval mass compressing the bladder anteriorally. Urinary anomalies commonly coexist.*

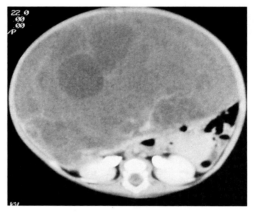

FIG. 17.70
Computed tomography of a mesenchymal hamartoma of the liver. In contrast to the neovascularization within a hepatic tumor, a hamartoma fails to show contrast enhancement.

creating a hematocolpos (Figs. 17.68, 17.69). Menstrual bleeding, unable to drain externally, creates a slowly expanding lower abdominal mass with pain that becomes worse every three to four weeks. Urinary anomalies are common and should be sought out during evaluation.

Abdominal Neoplasms

Hepatic enlargement shortly after birth may represent a subcapsular hematoma from birth trauma. Diffuse enlargement of the liver that develops in early infancy may be due to hemangioendothelioma; enlargement may be so severe that respiratory insufficiency results. Blood flow through the liver may create an audible bruit. Platelet trapping may result in thrombocytopenia. Hemangioendothelioma usually regresses with time without treatment; severe symptoms may require treatment with steroids, radiation or chemotherapy. Similarly, hepatic metastases from stage IV-S neuroblastoma regress completely without treatment in most cases. However, abdominal distention from hepatic enlargement may cause respiratory insufficiency sufficiently severe to require radiation therapy or chemotherapy. Mesenchymal hamartoma is the most commonly encountered benign hepatic tumor in infancy, creating homogeneous cystic areas on ultrasound and computed tomography (Fig. 17.70). Hepatoblastoma, primarily affecting infants under 2 years of age (Fig. 17.71), and hepatocellular carcinoma, primarily seen in preadolescents, represent the primary malignant hepatic tumors of childhood. Serum alpha fetoprotein levels are elevated in most cases, and this elevation is useful as a tumor marker to detect recurrence after resection. Hepatocellular carcinoma occurs more frequently in cases of pre-existing liver disease, such as biliary atresia.

Wilms' tumor is the most common intra-abdominal malignancy in childhood. Nearly all cases occur by the age of 6 years. In addition to a flank mass, hematuria and hypertension may be present. Children with aniridia and hemihypertrophy are considered to be at increased risk for the development of Wilms' tumor and should be monitored with semiannual ultrasound examinations. Intravenous urography (Fig. 17.72) and ultrasonography verify the presence of an intrarenal solid mass within the kidney. Ultrasound identifies the presence of tumor lying within the renal vein and inferior vena cava,

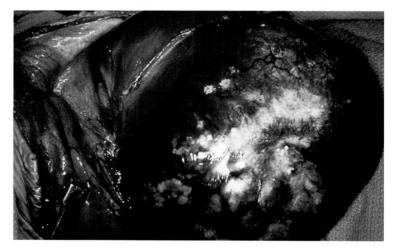

FIG. 17.71 *A large hepatoblastoma of the right lobe of the liver. Intravenous urography, computed tomography and ultrasonography all identify it as a hepatic tumor instead of one arising from the kidney or an adrenal gland.*

points of surgical significance. Wilms' tumor may arise in both kidneys (Fig. 17.73), a therapeutic challenge to excise the tumor yet leave the child with as much functioning renal mass as possible. Computed tomography may also identify nodal enlargement and liver nodules that may represent metastasis. Chest film and chest computed tomography help to identify metastases to the lung, the most common site. Children with clear cell sarcoma, previously considered to be a variant of Wilms' tumor but now considered a distinct neoplasm, frequently have bone metastasis and should receive a bone scan. Mesoblastic nephroma is an uncommon, relatively benign, variant of Wilms' tumor, and is present most frequently in newborn infants.

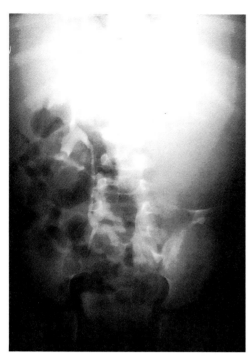

FIG. 17.72 A large Wilms' tumor has splayed the collecting system of the left kidney on intravenous urogram so that calyces are visible deep in the left iliac fossa. This distortion of the collecting system identifies a mass as arising from the kidney, one of the radiologic signs of Wilms' tumor.

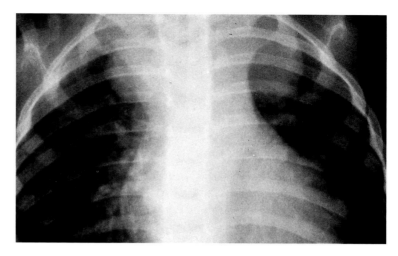

FIG. 17.74 An upper thoracic neuroblastoma, here seen in the right superior sulcus of the thorax, may produce unilateral Horner's syndrome.

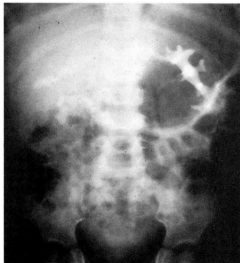

FIG. 17.73 Wilms' tumor arising in the lower poles of both kidneys. When possible, the surgical goal is conservative excision of tumor, leaving as much functioning kidney as possible.

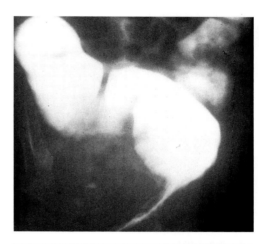

FIG. 17.75 A pelvic neuroblastoma causes compression of the rectum on barium enema study.

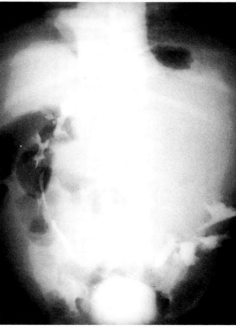

FIG. 17.76 Downward displacement of the entire kidney by a left adrenal neuroblastoma leaves the intrarenal collecting system anatomically intact but gives it a "drooping lily" appearance.

Neuroblastoma is the second most common solid tumor in childhood, exceeded only by brain tumors (Fig. 17.74). Tumors may arise in the adrenal glands, sympathetic ganglia, and organs of Zuckerkandl, and so may be found in the neck, chest, abdomen and pelvis (Fig. 17.75). Young children under 5 years of age are most commonly affected. Systemic symptoms, such as fever and failure to thrive, and remote effects of tumor, such as proptosis, opsomyoclonus, and ataxia, may predominate the clinical picture and the tumor may be relatively small or nonpalpable. More than 70 percent of children have metastases when first seen, accounting for the poor prognosis of neuroblastoma in general. Radiologic studies of an adrenal neuroblastoma reveal an extrarenal mass; inferior displacement of opacified calyces on intravenous pyelography give a characteristic "drooping lily" sign (Fig. 17.76). Because of the frequency of metastases, workup should include computed tomography of the chest and abdomen and bone scan. Laboratory findings have been found to have prognostic significance; sur-

vival is higher when serum ferritn is less than 150 ng/ml, neuron-specific enolase is less than 100 ng/ml, and the ratio of vanillylmandelic acid to homovanilic acid in the urine is greater than one. Stage IV-S neuroblastoma, a variant

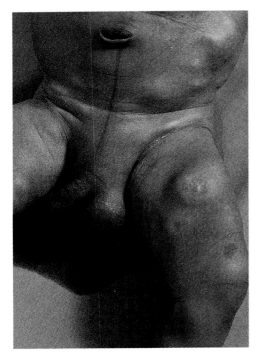

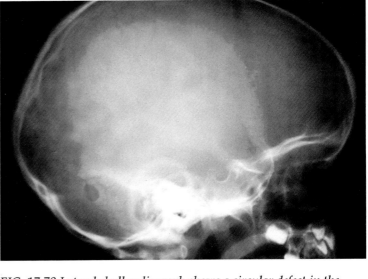

FIG. 17.77
Subcutaneous metas-
tasis in IV-S neurob-
lastoma give infants a
"blueberry muffin"
appearance. The
lesions generally
regress without
chemotherapy or radi-
ation therapy and the
survival rate exceeds
70 percent.

FIG. 17.79 Lateral skull radiograph shows a circular defect in the
occipital region of a patient who presented with a superficial dermoid
cyst over the occiput. The cyst extended through the defect into the
intracranial cavity.

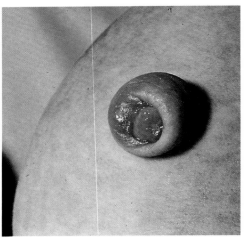

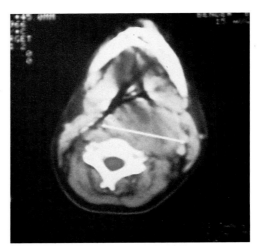

FIG. 17.78 A urachal
cyst abscess produces
a tender mass beneath
the umbilicus, which
also may become
enlarged and tender.

FIG. 17.80
Computed tomogra-
phy of the neck shows
a ganglioneuroma
lying below the
mandible distorting
the airway toward
the contralateral side.

of metastatic disease that often regresses completely without
therapy, is characterized by a localized primary tumor with
metastases to the liver, bone marrow, or skin (Fig. 17.77).

Non-Hodgkin's lymphoma involves abdominal sites in one-
quarter to one-half of all cases. It has a peak incidence of 5 to 8
years, and afflicts boys more often than girls. Pain is frequently
the earliest symptom and a mass may become palpable. The
tumor is located in the small bowel in the majority of cases
and may lead to intussusception. Tumors may arise in other
segments of the bowel, other organs, and retroperitoneum.
Non-Hodgkin's lymphoma grows rapidly but generally
responds promptly to chemotherapy, so aggressive workup
including biopsy is warranted.

In contrast to rhabdomyosarcoma of the trunk and extremities, those that involve the bladder, inguinal canal, and vagina
have commonly a nonalveolar histology and carry a good
prognosis. Ovarian tumors are varied in histology, including
both benign (cystic teratoma, follicular cyst) and malignant
histologies (teratocarcinoma, germ cell tumors, dysgermino-
ma). Germ cell tumors may be presacral in location and palpable only on rectal examination, causing no visible mass either
in the perineum or in the lower abdomen.

Inflammatory Masses

Adjacent loops of bowel and the omentum may localize perforated appendicitis in the right iliac fossa; appendicitis is discussed above as a cause of abdominal pain. An infected
urachal cyst causes a tender midline mass below the umbilicus
(Fig. 17.78). Cellulitis may involve the overlying skin and
umbilicus. Sonography shows a fluid collection anterior to the
bladder. Children with ventriculoperitoneal shunts may develop infected collections of fluid in the abdomen associated with
shunt infections. Fever and abdominal discomfort usually
resolve promptly following exteriorization of the shunt and
the administration of intravenous antibiotics. Persistence of
fever or symptoms suggest that an abscess has formed, either
from inadequate resolution of an infected fluid collection or
from intestinal perforation.

Crohn's disease may produce a tender right lower abdominal mass. Effective medical management leads to resolution of
the mass. Persistence or enlargement of the mass may indicate
fistula formation and abscess development. Ultrasound
detects a fluid collection that identifies an abscess, and may
show abnormal dilatation of the urinary tract from involve-

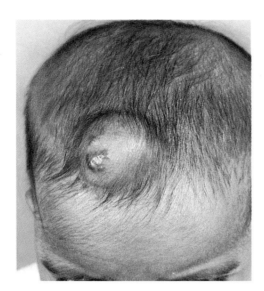

FIG. 17.81
Cavernous heman-
gioma of the scalp,
with overlying skin
involvement.

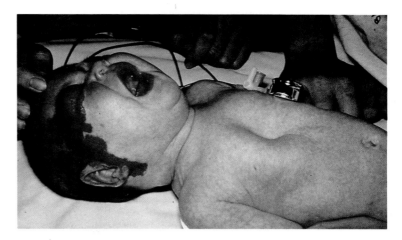

FIG. 17.82 Facial hemangioma covering the eye require intervention
with prednisone to hasten resolution and to avoid loss of slight from
amblyopia.

ment of the ureter in the inflammatory process. Contrast
enema and follow through of barium into the small bowel
define the extent of Crohn's disease, and may help define the
presence of fistulae.

HEAD AND NECK

The locations of head and neck lesions provide the most information regarding the probable diagnosis. Most are benign.
Physical examination should note the consistency and mobility of the mass, the presence of signs of inflammation, and any
abnormal drainage. Masses that impinge upon the airway or
compromise vision require urgent attention.

Skull, facial, and mandible films identify bone tumors and
superficial lesions that cause bony erosion (Fig. 17.79).
Children with lesions causing respiratory distress or dysphagia require x-ray views that show details of the airway and
soft tissue (Fig. 17.80) and endoscopic examination of the larynx, tracheobronchial tree, and esophagus. Other tests, such as
computed tomography and barium swallow, may provide
valuable information.

Most head and neck lesions require surgery: drainage of
abscesses, the evaluation and the relief of obstructive lesions,
diagnostic biopsy of lesions to exclude malignancy, and the
removal of benign lesions for cosmetic reasons. However,
many cases do not, including most cases of cervical adenitis,
torticollis, and hemangioma.

Scalp

Hemangiomas are common lesions in infancy, soft or firm in
consistency, bright red and elevated (Fig. 17.81). They blanch
when compressed, and reexpand when released. A capillary
hemangioma frequently involves the overlying skin. Large
lesions may cover extensive regions of the scalp and face (Fig.
17.82). However, most lesions involute spontaneously over a
period of four to six years, and expectant management leaves
surprisingly good cosmetic result. Lesions that cover the eyes
or occlude the airway require immediate intervention with
prednisone, radiation therapy, or tracheotomy to bypass an
obstruction.

Dermoid (or epidermal) cysts occur in regions of embryologic fusion. Hence they are frequently found at the corners

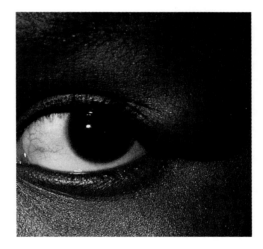

FIG. 17.83 Dermoid
cyst occurs common-
ly at the lateral cor-
ner of the eye, pic-
tured here, in the
eyebrow, anterior to
the ear, and in the
midline of the neck.

of the eye, along the sternocleidomastoid, or in the midline of
the face and neck (Fig. 17.83). They may be freely movable in
the subcutaneous tissue, or be fixed to the skin or underlying
skull. Those found in the preauricular area almost always have
a deep attachment to the origin of the helix cartilage. They
have a thin wall that contains keratin and, occasionally, hair.
Treatment is excision.

Face

Preauricular tags, cartilaginous remnants anterior to the ear,
are common minor anomalies which are thought not to have a
branchial cleft origin. Most are asymptomatic. Indications for
removal are cosmetic. Preauricular sinus tracts end blindly
beneath the skin, with hair or other epidermal elements at its
base, and are probably closely related to preauricular dermoid
cysts. Both have a tendency to infection, and complete
removal of any subcutaneous portion is necessary to prevent
recurrence.

Surgical lesions of the salivary glands are uncommon in
infancy and childhood. Hemangioma of the parotid, the most

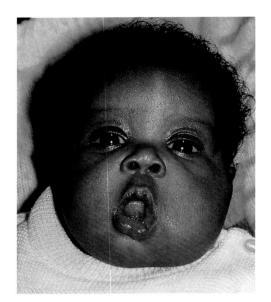

FIG. 17.84 A non-tender mass over the parotid in an infant identifies a parotid hemangioma. This lesion will involve over the next few years, and does not require excision.

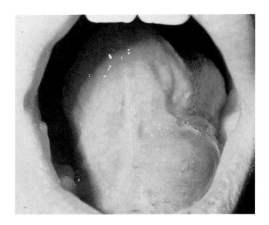

FIG. 17.85 A ranula arises in the floor of the mouth, created by congenital obstruction of the sublingual duct.

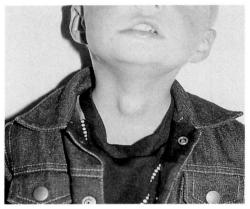

FIG. 17.86 Thyroglossal duct cyst produces a firm swelling in the midline of the neck. Its initial manifestation is sometimes a midline cervical abscess.

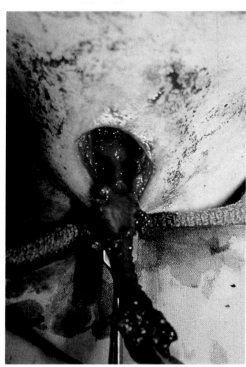

FIG. 17.87 The surgical specimen shows the thyroglossal duct as it courses from the lesion (pulled by the clamp), to the hyoid bone (swelling at the margin of the incision) and to the base of the tongue (in the depth of the incision).

common benign lesion, produces a unilateral swelling of the parotid within the first month of life (Fig. 17.84). It may increase in size over several months, but involutes over four to six years (like most hemangiomas of the face and neck). A cutaneous sentinel hemangioma provides positive identification, and biopsy is usually unnecessary. Parotid swelling from inflammatory causes, such as mumps, bacteria (usually Staphylococcus or gram-negative rods) and different causes of chronic parotiditis (chronic sialadentitis, sarcoidosis, and tuberculosis) cause tenderness and redness over the involved gland. The duct orifice may be red or "pouting" in appearance when an inflammatory cause is present.

Mouth

Tongue-tie (ankyloglossia inferior), common in infancy, usually disappears spontaneously or with sucking. A thick, stout frenulum may interfere with speech development. Division of the frenulum is a simple cure.

Ranula forms from obstruction of the sublingual duct, forming a pseudocyst in the floor of the mouth (Fig. 17.85). A large ranula may cause upper airway obstruction in infancy. Marsupialization of the pseudocyst is effective treatment.

Oral lymphangioma presents difficult problems in both short- and long-term management. It is the most common cause of macroglossia in infancy, although other causes, such as Beckwith's syndrome and hypothyroidism, must be considered. An oral lymphangioma appears as a raised, firm mass in the tongue and floor of the mouth, with tiny cysts over its surface. When extensive, they may obstruct the upper airway. Suppurative glossitis, a common occurrence, is treated by intravenous antibiotics. Subtotal glossectomy is recommended to prevent prognathism and to facilitate speech.

Lingual thyroid appears as a hill-like mass at the foramen cecum. An unusually large lingual thyroid may obstruct the airway in infants, but most present later in childhood as a "lump in the throat" when swallowing. The lingual thyroid, generally the only thyroid tissue present, produces insufficient thyroid hormone. Hypothyroidism may be present. Thyroid replacement becomes necessary after transoral excision, the treatment of choice.

Neck-Midline

Thyroglossal duct remnants, dermoid cysts, and enlarged lymph nodes comprise the common midline masses in the neck. During embryologic development, the thyroglossal duct arises from the foramen cecum, descends in the midline close to the hyoid, and gives rise to the thyroid gland upon reaching

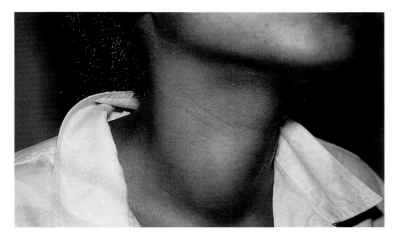

FIG. 17.88 Goiter in a 15-year-old girl, from Hashimoto's thyroiditis.

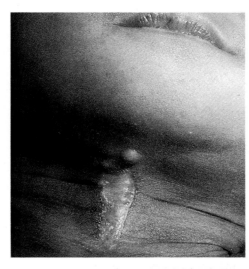

FIG. 17.89 Midline cervical cleft.

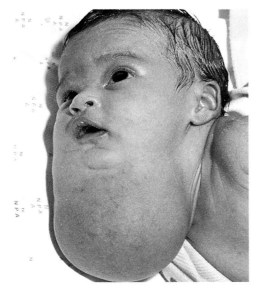

FIG. 17.90 Cystic hygroma involving the anterior triangle of the neck and the floor of the mouth. The cysts, which are large over the neck, are tiny and infiltrate the tongue and floor of the mouth, causing diffuse swelling that may compromise the upper airway.

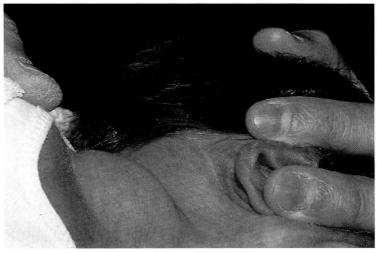

FIG. 17.91 Cystic hygroma extending from the posterior triangle.

the neck. Incomplete regression of the duct may cause a cyst to form anywhere along its course from foramen cecum to sternal notch, most commonly just below the hyoid (Fig. 17.86). It moves with swallowing and movement of the tongue, but these maneuvers do not distinguish a thyroglossal duct cyst with certainty. Infection may result from its communication with the oropharynx. To reduce the risk of recurrence after surgical excision, the entire cyst and duct must be removed to the level of the foramen cecum, including the midportion of the hyoid (Fig. 17.87).

Thyroid nodules occur in children as in adults (Fig. 17.88). However, benign nodules are much less common, and the possibility that a palpable nodule is malignant is considerably greater in a child than in an adult. More than half of solitary nodules in children are malignant, nearly all papillary carcinomas. Nodular Hashimoto's disease is the most common benign lesion. Thyroid scans are useful only in the identification of hyperfunctioning nodules, all of which are benign and are rarely seen in pediatrics. Fine-needle aspiration generally yields a diagnosis in solid lesions, and "cures" cystic ones, making ultrasound examination unnecessary. Total thyroidectomy is recommended for malignant thyroid lesions; lobectomy and isthmusectomy are recommended for benign lesions in which cancer cannot be ruled out.

Midline cervical cleft is a vertical streak of thinly epithelialized tissue in the anterior midline of the neck, probably the result of defective midline fusion of the branchial arches (Fig. 17.89).

Neck-Lateral Masses

Cystic hygroma occur most commonly in the neck and axilla (Figs. 17.90, 17.91). Most are discovered at birth; smaller lesions may be found later in infancy. Composed of fluid-filled, thin-walled cysts, they are soft and transilluminate brightly. Those in the neck may compress the trachea or spread into the floor of the mouth or tongue, thus causing upper airway obstruction. Complications include hemorrhage and infection.

Benign lymphadenopathy of one of the anterior cervical lymph nodes is by far the most common neck mass. Nearly all cases are due to nonspecific reactive hyperplasia to an infection in the ears, nose, mouth, throat, face or scalp. Enlarged reactive nodes are generally small (less than 2 cm in diameter), minimally tender, and high in the anterior cervical chain (most commonly the so-called tonsillar node near the angle of the jaw), and regress with resolution of the primary infection. Infection with the node itself makes the node more tender and

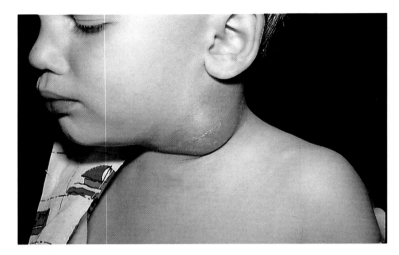

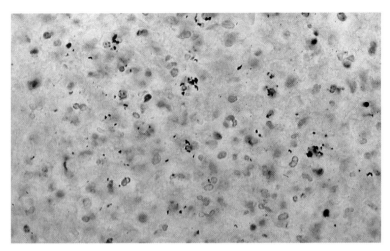

FIG. 17.92 Erythema and fluctuance identifies the presence of an abscess. An abscess may be present without fluctuance, however, from induration from surrounding inflammation.

FIG. 17.93 Warthin-Starry silver stain identifies the black-staining organisms associated with cat-scratch disease, seen on examination of an enlarged lymph node.

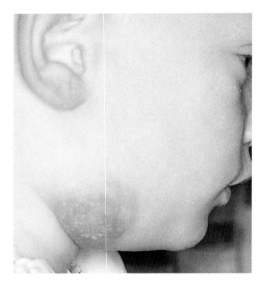

FIG. 17.94 The skin overlying a tuberculous lymph node is often discolored and may break down into a chronically draining sinus.

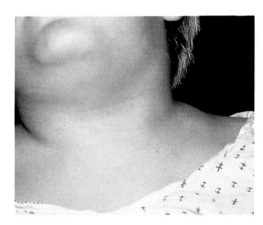

FIG. 17.95 Enlarged lymph nodes in unusual locations, such as in this patient with supraclavicular lymphadenopathy from non-Hodgkin's lymphoma, require excisional biopsy to rule out malignancy.

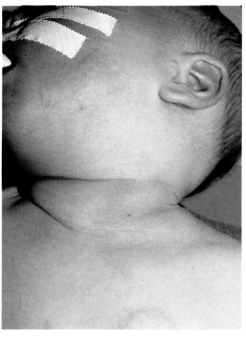

FIG. 17.96 Mucus may drain from a small punctum at the anterior border of the sternocleidomastoid, identifying it as the secondary opening of a second branchial cleft fistula. The primary opening lies in the tonsillar fossa.

enlarged, and the overlying skin becomes red. Early antibiotic therapy against staphylococcus and streptococcus may clear the infection. The development of fluctuance means suppuration has occurred and incision and drainage are required for cure (Fig. 17.92). Needle aspiration may indicate the presence of pus within an involved node that is firm and free from areas of fluctuance.

Causes of chronic cervical adenopathy include cat-scratch disease, atypical mycobacteria (mycobacterium avium-intracellulare scrofulum, or MAIS), and tuberculosis. Lymphadenopathy in cat-scratch disease arises 2 to 4 weeks after the animal scratch, which is usually healed and forgotten. Regression of node enlargement usually takes 2 to 4 weeks, but some cases may require months. When excised, silver stains reveal the cat-scratch organism (Fig. 17.93). Skin tests depend upon the availability of a reliable preparation of cat-scratch antigen.

Skin tests and chest films help to distinguish different causes of mycobacterial cervical adenitis. The most common cause is one of the MAIS complex. This form of mycobacterial infection is free from pulmonary involvement. Submandibular and preauricular lymph nodes typically are involved, and are remarkably free from pain or tenderness. The nodes are fixed

to surrounding tissues by perinodal inflammation. The overlying skin has a blue discoloration, and may break down to form a draining sinus. Excision of the node and sinus is curative, and no antituberculous chemotherapy is required. In contrast, adenitis from mycobacterium tuberculosis (Fig. 17.94) is com-

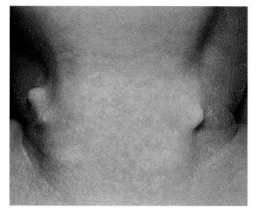
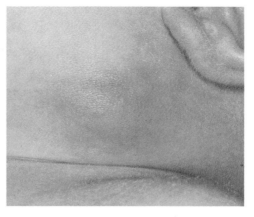
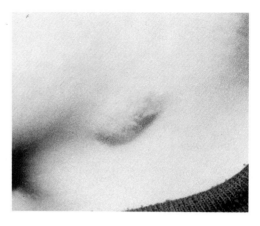

FIG. 17.97 Cartilaginous remnants from the second branchial cleft present as a mobile cyst beneath the anterior border of the sternocleidomastoid (left). In another patient (right), the cyst was infected, producing redness of the overlying skin.

FIG. 17.98 First branchial arch fistula, previously diagnosed as an infected lymph node. The location of the secondary opening is near the angle of the mandible.

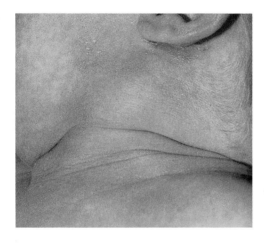

FIG. 17.99 The sternocleidomastoid in a newborn infant with torticollis may exist as a tight tendon-like cord, or swell and appear as a discrete tumor in the midportion of the muscle, pictured here.

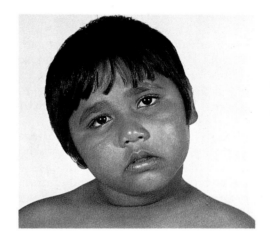

FIG. 17.100 Longstanding torticollis may cause permanent "wry-neck," facial shortening of the affected side of the face, and plagiocephaly.

monly complicated by coexisting chest disease, and antituberculous chemotherapy for active disease is necessary.

Painless cervical adenopathy is the most common presentation of Hodgkin's disease, and on occasion is the first manifestation of non-Hodgkin's lymphoma. Nodes involved with malignant lymphoma are enlarged, nontender, firm and rubbery. Malignancy should be considered when large, painless nodes without signs of inflammation are discovered, particularly low in the neck and in the supraclavicular regions (Fig. 17.95). Incisional biopsy becomes necessary when studies fail to confirm a definite diagnosis, or if enlargement continues despite treatment for a presumed infectious cause.

Branchial cleft remnants lead to the formation of cysts and fistulas in the lateral neck. A remnant of the second branchial cleft, the most common form, has an opening in the tonsillar fossa in the pharynx that runs along the anterior border of the sternocleidomastoid. A complete fistula drains mucus from a punctum located along this border (Fig. 17.96). When no cutaneous opening is present, a firm, mobile cyst forms. A neck abscess forms from superinfection (Fig. 17.97). Removal of the entire tract to the level of the primary opening in the tonsillar fossa prevents recurrence. First branchial cleft remnants, very rare, usually cannot be distinguished from an enlarged cervi-

cal node (Fig. 17.98). First branchial cleft fistulas lead from the external auditory canal to a point high in the neck at the angle of the mandible, very near branches of the facial nerve, a feature of obvious surgical importance.

Fibrous dysplasia of the sternocleidomastoid is the most common cause of torticollis in childhood. Two-thirds of children have a firm, painless tumor within the muscle (Figs. 17.99, 17.100), whereas the remainder have torticollis without the tumor. Daily exercises to force full rotation of the head upon the neck from side to side is effective management to correct torticollis in most children, with surgical division of the muscle in reserve for those who fail to respond. Neglected cases may lead to facial asymmetry and plagiocephaly.

CHEST WALL

The sternum is concave downward as well as side to side in pectus excavatum (funnel chest), the most common congenital deformity of the chest wall (Fig. 17.101). The concavity also involves the costal cartilages, and rotates to the right. Although infants with dyspnea exhibit sternal retractions and ultimately may develop a fixed deformity, the pectus excavatum arises frequently in children free from respiratory prob-

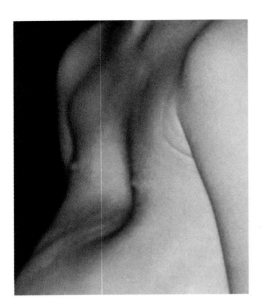

FIG. 17.101 Pectus excavatum (funnel chest) seldom creates cardiorespiratory symptoms, but psychologic consequences may be severe.

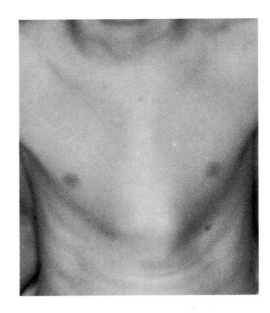

FIG. 17.102 The sternum projects like a keel in front of the anterior chest wall in pectus carinatum (pigeon chest). Like pectus excavatum, pectus carinatum produces no symptoms.

lems. The deformity arises gradually in infancy, and becomes more pronounced as the child grows. It fails to compromise significantly cardiorespiratory function in nearly all cases. Its appearance produces psychologic effects that may lead to withdrawal from activities that will expose the chest (such as swimming).

The sternum pushes forward like a keel in pectus carinatum (pigeon chest), with depression of the costal cartilages on either side (Fig. 17.102). A second form, "pouter pigeon chest," appears as a "Z" in profile: prominence of the manubrium, depression of the upper sternum, and protrusion of the lower sternum. The deformity first becomes obvious at age 3 to 4 years, and becomes increasingly apparent. There are no functional side effects.

Poland syndrome is a rare chest anomaly that includes unilateral absence of the second, third and fourth costal cartilages and ribs, with hypoplasia or absence of the overlying pectoralis muscles, subcutaneous tissue, breast and nipple (Fig. 17.103). The ipsilateral fingers may be short and webbed. Ectopia cordis may complicate sternal cleft, one of the features of pentalogy of Cantrell, discussed as an abdominal wall anomaly below. Complex congenital heart defects complicate ectopia cordis frequently; tetralogy of Fallot and ventricular diverticulum are common.

Along with the neck, the axilla is the most common site of cystic hygroma, which may communicate between the two regions. A chest film is necessary because the lesion may extend into the mediastinum.

Mastitis and abscess are the most common breast lesions in newborn infants. Nearly all cases of mastitis respond to warm compresses and antibiotics; failure of inflammation to resolve indicates the presence of an abscess that requires drainage. Localized breast masses in childhood are nearly always benign. Fibroadenomas, accounting for up to 90 percent of reported cases, form a mobile, smooth mass within the breast. Growth may produce lesions that replace a large portion of the breast, making a cosmetically pleasing excision difficult. Fibrocystic disease, another common disorder, primarily affects older adolescents. One to several firm, fixed masses become gradually prominent in a breast that has diffuse areas of cord-like thickening, which represent overgrowth of fibrous tissue. Size, consistency and tenderness of the masses change with different phases of the menstrual cycle, a characteristic of

the disease. Because the condition has an increased risk for breast cancer, breast self-examination should begin at an early age. Nipple discharge, unusual in childhood and adolescence, indicates the presence of intraductal papilloma, fibrocystic disease, or ductal ectasia. Cytologic examination of fine-needle aspiration from the mass provides a reliable means of diagnosis. Excisional biopsy should be avoided in prepubertal girls, as surgical damage to the small, immature breast will magnify as the breast increases in size at maturity, with potential disfigurement. Rapidly enlarging breast masses should be removed to avoid distortion of the architecture of the remaining breast tissue. Small lesions can be safely followed after confirmation of a benign diagnosis clinically or by fine-needle aspiration. Breast enlargement in boys is a common occurrence in the first two years after the onset of puberty; thereafter resolution is gradual and complete. Psychologic problems and social pressures justify subcutaneous mastectomies in boys with persistent enlargement or prominent breasts.

ABDOMINAL WALL
Gastroschisis and Omphalocele

Omphalocele and gastroschisis are the two major congenital abdominal wall defects of the newborn infant. In omphalocele the viscera herniates through the umbilical region of the abdomen, covered by peritoneum and amniotic membrane. The umbilical cord emerges from the sac that covers the herniated organs. In the most common form of omphalocele, the defect is placed centrally in the abdomen and contains liver, stomach and intestine (Fig. 17.104). Failure of the upper abdominal fold to form causes a defect in the epigastrium and lower chest; ectopia cordis with intracardiac malformation, sternal cleft and diaphragmatic hernia may be present in addition to omphalocele (pentalogy of Cantrell). Failure of the lower abdominal fold to form creates an omphalocele inferior to the umbilicus, associated with a number of lower body structures: spina bifida with myelomeningocele, imperforate anus, and cloacal exstrophy (caudal regression syndrome, Fig. 17.105). Chromosomal anomalies, cardiac defects, and other extra-abdominal anomalies occur commonly in large omphaloceles, and are the primary limitations of survival. The volume of herniated viscera may preclude primary closure of

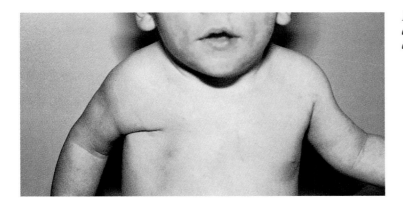

FIG. 17.103 Congenital unilateral absence of the anterior ribs, muscle and soft tissues characterize Poland syndrome, producing its typical appearance pictured here.

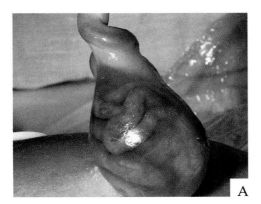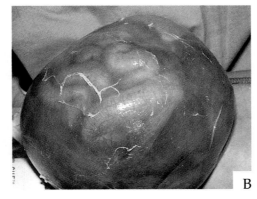

FIG. 17.104 **A**, small omphalocele with the umbilical cord attached to the apex of the sac. In the absence of chromosomal anomalies, other anomalies are rare and the ultimate prognosis is good. **B**, giant omphalocele containing liver, stomach and the intestines. Other anomalies are common, particularly cardiac, which affect prognosis.

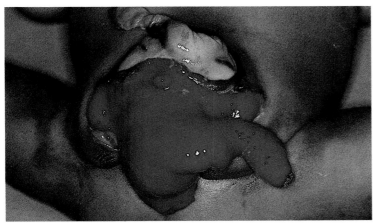

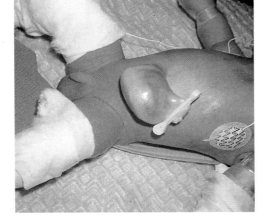

FIG. 17.106 A small omphalocele is easily reduced into the abdomen.

FIG. 17.105 Cloacal exstrophy consists of an omphalocele superiorly, below which the bladder is separated into halves by the exposed intestine. Both the proximal and distal bowel loops have prolapsed, producing the "elephant trunk" appearance.

the abdomen, making a staged closure using a silastic abdominal prosthesis necessary. With either approach, reduction of viscera may lead to respiratory insufficiency.

An umbilical defect less than 4 cm in diameter containing only loops of intestine represents a small omphalocele or hernia of the umbilical cord (Fig. 17.106). Those not associated with chromosomal anomalies are frequently free from any other anomalies. Repair is simple and gives a good cosmetic result.

The defect in gastroschisis is a hole to the right of the umbilical cord, which lies intact and separate from the defect (Fig. 17.107). Often a thick inflammatory membrane ("peel") covers the extruded intestine, which lies outside the abdomen without covering. The stomach and bladder, but not the liver, may also lie outside the body. The identification of organs which lie outside the body contour and the presence of a sac represent

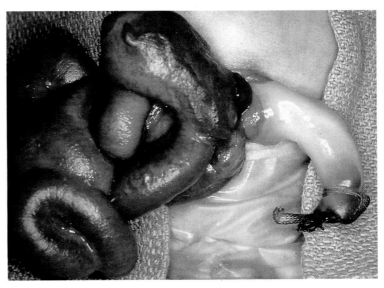

FIG. 17.107 The abdominal defect lies to the right of an intact umbilical cord, and the intestines lie exposed without a covering sac, free in the amniotic fluid. Both distinguish gastroschisis, here pictured, from omphalocele.

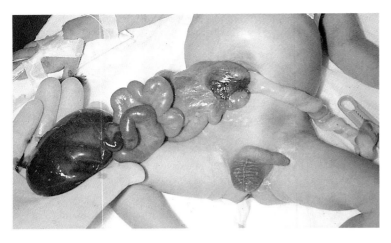

FIG. 17.108 Intrauterine volvulus of the cecum (purple in color) complicates this case of gastroschisis. Occurrence earlier in gestation may have led to absorption of the involved loop of bowel, and may have resulted in an atresia. Extraintestinal anomalies are rare in gastroschisis.

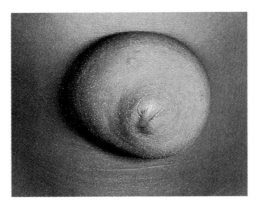

FIG. 17.109 Most infants with umbilical hernia will undergo spontaneous closure by age 3 to 4 years. Those that persist require repair.

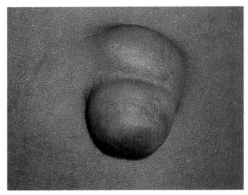

FIG. 17.110 Supraumbilical hernia, here seen as a crescent-shaped defect above an umbilical hernia, does not close spontaneously and requires repair.

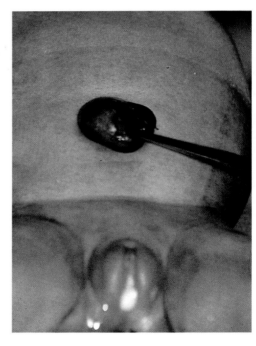

FIG. 17.111 Intestinal contents drain from the umbilicus through an omphalomesenteric fistula.

important differentiating signs on prenatal diagnosis. Intestinal atresias complicate gastroschisis in some cases, probably a result of inflammation induced by exposure to amniotic fluid in utero or volvulus (Fig. 17.108). Extraintestinal anomalies are uncommon. Some authors have suggested that gastroschisis may represent hernias of the cord that have ruptured in utero; these are similar in that both are largely free from associated anomalies. The right-sided location is a consequence of absence of the right umbilical vein in humans, leaving a relatively weak area at the base of the cord on the right side. Primary closure of gastroschisis is the preferred mode of management, but some may require a staged repair. Parenteral nutritional support is a frequent necessity, as slow recovery of intestinal function is characteristic.

Umbilicus

Most common of the minor umbilical anomalies is umbilical hernia (Fig. 17.109). It is six to ten times more prevalent in black children than in whites. Most close spontaneously, the majority within the first three years of life. They rarely incarcerate, and so repair is reserved for cases that do not close by three to four years of age. Resembling an umbilical hernia but actually situated superior to the umbilicus, a supraumbilical hernia does not resolve spontaneously and requires repair (Fig. 17.110). An umbilical granuloma forms following separation of the cord remnant in infants. Easily recognized as a friable polypoid mass emerging from a short stalk, it is treated by simple ligation. Drainage of intestinal contents signifies the presence of an omphalomesenteric fistula (Fig. 17.111), which represents a persistence of the communication between the embryonic midgut and the yolk sac. Division of the fistula is necessary to stop the drainage and to prevent volvulus. Drainage of urine indicates the presence of a patent urachus, which represents a remnant of the connection between the embryonic bladder and allantois. Its presence suggests the presence of bladder neck obstruction (such as posterior urethral valves), so a voiding cystourethrogram and cystoscopy should be performed.

Inguinal Hernia and Hydrocele

Inguinal hernia is one of the most common surgical conditions in infancy, with an incidence of 0.8 to 4.4 percent (Fig. 17.112). It is more prevalent among boys (exceeding its incidence in girls by six to one), and prematurely born infants (present in 7 to 17 percent). Inguinal hernia and hydrocele develop because the processus vaginalis remains open after birth. When fluid passes distal to the internal ring, a hydrocele forms. An intra-abdominal structure entering the processus, usually the intestine and commonly the ovary in girls, produces a hernia. Clinical features of inguinal hernia are familiar. A bulge

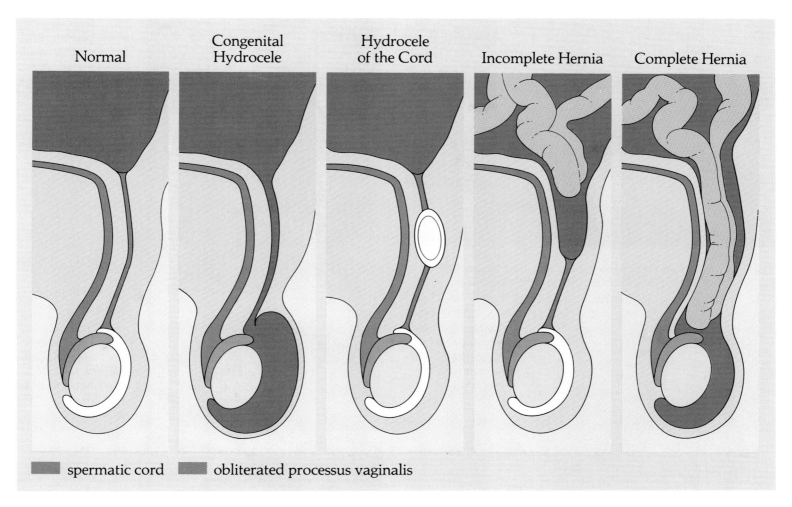

| Normal | Congenital Hydrocele | Hydrocele of the Cord | Incomplete Hernia | Complete Hernia |

■ spermatic cord   ■ obliterated processus vaginalis

FIG. 17.112 *Abnormalities of the processus vaginalis.*

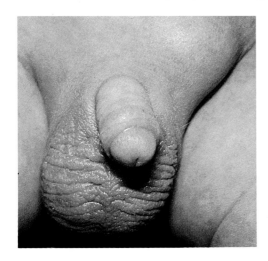

FIG. 17.113 *Incomplete inguinal hernia produces a bulge in the left groin, but does not extend into the scrotum.*

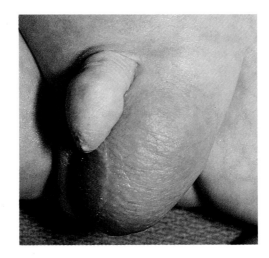

FIG. 17.114 *A complete inguinal hernia extends into the scrotum, obscuring the testis.*

appears in the groin that increases in size with crying and straining. It emerges through the external inguinal ring above and slightly lateral to the pubis (Fig. 17.113), and may extend into the scrotum (Fig. 17.114). It may disappear spontaneously with relaxation. Bowel within the hernia may transilluminate and thus may be confused with a hydrocele. A hernia extends above the pubis, whereas most hydroceles are situated distally, separated from the area of the external ring. A more proximally placed hydrocele in the spermatic cord (or canal of Nuk in girls) located near the ring may be clinically indistinguishable from an incarcerated hernia. Fluid in such a hydrocele cannot be decompressed through the processus into the abdomen, thus reinforcing the impression that it is an incarcerated her-

nia. A retractile or undescended testis may appear as a groin swelling and be confused with an inguinal hernia, so the position of both testes must be ascertained. An undescended testis may coexist with a hernia, a situation that requires orchidopexy in 5 percent of hernia repairs.

Demonstrating an inguinal hernia may be difficult. Stretching an infant supine on a bed with both legs extended and arms straight above the head usually causes the baby to struggle and strain. Familiar maneuvers in older children, who are examined while standing, include coughing, straining, and blowing up a balloon. Many surgeons proceed with repair even when these maneuvers fail, if the hernia has been identified previously by a pediatrician.

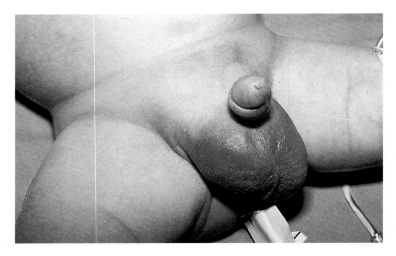

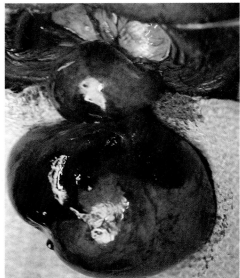

FIG. 17.116 Twisting of the spermatic cord in testicular torsion pulls the testis proximally, making it lie in a transverse axis. The dark, congested epididymis is seen overlying and to the left of the testis.

FIG. 17.115 Incarceration and strangulation of an inguinal hernia appears as redness and erythema overlying a firm groin mass.

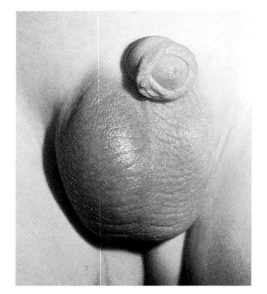

FIG. 17.117 A red, tender hemiscrotum may be due to torsion of the testis with gangrene, a surgical emergency.

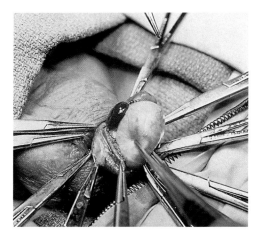

FIG. 17.118 The congested, twisted appendix testis contrasts with the normal pale pink testis. If the appendix testis can be identified through the scrotum, scrotal exploration is unnecessary.

Repair is mandatory because of the risk of incarceration; an inguinal hernia will not resolve spontaneously. The risk of incarceration is highest during the first months of life, approaching 30 percent during the first year; 69 percent of incarcerated hernias occur in infants before 1 year of age, and 27 percent occur in the first month. When the contents of the sac cannot be easily reduced into the intra-abdominal cavity, the hernia is considered to be incarcerated. Strangulation occurs when hernia contents become ischemic or gangrenous because of their constriction within the inguinal canal. Incarceration causes irritability, abdominal pain and vomiting. The groin bulge appears more tense and tender. The overlying skin becomes red and edematous (Fig. 17.115). Pain increases as hernia contents become ischemic. Intestinal obstruction leads to vomiting, which may be bilious or feculent. The stools may become bloody. The child may have fever, and the testis may swell. Plain films of the abdomen may show intestinal obstruction.

A number of conditions mimic an incarcerated hernia. Torsion of the testis pulls the exquisitely tender testicle upward toward the groin but rarely into the inguinal canal (Fig. 17.116). A hydrocele of the cord or canal of Nuk may closely resemble an incarcerated hernia, but is movable, is usually nontender, and has an upper limit to the swelling. Examination through the rectum reveals no bowel entering the internal ring, felt as abnormal thickening in the area of the groin. Sudden development of a hydrocele may cause discomfort and tenderness; this presentation may make its distinction from an incarcerated hernia difficult. Because of the risk of intestinal ischemia or gangrene, operation may be required when the diagnosis remains in question (Fig. 17.117). Torsion of an appendix testis does not compromise the testis, but may produce enough pain and overlying inflammation to cause confusion with true testicular torsion (Fig. 17.118). A congested appendix testis may appear as a "blue dot" through the scrotal skin.

Hydrocele arises most often in infancy; less commonly, later in childhood. It appears as a swelling in the scrotum that surrounds the testis (Fig. 17.119). It may fluctuate in size, becoming smaller at night during sleep. A number of features distinguish it from hernia, a sometimes difficult task. A hydrocele usually does not extend into the inguinal canal, unlike a her-

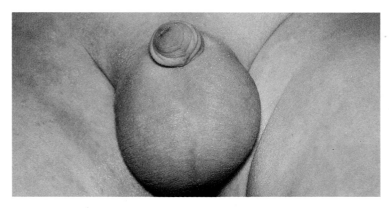

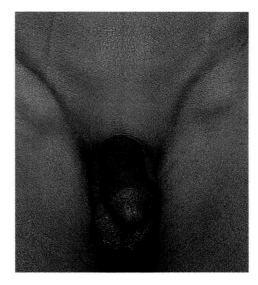

FIG. 17.120 Swelling lying below the inguinal ligament identifies femoral hernias, extremely rare in childhood.

FIG. 17.119 Bilateral congenital hydroceles. Groin swellings are absent, distinguishing them from hernias. The fluid collections may fluctuate in size, filling and emptying through a patent processus vaginalis. Spontaneous closure of the processus and absorption of fluid around the testis generally occurs, reserving hydrocelectomy for those that persist after age two years.

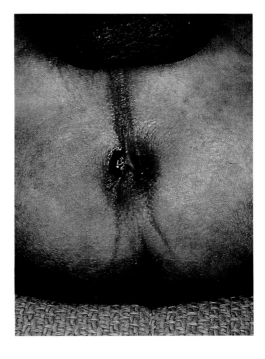

FIG. 17.121 A spot of meconium is visible beneath a "bucket handle" bridge of skin in an infant with a low imperforate anus.

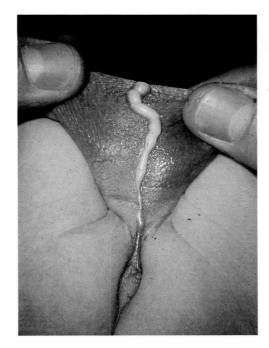

FIG. 17.122 In male infants, white mucus or black meconium may pass through a perineal fistula from a low imperforate anus into the scrotal raphe.

nia. A hydrocele is more mobile than a hernia and is not tender. A hallmark of a hydrocele is its brilliant transillumination. However, a gas-filled bowel in an infant may also transilluminate. Diagnostic aspiration of an inguinal mass should never be attempted. The processus vaginalis closes and the hydrocele resorbs during the first 12 to 18 months of life in most infants. Some surgeons believe that a hydrocele is in theory a potential hernia, and later may develop into one. However, most simple hydroceles do not develop into hernias, and hydrocelectomy can be deferred safely. Those that persist into childhood can be repaired, usually at 2 years of age.

Femoral hernias are extremely rare in childhood. Swelling is below the inguinal ligament, medial to the femoral artery (Fig. 17.120).

ANUS

A clinically obvious diagnosis, imperforate anus is detected immediately after birth, before vomiting takes place. There are three anatomic groups, based upon the relation between the end of the rectum and the levator ani muscle. In low imperforate anus, the rectum passes through the levator ani completely, and ends as a small opening in the anal region in the center of a prominent ridge (termed a "bucket handle" deformity; Fig. 17.121), or anterior to the anal structures as a perineal fistula. In males, the fistula may form within the scrotal raphe, and the meconium visible within it as a white or black line (Fig. 17.122). Because low lesions pass through the levator ani, prognosis for fecal continence is excellent after perineal anoplasty. High lesions fail to pass through the levator ani. No

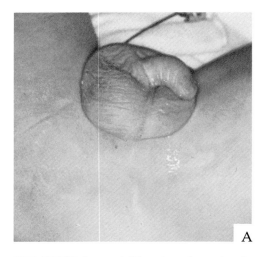 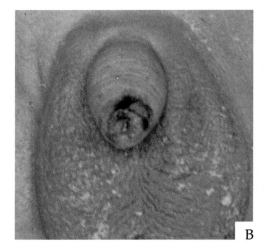 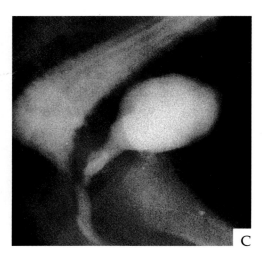

FIG. 17.123 **A**, no visible external opening forms in high imperforate anus. Absence of the intergluteal cleft is also seen commonly, frequently associated with sacral agenesis. **B**, meconium passes into the bladder or urethra through a rectal fistula and appears in the urine. **C**, retrograde urethrography demonstrates the rectourethral fistula.

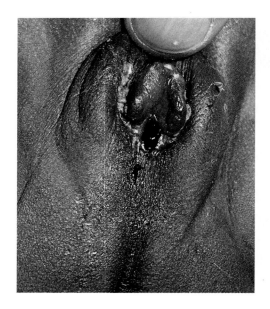 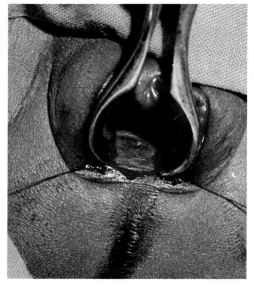

FIG. 17.124 A high imperforate anus communicates into the vagina. Meconium is passed through the vagina (left). Vaginoscopy reveals the fistula on the posterior wall of the vagina well above the hymen (right). A bicornuate uterus accompanies rectovaginal fistula in high lesions in girls.

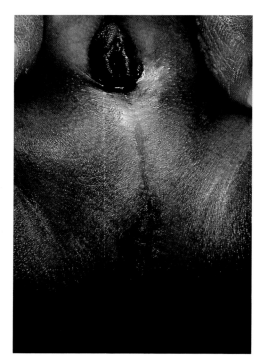

FIG. 17.125 Cloacal anomaly is the most complete expression of imperforate anus in girls, with urinary, genital and intestinal tracts converging into a single cloacal channel which exists as the sole perineal opening.

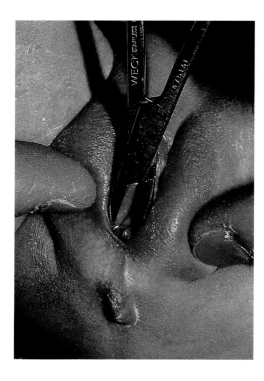

FIG. 17.126 An intermediate lesion passes partially through the levator ani, but fails to approach the perineum as closely as low lesions.

visible external fistula forms (Fig. 17.123). Most frequently, the rectum ends as a fistula into the prostatic urethra in boys, or into the vagina above the hymen in girls. Boys pass meconium or gas from the urethra; girls, from the vagina above the hymen (Fig. 17.124). A cloacal anomaly results when urethra, vagina and rectum join and exit the perineum as a single opening (Fig. 17.125). Babies with high lesions require a colostomy in the newborn period. The rectum is brought to the perineum when the child is bigger in a pull-through procedure. The prognosis for fecal continence in these children is guarded, and dependent partly on the quality of surgical reconstruction of levator ani and external sphincter musculature. Intermediate lesions are partially translevator (Fig. 17.126). For most, the surgical approach is the same as that for those with high imperforate anus. Because the rectum is partially translevator, they enjoy better fecal continence than those with high lesions. Many children with anorectal anomalies have associated anomalies, particularly those with high lesions. Anomalies may involve the sacrum and spine, the genitourinary tract and the spinal cord (tethered cord). Complete evaluation of a baby with imperforate anus must include studies that address these areas.

Anal fistula is a common problem among infants. It arises from an infected anal crypt along the dentate line, typically lateral in position (Fig. 17.127). A perirectal abscess develops, characteristically arising lateral to the anal verge. Incision and drainage, followed by warm sitz baths, lead to resolution of the abscess in the majority of cases, and recurrence is uncommon. Chronic drainage from the fistula, or the development of recurrent abscesses, requires fistulectomy. Although anal fistula may be a presenting sign of Crohn's disease and chronic granulomatous disease, nearly all cases presenting in infancy are idiopathic.

The cause of rectal prolapse is unknown in the vast majority of cases (Fig. 17.128). Inadequate perineal innervation and atrophy of the supporting musculature of the perineum explains rectal prolapse in children with spina bifida. Prolapse also occurs in cystic fibrosis, where the cause is less clear. Hookworm infestation can cause tenesmus and straining that can result in prolapse. Idiopathic rectal prolapse has a peak incidence in the second year of life, often brought on by an acute diarrheal illness or a severe episode of constipation. Incarceration is extremely rare, and the parents should be instructed how to reduce the prolapsed rectum. The condition resolves with resolution of diarrhea or effective dietary changes that address constipation. All such patients should undergo a sweat test to rule out cystic fibrosis. Refractory cases should undergo stool examination for ova and parasites, sigmoidoscopy and contrast study of the colon to check for the possible presence of polyps and worm infestation. Circumferential injection of a sclerosing solution such as 20 percent dextrose solution, into the submucosa is simple and effective treatment.

Anal fissure, another common problem among infants, is discussed as a cause of gastrointestinal bleeding above.

BIBLIOGRAPHY

Holder TM, Ashcraft KW: *Pediatric Surgery*. Philadelphia, Saunders, 1980.

Knight PJ, Reiner CB: Superficial lumps in children: what, when and why? 1983; *Pediatrics* 72:147-153.

Raffensberger JG: *Swenson's Pediatric Surgery*, ed 4. New York, Appleton-Century-Crofts, 1980.

Rickman PP, Soper RT, Stauffer UG: *Synopsis of Pediatric Surgery*. Stuttgart, Georg Thieme Verlag, 1975.

Sheldon CA, Martin LW: Pediatric surgery. *Surg Clin North Am* 1985;65:1059-1687.

Welch KJ, Randolph JG, Ravitch MM, et al: *Pediatric Surgery*, ed 4. Chicago, Year Book, 1986.

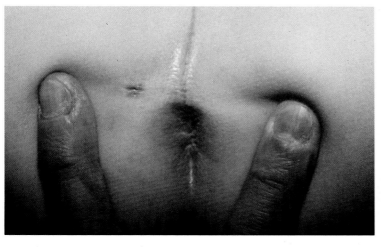

FIG. 17.127 *A punctum is visible to the left of the anus, the secondary opening of a fistula arising from an anal crypt within the anal canal. Recurrent abscesses arise from a well-formed fistula like this one, an indication for fistulectomy.*

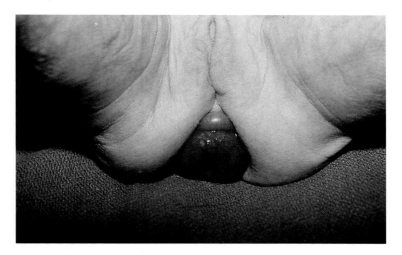

FIG. 17.128 *Although the cause of rectal prolapse is unknown in the majority of cases, all infants should undergo an evaluation for cystic fibrosis.*

PEDIATRIC AND ADOLESCENT GYNECOLOGY

Pamela Murray, M.D., M.H.P. ◆ Holly W. Davis, M.D. ◆ Melissa Hamp, M.D.

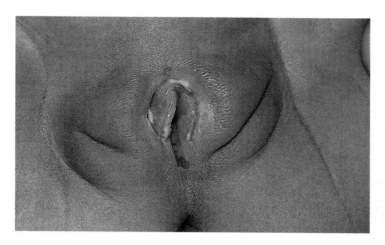

FIG. 18.1 Normal appearance of the genitalia in a newborn female. The labia majora are full and the thickened labia minora protrude between them. The mucosa is pink and a milky white discharge is seen, reflecting stimulation by maternal hormones. (Courtesy of Dr. Ian Holzman)

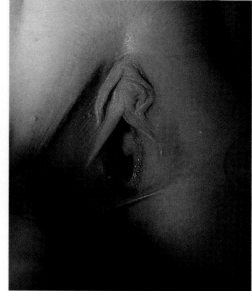

FIG. 18.2 Normal appearance of the genitalia of a 2-year-old female. The labia majora are flattened and the labia minora and hymen are thin and flat. The vaginal orifice is easily seen and the mucosa is thin, relatively atrophic, and reddish. Visualization was facilitated by use of the labial traction technique with the patient in the semisupine lithotomy position.

Pediatricians and other primary care physicians who treat children and adolescents are increasingly confronted with patients with gynecologic complaints. This trend stems in part from social changes, including earlier onset of sexual activity and consequent higher rates of pregnancy and sexually transmitted diseases (STDs) in the teenage population. In addition, there is increased media, public, and family discussion of sexual and gynecologic subjects. Young women and their mothers are less inclined to suffer silently the discomfort caused by reproductive system problems, including dysmenorrhea, abnormal uterine bleeding, and uncomfortable vaginal discharges. The increased survival of children with chronic illnesses represents another patient group in need of skilled and sensitive attention to the psychologic and physiologic aspects of their sexual development. There is also an increased interest among pediatricians in adolescent medicine. Practitioners are developing greater expertise and increasing their knowledge and understanding of the gynecologic conditions affecting adolescents such as vulvovaginitis, of the changing spectrum and epidemiology of STDs, of reproductive endocrinology, and of sexual abuse. An adolescent's first pelvic examination should no longer require transferring "well-child care" to a gynecologist. Accordingly, this chapter will emphasize normal anatomy, techniques of examination, and the pathologic conditions most commonly encountered: gynecologic trauma, inflammation, infections, and obstructing anatomic abnormalities that can be diagnosed on physical examination.

The reader is referred to Chapter 6 for a more detailed description of the approach to sexual abuse and an outline of specimen collection in the prepubertal female. Chapter 9 illustrates Tanner staging and discusses normal, delayed, and precocious puberty.

NORMAL FEMALE GENITALIA

Newborn and Prepubertal Periods

In the newborn female the physical appearance of the genitalia reflects stimulation by maternal hormones. The labia majora appear puffy and the thickened labia minora protrude between them (Fig. 18.1). Separation of the labia minora reveals thick, redundant hymenal folds that often hide the small central vaginal opening and urethral meatus. The mucosa is pink and moist, vaginal pH is acidic, and a milky discharge (physiologic leukorrhea) is seen. The phenomenon of withdrawal bleeding during the first week of life is not

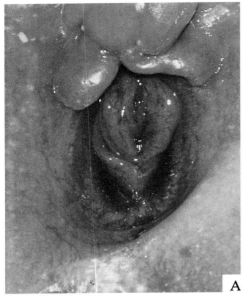

A

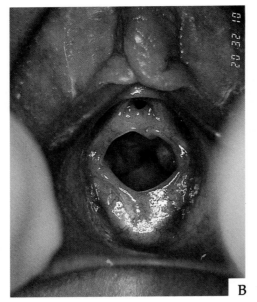

B

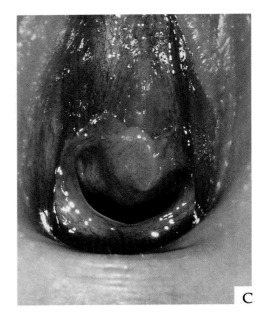

C

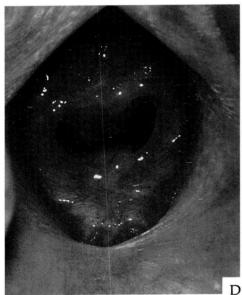

D

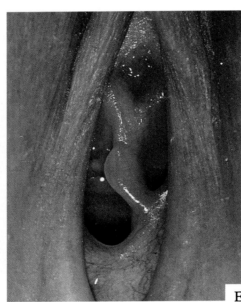

E

FIG. 18.3 Normal variations in hymenal configuration. **A**, redundant hymenal folds in a 12-month-old child. **B**, annular orifice of a 2 -year-old. Note the thin sharp edges of the membrane. **C**, crescentic hymenal orifice. **D**, crescentic orifice with septal remnants at 1 and 5 o'clock. **E**, septate hymen. See also Fig. 18.6. (**A, C, D**, and **E**, courtesy of Dr. Pat Bruno, Sunbury Community Hospital Center for Child Protection, Sunbury, PA. **B**, courtesy of Dr. John McCann, University of California at San Francisco)

uncommon. Breast development with palpable breast tissue, engorgement and, less commonly, a clear or cloudy discharge is observed in full-term neonates of both sexes (see Chapter 2, Neonatology). This gradually subsides over the first month of life as maternal estrogen levels fall. During this period, infants are at increased risk for developing breast inflammation and infection (see Chapter 12, Infectious Diseases).

Within 6 to 8 weeks the effect of maternal hormones on the female genitalia begins to abate; the labia majora lose their fullness and the labia minora and hymen gradually become thinner and flatter. Separation of the labia minora usually will expose the vaginal opening (Fig. 18.2). In fact the labia do not fully cover the vaginal vestibule (particularly when the infant or child is sitting) and thus offer incomplete protection from external sources of irritation. The mucosa is thin, relatively atrophic, and has a reddish hue. On first inspection, this normal red vascular appearance sometimes is mistaken for inflammation by observers unaccustomed to examining prepubertal genitalia. Vaginal pH is now neutral or alkaline and secretions are minimal. A series of physiologic changes also causes variations in the appearance of the hymenal tissues during childhood. The tissues remain relatively thick and

often are redundant during infancy (Fig. 18.3A), but by about 18 months the hymen is thin and translucent, with thin and smooth edges (see Figs. 18.2 and 18.3B–D). Between 3 and 4 years it becomes thickened and redundant again, only to progress through yet another phase by 6 to 7 years of age, and become thinner and somewhat more translucent. Finally, when the child enters puberty (reaching Tanner stage II), the hymen again thickens. The normal transverse diameter of the hymenal orifice is approximately 1 mm per year of age, although deviations of 2 to 3 mm in either direction are within normal limits. The appearance of the hymen is probably of greater significance in the diagnosis of sexual abuse than is the transverse diameter alone (see Chapter 6, Child Abuse and Neglect). The shape of the orifice also varies from patient to patient. It may be annular (Fig. 18.3B), crescent-shaped (Fig. 18.3C,D), irregular, or it may resemble a teardrop with the narrow portion formed by a notch to one side of the clitoris (see Fig. 18.6A,D). On rare occasions, a complete septum (Fig. 18.3E) or a fenestrated hymen may be seen.

From about 6 to 8 weeks of age and until puberty, the perineum, perivaginal tissues, and pelvic supporting structures are relatively rigid and inelastic. This factor increases the likeli-

	Newborn	Early Childhood	Late Childhood (7–10 yrs) Peripuberty (10–13 yrs)	Postmenarche (13+ yrs)
Ovary	Not palpable 0.1–0.2 cc	Pelvic brim 0.7–0.9 cc	w/in pelvis 2–10 cc	1.5x2.5x4 cm 15 cc
Uterine length (cm)	2.5–4.0	2.0–3.0	3.2–5.4	8.0 (nulliparous) (8x5x2.5)
Corpus:cervix ratio	3:1	2:1	1:1	2–3:1
Vaginal length (cm)	4	4–5	7–8.5	10–12
Hymen				
Orifice diameter (mm)	4	5	5–10	10
Thickness	Thick	Thin	Thickening	
Clitoris				
Width (mm)	5.0	2	2–4	$\leq$10
Length (mm)	10–15	3		15–20
Labia	Smooth	Smooth, flat	Progress through early Tanner stages until full & thickened	Tanner stages IV–V completed
Majora	Hairless	Hairless		Separation and differentiation of labia minora and majora
Minora	Prominent	Thin		
Vaginal secretions	White-clear, copious	Minimal	Physiologic leukorrhea	Physiologic leukorrhea may decrease
pH	5.5–7.0	6.5–7.5	4.5–5.5	3.5–5.0
Normal flora	Maternal enteric	Nonpathogenic flora including Staph and coliforms	Mixed vaginal flora	Lactobacilli
Hormonal influence	Maternal hormones	Minimal sex steroids	Low levels endogenous estrogen	High levels endogenous cyclic hormones

FIG. 18.4

hood of tearing as a result of trauma. Also during this period, the ovaries actually are intra-abdominal organs, being positioned above the pelvic brim until the onset of early puberty. Hence, ovarian disorders in the prepubertal years present with abdominal rather than pelvic symptoms and signs.

Peripubertal Period

With the onset of puberty the mons pubis begins to thicken and midline hair begins to form. Fat deposition fills out the labia majora. The labia minora thicken, become softer, and are more rounded. The clitoris enlarges slightly, and the urethra becomes more prominent. The hymen also becomes thicker as its central orifice enlarges. The vaginal mucosa thickens and softens, becomes moist and pink, secretions increase, and pH drops. Perineal and pelvic tissues become more elastic and the ovaries gradually descend into the pelvis. In the months preceding menarche, physiologic leukorrhea increases and

becomes noticeable. It consists of a white discharge containing mature epithelial cells and vaginal secretions stimulated by estrogen (see Fig. 18.25). The developmental aspects of gynecologic anatomy and physiology are summarized in Figure 18.4. The Tanner stages of pubertal development are presented in Chapter 9, Endocrinology.

GYNECOLOGIC EVALUATION

Examination of the Prepubertal Patient

INDICATIONS FOR EXAMINATION

Inspection of the external genitalia should be a part of every general physical examination. Careful attention to perineal inspection of female infants at the newborn, and 2-week, and 8-week visits facilitates early identification of major congenital anomalies. This is important because of a strong association between congenital anomalies of the external genitalia and

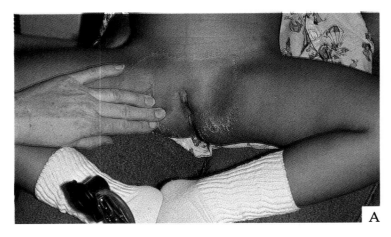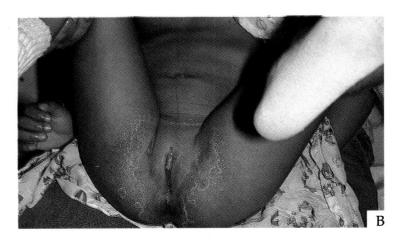

*FIG. 18.5 Optimal position for perineal inspection of the young pre-pubertal girl. **A**, frog leg position on the mother's lap. **B**, lithotomy position on the mother's lap.*

other genitourinary malformations that may require early intervention. Conversely, children in whom renal or urinary tract abnormalities have been identified should undergo careful examination of their genitalia, with the awareness that they may be at higher risk for genital abnormalities as well. Furthermore, children with known anatomic urinary tract abnormalities should have ultrasound evaluations of pelvic structures and the urinary tract as they enter puberty because the uterus, cervix and fallopian tubes, being derived from the Müllerian or paramesonephric ducts, are at greater risk for deformity. Routine inspection during well-child care visits allows early diagnosis of any new problems. The reluctance of some parents to express concern about possible genital disorders adds to the importance of such screening examinations.

Following the neonatal period, careful inspection of the external genitalia is recommended at each well-child visit. Speculum and routine pelvic examination are generally unnecessary until the onset of coital activity or until the later teens.

An exception to this rule would be the child or adolescent exposed to diethylstilbestrol (DES) in utero. These females have an increased risk of nonmalignant vaginal adenosis and other structural genital anomalies, of experiencing premature labor, and of developing vaginal adenocarcinoma in adolescence. They should begin special gynecologic and colposcopic evaluations under the care of a gynecologic colposcopist at age 14, at the time of menarche, or at the onset of any vaginal bleeding or discharge, whichever occurs first. As the first definitive link between DES and clear cell adenocarcinoma of the vagina was published in 1971, there should have been little use of DES in pregnancy after that date.

Patients presenting with certain complaints at acute care visits warrant inspection of the genitalia, and, on occasion, internal examination. These complaints include abdominal pain; dysuria, urinary frequency, urgency, incontinence, or enuresis; constipation or encopresis; perineal pruritus and/or pain; vaginal discharge or bleeding prior to menarche; and suspected or acknowledged sexual abuse.

TECHNIQUE OF EXAMINATION

Whether the patient is being seen for a routine checkup or for a specific problem, the gynecologic portion of the assessment should occur toward the end of the examination to avoid frightening the child at the outset. Careful evaluation of physi-

cal growth and secondary sex characteristics is important for patients with precocious puberty (see Chapter 9, Endocrinology) and for patients in the peripubertal and pubertal periods. All children with potential gynecologic problems deserve a thorough abdominal and inguinal examination.

Adequate preparation is important prior to the gynecologic assessment itself. In the case of patients being seen for routine checkups, the task is one of simple external inspection. In such instances, following abdominal and inguinal examination the physician generally can say to patients old enough to understand, "Now, I need to take a look at your bottom, and you can help me." The patient then can be shown how to help by getting into position. Drapes generally are unnecessary and often are perceived by the patient as threatening. Young infants can be assessed easily on an exam table after being positioned by the examiner. Older infants and toddlers tend to be more relaxed when examined on their mother's lap, with the mother assisting by gently holding the child in either the frog leg or lithotomy position (Fig. 18.5). Older preschool and young school-age children usually are able to be examined on the table in the frog-leg, lithotomy, or knee-chest position (see Chapter 6). The latter enables the best visualization of the vagina and may even permit inspection of the cervix because, on deep breathing, the orifice tends to open widely (Fig. 18.6A). This phenomenon also facilitates specimen collection. Although the knee-chest position is unacceptable to many patients who feel threatened by examination from behind, it can be very useful for selected school-age patients. Inspection is facilitated by use of good lighting. In the office setting, the otoscope provides both light and magnification, but prior to its use, the patient must be reassured that no speculum will be attached.

Once the patient is in position, visualization of the introitus, hymen, and lower portion of the vagina is facilitated by maneuvers that separate the labia. These include labial separation, which is achieved by pressing down and laterally with the index and middle fingers of both hands on the lower portion of the labia majora (Fig. 18.6B,C), and labial traction, which involves grasping the labia majora between thumbs and index fingers and gently pulling them down laterally and slightly toward the examiner (Fig. 18.6D and see Fig. 18.2). Excess traction should not be applied during these maneuvers, as it can result in tearing of labial adhesions if these are present.

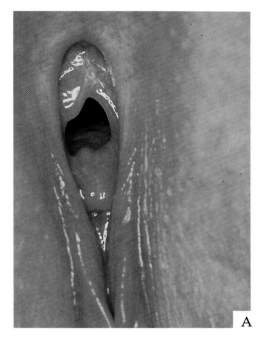

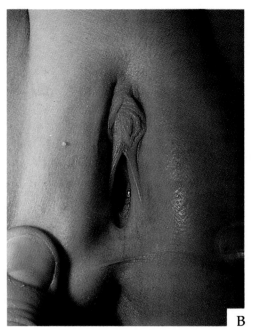

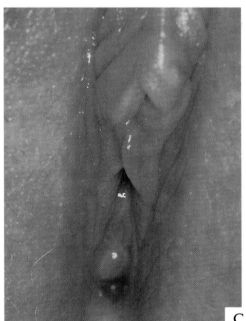

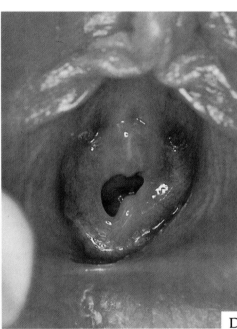

FIG. 18.6 *Perineal visualization in various positions and with different techniques of parting the labia.* **A,** *knee-chest position.* **B,** *semi-supine lithotomy position with labial separation. To facilitate visualization of the introitus and lower third of the vagina, the examiner can either press down and laterally on the labia majora with the index and middle fingers of both hands as shown here, or can gently grasp the labia majora between thumbs and index fingers and pull down laterally.* **C,** *supine frog-leg position with labial separation.* **D,** *supine frog-leg position with labial traction.* **A, C,** *and* **D** *are views of the same child, taken on the same day, and clearly show the variations in appearance using different positions and different techniques.* **B** *and Fig. 18.2 are two views of another child. (**A, C,** and* **D,** *courtesy of Dr. Mary Carrasco, Children's Hospital of Pittsburgh)*

These maneuvers should be explained first and the child reassured that the examiner is just going to look. If the patient so desires or if she is mildly anxious, she may place her hands beneath the examiner's, or the mother may be enlisted to perform the maneuver. Some girls prefer to separate their labia themselves.

If the patient is unusually anxious about the procedure and unable to be reassured, the exam should be deferred to a later date. At no time should an anxious struggling child be physically restrained and forced to undergo examination, as yield will be minimal and the experience traumatic.

On inspection the physician can readily ascertain the presence or absence of pubic hair; note the appearance and configuration of the labia majora, labia minora, clitoris, urethra, hymen, and vaginal orifice; observe the color of the mucosa and the presence or absence of rash or discharge; and visualize the distal vagina. Vaginoscopy is required only occasionally in the prepubertal child, and then only in those with spe-

cific problems. These include vaginal bleeding with or without evidence of trauma, discharges resistant to routine therapy, suspected vaginal foreign body, and suspected vaginal tumors. Because of the high potential for inflicting pain, especially if the patient moves suddenly, vaginoscopy generally is best performed under anesthesia. Heavy sedation may suffice in the child under 3 or 4 years of age but often is insufficient. Older school-age children may tolerate internal examination by a skilled examiner without sedation if preparation is careful. Again, a traumatic experience is to be avoided at all costs.

When specimens of vaginal secretions are required for cultures, wet mounts, or cytology, these can be collected easily and with little or no discomfort by use of small swabs (calcium alginate swabs on wire are optimal) premoistened with sterile nonbacteriostatic saline or via aspiration through a small, soft intravenous catheter (18- to 19-gauge). However, if collection is likely to be difficult because of pain or anxiety or because the orifice is very small, application of 2% Xylocaine®

FIG. 18.7

LABORATORY INVESTIGATIONS CONTRIBUTING TO THE DIAGNOSIS OF VULVOVAGINITIS WITH VAGINAL DISCHARGE

Saline wet mount	Yeast, *Trichomonas*, clue cells, inflammatory cells, pinworms, sperm
Gram's stain	Inflammatory cells, bacteria (GC), clue cells
Giemsa stain	Herpes
KOH	Yeast; "whiff test" for *Gardnerella* (can also be positive for *Trichomonas*)
Cultures	Routine culture for normal flora, nonvenereal pathogens, and *Gardnerella* Gonorrhea culture Culture in stool transport media for enteric bacteria, especially *Shigella* Viral culture for herpes *Chlamydia* culture (note: Chlamydiazyme® is inaccurate in prepubertal patients) *Mycoplasma* and *Ureaplasma* cultures
Pap smear	Human papilloma virus, herpes simplex virus, fungi, *Trichomonas*, inflammation, cell maturation index
Perianal Scotch® tape test	Pinworms and eggs
Blood	Rapid plasma reagin for syphilis, HIV titers, hepatitis serology
Urine	Urinalysis and urine culture
Urethral cultures	*Chlamydia*, gonorrhea, *Trichomonas*

ointment to the perineal and hymenal area 5 minutes beforehand is often beneficial. The patient should always be prepared for the procedure with simple and truthful explanations. It is often helpful to let her handle a swab or catheter and touch herself with it. If an appointment has been made for a child with vaginal discharge or perineal or urinary complaints, it is advisable to ask the family to not bathe the patient or apply any creams for at least 12 hours before the exam.

Routine bacterial cultures, including those for gonococci, can be collected from any visible discharge on the perineum; however, chlamydia cultures must contain superficial cells from the vaginal wall. Herpes cultures should be obtained from vesicles or ulcers. If no discharge is present on the perineum and specimens must be collected because of history of discharge or suspicion of sexual abuse, a small, premoistened swab or soft 18- to 19-gauge catheter is inserted gently through the vaginal opening with care taken to avoid contact with the hymen (as this is exquisitely sensitive). When a discharge is present, it can be gently aspirated through a catheter. In the absence of discharge, sterile nonbacteriostatic saline can be instilled slowly and then aspirated back. Dry cotton-tipped swabs are best avoided, as they tend to abrade the thin vaginal mucosa of the prepubertal child. Further, by using a soft catheter, enough material can be obtained via aspiration for multiple culture swabs and smears. Chlamydia cultures, however, must include cellular material directly from the mucosal surface, necessitating use of a saline-moistened calcium alginate or Dacron® swab. Figure 18.7 lists the specimens that should be considered in evaluating patients with vaginal discharge.

Patients with precocious puberty, suspected abdominal masses, suspected vaginal foreign body, and/or abdominal pain should undergo rectal bimanual examination (vaginal bimanual is virtually never necessary). In most cases this can be accomplished readily in the office, with good preparation of the patient along the lines described previously. If the patient is unable to cooperate, the procedure should be deferred and an examination under anesthesia considered, if clinical circumstances or the results of ancillary studies such as sonography or CT scan warrant it.

Examination of the Adolescent or Pubertal Patient

INDICATIONS FOR EXAMINATION

A pelvic examination is indicated for any postmenarchial adolescent as part of the evaluation of numerous complaints and concerns. These include abnormal vaginal discharge; pelvic, abdominal or perineal pain or dysuria; severe dysmenorrhea, amenorrhea, oligomenorrhea, polymenorrhea or abnormal uterine bleeding; sexual contact with a partner with suspected or confirmed STD; suspected sexual abuse; concerns with pubertal development, including absence of secondary sex characteristics by age 14, no menarche by age 16, hirsutism and/or masculinization, abnormal sequence of pubertal development or anatomic genital anomalies; and history of DES exposure. Pelvic examination should also be a part of routine health care for sexually active adolescent girls and should be given serious consideration when requested by the patient. The nature of the initial experience of this procedure may greatly affect a young woman's comfort with her body and the ease with which she experiences routine gyne-

COMPLETE HISTORY IN AN ADOLESCENT WITH GYNECOLOGIC CONCERNS

Home	Who lives there and quality of relationships; sources of conflict and support
Education	School, grades, curriculum, repeated grades, goals, behavioral or learning difficulties. If working—type, occupational hazards, hours
Activities	Exercise, nutrition and eating patterns, peer activities, friends
Drugs	Caffeine, cigarettes, alcohol, marijuana, crack, cocaine, pills, etc.
Suicide	Depression, psychiatric history, losses
Abuse	Physical, sexual, emotional, dating/relationship violence

Obstetric and gynecologic history:

Menstrual history	Menarche—age Cycles—length, duration, quantity of flow, use of pads/tampons Last menstrual period (LMP) Dysmenorrhea Premenstrual symptoms (PMS) Abnormal bleeding and other irregularities Mittelschmerz, mid-cycle spotting
STD history	Herpes, GC, Chlamydia, syphilis, PID, pubic lice ("crabs"), HIV, HPV (venereal warts)
PAP history	Abnormal smears, colposcopy, biopsies, treatments, followup
Urologic history	History of urinary tract infection or kidney problems
DES exposure	Abnormal bleeding, discharge
Vaginal discharge	Abnormal bleeding, pelvic pain, color, odor, quantity, pruritus
Obstetric history	Previous pregnancies and outcome
Sexual history	Sexual experience and age of onset Sexual practices Sex of partner(s) Number of partners Satisfaction with sexual experience Sexual problems with self or partner Contraceptive history: current and past methods, satisfaction, consistency of use, and problems
Family history	Disease or death caused by alcohol, drugs, cigarettes Gynecologic or obstetric problems Age of child-bearing Endocrine problems (especially thyroid) Bleeding problems (especially ob-gyn-related) Congenital malformations, mental retardation and reproductive loss

FIG. 18.8

cologic care throughout her adult life. It is helpful to ask about previous pelvic exam experiences to avoid repeating any prior emotional or physical trauma. The examiner's approach should be sympathetic, unhurried, and sensitive to the modesty of the patient. A thorough and directed history is to precede the examination. A comprehensive outline is suggested in Figure 18.8.

Prior to the exam, adequate time should be made available to interview all young women alone to provide an opportunity to ask questions about voluntary and involuntary sexual activity and explore other concerns that also may be difficult to discuss in the presence of a parent. A similar opportunity should be given to the parent to express any particular concerns or worries that they have been reluctant to share in their daughter's presence.

TECHNIQUE OF EXAMINATION
Successful examination depends on adequate patient preparation and use of appropriate instruments. For virginal adolescents, the narrow-bladed Huffman speculum (½ " x 4½ ") is recommended. While long enough to expose the cervix, its narrow blades are inserted easily through the virginal introitus. Most

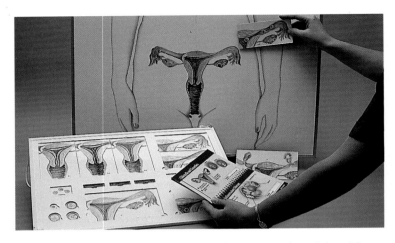

FIG. 18.9 Anatomic drawings are useful in preparation of the adolescent patient for examination and in gynecologic education.

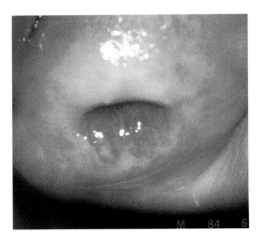

FIG. 18.10 Normal nulliparous cervix. The surface is covered with pink squamous epithelium that is uniform in consistency. The os is small and round. A small area of ectropion is visible inferior to the os. (Courtesy of C. Stevens)

sexually active adolescents can be examined with the straight-sided Pedersen (1" x 4½ ") speculum. The Huffman speculum should be considered as an alternative for a first pelvic exam or for particularly anxious patients. The duck-billed Graves speculum (1⅜ " x 3¾ ") is useful in parous patients. Gloves should be available in the examining room, and worn by the practitioner for both external and internal examinations.

The older teenager will generally prefer not to have her mother present during the pelvic examination. However, if she wishes her mother to remain, this should be respected. In general, and particularly with a male examiner, the presence of a chaperone (such as a nurse or an aide) is recommended for propriety as well as to facilitate the handling of specimens.

Before beginning, the examiner should carefully explain the various parts of the examination–inspection of the external genitalia, speculum examination of the vagina and cervix, and bimanual palpation. Use of anatomic drawings and/or models can be quite helpful and educational (Fig. 18.9).

The patient should be shown the speculum and be allowed to touch it if she so desires. Patients experiencing their first pelvic exam should be reassured that only the blades of the speculum will be inserted. Comparing the size of an open speculum to a finger or tampon often is reassuring. Both plastic and metal specula can be moistened with warm water to increase comfort and ease of insertion. This does not compromise specimen collection. If only a single size of disposable plastic specula is routinely used at a facility, it is important to have a back-up supply of smaller metal specula.

Before and during the examination, the examiner should talk to the patient to explain what she or he is seeing and to provide reassurance and education. Maintaining a dialogue throughout the procedure also usually helps the patient to relax. Conversation can be used to confirm normal anatomic findings, and to provide the patient with examples of a correct and comfortable vocabulary describing her reproductive anatomy and function. A hand mirror held by the patient is often useful for similar reasons. The patient should be told that she will have "a feeling of pressure," not pain, during speculum insertion and should be reminded to breathe at a regular rate. Tensing abdominal or pelvic muscles can produce discomfort and make the examination more difficult to perform. The patient should empty her bladder before the start of the pelvic examination. A urine specimen can be collected at this time.

With the patient in the lithotomy position, the external genitalia are inspected first. Pubic hair pattern and clitoral size are

assessed. The presence of vulvar lesions or of vaginal discharge on the perineum should be noted. The introital opening is inspected and its edges palpated for any swellings in the regions of Bartholin's glands. The urethral opening is then inspected, and if erythema or discharge is noted, the urethra is gently stripped with a gloved finger along the vaginal roof. Any purulent material obtained should be cultured. Note: swabs used to obtain chlamydia cultures from the urethra and any other sites must have direct contact with the mucosal surface, rather than the discharge itself.

The examiner then should gently insert the index finger into the vagina to assess the size of the introital opening and to locate the cervix. Vaginal muscle tone can be assessed by asking the patient to "tighten her muscles" around the examiner's finger. Conscious relaxation can be practiced by asking the patient to relax those same muscles and to push her buttocks onto the examining table. With the index finger partially withdrawn but gently pressing on the vaginal floor, the speculum (premoistened with warm water, not lubricant) is inserted over the finger into the vagina. Excess pressure on the anterior vaginal wall, and hence on the urethra, is to be avoided.

With the speculum in place the vaginal walls are inspected for erythema, lesions, or the presence of discharge. Visible vaginal secretions from the posterior vaginal pool should be sampled with a cotton swab and placed in a small amount of normal saline for wet mount and KOH examination. The cervix is then inspected. Any vaginal pool secretions and cervical mucus should be removed from the cervical surface, using cotton swabs, prior to inspection of the cervix or sampling of cervical secretions. The normal nulliparous cervix usually has a small round os and is covered with squamous epithelium that is pink and uniform in consistency (Fig. 18.10). Cervical lesions (cysts, warts, polyps, vesicles) should be noted. An ectropion (or eversion) of the endocervical columnar epithelium onto the cervical surface is common in adolescents, and not abnormal (Fig. 18.11). Ectropion should be distinguished from cervicitis, the latter being suggested by the presence of erythema, friability, and mucopurulent cervical discharge (see Fig. 18.41B). If the endocervical epithelium extends onto the vaginal walls or if the cervical shape is abnormal or hypoplastic, this raises the possibility of in utero DES exposure, and gynecologic referral is warranted.

Cervical specimens are then collected. First, a Pap smear is obtained by rotating a wooden Ayre® spatula circumferentially around the cervical os. The entire squamocolumnar junction

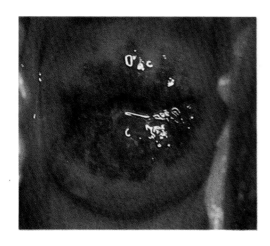

FIG. 18.11
Ectropion. Columnar mucosal cells usually found in the endocervical canal have extended out into the surface of the cervix creating a circular raised erythematous appearance. Note the normal nonpurulent cervical mucus. This normal variant is not to be confused with cervicitis. (Courtesy of Dr. E. Jerome)

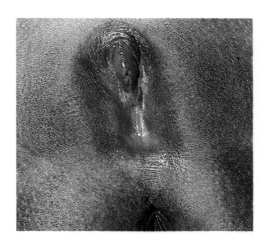

FIG. 18.12
Labial adhesions. Agglutination and adhesion of the labia minora, as a result of healing following erosion or inflammation, produce the appearance of a smooth flat surface overlying the introitus, divided centrally by a thin lucent line. (Courtesy of Dr. D. Lloyd)

should be gently scraped. A sample from the endocervical canal is collected with a cotton swab or, preferably, a cytobrush. Each sample is smeared onto a labeled glass slide according to laboratory protocol and treated immediately with fixative. Pap smear results may be uninterpretable in the presence of inflammation, bleeding, or inadequate fixation. Ideally, Pap smears collected for screening for cervical dysplasia should be deferred until infections are treated and menstrual bleeding has finished. Concerns with patient compliance and followup, or urgent clinical needs may justify collection of Pap specimens at less optimal times. Sometimes, Pap smear results can contribute to the diagnosis of abnormal bleeding or chronic cervicitis when problems are caused by infection with HPV, HSV, *Trichomonas*, or by dysplasia itself.

For routine sexual health care, or for evaluation of pain, bleeding, or discharge from the cervix, specimens should be obtained to determine the presence of infection. A saline wet mount for microscopic evaluation in the office can be prepared by placing a sample of cervical discharge into a small amount (1 ml) of saline or by placement directly onto a slide with a drop of saline. Gonorrhea cultures are obtained from the endocervical canal. A sterile swab is inserted into the canal and rotated for at least 10 seconds. The swab is then placed immediately into a selective transport or culture medium. Either medium must be at room temperature before inoculation. It is possible, but less than ideal, to grow gonorrhea from routine culture specimens. Gonorrhea-specific media prevent bacterial overgrowth by other species and allow a longer transport time. Chlamydia cultures or ELISA assays (of which Chlamydiazyme® is perhaps the best known) require mucosal surface cells because the pathogen is an obligate intracellular organism. Dacron® swabs or cytobrushes are placed in the endocervical canal and thoroughly rotated in order to obtain the necessary cellular material. After these routine specimens are obtained, the examination may continue using lubricant or acetic acid as needed.

The speculum is then removed and the bimanual (vaginal–abdominal) examination is performed. The examiner should note the size, consistency, position, and mobility of the uterus, and should check for tenderness on cervical or fundal motion. The adnexa should be palpated for enlargement or tenderness. A recto-vaginal examination using the index and middle finger is then performed to confirm the vaginal–abdominal examination, to palpate the cul-de-sac, and to examine a retroflexed uterus.

Once the examination has been completed, the patient should be helped out of the lithotomy position, given tissues to wipe away any lubricant or discharge, and allowed privacy to get dressed. During this time the examiner can review the wet mount and KOH preparation. With this additional information, the practitioner can now review the presenting problems and subsequent findings with the patient. Use of printed pictures or line drawings will enhance the patient's understanding of the discussion (see Fig. 18.9). They also provide an opportunity to encourage communication between the young woman and her parent, as appropriate to the circumstance.

GENITAL TRACT OBSTRUCTION
Labial Adhesions

The most common form of vaginal obstruction in prepubertal patients is that produced by "fusion" of the labia minora as a result of labial adhesions. On inspection one finds a smooth, flat membrane with a thin lucent central line overlying the introitus. It is postulated that inflammation and erosion of the superficial layers of the mucosa—whether due to infection, dermatitis, or mechanical trauma—result in agglutination of the apposed labia minora by fibrous tissue upon healing. The process typically begins posteriorly and extends forward. In most cases the fused portion is less than 1 cm in length but, on occasion, it can extend to cover the vaginal vestibule and, rarely, the urethra (Fig. 18.12). Even when fusion is extensive, urine flow and vaginal secretions are able to exit through the opening anteriorly. While most patients with labial fusion are asymptomatic, some present with symptoms of lower urinary tract inflammation.

The problem readily responds to application of estrogen cream along the line of fusion twice daily for 2 weeks followed by nightly application for an additional week, if necessary. After the labia have separated, lubricant should be applied nightly for several months to prevent recurrence. The patient's mother should be informed that topical estrogen may cause transient hyperpigmentation of the labia and the areolae and an increase in breast tissue, but that these changes will regress once therapy is completed. An estrogen withdrawal bleed (similar to that seen in the neonate) occasionally occurs. Removal of irritants, treatment of infections, and instructions on good perineal hygiene also tend to prevent recurrence.

Manual separation of fused labia is painful, traumatic, and is frequently followed by a recurrence of fusion. Hence, this practice should be abandoned. True fusion—adhesions present in the first months of life or adhesions that do not respond to the prescribed therapy—require further evaluation for abnormalities in sex differentiation.

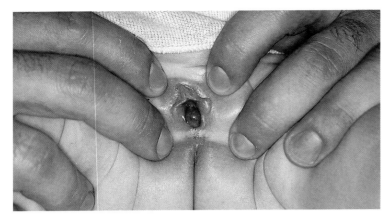

FIG. 18.13 *Imperforate hymen with neonatal hematocolpos. A dark purplish bulge at the introitus was noted by the mother during a diaper change.*

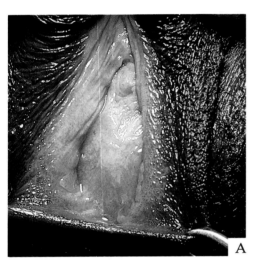

A

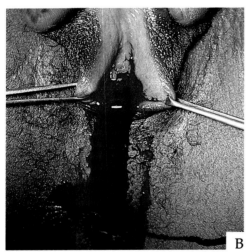

B

FIG. 18.14 *Imperforate hymen/hematocolpos. The adolescent presented with a 2-month history of intermittent crampy lower abdominal pain, which had acutely worsened. She had well-developed secondary sex characteristics but was premenarchial by history. A, examination revealed midline fullness and tenderness of the lower abdomen and a smooth bulging mass at the introitus. B, incision of the imperforate membrane just inside the hymenal ring allowed the accumulated menstrual blood and vaginal secretions to drain. (Courtesy of Dr. D. Lloyd)*

Imperforate Hymen

The anomaly referred to as imperforate hymen consists of an imperforate membrane located just inside the hymenal ring. This is the most common truly obstructive abnormality. It is frequently missed on the newborn examination because of the redundancy of hymenal folds. However, it may become evident by 8 to 12 weeks of age on careful perineal inspection, being seen as a thin, white transparent hymenal membrane that bulges when the infant cries or strains. Occasionally, young infants with this anomaly have copious vaginal secre-

CAUSES OF GENITAL TRACT OBSTRUCTION

Labial adhesions (partial obstruction)

Labial fusion

Imperforate hymen

Vaginal atresia (failure to canalize the vaginal plate)

Vaginal (with or without uterine) agenesis, including Mayer-Rokitansky-Kuster-Hauser syndrome (Müllerian aplasia); congenital absence of vagina and uterus

Transverse vaginal septum at the junction of upper third and lower two thirds of vagina

Longitudinal vaginal septum

Androgen insensitivity (testicular feminization syndrome)

Absence of cervix and/or uterus

Obstructing Müllerian malformations, with elements of duplication, agenesis, and/or incomplete fusion

FIG. 18.15

tions secondary to stimulation by maternal hormones, and as a result develop *hydrocolpos*. In such cases, the infant may be noted to have midline swelling of the lower abdomen (especially noticeable when the bladder is full), which feels cystic on palpation. Perineal inspection reveals a whitish, bulging membrane at the introitus. The cystic mass may also be palpable on rectal examination. In the presence of a neonatal withdrawal bleed or trauma, a *hematocolpos* may develop. This presents as a red or purplish bulge (Fig. 18.13). Treatment consists of incision of the membrane to allow drainage, followed by excision of redundant portions.

If undetected in infancy, the patient with an imperforate hymen usually presents in late puberty with *hematocolpos*. The major complaint is one of intermittent lower abdominal and low back pain, which rapidly progresses in severity and duration. If an imperforate hymen is not diagnosed promptly, difficulty in urination and defecation ensues and a lower abdominal swelling may become noticeable. On occasion, acute urinary retention may prompt the visit. The patient has well-developed secondary sex characteristics, but is premenarchial by history. Perineal inspection reveals a thick, tense, bulging membrane, often bluish in color, at the introitus (Fig. 18.14A). A low cystic swelling is palpable anteriorly on rectal examination. Operative excision allows drainage of the accumulated blood and vaginal secretions (Fig. 18.14B). Other hymenal abnormalities may allow menstrual blood to flow, but may present with difficulty initiating intercourse. Because hymens are not of müllerian origin, imperforate hymens are not associated with other genitourinary abnormalities.

Other forms of genital tract obstruction (Fig. 18.15) are rare. Partial or complete obstruction can present with a wide range of signs and symptoms. Symptoms may include vaginal, pelvic or abdominal pain which is often cyclic; primary amenorrhea or irregular vaginal bleeding; urinary tract symptoms;

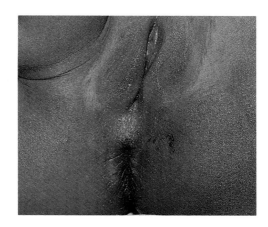

FIG. 18.16
Superficial blunt trauma. Healing abrasions are seen in this patient who was a victim of sexual abuse.

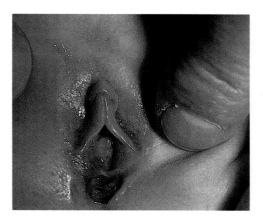

FIG. 18.17
Superficial penetrating injury. This infant presented with a chief complaint of blood spotting on the diaper. Inspection revealed a perineal tear just posterior to the hymenal ring, with no evidence of internal extension on vaginoscopy under anesthesia. Sexual abuse was suspected.

and difficulty initiating intercourse or dyspareunia. Clinically, a vaginal, pelvic or abdominal mass may be found, reflecting hydro- or hematocolpos, pyohematocolpos or hematometra.

It is important to note, however, that early routine genital inspection in most cases will reveal the absence of a vaginal orifice, enabling early delineation of the anomaly and thus facilitating treatment. Genital abnormalities of Müllerian origin are often accompanied by renal defects; hence, an evaluation of Müllerian abnormalities should include investigation of both the genital and urinary systems.

GENITAL TRAUMA

As mentioned earlier the genital structures and pelvic supporting tissues of the prepubescent girl not only are smaller but also are considerably more rigid than those of the adolescent or adult female. This inelasticity significantly increases the risk of tearing with either blunt or penetrating trauma and of internal extension of injury, especially in cases of penetrating injury. Appropriate assessment and management necessitate appreciation of this factor along with recognition that serious internal injuries of the vagina, rectum, urethra, bladder, and peritoneal structures may underlie deceptively mild external abnormalities. Careful attention must be given to vital signs, abdominal examination and evaluation of the urethra, hymen, lower vagina, perineal body, and rectum.

Clues to internal extension of injury include hymenal tears, vaginal bleeding and/or vaginal hematoma, tears of the perineal body, inability to urinate or gross hematuria, and abnormal sphincter tone or rectal bleeding. When injuries have extended to involve peritoneal structures, lower abdominal tenderness is seen, and at times is associated with signs of hypovolemia. Direct tenderness may range from mild to marked and may or may not be accompanied by rebound tenderness. Occasionally, a palpable mass can be appreciated.

Adolescents, in contrast, are more likely to have contusions than tears and are much less likely to have internal extension of injury unless the applied force is very great.

The role of the primary care or emergency physician is one of assessing the patient's general status and determining the likely extent and cause of the injury. This can be accomplished largely with a good general examination, careful perineal inspection, and urinalysis. The physician must at all times be sensitive to the patient's physical discomfort and emotional distress, providing emotional support whenever possible. Patients should also be protected from having to undergo multiple examinations, a particular risk in teaching hospitals.

When external inspection suggests that the prepubertal pa-

tient's injury is more than superficial, internal examination under anesthesia (by a pediatric surgeon or gynecologist) should be arranged. This enables meticulous inspection, wound exploration and repair under optimal conditions without traumatizing the child further.

Most adolescents are able to tolerate inspection and internal examination as outpatients. However, if injuries are severe or if the postmenarchial patient is too anxious to undergo pelvic examination when indicated, examination under anesthesia is the better course.

Superficial Perineal Injuries

The majority of cases of superficial perineal trauma are the result of mild, blunt force incurred via straddle injury, minor falls, and sexual abuse. Patients with accidental injuries that result in pain, swelling, or bleeding are rapidly brought to medical attention. A clear history of the preceding incident (often witnessed) is usually given, and findings fit the reported mechanism of injury. Accidentally incurred superficial abrasions may not be noticed by parents until the child cries on urination or complains of dysuria. As noted in Chapter 6, victims of sexual abuse may present with a chief complaint of abuse, but more often they complain of unexplained bleeding or pain with no history of trauma.

Typical lesions include superficial abrasions, mild contusions, and occasionally superficial lacerations (Fig. 18.16). The latter are found most frequently at the junction of the labia majora and minora and usually are only 1 to 3 mm deep. Accidental straddle injuries result in the crushing of the perineal soft tissues between the pubis and the object on which the patient falls or bumps herself. Hence, these tend to produce contusions or tears in and around the area of the clitoris and the anterior portions of the labia majora and minora (see Fig. 18.18). Minor falls onto or scrapes against sharp objects tend to produce simple perineal and vulval lacerations. As in cases of mild blunt trauma, the junction of the labia minora and majora is the site most frequently involved; however, tears of the labia majora or perineal body are not uncommon (Fig. 18.17).

Whether blunt or penetrating, when injuries are truly superficial, bleeding if present at all tends to be scant. The exception to this is a penetrating injury involving the corpus cavernosum of the labia majora, in which case hemorrhage may be profuse. Patients may experience mild perineal discomfort and pain on urination, but otherwise are asymptomatic. Most of these injuries can be managed supportively with topical bacteriostatic ointment, sitz baths, and careful perineal cleansing. Application of the ointment prior to urinating relieves

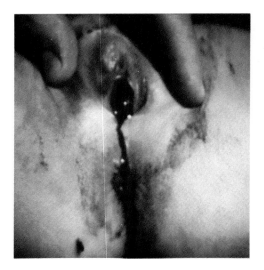

FIG. 18.18 Moderate genital trauma. Following a straddle injury on a diving board, this 9-year-old girl presented with vaginal bleeding. Inspection disclosed a hematoma of the anterior portion of the right labium majora and contusions of the introitus and a hematoma protruding through the vaginal opening. A small superficial laceration is present on the left, between the labia majora and minora, and another on the right between the superior portion of the introitus and the labium minora. At vaginoscopy under anesthesia a vaginal tear involving the right lateral wall was found. (Courtesy of Dr. K. Sukarochana)

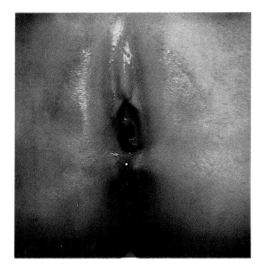

FIG. 18.19 Moderate blunt trauma. This 6-year-old girl presented with painless vaginal bleeding, which had soaked three sanitary pads in 2 hours. External inspection revealed a superficial tear of the anterior portion of the perineal body, a small hematoma to the right of the introitus, and blood trickling through the vaginal orifice. Examination under anesthesia disclosed a tear of the lateral vaginal wall. Sexual abuse was strongly suspected. (Courtesy of Dr. K. Sukarochana)

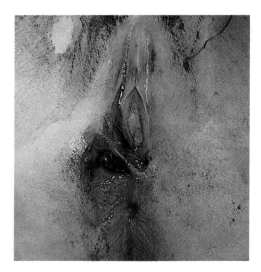

FIG. 18.20 Moderately severe penetrating genital trauma. This youngster fell while roller skating and slid on her bottom for several feet, tearing her perineum on an object projecting up from the ground. A laceration involving the right labia majora and minora and extending through the perineal body to the anus is evident on inspection. The patient complained of only minor discomfort. Examination under anesthesia revealed vaginal and rectal extension of the tear with complete transection of the external anal sphincter. The peritoneum was intact.

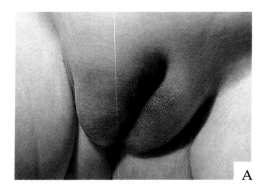

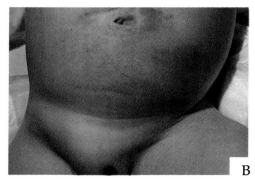

A   B

FIG. 18.21 Severe blunt perineal trauma. Following a fall from a height in which she had landed on her bottom, this young child presented with (A), labial contusions and hematomas, lower abdominal tenderness, and signs of hypovolemia. The force of the fall ruptured pelvic vessels, resulting in retroperitoneal bleeding that (B), ultimately extended along the anterior abdominal wall. These photographs were taken several days after the injury. (Courtesy of Dr. Marc Rowe, Children's Hospital of Pittsburgh)

dysuria as does urinating in a tub of water. If urinary retention continues to be a problem, use of a topical anesthetic ointment may be necessary for the first day or two. Deeper tears of the labia majora necessitate control of bleeding vessels and suturing under anesthesia.

Moderate Genital Trauma

Moderately forceful blunt trauma often results in perineal tears and in venous disruption and hematoma formation. Hematomas of the perineum appear as tense round swellings with purplish discoloration, which are tender on palpation (Fig. 18.18). When large, these may cause intense perineal pain. Those located in the periurethral area may interfere with urination. Moderate blunt force also can produce submucosal tears and vaginal mucosal separation with resultant vaginal bleeding or vaginal hematoma formation (Figs. 18.18, 18.19). In some cases, the associated external injuries can be deceptively mild (Fig. 18.19). Vaginal hematomas are the source of

significant pain that usually is perceived as perineal and/or vaginal, but at times is referred to the rectum or buttocks. Inspection through the vaginal orifice reveals a bluish swelling involving one of the lateral walls. This also may be evident as a tender swelling anterolaterally on rectal examination.

Moderate penetrating injuries result primarily from falls onto sharp objects ("picket fence injury"), rape, sexual molestation with phallic-shaped objects, and occasionally auto accidents. Lesions include perineal tears that extend into the vagina, rectum, or bladder but do not breach the peritoneum. While many patients present with external lacerations that obviously are extensive on inspection (Fig. 18.20; see also Chapter 6), a significant proportion have deceptively minor external injuries. It is important to bear in mind that, in the absence of associated hematomas, extensive tears may produce little pain. Furthermore, while most such injuries result in moderate bleeding, some patients have remarkably little blood loss.

Whether the mechanism of injury involves blunt force or penetration, when physical findings include bleeding through

CAUSES OF NONINFECTIOUS VULVOVAGINITIS AND DYSURIA

Condition	Historical Clues
Poor hygiene	Infrequent bathing, hand washing and clothing changes; soiled underwear, toilet independence
Poor perineal aeration	Tight clothing, nylon underwear, tights and leotards, wearing wet bathing suits for long periods, hot tubs, obesity
Frictional trauma	Tight clothing, sports, sand from sandbox play, excessive masturbation or sexual abuse, obesity
Chemical irritants	Bubble bath, harsh or perfumed soaps or detergents, powder, water softeners, perfumed and dyed toilet paper, ammonia; douches and feminine hygiene products in adolescents
Contact dermatitis	Poison ivy, topical creams or ointments
Vaginal foreign bodies	Wiping habits, excessive masturbation or self-exploration, sexual abuse
Parasites, insect bites, infestations	Home environment, pets, sandboxes, travel
Medication-related	Topical steroid or hormone creams, antibiotics, chemotherapy
Generalized skin disorders	History of pruritis, chronic skin lesions, prior diagnosis
Anatomic anomalies	Vesicovaginal fistulas, rectovaginal fistulas, ectopic ureters, spina bifida
Long-term effect of diethylstilbestrol	Maternal history
Neoplasms	Discharge bleeding
Systemic illness: Steven-Johnson syndrome, Crohn's disease with perineal fistulas	Prior infection or medication use, evidence from other physical findings, including short stature, abdominal pain, diarrhea
Pelvic appendiceal abscess	History of fever, anorexia, vomiting, progression of periumbilical to right lower quadrant pain

FIG. 18.22

the vaginal orifice, a vaginal hematoma, rectal bleeding, rectal tenderness or abnormal sphincter tone, gross hematuria or inability to urinate, internal extension of injury is probable. All such patients warrant exploration and repair in the operating room. This obviates the need for extensive examination in the office or emergency department.

Severe Genital Trauma

Severe falls from heights onto flat surfaces can produce major perineal lacerations simulating penetrating injury. In addition, occasionally they can cause disruption of pelvic vessels, mesentery, and intestine, with or without pelvic fracture (Fig. 18.21). Similarly, severe penetrating injury may produce tears that extend through the cul-de-sac, rupturing pelvic vessels and tearing intra-abdominal structures. While external injuries in these cases usually are extensive and associated with significant bleeding, they can be incredibly minor in appearance, particularly when penetration is the source. These children will complain of lower abdominal and perineal pain, which may radiate down one leg. Abdominal examination should reveal at least mild direct tenderness with some guarding and possibly mild rebound tenderness early on. Patients with pelvic bleeding will ultimately have signs of hypovolemia (at a minimum, they will exhibit tachycardia with widened pulse pressure) although these signs may not be evident immediately following the injury. Any patient with clinical signs of peritoneal extension of genital trauma warrants prompt hemodynamic stabilization followed by surgical exploration and repair.

NONTRAUMATIC VULVOVAGINAL DISORDERS

Prepubertal "Vulvovaginitis"

Strictly defined, vulvovaginitis denotes an inflammatory process involving both the vulva and the vagina. In practice, however, the term is used less precisely to refer to patients who describe symptoms of dysuria, vulvar pain or itching, or vaginal discharge, but who often lack signs of inflammation or who have evidence of vulvar inflammation without vaginal involvement.

Vulvovaginitis is relatively common in prepubertal girls and accounts for a large majority of genital complaints prior to menarche. Its frequent occurrence is explained in part by the fact that the labia do not fully cover and thus do not completely protect the vaginal vestibule from friction and external irritants, especially when the child is sitting or squatting. Additionally, the unestrogenized vaginal epithelium is thin, relatively friable, and more easily traumatized. Transient irritation without discharge is common in the young child because of exposure to chemical irritants (e.g., bubble bath, deodorant soaps, or harsh soaps and detergents), inconsistent hygiene and poor aeration. Finally, young children are less careful than older children and adults about cleansing their perineum and avoiding contamination with stool.

Causes of vulvovaginitis are protean and perhaps most easily classified into noninfectious and infectious subgroups, with the latter subclassified into nonsexually transmitted and sexually transmitted infections. Figure 18.22 presents the most

INFECTIOUS CAUSES OF PREPUBERTAL AND PUBERTAL VULVOVAGINITIS

Non-Sexually Transmitted Pathogens

Bacterial respiratory and/or skin pathogens
Group A beta-hemolytic streptococci*
Streptococcus pneumoniae*
Haemophilus influenzae*
Neisseria meningitidis
Staphylococci

Viral pathogens
Varicella-zoster virus
Herpes simplex types 1 and 2
Adenoviruses*
Echoviruses*
Measles virus

Gastrointestinal pathogens
Candida species*
Shigella species*
Enterobius vermicularis
Yersinia species

Sexually Transmitted Pathogens

Bacterial pathogens
Chlamydia trachomatis*
Gardnerella vaginalis
Neisseria gonorrhoeae*
?Genital mycoplasmas
Treponema pallidum

Protozoa
Trichomonas vaginalis*

Viral pathogens
Herpes simplex types 1 and 2
Human papilloma virus

Parasites
Phthirius pubis (lice)
Sarcoptes scabiei

Sexually Transmitted Pathogens Not Usually Associated with Vulvovaginitis

Bacterial pathogens
Calymmatobacterium granulomatis
  (granuloma inguinale or
  Donovanosis)
Group B streptococci
Haemophilus ducreyi (chancroid)

Protozoa
Cryptosporidium

Viral pathogens
Cytomegalovirus
Epstein-Barr virus
Hepatitis A virus
Hepatitis B virus
HIV types 1 and 2
Poxvirus (molluscum contagiosum)

Conditions in which vaginal discharge is prominent

FIG. 18.23

common causes of noninfectious vulvovaginitis with specific historical clues suggestive of each condition. Figure 18.23 presents the major infectious causes. Nonsexually transmitted bacterial pathogens and the herpes simplex viruses often are spread to the vulvovaginal area from another site (e.g., nose, throat, skin, or GI tract) by the patient's hands, whereas involvement with other viral organisms is more often a part of systemic infection. Candida emerges as a pathogen in the peripubertal period and is seen more commonly in children who are receiving systemic antibiotics or steroids, are using topical steroid hormone creams, or have underlying diabetes mellitus. Vulvovaginitis due to sexually transmitted pathogens is almost always acquired through sexual contact. Specific conditions are discussed in the ensuing sections.

In contrast to adolescents and adults, prepubertal girls are at less risk for internal extension of vulvovaginal infections (cervicitis and pelvic inflammatory disease) as the unestrogenized genital tract does not support the ascent of infection through the uterus and fallopian tubes.

The evaluation of these patients must include questions not only related to symptoms and duration of problems, but also questions about recent respiratory, gastrointestinal, and urinary tract infections; type of clothing worn and soiling, soaps and bathing, laundry detergents, medications and topical agents, and recent activities; concurrent abdominal pain; and possible sexual contact. Developmental, behavioral, environmental, and medical histories may contribute to a diagnosis and aid in the formulation of a therapeutic plan.

Physical assessment must include determination of degree of pubertal development, inguinal, abdominal, and often rectal examination, along with careful perineal and vaginal inspec-

tion. The degree and extent of inflammation and excoriation should be documented. Underwear should be checked for fit, cleanliness, and signs of discharge, stool, and urine. When patients are seen by appointment for vulvovaginal complaints, the parents should be asked to neither bathe nor apply creams to the child for 12 to 24 hours before the evaluation; otherwise, many children with a history of discharge will have none when examined.

The presence of a vaginal discharge necessitates specimen collection (see Fig. 18.7 and see section on Examination of the Prepubertal Patient). Urine should be collected for urinalysis and culture. If a vaginal foreign body is suspected, rectal examination and vaginoscopy are indicated.

Vulvovaginal Complaints in Adolescents

Among sexually active adolescent females, infectious processes are the major source of vulvovaginal inflammation, and sexually transmitted pathogens are the predominant offending organisms. The clinical manifestations of some of these disorders in adolescent girls can be very similar to those seen in prepubertal children although estrogenization and maturation of the genital tract alter its pathophysiologic response, favoring upward spread of some infectious processes, particularly those of gonorrhea and Chlamydia. As a result, subclinical infection, cervicitis, and pelvic inflammatory disease, in addition to vulvovaginitis, are significant concerns following menarche.

Clinically, vulvar lesions, vaginal discharge, odor, pruritus, and dysuria are common presenting problems in adolescents, but dyspareunia, pelvic pain, fever, and irregular bleeding may be prominent complaints as well. These symptoms are

CLINICAL AND LABORATORY FEATURES OF DISORDERS CAUSING VAGINAL DISCHARGE IN ADOLESCENTS

	Physiologic	Candida	Chlamydia	Gonorrhea	Trichomonas	Gardnerella	HPV
Appearance of discharge	White, gray or clear, flocculent	White, curdlike, with adherent plaques	Mucopus at cervix, +friable cervix with bloody discharge	Mucopus at cervix, white, yellow or greenish discharge	Gray, yellow or green; sometimes frothy, malodorous	Gray, white; homogeneous	White or clear, generalized or localized inflammation
Amount	Variable	Variable	Scant to variable	Scant to variable	Large	Large	Scant
Vulvar and vaginal inflammation	None	Usual	Not usual; with or without Bartholin's gland abscess	Variable; with or without Bartholin's gland abscess	Occasional	Rare	Common, evidence of HPV with acetic acid wash or overt condylomata
pH of discharge	≤4.5	≤4.5	≤4.5	≤4.5	≥4.5	≥4.5	≤4.5
Microscopy	Epithelial cells, few WBCs, lactobacilli	↑WBCs, + KOH with pseudo-hyphae and budding yeast	↑WBCs	↑WBCs	↑WBCs, motile trichomonads (in saline prep) in 60–70% of symptomatic patients; trichomonads in urine	Few WBCs + clue cells in saline prep	Moderate ↑WBCs
Predisposing or concurrent factors	Secretion of estrogen	Menstruation, broad spectrum antibiotics, diabetes, local heat and moisture, pregnancy, OCPs, AIDS, topical steroid or hormone creams, immune deficiencies	Infection with Gardnerella, gonorrhea	Often accompanied by Chlamydia, symptoms often develop toward the end of a menstrual period	Other STDs	Previous Gardnerella vaginalis infection	Abnormal PAP smear, other STDs; history of genital warts or recurrent unexplained vulvovaginitis
Other clinical signs and symptoms	None	Itching prominent, may have dysuria	Urethritis, with or without PID	Pharyngitis, with or without PID, proctitis, urethritis	Vulvar itching and burning prominent, dysuria, pelvic discomfort	None	Visible external or flat warts, chronic low-grade vulvovaginitis, fissures, failure of other therapies
Whiff test (+ amine odor on addition of 10% KOH)	Negative	Negative	Negative	Negative	Sometimes positive	Positive	Negative

FIG. 18.24

relatively nonspecific and may represent the final common pathway of different etiologic agents of irritation, infection, or infestation.

In addition to identification of specific etiologic agents, a major goal of evaluation is to differentiate vulvovaginal or cervical processes from upper tract disease (e.g., pelvic inflammatory disease, adnexal torsion or cysts, or normal or abnormal pregnancy), and from intra-abdominal processes (e.g., appendicitis, endometriosis, or tumors). Hence, a complete pelvic examination is necessary when evaluating adolescents with vulvovaginal complaints. The presence of systemic signs and symptoms and of abnormalities on bimanual pelvic examination suggests processes involving the uterus and adnexal and peritoneal structures. In contrast, isolated vulvovaginal disorders rarely are accompanied by such findings. In the majority of cases, careful history inspection, "bench" lab tests (such as wet mount, KOH prep, and Gram's stain), and selected cultures will provide a specific diagnosis on which to base treatment decisions. Some of the clinical and laboratory features of various etiologic agents of vaginal discharge are presented in Figure 18.24.

PHYSIOLOGIC LEUKORRHEA

Physiologic leukorrhea, though manifest as a vaginal discharge, is in actuality a normal phenomenon and not a form of vulvovaginitis. It is produced in response to estrogen stimulation, and thus it is seen in the newborn period and recurs in the 6–12 months preceding the onset of menses. The discharge consists of normal cervical and vaginal secretions along with desquamated vaginal epithelial cells. It is clear or

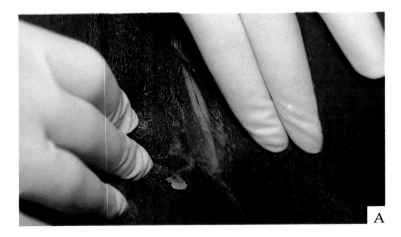

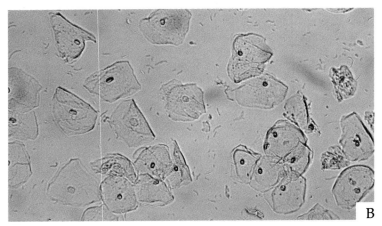

FIG. 18.25 Physiologic leukorrhea. **A**, the clinical appearance of this milky discharge is seen on the perineum of this normal adolescent. The discharge is produced in response to estrogen stimulation and is most evident in the newborn and peripubertal periods. **B**, on microscopy the discharge is found to contain sheets of estrogenized vaginal epithelial cells. There is no predominant flora and leukocytes are not increased.

ORGANISMS THOUGHT TO CONSTITUTE NORMAL OR NONPATHOGENIC VAGINAL FLORA

Aerobes and Facultative Anaerobes

Branhamella catarrhalis	Lactobacillus
Candida albicans and other yeasts*	*Klebsiella* species
	Mycoplasmas*
Corynebacterium species	*Neisseria sicca*
Diphtheroids	*Proteus* species
Enterococcus	*Pseudomonas* species
Escherichia coli	*Staphylococcus* species
*Gardnerella vaginalis**	*Streptococcus* species
Haemophilus species	

Anaerobes

Bacteroides species
Clostridium species
Peptococcus species
Peptostreptococcus species

Mycoplasma hominis, Ureaplasma urealyticum, Candida species and *Gardnerella vaginalis* can constitute normal flora in asymptomatic women; however, they may be responsible for genital tract infections as well.

FIG. 18.26

milky, relatively thin, odorless, and nonirritating (Fig. 18.25). When dried on a diaper or underwear it may appear yellow or brown. Perimenarchial patients often present with complaints of discharge because they and their mothers are not aware that the secretions are normal. These children are otherwise asymptomatic.

Examination reveals good pubertal development and a normal perineum and distal vagina with the typical discharge. Diagnosis is confirmed by findings on wet prep, which disclose estrogenized epithelial cells with no increase in leukocytes (Fig. 18.25B). (As a general rule, there should be no more than one polymorphonuclear leukocyte for every vaginal epithelial cell.) Treatment consists of reassurance and education.

Noninfectious Vulvovaginitis

Clinical findings of noninfectious vulvovaginitis vary considerably depending on cause. Although the physical examination often is unimpressive, patient and parental concern with the symptoms may be great. In some patients the vulva and vagina appear normal while in others varying degrees of inflammation or irritation are present, at times accompanied by signs of excoriation. Vaginal discharge is unusual, however, and vaginal cultures grow normal or nonspecific flora (Fig. 18.26). These disorders are quite common in prepubertal children but are relatively infrequent following menarche. Symptoms are similar

for most etiologies: perineal itching, external or contact dysuria, and occasionally vaginal discharge.

IRRITATION SECONDARY TO POOR HYGIENE
Poor perineal hygiene is one of the most common causes of irritation. Examination typically reveals mild nonspecific vulvar irritation. Pieces of stool and toilet paper may be seen adhering to the perineum and perianal areas, and smegma may be found around the clitoris and labia (Fig. 18.27). Frankly feculent vaginal discharge should lead to the consideration of a rectovaginal fistula. Underwear is often dirty. Coliforms tend to predominate on vaginal culture when lower vaginal inflammation is associated. The search for other causes is unrewarding, and symptoms resolve with a regimen of sitz baths and careful cleansing after urination and defecation. Failure to improve should lead to suspicion of treatment noncompliance or of the possibility of sexual abuse.

MACERATION SECONDARY TO POOR PERINEAL AERATION
Moisture, whether from normal secretions, perspiration or swimming, when unable to evaporate, promotes maceration and inflammation of perineal tissues. Obesity, wearing tight clothing or tights over nylon underwear, and sitting for long periods in a wet bathing suit are common predisposing factors to this form of vulvar irritation. Patients with urinary inconti-

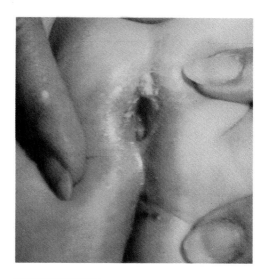

FIG. 18.27 Poor perineal hygiene. Despite prior cleansing by a nurse for a "clean-catch" urine, the initial specimen contained numerous white cells and debris. When the perineum was rechecked, the infant was found to have copious amounts of smegma adhering to the clitoris and labia minora. Urine obtained after thorough recleansing was normal.

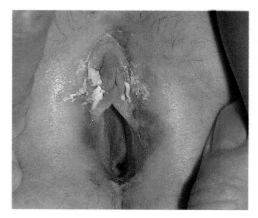

FIG. 18.28 Maceration secondary to poor perineal aeration. This child's chief complaint was one of dysuria. On examination the inner surfaces of the labia were found to be macerated and mildly inflamed. Adherent smegma suggested poor perineal hygiene as well.

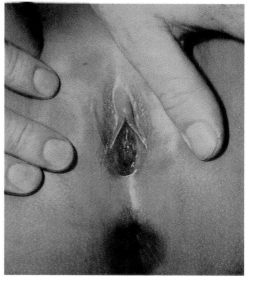

FIG. 18.29 Nonspecific inflammation characteristic of chemical irritant vulvovaginitis.

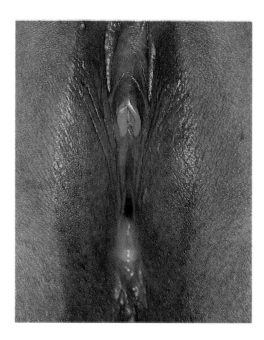

FIG. 18.30 Frictional trauma (nonspecific thickening of the vulvar skin). This patient's labial skin is thickened and mildly irritated. She had a history of recurrent vaginal foreign bodies and was strongly suspected to be a victim of chronic sexual abuse. (Courtesy of Dr. K. Sukarochana, Children's Hospital of Pittsburgh)

nence, a vesicovaginal fistula or ectopic ureter can also present with these findings. A history of a chronically wet perineum and the smell of urine on the child's underclothes should lead one to consider these possibilities. Nonspecific inflammation, often with frank maceration, will be the predominant physical finding (Fig. 18.28).

When maceration occurs, secondary infection is common, and some patients have associated intertrigo. Attention to perineal hygiene and drying, weight loss (when appropriate), avoidance of tight clothing and treatment of secondary infection are the mainstays of management.

CONTACT DERMATITIS, ALLERGIC VULVITIS

Allergic vulvitis should be considered in patients whose most prominent symptom is pruritis, although scratching and excoriation may result in secondary burning and dysuria. When patients are seen in the acute phase, inspection of the labia and vestibule reveals a microvesicular papular eruption that tends to be intensely erythematous and somewhat edematous. Excoriated scratch marks are common and place the patient at risk for secondary infection. When the process has become chronic, the vulvar skin has an eczematoid appearance with cracks, fissures, and lichenification. Topical ointments, creams and lotions, perfumed soaps and toilet paper,

and poison ivy are common causative factors in prepubertal children, while in adolescents, feminine hygiene products, douches, and perfumed sanitary pads may be responsible.

CHEMICAL IRRITANT VULVOVAGINITIS

Many of the agents capable of causing allergic vulvitis can also act as chemical irritants. Bubble bath, harsh soaps, laundry detergents, water softeners, and perfumed or dyed toilet paper are common offenders. Furthermore, prior to toilet training, children whose diapers are changed infrequently may develop irritation due to ammonia, produced when the organisms in stool split the urea in urine. Itching and dysuria are prominent symptoms, and examination usually discloses mild nonspecific inflammation (Figure 18.29), at times associated with signs of scratching. On occasion, findings are normal. Diagnosis is dependent on history (see Fig. 18.22).

FRICTIONAL TRAUMA

Frictional trauma may be the source of superficial abrasive changes and, when chronic, may result in lichenification or even atrophic skin changes (Fig. 18.30). Wearing tight clothing, certain sporting activities (especially long-distance bicycle riding and long-distance running), sand from sand boxes, and excessive masturbation are the major predisposing factors.

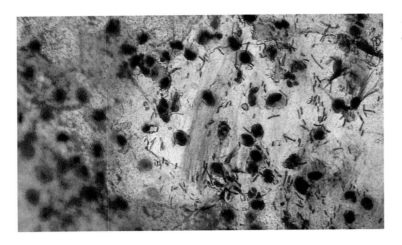

FIG. 18.31 *Sympathetic purulent vaginal discharge. This photomicrograph shows numerous leukocytes and epithelial cells, with mixed flora. The patient presented with vomiting, anorexia, lower abdominal pain and a purulent vaginal discharge, and was found to have a pelvic appendiceal abscess. The vaginal discharge was the result of sympathetic inflammation.*

Although itching and/or mild discomfort are the major symptoms, dysuria may be prominent in acute cases.

SYMPATHETIC INFLAMMATION AND FISTULAS
Appendicitis with Pelvic Appendiceal Abscess

Preschool and young school-age children with appendicitis often do not come to medical attention until after appendiceal rupture has occurred. Females with a pelvic appendix who wall off the rupture in a periappendiceal abscess may develop a copious purulent vaginal discharge due to sympathetic inflammation of the vaginal wall. On microscopy, the discharge contains numerous leukocytes, epithelial cells, and mixed flora (Fig. 18.31). The antecedent clinical course consisting of anorexia, nausea, and vomiting and initial periumbilical abdominal pain later localized to the right lower quadrant suggests the diagnosis. Direct and percussion tenderness on abdominal examination is more marked on the right, and a tender cystic mass often is palpable on rectal examination. The fact that the unestrogenized genital tract of the prepubertal girl does not promote the ascent of sexually transmitted infections eliminates pelvic inflammatory disease from the differential diagnosis.

Fistulas

Patients with *vesicovaginal fistulas* and *ectopic ureters* can present with symptoms of vulvovaginitis. Patients have a history of a constantly wet perineum. Nonspecific inflammation and maceration are the predominant physical findings (see Figure 18.28 and Chapter 14, Urologic Disorders).

Rectovaginal fistulas also can cause vulvovaginal inflammation, but the presence of a grossly feculent vaginal discharge usually makes diagnosis relatively easy. When rectovaginal fistulas are neither congenital nor post-traumatic in origin, or when a perianal fistula is found, inflammatory bowel disease should be considered.

VAGINAL FOREIGN BODY

The hallmark of a vaginal foreign body is the presence of a profuse, foul-smelling, brownish or blood-streaked vaginal discharge. The majority of patients are in the 3 to 8 year age group. While wads of toilet tissue, paper, or cotton are the materials found most often, all types of small objects have been retrieved. There may be a long noninflammatory latency period for inert objects. The objects most commonly found in adolescents are forgotten tampons or retained condoms. Objects made of hard materials often are palpable on rectal examination. Since radiopaque objects generally are palpable,

radiographs are unnecessary. Results of Gram's stain, wet prep, and culture are nonspecific. Vaginoscopy is diagnostic and, when tolerated, it provides access for extraction which is curative, once secondary infections are treated. Vaginal lavage with lukewarm saline also can help in removal of paper from young children, although extraction of other objects often must be done under general anesthesia.

Shigella vaginitis in prepubertal patients and necrotic tumors produce a discharge that is clinically indistinguishable from that of a vaginal foreign body.

When a prepubertal patient is found to have a vaginal foreign body, it is important to obtain a detailed behavioral history of the child in addition to a family psychosocial history, as the problem often is recurrent and may be the result of disturbed behavior by the patient or of chronic sexual abuse.

Infectious Vulvovaginitis

In contrast to most of the primarily noninfectious forms of vulvovaginitis, vaginal discharge is usually a prominent part of the clinical picture of infectious vulvovaginitis in all age groups. While some pathogens produce a fairly characteristic-looking discharge, not all patients present with this classic picture, and the discharge seen with many pathogens often is nonspecific in appearance. Furthermore, in the case of sexually transmitted infections, more than one pathogen may be present. For these reasons, careful attention to smear and culture techniques is important.

There are two major subgroups of vulvovaginal infection. In the first subgroup genital involvement is secondary, being either part of a systemic infection or the result of transfer of the pathogen from another primary site such as the skin, or the respiratory, gastrointestinal, or urinary tracts via contaminated fingers or proximity. Infection at the primary site may precede or coexist with genital infection, and in some cases colonization of another site, without overt infection, appears to predispose. This nonvenereal infectious vulvovaginitis is not uncommon in prepubertal patients, although it is rare in adolescents because the mature female genital tract does not support these types of pathogens.

The second subgroup of infectious vulvovaginitis consists of those infections due to venereal pathogens. Both prepubertal and postmenarchial patients can present with vulvovaginitis when infected with these organisms. After puberty, however, patients can present with other clinical pictures as well, including cervicitis (with or without vulvovaginal inflammation) and salpingitis. Figure 18.32 enumerates the possible clinical

MAJOR CHARACTERISTICS OF THE MOST COMMON SEXUALLY TRANSMITTED DISEASES AND DIAGNOSTIC MEASURES

	Herpes Simplex	HPV	HIV	Trichomonas	Gonorrhea	Chlamydia	Syphilis
Possible clinical findings	Vulvar skin lesions, vulvitis, vaginitis, cervicitis; may be normal	Nonspecific vulvovaginal inflammation, subclinical lesions revealed by acid wash, vulvar, vaginal, and/or cervical condylomata	See Fig. 16.51	Vaginitis, vulvitis, vaginal and/or cervical petechiae	May be normal, cervicitis, salpingitis, vaginitis, vulvitis, occasionally proctitis, pharyngitis, or urethritis	Often normal, cervicitis, salpingitis, occasionally vaginitis and vulvitis; occasionally urethritis	Primary—vulvar, vaginal, or cervical chancre; secondary—condylomata lata involving vulva with or without generalized exanthem
Incubation period	3–14 days	1–3 months (up to 9 months)	Acute flu-like viral illness (several weeks); AIDS (variable—up to 10 years)	3–30 days	2–7 days	7–21 days (?)	Primary (15–90 days); secondary (6 weeks–6 months); tertiary (2–20 years)}
Infectivity	75–80%	60–70%	Varies with infecting behavior	70–90% for male-to-female transmission, less for female-to-male	100% male-to-female; 25% female-to-male	45%(?) male-to-female	10% single encounter; 30% after 1 month of sexual activity
Duration	Primary (2–3 weeks); Secondary (7–12 days)	Variable	Acute infection (2–3 weeks); asymptomatic phase (months); symptomatic (not AIDS) (months–years); AIDS (months–several years) (fatal)	Self-limiting in many males; persistent in most females until treated	Until treated	Until treated	Primary (2–6 weeks); secondary (2–6 weeks) may recur; tertiary persists until treated
Recurrence	60% (HSV - 1); 90% (HSV - 2) (within 1 year)	Variable	Persistence	With reinfection	With reinfection	With reinfection	With reinfection
Routine diagnostic techniques	Rapid diagnostic tests, Tzanck prep, culture, PAP smear	Inspection, PAP smear, acetic acid wash, colposcopy	ELISA, Western blot, viral culture	Wet prep, urinalysis, PAP smear	Cervical culture, oral or rectal culture, Gram's stain	Antigen detection by ELISA–Chlamydiazyme, or direct immuno-fluorescence, tissue culture	Dark-field microscopy, serologic tests including VDRL, RPR, and FTA
Pre- or perinatal transmission	Yes—can cause skin, CNS, and disseminated infection	Yes—can cause laryngeal papillomas	Yes, and postpartum via breast milk	Yes—may have neonatal vaginal discharge or asymptomatic colonization	Yes—can cause conjunctivitis, septicemia, meningitis	Yes—can cause conjunctivitis and/or pneumonia	Yes, and postpartum via breast milk
Partner evaluation	Inspection	Inspection and acetic acid wash	Antibody test	Antimicrobial Rx	Cultures and antimicrobial Rx	Specimen collection and antimicrobial Rx	Serologic and clinical antimicrobial Rx

FIG. 18.32

features seen in adolescent girls with sexually transmitted infections, and summarizes other major epidemiologic characteristics and appropriate diagnostic measures. Regardless of age, the most frequent mode of transmission of venereal infection is sexual contact. The majority of these infections in prepubertal patients are the result of sexual abuse, although in a minority of cases transmission occurs pre- or perinatally as a result of sex play with other children or, rarely, as a result of consensual sexual activity in perimenarchial girls (see Chapter 6). Hence, when venereal disease is found in the prepubertal child, the possibility of sexual abuse must be investigated. In adolescence, consensual sexual activity is the major mode of acquisition of infection by sexually transmitted pathogens, although sexual abuse remains a significant possibility. These factors necessitate obtaining a confidential history of sexual activity and case findings of sexual partners. *It also should be borne in mind that the presence of one venereal pathogen in any child or adolescent should prompt investigation for others, as multiple infections are common* (see section on Genital Infections Due to Sexually Transmitted Pathogens).

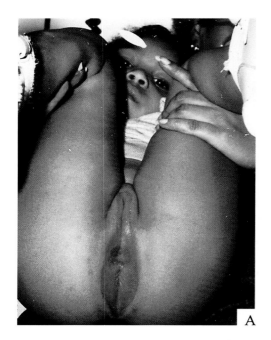

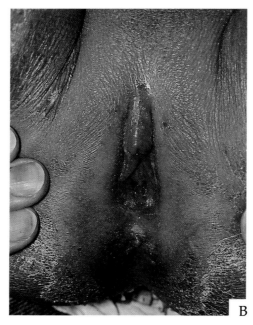

FIG. 18.33 *Streptococcal vulvovaginitis.* **A**, in this child the area of inflammation was sharply circumscribed and extended from the vulva to the perianal area. **B**, in this patient, who presented late in the course of a case of scarlet fever, vulvar inflammation is still evident and desquamation has begun.

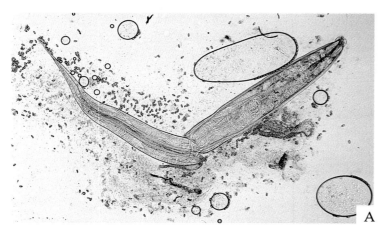

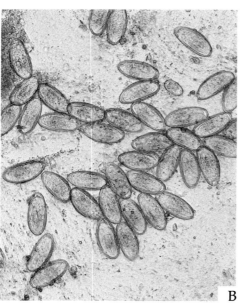

FIG. 18.34 *Pinworms (Enterobius vermicularis). On this wet mount (**A**), a mature worm is shown surrounded by eggs, which are shown more clearly at higher power (**B**). Patients with intestinal infestation may have vulvovaginal symptoms, either as a result of scratching and excoriation or of migration of the worms into the vagina.*

sion. *Streptococcus pneumoniae* and *Haemophilus influenzae* frequently have proven to be the cause of purulent vaginal discharge, with associated vulvitis and vaginitis, either following or concurrent with upper respiratory tract infection. The most dramatic form of bacterial vulvovaginitis due to a primary respiratory (or skin) pathogen is that due to group-A beta-hemolytic streptococcus. This infection may be associated with streptococcal nasopharyngitis or scarlet fever, or it may occur in apparent isolation, although throat culture is often positive for strep even in the absence of pharyngeal or upper respiratory symptoms. The onset of vulvovaginal symptoms is abrupt, with severe perineal burning and dysuria. Inspection reveals intense erysipelas-like erythema of the vulva, distal vagina, and perianal area (Fig. 18.33A). The involved skin weeps serous fluid. Most patients have a serosanguineous or grayish-white vaginal discharge, and about one-third will have vaginal petechiae. Gram's stain may be unrevealing, but culture of perineal skin and/or discharge is positive. Desquamation ensues with recovery (Fig. 18.33B).

Impetigo and folliculitis may occur in the vulvar area of patients of any age and generally is secondary to poor hygiene, excessive sweating, and/or mechanical irritation. Simultaneous involvement of the buttocks or other skin sites is common (see Chapter 12, Infectious Diseases).

Some persons with increased androgens due to congenital adrenal hyperplasia or polycystic ovarian syndrome, children with a familial predisposition to keratosis pilaris, and patients with Down syndrome may be especially prone to developing folliculitis and/or impetigo.

Viral pathogens also have been linked to vulvovaginitis in young children. Varicella is perhaps the most common, with pruritus and dysuria as its most prominent symptoms. Inspection reveals typical lesions involving the perineum and/or vagina (see Chapter 12). Adenovirus has been reported to cause vulvovaginitis with a serous discharge in association with pharyngitis, conjunctivitis, and an exanthem, whereas echovirus has been found to cause a thick, clear vaginal discharge concurrently with gastroenteritis.

VULVOVAGINITIS DUE TO NONSEXUALLY TRANSMITTED PATHOGENS

Vulvovaginitis Due to Respiratory and/or Skin Pathogens
Bacterial respiratory pathogens can cause vulvovaginitis in prepubertal patients, presumably as a result of orodigital transmis-

Vulvovaginitis Due to Gastrointestinal Pathogens
Shigella. In recent years a distinct form of vulvovaginitis due

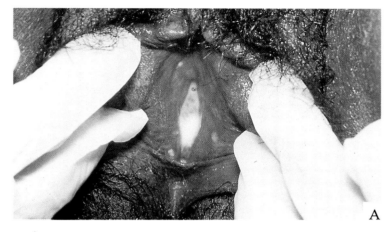

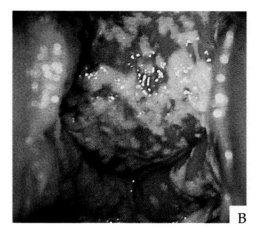

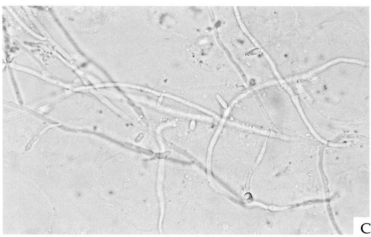

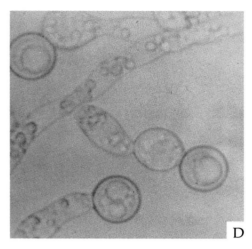

FIG. 18.35 Candida vulvovaginitis and cervicitis. **A**, the vulva is intensely hyperemic and a thick cheesy white discharge covers the urethra, entroitus, and hymenal area. **B**, whitish plaques may be seen on the perineum and vaginal mucosa, and occasionally on the cervix in adolescents. A whitish cheesy or creamy vaginal discharge may be noted as well. **C** and **D**, these low- and high-power wet mount specimens contain pseudohyphae and budding yeast. (**A**, courtesy of Dr. B. Cohen, **B** and **D**, courtesy of Dr. Ellen Wald, Children's Hospital of Pittsburgh)

to *Shigella* species has been identified in premenarchial patients. The majority of patients have no overt gastrointestinal symptoms, although approximately one-third of cases have had associated diarrhea. It is thought that the neutral or alkaline pH of the vaginal mucosa in young children may predispose to infection with this organism.

The predominant complaint is chronic vaginal discharge, although some have dysuria. Most patients have been otherwise asymptomatic. A greenish-brown, often blood-streaked, purulent, and foul-smelling vaginal discharge is seen on inspection, along with vulvar and vaginal erythema. The clinical appearance of the discharge is indistinguishable from that seen with a vaginal foreign body. Gram's stain reveals polymorphonuclear leukocytes and a predominance of gram-negative rods. Culture is diagnostic. Without treatment it may persist for months.

Pinworms. Intestinal infestation with pinworms (*Enterobius vermicularis*) is primarily associated with perianal pruritus. However, the worms may crawl forward into the vagina bringing enteric flora with them and depositing eggs. Vaginal infection and discharge may result. Even without this, scratching may produce excoriation and secondary dysuria. In such patients (usually young children) a history of preceding perianal pruritus can generally be elicited. Inflammatory changes are nonspecific. Pinworm ova and/or adult worms may be found on wet mount of vaginal secretions (Fig. 18.34). In the occasional patient with associated vaginal discharge, culture is positive for enteric pathogens. When pinworm infestation is suspected despite negative vaginal smears, the perianal Scotch® tape test should be performed by the mother during the night for the highest yield.

Vulvovaginitis Secondary to Urinary Tract Infection
On occasion, a primary urinary tract infection may produce secondary vulvovaginal inflammation and masquerade as primary vulvovaginitis. The postulated mechanism is repetitive vulvar and vaginal contamination with infected urine and, in fact, passage of part of the urinary stream into the vagina has been demonstrated during voiding cystourethrography. Vulvar itching and burning, and dysuria are major complaints.

When cystitis is the primary infection, frequency, urgency, and hesitancy typically are associated. In primary pyelonephritis these symptoms are often absent, but fever, gastrointestinal symptoms, flank pain, and/or costovertebral angle tenderness may be found. Perineal inspection discloses nonspecific inflammation or maceration, usually without discharge (see Figs. 18.28 and 18.29). Urine and vaginal cultures are positive for the same pathogen.

Candida Vulvovaginitis
Candida species are one of the more common sources of nonvenereal infectious vulvovaginitis after puberty. It is rare in the healthy prepubertal child. Predisposing factors include recent antibiotic intake, poor perineal ventilation, diabetes mellitus, immunodeficiency, pregnancy, and the use of oral contraceptives. Pruritus and contact dysuria are the most prominent symptoms. Examination usually discloses diffuse intense erythema of the vulva associated with a thick cheesy discharge (Fig. 18.35A). Excoriations from scratching also may be noted. Satellite lesions on the perineum are common, and on occasion whitish plaques may be seen on external genital structures. In many cases, signs of perianal dermatitis and intertrigo are found in association with vulvovaginal involvement.

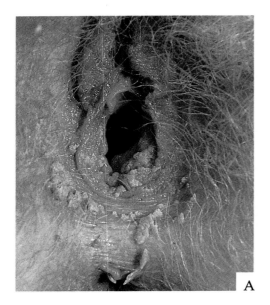

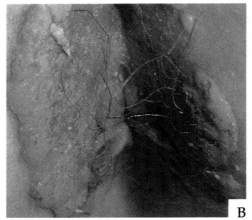

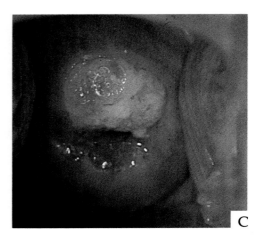

FIG. 18.36 Condylomata acuminata. These sexually transmitted viral warts (**A**) tend to be discrete early on, but (**B**) with evolution become confluent. **C**, adolescents have a significant risk of developing vaginal and cervical lesions. (**A** and **C**, courtesy of Dr. E. Jerome, **B**, courtesy of Dr. M. Sherlock)

Inspection of the lower third of the vagina in young patients and speculum examination in adolescents may reveal a thick white discharge of creamy or cheesy consistency: whitish plaques may adhere to the vaginal mucosa or to the cervix in adolescents (Fig. 18.35B). A KOH or wet prep will confirm the presence of budding yeast and pseudohyphae, and possibly an increase in inflammatory cells (Figs. 18.35C,D).

Topical application of antifungal cream with instillation into the lower vagina is the treatment of choice. In sexually active adolescents, careful consideration must be given to the possibility of pregnancy before prescribing antimicrobials or any other medication. In patients with recurrences, predisposing factors, such as medications, should be considered. An infected male partner with subacute or chronic monilial balanitis may be the source of recurrences in sexually active patients, although this infection is not generally transmitted sexually.

GENITAL INFECTIONS DUE TO SEXUALLY TRANSMITTED PATHOGENS

The number of pathogens recognized as being transmitted by intimate sexual contact has mushroomed in the past two decades (see Fig. 18.23). The "sexual revolution" and the consequent rise in prevalence of venereal disease and neonatal infections have stimulated extensive research, leading to the recognition of an increasing array of pathogens and to a better understanding of their pathophysiology and the clinical pictures they produce (see Fig. 18.32). It also has made the evaluation of patients with STDs considerably more complex. The majority of infections are manifested by external lesions and/or vulvovaginal inflammation with vaginal discharge. However, while some infections produce relatively specific clinical findings, many are characterized by nonspecific signs and symptoms that appear to represent a final common pathway of a number of different etiologic agents of irritation, infection, or infestation. Several pathogens can induce two or three different clinical pictures (or a mixed picture) in adolescents. Furthermore, the high frequency of multiple simultaneous infections adds to the complexity, and necessitates more extensive laboratory evaluation. The clinical approach to these patients must not only be sensitive and individualized, but also must differ considerably depending on whether or not the patient is premenarchial or postmenarchial.

Approach to Sexually Transmitted Infections in Prepubertal Patients

Prior to menarche, lack of estrogenization inhibits ascent of infection and subclinical infection is probably unusual if not rare. Hence, manifestations of venereal infection are confined to the vulva and lower vagina. As a result, external inspection of the perineum and lower vagina and laboratory evaluation of samples of vaginal discharge are sufficient for identification of pathogens and for institution of therapy. This does not complete the assessment, however, for whenever venereal disease is identified in a prepubertal patient, *sexual abuse must be considered as the probable source.* This necessitates obtaining an extensive psychosocial history and initiating a thorough investigation to find the person responsible for transmitting the infection to the child (see Chapter 6).

Approach to STD in Pubertal Patients

Presenting complaints of vulvovaginitis in pubertal patients include vulvar lesions, vaginal discharge, odor, pruritus or perineal discomfort, and dysuria; but these symptoms also may be associated with pelvic pain, dyspareunia, fever, and irregular bleeding. This is not the only clinical picture seen, however. A number of pathogens involve only the lower genital tract (e.g., they do not produce salpingitis), but, in contrast to the picture seen in younger patients, they may produce more extensive vaginal inflammation and may involve the cervix as well. Herpes simplex, *Trichomonas vaginalis* and human papilloma viruses are prime examples. Infection with *Neisseria gonorrhoeae* or *Chlamydia trachomatis* may be both asymptomatic and inapparent on examination, or may result in cervicitis, which usually is characterized by cervical inflammation and friability, with a mucopurulent discharge (see Fig. 18.41B). Cervicitis, too, may be largely silent clinically, or it may be accompanied by vulvovaginitis with vaginal discharge or, with ascent of infection to the upper tract, may be associated with salpingitis (see Figs. 18.24 and 18.32).

Hence, a complete pelvic examination is necessary when evaluating adolescents for vulvovaginal complaints and for the possibility of STD. Following inspection of the perineum, the vaginal mucosa and the cervix must be visualized and their appearance assessed for signs of erythema, friability, focal lesions, and mucopurulent discharge. To differentiate a true cervical discharge from normal pooled vaginal secretions adhering to the cervix, visible discharge should be removed gently with cotton swabs before inspection. Cervical secretions should be sampled (for wet prep and cultures) by insertion of a swab into the os. The finding of cervicitis with a mucopurulent cervical discharge suggests gonorrhea or chlamydial infection or both, and necessitates an attempt either to identify or to rule out upper tract involvement via bimanual examination. Cervical motion and uterine tenderness and/or a tender, palpable adnexal mass with or without systemic signs and symptoms, suggests this possibility (see section on Pelvic Inflammatory Disease).

A number of additional considerations are important in evaluating postpubertal patients suspected of having an STD. A sexual history, obtained in confidence, is essential, and while consensual activity is common in adolescence, it must be remembered that these patients may be victims of sexual abuse including incest, sexual harassment, and date rape. Sexual partners should be evaluated and treated whenever an STD is identified; otherwise reinfection is probable.

It is also important to recognize that adolescent girls with asymptomatic cervical infections may serve as silent reservoirs of venereal pathogens. This phenomenon is quite significant in the epidemiology of STDs. Hence, female partners of men known to have gonorrhea or nongonococcal urethritis should be cultured and treated appropriately. The patient and partner must be advised to abstain from sexual intercourse until the course of treatment is completed. They also should be seen in followup for test of cure, and once cured should be seen at least every 6 months for STD surveillance because of the significant incidence of recurrent (and often subclinical) infection.

The importance of aggressive case finding, diagnosis, and treatment cannot be overemphasized because of the potential, not only for spread to others, but also for major sequelae that include ectopic pregnancy and infertility as a result of smoldering or recurrent acute upper tract disease. Finally, it is the physician's responsibility to provide education regarding STDs. Patients should understand how the disease was contracted and how to prevent recurrence. Good hygiene and use of condoms and spermicides should be encouraged. Education should include discussion of responsible sexuality, including use of contraceptives and safer sex practices, as appropriate to the patient.

Surface Infestations and Perineal Lesions

Parasitic infestations. Two parasitic infestations, scabies and pubic lice, may be transmitted via sexual contact and may present with symptoms of vulvar and inguinal pruritus and irritation. Sexual transmission is more likely in adolescents than in young children, who may acquire the parasites by close nonsexual contact. Development of pubic hair is necessary for acquisition of pubic lice. Meticulous inspection of the pubic area for nits and adult lice ("crabs") may be necessary to discover early infestations. The clinical findings of both disorders are presented in Chapter 8.

Human Papilloma Virus. The human papilloma virus (HPV) has emerged as the most prevalent sexually transmitted pathogen found in adolescent females. Genital or venereal warts, also called condylomata acuminata are no longer an isolated nuisance, being but one manifestation of a spectrum of lower genital tract diseases caused by HPV. The virus recently has been implicated in a critical role in the development of cervical intraepithelial neoplasia (CIN) or dysplasia, and is believed to be a cofactor or precursor of invasive carcinoma of the cervix and, similarly, carcinoma of other genital tissues in both males and females.

Transmission is usually via sexual contact in adolescents, although it is thought that close family contact may be responsible for some cases in young children. Passage to neonates during delivery also has been documented and can result in subsequent development of laryngeal papillomata. Vaginal involvement is uncommon in the prepubertal child but, when present, it is often accompanied by a vaginal discharge.

Condylomata may emerge following subclinical, acute, or chronic nonspecific vulvovaginal inflammation incited by the virus in both pre- and postpubertal females. In most cases, the lesions are asymptomatic, although pruritis is reported by some patients. However, when the warts are traumatized or become secondarily infected, pain may be a complaint. In rare cases, rapid growth is followed by necrosis, and the patient presents with a weeping mass of warts and foul-smelling discharge, which necessitates histologic examination to rule out malignancy.

Generally, the warts appear as fleshy, rounded or ragged papules, often located at the posterior edge of the introitus and/or in the perianal region. Lesions may be discrete early on (Fig. 18.36A), but with evolution they tend to become confluent (Fig. 18.36B). The warts can also be flat, or even subclinical. While most lesions involve the perineum and perianal areas, vaginal and cervical involvement also are common in adolescents (Fig. 18.36C). Hence, when vulvar condylomata are found in postmenarchial patients, inspection of the vagina and cervix should be undertaken and a cervical Pap smear obtained. The virus also can infect other mucous membranes including the anus, urethra, mouth, larynx and conjunctiva.

Clinical diagnosis is made by careful inspection of external genitalia, vagina, and cervix (in adolescents), and perianal areas for visible warts. Examination of genital tissue after washing or soaking with 5 percent acetic acid (household vinegar) for up to 5 minutes reveals subclinical lesions, although this may cause mild but usually well-tolerated discomfort in some patients. Acetic acid causes proliferating and immature epithelium to turn white because of disordered orientation of intracellular fibers. Most normal tissues retain a pink color. Other causes of aceto-white changes include injury, contact dermatitis, candidiasis, folliculitis, allergic excoriation.

HPV infection is identified cytologically on the Pap smear by characteristic changes, including koilocytosis which is pathognomonic for HPV infection. DNA hybridization has identified more than 60 subtypes of the virus, many of which are site- and pattern-specific in their disease expression. Viral Paps and DNA probes are used for identification of subtypes, but the clinical utility of these tests is not yet known. Patients with cervical lesions merit gynecologic referral for colposcopy and definitive treatment because of the potential of these lesions to undergo malignant transformation. A rapid increase in warty tissue may be associated with pregnancy or HIV infection.

Molluscum contagiosum. These sharply circumscribed, waxy papular umbilicated lesions caused by a pox virus can be spread as a result of sexual contact, in which case lesions will be found predominantly on the labia, mons pubis, buttocks, and lower abdomen. This mode of spread is much more likely in the adolescent than in the young child. The clinical characteristics of molluscum lesions are presented in Chapter 8.

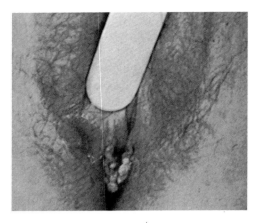

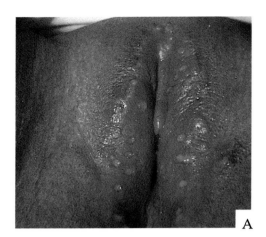

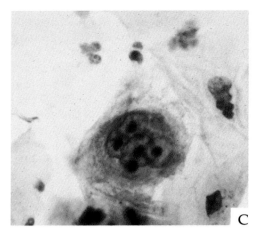

FIG. 18.37 Primary syphilis. This luetic chancre was painless and indurated on palpation. The base is smooth and the margins are rolled. This patient also has condylomata acuminata. (Courtesy of Dr. Ellen Wald, Children's Hospital of Pittsburgh)

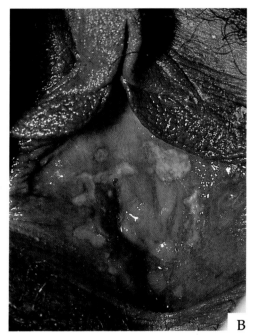

FIG. 18.38 Herpes simplex. **A**, this prepubertal child presented with intense dysuria and perineal pain and had numerous thick-walled vesicular lesions over her perineum. **B**, the ulcerative phase of herpetic vulvitis is seen in this adolescent patient, who also must be checked for possible vaginal and cervical involvement. **C**, Wright-Giemsa stain of scrapings from the base of an herpetic ulcer demonstrates a typical multinucleated giant cell, with viral inclusions. (**C**, courtesy of Dr. Ellen Wald, Children's Hospital of Pittsburgh)

Syphilitic chancre. Primary syphilis should be considered in any patient presenting with a genital ulcer. The typical syphilitic chancre is painless and indurated, with rolled margins and a smooth base (Fig. 18.37). However, atypical lesions are common and thus, all suspicious ulcers should prompt investigation by darkfield examination of scrapings and by reagin serologic tests (VDRL or RPR). The latter test may be negative early in the disease course and therefore, should be repeated at 1- and 3-month intervals if syphilis is strongly suspected. Positive reagin tests should always be confirmed by a fluorescent treponemal antibody (FTA) test.

Bartholin's gland abscess. This problem presents as a unilateral red, hot, tender mass at the posterior margin of the introitus at the base of a labia majorum (see Fig. 18.41A). It is generally seen in adolescents with gonorrhea, but it can occur in younger patients infected with the gonococcus, and it is increasingly associated with Chlamydia. When such a mass is encountered, material expressed from the abscess should be cultured, because other agents such as streptococci and vaginal anaerobes also have been documented as pathogens. A full evaluation for STDs, including cervical swabs, may be necessary for organism identification. Treatment is based on Gram's stain and culture results. Occasionally, incision and drainage are required.

Lower Tract Disease

A number of sexually transmitted infections that are manifest as vulvovaginitis in the prepubertal patient produce findings limited to the lower genital tract (e.g., vaginitis and cervicitis) in the adolescent. A discussion of these infections follows. Their upper tract manifestations will be discussed later in the section on Pelvic Inflammatory Disease.

Genital herpes. Herpes simplex type 2 and less commonly type 1 have been confirmed as genital pathogens in both pubertal and prepubertal girls. In adolescents, genital infection is acquired almost exclusively by sexual or intimate contact with infected mucosal surfaces. In prepubertal children, vulvar involvement can also result from sexual contact, but more often results from spread from another infected site, such as the lip, mouth, or an herpetic whitlow. It has also been acquired from parents with herpes labialis who fail to wash their hands properly before changing diapers. Most infections are symptomatic but, occasionally, individuals have no symptoms. An antibody response, with or without symptoms, can be produced within a few days.

Patients with primary infection frequently have systemic symptoms of fever, malaise, and myalgia, in addition to severe perineal pain and dysuria. Tender inguinal adenopathy usually is prominent but may not develop for several

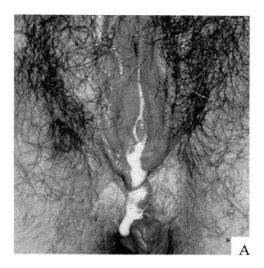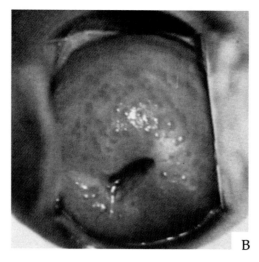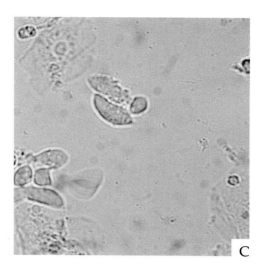

FIG. 18.39 Trichomonas. *A*, T. vaginalis *produces a profuse acrid-smelling watery discharge that usually is visible on perineal inspection. In some cases it is homogeneous, while in others it is bubbly. Vulvar pruritus often is intense.* **B**, *the vaginal mucosa is inflamed and often speckled with petechial lesions. In adolescents petechial* hemorrhages may also be found on the cervix, resulting in the so-called "strawberry cervix." **C**, microscopic examination of a wet mount reveals multiple motile trichomonads. A sperm is seen in the upper portion of the picture. (**A** and **B**, courtesy of Dr. Ellen Wald, Children's Hospital of Pittsburgh)

days. Perineal inspection reveals single or clustered vesicular lesions and/or ulcers on erythematous and edematous bases (Fig. 18.38A). Acute ulcerations are typically covered by yellow exudate and may be quite extensive (Fig. 18.38B). A copious, foul-smelling, watery, yellow vaginal discharge may be seen as well. Associated sterile pyuria may be a feature. Dysuria may be so severe as to cause acute urinary retention. The ulcerative phase gradually resolves as the lesions heal within a period of 14 to 28 days. Following primary infection, a persistent subclinical infection is established in the lumbosacral ganglia.

Diagnosis can usually be made on the basis of clinical appearance, but is confirmed by finding multinucleated giant cells on cytologic smears obtained by scraping the base of a lesion, smearing the specimen on a glass slide, and staining it with Wright-Giemsa stain (Fig. 18.38C). Viral culture of a fresh, and, ideally, vesicular lesion also is confirmatory. Rapid diagnostic tests that provide results within hours are now available.

Recurrences are common and generally are milder, of shorter duration, and only locally symptomatic. Possible triggers of recurrence include fever, menstruation, emotional stress, and friction. Occasionally, prodromal tingling, pain, burning, or hyperesthesia is noticed in the area where vesicles ultimately recur. The interval between episodes varies widely.

Postmenarchial patients with vulvar herpetic lesions require speculum examination to look for the presence of herpes cervicitis, which is characterized by ulceration, friability, and a serosanguineous discharge. Occasionally, herpetic ulcers are found on the vaginal mucosa as well. Patients with cervical involvement should be referred for followup pelvic examination and periodic Pap smears because of the association between herpetic infection and development of cervical dysplasia. Additionally, because of the risk of transmitting the virus to the newborn during vaginal delivery, pregnant young women with a history of genital herpes should have serial cultures during the last trimester. If evidence of active infection is present, elective cesarean section is recommended.

Trichomonas. T. *vaginalis* is a flagellated protozoan. It has been found in the vaginal discharge of newborns delivered of mothers infected at the time of delivery, but thereafter it tends to be an unusual finding until the peripubertal period. This is thought to be due to the unfavorable alkaline environment of the unestrogenized vaginal mucosa. Beyond the neonatal period it is acquired almost exclusively by sexual contact, often in concert with other sexually transmitted pathogens. Although infection is occasionally asymptomatic in adolescents, the majority of patients have vulvar pruritus, burning, and dysuria, in association with a profuse vaginal discharge. The latter may be watery, yellow-gray, or green. In some cases it is bubbly; in others it is homogeneous. The discharge frequently has a foul acrid odor. Affected adolescents may complain of pelvic pain or heaviness.

On inspection the vulva may be hyperemic and occasionally edematous, but the degree of inflammation is highly variable. Because the discharge is profuse, it tends to be present on the perineum (Fig. 18.39A). It pools in dependent portions of the vagina and coats the vaginal walls. The vaginal mucosa is erythematous, and punctate petechial lesions may be noted. In the adolescent these hemorrhagic areas may involve the cervical mucosa, producing the so-called "strawberry cervix" (Fig. 18.39B). This organism does not ascend to infect the upper genital tract.

Diagnosis is made by finding mobile trichomonads on microscopic examination of a saline wet mount (Fig. 18.39C). On close observation, whiplike flagellar movements are noted. Leukocytes are usually seen in increased numbers and may surround the organisms, making detection more difficult. Dilution of a densely cellular discharge may make it easier to see the organisms moving. The slide must be examined soon after preparation, as drying makes it uninterpretable. A positive whiff test (release of amine odor on addition of 10 percent KOH to a drop of discharge) is also common. Trichomonads may also be found in urine specimens.

Metronidazole has been shown to be effective for treatment, but should be avoided in pregnant patients because of its ter-

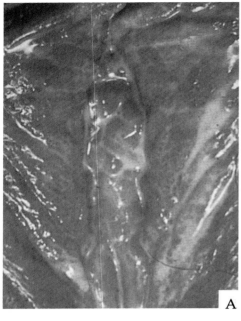
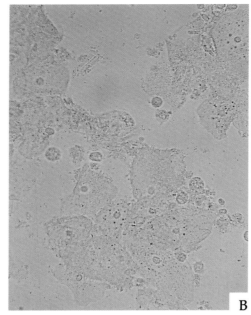

FIG. 18.40 *Gardnerella vaginalis.* This surface pathogen is thought to act in concert with vaginal anaerobes to produce this form of vulvovaginitis. *A,* the major symptom is one of a malodorous homogeneous vaginal discharge. *B,* characteristic "clue cells" are seen on wet mount and consist of vaginal epithelial cells covered with adherent refractile bacteria. Since the organism is noninvasive, leukocytes are not increased. (*A,* courtesy of Dr. Ellen Wald, Children's Hospital of Pittsburgh)

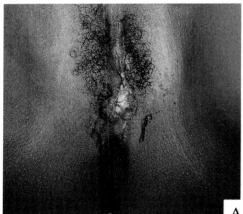
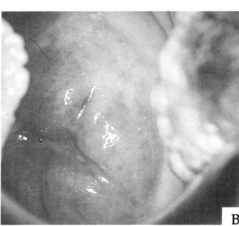
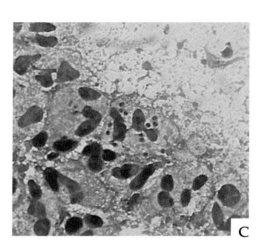

FIG. 18.41 Gonorrhea. *A,* vulvar inflammation, edema, and a purulent vaginal discharge are seen in this peripubertal child who was a victim of sexual abuse. She also has a unilateral Bartholin's gland abscess. *B,* adolescents are vulnerable to ascent of infection and usually have findings of cervical inflammation with mucopurulent discharge. *C,* on Gram's stain the vaginal discharge from the patient in *A* is found to contain sheets of leukocytes, many of which contain gramnegative intracellular diplococci. This test is highly reliable for prepubertal patients, but adolescents have a significant incidence of false negatives. (*B,* courtesy of Dr. L. Vontver)

atogenic potential. Sexual partners usually are asymptomatic but, occasionally, have symptoms of urethritis. They should be treated whether or not they have symptoms.

Gardnerella vaginalis. Recent studies have confirmed *Gardnerella vaginalis* as a pathogen and as a significant source of vulvovaginitis both before and after menarche. *Gardnerella* is a gram-negative facultative anaerobe which was previously known as both *Corynebacterium vaginale* and *Haemophilus vaginalis.* It is now thought that the organism acts in concert with vaginal anaerobes to produce the clinical syndrome, and that many cases of vaginitis previously thought to be nonspecific are caused by *Gardnerella.* The major presenting symptom in all groups is a vaginal discharge with a noticeable odor. Some prepubertal patients have vulvar inflammation and discomfort, but adolescents may have little in the way of vulvovaginal irritation, and the cervix and upper tract are spared. It is as yet unclear whether *Gardnerella* in prepubertal patients is acquired primarily through sexual contact or by other means.

On inspection, discharge is frequently present on the perineum (Fig. 18.40A) and may be seen adhering to the vaginal walls, which do not appear to be inflamed. Generally the discharge is thin and homogeneous in consistency, grayish-white in color, and malodorous. In adolescents, the vaginal pH is elevated to 4.5 or above. Addition of 10 percent KOH to a sample of the discharge produces a noticeable amine odor (positive "whiff test"). A saline wet prep usually reveals characteristic "clue cells," vaginal epithelial cells covered with adherent refractile bacteria (Fig. 18.40B). On Gram's stain the cells appear studded with gram-negative or gram-variable rods. When clue cells are present, a routine vaginal culture is unnecessary for diagnosis. If clue cells are absent but clinical suspicion of *Gardnerella* is high, a culture is recommended. Because *G. vaginalis* is a surface pathogen and thus is rarely associated with evidence of tissue invasion, leukocytes should not be seen in increased numbers. If they are, additional pathogens should be sought and are often found. In cases of recurrent infection, patients as well as their sexual partners should

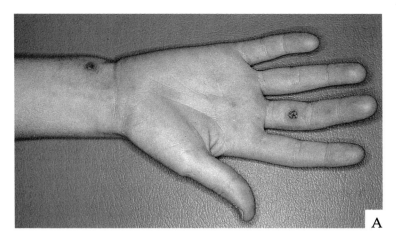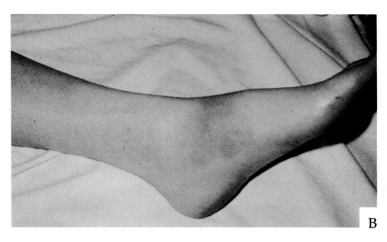

FIG. 18.42 Disseminated gonococcal infection. **A**, these pustular skin lesions with erythematous halos are characteristic of disseminated gonorrhea, which may occur at any age. **B**, tenosynovitis and monoarticular arthritis are commonly seen in association with skin lesions in disseminated disease. (**A**, courtesy of Dr. Ellen Wald, Children's Hospital of Pittsburgh)

receive 1 week of therapy with metronidazole.

Gonorrhea. The gonococcus is no longer the most frequently identified venereal pathogen in either prepubertal or postmenarchial patients, because of increasing incidence and detection of other agents, particularly *Chlamydia* and HPV. However, the incidence of gonorrhea in the population dropped only slightly in the 1980s. The major complaint is vaginal discharge. Prior to menarche the child may be otherwise asymptomatic, but most experience some degree of vulvar discomfort, pruritus, or dysuria. Symptomatic adolescents without upper tract extension can have a similar picture, but are more likely to have lower abdominal pain. Inspection reveals inflammation and sometimes edema of the vulva and a profuse purulent discharge that usually is greenish yellow, but also can be creamy, yellow, green, or white (Fig. 18.41A). Inspection of the vaginal mucosa in younger children reveals the lower portion to be inflamed. In adolescents, the vaginal mucosa can appear normal, but the cervix usually is erythematous and friable, with purulent material seen draining through the os (Fig. 18.41B). Patients in this age group also may have evidence of urethritis manifested by erythema, edema, and tenderness of the urethra. When the latter findings are present, purulent material can be expressed by pressing along the length of the urethra through the anterior vaginal wall. A sample of this material should be sent for culture.

Laboratory studies are essential for accurate diagnosis. In prepubertal patients a Gram's-stained smear of the vaginal discharge will be reliably positive for large numbers of leukocytes and gram-negative intracellular diplococci and is adequate for initiation of treatment (Fig. 18.41C). Culture is important to detect the few cases with false negative Gram's stain, to determine antimicrobial sensitivity, and for medicolegal confirmation. Since simultaneous throat and anal cultures commonly are positive (despite the absence of anorectal or pharyngeal symptoms), these sites should also be cultured when gonorrhea is suspected or confirmed. They may, in fact, be positive when the vaginal culture is negative. Both tonsils and the posterior pharyngeal wall should be swabbed in obtaining the throat specimen, and the rectal swab should be inserted no more than 1 to 2 cm past the anal orifice to avoid

fecal contamination. Culture swabs should be placed immediately on appropriate transport medium or plated promptly on Thayer-Martin culture plates to maximize the chance for positive results.

In adolescents with symptomatic gonorrhea, Gram's stain of the mucopurulent cervical discharge will reveal a predominance of leukocytes that may contain gram-negative intracellular diplococci. When results are positive, this is specific and treatment may be instituted. The incidence of false negative Gram's stains is significant, however. False positives also may be encountered in asymptomatic women colonized by *Neisseria* species. Cultures are thus essential. Recent studies of women with culture-proven gonococcal cervicitis have shown concurrent chlamydial infection in up to two-thirds of these patients. Thus, when purulent cervicitis is found, specific specimens for detection of *Chlamydia* should also be obtained and treatment for both pathogens begun.

On occasion, patients with gonorrhea may develop *disseminated gonococcal infection* via hematogenous spread. This phenomenon may occur at any age. It is more common in adolescent girls with asymptomatic (and therefore, untreated) endocervical infection, in males with asymptomatic urethral infection, and in patients of both sexes and all ages with silent anal or pharyngeal infections. Yet it also can be seen in patients with symptomatic vulvovaginitis, cervicitis, or urethritis. In postmenarchial females, symptoms are more likely to develop during a menstrual period or during pregnancy.

The clinical picture often has two stages. Initially fever and chills are prominent, and the patient is intermittently bacteremic. During this stage, which lasts 2 to 5 days, polyarthralgias are experienced (involving knees, wrists, ankles, elbows, and hands), and characteristic skin lesions often appear. The latter begin as small erythematous papules or petechiae that usually evolve to form pustules surrounded by red halos (Fig. 18.42A). Later, these may necrose centrally. Lesions often contain gram-negative diplococci, but usually are culture-negative. If not diagnosed and treated promptly, patients progress to a second phase, characterized by monoarticular arthritis with effusion, or tenosynovitis (Fig. 18.42B). In up to 50 percent of these cases, culture of joint aspirates will be positive. Specialized techniques to isolate cell-wall-deficient organisms further increase culture yield. Myocarditis, pericarditis, endocarditis, and meningitis also may yield from hematogenous seeding.

Chlamydia trachomatis. Chlamydia has replaced gonorrhea as the most common sexually transmitted pathogen causing cervicitis and upper genital tract disease. Its high prevalence (up to 25 percent) in adolescent populations and its serious sequelae make its proper diagnosis and treatment an important aspect of adolescent sexual health care. When compared with gonococcal infection, its transmission rate for a single episode of intercourse is lower, but its prevalence and persistence are higher, being greatest in sexually active 15- to 21-year-old persons. Forty-five percent of female partners of males infected with *Chlamydia* are infected as well.

Chlamydia are unique microorganisms. They are obligate intracellular parasites which cannot be cultivated on artificial media, and which depend on their cellular hosts for high energy ATP and other nutrients. Identification has become more accessible with ELISA (Chlamydiazyme), tissue culture, and monoclonal antibody techniques, but it is still a relatively expensive laboratory procedure. Specimens must be appropriately collected and transported. *Chlamydia* cultures are the gold standard, and must be used for prepubertal evidentiary and rectal specimens. For all collections, cell scrapings are necessary rather than secretions or discharge because of the intracellular nature of the organism. Swabs or cytologic brushes are acceptable for specimen collection. External mucus and debris should be removed first. A Dacron® swab with a plastic shaft should be used for culture, as cotton swabs may interfere with recovery of the organism from tissue culture. Calcium alginate-tipped swabs may produce false positive Chlamydiazyme results when specimens are not processed shortly after collection. Serologic tests are not useful, except for confirmation of lymphogranuloma venereum caused by specific immunotypes. Tests of cure are not reliable for several weeks after treatment and are not recommended by the Centers for Disease Control (CDC). Because of the high cost of all detection methods, diagnostic procedures are often eliminated and treatment is begun empirically. Reinfection is common.

Prepubertal females tend to have vulvovaginitis with vaginal discharge which may be thin or serous, white or yellowish-brown. It may be intermittent or persistent and usually is associated with vulvular pruritis. Co-infection with *N. gonorrhoeae* is common and many of the first *Chlamydia* infections discovered in premenarchial girls were the result of culture of discharge which persisted after appropriate therapy for gonorrhea.

Adolescent females present with symptoms of both cervical and urethral infection. Pelvic or abdominal pain, spotting or irregular vaginal bleeding, or vaginal discharge may accompany infection. A picture indistinguishable from that of symptomatic gonorrhea, with purulent vaginal discharge, perineal irritation, and findings of cervicitis with mucopurulent discharge also can be seen (see Fig. 18.41B). Endometritis is common with cervicitis, even in the absence of classic symptoms of pelvic inflammatory disease, and Bartholin's duct infections are not uncommon. Asymptomatic *Chlamydia* infection in both females and males is common, if not usual.

On examination of the cervix, the presence of yellow-green mucopus, cervical ectopy, and erythema are all associated with *Chlamydia* infection. Often the cervix is friable, bleeding during the minimal manipulation necessary to obtain specimens. When seen as an isolated infection, on Gram's stain the cervical discharge is found to contain increased numbers of leukocytes without intracellular organisms. Microscopic evidence of other infections (e.g., *Gardnerella, Trichomonas*) does not decrease the likelihood of *Chlamydia* co-infection and should not deter the practitioner from treating for *Chlamydia* if suggested otherwise by the history or physical findings. Patients commonly have simultaneous infection with the gonococcus and *Chlamydia*—hence the rationale for culturing for both organisms and covering for both with treatment, when purulent cervicitis is found on examination.

Chlamydia can produce acute urethral syndrome in postpubertal patients as well. Dysuria, urgency, and frequency may or may not be accompanied by physical signs of urethral discharge, meatal redness, and swelling. Pyuria may exist in the absence of bacteriuria. Urethral specimens for *Chlamydia* must be collected by inserting a thin Dacron® swab 2 cm into the urethra and rotating it 360° before withdrawal. Rectal infection exists in both heterosexual and homosexual populations. Pharyngeal infection is rarely detected. A careful sexual history may reveal possible extragenital sites of infection, but treatment at other sites is not known to differ, as it may with extragenital gonorrhea.

Genital Mycoplasmas

Mycoplasma hominis, M. genitalium and *Ureaplasma urealyticum* are the three species of mycoplasma implicated in genital infections of females and males. The organisms may be cultured from vaginal specimens of neonates and sexually active women in the absence of disease, but colonization in the prepubertal girl is rare. Mycoplasmas also have been cultured from polymicrobial upper genital tract infections, but it remains unclear whether they are initiators of ascending infections, or whether they behave as normal bacterial flora accompanying the primary ascending infection of gonorrhea or *Chlamydia*, becoming pathogenic once relocated in the fallopian tubes. Mycoplasmas have been found causative in some cases of acute urethral syndrome.

The currently widespread practice of broad spectrum antimicrobial treatment of STDs to include *Chlamydia*, and the general unavailability of laboratory confirmation of mycoplasma involvement in infection have made it difficult to further understand the role of this bacterium. This broad spectrum therapy, however, has provided treatment for problems that might have persisted due to an inability to establish a precise diagnosis. While routine cultures for mycoplasma are not justified, they should be considered for infections resistant to documented therapy in the absence of reinfection by an untreated partner.

Human immune deficiency virus (HIV). Acquired immune deficiency syndrome (AIDS) and other manifestations of HIV infection are discussed in Chapter 4, Allergy and Immunology. The adolescent history outlined previously (see Fig. 18.8) should identify teenagers at risk of acquiring HIV infection. In an attempt to reduce subsequent transmission and treat infection early, confidential HIV testing is to be encouraged for teens at risk of exposure to the virus. The definition of moderate to high risk has been regularly changing as an understanding of the disease, its epidemiology, and treatment opportunities evolve. Reliable sources of such information (e.g., the CDC) should be regularly consulted.

From the gynecologic perspective, a number of infections may present differently in the HIV individual. These include infections with *Candida*, human papilloma viruses, herpes simplex, and molluscum contagiosum. In such cases the disease may be unusually severe, may present atypically, or may be resistant to treatment.

Pelvic Inflammatory Disease

An important complication of lower genital tract infection in the postmenarchial female is pelvic inflammatory disease (PID). PID results from ascending spread of a cervical infection that may or may not have been symptomatic. Though classically attributed to gonorrhea, PID is being increasingly recognized as a polymicrobial infection. Initiating pathogens implicated include *N. gonorrhoeae, C. trachomatis,* and *M. hominis.* A number of other organisms which are considered normal vaginal or enteric flora are potentially pathogenic given the right circumstances. Among these are *Bacteroides* species, other anaerobic gram-positive bacilli and cocci, and aerobes including streptococcal species, *E. coli, Klebsiella,* and *Proteus* species (see Fig. 18.26). The majority of cases of salpingitis may be due to mixed anaerobic and aerobic infection, although the classically recognized venereal pathogens may play the important initiating role.

Risk factors for developing upper tract infection include adolescence, multiple sexual partners, use of an IUD, and previous PID. Because menstruation facilitates ascent of pathogenic organisms from the cervix to the uterus and fallopian tubes, the time of onset of symptoms is often during or shortly after a menstrual period. Long-term morbidity includes an increased incidence of ectopic pregnancy, decreased fertility, and chronic pelvic pain. These sequelae are secondary to tubal occlusion and scarring of pelvic structures. It is estimated that for every episode of PID there is an additional 15 percent chance of subsequent fertility problems.

The "textbook" picture of acute PID is that of a sexually active female who abruptly develops a high fever and shaking chills in association with intense lower abdominal pain. Nausea and vomiting are common. The patient appears acutely ill and uncomfortable, and may have pain on walking with an antalgic gait. On abdominal examination there is prominent lower abdominal tenderness and guarding with rebound. Cervical visualization discloses signs of cervicitis with mucopurulent discharge. Bimanual palpation elicits extreme pain on cervical motion and reveals marked tenderness of the fundus and adnexa. Adnexal enlargement, if present, suggests abscess formation. The sedimentation rate is markedly elevated, and there is a pronounced leukocytosis with a left shift on CBC and differential.

This picture is seen most often in the first episode of PID and has the highest likelihood of being associated with positive cultures for *N. gonorrhoeae.* Yet even with this "classic" picture (which constitutes a relatively small percentage of cases), errors in diagnosis are not uncommon and gynecologic consultation should be strongly considered when PID is suspected.

More commonly, the onset of symptoms is insidious and the clinical picture more subtle. This is particularly likely with nongonococcal PID. Fever may be absent or low grade; the abdomen and pelvis may be only mildly tender; and blood work is often normal. In such cases diagnosis can be particularly difficult, requiring considerable suspicion and a readiness for obtaining cultures on the part of the clinician. Lower abdominal or pelvic pain, cervical motion tenderness, and some evidence of lower genital tract inflammation usually are present. However, some cases of chronic PID may not fit even this milder picture. A low-grade tubal infection may produce more in the way of adnexal findings and few, if any, uterine signs.

Diagnosis is complicated by the fact that there is a wide range in severity of the clinical picture and by a lack of clear diagnostic guidelines for PID, especially mild infection.

Furthermore, acute salpingitis may mimic a number of other disorders, including ectopic or intrauterine pregnancy; appendicitis or appendiceal abscess, in cases with right-lower-quadrant abdominal pain and tenderness; torsion or hemorrhage of an ovarian cyst; septic abortion; endometriosis; pyelonephritis; cholecystitis; and pelvic tumors, inflammatory and irritable bowel disease, and severe dysmenorrhea.

The adolescent with right-lower-quadrant abdominal pain can be particularly challenging diagnostically. Figure 18.43 summarizes clinical findings which may aid in distinguishing among the many potential causes. Figure 18.44 illustrates some of the ultrasound findings in disorders that may cause pelvic or right-lower-quadrant abdominal pain.

Because of the potentially devastating long-term sequelae of PID, aggressive and largely empiric antimicrobial therapy is warranted. Treatment should include antibiotics which cover the common organisms in accordance with current CDC recommendations. Polymicrobial coverage is prescribed from the time of diagnosis even if presumptive at that time. **Patients suspected of having an abscess, patients in whom the diagnosis is uncertain, and those patients with manifestations of toxicity, pregnant, or unable to comply with outpatient treatment should be admitted for parenteral treatment.** Many physicians admit all adolescents with PID. If treated as an outpatient, it is mandatory that the patient with PID be reexamined within 24 to 48 hours to document improvement. If no such improvement occurs, she should be admitted and treated parenterally. In addition to antibiotic resistance, failure to improve promptly on therapy raises the possibility of complications such as abscess formation, the development of a tubo-ovarian complex, or of a missed diagnosis of ectopic pregnancy, miscarriage or appendicitis. Additional procedures such as culdocentesis or laparoscopy may be helpful, along with serial reexamination in questionable cases. Sonography also is of use in evaluating masses and suspected tubo-ovarian complexes.

Perihepatitis (Fitz-Hugh-Curtis syndrome). One of the more acute complications of PID, seen in 5 to 20 percent of cases, presents as right-upper-quadrant pain caused by perihepatitis. The infection probably ascends from the fallopian tubes along the paracolic gutters to the right upper quadrant, resulting in inflammation of the liver capsule and adjacent peritoneum.

The clinical picture is one of sudden onset of severe pleuritic right-upper-quadrant pain which may be referred to the right shoulder, and which is associated with chills, fever, nausea, and vomiting. Although in the majority of cases the pain develops simultaneously with pelvic symptoms of PID, it may present in the course of an asymptomatic ascending lower tract infection before genital tract signs emerge, or later in the course of a partially treated infection. Upper abdominal pain may be so severe that the patient remains unconcerned about lower abdominal and pelvic complaints.

Right-upper-quadrant tenderness and guarding are the major physical findings; peritoneal signs may be present. Gynecologic examination in most instances will disclose findings of purulent cervicitis and PID. *N. gonorrhoeae* and *C. trachomatis* are the major pathogens associated with this syndrome. When nongonococcal in origin, the predisposing salpingitis may be silent.

The sedimentation rate is elevated, but there are only minimal abnormalities of liver function tests. Although usually not necessary, ultrasound examination of the right upper quadrant

PERTINENT CLINICAL CHARACTERISTICS OF DISORDERS CAUSING RIGHT-SIDED ABDOMINAL PAIN IN ADOLESCENT FEMALES

	PID	Ovarian Torsion	Ovarian Cyst	Ectopic Pregnancy
Location and quality of pain	Mid and lateral pelvic, usually bilateral; can be vague, dull, crampy or sharp	Unilateral RLQ or LLQ (R:L, 3:2); colicky	RLQ or LLQ, colicky, but usually asymptomatic	Lateral pain; colicky; +/− uterine cramping
Onset	GC—immediately post-menstrual and rapid; *Chlamydia*—gradual over days to months	Sudden	Gradual	Gradual with sudden exacerbation
History	Unprotected sexual intercourse; previous PID or STDs; multiple partners	+/− history of similar pain with resolution; increased ovarian size, anatomic variation may predispose	Midcycle or luteal phase; physiologic rupture causes Mittelschmerz of 24–48 hours' duration	Amenorrhea (75%); +/− pregnancy signs and symptoms
GI symptoms (vomiting/ diarrhea)	Nausea; vomiting; anorexia; not necessarily present	Vomiting with onset of pain (25%)	Rare	GI symptoms secondary to pregnancy or severe secondary to rupture and peritonitis
Masses	Occasional; if present, consider tubo-ovarian complex or ectopic pregnancy	Usually present; increased size secondary to edema	Often palpable if not physiologic cyst	Adnexal mass palpable in 50% of cases
Physical exam and lab findings	Cervical motion and adnexal tenderness; clinical and lab evidence of cervicitis; vaginal bleeding; +/− discharge; +/− RUQ pain; perihepatitis; + cervical cultures for gonorrhea or *Chlamydia*	Tender adnexa; +/− guarding or peritonitis	Unilateral cystic adnexal mass; x-ray rules out dermoid	Normal uterus; unilateral or bilateral adnexal tenderness; + pregnancy test in most, but inadequate; beta HCG doubling; drop in Hct. with rupture
Ultrasound findings	Usually normal; tubo-ovarian complex in minority	Usually solid ovarian mass	Cyst > 3 cm; +/− fluid in cul-de-sac—frequent incidental finding on U/S	Tubal mass; vaginal probe may enhance detection

FIG. 18.43

should demonstrate a normal liver, bile duct, and gallbladder. Laparoscopic findings of purulent and fibrinous peritonitis of the capsule and hemorrhagic areas of adjacent parietal peritoneum are diagnostic, but laparoscopy is rarely indicated for this condition.

Major differential diagnostic considerations include viral and drug-induced hepatitis; hepatitis secondary to bacteremia; pneumonia, pleuritis and pleurodynia; subphrenic abscess, and acute cholecystitis. Perforated gastric or duodenal ulcers and pancreatitis may cause right-upper-quadrant pain but are more likely to cause burning epigastric pain or boring epigastric pain, respectively.

PREGNANCY

The pregnancy rate for adolescents in the U.S. is approximately 110/1,000 for 15- to 19-year-old females per year. It remains one of the highest among industrialized countries. While the birth rate of 15- to 19-year-olds has declined slightly since 1974, the rate of pregnancies among younger adolescents (below age 15) has increased.

Sexual activity among teenagers has dramatically increased since the early 1970s, with a greater percentage of young women of all ages reporting having had sexual intercourse. A larger number of unplanned teenage pregnancies occur in the

	Inflammatory Bowel Disease	Appendicitis	Irritable bowel/ Constipation	Dysmenorrhea	IUP
Location and quality of pain	LLQ, crampy	Periumbilical cramping changing to RLQ cramping, burning or sharp pain	LLQ; crampy or colicky	Suprapubic; mid-abdominal; lower back; dull cramping	Midline fullness
Onset	Gradual; weeks to months with exacerbations	Gradual over hours to days	Long history of GI problems; months to years	Periodic, evolving over hours	Gradual over weeks or months
History	Weight loss or growth failure, rashes, arthritis, fever	Usually no prior pain	Constipation, diarrhea distension common; + family Hx; increases with stress	If unusual pattern of severity, consider congenital abnormalities or obstruction, threatened abortion or ectopic pregnancy	Amenorrhea, pregnancy signs and symptoms
GI symptoms (vomiting/ diarrhea)	Increased stool frequency, nocturnal stools, sometimes bloody diarrhea	Vomiting may follow onset of pain; anorexia	Long intermittent history of alternating diarrhea and constipation	Diarrhea, flatulence or vomiting not uncommon	Nausea with vomiting, worse in morning
Masses	Unusual, except with chronic complicated disease	Rare	Feces	None	Midline pelvic; abdominal mass palpable above
Physical exam and lab findings	Recto-abdominal tenderness; hematologic abnormalities; stool heme +	↑WBCs, fever, evolving peritoneal signs	Occasional tender colon, usually normal	Normal	+Serum pregnancy test 8-10 days after conception; + urine test 10-14 days
Ultrasound findings	Normal	Appendix frequently visible	Normal	Normal	Gestational sac after 6-8 weeks

6 months following first intercourse, and the average delay in seeking contraceptive counseling is almost 1 year after initiating sexual activity. Some of the same factors that delay the education and medical counseling needed to effectively prevent pregnancy also influence the delay in diagnosis of pregnancy and subsequent medical care.

Given the frequency of teenage pregnancy, the practitioner who cares for sexually active adolescents should have some familiarity with the diagnosis of pregnancy.

In the first trimester, patients often experience fatigue, mood swings and food cravings. Increased facial oil gland activity and chloasma (darkening of facial pigmentation) may be noted. At about 5 weeks gestation, breast tenderness and swelling and darkening and increased sensitivity of the nipples develop. Nausea and vomiting, especially in the morning, tend to begin at about 6 weeks gestation. If a pregnant adolescent is examined between the sixth and eighth weeks, **Hegar's sign** (softening of the lower corpus), **Chadwick's sign** (bluish discoloration of the cervix), and **Goodell's sign** (softening of the cervix) may be noted. Ultrasonography can detect the fetus after the sixth week of pregnancy.

In the second and third trimesters, breast enlargement increases as do abdominal girth and weight. Normal vaginal discharge increases as well. On examination, congestion of the

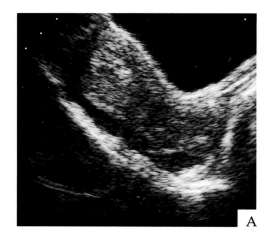
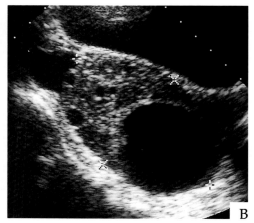

FIG. 18.44 Ultrasound findings in the diagnosis of pelvic or abdominal pain. *A*, this image shows an abnormal amount of fluid in the cul-de-sac released from a ruptured ovarian cyst in a 15-year-old with left lower quadrant and midline pelvic pain. *B*, in a 12-year-old female with a 4-day history of colicky right lower quadrant pain, ultrasound demonstrates a single large abnormal cyst and multiple small physiologic cysts. Operative diagnosis was right ovarian torsion. The ovary was not salvageable and was removed.

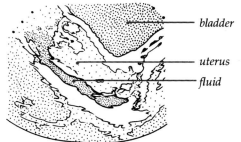
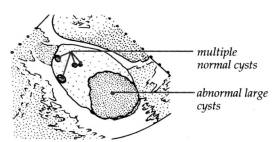

vaginal mucosa is seen. The uterus is palpable as a midline mass, with its dome at the pelvic brim at about 12 weeks; midway between the pelvic brim and the umbilicus at 16 weeks; and at the level of the umbilicus at 20 weeks. Fetal heart tones become detectable with Doppler between 12 and 14 weeks, and fetal movements are perceptible between 16 and 20 weeks gestation.

Current laboratory pregnancy tests give us the opportunity to diagnose pregnancy earlier and with greater reliability. Serum radioimmune assay is positive 24 to 48 hours after implantation (about 7 days after conception). A first-morning specimen of concentrated urine with a specific gravity greater than 1.020 will give a positive result on a sensitive urine ELISA assay for an intrauterine pregnancy 8 to 10 days following conception.

Home pregnancy tests are variable in their sensitivity—some may not give a positive result on a first-morning specimen until 14 to 21 days post-conception. Despite improvements, false positive and false negative results still are encountered. Causes of false negative findings include testing too early (see above) or too late (after 16–20 weeks), dilute urine (specific gravity <1.020), adulterated urine, ectopic pregnancy or an impending or missed abortion. False positive pregnancy tests can occur in adolescents with hydatidiform moles or malignancies, following abortion or during a mid-cycle LH surge.

It must be noted that pregnancies are dated from the last normal menstrual period and not from conception, which occurs 2 weeks later. This may confuse patients, parents, and boyfriends, and should be clarified to minimize confusion, to facilitate decision making, and to clarify paternity.

BIBLIOGRAPHY

Altchek A: Vulvovaginitis, vulvar skin disease and pelvic inflammatory disease. *Pediatr Clin North Am* 1981;28:397–432.

Amsel R, Totten PA, et al: Nonspecific vaginitis. *Am J Med* 1983;74:14–22.

Bacon JL: Pediatric vulvovaginitis. *Adolesc Pediatr Gynecol* 1989;2:86–93.

Barr RG: Abdominal pain in the female adolescent. *Pediatr Rev* 1983;4(9)281-289.

Braverman PK, Strasburger WB: Why adolescent gynecology? *Pediatr Clin North Am* 1989;36:471–487.

Buck HW, et al: *Genital human papilloma virus (HPV) disease. Diagnosis, management and prevention.*Rockville, MD American College Health Association, 1989.

Centers for Disease Control: 1989 sexually transmitted diseases treatment guidelines. *MMWR* 1989;38:1-43.

Corey L: Diagnosis and treatment of genital herpes. *JAMA* 1982;248:1041–1049.

Cowell CA: The gynecologic examination of infants, children, and young adolescents. *Pediatr Clin North Am* 1981;28:247–266.

Cowell CA (ed): *Pediatric and Adolescent Gynecology.* Philadelphia, WB Saunders, 1981.

Davis AJ, O'Boyle EA, Reindollar RH: Human chorionic gonadotropin in pediatric and adolescent gynecology. *Adolesc Pediatr Gynecol* 1989;2:207–215.

Dewhurst J: Genital tract obstruction. *Pediatr Clin North Am* 1981;28:331–344.

Droegemueller W, Herbst AL, Mishell DR, Stenchever MA: *Comprehensive Gynecology.* St. Louis, CV Mosby, 1987.

Edmonds DK: *Dewhurst's Practical Paediatric and Adolescent*

Gynaecology, ed 2. London, Butterworths, 1989.

Emans SJ: Vulvovaginitis in the child and adolescent (abstr.) Pediatr Rev 1986;8:(1):12-19.

Emans SJ, Goldstein DP: Pediatric and Adolescent Gynecology, ed 3. Boston, Little, Brown, 1990.

Eschenback DA: Vaginal infection. Clin Obstet Gynecol 1983;26:186–202.

Gidwani GP: Endometriosis: more common than you think. Contemp Pediatr 1989;6:99–110.

Greydanus DE, Shearin RB: Adolescent Sexuality and Gynecology. Philadelphia, Lea & Febiger, 1990.

Hammerschlag MR, Rosner I, Alpert S, et al: Microbiology of the vagina in children: normal and potentially pathogenic organisms. Pediatrics 1978;62:57–62.

Hatcher RA, Quest F, Stewart F, et al: Contraceptive Technology, ed 14. New York, Irvington, 1988.

Heller RH, Joseph JM, Davis HJ: Vulvovaginitis in the premenarchial child. J Pediatr 1969;74:370–377.

Holmes KK, Mardh P, Sparling PF, Wiesner PJ: Sexually Transmitted Diseases, ed 2. New York, McGraw-Hill, 1990.

Holmes KK, Stamm WE: Chlamydial genital infections: a growing problem. Hosp Pract 1979;Oct:105–117.

Huffman JW: The Gynecology of Childhood and Adolescence, ed 2. Philadelphia, WB Saunders, 1981.

Jay SM, Bridges CE, Gottlieb AA, DuRant RH: Adolescent contraception. Adolesc Pediatr Gynecol 1988;1:83–95.

Jacobson L, Westron L: Objectivized diagnosis of acute pelvic inflammatory disease. Am J Obstet Gynecol 1980;138:905–1008.

Kaufman RH, Friedrich EG, Gardner HL: Benign Diseases of the Vulva and Vagina. Chicago, Year Book, 1989.

McAnarney ER, Hendee WR: Adolescent pregnancy and its consequences. JAMA 1989;262:74–77.

McAnarney ER, Hendee WR: The prevention of adolescent pregnancy and childbearing. JAMA 1989;262:78–82.

Nuovo GJ, Richard RM: Human papilloma virus: a review, in Mishell DR, Kirschbaum TH, Morrow CP (eds): The Year Book of Obstetrics and Gynecology. Chicago, Year Book, 1989.

Paradise JE, Campos JM, Friedman HM, Frishmuth G: Vulvovaginitis in premenarchial girls: Clinical features and diagnostic evaluation. Pediatrics 1982;70:193–198.

Peter G, Hall CB, Lepow ML, Phillips CF: Report of the Committee on Infectious Diseases. Elk Grove Village, IL, American Academy of Pediatrics, 1988.

Pheifer TA, Forsyth PS, Durfee MA et al: Nonspecific vaginitis role of H. vaginalis and treatment with Metronidazole. N Engl J Med 1978;298:1429–1434.

Shafer MA, Irwin CE, Sweet RL: Acute salpingitis in the adolescent female. J Pediatr 1982;100:339–350.

Shulman LP, Elias S: Developmental abnormalities of the female reproductive tract: pathogenesis and nosology. Adolesc Pediatr Gynecol 1988;1:230–238.

Speroff L, Glass RH, Kase NG: Clinical Gynecologic Endocrinology and Infertility, ed 4. Baltimore, Williams & Wilkins, 1989.

Stamm WE, Guinan ME, Johnson C, et al: Effect of treatment regimens for Neisseria gonorrhoeae on simultaneous infection with Chlamydia trachomatis. N Engl J Med 1984;310:545–549.

Strasburger VC (ed): Adolescent gynecology. Pediatr Clin North Am 1989;36(3).

Treatment of Sexually Transmitted Diseases. Med Lett 1990;32(810):5–9.

Wright VC, Lickrish GM: Basic and Advanced Colposcopy: a Practical Handbook for Diagnosis and Treatment. Houston, Biomedical Communications, 1989.

Zuckerman B, Weitzman M, Alpert J (eds): Children at risk: Current social and medical challenges. Pediatr Clin North Am 1988; 35(6).

19

PEDIATRIC OPHTHALMOLOGY

Kenneth P. Cheng, M.D. ◆ Albert W. Biglan, M.D. ◆ David A. Hiles, M.D.

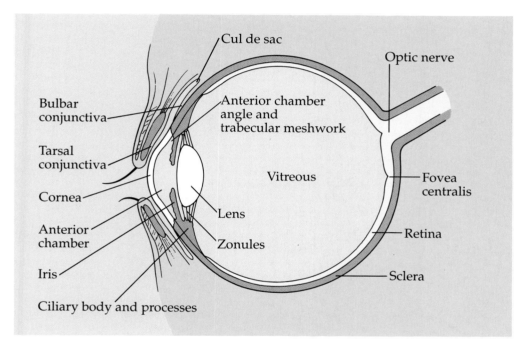

FIG. 19.1 Globe and surrounding structures.

FIG. 19.2 Normal fundus. Posterior pole of fundus with normal optic disc and retinal vasculature. The macula is visualized as an area of increased pigmentation surrounded by retinal vessels. The fovea centralis or center of the macula is maintaining fixation on the end of a vertical fixation target.

Over the past three decades pediatric ophthalmology has become established as a distinct sub-specialty of ophthalmology.

Common problems encountered include refractive errors, strabismus, amblyopia, and infections or trauma that involve the eye and/or its surrounding tissues. Other problems encountered include ocular complications of systemic disease, developmental and genetic conditions and neoplasms affecting the globe and orbits.

ANATOMY OF THE VISUAL SYSTEM

The visual system is conveniently separated into three principal parts: the globe and surrounding structures (Fig. 19.1), the visual pathways, and the visual or calcarine cortex.

The eyelids provide protection for the globe and assist in even distribution of the tear film over the cornea to provide a clear, undistorted optical system for focusing light. The crystalline lens complements the cornea's refracting power with its ability to adjust the focal length of the optical system so that incoming light from objects at any distance may be clearly imaged on the retina. During the first 2 to 3 months of life, children develop the ability to focus images at any range. Light is focused on the macula, the portion of the retina responsible for the central field of vision (Fig. 19.2). The retina contains the sensory receptors; the rods and cones. The fovea centralis is the center of the macula and it has the greatest concentration of cones and, therefore, has the greatest potential for visual acuity.

Light falling on the fovea and peripheral retina is converted into nerve impulses by the rods and cones. Nerve fibers emanate from the ganglion cell layer of the retina, coalesce to form the optic nerve and synapse in the lateral geniculate body. Fibers from the temporal retina travel without crossing

FIG. 19.3 Visual field.

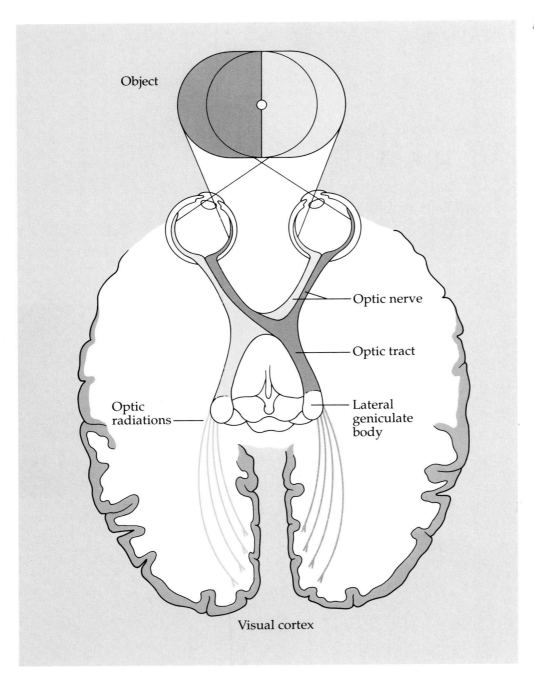

Object

Optic nerve

Optic tract

Lateral geniculate body

Optic radiations

Visual cortex

at the chiasm to the ipsilateral visual cortex (Fig.19.3). Nerve fibers from the nasal retina will decussate at the chiasm and are directed toward the contralateral visual cortex. This decussation of nerve fibers causes portions of each retina to image a different part of the visual field. For example, if an object is seen off to the person's left, the image is received by the nasal retina of the left eye and the temporal retina of the right eye. Similarly, if the object is off to the person's right, the image will fall on the nasal retina of the right eye and the temporal retina of the left eye. The temporal retina images objects in the contralateral visual field and the nasal retina images objects in the ipsilateral visual field. Because of the decussation of nasal retinal fibers, the right visual cortex will therefore receive images from the left visual field and the left visual cortex will receive images from the right visual field.

Lesions of the visual pathways will produce predictable patterns of visual field loss; for example, a left homonymous hemianopsia is produced by a lesion of the right occipital cortex. Visual field defects which respect or do not extend across the vertical midline suggest pathology involving the intracranial portion of the visual system.

The visual field can be arbitrarily divided into the central field of vision and the peripheral field. The macula is responsible for the central field. A physiologic blind spot is found about 10 to 15 degrees temporal to central fixation (the fovea) and represents the area of the field that corresponds to the optic nerve head (optic disc). Precise measurement of the visual field of each eye can be obtained in a cooperative child or adult using a Goldmann visual field perimeter. This test requires steady fixation and concentration for roughly 30 minutes. In young children, it is impractical to attempt this tedious measurement. Young patient's visual fields are assessed by observation of the child's eyes fixating on small targets brought into the peripheral field of vision in each quadrant of the visual field. Visual fields may be also assessed using a confrontation method where the child fixates on the examiner's nose and is asked to count the examiner's fingers as they are presented in each quadrant of the visual field.

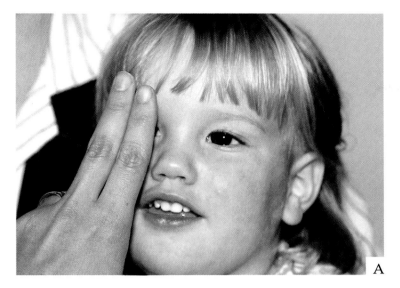

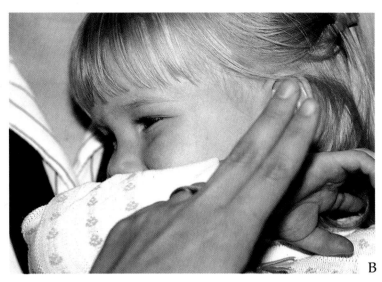

A

B

FIG. 19.4 Test for central fixation. **A,** alert infant seated on mother's lap with one eye covered. Infant is content to fix and follow with normal eye. **B,** cover (in this case, fingers) is then transferred to normal

eye, occluding that eye. The infant now becomes disturbed, pushes hand away, and moves head to see.

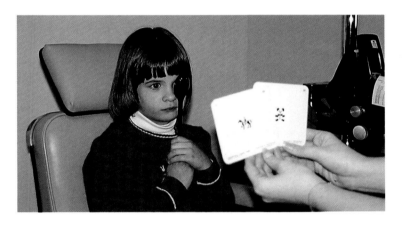

FIG. 19.5 Visual acuity testing with the Allen object recognition cards. Recognition of each figure at a distance of 20 feet is equivalent to a visual acuity of 20/30. The visual acuity is quantitated as the number of feet at which each figure may be recognized over 30 (e.g., 5/30, 15/30, 20/30).

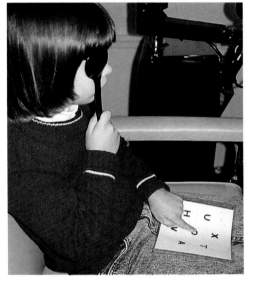

FIG. 19.6 The Sheridan-Gardiner visual acuity test presents letters of decreasing size to a child who matches the figure presented to one on a card held on his or her lap. This test provides an accurate assessment of visual acuity for children who have not yet mastered reading the alphabet.

EVALUATION OF VISION

The most valuable test for assessment of visual function is measurement of visual acuity. Selection of a test to measure it will depend on the patient's age and level of development.

The evaluation of vision in a young infant utilizes the fixation reflex. This reflex develops during the first month or two of life. A 3-month-old infant may be expected to steadily fixate and begin to follow a face, toy, or penlight. By age 5 to 6 months, a child should be able to follow a fixation target into all fields of gaze. The level of vision can be estimated by the quality and intensity of the fixation response. If the visual acuity is normal, central fixation will be steady and maintained (CSM) on objects. If visual acuity is profoundly decreased, the quality of fixation may be eccentric or wandering in nature (ECC) (Fig. 19.4). Central, steady, maintained fixation (CSM) equates to visual acuity of 20/200 or better. Eccentric fixation usually means that the visual acuity is decreased to the 20/800 range.

The Allen object recognition cards, cards with simple pictures of common objects, are a useful method for assessing

visual acuity in a 2½- to 3½-year old child who is not able to comprehend the E game or recognize Snellen letters. To perform this test, one eye is occluded and picture cards are individually presented at increasing distances until the patient recognizes the cards at 20 feet, or he or she fails to recognize cards that are presented (Fig. 19.5). The visual acuity is quantitated as the number of feet at which a picture equal to 20/30 visual acuity can be recognized (e.g., 5/30, 15/30, 20/30). This is a measurement of recognition visual acuity. Although use of isolated targets is not ideal for detection of amblyopia, comparison of vision between the eyes will detect most cases of amblyopia and other defects in visual acuity.

The Sheridan-Gardiner or HOTV visual acuity tests are easy to administer tests which more accurately measure visual acuity. In the HOTV test the letters H,O,T, and V are individually presented on cards and the child matches the letter with a corresponding letter on a card that is held on the lap (Fig. 19.6).

Another commonly used test to measure the visual acuity in 3½-year-olds, is the "E game." The letter "E" in decreasing size is presented to the child rotated in an up, down, right, or left

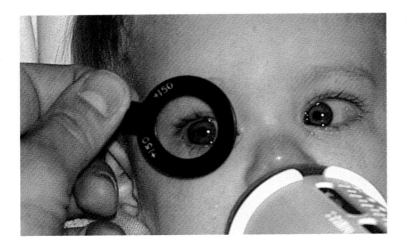

FIG. 19.7 *The examiner is viewing light emanating from the retina through the retinoscope. A lens is held in front of the patient's eye to neutralize refractive errors.*

orientation and the child indicates the direction of the crossbars of the E by pointing.

The "gold standard" for measurement of visual acuity is the presentation of a full line of Snellen letters. This presentation is best achieved with a wall chart or by projection of the letters onto a standardized reflective surface. Because dim illumination increases measured visual acuity in eyes that have amblyopia, testing should be performed in a well-illuminated, glare-free room.

Normal values for visual acuity will depend on the patient's age and the visual acuity test used. A child at 6 months of age should have a visual acuity of 20/60 to 20/100. A child who is 3 years old can be expected to have an acuity in the range of 20/25 or 20/30 using the "E game" or a recognition target test. With further maturation, a 5 to 7-year-old child will have visual acuity of 20/20 to 20/25 as tested with a full line presentation of Snellen letters. All children over age 8 should be able to achieve 20/20 corrected visual acuity. Those who cannot should be referred for evaluation to explain the reason for the defective vision.

The visual pathways coalesce in the visual cortex. Electrical impulses in the visual cortex produced by light stimulation of the retina can be measured by placement of sensitive electrodes on the overlying scalp. This is termed the visually evoked response (VER). The pattern visual evoked potential (PVEP) is generated with a CRT monitor that produces an alternating checkerboard stimulus which can be controlled to produce a pattern of checks that may be increased or decreased in size. This test can be used to estimate visual acuity. Caution must be used in interpreting this test, however, since children and adults with known 20/20 vision can suppress the visually evoked response. Additionally, children who have significant decreases in their visual acuity may give a VER response that overestimates the visual acuity.

It is recommended that visual screening be conducted as part of well-child care at regularly scheduled intervals in the pediatrician's or family practitioner's office. In infancy, the response of each eye to a fixation target should be recorded. Beginning at age three, quantitation of the visual acuity using either Allen cards, the "E" game, or an HOTV chart should be completed. Later, a Snellen visual acuity test should be performed by the office staff or physician and the results should be routinely recorded as part of the patient's medical record. If the physician has special concerns, referral to an ophthalmologist for examination may be appropriate.

Once children enter school, some state laws require that visual acuity be measured at 1- to 2-year intervals. Children who fail these exams (VA <20/40 in either eye) are referred to eye care specialists for further evaluation.

REFRACTIVE ERRORS

Subnormal visual acuity may be the result of an error in the refractive power of the eye. This may be due to variation in the curvature of the cornea or lens or variation in the axial length of the eye. If visual acuity is improved by looking through a pinhole held in front of an eye a refractive error is the cause for the decrease in visual acuity. The pinhole eliminates the off-central rays of light that require refraction. Squinting serves the same purpose and will partially compensate for refractive errors. Those patients who do not have an improvement in visual acuity with a pinhole usually have ocular pathology.

Determination of the refractive state of the eye is part of a comprehensive ophthalmic evaluation. In children, refraction is aided by the use of drugs that temporarily inhibit accommodation and cause pupillary dilatation. Thirty minutes after such cycloplegic-mydriatic agents as cyclopentolate or tropicamide are instilled, accommodation is paralyzed and the pupil is dilated. A retinoscope is used to project a beam of light into the eye to illuminate the retina. The light is then reflected back through the pupil. The quality and character of the reflected light is neutralized by placement of appropriate lenses in front of the eye and the refractive error is accurately and objectively measured (Fig. 19.7).

Low levels of hypermetropia (farsightedness) in the range of +1.50 to +2.00 diopters are normal during childhood and are easily compensated for by the focusing mechanism of the lens, accommodation. The amount of hypermetropia normally increases until age 6 years and then decreases. Under normal circumstances, emmetropia, or no refractive error, is achieved.

REFRACTIVE ERRORS

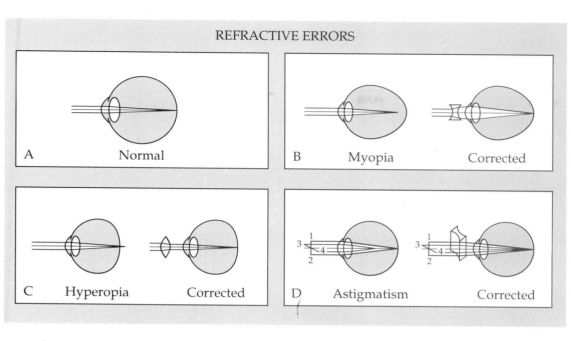

A   Normal

B   Myopia   Corrected

C   Hyperopia   Corrected

D   Astigmatism   Corrected

FIG. 19.8 In the normal or emmetropic eye light from a distant object is focused on the retina. In a myopic eye it is focused in front of the retina, in a hyperopic eye it is focused behind the retina, and in an astigmatic eye light in different meridians is brought to focus either in front of or behind the retina.

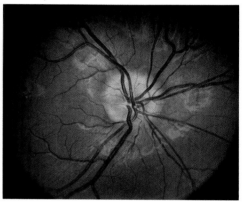

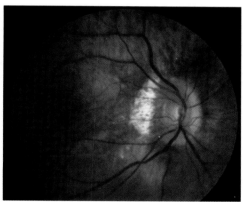

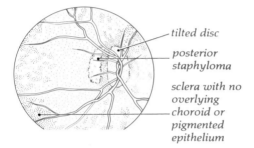

tilted disc

posterior staphyloma

sclera with no overlying choroid or pigmented epithelium

FIG. 19.9 Funduscopic view of a pseudopap-illedema in a hypermetropic child. Vessels are normal-sized; hemorrhages, exudates, and edema are absent.

FIG. 19.10 Opthalmoscopic view of a myopic eye. Thinning of retinal pigment epithelium, a tessellated fundus appearance, macular cracks in Bruch's membrane (Fuch's spot), temporal crescents, and posterior staphyloma are evident.

If excessive axial growth of the eye occurs, myopia (nearsightedness) develops. A patient's refractive error is for the most part genetically predetermined. The effect that environment has on refractive error remains unclear (Fig. 19.8A–D).

The optical image formed by a hypermetropic eye is in focus behind the retina. By changing the shape of the lens with accommodation, the image can be brought into focus on the retina. If a large amount of hypermetropia is present (+4.00 diopters or more), fatigue, headaches, asthenopia, and blurring of vision, especially at near, may occur. Hypermetropia greater than +5.00 or +6.00 diopters may cause ametropic amblyopia. When this occurs, glasses are prescribed to correct the child's refractive error and stimulate the development of normal vision. If large hypermetropic refractive errors are not treated by the age of 6 to 8 years, the resultant amblyopia may be irreversible. The optic discs in eyes with large degrees of hyperopia may have an appearance simulating papilledema (Fig. 19.9).

Myopia (nearsightedness) is frequently due to an increase in axial length of the eye in reference to the optical power of the eye. Children are who myopic can see near objects clear-ly; objects at distance are blurred and cannot be brought into focus. High degrees of myopia ranging from –8.00 to –20.00 diopters may be associated with systemic conditions such as Stickler syndrome, a condition associated with increased axial length of the eye. Myopia is inherited as a multifactorial trait.

Lengthening of the globe may be associated with retinal thinning, peripapillary pigment crescents, staphylomas (a focal area of bulging of the posterior globe wall), and decreased macular function with poor visual acuity. The optic nerve may appear to enter the eye at an angle (Fig. 19.10).

Myopia or nearsightedness may be present at birth but usually develops with growth spurts that occur between 8 and 10 years of age. The amount of myopia present usually increases until growth is completed.

In astigmatism the refractive power of the eye is different in different meridians. This produces a blurred retinal image for objects at any distance. Astigmatism occurs when the cornea, lens or retinal surface has a toric shape rather than a spherical one. This may be likened to the two different curves that give a football its characteristic shape. Bulky masses in the lids

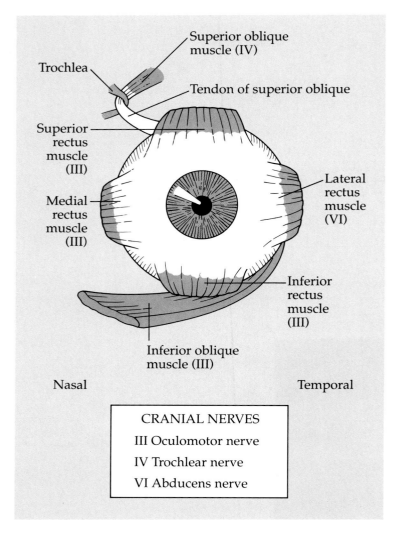

FIG. 19.11 *Innervation of extraocular muscles.*

Diagram labels:
Superior oblique muscle (IV)
Trochlea
Tendon of superior oblique
Superior rectus muscle (III)
Lateral rectus muscle (VI)
Medial rectus muscle (III)
Inferior rectus muscle (III)
Inferior oblique muscle (III)
Nasal
Temporal

CRANIAL NERVES
III Oculomotor nerve
IV Trochlear nerve
VI Abducens nerve

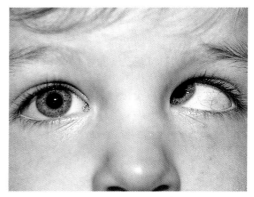

FIG. 19.12 Infantile esotropia with decentered corneal light reflexes.

FIG. 19.13 This deviation is due to an overacting left inferior oblique muscle or elevation in adduction associated with esotropia.

such as chalazions or hemangiomas may compress the cornea and induce astigmatic refractive errors.

Anisometropia refers to the condition where one eye has a different refractive error than the other. Usually the eye with the least amount of hyperopia will be the dominant or preferred eye. The fellow eye may be suppressed and frequently will develop amblyopia. Anisometropia may occur with hyperopia, myopia, astigmatism, aphakia (absence of the lens), or a combination of these refractive errors. If the degree of anisometropia is large, the optical properties of the required correcting lenses produce a difference in image size between the two eyes. This is called aniseikonia.

STRABISMUS

Misalignment of the visual axes is referred to as strabismus. Strabismus may be congenital or acquired and it occurs in 1 to 4 percent of the population. It may occur on a hereditary basis. Strabismus may be due to poor vision or it may be due to a "motor" component defect such as a cranial nerve palsy or a neurologic disorder which interferes with conjugate movement of the eyes.

An abnormal head posture may be a sign of strabismus. These postures are usually observed in children who have good binocular function. Head postures are used to compensate for double vision caused by horizontal, vertical, or cyclovertical muscle palsies. In a patient with nystagmus, a head posture may be used to place the eyes in the null point or direction of gaze where the amplitude of nystagmus is the least.

Voluntary and reflex movement of the eyes is mediated via the extraocular muscles. These muscles are coordinated in their saccadic and pursuit movements by centers in the frontal and occipital areas of the cerebral cortex with modification by the cerebellum. Saccades are voluntary movements used to move the eyes to the object of regard. These are rapid eye movements. Pursuit or following movements are used to track or follow moving objects. These are slow eye movements.

The third, fourth, and sixth cranial nerve nuclei, located in the brain stem, are the centers responsible for innervating the extraocular muscles. In addition to innervation of the inferior oblique, medial, inferior and superior recti, the third cranial nerve is responsible for innervation of the levator muscle, pupillary constriction and accommodation of the lens. The fourth cranial nerve provides innervation to the superior oblique muscle and the sixth cranial nerve supplies the lateral rectus muscle (Fig. 19.11).

Simultaneous fixation with the use of both eyes together has the advantage of producing stereoacuity or an enhancement of the perception of depth. To achieve this, the eyes must be aligned and their movement coordinated. Control of conjugate movement of the eyes is a complex reflex arc that involves the

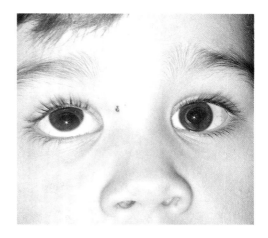

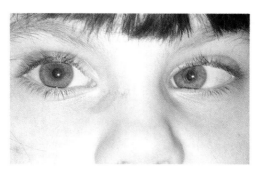

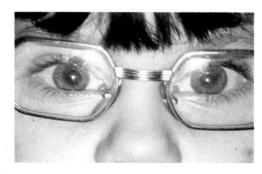

FIG. 19.15 The child at left has esotropia with a high degree of hypermetropia. At right we see that corrective glasses have reduced the hypertropia, and her esotropic eye has returned to orthophoria.

FIG. 19.14 Dissociative vertical deviation, an upward drifting of an eye without symptoms or the presence of a hypodeviation of the other eye.

visual images projected on each retina and the controlling centers located in the brain stem and higher cortical centers. Information is relayed to the muscles that move the eyes through the third, fourth and sixth cranial nerve nuclei and their efferent pathways.

VERSIONS

Eye movements are tested by moving the eyes right, left, up, down, up and right, down and right, up and left, and down and left. This tests the function of each of the extraocular muscles and its counterpart or yoke muscle in the fellow eye. A duction is the movement of a single eye. Versions refer to movement of both eyes together in conjugate gaze. The eyes should be parallel and they both should be aligned on the object of fixation as they move. Normal version movements should be present by 4 months of age.

Vergence movements consist of convergence or divergence of the eyes. Vergences are well established by 6 months of age. Convergence of the eyes, coupled with accommodation and miosis of the pupil, is referred to as the near response. Convergence facilitates alignment of the eyes at near.

PHORIAS AND TROPIAS

If strabismus is present, it may be manifest, a *tropia*, or may be held latent by sensory fusion, a *phoria*. When the fusion of a patient with a phoria is interrupted by placing an occluder in front of one eye, the eye will seek a position of rest and will deviate from the visual axis of the fellow eye. When the eye is uncovered and binocular vision is re-established, the fusion response will assist in the realignment of the eyes on the object of regard. A phoria may produce symptoms of intermittent double vision, fatigue, blurring or movement of objects. Phorias become symptomatic at times of fatigue or illness, or at the end of the day.

A tropia is a constant or intermittently present ocular deviation. The fusion mechanism is unable to maintain alignment of the eyes on an object of fixation. The deviation may occur in one or all positions of gaze. Phorias and tropias are classified according to the pattern of the eye deviation. The prefixes eso and exo classify horizontal strabismus, hyper and hypo are used for vertical deviations, and incyclo and excyclo for torsional deviations.

Esodeviations

An esodeviation is a convergent deviation of the eyes. The deviation may be latent, a phoria (esophoria) or it may occur as a manifest deviation, a tropia (esotropia). Common esodeviations seen in children are infantile esotropia, accommodative esotropia, esotropia due to sixth cranial nerve palsy, and Duane's syndrome.

INFANTILE ESOTROPIA

The most common esodeviation in children is infantile of "congenital" esotropia (Fig. 19.12). There is frequently a family history of infantile esotropia and the eyes will be crossed at birth or shortly thereafter. The angle of esodeviation is large and constant. Defects in abduction may appear to be present and differentiation from sixth cranial nerve palsy may be difficult. Cross-fixation is usually present with the adducted right eye used for vision to the left and the adducted left eye used for vision to the right. Children with this condition usually have good visual acuity and are otherwise systemically and neurologically normal.

Infantile esotropia requires surgical correction. Following correction, the ocular alignment remains unstable and inferior oblique overaction or dissociated vertical deviations may frequently develop. Inferior oblique overaction is seen as an elevation of one or both eyes in adduction (Fig. 19.13). Dissociated vertical deviation (DVD) (Fig. 19.14) is an upward and outward "floating" movement of one or both eyes which becomes prominent with fatigue or inattention.

ACCOMMODATIVE ESOTROPIA

Uncorrected hyperopia stimulates accommodation to obtain clear vision. With accommodation, the synkinetic near response, which includes miosis, accommodation and convergence of the eyes, will occur. If the fusion mechanism is unable to diverge the eyes to compensate for the convergence, esotropia will result. If an esodeviation is associated with a modest degree of farsightedness, treatment of the hyperopia is indicated. In patients with pure accommodative esotropia, this measure alone may completely correct the deviation (Fig. 19.15). More often than not, a residual esodeviation will remain and if this is large, surgical correction may be recommended.

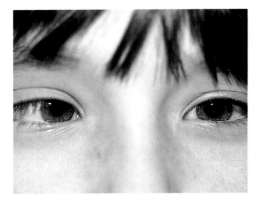
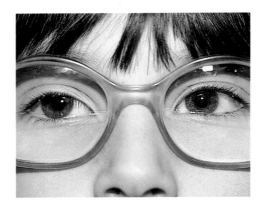
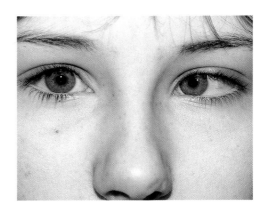
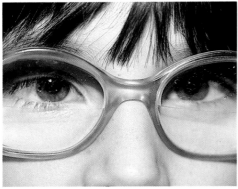
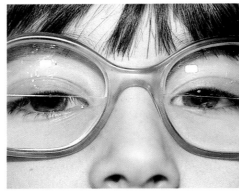
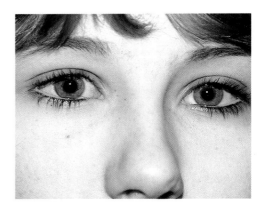

FIG. 19.16 This child displays hypermetropia and esotropia when fixing at distance, and even greater esotropia in near range (top left). When glasses were prescribed (top right), correction of hypermetropia occurred,

and her eyes straightened at distance. However, her near esotropia remained (bottom left). Bifocals were then prescribed, and the near esotropia was corrected (bottom right).

FIG. 19.17 The girl at top shows nonaccommodative esotropia, an esotropia which could not be corrected with glasses or miotics. Surgery was performed, and the 1-week postoperative photograph at bottom shows reduced esotropia with normal alignment.

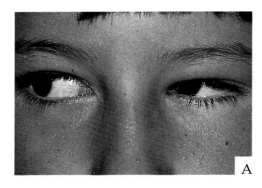
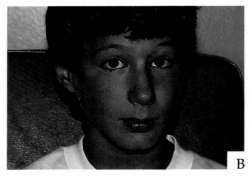
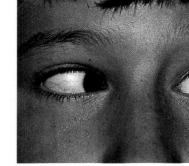

FIG. 19.18 Left Duane's syndrome. **A,** right gaze. While the left eye is noted to move into adduction, retraction of the globe is noted along with narrowing of the palpebral fissure. The globe retraction and lid changes are due to co-contraction of the medial rectus and lateral rectus muscles on the involved side. **B,** fixation target directly in front of patient. The patient is noted to maintain a slight left head turn in

order to maintain normal alignment of the eyes with the affected left eye held slightly in adduction. If the patient's head is forced out of the slight left head turn the left eye would become slightly esotropic. **C,** left gaze. The affected left eye is seen to have an absence of abduction due to aberrant innervation of the lateral rectus muscle.

In another form of accommodative esotropia the ratio between accommodative convergence and accommodation (AC/A ratio) may be abnormally high, producing excessive convergence when focusing on near objects. In high AC/A ratio accommodative esotropia the esodeviation with near vision will be greater in magnitude than it is with distance vision (Fig. 19.16).

NONACCOMMODATIVE ESOTROPIA
Children may develop an esodeviation that is not associated with a hypermetropic refractive error (Fig. 19.17). These nonac-

commodative esodeviations may be associated with poor vision, trauma, prematurity, aphakia, or high myopia.

OTHER CAUSES OF ESOTROPIA
Unilateral or bilateral *sixth cranial nerve palsy* will cause deficient abduction and an esodeviation. In sixth nerve palsy, the esotropia will increase with gaze directed toward the side of the palsy. Patients may display a head turn toward the side of the palsy in order to hold the involved eye in adduction and maintain binocular vision. Sixth cranial nerve palsies in children may be associated with increased intracranial pressure,

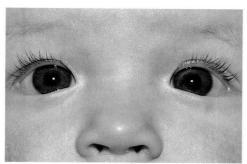

FIG. 19.19 Top: this infant has pseudos-trabismus, caused by a flat nasal bridge, wide epicanthal folds, and closely placed eyes. Bottom: the characteristics of pseudo-strabismus are illustrated.

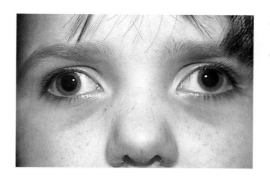

FIG. 19.20 Exotropia, a divergent deviation of the eyes.

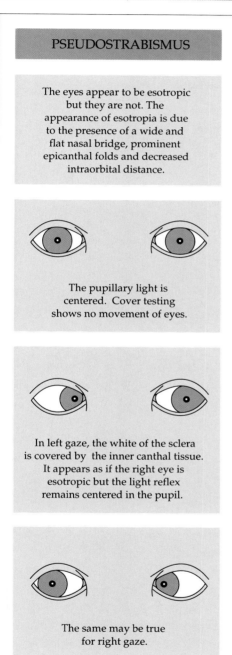

PSEUDOSTRABISMUS

The eyes appear to be esotropic but they are not. The appearance of esotropia is due to the presence of a wide and flat nasal bridge, prominent epicanthal folds and decreased intraorbital distance.

The pupillary light is centered. Cover testing shows no movement of eyes.

In left gaze, the white of the sclera is covered by the inner canthal tissue. It appears as if the right eye is esotropic but the light reflex remains centered in the pupil.

The same may be true for right gaze.

Duane's syndrome is a congenital unilateral or bilateral defect characterized by inability to abduct an eye. This may be accompanied by an up or down shoot of the eye and narrowing of the lid fissure on attempted adduction. In attempted abduction, the palpebral fissure widens. Duane's syndrome is caused by a malformation of the cranial nerve nuclei producing co-innervation of the medial and lateral rectus muscles. The lateral rectus muscle does not contract with abduction and paradoxically co-contracts along with the medial rectus on adduction. Patients with Duane's syndrome may be esotropic and have a head turn toward the involved side analogous to those seen with a sixth cranial nerve palsy. The changes in lid position and vertical deviations help to differentiate the two conditions (Fig. 19.18).

PSEUDOSTRABISMUS

Pseudostrabismus is seen in infants with prominent epicanthal folds, closely placed eyes, and flat nasal bridges. When these facial features are present, the white of the sclera between the cornea and inner canthus may be frequently obscured, giving the optical illusion that the eyes are esotropic (Fig. 19.19). Observation of symmetrical corneal light reflexes or cover testing will confirm or exclude the presence of a true deviation.

Exodeviations

When the visual axes are divergent, an exodeviation is present (Fig. 19.20). Many children with exodeviations will have family histories of strabismus. Exodeviations may also be acquired due to oculopathology or cranial nerve paralysis. An exodeviation may be controlled by fusion (*exophoria*), be manifest intermittently (*intermittent exotropia*), or be constant (*exotropia*). Intermittent exodeviations become manifest with fatigue, daydreaming, or illness. Patients with exodeviations will frequently squint one eye in bright light and may complain of discomfort at night or when tired.

If there is a defect in visual acuity, the decreased visual stimulation may produce a sensory deviation. Generally speaking, if the onset of decreased vision occurs after the age of 4 years, an exodeviation will occur; however, if sensory input to the eye is decreased before the age of 2 years, an esodeviation usually occurs.

Exodeviations may be simulated in patients with widely spaced eyes (hypertelorism) or in those whose maculae are temporally displaced, as may occur in retinopathy of prematurity. When the macula is displaced temporally, the eye will

trauma, tumor, or antecedent viral illness. In benign or "postviral" cases, the lateral rectus function may return fully over a 6-month period. If improvement does not occur, if the deviation increases, or if a gaze palsy develops, suspicion should be raised that a pontine glioma is the cause for the sixth nerve paralysis.

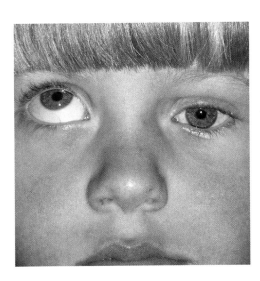

ANGLE KAPPA

Positive angle kappa produces an appearance of exotropia. This appearance is caused by a temporal displacement of the fovea, usually due to cicatricial changes of the retina after retinopathy of prematurity.

The left eye appears exotropic. Cover testing shows no movement of the eyes.

Normal vascular pattern

Fovea

Straightened vessels due to resolved R.O.P.

Temporal retinal cicatricial changes after resolution of stage 3 R.O.P. have caused the fovea to be displaced temporalward.

Angle Kappa

The fovea has been displaced and retains fixation. The eye therefore rotates outward to focus light on the fovea. The eye appears exotropic but is not.

FIG. 19.21

THIRD CRANIAL NERVE PALSY

A patient with left third cranial nerve palsy will not have a Bell's phenomenon on the affected side. The forced opening of tightly closed eyelids will reveal an upward, slightly outward movement of the eye under the closed eyelids (normal Bell's response). The patient with a third cranial nerve palsy cannot elevate or adduct the eye. The eye, when opened or under forced eyelid closure, is not elevated.

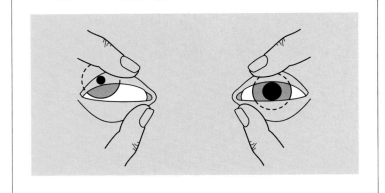

FIG. 19.23

rotate outward to align its visual axis on the fixation target. This will simulate an exodeviation. The term positive angle kappa is used to describe this condition (Fig. 19.21).

CONVERGENCE INSUFFICIENCY
Convergence insufficiency describes an exodeviation in which the size of the deviation is greater in the near range than at distance. This infrequently occurring pattern will cause double vision at near and difficulty with reading. To test for convergence insufficiency, a child is asked to fixate on a target with detail as the target is brought progressively closer. Normally, a child should be able to converge to a point 10 cm from the nose. If the eyes converge, then break their alignment and diverge at a distance greater than 10 cm from the eyes, the patient should be evaluated for convergence insufficiency.

THIRD (OCULOMOTOR) CRANIAL NERVE PALSY
The third cranial nerve innervates the medial rectus muscle. In third nerve paralysis the action of the lateral rectus muscle, innervated by the sixth cranial nerve, is unopposed and produces an exodeviation. The third nerve also innervates the superior and inferior recti, and the inferior oblique muscles, the levator palpebrae superioris which elevates the lid, the cil-

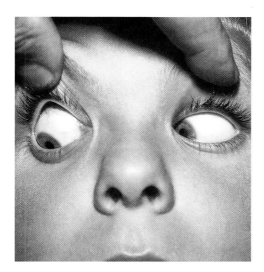

FIG. 19.24 Left fourth nerve palsy with an inability to depress the involved eye in adduction. Abnormal head posture is common, as is overaction of the direct antagonistic inferior oblique muscle.

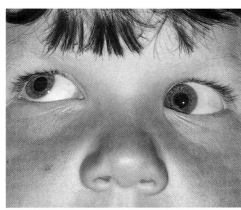

FIG. 19.25 Brown syndrome, an inability to elevate an eye in adduction due to a tight superior oblique tendon.

HIRSCHBERG TEST FOR OCULAR ALIGNMENT

A penlight is held 1 meter from the eyes. The pupillary light reflex is observed and its relationship to the center of the pupil is noted.

Normal Corneal Light Reflex
The reflexes are symmetrical and slightly displaced nasal to the center of the pupils.

Left Estropia
The reflex is displaced temporal to the center of the pupil.

Left Exotropia
The corneal light reflex is displaced nasal to the center of the pupil.

FIG. 19.26

iary muscle which is responsible for accommodation of the lens, and the iris sphincter muscle which produces miosis of the pupil. In the presence of a complete third cranial nerve palsy, the eye will assume a down and outward position, the eyelid will be ptotic, and the pupil will be enlarged (Fig. 19.22). Elevation of the eye with forced eyelid closure (Bell's phenomenon) is typically absent in patients with a third cranial nerve palsy (Fig. 19.23). The most common causes for third cranial nerve palsy in children are trauma and tumor.

Vertical Deviations

Isolated vertical misalignment of the eyes is uncommon. Vertical deviations may occur in only one field of gaze or they may be concomitant and equal in all fields of gaze. Vertical deviations may have a cyclotorsional component and be associated with a head tilt or head posture to eliminate double vision. All patients with torticollis should be evaluated for cyclovertical muscle palsies.

The most common cyclovertical deviation is due to a palsy of the fourth cranial (trochlear) nerve (Fig. 19.24). The eye is excyclorotated and the head is tilted to the shoulder opposite the side of the paretic superior oblique muscle. Other features are elevation of the eye and difficulty depressing the eye in adduction.

Brown's syndrome describes an isolated motility disorder in which there is an inability to elevate the eye when it is adducted (Fig. 19.25). This may be due to a defect in the superior oblique tendon as it passes through the trochlea or due to a congenital anomaly of the superior oblique tendon.

Abnormalities of extraocular muscle innervation rarely cause vertical deviations. Double elevator palsy is an inherited unilateral or bilateral condition in which there is hypotropia and limitation of elevation of the involved eye. To achieve binocularity, patients will tilt their chin up and position their head back. Ptosis is frequently present.

Additional causes of vertical deviations include myasthenia gravis, thyroid ophthalmopathy, external ophthalmoplegia, orbital fractures with muscle entrapment and orbital disease with intraorbital masses.

Tests for Strabismus

The type and degree of ocular misalignment may be estimated using the corneal light reflex test or *Hirschberg test*. The patient fixates on a penlight held at 1 m. Using the pupil as a point of reference, if the light reflex is displaced temporarily an esotropia is present. If the light reflex is displaced nasally in comparison to the other eye, an exodeviation is present (Fig. 19.26). This test only estimates ocular alignment. The most accurate test to measure defects in alignment of the eyes is the prism and alternate cover test.

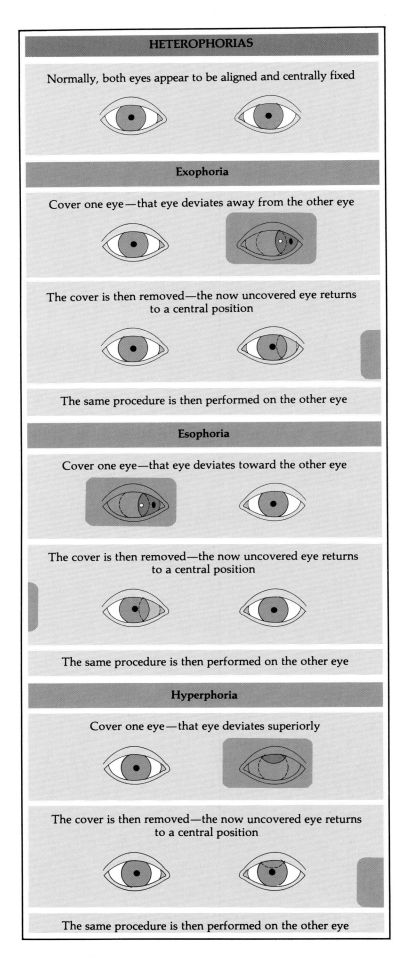

FIG. 19.27 The cover-uncover test for heterophorias.

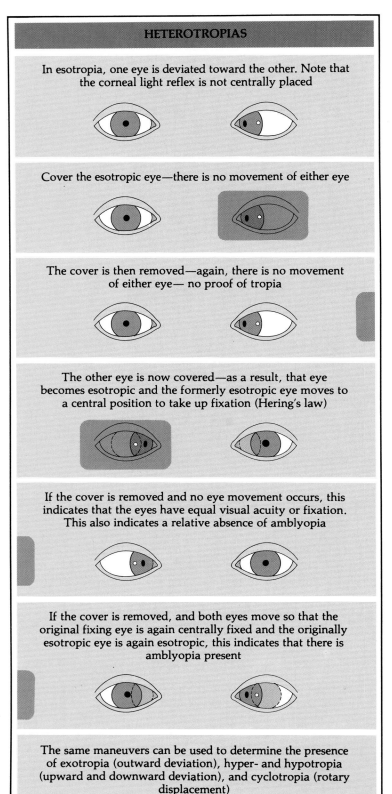

FIG. 19.28 The cover-uncover test for heterotropias.

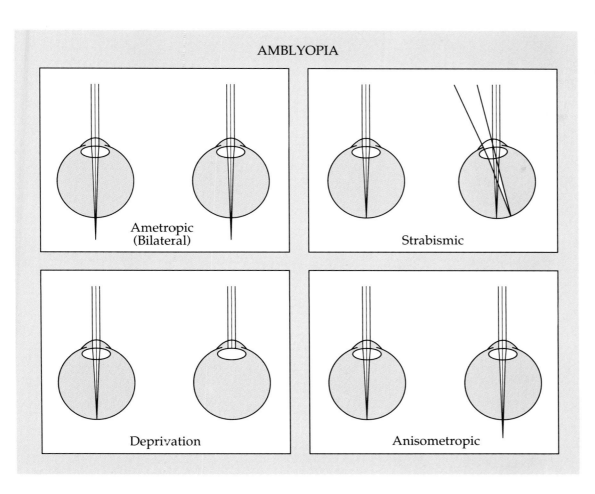

AMBLYOPIA

Ametropic (Bilateral)

Strabismic

Deprivation

Anisometropic

FIG. 19.29 Amblyopia is produced either by the absence of a focused retinal image (ametropic, deprivation, or anisometropic) or by suppression (strabismic).

The *cover test* requires vision in each eye and use of a target that stimulates accommodation. Cover testing is performed while the patient maintains fixation on targets at 20 feet and at 13 to 14 in. The *cover-uncover test* is used to detect phorias. This test is performed by placing a cover over one eye and disrupting fusion or binocularity. As the cover is removed the previously covered eye is observed. If the eye does not move, this indicates that both eyes are aligned on the object at that distance; orthophoria is present. If the eye deviates while covered and then moves to regain fusion and assume fixation as the cover is removed, a phoria exists. The test is then repeated covering and uncovering the other eye (Fig. 19.27).

The second component of the cover test is performed by covering one eye and observing the movement of the other. If neither eye moves as the eyes are alternately covered, the eyes are both aligned on the fixation target and the term orthophoria is used. No deviation is present in this case. If a tropia and a fixation preference are present, a fixation movement will occur when the deviating eye is uncovered, and when the cover is transferred back the previously deviating eye will again deviate behind the cover (Fig. 19.28). If a deviation is well controlled by fusion (a phoria) and is small in size, it may be safely observed if there are no symptoms and the fundus is normal. When a tropia is present, either constantly or intermittently, after 3 months of age, referral to an ophthalmologist is indicated.

AMBLYOPIA

Amblyopia is a decrease in vision in one or both eyes for which no organic cause can be detected. Amblyopia is caused by form deprivation, or the absence of stimulation of the immature visual system by a focused retinal image, or by strabismus, due to abnormal binocular interaction. Visual deprivation amblyopia may be caused by a corneal opacity, a dense cataract, high hyperopia or anisometropia (Fig. 19.29).

In anisometropic amblyopia, an image is clearly focused on the fovea of one eye, but in the other eye the image is out of focus. The blurred retinal image is suppressed by the child's immature visual system. In high hyperopia, ametropic amblyopia may occur if the child does not or cannot accommodate to produce a focused retinal image to stimulate the visual system. Patients with strabismic amblyopia have suppression of the second image produced by the deviating eye.

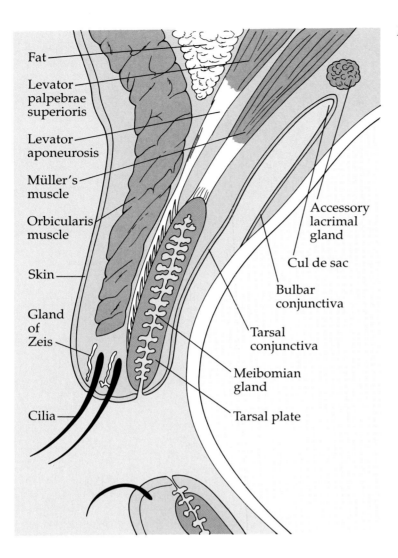

FIG. 19.30 Eyelids and adnexae.

Fat

Levator palpebrae superioris

Levator aponeurosis

Müller's muscle

Orbicularis muscle

Skin

Gland of Zeis

Cilia

Accessory lacrimal gland

Cul de sac

Bulbar conjunctiva

Tarsal conjunctiva

Meibomian gland

Tarsal plate

The severity of the visual loss produced by amblyopia is determined by the nature of the visual deprivation, the age of onset, its consistency, severity, and duration. If a patient is suspected of having amblyopia, careful measurement of visual acuity is performed in a well-illuminated room. Suspicion will be heightened if there is a coexistent deviation or there is evidence of an opacity that interferes with visualization of the fundus. Patients who are suspected of having amblyopia, should be promptly referred to an ophthalmologist. Amblyopia responds best to treatment when treatment is begun early in life. Treatment is rarely effective after 8 years of age.

DISEASES OF THE EYES AND SURROUNDING STRUCTURES

Eyelids and Adnexae - Anatomy of the Eyelid

The eyelid is composed of skin and its related appendages, glands that contribute to the tear film and muscular structures that permit the eyelid to open and close (Fig. 19.30).

Conditions affecting the eyelid will be related to these anatomic structures.

Telecanthus refers to an increase in the distance between the inner canthus of each eye (Fig. 19.31). Telecanthus can be due to the hereditary transmission of facial features or mid-line embryonic defects, or related to a syndrome such as Komoto's (Fig. 19.32). This inherited syndrome consists of telecanthus, epicanthus inversus, blepharophimosis (horizontal shortening of the lid fissure), and ptosis. Hypertelorism refers to an increase in the distance between the nasal walls of the orbits. This is usually associated with telecanthus.

Blepharoptosis or ptosis is a unilateral or bilateral decrease in the vertical distance between the upper and lower eyelids (palpebral fissure) due to dysfunction of the levator muscle (Fig. 19.33). Congenital blepharoptosis is frequently transmitted as an autosomal dominant trait with variable penetrance. Other causes for blepharoptosis include ocular inflammation, chronic irritation of the anterior segment of the eye, chronic use of topical steroid eyedrops, third valve palsy, and trauma. Ptosis may be severe enough to cause visual deprivation and amblyopia.

The *Marcus Gunn jaw winking phenomenon* is caused by a misdirection of the motor division of the fifth cranial nerve to

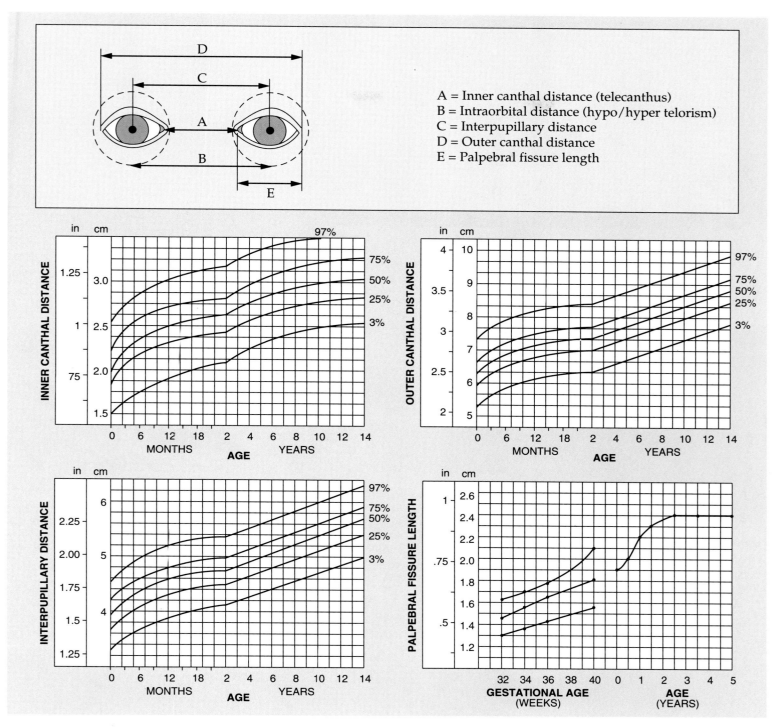

FIG. 19.31 Normal adnexal measurements.

A = Inner canthal distance (telecanthus)
B = Intraorbital distance (hypo/hyper telorism)
C = Interpupillary distance
D = Outer canthal distance
E = Palpebral fissure length

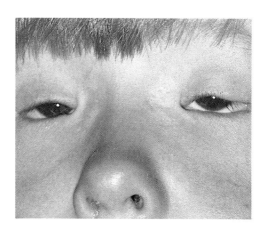

FIG. 19.32 Komoto syndrome, a combination of blepharophimosis, ptosis, epicanthus inversus, and telecanthus.

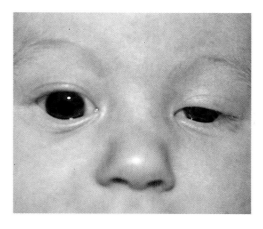

FIG. 19.33 Unilateral congenital ptosis with lid covering pupil.

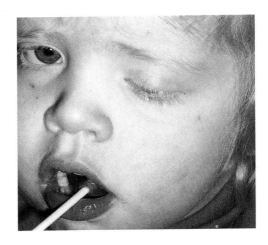

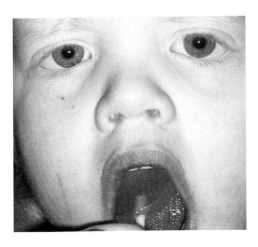

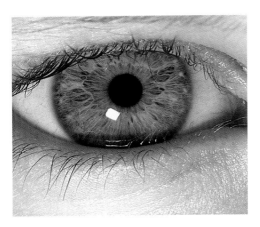

FIG. 19.34 At left, the toddler exhibits the Marcus Gunn jaw-winking syndrome with

ptosis, while at right he shows a wide open ptotic lid with movements of the jaw.

FIG. 19.35 Districhiasis, a double row of lashes. One row, directed toward the cornea, arises from the meibomian gland orifices. The second row is directed outward in the normal position.

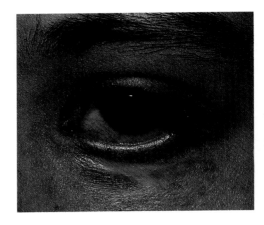

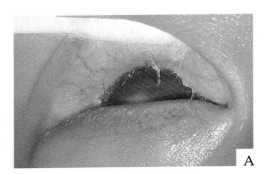

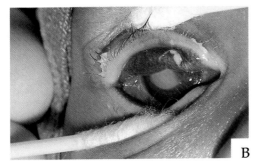

FIG. 19.36 Ectropion of the left lower lid due to scleroderma. The lower eyelid skin has become contracted, causing eversion of the lower eyelid.

FIG. 19.37 Congenital entropion of the right upper lid. The lid is inverted and the lashes and skin rest on the corneal surface. This case is caused by a congenital horizontal kink in the upper tarsal plate. A, the eyelid is propped up with a cotton-tipped applicator displaying the area of skin inverted against

the eye. The Betadine® prep solution has not coated the affected area of the lid. B, with the upper lid everted and the lids held widely open, extensive corneal scarring due to the abrasion caused by the inverted skin and lashes is seen.

the ipsilateral levator muscle of the eyelid (Fig. 19.34). With jaw movement to the ipsilateral side the eyelid droops and when the jaw is moved to the contralateral side the eyelid elevates. The eyelid "winks" with chewing or feeding. This condition represents a curiosity and is not associated with other neurologic abnormalities.

Trichiasis is the term used to describe misdirected eyelashes that irritate the cornea or conjunctiva. It can be caused by chronic inflammation of the eyelids, entropion, eyelid trauma or inflammatory conditions with scarring of the conjunctiva, such as Stevens-Johnson syndrome.

Districhiasis describes a condition where there is an accessory row of eyelashes (cilia) along the posterior border of the eyelid (Fig. 19.35). Eyelid eversion or ectropion will frequently co-exist because of defects in the tarsal plate. This condition is inherited as an autosomal dominant condition but it may also be a sequela of severe ocular inflammation.

Ectropion is an outward rotation of the eyelid margin. If severe, ectropion can lead to problems of corneal exposure. Ectropion may be congenital or caused by any condition (trauma, scleroderma) causing the eyelid skin to contract and evert the eyelid (Fig. 19.36). Ectropion may occur after seventh cranial nerve palsy with paralysis of the facial musculature.

Entropion is an inverted eyelid with the lashes rubbing against the conjunctiva or cornea. This may be present at birth and is associated with a horizontal kink in the tarsus, or it may occur with severe blepharospasm, inflammation or trauma. If severe, the abrasion of the cornea by the lashes can cause permanent corneal scarring (Fig. 19.37).

Epiblepharon, a single row of lashes rotated up against the globe, is usually observed during the first year of life (Fig. 19.38). Facial tissue anterior to the eyelid pushes the medial third of the eyelid upward and rotates the soft lashes in toward the eye. This defect corrects itself spontaneously by 1

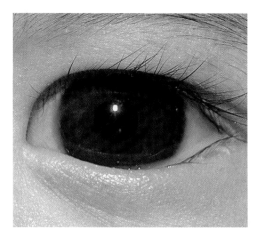

FIG. 19.38 In epiblepharon, the eyelashes are rotated upward against the globe in the medial third of the eyelid.

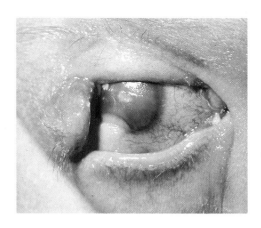

FIG. 19.39 Goldenhar syndrome with eyelid coloboma and corneal limbal dermoid.

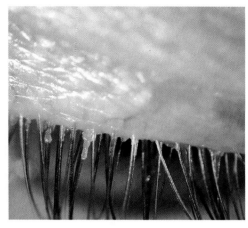

FIG. 19.40 Thickened lids with crusts around lashes in a patient with blepharitis.

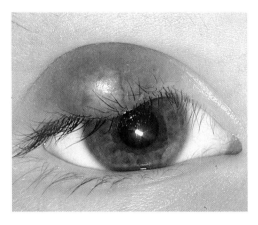

FIG. 19.41 Acute hordeola of the eyelid with swelling, induration, and purulent matter pointing externally.

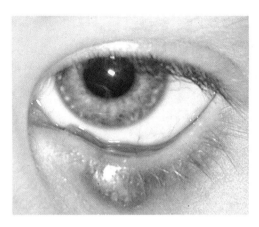

FIG. 19.42 Chalazion, a painless lid mass pointing externally or internally.

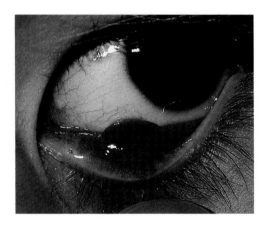

FIG. 19.43 Chalazion of the left lower lid pointed internally. A pyogenic granuloma consisting of a vascularized mound of conjunctival tissue has developed over the chalazion due to spontaneous rupture of the chalazion to the conjunctival surface.

year of age. Corneal abrasion usually does not occur because of the soft texture of the infant's eyelashes.

Congenital *eyelid colobomas* are defects or notches in the eyelid margin caused by failure of fusion of embryonic fissures early in development. These may be isolated defects or associated with conditions such as Goldenhar syndrome (Fig. 19.39). Goldenhar syndrome consists of eyelid colobomas, vertebral anomalies, corneal limbal dermoids, and preauricular skin tags.

Ankyloblepharon is a fusion of the upper and lower eyelid margins. This may range from a few thin strands of tissue to complete fusion of the lids.

Children frequently have a low-grade inflammation of the eyelid margin, chronic blepharitis, due to staphylococcus infection. Blepharitis may be associated with seborrhea or allergies and occurs commonly in children with Down syndrome. Symptoms include itching, light sensitivity, and irritation of the lids. The lashes may be matted and adherent in the morning. This chronic problem causes thickening of the eyelid and misdirection of the eyelashes to the point where they may invert and irritate the cornea and/or conjunctiva (Fig. 19.40). Complications include ulceration of the lid margin, abscess or hordeolum formation, chronic conjunctivitis, and keratitis.

A *hordeolum* is a staphylococcal infection involving the glands of Zeis at the base of the follicles for the cilia (Fig. 19.41). This produces painful swelling and erythema of the eyelid. A purulent discharge may be seen and spontaneous resolution frequently occurs. Preseptal cellulitis may occur as a complication.

A *chalazion* is a chronic granulomatous inflammation of the meibomian glands within the tarsal place. There will be painful swelling and redness of the eyelid due to distention of the gland and the inflammatory response caused by the retained glandular secretions. The gland may spontaneously rupture either to the conjunctival surface or externally to the skin (Figs. 19.42, 19.43). Spontaneous resolution may occur; however, tissue reaction may persist and leave a firm mass within the lid.

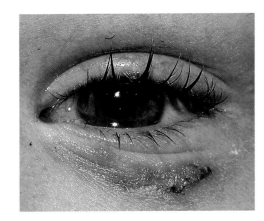

FIG. 19.44 Primary herpes simplex infection involving the periocular area. Primary infection is frequently associated with a mild diffuse keratoconjunctivitis; dendritic forms are uncommon.

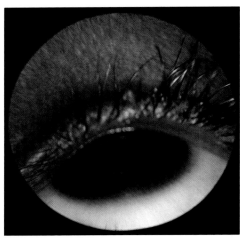

FIG. 19.45 Infestation of the eyelashes with the crab louse Phthirus pubis. The lid margin has a crusty appearance due to the presence of adult organisms and eggs adherent to the eyelashes. The salivary material of the parasites results in toxic and immunologic reactions that will cause itching and burning of the eyes.

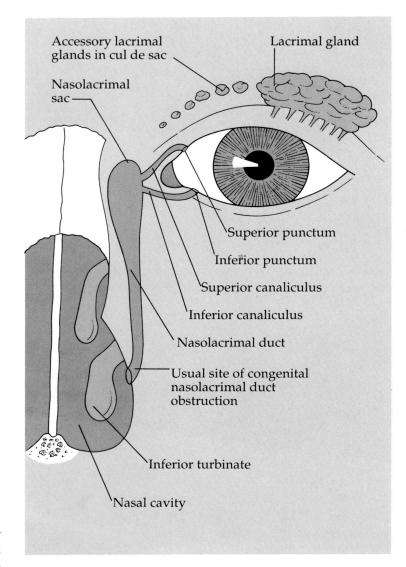

FIG. 19.46 Lacrimal secretory and collecting system.

Primary herpes simplex infection may affect the periocular skin (Fig. 19.44). This is characterized by small skin vesicles, frequently unilateral, with an associated mild conjunctivitis and punctate keratitis. Varicella produces eyelid swelling and vesicular skin eruptions, usually without scarring. Conjunctival vesicles and keratitis may also occur. Herpes zoster is uncommon in children. A lesion on the tip of the nose indicates involvement of the ophthalmic division of the maxillary nerve and possible involvement of the eye with keratouveitis and glaucoma. Another common eyelid lesion found in children is caused by *molluscum contagiousum. Molluscum* is characterized by elevated, 1 to 2 mm umbilicated lesions of the eyelid skin. If the lesions involve the eyelid margin, they may cause an associated keratoconjunctivitis (see Chapter 8, Dermatology).

Phthiriasis or infestation of the lashes with the crab louse *Phthirus pubis* is manifested as a crusty appearance of the lid margin. Closer inspection will reveal egg cases and the adult louse (Fig. 19.45).

Lacrimal Gland and Nasolacrimal Drainage System

Reflex tears are produced by the lacrimal gland, whereas the basal secretion of tears comes from the accessory lacrimal glands (Fig. 19.46). The secretions from the glands of Zeis and the meibomian glands contribute to the tear film. During the first month of life the eye remains moist, but reflex tearing or tearing due to emotion does not occur until the second month of life.

Disorders of the lacrimal gland are rare in children. Acute dacryoadenitis may occur with viral infections, most frequently mumps. Chronic diseases such as sarcoid, Hodgkin's disease, leukemia and mononucleosis may produce lacrimal gland swelling with a palpable mass in the upper outer portion of the orbit (Fig. 19.47).

The tears are drained from the eye by the superior and inferior punctae which connect to the superior and inferior canaliculae (see Fig. 19.46). The canaliculae may unite before they enter the nasolacrimal sac or they may enter the sac separately. The medial canthal tendon is anterior to the nasolacrimal sac. The sac is connected to the nasolacrimal duct, which is located in the nasal bone. The distal portion of the nasolacrimal duct enters the nasal antrum, beneath the inferior turbinate.

Stenosis or obstruction of the nasolacrimal duct is present in 30 percent of newborns (Fig. 19.48). Signs include tearing and mucopurulent discharge which usually begin 3 to 5 weeks following birth. A helpful diagnostic technique is to apply gentle pressure over the nasolacrimal sac to cause reflux of tears and mucopurulent material from the sac. Spontaneous resolution of the obstruction is common before 6 months of age. If the

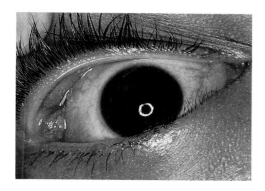

FIG. 19.47 Dacryoadenitis. The lacrimal gland has become swollen and inflamed, and is visible beneath the lateral aspect of the upper eyelid. The swelling is frequently accompanied by symptoms of pain and tenderness.

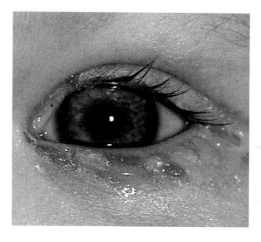

FIG. 19.48 Unilateral stenosis of the left nasolacrimal duct with mucopurulent discharge and tearing.

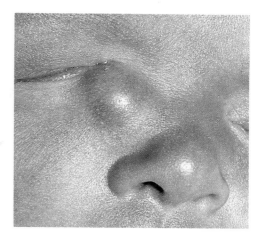

FIG. 19.49 Congenital nasolacrimal sac mucocele presents shortly after birth as a bluish mass below the medial canthal tendon.

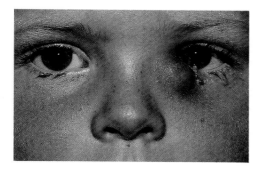

FIG. 19.50 Acute dacryocystitis caused by bacterial infection of the nasolacrimal sac associated with nasolacrimal duct obstruction. The infection of the nasolacrimal sac has spread to the surrounding tissues producing a cellulitis.

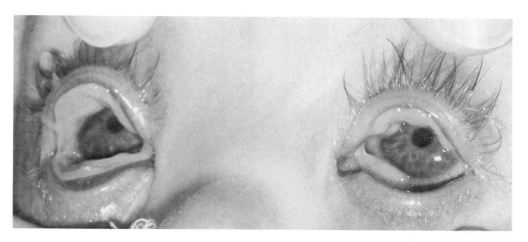

FIG. 19.51 Ophthalmia neonatorum, a hyperacute bacterial conjunctivitis, with thick purulent discharge and red swollen lids.

obstruction has not cleared by this age spontaneous resolution is much less likely, and the patient should be referred for probing of the nasolacrimal duct.

If both the nasolacrimal duct and the canaliculae entering the sac are obstructed at birth, a bluish swelling will occur over the nasolacrimal sac (congenital nasolacrimal sac mucocele) (Fig. 19.49). Other congenital defects of the nasolacrimal collecting system include absence of the puncta and fistulae from the nasolacrimal sac to the overlying skin.

Obstruction of the nasolacrimal system may also occur secondary to infections such as trachoma, tuberculosis, or fungal infections. Dacryocystitis may spread to the surrounding tissues, producing a periorbital cellulitis. Acute dacryocystitis is usually due to a bacterial infection that involves the nasolacrimal sac and collecting system (Fig. 19.50).

Conjunctiva

The conjunctiva is a mucous membrane that covers the posterior aspect of the eyelids. It is reflected into the cul-de-sac and extends onto the globe where it fuses to the sclera at the corneal scleral limbus. Conjunctiva has goblet cells which contribute mucin to the tear film. When the eyelids are closed, the oxygen supplied by the blood vessels of the conjunctiva is responsible for maintaining oxygenation of the cornea. Conjunctivitis refers to inflammation of the conjunctiva. Infections of the conjunctiva may be bacterial or viral.

The etiology of neonatal conjunctivitis is related to the time of onset. Neonatal conjunctivitis occurring within the first day or two of life usually is due to the use of Credé prophylaxis. One percent silver nitrate solution may cause a mild chemical conjunctivitis which spontaneously resolves within 1 or 2 days. Neonatal conjunctivitis occurring 2 to 4 days after birth and accompanied by a copious purulent discharge, either with or without corneal involvement, usually is due to gonococcus (Fig. 19.51). Infectious neonatal conjunctivitis occurring after 8 days (but before 2 weeks) and accompanied by a watery discharge is often due to Chlamydia. Conjunctivitis is usually contracted following early rupture of membranes or during passage through the birth canal.

Conjunctiva has a limited variety of responses to infection or inflammation. Inflammation of the conjunctiva results in the formation of follicles or papillae. A follicle is an aggregate of lymphocytes with an avascular center and a peripheral vascu-

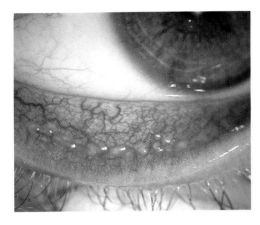

FIG. 19.52 Follicular conjunctivitis of viral origin.

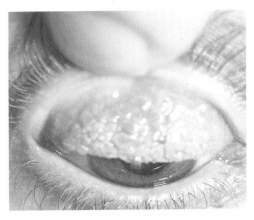

FIG. 19.53 Papillary conjunctivitis of bacterial or allergic origin.

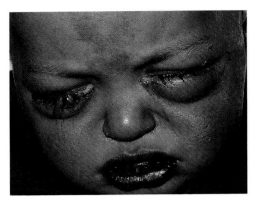

FIG. 19.54 Acute bacterial conjunctivitis. Copious amounts of mucopurulent discharge have made the upper and lower eyelids adherent to each other. Chemosis of the upper and lower lids may also make opening of the eyelids difficult.

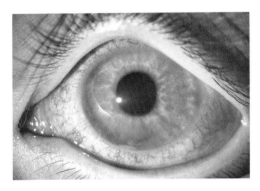

FIG. 19.55 Viral conjunctivitis with hyperemia and a thin watery discharge.

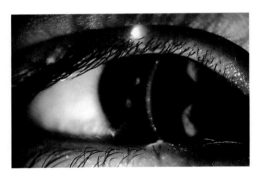

FIG. 19.56 Subepithelial infiltrates of epidemic keratoconjunctivitis caused by adenovirus. The beam of the slit-lamp light is used to demonstrate corneal subepithelial infiltrates (small white opacities). Only severe adenoviral keratoconjunctivitis produces subepithelial infiltrates. These may persist for months, causing symptoms of glare and blurring of vision.

lar network (Fig. 19.52). Newborns will seldom develop follicles because lymphoid tissues have not yet developed.

Papillae are small, raised nodules with a central vascular core (Fig. 19.53). They may be located on the tarsal surface of the upper and lower eyelids. Papillae may become large, measuring 1 to 2 mm in diameter if inflammation is chronic. Papillae are the conjunctiva's response to bacterial or allergic conjunctivitis. Giant papillae may be produced by the continuous irritation caused by a contact lens.

Bacterial conjunctivitis may be acute or chronic. Acute conjunctivitis is painful with lid edema and keratitis. The bulbar conjunctiva will swell (chemosis) and become hyperemic (injection). Corneal ulceration may occur as a complication. Acute bacterial conjunctivitis is usually due to staphylococcus, pneumococcus, or *Haemophilus* infections. Mucopurulent discharge is associated with tearing and the eyelids may be stuck together on awakening (Fig. 19.54).

Chronic bacterial conjunctivitis results from bacterial toxins of *Staphylococcus aureus, Proteus, Moraxella* or, in third world countries, trachoma. A foreign body sensation may be experienced and the eyes may be hyperemic with a chronic, mucopurulent or watery discharge. Papillary hyperplasia and thickening of the conjunctiva may also occur.

Viral conjunctivitis usually is caused by various strains of adenovirus (Fig. 19.55). The eyes are extremely light sensitive due to subepithelial infiltrates of the cornea (Fig. 19.56). Signs include copious tearing with a watery or thin mucopurulent discharge, conjunctival redness, and preauricular lymph node enlargement. Viral conjunctivitis is self-limited and will usually resolve in 7 to 10 days depending on the viral strain. This form of viral conjunctivitis is highly contagious.

Allergic conjunctivitis occurs as a hypersensitivity response to dust, pollen, animal dander, or other airborne allergens. The eyes will exhibit copious tearing, itching, and photophobia. The eyelids and palpebral conjunctiva are hyperemic and edemetous (see Chapter 4, Allergy/Immunology). Acute chemosis may cause a startling collection of serous discharge under the conjunctiva so that the conjunctiva may protrude between the eyelids to the extent of obscuring the cornea. This is usually self-limited and resolves within several hours. Allergic conjunctivitis may become chronic with repeated exposure to the allergen. In cases of chronic allergic conjunctivitis, the conjunctiva becomes pale and boggy and demonstrates a papillary reaction. Complications include keratitis and, rarely, iritis.

Subconjunctival hemorrhages may occur spontaneously or they may be secondary to trauma (Fig. 19.57). These present as a striking bright red discoloration underneath the bulbar conjunctiva. The size and configuration of the hemorrhage will depend on the amount and location of the blood between the conjunctiva and the globe. Spontaneous resolution occurs within 1 to 2 weeks.

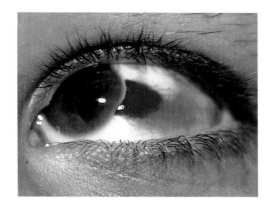

FIG. 19.57 Subconjunctival hemorrhage secondary to blunt ocular trauma.

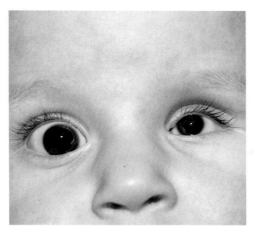

FIG. 19.58 Unilateral microcornea and microphthalmos.

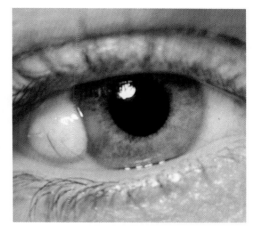

FIG. 19.59 Corneal-limbal dermoid, often associated with Goldenhar syndrome.

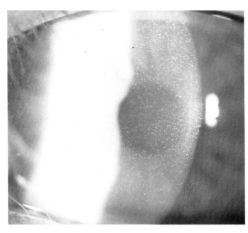

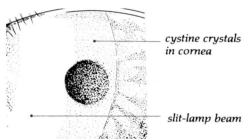

cystine crystals in cornea

slit-lamp beam

FIG. 19.60 Cystinosis of the cornea with deposition of L-cystine crystals in the stroma.

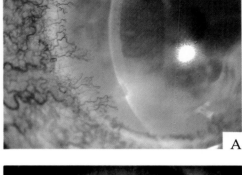

A

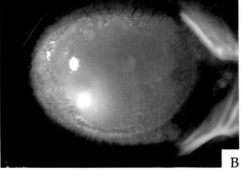

B

FIG. 19.61 Bacterial corneal ulcer. **A,** the conjunctiva displays a marked inflammatory response with injection, most prominent in the quadrant nearest the corneal ulcer. The ulcer is visualized in the slit beam as a small white infiltrate of the corneal stroma. There is an overlying epithelial defect. **B,** the epithelial defect is easier to visualize after the application of fluorescein dye. The dye is taken up by the corneal stroma in the area of the epithelial defect. The areas of abrasion will fluoresce with cobalt blue light illumination.

Cornea

Developmental anomalies of the cornea include sclerocornea, Rieger's syndrome, microcornea, and corneal dermoid.

Sclerocornea, present at birth, is a rare condition in which the cornea is white and resembles sclera. Rieger's syndrome, a variant of anterior segment dysgenesis, is a dominant hereditary disorder that affects development of the anterior segment of the eye. Features include hyperplasia of the iris stroma, pupillary anomalies, anomalies of the trabecular meshwork, and early-onset glaucoma. Microcornea, whether an isolated anomaly or associated with glaucoma, cataracts, iris abnormalities, or anterior segment dysgenesis, is present when the corneal diameter is 9 mm or less (Fig. 19.58).

The developmental abnormalities mentioned require further tests to exclude glaucoma. If the anterior segment of the eye is severely disorganized, the cornea is opaque, or glaucoma exists, surgical reconstruction and repair are indicated. The prognosis for vision is guarded for severe cases.

Corneal dermoids occur at the limbus, grow slowly, and may encroach upon the visual axis or cause high degrees of astigmatism (Fig. 19.59). They are composed of fibrolipoid tissue containing hair follicles and sebaceous glands.

The cornea is also the site of many systemic diseases. Hurler syndrome, a mucopolysaccharidosis, produces clouding of the cornea. The cornea, clear at birth, develops an opacification by 2 to 3 years of age. Pigmentary retinopathy and optic atrophy coexist.

Cystinosis, seen in the early months of life, involves the deposition of L-cystine in the cornea. This may be seen as a very subtle haze of the cornea. Slit-lamp examination is necessary to clearly visualize the corneal deposits. (Fig. 19.60).

Corneal inflammations are associated with bacterial, viral, mycotic, and allergic diseases. Corneal ulcers are caused by the invasion of bacterial organisms into the corneal stroma, leading to abscess formation (Fig. 19.61A,B). The infection may involve the entire cornea and result in visual impairment, corneal perforation, and loss of the globe. Bacteria commonly

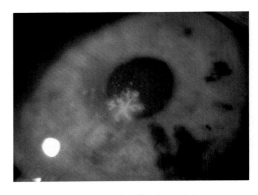

FIG. 19.62 Herpes simplex keratitis. Infection of the corneal epithelium with herpes simplex virus produces a pattern of fluorescein staining that resembles a neuronal dendrite. The surrounding area may be hazy due to epithelial and stromal edema and infiltration. Conjunctival injection is typically present.

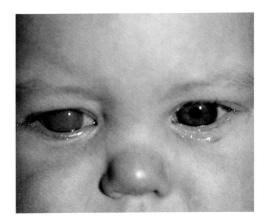

FIG. 19.63 Congenital glaucoma. The right cornea is hazy and opaque due to corneal edema. Breakdown of the corneal epithelium has caused ocular irritation and the conjunctiva is slightly injected. Epiphora is present due to reflex tearing caused by the increased intraocular pressure.

involved include staphylococcus, pneumococcus, *Moraxella, Pseudomonas aeruginosa, Escherichia coli,* and *Klebsiella pneumoniae*. Appropriate smears and cultures are obtained as soon as the diagnosis is suspected.

Herpes simplex, a severe viral infection of the cornea, may be transmitted from active herpes in the maternal birth canal, or may result from direct contact with infected individuals. Primary herpes is a unilateral lesion associated with regional lymphadenopathy. A few weeks after infection, half of all patients will develop a punctate or typical dendritic keratitis (Fig. 19.62). This is best seen using a fluorescein stain and a cobalt blue filter over a pen light.

Recurrent herpes kertitis occurs in 25 percent of infected individuals. The lesions may have a typical appearance of branching dendrites. Recurrences may be complicated by stromal keratitis, keratouveitis, and anesthesia of the cornea. Stromal disease is a serious complication reducing visual recovery due to corneal vascularization and scarring. Patients with a history of herpes keratitis must be evaluated by an opthalmologist for any episode of conjunctivitis.

Phlyctenular or nodular keratoconjunctivitis occurs in response to an allergy. Phylctenular lesions are small, pinkish-white nodules in the center of hyperemic areas of conjunctiva at the limbus which may evolve into microabscesses. Healing occurs in 10 to 14 days without scarring. Symptoms consist of itching, tearing, and irritation. A mucopurulent discharge may occur if secondary infection is present. Patients with corneal phlyctenulosis have more severe symptoms of pain, light sensitivity, and tearing.

Anterior Chamber

The term "anterior chamber" refers to the fluid-filled space between the cornea and the iris diaphragm. The aqueous is an optically clear fluid which provides nutrition for the corneal endothelial surface. The aqueous fluid is secreted by the ciliary processes, reaches the anterior chamber by passing through the pupillary space and leaves via the trabecular meshwork in the periphery of the anterior chamber angle.

GLAUCOMA

The incidence of infantile or congenital glaucoma is approximately 1 in 12,500 births. The inheritance of congenital glaucoma is multifactorial; parents of an affected child have a 5 percent chance of having another child with glaucoma, and an affected parent has a 5 percent chance of having an affected child. Two thirds of all patients are male. Glaucoma can present at birth, but more commonly it has its onset during the first several weeks or months of life. An embryonic defect in the development of the trabecular meshwork or filtration area of the eye has been hypothesized as the cause.

Infants with glaucoma have corneal edema, which gives the cornea a hazy or cloudy appearance. Corneal edema may produce an irregular corneal light reflex or dull the red reflex. Initially, the edema may be limited to the epithelium but stromal edema may follow (Fig. 19.63). As this increases, Descemet's membrane may rupture and produce Haab's striae (Fig. 19.64).

A break in Descemet's membrane may produce a corneal opacity or, if edema is not present, it may be visualized against the red reflex when viewed with a slit lamp or direct ophthalmoscope. Breaks in Descemet's membrane can produce irregular astigmatism. Glare from the scatter of light produced by the epithelial and stromal edema is responsible for photophobia and blinking. Breakdown of the corneal epithelium may produce squinting and bleph-arospasm.

For children less than 2 years of age, an increase in corneal diameter indicates increased intraocular pressure (Fig. 19.65). An infant's horizontal corneal diameter is normally 9.5 mm and this increases over the first 2 years of life to a normal corneal diameter of 11.5 mm. In addition to enlargement of the corneal diameter, chronic elevated intraocular pressure may also produce enlargement of the entire eye. This produces an increase in axial length and myopic refractive error. A rapid

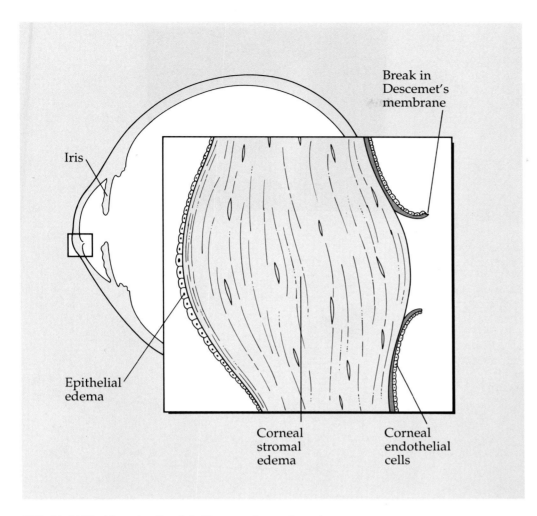

FIG. 19.64 Haab's striae (break in Descemet's membrane).

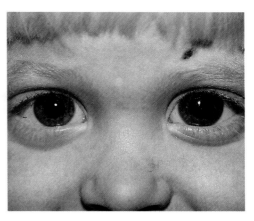

FIG. 19.65 Congenital glaucoma. This patient has corneal asymmetry due to glaucoma in the left eye. The horizontal corneal diameter is 11.0 mm in the right eye and 13.5 mm in the left eye. The entire left eye has become enlarged and the axial length is greater than normal. The increase in axial length of the left eye has produced a myopic refractive error.

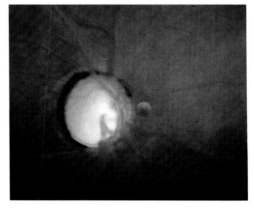

FIG. 19.66 Glaucomatous optic atrophy. In glaucoma, excavation extends to the disc edge in contrast to the cupped disc seen in myopia where a normal rim of tissue exists. Retinal vessels emerge from under the disc edge.

increase in myopia may be a sign of glaucoma. The anterior chamber in infancy is shallow when compared to older children and another sign of congenital glaucoma is an anterior chamber which is deeper than normal.

Epiphora, or tearing, is a sign of glaucoma and is differentiated from nasolacrimal duct obstruction by the presence of rhinorrhea. When the nasolacrimal duct is obstructed, rhinorrhea is absent.

The optic nerve damage caused by elevated intraocular pressure is reflected in the degree of enlargement of the optic cup (Fig. 19.66). Asymmetry of the cup/disc ratio between the eyes or an increase in cup/disc ratio to greater than 0.5 are indicators of glaucoma. Enlargement of the optic cup is reversible in infants and young children but is usually permanent in adults. Enlargement of the optic cups without glaucoma may be inherited; examination of family members may be of value.

Elevation of intraocular pressure is the hallmark of congenital glaucoma. Normal intraocular pressure (IOP) in infants and young children is less than 20 mm Hg. Pressures greater than 25 mm Hg strongly suggest glaucoma.

Precise measurement of pressure is difficult in children. An estimate of the intraocular pressure may be obtained by palpating the globes with fingertips over closed eyelids. More precise measurements are obtained with a hand-held Schiotz tonometer or an applanation tonometer. These procedures and decisions regarding the management of the pressure may require an examination that is conducted under general anesthesia. Unfortunately, some anesthetic agents alter intraocular pressure.

Glaucoma may occur with congenital ocular malformations such as aniridia or mesodermal (iridocorneal) dysgenesis, in systemic syndromes, or after trauma. Sturge-Weber syndrome, neurofibromatosis, Lowe syndrome, Rubinstein-Taybi syndrome, and the congenital rubella syndrome are associated with congenital glaucoma. Patients with chronic uveitis frequently develop glaucoma and 8 percent of children who have cataract surgery will develop glaucoma following surgery.

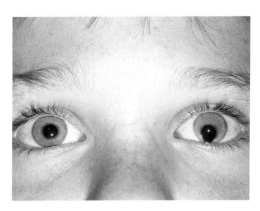

FIG. 19.67 Typical unilateral coloboma in an otherwise normal left eye.

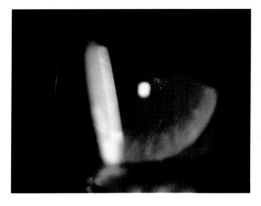

FIG. 19.68 Aniridia. Iris structures are only present as rudimentary findings and the red reflex fills the entire corneal diameter. The edge of the lens is visible peripherally and early cataractous lens changes are present centrally.

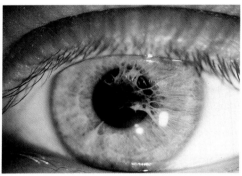

FIG. 19.69 Persistent pupillary membranes. Hyperplasia of the mesoderm of the anterior layer of the iris has caused iris strands to become adherent to the anterior lens surface. The lens is clear and these are visually insignificant.

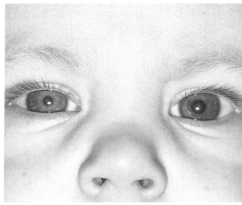

FIG. 19.70 Horner's syndrome (right side) with iris heterochromia. The right upper lid is slightly ptotic and the right lower lid is slightly higher than its mate. Anisocoria is present. The right pupil is smaller than the left. The iris on the side affected by Horner's syndrome is lighter in color than the other.

Iris

A *coloboma* results from failure of fusion of the embryonic fissure of the optic cup anywhere from the optic disc to the iris (Fig. 19.67). The defect is usually inferior and nasal in location and it may involve any ocular structure.

Colobomas occur either as isolated defects or in association with systemic syndromes. Iris colobomas occur in the CHARGE association, cat-eye syndrome, Rieger's syndrome, and the facio-auriculo-vertebral anomalies. Isolated colobomas may be inherited as a dominant trait.

Aniridia, an apparent absence of the iris, is due to failure of the mesoderm to grow outward from the iris root during the fourth month of gestation. The pupil appears the same size as the cornea and iris structures are present as only rudimentary findings (Fig. 19.68). A fibrovascular membrane can form between the rudimentary iris and the trabecular meshwork and cause glaucoma.

Hypoplasia of the macula occurs in patients with aniridia, and visual acuity is decreased to the 20/400 level. Associated defects include corneal opacities, lens dislocations, and cataracts. Affected patients have photophobia and nystagmus.

An autosomal-dominant inheritance pattern is present in two thirds of all patients. It is estimated that 1 to 70 patients with sporadic aniridia will have Wilms' tumor and 90 percent of these will occur before age 3. Other genitourinary defects and mental retardation may occur and many of these patients have abnormalities of the 11 p chromosome.

Persistent pupillary membranes are due to hyperplasia of the mesoderm of the anterior layer of the iris and are a frequent finding in children born prematurely (Fig. 19.69). Instead of

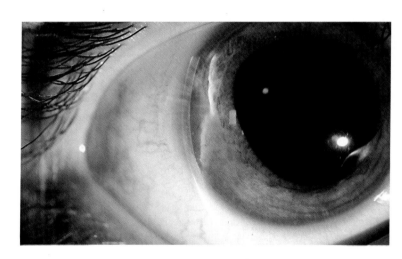

FIG. 19.71 Juvenile xanthogranuloma (JXG). The ocular lesion of JXG is visualized as a fleshy, yellow-brown tumor on the surface of the iris. The lesions are vascular, bleed easily, and can cause spontaneous hyphemas.

terminating at the pupillary margin, iris strands with accompanying blood vessels encroach on the pupillary space or adhere to the anterior lens surface. They are rarely visually significant.

Heterochromia iridis, or asymmetry in the color of the iris, if isolated, is visually insignificant. Heterochromia may occur in

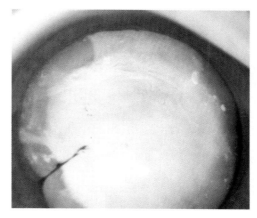
FIG. 19.73 Total cataract with no visible fundus details.

DIFFERENTIAL DIAGNOSIS OF LEUKOCORIA

Angiomatosis retinae
Cataracts
Coats' disease
Colobomas
Congenital retinal fold
High myopia
Incontinentia pigmenti
Medulloepithelioma
Myelinated nerve fibers
Persistent hyperplastic primary vitreous
Retinal detachment
Retinal dysplasia
Retinoblastoma
Retinopathy of prematurity
Toxocariasis
Uveitis
Vitreous hemorrhage

FIG. 19.72

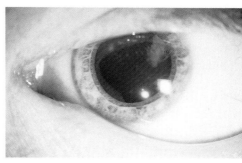
FIG. 19.74 Spoke-like cortical cataract of Down syndrome. The lens opacification does not affect the visual axis and is visually insignificant. Lens opacification such as this may rapidly progress and produce visual loss.

congenital Horner's syndrome, the eye with Horner's syndrome being lighter in color. Heterochromia may also occur secondary to inflammation, or following intraocular surgery or ocular trauma. Trauma may cause the affected iris to become darker than the fellow iris as late as many years after the incident (Fig. 19.70).

The iris may provide signs which aid in the diagnosis of systemic conditions. Patients with neurofibromatosis may have multiple small melanocytic iris nevi, Lisch nodules, on the surface of the iris (see Chapter 15, Neurology). These may be identified with magnification provided by the direct ophthalmoscope. Other ocular findings associated with neurofibromatosis include plexiform neurofibromas of the lids, thickened corneal nerves, congenital glaucoma, and optic nerve gliomas.

Patients, usually less than 1 year of age, with *juvenile xanthogranuloma (JXG)* may develop unilateral asymptomatic fleshy, yellow-brown tumors on the surface of the iris (Fig. 19.71). These vascular lesions bleed easily and may produce a spontaneous hyphema.

Brushfield spots are found in patients with Down syndrome. The spots consist of tiny areas of normal iris stroma which are surrounded by rings of mild iris hypoplasia. Brushfield spots give the iris a speckled appearance.

Lens

The lens may be affected by developmental, hereditary, syndrome-related, inflammatory, metabolic, or traumatic conditions. This can result in the development of a cataract, an opacification of the crystalline lens, which may be either partial or complete. The lens may also be dislocated from its supporting zonulae or subluxated.

CATARACTS

Leukocoria refers to the white pupillary reflex produced by reflection of light from a light-colored intraocular mass or structure. Several conditions of variable severity and prognosis produce leukocoria (Fig. 19.72). Examination with a penlight, the plus lens of a direct ophthalmoscope, or a slit-lamp biomicroscopy will help to differentiate lens opacification from other forms of leukocoria.

Cataracts have variable morphology. Those with opacification of the posterior aspect of the lens and a clear nucleus and anterior lens capsule may be difficult to differentiate from retinal detachment or retrolental membranes of retinopathy of prematurity.

Congenital or infantile cataracts may be unilateral or bilateral and the extent of opacification may be complete or partial (Fig. 19.73). Bilateral cataracts usually arise early in infancy and, if not treated early, may produce severe visual deprivation accompanied by poor fixation and nystagmus. Visually significant unilateral cataracts are associated with severe deprivation amblyopia and strabismus.

Opacification of a child's lens may be due to heredity (autosomal dominant), chromosomal disorders (Trisomy, 13, 18, and 21) (Fig. 19.74), inflammation (iritis and uveitis), infection (TORCH), metabolic disorders (galactosemia and disorders of calcium and phosphorous metabolism), exposure to toxins, vitamin deficiencies (Vitamins A and D), systemic syndromes

SYNDROMES ASSOCIATED WITH CATARACTS

Albright's hereditary osteodystrophy
Alport's syndrome
Cat-eye syndrome
Cerebro-oculo-facial-skeletal syndrome
Chondrodysplasia punctata (Conradi-
 Hünermann syndrome)
Cockayne's syndrome
Congenital ichthyosis
Conradi's syndrome
Craniofacial syndromes (Apert
 and Crouzon's syndromes)
Down syndrome (trisomy 21)
Edward's syndrome (trisomy 18)
Hallgren's syndrome
Hallermann-Streiff syndrome
Ichthyosis
Incontinentia pigmenti

Kneist syndrome
Lantieri syndrome
Lawrence-Moon-Bardet-Biedel syndrome
Lowe syndrome
Marinesco-Sjögren's syndrome
Marshall's syndrome
Myotonic dystrophy
Osteogensis imperfecta
Patau's syndrome (trisomy 13–15)
Progeria
Rothmund-Thompson syndrome
Robert syndrome
Rubinstein-Taybi syndrome
Smith-Lemli-Opitz syndrome
Stickler syndrome
Turner syndrome
Zellweger syndrome

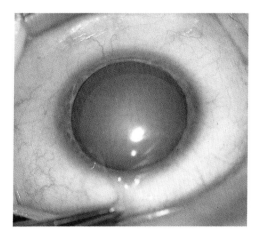

FIG. 19.76 A microspherophakic cataractous lens in rubella syndrome.

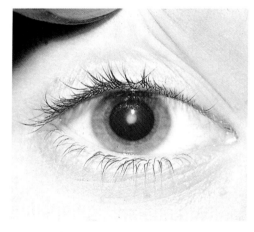

FIG. 19.77 Anterior polar cataract. This type of lens opacity is a developmental abnormality which in most cases remains stable and rarely affects vision.

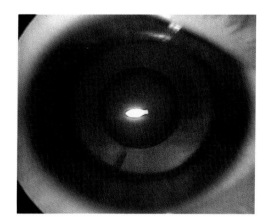

FIG. 19.78 Lamellar cataract with riders, surrounded by a clear cortex.

with cataracts (Fig. 19.75), ocular conditions producing retinal detachment, radiation exposure, and trauma. Roughly one third of pediatric cataracts are hereditary, one third are syndrome or disease related, and one third remain as "due to undetermined causes."

The presence of ocular anomalies will frequently identify a developmental defect as being the cause for the cataract. *Microphthalmia*, the globe being smaller than normal, may be caused by ocular disease or inflammation, or it may be present as a developmental defect (see Fig. 19.58). Eyes with persistent hyperplastic primary vitreous (PHPV) are usually microphthalmic and frequently have cataracts.

The morphology of the lens opacification may provide a clue to the etiology of a congenital cataract if opacification is not complete. During the process of development, the lens cells lay down fibers which grow out from the peripheral lens to the anterior and posterior lens surfaces. These will form

sutures. Because of this, the gestational age at the time of cataract development will determine the location of the opacity. For example, the nuclear cataracts of rubella syndrome (Fig. 19.76), indicate infection early in gestation, while a zonular or lamellar cataract represents an insult to the lens occurring later in lens development. A zonular or lamellar cataract is one with radial spokes of opacity either in the anterior or posterior lens substance. If the zonules coalesce, the term lamellar cataract is used.

Small central opacities on the anterior or posterior poles of the lens, polar cataracts, are developmental abnormalities which remain stable and rarely affect vision (Fig. 19.77). Lamellar or zonular cataracts have a normal, transparent central nucleus, an affected lamellar zone, and a clear outer layer of cortex. Riders or radial extensions frequently are present (Fig. 19.78). Zonular cataracts may be autosomal dominant, be associated with vitamin A and D deficiency, or follow hypocal-

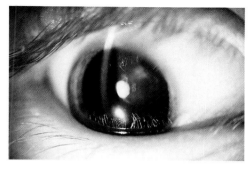

FIG. 19.79 Cataract of galactosemia. Early lens changes cause the nucleus of the lens to have an "oil droplet" configuration due to the accumulation of dulcitol, a metabolic product of galactose, within the lens. The resultant osmotic gradient draws water into the lens, producing the opacification. Early lens changes in galactosemia are reversible.

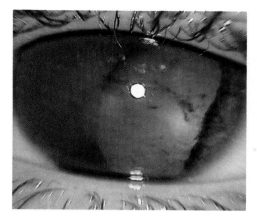

FIG. 19.80 A traumatic, dislocated cataractous lens.

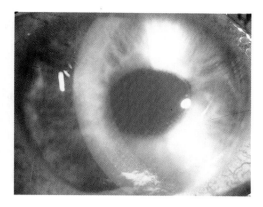

FIG. 19.81 Iritis with circumcorneal ciliary flush.

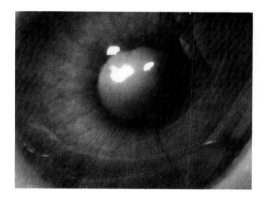

FIG. 19.82 Yellow cyclitic membrane behind a clear lens in a soft phthisical eye.

cemia. Multicolored flecks may be seen in hypoparathyroidism or myotonic dystrophy and an oil droplet configuration is seen in galactosemia (Fig. 19.79).

If a child's history is negative for trauma, the family history is unremarkable, the general physical examination fails to uncover a systemic syndrome or chromosomal abnormality, and ocular examination is not helpful in determining the etiology of a cataract, then a focused laboratory evaluation to determine the cause of the cataract may be undertaken. The most common metabolic disorders causing congenital cataracts are hypoglycemia and hypocalcemia. Laboratory evaluation for galactosemia and galactokinase deficiency should include blood tests for galactose and galactose-1-phosphate, as well as examination of the urine for reducing substances. Examination of the urine for protein and amino acids will identify patients with Lowe (oculo-cerebro-renal) syndrome and a urine nitroprusside test will diagnose homocystinuria. Screening tests for congenital TORCH infections and syphilis also should be performed.

Positional abnormalities of the lens may occur. A partial dislocation of the lens is referred to as subluxation. A dislocated lens, ectopia lentis, may cause a profound decrease in vision by producing a large refractive error and amblyopia. Ectopia lentis may be bilateral and inherited or it may be unilateral and due to trauma (Fig. 19.80).

Simple ectopia lentis is a bilateral, symmetric condition with an autosomal dominant inheritance pattern. Bilateral superotemporal lens dislocation is present in 50 to 80 percent of patients with Marfan syndrome. Ninety percent of patients with homocystinuria will have an inferior lens dislocation, and patients with the Weill-Marchesani syndrome may have dislocation of their microspherophakic lenses.

Uvea

Inflammation of the uveal tract (iris, ciliary body, and choroid) has many potential causes, including infections (toxoplasmosis, herpes zoster and simplex, and Lyme disease), collagen vascular disease (most frequently JRA and sarcoidosis), and trauma. In the majority of children, the etiologic agent cannot be determined. Advanced retinoblastoma may also present with signs that suggest uveitis.

Involvement of the iris alone (iritis or anterior uveitis) produces pain, ciliary injection (conjunctival redness in the circumlimbal area), tearing, photophobia, and decreased vision. Synechiae, adhesions between the iris and lens or peripheral cornea, may produce corectopia, an abnormally shaped pupil. Inflammatory reaction in the anterior chamber may be viewed with the aid of a slit-lamp as inflammatory cells and fibrin or protein (flare) in the aqueous fluid. If marked, this may give the eye a dull or "glassy" appearance (Fig. 19.81). Clumps of inflammatory cells may adhere to the posterior corneal surface forming keratic precipitates (KP).

Because iritis may be present without signs and symptoms, children with JRA should have periodic screening ophthalmic examinations. Children with polyarticular disease should be examined annually and those with positive antinuclear antibodies and pauciarticular disease, who are more likely to develop ocular complications, should be examined three to four times a year (see Chapter 8, Rheumatology).

Pars planitis or intermediate uveitis is an idiopathic, bilateral inflammation of the pars plana or pars ciliaris portions of the ciliary body. Symptoms include light sensitivity, "floaters," and blurring of vision. Inflammatory cells in the anterior vitreous can make visualization of the retina with the direct ophthalmoscope difficult. If the inflammation is severe, it may produce leukocoria. Most cases are self-limited; however, chronic courses with exacerbations and remissions may produce visual loss due to cataracts, optic nerve inflammation, and cystoid macular edema. Retinal detachment due to membrane formation and phthisis bulbi may occur in advanced cases (Fig.19.82).

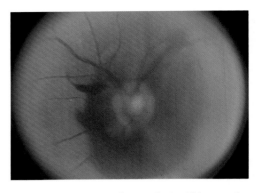

FIG. 19.83 Vitreous hemorrhage. Dispersed red blood cells in the vitreous have made it hazy. The diffraction of light will cause blurred vision. Fluid levels often are visible and collections of blood may appear to "float" within the eye.

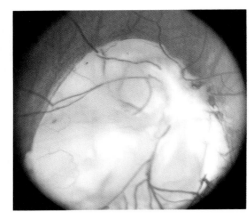

FIG. 19.84 Coloboma of optic nerve, retina, and choroid. Yellow-white sclera is visible,

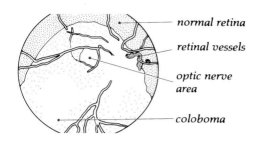

and retinal vessels can be seen coursing through the coloboma.

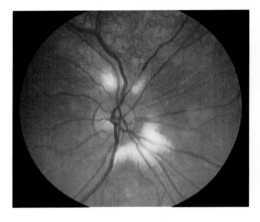

FIG. 19.85 Myelinated nerve fibers. Myelination of the optic nerve fibers may continue beyond the optic disc to include the retinal nerve fibers. This is visible as yellow-white flame-shaped patches oriented with the retinal nerve fibers. Myelinated nerve fibers may produce the clinical sign of leukocoria.

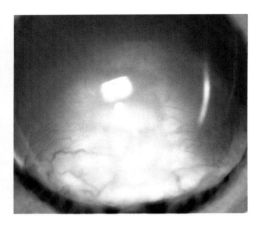

FIG. 19.86 Persistent hyperplastic primary vitreous presenting as a dense fibrovascular retrolental mass with microspherophakia,

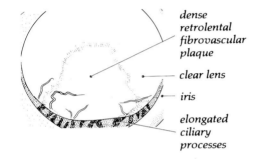

microphthalmia, and elongated ciliary processes.

Posterior uveitis (inflammation of the posterior vitreous, retina, and/or choroid) can be caused by infection but, frequently, the precise etiology is undetermined. Infection of the retina by protozoa, fungi, and viruses may produce an intense inflammatory response in the vitreous, rendering it hazy or opaque. Leukocoria may be produced if extensive retinal involvement is present.

Vitreous

VITREOUS HEMORRHAGE

Trauma, be it penetrating, concussive, or due to the shaken baby syndrome, is the most common cause of vitreous hemorrhage. Vitreous hemorrhage may occur with hemorrhagic disease of the newborn (hypoprothrombinemia) or in advanced stages of retinopathy of prematurity. Patients with a subarachnoid hemorrhage may develop vitreous hemorrhage (Terson's syndrome), and vitreous hemorrhage may also occur in patients with leukemia.

Blood in the vitreous, if located centrally or posteriorly, may be visible with the direct ophthalmoscope. If the vitreous is liquid, the hemorrhage may appear to "float" inside the eye (Fig. 19.83). Blood in the vitreous may produce leukocoria as it organizes and becomes yellow and then gray in color.

Retina

DEVELOPMENTAL ABNORMALITIES

Colobomas

Retinal colobomas are caused by a defect in closure of the embryonal fissure of the optic cup. They may occur unilaterally or bilaterally. Large colobomas are manifest as an absence of the retina and choroid with or without marked excavation of the optic disc (Fig. 19.84). There is usually a ring of pigment around the coloboma. Leukocoria may be produced by the yellow-white reflection of the underlying sclera. Using a direct ophthalmoscope, an occasional vessel may be seen bridging the area of the coloboma. The coloboma and retina will be at a different plane of focus when visualized with the ophthalmoscope.

Colobomas may occur in otherwise normal eyes or in association with microphthalmia or retinal detachment. If the optic

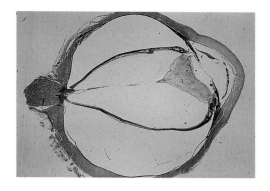

FIG. 19.87 Pathologic section of persistent hypoplastic primary vitreous (PHPV). (Courtesy Dr. B.L. Johnson)

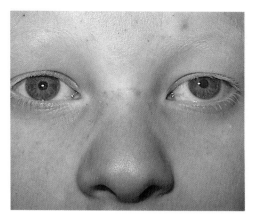

FIG. 19.88 Albinism, characterized by white hair, pale skin, and translucent irides.

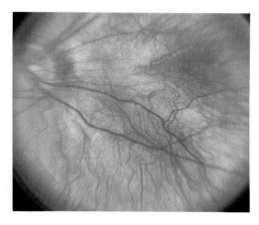

FIG. 19.89 Ophthalmoscopic view of a patient with albinism demonstrates a pale fundus, poor macular development, and prominent choroidal vasculature.

disc and macula are not involved, visual acuity may be normal. Colobomas may be inherited as isolated anomalies or they may be associated with chromosomal defects (trisomy 13) or other syndrome-related entities (CHARGE association).

Myelinated Nerve Fibers

Prior to birth, myelination of the optic nerve begins in the central nervous system, progresses peripherally, and usually stops at the optic disc before birth. Myelination may continue beyond the optic disc to include the retinal nerve fiber layer. Once completed, the process remains stationary. Myelinated fibers are oriented with the retinal nerve fibers and are easily seen with the direct ophthalmoscope as yellow-white flame shaped patches overlying the sensory retina and choroid (Fig. 19.85). The macula is rarely involved and normal vision is usually present, although scotomas corresponding to the areas of myelination may be found on visual field examination.

Persistent Hyperplastic Primary Vitreous (PHPV)

PHPV occurs as a unilateral defect in the involution of the primary vitreous during the seventh month of gestation. Eyes with PHPV are usually microphthalmic. PHPV may be associated with cataracts, intraocular hemorrhage, glaucoma, and retinal detachment. Eyes with advanced PHPV can become phthisical (Figs. 19.86, 19.87).

Albinism

Albinism refers to conditions involving deficiencies of melanin in the skin and/or eye (Fig. 19.88). The loss of pigmentation may predominantly affect the eye (ocular albinism), be generalized to the skin and eye (oculocutaneous albinism), or occur in conjunction with a systemic syndrome such as Chediak-Higashi or Hermansky-Pudlak syndrome.

Ocular albinism occurs as an X-linked or autosomal recessive trait. Photophobia is frequently a symptom. The loss of cutaneous pigmentation may be mild. Patients will have iris transillumination defects in which the red reflex is seen through multiple punctate defects in the iris. Absence of pigment in the retinal pigment epithelium layer of the retina will make the fundus appear a lighter yellow-orange color than usual. The macula and fovea are hypoplastic and visual acuity is decreased (Fig. 19.89). Albinism must be included in the differential diagnosis of an infant with nystagmus.

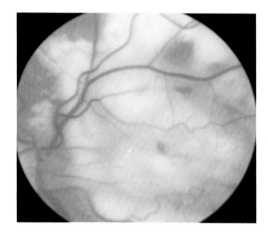

FIG. 19.90 Ophthalmoscopic manifestations of Coats' disease. Peripheral telangiectasis along the course of the retinal veins leads to exudation giving the retina a yellow/white appearence

Ocular pigmentary abnormalities may also occur in a milder form, albanoidism. Such patients have iris transillumination defects, fundus hypopigmentation, and photophobia. Their maculas, however, are less severely affected or are normal. Because of this, nystagmus is uncommon and visual acuity is normal or only minimally reduced. Albanoidism is inherited as an autosomal dominant with incomplete penetrance.

Coats' Disease (Retinal Telangiectasis)

Coats' disease occurs unilaterally in males younger than 18 years of age. The most common age at diagnosis is between 8 and 10 years. Peripheral retinal vessel telangiectasis and aneurysmal dilation lead to extensive areas of exudation, giving the retina a yellow-white appearance which may produce leukocoria (Fig. 19.90). The macula is a common site for exudation to collect; when this occurs, visual loss is profound.

Retinitis Pigmentosa

Retinitis pigmentosa (RP) is a pigmentary retinopathy characterized by visual field loss, night blindness, and a depressed or extinct electroretinogram (ERG). Symptoms of visual loss may be present in childhood, but usually do not become apparent until the second or third decade of life. Poor night vision is the earliest symptom, followed by progressive loss of peripheral visual field and, finally, loss of central vision. The rate of progression of visual loss varies for each pedigree and may ultimately be mild or severe.

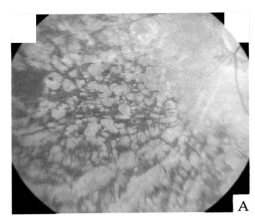

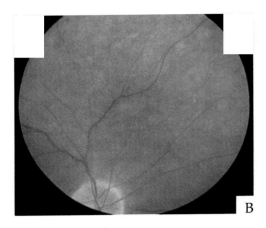

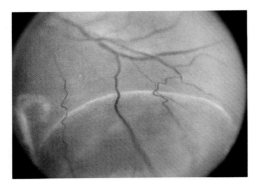

FIG. 19.91 **A,** retinitis pigmentosa, characterized by retinal pigment disposition, narrow arterioles, and a pale disc. **B,** early fundus signs of retinitis pigmentosa. The optic disc has a waxy pallor and the retinal arterial system is sclerotic. Early pigment deposition is seen in the midperipheral retina (top). In children pigmentary changes may not be as advanced or as noticeable as in adults.

FIG. 19.92 Retinal detachment. The inferior retina is detached and a demarcation line between the attached and detached retina is visible. Fluid beneath the detached sensory retina will shift with movement of the eye and cause the detached retina to move or undulate.

The retinal pigment epithelial changes include deposition of pigment in a perivascular pattern. Pigment deposition in the midperipheral retina gives a characteristic "bone spicule" pattern late in the course of the disease (Fig. 19.91A). Early in the disease, the optic nerve may have a waxy pallor and the retinal arteries may be attenuated (Fig. 19.91B).

Systemic disease entities are associated with RP. Patients with sensorineural hearing loss should be examined for the associated presence of retinitis pigmentosa (Usher's syndrome and Hallgren's syndrome). Renal diseases including Fanconi's syndrome, cystinuria, cystinosis, and oxalosis may be associated with pigmentary retinal changes, as may the mucopolysaccharidoses, Refsum's disease, and syphilis.

RETINAL DETACHMENT

Trauma is the most common cause of retinal detachment in children. Leukocoria occurs when the detached retina is in apposition to the lens. Retinal detachments, if located posteriorly, may be viewed with the direct ophthalmoscope as elevations of the retina (Fig. 19.92). The detached retina may move or undulate with eye movement.

RETINOPATHY OF PREMATURITY

Retinopathy of prematurity (ROP) is characterized by abnormalities in the developing retinal vascular system. Mild forms affect the peripheral retina at the junction between the vascularized and immature avascular retina. These changes can be observed using an indirect ophthalmoscope. Severe forms produce fibrovascular proliferations that extend into the vitreous and cause traction which may lead to detachment of the retina (Fig. 19.93). A white fibrovascular mass may occupy the retrolental space (retrolental fibroplasia) and produce leukocoria.

In 75 percent of patients, ROP is bilateral and symmetric. Retinopathy of prematurity primarily affects the ill, premature infant whose birthweight in less than 1,600 g or who has been exposed to more than 30 days of supplemental oxygen. Because early phases of this disease are treatable, programs to screen neonates who are at risk for developing this condition are necessary.

RETINITIS AND RETINOCHOROIDITIS

Inflammation of the retina and choroid is most commonly the result of viral, protozoal, fungal, or bacterial infection. The final common pathway for recovery or resolution of retinal inflammation is the production of a pigmented chorioretinal scar. The characteristics and location of these scars will frequently be diagnostic for the infecting agent. In many cases, however, isolated chorioretinal scars will be present which do not suggest any particular disease.

A rare cause of retinochoriditis is sympathetic ophthalmia. Sympathetic ophthalmia occurs after an injury of one eye, the "exciting" eye, followed by a latent period and the development of uveitis in the uninjured eye, the "sympathizing" eye. Sympathetic ophthalmia may occur as early as 10 days after the original injury but may also have a delayed onset, years after the incident. The etiology of sympathetic ophthalmia is unknown.

TORCH INFECTION
Toxoplasmosis

Toxoplasmosis, a protozoal infection of the retinal cells, is most often considered to be congenital in origin with transplacental transmission. Eighty percent of neonates severely affected by toxoplasmosis will have retinochoroiditis. Involvement is bilateral and often includes the macula. The retinal lesions may develop after birth and most are inactive when first diagnosed. These lesions characteristically occur as multifocal pigmented chorioretinal scars. Inactive lesions may reactivate anytime throughout life with active inflammation developing adjacent to areas of scarring. This is seen as a white fluffy response that may extend into the vitreous overlying the lesion (Fig. 19.94).

Rubella

Exposure to Rubella virus during the first trimester of pregnancy may result in an intrauterine infection manifested as the congenital rubella syndrome. Ocular findings include microphthalmia, microcornea, anterior uveitis, iris hypoplasia, nuclear or complete cataracts, corneal opacification, and glaucoma. The retinopathy of rubella syndrome is a diffuse "salt and pepper" retinopathy that develops early in childhood and

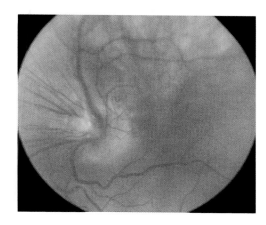

FIG. 19.93 Retrolental fibroplasia with temporal tugging of the disc.

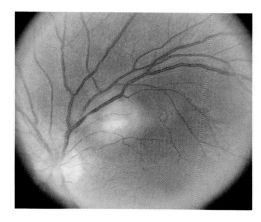

FIG. 19.94 Acute, recurrent, toxoplasmic chorioretinal inflammation adjacent to a healed pigmented lesion.

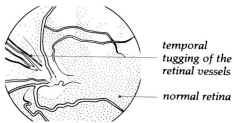

temporal tugging of the retinal vessels

normal retina

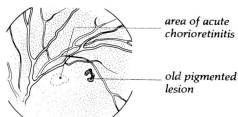

area of acute chorioretinitis

old pigmented lesion

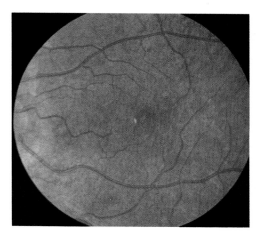

FIG. 19.95 Pigmentary retinopathy in rubella syndrome.

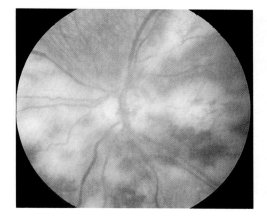

FIG. 19.96 Retinitis, with obvious hemorrhages and perivascular yellow-white exudates secondary to cytomegalic inclusion disease.

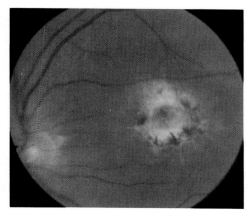

FIG. 19.97 A retinal toxocariasis lesion appears as a white elevated mass with surrounding pigmentation.

does not affect vision. The pigmentary changes may be similar in appearance to those of syphilis, retinitis pigmentosa and Leber's congenital amaurosis (Fig. 19.95).

Cytomegalovirus
Cytomegalovirus (CMV) infection produces a bilateral retinochoroiditis manifested as multiple, yellow-white, fluffy retinal lesions (Fig. 19.96). Hemorrhage is a prominent feature. Other ophthalmic manifestations include microphthalmia, uveitis, cataracts, optic disc atrophy, strabismus, and nystagmus.

CMV retinitis may be an opportunistic infection occurring in patients who are immunosuppressed due to immunodeficiency disorders or who are receiving immunosuppressive drugs. Retinal inflammation, edema, and hemorrhage may be extensive and rapidly progressive in these patients.

Herpes Simplex Virus
Herpes simplex virus (HSV) infection may involve the anterior segment of the eye, with conjunctivitis and/or keratitis, or, when disseminated in the perinatal period, retinochoroiditis.

Retinal involvement with disseminated HSV is severe, with extensive inflammatory reaction producing yellow-white exudates and retinal necrosis.

Syphilis
Congenital syphilis may cause bilateral chorioretinitis resulting in a "salt and pepper" fundus appearance. Differentiation of the retinopathy of congenital syphilis from retinitis pigmentosa may be difficult. Syphilis may also cause interstitial keratitis, anterior uveitis, glaucoma, and optic nerve atrophy.

Toxocariasis
Toxocara canis larvae infect children from 2 to 9 years of age. When the eye is involved a white, elevated chorioretinal granuloma develops (Fig. 19.97). Chronic unilateral uveitis with opacification of the vitreous overlying the granuloma may occur. Inflammation in ocular toxocariasis occurs only after the organism dies. Externally, the eye does not appear to be inflamed. With extensive inflammation, fibrotic preretinal membranes may develop and produce retinal detachment. Differentiation from retinoblastoma may be difficult.

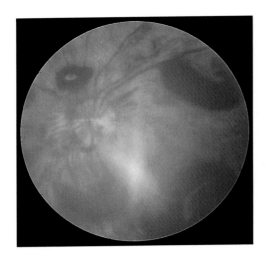

FIG. 19.98 Shaken baby syndrome. Multiple retinal hemorrhages are present in the posterior fundus. There are small flame-shaped hemorrhages within the nerve fiber layer that follow the pattern of the retinal vessels. More extensive areas of hemorrhage have broken through to the preretinal space and are seen as areas of blood that obscure the retina. A Roth spot, a hemorrhage with a white center, is visible just above the optic disc. The white reflection from the camera flash is visible due to dispersed RBCs within the vitreous.

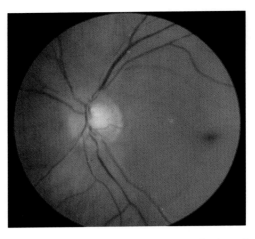

FIG. 19.99 Central retinal artery occlusion. A cherry-red spot is visible in the fovea. This sign is due to edema and opacification of the ganglion cell layer of the retina surrounding the fovea.

Calcification is rare in toxocariasis as opposed to retinoblastoma. The diagnosis is confirmed by enzyme linked immunosorbent assay (ELISA) for *Toxocara canis* on blood and/or intraocular fluid.

BACTERIAL ENDOCARDITIS

"Cotton-wool" spots frequently develop in patients with bacterial endocarditis and septic emboli. These represent infarction of the nerve fiber layer of the retina and appear as white, irregular lesions with indistinct borders. Cotton-wool spots may be seen in any condition that produces retinal ischemia, such as hypertension and diabetes, or in patients with AIDS. Intraretinal hemorrhages occur with septic emboli and are flame-shaped or dot-blot in nature. If the hemorrhage has a white center, from the accumulation of leukocytes, the term Roth spot is used. Roth spots are not specific for bacterial endocarditis. They may occur in leukemia or the shaken baby syndrome (Fig. 19.98). Conjunctival petechiae may be seen with septic embolic phenomenon; however, they may also be seen after a cardiovascular bypass procedure without infection.

Emboli to the eye may cause a central or branch retinal artery obstruction. Occlusion of the central retinal artery causes a sudden loss in vision, loss of the pupillary direct light reflex, absence of venous pulsations, and the development of a cherry-red spot in the fovea. Edema and opacification of the ganglion cell layer surrounding the fovea produces this sign (Fig. 19.99).

LEUKEMIA

Patients with acute lymphoblastic, myelogenous, or monocytic leukemia may develop flame-shaped intraretinal hemorrhages. These are usually visible with the direct ophthalmoscope. The presence of hemorrhage is not correlated with anemia or thrombocytopenia. Leukemic infiltration may also occur in the retina as a perivascular infiltrate, in the choroid, or in the optic disc producing disc swelling and a papilledemalike appearance. Leukemic involvement of the orbit may be difficult to distinguish from bacterial cellulitis.

DIABETES

The most common ocular finding in young diabetics is lenticular myopia. This occurs in patients who have had a rapid rise in blood glucose. Sorbitol accumulates within the lens as a metabolic product, increasing the lens osmolarity, thus causing the lens to swell and produce myopia. After the blood sugar returns to normal, myopia may continue to persist for several weeks. Children with diabetes rarely develop cataracts.

The earliest sign of background diabetic retinopathy (BDR) is the presence of microaneurysms (tiny discrete red spots). Small retinal hemorrhages, cotton-wool spots, venous dilatation, and hard exudates (small, discrete, yellow lesions) may also be seen. The occurrence of background diabetic retinopathy is related to the duration of diabetes and it is rarely seen within 3 years following diagnosis. The prevalence of retinopathy increases to 90 percent in patients who have had juvenile onset diabetes for greater than 15 years. Children do not develop the proliferative diabetic retinopathy which is seen in adults.

SICKLE CELL RETINOPATHY

The ocular abnormalities of the hemoglobinopathies are caused by intravascular sickling, hemostasis and thrombosis. Retinal findings occur in the peripheral fundus and are difficult to visualize with the direct ophthalmoscope. Retinal complications occur most frequently in patients with SC and S thal disease. Patients with sickle cell disease (Hb SS) are less frequently affected. The decreased hematocrit may provide protection to the retinal vasculature. Rarely, patients with the milder hemoglobinopathies, AS and AC, may have retinal findings.

Retinal findings may be divided into nonproliferative and proliferative changes. Proliferative changes include arteriolar occlusions which lead to arteriole-venous anastomosis causing areas of retinal nonperfusion. Neovascularization occurs at the edge of these areas of nonperfusion, in the form of a gossamer vascular network (a seafan), and often leads to vitreous hemorrhage, traction, and retinal detachment (Fig. 19.100A). The disease process is similar to that seen in retinopathy of prematurity.

Nonproliferative changes include refractile or iridescent deposits, black sunburst lesions, and salmon patch hemorrhages. Refractile deposits are sequelae of old reabsorbed hemorrhages. Sunburst lesions are areas of perivascular retinal pigment epithelial hypertrophy and pigment migration (Fig.

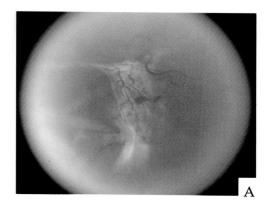
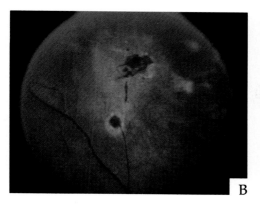
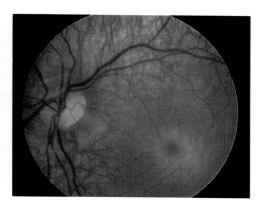

FIG. 19.100 Sickle cell retinopathy. **A,** neo-vascularization or growth of fragile blood vessels into the vitreous in the midperipheral retina. The white fibrous tissue present is due to the proliferation of fibroglial elements. This produces traction on the retina, which

may subsequently lead to retinal detachment. **B,** the black sunburst lesions are areas of perivascular retinal pigment epithelial hypertrophy with pigment migration. This finding is an example of nonproliferative change.

FIG. 19.101 Tay-Sachs disease. Because the perifoveal area has many retinal ganglion cells and the fovea has none, the fovea retains its orange-red color but it is surrounded by retina that is whitish in color. This produces the "cherry-red spot" in the macula.

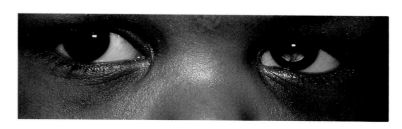

FIG. 19.102 Leukocoria. The patient's left eye has a white pupillary reflex produced by reflection of light from a retinoblastoma. Leukocoria is the most common presenting sign (60 percent) of retinoblastoma.

19.100B). Salmon patch lesions represent areas of intraretinal hemorrhage. Parafoveal capillaries and arterioles may become occluded and produce decreased visual acuity in sickle cell retinopathy. Segmentation of the conjunctival blood vessels produces comma-shaped capillaries ("comma sign").

METABOLIC DISEASES

The *mucopolysaccharidoses (MPS)* are syndromes caused by inherited defects in the lysosomal enzymes which degrade acid mucopolysaccharide. All of the mucopolysaccharidoses are transmitted as autosomal recessive traits except Type 2 (Hunter's), which is X-linked recessive. A common ocular finding is retinal pigmentary degeneration, which closely resembles retinitis pigmentosa. Optic atrophy also occurs, as does corneal clouding due to stromal infiltration.

The *sphingolipidoses* are caused by a deficiency of the lysosomal enzymes responsible for the degeneration of sphingolipids. Tay-Sachs disease (GM 2 Type 1 gangliosidosis) and Nieman-Pick disease are the two most common sphingolipidoses. Sphingolipids will accumulate in the retinal ganglion cells, giving a whitish appearance to the retina. Because the parafoveal area has many retinal ganglion cells and the fovea none, the fovea has its normal orange red color, whereas the retina peripheral to the fovea is white. This produces a "cherry-red spot" in the macula (Fig. 19.101).

The *mucolipidoses* are caused by abnormal glycoprotein metabolism. These have clinical findings of some of the sphingolipidoses and some of the mucopolysaccharoidoses. The ocular findings include corneal epithelial edema, retinal pigmentary degeneration, macular cherry-red spots, and optic atrophy.

Cystinosis represents a defective transport mechanism for cystine within the lysosomes, which cause intralysosomal accumulation of cystine. Patients develop "salt and pepper" changes of the retinal pigment epithelium and areas of patchy

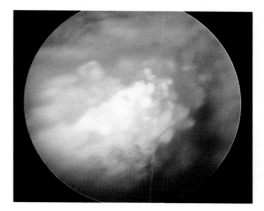

FIG. 19.103 Retinoblastoma. The tumor mass of retinoblastoma usually is elevated and yellow or white in color. Dilated feeding vessels of the tumor may be visible. Seeding into the vitreous from the tumor may produce a cloudy vitreous.

depigmentation with irregularly distributed pigment clumps. These changes do not produce loss of vision. Photophobia is due to the accumulation of corneal crystals.

RETINOBLASTOMA

Retinoblastoma is the most common intraocular malignancy of childhood. It occurs with a frequency of between 1 in 14,000 to 1 in 20,000 births. The most common age of diagnosis is between 1 and 1½ years with 90 percent of cases presenting prior to age 3 years. The most common presenting signs of retinoblastoma are leukocoria (60 percent) and strabismus (22 percent) (Fig. 19.102). One third of cases are bilateral. The tumor may present as an elevated, round, white or yellow mass (Fig. 19.103). Retinoblastoma may be multicentric, with several tumor masses arising within the same eye. Seeding into the vitreous may occur, producing a cloudy vitreous. A frequent feature of retinoblastoma is the presence of calcification within the mass.

Great advances have occurred in the understanding of the genetics of retinoblastoma. Retinoblastoma may be transmitted in an autosomal dominant inheritance pattern. Sixty per-

FIG. 19.104
Swinging flashlight test.

MARCUS GUNN PUPIL

To Perform Test:
Shine a bright light into each pupil for about 3-4 seconds. Alternate back and forth. Look for pupil to dilate, instead of constrict, with light.

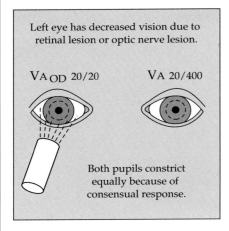

Left eye has decreased vision due to retinal lesion or optic nerve lesion.

VA OD 20/20   VA 20/400

Both pupils constrict equally because of consensual response.

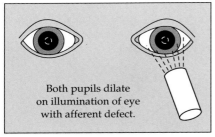

Both pupils dilate on illumination of eye with afferent defect.

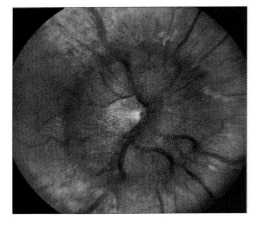

Fig. 19.105 Acute papilledema, characterized by blurred disc edges, an absent physiologic cup, and intraretinal exudates.

Optic Nerve

The optic nerve relays information from each eye to the brain. Its function is assessed by measuring visual acuity, visual fields, color vision, and the pupillary response. Visualization and assessment of the morphology of the optic disc with the direct ophthalmoscope provides valuable information regarding the function of the nerve.

COLOR VISION

Change in color vision, in particular the ability to perceive red, is an early feature seen in disorders that compromise the function of the optic nerve. Patients may complain of subjective changes in color perception or they may demonstrate defects in color vision on objective tests.

An easy test to assess color vision is to judge color comparison between the two eyes. The patient is asked to look at a red object first with one eye, then with the other, and is asked whether it is more red with one eye or the other. A subjective desaturation of red in one eye is an indication of dyschromatopsia and a potential optic nerve disorder. If the patient reports that the object is only 50 percent as red to one eye as compared to the other the results would be recorded as a red desaturation of 50 percent. In children it is valuable to present the object to the "normal eye" first with the question "If this is $1.00 of red, how much red is it now?" offering a comparison with the fellow eye. A similar comparison may be performed for brightness by shining a light first into one eye and then into the other. The sense of brightness will also be decreased in the presence of optic nerve disease. Formal assessment of color vision is performed using color plates such as the Hardy-Rand-Rittler or Ishihara color plates. Patients with heritable congenital color vision defects will be equally affected in both eyes. Patients with asymmetric optic nerve disease (optic neuritis, tumor, toxic optic neuropathy) will have asymmetrically decreased color vision, especially for the red hues.

PUPILS

Assessment of the pupils for size, shape, position and reactivity is an important part of the neurologic and ophthalmic evaluation. Neurologic abnormalities that effect the pupil include defects of the afferent pathway (the optic nerve and visual system), the parasympathetic pathway (for pupillary constriction), and the sympathetic pathway (for pupillary dilation).

Afferent Pupillary Defects

In a normal patient, shining a penlight in one eye causes both pupils to constrict. Pupillary constriction in the illuminated eye is the direct response and the constriction in the fellow eye is the consensual response. The pupils are normally equal in size even if one eye is blind; each eye receives equal pupillary innervation.

The swinging flashlight test is used to assess optic nerve function (Fig. 19.104). If an afferent pupillary defect (APD) is present, the term Marcus Gunn pupil is used. A penlight is used to illuminate one eye and then the other. The pupil of the illuminated eye is observed. If both eyes have equal afferent input, then illumination of either eye should produce equal constriction of the pupils. Normally, after shining a light in one eye the response will be initial constriction of both pupils followed by a small dilation. If the light is then swung quickly to the fellow eye the response will be the same. When there is a decrease in afferent input for pupillary constriction on one

cent of patients with the disease have a family history of retinoblastoma. Penetrance is high (60 to 90 percent) but incomplete. Sporadic cases occur as either somatic mutations in 75 percent of patients or as germinal mutations which may be passed on to offspring. These sporadic cases are almost always unilateral and the hereditary forms are usually bilateral; however, a patient with a unilateral tumor may have heritable disease. Current research is making it possible to determine which patients with unilateral tumors have the hereditary form of the disease and which patients do not (see Chapter 1, Genetics).

side, when the light is switched to the affected eye, constriction will either be absent or decreased and the pupils will dilate. The critical observation is that when the affected eye is illuminated a gradual dilation of the pupils occurs as compared to the response of the normal eye. It is important to have the patient maintain fixation on a distant object since accommodation will cause constriction of the pupils and may lead to misinterpretation of the findings.

An afferent pupillary defect (APD) indicates disease affecting the optic nerve. Unilateral or bilaterally asymmetric optic nerve disease will always cause a relative afferent pupillary defect. Mild optic nerve disease producing minimal or no objectively measurable decrease in visual acuity will still produce an APD, whereas a retinal defect must be profound in order to produce an APD. Afferent pupillary defects are not seen with dense cataracts, refractive errors, cortical lesions or functional visual loss. Amblyopia may produce a subtle APD.

Anisocoria

Lesions of the parasympathetic or sympathetic system cause pupillary constriction or dilation and produce pupils that are unequal in size, anisocoria, if unilateral or asymmetric. Pupillary involvement in third nerve palsy is usually accompanied by ptosis and disturbances in ocular motility. In cases of brain stem herniation and basil meningitis, however, pupillary dilation may be the only sign of the third nerve palsy. Pharmacologic mydriasis may occur with minimal exposure to atropine, cyclopentolate, or other parasympatholytic agents. Pharmacologic miosis will occur with phospholine iodide or pilocarpine. Pharmacologic testing with 1 percent pilocarpine is useful for differentiating pharmacologic mydriasis from third cranial nerve palsy; pupillary constriction will occur in third nerve palsy and will not occur with pharmacologic mydriasis.

A lesion at any point along the sympathetic pathway for pupillary constriction results in Horner's syndrome. The classic triad of findings includes ptosis, miosis, and anhidrosis. The anisocoria of Horner's syndrome is more apparent in dim illumination and the affected pupil will show a lag in dilation upon dimming of the lights. The light and near pupillary reactions are intact. Paresis of Mueller's muscle of the lid leads to the mild upper lid ptosis. The lower eyelid on the affected side may rest 1 mm higher than the fellow lid and the narrowed palpebral fissure gives the appearance of enophthalmos (see Fig. 19.70). Anhidrosis of the ipsilateral side of the body, side of the face, or forehead may be present depending upon the site of the innervation defect. A characteristic of congenital Horner's syndrome is the development of iris heterochromia with the affected iris being lighter in color.

The sympathetic pathway for pupillary constriction involves three neurons. The location of first-order neuron lesions is in the brain stem and spinal cord, examples being cervical trauma or demyelinating disease. Preganglionic, or second-order neuron lesions, occur within the chest or neck (e.g., neuroblastoma arising in the sympathetic chain). Congenital Horner's syndrome caused by birth trauma to the brachial plexus is another cause for a second-order neuron lesion. Third-order neuron lesions, postganglionic in reference to the superior cervical ganglion, are usually benign; however, extracranial or intracranial tumors of the nasopharynx or cavernous sinus may produce such lesions. More common causes for a postganglionic Horner's syndrome are migraine variants such as cluster headache.

Physiologic Anisocoria

Approximately 20 percent of the population has a perceptible anisocoria. The degree of anisocoria may vary from day to day but usually the difference in pupil size is 1 mm or less. The magnitude of anisocoria remains the same in bright or dim illumination; however, in some cases the anisocoria may be more apparent in dim light than in bright light, thereby simulating Horner's syndrome. Differentiating physiologic anisocoria from Horner's syndrome may be difficult. In physiologic anisocoria, there is no dilation lag. Pupils with physiologic anisocoria dilate after the instillation of 4 percent cocaine, whereas a Horner's pupil will fail to dilate.

Optic Neuritis

Inflammation of the optic nerve may occur either as a papillitis, referring to the intraocular form in which optic disc swelling is present, or as a retrobulbar neuritis, in which the optic disc appears normal and inflammation of the optic nerve occurs posterior to the globe. Vision loss may be sudden and profound and accompanied by complaints of pain in or behind the eye which may be accentuated by movement of the eyes. An afferent pupillary defect will be present if the condition is unilateral or if it is bilateral and asymmetric. Visual fields will usually show a cecocentral scotoma, an area of vision loss located in the central visual field.

The optic disc, if affected, may show swelling of the peripapillary nerve fiber layer and elevation. Small vessels at the optic disc margin may hemorrhage or become obscured by edema.

Optic neuritis in children is frequently bilateral and usually follows mumps, measles, chicken pox, or meningoencephalitis. Collagen vascular disease, particularly SLE and sarcoidosis, may be associated with optic neuritis. Syphilis and tuberculosis also cause optic neuritis. Visual acuity gradually improves one to four weeks after onset and usually returns to normal over several months.

PAPILLEDEMA

Increased intracranial pressure (ICP) is transmitted to the optic nerves via the CSF and subarachnoid space and causes papilledema. The axoplasmic flow from the retinal ganglion cells to the cells in the lateral geniculate nucleus is blocked and causes the optic disc to swell. The degree of disc swelling may be asymmetric; however, increased intracranial pressure rarely causes papilledema in only one eye. Ophthalmoscopic signs include blurring of the disc margin and disc edema. The disc may be hyperemic due to telangiectasia of the superficial capillaries on the disc and small hemorrhages may appear on the disc margin (Fig. 19.105). Visual acuity is normal unless hemorrhage and edema involve the macula. Patients complain of transient obscurations of vision. The visual fields may show an enlarged blind spot and the pupillary response and color vision are normal.

If papilledema is chronic, elevation of the optic disc may persist but the hemorrhages and exudates seen in the acute phase resolve. When the condition is prolonged, optic nerve atrophy will occur.

PSEUDOPAPILLEDEMA

Pseudopapilledema occurs in eyes with high hyperopia or optic disc drusen (see Fig. 19.9). The disc is not hyperemic, the vessels of the disc margin remain visible, and there is no nerve fiber layer swelling. There may be anomalous branching and

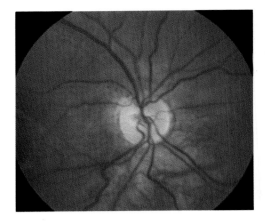

FIG. 19.106 *Optic atrophy, characterized by a sharply demarcated, pale yellow-white disc, with an absence of small vessels and disc substance.*

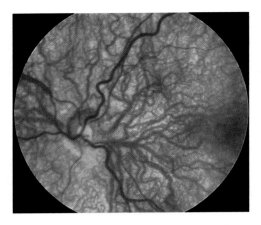

FIG. 19.107 *Optic nerve hypoplasia. A pigment crescent surrounds the hypoplastic nerve. This corresponds to the scleral opening for a normal-sized optic nerve and is termed the "double ring sign." In this patient the pattern of the retinal vasculature also is abnormal, as is the retinal pigmentation.*

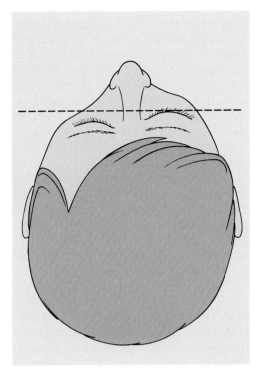

FIG. 19.108 *Blowout fracture of inferior orbital wall and dislocation of zygoma (left side).*

tortuosity of the retinal vessels and the physiologic cup is usually absent. The disc borders may be irregular. Hemorrhages, exudate, cotton-wool spots, and venous congestion do not occur. Spontaneous venous pulsations are not present in 20 percent of the normal population. If they are present, they are an indication that the disc swelling is pseudopapilledema and not caused by increased intracranial pressure. Central visual acuity is normal.

OPTIC DISC ATROPHY

Optic nerve atrophy causes the optic disc to lose its reddish-orange color. The lamina cribrosa may become visible with enlargement of the optic cup, leaving a "pinholed" appearance (Fig. 19.106). As the disease process continues, the disc eventually becomes white in color, visual acuity decreases and visual field defects emerge.

Optic atrophy may occur as a sequela of papilledema, optic neuritis, compressive lesions of the optic nerve or chiasm, trauma, hereditary retinal disease, or glaucoma. Optic atrophy may also be inherited as a recessive or dominant trait. Atrophy may occur as a component of a generalized neurologic condition, such as Behr's optic atrophy with cerebellar ataxia, hypotonia, and mental retardation. Leber's optic atrophy occurs in late adolescence or early adulthood, with acute disc edema being rapidly followed by progressive bilateral optic atrophy.

DEVELOPMENTAL ANOMALIES OF THE OPTIC NERVE

Developmental anomalies of the optic nerve include colobomas, tilted discs, and optic nerve hypoplasia (see Figs. 19.9, 19.84). The level of visual acuity is related to the type and extent of the defect.

Hypoplasia of the optic nerve occurs either unilaterally or bilaterally. The optic disc is smaller than normal and will have a yellow-white ring which corresponds to the scleral opening for a normal-sized optic nerve. The term "double ring sign" is

used to describe the ring with its surrounding pigment crescent. The retinal vessels are normal in size but may appear crowded as they leave the optic disc (Fig. 19.107). Visual acuity will be related to the degree of hypoplasia and an afferent pupillary defect may be present if the degree of involvement is asymmetric. Optic nerve hypoplasia is associated with midline central nervous system abnormalities, including absence of the septum pellucidum (DeMorsier's syndrome). Children with optic nerve hypoplasia should be examined for abnormalities in pituitary and hypothalamic function.

Orbit

Clinical signs of orbital disease are proptosis and restriction in ocular motility, compression of the optic nerve, optic disc swelling, changes in refraction, and retinal striae. Retinal striae appear as radial lines on the retinal surface and are caused by compression of posterior portion of the globe.

Orbital disease or trauma may cause orbital asymmetry with displacement of the globe (Fig. 19.108). Posterior (enophthalmos) or anterior (exophthalmos) displacement of the globe in orbital disease may be subtle. Comparison of the position of the globes in relation to the lateral orbital rims, looking especially for asymmetry, is a valuable clinical test. The Hertel exophthalmometer is an instrument used to compare the position of the globes in relation to the lateral orbital rim (Fig. 19.109). Palpation of the globes over closed eyelids, gently retropulsing the globe into the orbit, may reveal the character of an orbital mass. Ocular rotations are tested looking for restrictions in motility. Other adjuncts to the clinical examination include A and B scan ultrasonography and computerized tomography, and magnetic resonance imaging of the orbit.

The most common orbital disease in childhood is cellulitis (see Chapter 22, Otolaryngology). Capillary hemangioma and

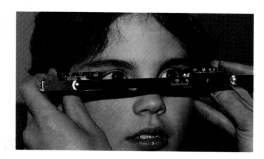

FIG. 19.109 The Hertel exophthalmometer measures the anterior to posterior distance from the corneal surface to the lateral orbital rim. A base measurement, the distance between the two lateral orbital rims, is recorded so that progression or regression can be determined by comparable serial measurements.

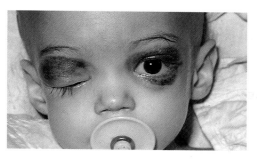

FIG. 19.110 Neuroblastoma. Neuroblastoma metastatic to the orbit may present with an abrupt onset of unilateral or bilateral proptosis and ecchymosis of the eyelids. Neuroblastoma is the most common lesion to metastasize to the orbit in childhood.

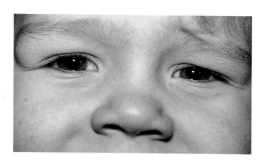

FIG. 19.111 Dermoid cyst. These cysts present as smooth, painless, mobile, subcutaneous, round or oval masses. Dermoid cysts are most frequently located in the lateral brow area adjacent to the zygomaticofrontal suture. Although benign, if they are ruptured by trauma, an intense inflammatory reaction with scarring in the area may occur.

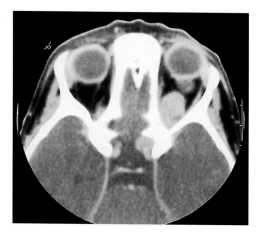

FIG. 19.112 Optic nerve glioma. Its presence may cause a gradual onset of painless proptosis. Children seldom complain of monocular visual loss, and the discovery of a profound loss of vision may be the presenting sign of an optic nerve glioma. In children, optic nerve gliomas are benign lesions which may, however, extend to the optic chiasm or intracranially.

lymphangioma are the most common benign primary orbital tumors of childhood. Orbital capillary hemangiomas present shortly after birth, enlarge over the first 6 months of life and then begin to regress. Lymphangiomas may involve the conjunctiva, lids, or orbit. These tumors may rapidly enlarge during upper respiratory tract infections. Sudden enlargement may occur after hemorrhage within the lesion.

Rhabdomyosarcoma is the most common primary orbital malignancy in childhood. This tumor should be a consideration in any child between the ages of 7 and 8 years who has rapidly progressing unilateral proptosis. The tumor mass may be palpable in the upper eyelid area or it may be located deeper in the orbit.

The most common metastatic lesion to the orbit in childhood is neuroblastoma. This tumor presents with an abrupt onset of proptosis and ecchymosis which may be bilateral (Fig. 19.110). Metastasis in neuroblastoma typically occurs late in the course of the disease when the primary tumor can easily be detected in the abdomen.

Dermoid and epidermoid cysts are relatively common. These benign masses are usually located anterior to the orbital septum but may extend posteriorly into the orbit. These cysts present as smooth, painless, freely movable round or oval masses and are usually located in the lateral brow area, adjacent to the zygomaticofrontal suture (Fig. 19.111). They may, however, be found in close proximity to any bony suture. These cysts contain dermal and epidermal elements that have become isolated from the skin during the course of embryonic development. If ruptured by trauma, an intense inflammatory reaction occurs.

Optic nerve gliomas are tumors that occur in children younger than 10 years of age. One third of children will have a history of neurofibromatosis. The presenting sign may be loss of vision or painless proptosis. An afferent pupillary defect and optic atrophy are usually present. Papilledema may also occur. Strabismus may be present due to decreased visual acuity (Fig. 19.112).

Plexiform neurofibromas are also seen in association with neurofibromatosis. They occur within the orbit or within the upper lid tissue. This will cause a fullness and ptosis of the lateral portion of the eyelid causing an "S-shaped" upper lid deformity.

Orbital pseudotumor is a unilateral or bilateral orbital inflammatory process affecting the structures within the orbit. Children with pseudotumor will have signs of headache, fever, lethargy, orbital pain, proptosis, lid erythema, conjunctival injection, and restricted ocular motility causing diplopia. The extraocular muscles and their tendons may be thickened. Orbital pseudotumor is a benign condition; however, recurrent tumor with scarring and fibrosis may cause restriction of ocular motility and optic nerve atrophy. Orbital pseudotumor must be differentiated from leukemia. The most common form of leukemia that affects the orbit is acute lymphoblastic leukemia.

OCULAR TRAUMA

In the evaluation of children with orbital or periocular trauma, one must presume that a serious ocular injury has occurred even if only minimal external signs exist. Prior to any evalua-

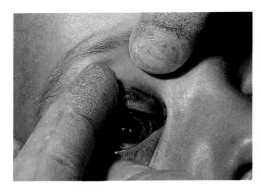

FIG. 19.113 Canalicular laceration. This patient experienced a laceration of the upper canaliculus. Simple apposition of the wound edges in this case will not approximate the cut ends of the canaliculus. Silastic tubes are used to splint the canaliculus during the healing process.

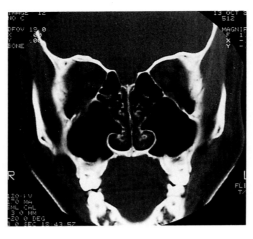

FIG. 19.114 Blowout fracture at the right orbit (coronal CT scan). Protruding through the fracture in the orbital floor into the maxillary sinus is orbital fat. The inferior rectus muscle is potentially entrapped within the fracture site.

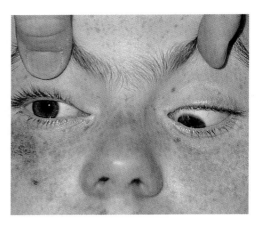

FIG. 19.115 Blowout fracture of the right orbit leading to the inability to depress the right eye.

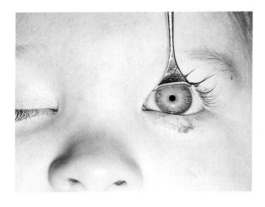

FIG. 19.116 A Desmarre lid retractor may be used to gently open the eyelids of an uncooperative child or in cases of trauma or preseptal cellulitis in which lid swelling makes opening of the lids for globe examination difficult.

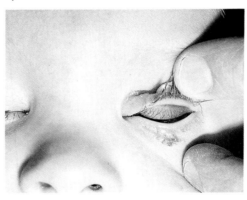

FIG. 19.117 The upper eyelid may be easily everted by placing a cotton swab at the upper edge of the tarsal plate. The lashes are then gently grasped and pulled anteriorly and upward to evert the lid over the cotton swab. The tarsal conjunctiva may be inspected for the presence of a foreign body.

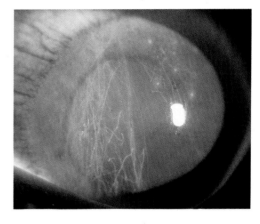

FIG. 19.118 Corneal abrasions stained with fluorescein dye and viewed under blue light. The abrasions appear green in the area of corneal epithelial loss.

tion on manipulation of the patient, an assessment of visual acuity must be performed. This provides information regarding the severity and nature of the trauma, as well as recording data which may be of medicolegal importance.

The anatomy of a laceration of the eyelid will dictate the measure required for repair. The presence of orbital fat indicates penetration of the lid and entrance into the orbit. Additionally, evaluation of the laceration must include the degree of involvement of the lid margin, loss of tissue, injury to the medial and lateral canthal tendons and injury to the canaliculi of the nasolacrimal drainage system (Fig. 19.113). Each of the above injuries requires a special technique for repair.

Patients who have sustained blunt orbital trauma should be evaluated for a fracture of the orbital floor or the medial wall of the orbit. Signs of a fracture with entrapment of one of the extraocular muscles include enophthalmos, diplopia, restricted gaze, and paresthesias in the distribution of the infraorbital nerve. Fractures may be isolated to the floor or they may extend to the orbital rim (Fig. 19.114). If subcutaneous air or orbital emphysema is present, the fracture has permitted communication with the sinuses. Intraorbital edema or hemorrhage within extraocular muscle may also restrict ocular motility. The most commonly involved muscles are the inferior and medial rectus muscles (Fig. 19.115).

Conjunctival lacerations may appear greatly disproportionate to their degree of severity. On the other hand, a small penetration of the conjunctiva may indicate a penetrating injury to the globe.

The use of a topical anesthetic such as tetracaine or proparacaine will anesthetize the cornea and permit a close examination of the cornea and surrounding conjunctiva for foreign bodies. A Desmarre lid retractor may be helpful in exerting gentle pressure to open the lids of uncooperative children or if swelling of the lids makes examination difficult (Fig. 19.116). The lids may also be everted over a cotton swab to inspect the underside of the lids (Fig. 19.117). The presence of a foreign body under the upper eyelid will cause vertical epithelial abrasions on the underlying corneal surface (Fig. 19.118). Corneal abrasions cause extreme pain and photophobia. The use of sodium fluorescein dye applied to the conjunctival cul-de-sac and examination with a cobalt blue filtered light will aid in the

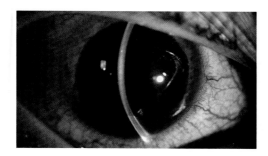

FIG. 19.119 Hyphema. Red blood cells within the anterior chamber have settled into the inferior anterior chamber angle.

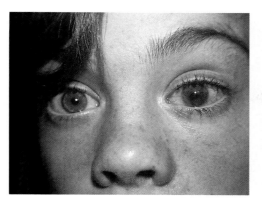

FIG. 19.120 A complication of hyphema is corneal blood staining. This patient's left cornea has an area of brown staining inferiorly due to prolonged presence of blood within the anterior chamber.

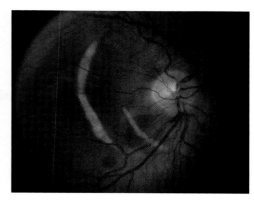

FIG. 19.121 Blunt trauma to the eye has caused a rupture of the choroid. This is visualized as white concentric rings around the optic disc where, beneath the retina, the choroid has separated, making the underlying sclera visible.

detection of superficial epithelial abrasion. The dye will stain areas which are missing epithelium. When possible, examination should be conducted with magnification as provided by a slit lamp or magnifying glass.

Blunt trauma to the eye may cause iritis or an anterior uveitis. Patients will complain of dull eye pain and light sensitivity. Signs of iritis include miosis of the pupil, tearing, and ciliary injection. With severe blunt trauma, the iris may be avulsed from its insertion (iridodialysis) or the iris and ciliary body may be avulsed (cyclodialysis). Eyes that receive blunt trauma may develop traumatic angle recession and glaucoma years after the incident.

An injury to the globe may cause bleeding from the small vessels of the peripheral portion of the iris or the ciliary body. Blood, which is heavier than aqueous fluid, will usually settle out in the inferior portion of the eye, causing a hyphema (Fig. 19.119). While the red blood cells are dispersed throughout the aqueous fluid, vision may be dramatically decreased. The blood may remain fluid and shift with changes in head position or it may clot. Complications following a hyphema include rebleeding, glaucoma, and blood staining of the cornea (Fig. 19.120). In the latter case, concurrent increased intraocular pressure will increase the risk of developing blood staining. The opacification of the cornea may resolve over several months to resolve. In children, this may cause amblyopia.

Immediate or delayed opacification of the lens may occur with penetration of the lens capsule. Blunt trauma may disrupt the lens zonules and dislocate the lens (see Fig. 19.80).

All eyes receiving trauma must have an examination of the fundus using a direct or indirect ophthalmoscope. Blunt trauma may cause a macular hole or a rupture of the choroid. A choroidal rupture is visualized as a white concentric ring around the optic disc where the underlying sclera has become visible (Fig. 19.121).

Trauma may produce retinal hemorrhages which are limited to the retina or which extend into the vitreous. Crushing injury to the chest may raise intrathoracic pressure with transmission to the retina causing hemorrhages. Purtcher's retinopathy includes retinal hemorrhages, cotton-wool spots, retinal edema, and fat emboli. Terson's syndrome is the transmission of subarachnoid hemorrhage to the optic nerve and disc and results in vitreous and retinal hemorrhages. Infants with the shaken baby syndrome may have extensive intraretinal hemorrhages accompanying their intracranial injuries and the severity of intraocular hemorrhage may correlate with the severity of intracranial injury.

In cases of penetrating injury to the eye, the key to examination is to be brief and gentle so as not to extend the injury by causing expulsion of intraocular contents. Immediately after identifying an ocular injury as penetrating, further examination should be limited and conducted in the operating room under general anesthesia. Topical medications should not be applied to the eye, and the eye should be protected at all times with a shield. Penetrating injuries caused by projectiles or foreign bodies may produce very subtle findings. In cases where the index of suspicion is high, appropriate evaluation may include plain film x-ray imaging studies including CT or MRIs or scans. If the potential intraocular foreign body is metallic, NMR scanning is contraindicated.

BIBLIOGRAPHY

Harley RD (ed): *Pediatric Ophthalmology*, ed 2. Philadelphia, WB Saunders, 1983.

Helveston EM, Ellis FD: *Pediatric Ophthalmology Practice*. St. Louis, CV Mosby, 1980.

Isenberg SJ: *The eye in infancy*. Chicago, Yearbook Medical Publishers, 1989.

Miller NR: *Clinical Neurophthalmology*, ed 4. Baltimore/London, Williams and Wilkins, 1985.

Renie WA: *Goldberg's Genetic and Metabolic Disease*, ed 2. Boston/Toronto, Little Brown, 1986.

Taylor D (ed): *Pediatric Ophthalmology* Boston, Blackwell Scientific Publications, 1990.

Von Noorden GK: *Binocular Vision and Ocular Motility*, ed 4. St. Louis, CV Mosby, 1989.

Von Noorden GK: *Von Noorden's-Maumanee's Atlas of Strabismus*, ed 4. St. Louis, CV Mosby, 1983.

Yanoff M, Fine BS: *Ocular Pathology*, ed 3. Philadelphia, JB Lippincott, 1989.

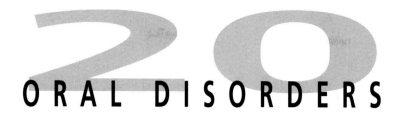

ORAL DISORDERS

M. M. Nazif, D.D.S., M.D.S. ◆ Holly Davis, M.D. ◆ D.H. McKibben, D.M.D., M.D.S. ◆ Mary Ann Ready, D.M.D.

FIG. 20.1 Diagrammatic representation of a molar shows the enamel, dentin and pulp, the periodontal membrane, the entrance of the neurovascular bundle through the root apices, as well as the bony supporting structures.

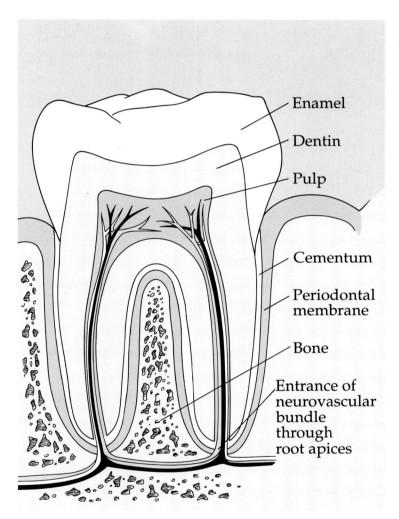

Enamel

Dentin

Pulp

Cementum

Periodontal membrane

Bone

Entrance of neurovascular bundle through root apices

NORMAL ORAL STRUCTURES

The oral cavity, including the teeth, gingivae, and periodontal ligaments, is in a constant state of evolution during infancy and childhood. From the early teething stage, through the eruption and exfoliation of the primary dentition, and finally to the eruption of all permanent teeth, the oral cavity provides one of the most visible signs of development.

To facilitate understanding of this chapter and communication when consulting dentists, a review of basic terminology is in order. Each tooth is composed of an outer protective enamel layer, an inner layer of dentin consisting of tubules, which are thought to serve a nutritional function, and a central neurovascular core termed the pulp. The roots of the teeth are anchored in the sockets of the alveolar processes of the mandible and maxilla by an encompassing periodontal membrane or ligament. The neurovascular supply to the root apex also passses through this structure. The bony processes between the teeth are referred to as the interdental septae (Fig. 20.1).

Following eruption, the visible portions of teeth are referred

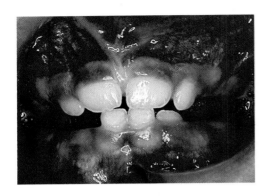

FIG. 20.2 Early primary dentition. The mandibular and maxillary central and lateral incisors are the first to erupt.

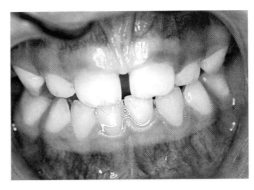

FIG. 20.3 Full primary dentition. By age 3, all 20 primary teeth have erupted.

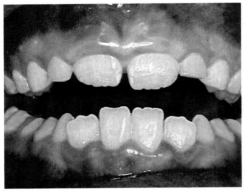

FIG. 20.4 Mixed dentition. This transitional stage from primary to permanent dentition begins at age 6 and lasts for about 6 years.

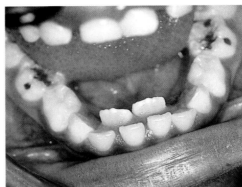

FIG. 20.5 Abnormal eruption patterns frequently occur in the early mixed dentition phase. One example is shown here, with the eruption of the permanent central incisors behind the primary teeth.

to as the crowns, and the interface between them and the gingivae is termed the gingival crevice. Finally, the portions of the gingivae located between teeth are called interdental papillae.

Normal Oral Cavity in the Newborn

The lips of an infant reveal a prominent line of demarcation at the vermilion border. The mucosa may look wrinkled and slightly purple at birth, but within a few days it exhibits a dryer appearance, with the outer layer forming crusty "sucking calluses." This callus formation affects the central portion of the mucosa and persists for only a few weeks.

The maxillary alveolar arch is separated from the lip by a shallow sulcus. In the midline, the labial frenulum extends posteriorly across the alveolar ridge to the palatine incisive papilla. Two lateral miniature frenula are also evident. The alveolar ridge peaks anteriorly and gradually flattens as the ridge extends posteriorly, forming a pseudoalveolar groove medial to the ridge along its palatal side. This flattened appearance is seen in young infants, and gradually disappears with the growth of the alveolar process and the formation and calcification of posterior tooth buds. The mandibular alveolar ridges also peak anteriorly and flatten posteriorly. The mandibular labial frenulum connects the lower lip to the labial aspect of the alveolar ridge. Careful visual inspection and palpation of the ridges should confirm the presence and location of tooth buds. Anterior tooth buds are located on the labial side of the alveolar ridges, while posterior tooth buds are often

located closer to the crests of the alveolar ridges. Palatal morphology and color are variable. The tongue and the floor of the mouth differ only slightly from those of older children.

Normal Primary Dentition

Development of the alveolar bone is directly related to the formation and eruption of teeth, and normal patterns of dental development occur symmetrically. At approximately 6 months of age, the mandibular central incisors erupt. This stage is often preceded by a period of increased salivation, local gingival irritation, and irritability. These symptoms may vary in intensity, but they respond well to oral analgesics and usually subside when the last primary tooth erupts into the oral cavity. Other symptoms such as fever or diarrhea have never been proven to be directly related to teething. The lower incisors are soon followed by the maxillary central incisors and the maxillary and mandibular lateral incisors (Fig. 20.2). By the end of the first year, all eight anterior teeth are usually visible. At 2 years, all primary teeth have erupted with the exception of the second primary molars, which erupt shortly thereafter. By the age of 3 years, the primary dentition is fully present and functional (Fig. 20.3).

Any variation in the time and sequence of eruption in an otherwise normal infant may call for early dental referral. In most instances, careful observation is the best course of action. For example, delayed eruption of primary teeth for up to 8 months is occasionally observed and is considered a normal

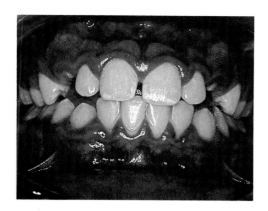

FIG. 20.6 *The earliest stage of permanent dentition begins with the eruption of the 6-year molars and central incisors. The cuspids and second molars are the last to erupt.*

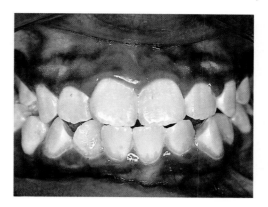

FIG. 20.7 *Gingivitis during puberty. The gingival tissues are mildy erythematous and edematous, and tend to bleed easily with brushing. Hormonal changes and inattention to careful dental hygiene are thought to be contributory.*

variation. Rarely, retarded eruption is associated with Down syndrome, hypothyroidism, hypopituitarism, achondroplastic dwarfism, osteopetrosis, rickets, or chondroectodermal dysplasia. A significant variation affecting a single tooth or only a few teeth should be carefully investigated, as well.

Spacing (extra space between teeth) during this stage is normal and desirable, and often indicates that more space is available for the larger permanent teeth. The completed primary dentition establishes a baseline which dictates to a great extent the future alignment of permanent teeth and the future relationship between the maxillary and mandibular arches.

During most of the primary dentition stage, the gingiva appears pink, firm, and not readily retractable. A well-defined zone of firmly attached keratinized gingiva is present, extending from the bottom of the gingival sulcus to the junction of the alveolar mucosa. Rarely, local irritation may develop into acute or subacute pericoronitis, with elevated temperature and associated lymphadenopathy (see Fig. 20.49). Topical and/or systemic therapy may be required for treatment; however, lancing the gingiva to relieve such symptoms is not usually indicated.

NORMAL MIXED DENTITION

This stage of development begins with the eruption of the first permanent molars at about 6 years of age and continues for approximately 6 years. During this period, the following teeth erupt from the gums in this sequence: mandibular central incisors, maxillary central incisors, mandibular lateral incisors, maxillary lateral incisors, mandibular cuspids, maxillary and mandibular first premolars, maxillary and mandibular second premolars, maxillary cuspids, and mandibular and maxillary second molars (Fig. 20.4).

The mixed dentition during this stage undergoes certain physiologic changes including root resorption followed by exfoliation of primary teeth, eruption of their successors, and eruption of the posterior permanent teeth. During the period of root resorption of primary teeth, and for several months following the eruption of permanent teeth, these are relatively loosely imbedded in the alveolar bone and more vulnerable to displacement with trauma. Other minor complications may occur during resorption and exfoliation of primary teeth and eruption of permanent teeth. Gingival irritation can occur as a result of increased mobility of primary teeth, but usually disappears spontaneously when the tooth is lost or extracted. Two transient deviations of eruption pattern may occur: the mandibular incisors may erupt in a lingual position behind the primary incisors ("double teeth") (Fig. 20.5), and the maxillary incisors may assume a widely spaced and labially inclined position ("ugly duckling" stage). Finally, the occlusal surfaces of newly erupted permanent teeth are relatively "rough" (see Figs. 20.4 and 20.41), facilitating plaque accumulation which increases the risk of staining, gingivitis, and possibly the formation of caries.

Normal Early Permanent Dentition

This stage marks the beginning of a relatively quiescent period in dental development. Activities are limited to root formation of a few permanent teeth and the calcification of the third molars. By this time the length and width of the dental arches are well-established (Fig. 20.6); however, the jaws will undergo a major growth spurt during puberty which will alter their size and relative position. The gingiva begins to assume adult characteristics, becoming firm, pink in color, with an uneven, stippled surface texture and a thin gingival margin. Puberty is occasionally associated with gingivitis, thought secondary in part to hormonal changes (Fig. 20.7). The gingivae become mildly edematous and erythematous, and bleed with brushing (the common chief complaint). Inattention to careful dental hygiene may also contribute to development of this disorder, which necessitates good oral hygiene for control.

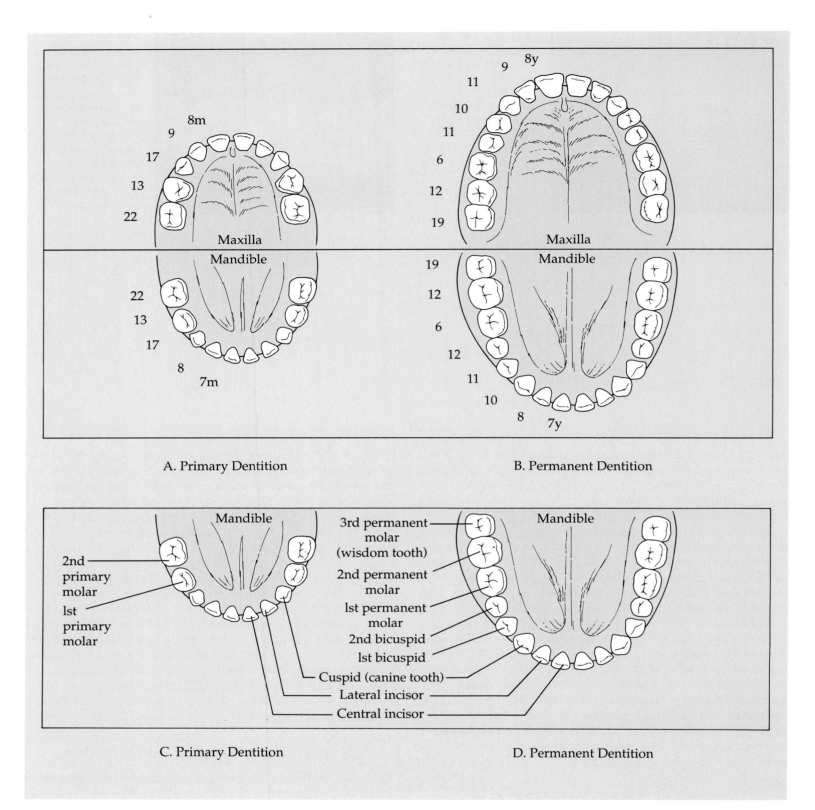

FIG. 20.8 Artist's illustrations of the primary and permanent dentition. **A** and **B,** the numbers represent the average age of eruption for the teeth indicated in months for the primary teeths and years for the permanent dentition. **C** and **D,** the names of specific teeth in the primary and permanent dentition are shown.

In Figure 20.8, the primary and permanent dentition are presented diagrammatically.

Harmful Oral Habits

Children often develop sucking habits, using thumb, finger(s), or objects. Thumb and finger sucking begins prenatally and is considered a normal behavior pattern. However, if the habit persists beyond the late primary dentition stage of dental arch development (5 years), the extrinsic forces applied by the sucking action can produce pathologic changes in the child's normal arch growth. These deviations range from minor, reversible changes to gross malformations in the dental arches producing significant anterior open-bites and/or posterior

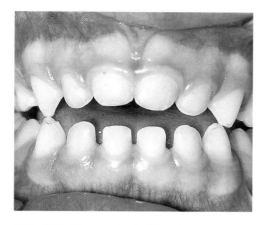

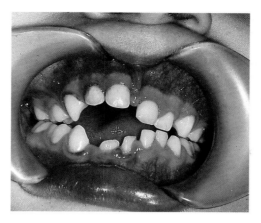

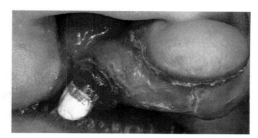

FIG. 20.9 Changes in the bite often occur as the result of prolonged digit-sucking. This child's upper arch has been narrowed and an anterior open-bite is developing.

FIG 20.10 A 2-year-old with a prolonged pacifier-sucking habit has severe deformity of the alveolar arches and teeth due to the extrinsic force of the pacifier-sucking action.

FIG. 20.11 A natal tooth associated with cleft palate. Extraction is only necessary if it is of abnormal morphology or causes feeding difficulties.

crossbites. The degree of changes depends on the duration and the frequency and intensity of the sucking habit (Fig. 20.9).

BOTTLE AND PACIFIER HABITS

The forces produced by prolonged use of bottles and pacifiers can first cause dental malocclusions and may, if the habit persists, worsen the resulting deformity with the involvement of adjacent jaw structures. Usually, if the child is weaned from the bottle and pacifier by the age of 18 months, no permanent changes in bite development can be expected. The longer any force is applied, the greater the risk that the distortion in the dental arches and adjacent bony structures will not self-correct (Fig. 20.10).

Hence, the use of bottles and pacifiers should be discouraged by the age of 18 months. After this age, changes in the oral structures have been noted and are more likely to be permanent. Counseling parents from the neonatal period not to put their infants to bed with a bottle, but rather hold them during all feedings, is probably one of the best ways to prevent later difficulties with weaning. Such practices also prevent the development of nursing-bottle caries.

THERAPY

Clinical management of harmful oral habits should be customized to the child's age. Obviously, harsh measures to discourage digit sucking in a 2-year-old are not justified, and may be counterproductive. In fact, children who receive frequent criticism for thumb sucking are probably more likely to cling to the habit than are those whose families ignore it. However, when the habit persists until the age of reason, calm discussions with the child concerning feelings related to the sucking, and the physical damage possible if it continues, often produce the desired results. When a child has expressed a strong will to cease sucking, but is unable to accomplish this goal without help, appliance therapy by a dental professional may

be indicated. Referral for oral evaluation and consultation is appropriate after the child has passed the appropriate age of the behavior pattern involved, i.e., over 5 years of age for digit sucking habits, or 18 months for pacifiers.

NATAL AND NEONATAL ABNORMALITIES

Natal and Neonatal Teeth

Teeth present in the oral cavity at birth are called natal teeth, while those erupting during the neonatal period are called neonatal teeth. The incidence of natal teeth has been reported to be approximately 1 in 2,000 births. Though seen in normal infants, this anomaly is more frequent in patients with cleft palate (Fig. 20.11) and is often associated with the following syndromes: Ellis-van Creveld, Hallermann-Streiff, and pachyonychia congenita. The vast majority of such teeth are true primary teeth, but occasionally they are supernumerary. Some are abnormal, with either hypoplastic defects or poor crown or root development. Natal teeth may cause feeding problems for both the infant and mother. Ulceration of the ventral surface of the tongue by sharp tooth edges (Riga-Fede disease) may develop if natal teeth remain in the oral cavity. This condition is usually transient, but in persistent cases symptomatic treatment or extraction of such teeth may be indicated. Most normal-appearing natal teeth can be retained, but those that are supernumerary, abnormal, or very loose may have to be removed.

Gingival Cysts in the Newborn

Gingival cysts of the oral cavity are small, single or multiple superficial lesions which are formed by tissues trapped during embryologic growth and occur in about 80 percent of newborn

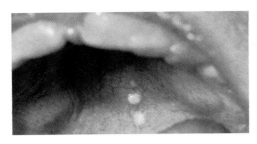

FIG. 20.12 Gingival cysts. The small, whitish cystic lesions along the midpalatine raphe are called Epstein pearls.

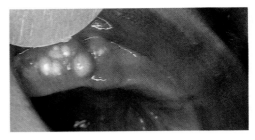

FIG. 20.13 Gingival cysts. The firm, grayish white mucous gland cysts on the buccal aspect of the alveolar ridges are called Bohn nodules.

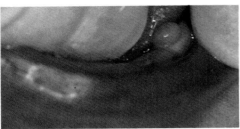

FIG. 20.14 Dental lamina cyst. The cysts are found on the alveolar ridge and usually occur singly.

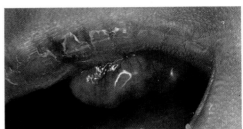

FIG. 20.15 Congenital epulis. This 4-day-old patient presented with a benign tumor of the anterior maxilla that affected both jaws.

infants. They are asymptomatic, do not enlarge, seldom interfere with feeding, and usually exfoliate within a few weeks.

Three types of cysts exist:

1. Epstein pearls are keratin-filled cystic lesions lined with stratified squamous epithelium. They appear as small, whitish lesions along the midpalatine raphe and contain no mucous glands (Fig. 20.12).

2. Bohn nodules are mucous gland cysts, often found on the buccal or lingual aspects of the alveolar ridges and, occasionally, on the palate. They are multiple, firm, and grayish white in appearance. Histologically, they show mucous glands and ducts (Fig. 20.13).

3. Dental lamina cysts are found only on the crest of the alveolar mucosa. Histologically, these lesions are different since they are formed by remnants of dental lamina epithelium. They may be larger, more lucent, and fluctuant than Epstein pearls or Bohn nodules, and are more likely to occur singly (Fig. 20.14).

Congenital Epulis in the Newborn

This benign, soft-tissue tumor is seen on the alveolar mucosa at birth or shortly after. It is usually found on the anterior maxilla as a pedunculated swelling (Fig. 20.15), but may appear on the mandible or occasionally on both jaws. The mass is firm on palpation, and the overlying mucosa appears normal. Histologically, sheets of large granular cells are seen. Differential diagnosis should include rhabdomyoma and melanotic neuroectodermal tumor of infancy. The lesion is amenable to conservative surgical excision, and recurrence is infrequent.

Melanotic Neuroectodermal Tumor of Infancy

This benign yet aggressive tumor occurs during the first year of life, and is often found on the anterior maxilla in association with unerupted or erupted teeth. It often bulges and destroys the alveolar bone, thus displacing the associated primary tooth. The tumor mass is grayish blue, firm on palpation, and spherical in shape (Fig. 20.16). Careful surgical removal is effective, and recurrence is unusual.

DEVELOPMENTAL ABNORMALITIES
Soft-Tissue Abnormalities

GEOGRAPHIC TONGUE
(BENIGN MIGRATORY GLOSSITIS)
This painless condition is characterized by inflamed, irregularly shaped areas on the dorsum of the tongue which are devoid of filiform papillae. Lesions are red, slightly depressed, and bordered by a whitish band (Fig. 20.17). Spontaneous healing followed by the formation of similar lesions elsewhere on the tongue results in a migrating appearance. Etiology is unknown; however, strong association with stress and allergies is suspected. Although benign, the course of this disorder may be prolonged for months, and it may recur.

ABNORMALITIES OF THE FRENULA
During embryonic life, the maxillary labial frenulum extends as a band of tissue from the upper lip over and across the alveolar ridge and into the incisive (palatine) papilla. Postnatally, as the alveolar process increases in size, the labial frenulum separates from the incisive papilla and becomes relatively smaller. With the eruption of primary and later permanent teeth, the frenulum attachment moves apically and further atrophies as a result of vertical growth of the alveolar process. The developmental gap (diastema) between the maxillary central incisors tends to close with the full eruption of the maxillary permanent canines. Occasionally, the maxillary frenulum fails to atrophy and the diastema persists (Fig. 20.18). The mandibular midline frenulum only rarely maintains a lingual extension and therefore only rarely causes a diastema between the mandibular central incisors.

The lingual frenulum extends almost to the tip of the tongue in early infancy and then gradually recedes. Occasionally, ankyloglossia (tongue tie) is seen, but this is rarely associated with feeding or speech difficulties. Various surgical procedures have been advocated to correct this condition. In general, frenulectomy is seldom indicated and should be recommended only after appropriate justification (Fig. 20.19). Congenital anomalies may include an enlarged frenulum, labiolingual frenulum extensions, or supernumerary frenula as seen in orofaciodigital syndrome (Fig. 20.20).

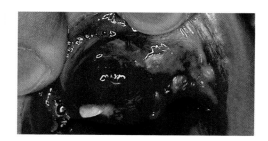

FIG. 20.16 Melanotic neuroectodermal tumor. This benign but locally aggressive tumor of the anterior maxilla has produced elevation of the lip and displaced a primary tooth.

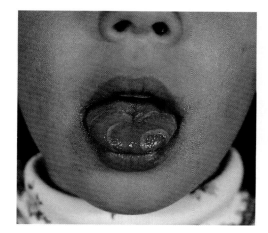

FIG. 20.17 Characteristics of benign migratory glossitis (geographic tongue), a chronic and often recurring condition affecting the filiform papillae of the tongue. Lesions are red, slightly depressed, and are bordered by a whitish band.

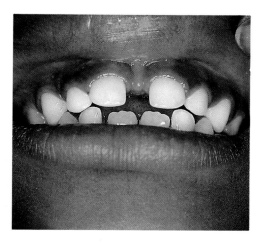

FIG. 20.18 Large diastema (excessive spacing) between the front teeth secondary to an inferiorly positioned maxillary frenum.

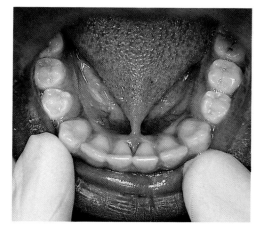

FIG. 20.19 Ankyloglossia. The extremely short lingual frenulum with a high insertion point on the gingival margin, seen in this child, is an indication for surgical intervention.

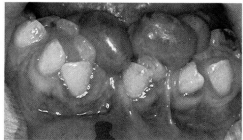

FIG. 20.20 Multiple hyperplastic frenula are seen in this patient with orofaciodigital syndrome. These frenula interfered with the eruption of teeth, causing rotations and crowding.

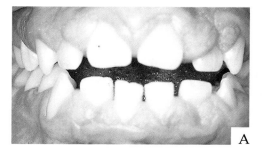

A

FIG. 20.21 Phenytoin-induced gingival overgrowth. *A,* a typical gingival response (hyperplasia) to chronic phenytoin ingestion. Similar gum changes can result from

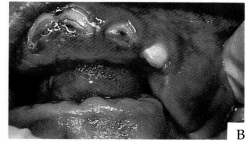

B

cyclosporine therapy. *B,* severe overgrowth. The firm hyperplastic gingival tissues have completely covered the posterior teeth and are interfering with mastication.

GINGIVAL HYPERPLASIA

Generalized gingival hyperplasia is a fairly common nonspecific pathologic entity. This disorder is frequently a complication of drug therapy as is seen with phenytoin and cyclosporine. Gingival hyperplasia may also be idiopathic or genetically transmitted as in familial fibromatosis. Differentiation of various types of hyperplasia must be based on thorough physical evaluation and appropriate medical history. Histopathologically, it is impossible to differentiate between these various disorders; therefore, the final diagnosis and recommendations for therapy should be based on all available clinical data and an appropriate dental consultation.

Phenytoin-Induced gingival Hyperplasia

The administration of phenytoin over a period of time frequently causes generalized hyperplasia of the gingivae (Fig. 20.21A,B). The gingiva may become secondarily inflamed, edematous, and boggy, especially if proper oral hygiene is not practiced. The severity is often related to the degree of local irritation, stemming from poor oral hygiene, mouth breathing, caries, or poor occlusion (alignment). As hyperplasia tends to recur following surgical excision, gingivectomy is usually reserved for those patients whose overgrowth interferes with function and for those whose therapy has been discontinued.

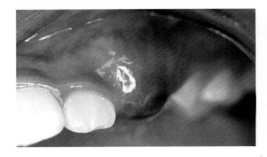

FIG. 20.22 Eruption hematoma. A bluish, fluid-filled fluctuant swelling can be seen over the crown of an erupting maxillary cuspid. The lesion resolved without treatment when the tooth erupted.

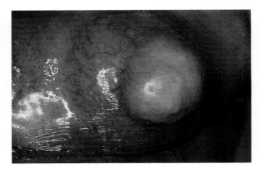

FIG. 20.23 A mucocele on the lower lip with the characteristic translucent coloration secondary to fulid retention.

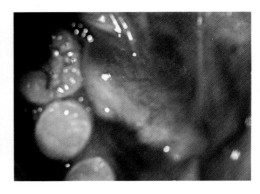

FIG. 20.24 Ranula. The bluish, fluctuant swelling in the floor of the mouth is a retention cyst associated with trauma to a salivary duct.

Cyclosporine-Induced Gingival Hyperplasia

Cyclosporine has been used primarily in treating patients following organ transplants. The drug has been demonstrated to directly increase cellular growth of gingival fibroblasts. It also increases the production and retention of collagen. Further, this agent's immunosuppressive action may predispose gingival tissues to invasion by microorganisms, thereby increasing inflammatory changes. While meticulous oral hygiene reduces inflammation, it has no significant affect on the degree of hyperplasia.

Fibromatosis Gingivae

This rare genetically-determined condition may be clinically evident at birth and, in such instances, may prevent or slow subsequent dental eruption. The clinical manifestations include the generalized presence of firm fibrous tissue that extends around the crowns of involved teeth. Inflammation, when present, is usually secondary.

Surgical excision of excessive tissues is usually indicated, but recurrence is a distinct possibility.

Idiopathic Gingival Hyperplasia

Different types of patients, often with significant systemic illnesses or syndromes, may manifest generalized gingival enlargements. These may primarily involve the gingival tissues or may sometimes be related to underlying thickening of cortical bone, which causes gingival hyperplasia by impeding dental eruption. Each of these cases must be evaluated individually for possible etiology, and appropriate treatment.

ERUPTION CYSTS (ERUPTION HEMATOMA)

An eruption cyst is a fluid-filled swelling, nontender in the vast majority of cases, over the crown of an erupting tooth. When the follicle is dilated with blood, the lesion takes on a bluish color and is termed an eruption hematoma (Fig. 20.22). Although the eruption cyst is a superficial form of dentigerous cyst, it rarely impedes eruption, and surgical exposure of the crown is seldom necessary. Very rarely such a cyst may become secondarily infected. In such cases, patients complain of headache or facial pain, and the cyst is tender on palpation. Incision and drainage are required when infection has developed.

MUCOCELE AND RANULA

A mucocele is a painless translucent or bluish lesion of traumatic origin, most often involving minor salivary glands of the lower lip (Fig. 20.23). The lesion may alternately enlarge and shrink. The treatment of choice is surgical excision of the lesion and the associated minor salivary gland.

A simple ranula is a retention cyst, in the floor of the mouth, which is confined to sublingual tissues superior to the mylohyoid muscle. It appears clinically as a bluish, transparent, thin-walled fluctuant swelling (Fig. 20.24). Herniation of the ranula through the mylohyoid muscle results in a cervical or plunging ranula that becomes more apparent in the oral cavity with the muscle contraction associated with jaw opening. Simple incision and drainage of the ranula is not an acceptable treatment since healing is followed by recurrence. Marsupialization by suturing the edges of the opened cystic wall to the mucous membrane is the recommended treatment. The plunging ranula must be removed in its entirety along with the associated salivary gland to avoid recurrence.

SALIVARY CALCULUS (SIALOLITHIASIS)

Formation of a salivary calculus is rare in the pediatric population, but when it does occur it may affect either Wharton's or Stenson's duct (Fig. 20.25A). Partial obstruction of the duct results in pain and enlargement of the gland, especially at mealtime. While palpation of the stone may be possible, dental radiographs confirm the diagnosis and give appropriate information about its size and location (Fig. 20.25B). Larger salivary stones wedged within the ducts may cause localized irritation and secondary infection. If the calculus cannot be manipulated through the duct, surgical intervention may be necessary.

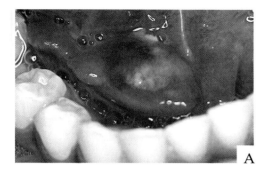

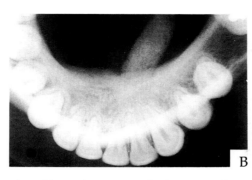

FIG. 20.25 Salivary calculus. **A,** this sialolith obstructing a salivary duct is observed in the floor of the mouth. **B,** a dental radiograph of the sublingual space reveals the size and location of the salivary calculus.

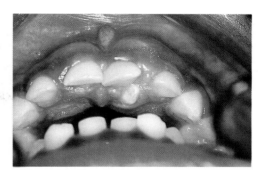

FIG. 20.26 Hyperdontia. Erupted supernumerary tooth lingual to the maxillary central incisor in the deciduous dentition.

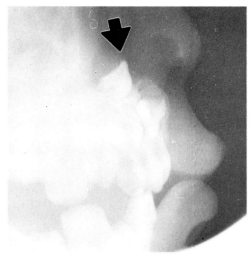

FIG. 20.27 Supernumerary nasal tooth. A lateral radiograph of the maxilla shows a supernumerary tooth erupting through the floor of the nasal cavity in a child with cleft palate who presented with recurrent epistaxis.

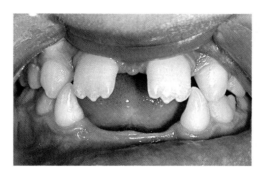

FIG. 20.28 Hypodontia. The congenital absence of teeth is seen in this patient with hereditary ectodermal dysplasia. This phenomenon may be an isolated anomaly or a manifestation of several syndromes.

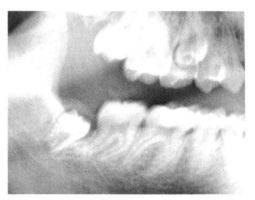

FIG. 20.29 A microdont can be seen on this panoramic radiograph near the second molar. Microdonts are often seen in the maxillary lateral incisor region.

Hard-Tissue Abnormalities

HYPER- AND HYPODONTIA

Variations in tooth number include both hyper- and hypodontia. Supernumerary teeth occur in about 3 percent of the normal population, but patients with cleft lip and/or cleft palate and cleidocranial dysostosis have a significantly higher incidence. The most common site is the anterior palate (Fig. 20.26). Supernumerary teeth may have the size and morphology of adjacent teeth or may be small and atypical in shape. They may erupt spontaneously or remain impacted. Early consideration of removal is justified due to complications such as impeded eruption, crowding, or resorption of permanent teeth; cystic changes; or ectopic eruption into the nasal cavity, the maxillary sinus, or other sites (Fig. 20.27).

Congenital absence of teeth is more often seen in the permanent dentition than in the primary. Most frequently missing are third molars, second premolars, and lateral incisors. Hypodontia is frequently associated with several ectodermal syndromes such as anhidrotic ectodermal dysplasia and chondroectodermal dysplasia (Fig. 20.28).

ALTERATION IN SIZE AND SHAPE

Teeth that are smaller or larger than normal are termed microdonts and macrodonts, respectively. These teeth are genetic anomalies. They are clinically significant when a discrepancy in tooth size and dental arch length results in severe crowding or spacing of the teeth. Size abnormalities are often localized to one tooth or to a very small group of teeth (Fig. 20.29).

Variations in shape also result from the joining of teeth or tooth buds. Fusion is the joining of two tooth buds by the dentin. Concrescence is the joining of the roots of two or more teeth by cementum. Gemination (twinning) results from the

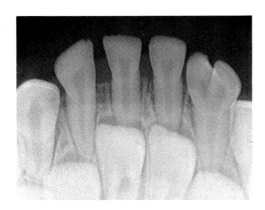

FIG. 20.30
Radiograph demon-
strates gemination
(twinning), the
incomplete division of
a tooth bud resulting
in a tooth with a large
notched crown and a
single root.

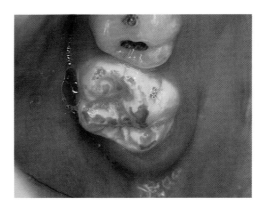

FIG. 20.31
Hypocalcification.
This 6-year-old
patient exhibits early
signs of hypocalcifi-
cation of his perma-
nent molars. Chalky
white spots indicate
poor calcification of
the enamel.

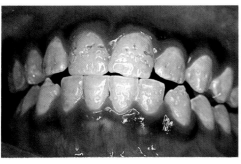

FIG. 20.32
Amelogenesis imper-
fecta, hypoplastic
type. This process
results in generalized
pitting of the enamel.

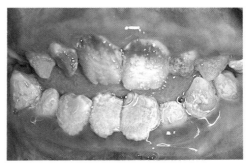

FIG. 20.33
Amelogenesis imper-
fecta, hypocalcified
type. The enamel
defects result in dis-
coloration and ero-
sion due to errors in
the mineralization
stage of tooth devel-
opment and sec-
ondary staining.

incomplete division of one tooth bud, resulting in a large crown with a notched incisal edge and a single root (Fig. 20.30).

HYPOPLASIA AND HYPOCALCIFICATION

Numerous local and systemic insults are capable of causing the enamel defects of hypoplasia and hypocalcification. The most common etiologic factors are local infections such as an abscessed primary tooth, which, when not diagnosed and treated promptly, may damage the enamel of its developing permanent counterpart. Other causes include systemic infections with associated high fever; trauma such as intrusion of the primary tooth; and chemical injury, of which excessive ingestion of fluoride is an example. Other etiologic factors include nutritional deficiencies, allergies, rubella, cerebral palsy, embryopathy, prematurity, and radiation therapy. Hypoplasia results from an insult during active matrix formation of the enamel, and clinically manifests as pitting, furrowing, or thinning of the enamel (see Fig. 20.32). Hypocalcification results from an insult during mineralization of the tooth, and is seen as opaque, chalky, or white lesions (Fig. 20.31).

HERITABLE DEFECTS OF ENAMEL AND DENTIN
Amelogenesis Imperfecta

Amelogenesis imperfecta is the term used to describe a group of genetically determined defects that involve the enamel of primary and permanent teeth without affecting dentin, pulp, or cementum. While the types of amelogenesis imperfecta are numerous, the major defect in each is hypoplasia, hypomaturation, or hypocalcification. The hypoplastic type results in thin, pitted, or fissured enamel (Fig. 20.32). Hypomaturation manifests as discolored enamel of full thickness but decreased hardness which tends to chip away slowly, exposing underlying dentin. Radiographic evaluation will demonstrate the decreased density of enamel. Hypocalcified enamel is chalky, variable in color, and quickly erodes away (Fig. 20.33). Depending on the type of amelogenesis imperfecta, inheritance may be autosomal-dominant, autosomal-recessive, or X-linked.

Dentinogenesis Imperfecta

Dentinogenesis imperfecta results in dentin defects, and is usually inherited as an autosomal-dominant trait. The most common manifestation is opalescent dentin, which may be associated with osteogenesis imperfecta. The teeth are blue to pinkish brown in color and have an opalescent sheen (Fig. 20.34). Despite normal enamel morphology, there is rapid attrition or wearing down of the crowns. The roots are shortened and the pulp cavities are calcified. Primary teeth are more severely affected than the permanent, although permanent teeth are fracture prone.

DISCOLORATION

Three major types of tooth discoloration are frequently observed: (1) discoloration from stains that adhere externally to the surfaces of the teeth (extrinsic); (2) discoloration from various pigments that are incorporated into the tooth structure during development (intrinsic); and (3) intrinsic discoloration secondary to hereditary defects, which was discussed above.

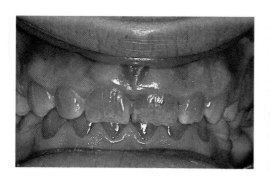

FIG. 20.34 Dentinogenesis imperfecta. The bluish opalescent sheen on several of these teeth results from genetically defective dentin. This condition may be associated with osteogenesis imperfecta.

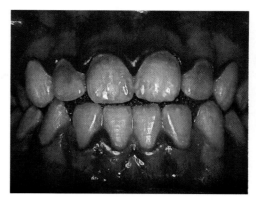

FIG. 20.35 Extrinsic discoloration. The green stain seen on the gingival third of the incisors is associated with poor oral hygiene.

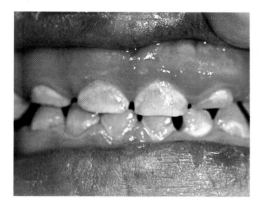

FIG. 20.36 Hepatic discoloration. Generalized intrinsic discoloration of the primary teeth is seen in this patient with biliary atresia.

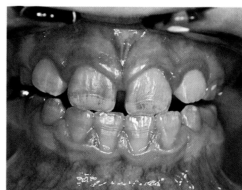

FIG. 20.37 Tetracycline discoloration. The severe discoloration seen in this patient is due to tetracycline administration during calcification of the permanent teeth.

Extrinsic Discoloration

Extrinsic discoloration is primarily limited to patients with poor oral hygiene, those receiving certain medications, those who heavily consume stain-containing foods or drinks, or those who smoke or chew tobacco or other substances. It occurs more often at certain locations, especially on the gingival third of the exposed crown. Diagnosis requires appropriate medical, dental, and dietary histories with emphasis on oral hygiene, food and drug intake, and tobacco habits. Treatment includes scaling, dental prophylaxis and polishing, and the practice of regular oral hygiene. The use of abrasive toothpaste can cause excessive wear of the enamel and should be avoided.

Brown/black stain on the lingual surfaces of anterior as well as posterior teeth is most common among young children who are taking liquid oral iron supplements and among adolescents who are smokers and tea drinkers. Green stain on the labial surfaces of the anterior maxillary teeth is common among children with poor oral hygiene. The source is usually chromogenic bacteria and fungi (Fig. 20.35). Orange/red stain is unusual, but when it does occur it can be found around the gingival third of the exposed crown. This stain often results from antibiotic intake, which causes a temporary shift in the oral flora.

Intrinsic Discoloration

Intrinsic discoloration is usually induced during the calcification of dentin and enamel by excessive levels of the body's natural pigments such as hemoglobin and bile or by pigments introduced by the intake of chemicals such as fluorides or tetracyclines. Occasionally, *isolated* intrinsic discoloration takes place as a result of pulpal necrosis, pulpal calcification, or internal resorption.

HEPATIC DISCOLORATION

Generalized intrinsic discoloration of primary teeth is seen in patients with advanced hepatic disease associated with persistent or recurrent jaundice and hyperbilirubinemia (Fig. 20.36). The intensity of the discoloration varies and may be somewhat related to the severity of the hepatic disorder. The color ranges from brown to grayish brown and usually has no clinical significance unless it is associated with significant hypoplasia of the dentition.

TETRACYCLINE DISCOLORATION

Teeth stained as a result of tetracycline therapy may vary in color from yellow to brown to dark gray. Staining occurs when the tetracycline is incorporated into calcifying teeth and bone. Both the enamel and, to a greater degree, the dentin that are calcifying at the time of intake incorporate tetracycline into their chemical structures. The severity of discoloration depends upon the dose, duration, and type of tetracycline administered. The initial yellow or light brown pigmentation tends to darken with age (Fig. 20.37). Tetracyclines readily cross the placenta, so staining of primary teeth is possible if tetracycline is taken during pregnancy. Therefore, tetracycline should not be prescribed to pregnant women or to children under 10 years of age.

ERYTHROBLASTOSIS FETALIS

Children born with congenital hemolytic anemia due to Rh incompatibility may exhibit distinct discoloration of their primary teeth due to the deposition of bilirubin in the dentin and enamel during primary tooth development. The color ranges from green to blue to orange. No treatment is indicated unless discoloration is associated with significant hypoplasia or hypocalcification. The permanent dentition is usually not affected.

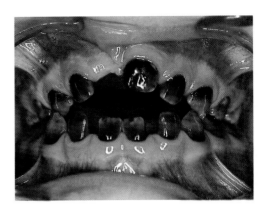

FIG. 20.38 The reddish-brown tooth discoloration associated with porphyria.

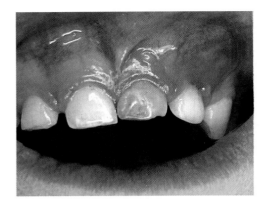

FIG. 20.39 Isolated intrinsic discoloration. The central incisor is discolored secondary to trauma. Often such a change is a manifestation of pulpal necrosis.

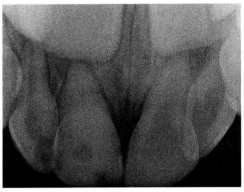

FIG. 20.40 Radiographic evidence of dystrophic calcification of the pulp and root canal of the upper right primary central incisor.

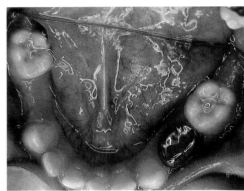

FIG. 20.41 The occlusal surfaces of newly erupted molars exhibit varying degrees of pit and fissure depth. The morphology of these patterns make these teeth more prone to early decay.

PORPHYRIA

This hereditary disturbance of porphyrin metabolism may produce a distinct reddish or brownish discoloration of the primary and permanent teeth secondary to deposition of porphyrin in developing teeth (Fig. 20.38).

ISOLATED INTRINSIC DISCOLORATION

Teeth with necrotic pulps develop an opaque appearance with discoloration ranging from light yellow to gray (Fig. 20.39 and see Fig. 20.46B). Such teeth may develop abscesses, periapical cystic lesions, or chronic fistulas. Pulpal calcification (Fig. 20.40) is often associated with a localized yellow discoloration. Internal resorption manifests clinically as a pink discoloration secondary to loss of dentin thickness.

CARIES

The interaction of microorganisms, especially *Streptococcus mutans*, and fermentable carbohydrates results in acid demineralization of susceptible enamel. Caries are seen as yellowish-brown to gray defects in the enamel surfaces of affected teeth (see Fig. 20.42). Untreated carious destruction progresses through the enamel and dentin, and with bacterial contamination of the pulp ultimately renders the pulp necrotic. The deep pits, fissures, and grooves characteristic of the surfaces of newly erupted teeth are at increased risk for developing carious lesions (Fig. 20.41 and see Fig. 20.4). Sealing these defects with plastic bonding agents may prevent the initiation of caries. Other preventive methods include brushing and flossing on a daily basis (beginning with eruption of the first tooth) to remove bacteria-containing plaque, implementation of systemic fluoride via the water supply or prescribed supplements, and control of the frequency of intake of fermentable carbohydrates, especially those high in sugar content and adhesiveness.

Nursing bottle caries involve the primary dentition of the child who is habitually put to bed with a bottle containing milk or another cariogenic (sugar-containing) liquid. This form of caries was originally associated with bottle-feeding only; however, an association with frequent and prolonged nocturnal breast-feeding has become apparent. Carious lesions initially develop on the maxillary incisors, and later on the molars and cuspids (Fig. 20.42A,B). The mandibular incisors are spared by the protective position of the tongue during nursing. The deleterious effect of nocturnal nursing is due not only to the frequency of carbohydrate intake but also to the decreased rate of swallowing and salivation during sleep. Brushing before bedtime and after any nocturnal feedings is especially important in prevention.

INFECTIONS
Viral Infections

HERPETIC GINGIVOSTOMATITIS

Primary herpetic gingivostomatitis, caused by herpes simplex, type I, is an extremely painful disease that affects children, especially those between the ages of 6 months and 3 years. The vesicular lesions of the lips, tongue, gingivae, and oral mucosa are preceded by fever, headache, regional lymphadenopathy,

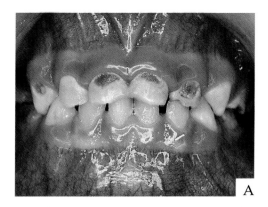

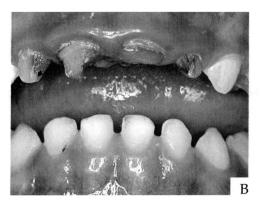

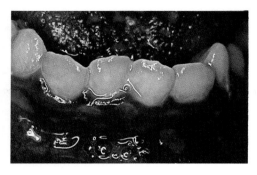

FIG. 20.42 Nursing bottle caries. **A,** a typical pattern, with the upper incisors being the first involved. **B,** when badly neglected, se-vere tooth erosion occurs and periapical abscesses may develop.

FIG. 20.43 Herpetic gingivostomatitis. The ulcerations seen on the oral mucosa were preceded by fever, headache, and hymphadenopathy. Note the erythematous halos around the ulcerations.

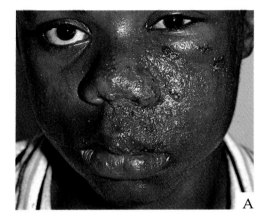

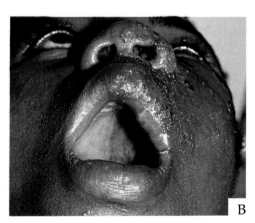

FIG. 20.44 Herpes zoster. This patient's infection involved the trigeminal nerve, including the nasociliary branch. Both the extraoral **(A)** and the intraoral **(B)** lesions stop at the midline.

and gingival hyperemia and edema. These lesions tend to rupture quickly, leaving shallow ulcerations covered by a gray membrane and surrounded by an erythematous halo (Fig. 20.43). The inflamed gingivae are friable and bleed easily. Lesions heal spontaneously in 1 to 2 weeks without scarring. Since inflammation makes brushing too painful, oral hygiene should be maintained using a preparation such as chlorhexidine or glycerin and peroxide (in very young children) to decrease the incidence of secondary infection. A bland diet and rinsing with viscous lidocaine (in children older than 6 or 7 years) or a solution of equal parts of Benadryl® and Maalox®, in addition to use of oral analgesics, are indicated to minimize and control pain. In some severe cases, codeine may be required. The use of systemic acyclovir may be indicated in cases with moderate to severe involvement. Topical application of the same drug can be helpful in milder cases.

Recurrent infections due to reactivation of latent herpes simplex virus are fairly common. Lesions are few in number and more localized; systemic symptoms are absent unless the host is immunocompromised. Lesions are usually located on the lips, with prodromal symptoms of itching and burning preceding the development of thin-walled vesicles which rupture and become crusty in appearance (see Chapter 12, Infectious Diseases). When intraoral lesions occur, they manifest as small vesicles in a localized group on mucosa that is tightly bound to periosteum.

HERPES ZOSTER (SHINGLES)
Herpes zoster results from activation of the varicella zoster virus and inflammation of the dorsal root or extramedullary cranial nerve ganglion. While the disease is seen in otherwise healthy children, it is more likely to occur in the severely debilitated or immunosuppressed child. The patient presents with a prodrome of malaise, fever, headache, and tenderness along the affected dermatome that may last a few to several days. This is followed by the extraoral formation of painful grouped vesicular lesions which rupture to form ulcerations. The oral cavity also may be affected with erosions following a unilateral distribution of maxillary and mandibular divisions of the trigeminal nerve (Fig. 20.44).

RECURRENT APHTHOUS ULCERS (CANKER SORES)
Aphthous ulcers are similar in appearance to herpetic ulcers but are not of viral origin. Precipitating factors include trauma, stress, sunlight, endocrine disturbances, hematologic disorders, and allergies, alluding to a multifactorial etiology. Onset is usually during adolescence or young adulthood. Unlike herpetic lesions, these ulcerations are not preceded by vesicle

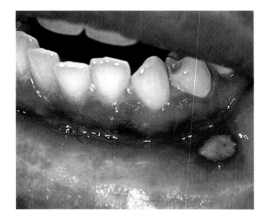

FIG. 20.45 Recurrent aphthous ulcers. The ulceration seen on the labial mucosa is surrounded by a characteristic erythematous halo.

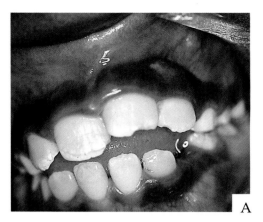

FIG. 20.46 Dental abscesses. **A,** a small abscess above the left upper lateral incisor developed following an injury in which the patient had chipped that tooth and his central inciser. **B,** this abscess above the right central

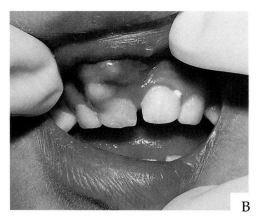

incisor has ruptured through the gingiva and begun to drain. The tooth is discolored as a result of pulp necrosis stemming from an injury 2 years earlier.

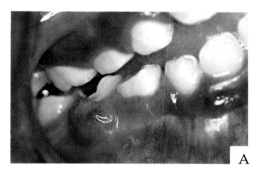

FIG. 20.47 **A,** a deep neglected cavity in this mandibular molar predisposed to development of a periapical abscess which, following rupture, resulted in formation of a gingival granuloma. **B,** left untreated such abscesses

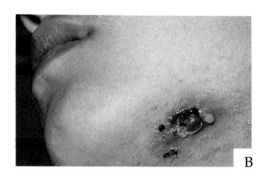

can be responsible for this type of extraoral lesion in which infection has spread by way of a fistulous tract to the skin. Extraction of the offending tooth is necessary for resolution of the extraoral lesion.

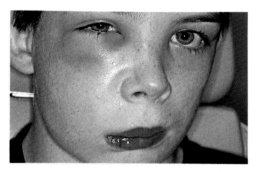

FIG. 20.48 Facial cellulitis associated with an abscessed maxillary tooth. Hospital admission for intravenous antibiotics, incision and drainage, and extraction of the abscessed tooth was necessary.

formation. They are extremely painful, and have a pseudomembrane and an erythematous halo (Fig. 20.45). They can vary in size, number, and distribution. Small aphthae may coalesce into larger lesions. While any oral mucosal surface may be involved, freely movable mucosa is more frequently involved than tightly bound. Lesions heal in 1 to 2 weeks without scarring.

Bacterial Infections

Odontogenic infections are caused by both aerobic and anaerobic microorganisms. Streptococci and staphylococci are isolated most frequently; however, any oral flora or opportunistic microorganism may be involved.

DENTAL ABSCESSES
Abscesses are most common in children with neglected dental caries due to poor dental hygiene and irregular dental care. Once caries extend to the pulp, infection and pulpal necrosis ensue, setting the stage for formation of a periapical abscess.

Children with traumatized teeth may go on to develop abscesses if the resulting pulpal hyperemia is so extreme that it causes pressure necrosis, or if the neurovascular bundle is severed.

Periapical abscesses require either endodontic therapy or extraction of the offending tooth. The potential for complications makes early diagnosis important, yet frequently this does not occur because often symptoms are insidious in onset and progression, and nonspecific in nature. This is in part due to the fact that in young children the alveolar processes of the mandible and maxilla are fenestrated anteriorly, facilitating early decompression of the abscess through the alveolus and gingiva. Patients may complain of headaches as the abscess enlarges and pressure builds up, then of abdominal pain following decompression as the draining pus is swallowed causing gastric irritation. Later in childhood abscessed maxillary teeth may intermittently decompress through the floor of a maxillary sinus, producing recurrent sinus infections. Other presenting symptoms may include anorexia, avoidance of chewy foods, halitosis, toothaches, a sensitive tooth or facial

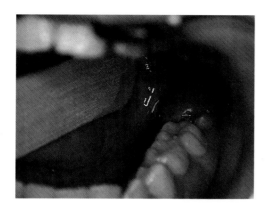

FIG. 20.49 Pericoronitis involving a partially erupted molar. Food particles and bacteria have become trapped under the residual overlying gingiva, resulting in inflammation and abscess formation. This condition can occur with any molar eruption, but is most common with partially erupted third molars (wisdom teeth).

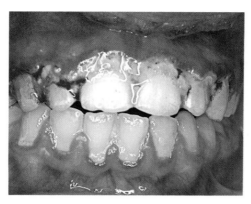

FIG. 20.50 Acute necrotizing ulcerative gingivitis. The infected gingiva exhibits localized necrosis, hemorrhage, and is covered with pseudomembranes.

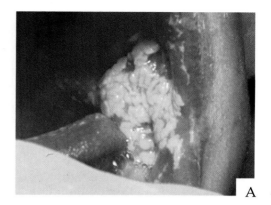

A

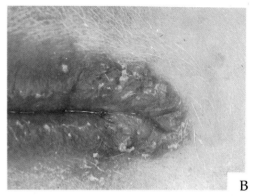

B

FIG. 20.51 Candidiasis. A, involvement of buccal mucosa with white plaque. B, mucocutaneous infection of the commissures of the lips.

swelling. Nonspecific complaints and complaints of referred pain are more common than a toothache in children, some of whom have no overt symptoms but report feeling better following treatment.

On physical examination one may find localized gingival swelling and/or erythema, a gingival abscess, a fistula or a granuloma (Figs. 20.46, 20.47). On occasion there is increased sensitivity to percussion. Left untreated, a periapical abscess of a primary tooth may damage the underlying developing tooth bud. Abscesses may also result in formation of an apical granuloma or a radicular cyst, or they may rupture and spread through the adjacent soft tissues to create a fistula, which drains through the skin (Fig. 20.47B), or cause facial cellulitis (Fig. 20.48). More ominously the infection may track through lateral pharyngeal, retropharyngeal, or sublingual spaces, threatening the airway and causing sepsis and/or mediastinitis. Rarely, septic thrombosis of the cavernous sinus may result from neglected infections that rupture into the maxillary sinus.

PERICORONITIS

Pericoronitis is a bacterial infection of the gingival soft tissue surrounding the crown of a partially erupted tooth. This occurs when food particles and plaque become trapped under the residual gingiva, stimulating bacterial growth and abscess formation. The third molars are most commonly involved. Symptoms include localized pain and tenderness, and occasionally fever and malaise. Erythema and edema are readily apparent on examination (Fig. 20.49) and an enlarged tender submandibular node is often found.

ACUTE NECROTIZING ULCERATIVE GINGIVITIS (VINCENT'S INFECTION, TRENCH MOUTH)

This is a fusospirochetal infection caused by fusiform bacilli and *Borrelia vincentii* which is seldom seen before the age of 10. Patients experience abrupt onset of fever, malaise, severe mouth pain and anorexia. The gingivae are reddened, edematous, and friable with necrotic punched-out craters in the interdental papillae. Occasionally the palate and tongue are affected as well. Involved areas hemorrhage readily and become covered with a pseudomembrane (Fig. 20.50). The breath is fetid, and cervical and submandibular nodes are enlarged and tender. Treatment generally consists of gentle dental prophylaxis followed by improved oral hygiene measures and topical peroxide applications. In most cases resolution occurs within several days without the use of antibiotics. Occasionally, secondary infection or severe involvement may necessitate the use of antibiotics; penicillin is then the antibiotic of choice.

Fungal Infections

CANDIDIASIS (MONILIASIS, THRUSH)

Candidiasis results from the opportunistic pathogen *Candida albicans*. This infection is seen in infants, in children with underlying systemic diseases, in immunosuppressed children, or in those on antibiotic treatment. Common sites of involvement are the buccal mucosa, tongue, palate, and the commissures of the lips. The intraoral lesions of acute infection are soft, elevated, creamy white plaques which do not scrape off easily (Fig. 20.51). Chronic candidiasis, usually seen in the immunocompromised host, can result in marked hypertrophy

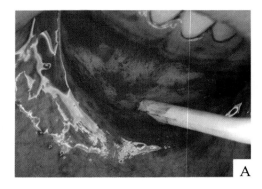

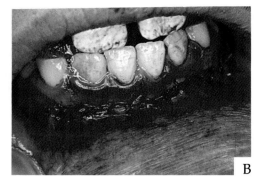

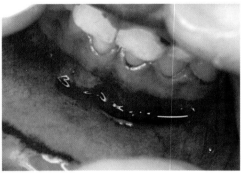

FIG. 20.52 Degloving injury, before (**A**) and after (**B**) repair. Such an injury to the oral mucosa requires immediate inspection, irrigation, approximation, and suturing.

FIG. 20.53 This laceration of the oral mucosa—deep and not well-approximated—requires immediate treatment.

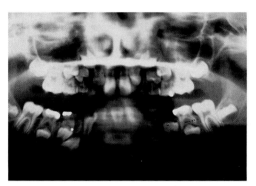

FIG. 20.54 A panographic radiograph shows bilaterally fractured mandibular condyles as a result of a blow to the chin.

and fissuring of the mucosa of the tongue. While culturing is difficult and not reliable, diagnosis may be made on the basis of clinical findings or examination of a KOH preparation. Treatment consists of local application of nystatin (miconazole or ketoconazole for severe or chronic cases), and control of the underlying causes, including sterilization of nipples used for formula feedings.

TRAUMA

Trauma to Soft Tissues

A variety of soft-tissue injuries including lacerations, contusions, abrasions, perforations, avulsions, and burns may occur. It is important to recognize that while soft tissue injuries may occur in isolation, they often are associated with injuries of teeth and supporting bones. Hence, any assessment of a soft-tissue injury must include careful attention to the teeth and underlying structures. The injured area should be cleansed of blood clots, debris, and foreign material, then carefully examined to determine the extent of tissue involvement. Mechanical debridement of any ragged, necrotic, or beveled margins may be necessary. Appropriate tetanus prophylaxis should also be considered. Saline rinses, careful attention to oral hygiene and soft diet are mainstays of management of soft tissue injuries.

ABRASIONS
Superficial abrasions usually heal without complications. Extensive abrasions should be covered with a water-soluble medicated gauze following irrigation. Extensive deep abrasions may require skin grafting.

CONTUSIONS
A contusion, or bruise, usually requires no treatment, and healing proceeds favorably in most instances. Contusions are often associated with underlying injuries; therefore, a careful examination of adjacent structures is indicated.

PERFORATIONS
These small deep wounds caused by sharp objects are fairly common in children, especially as a result of falls with such an object in the mouth. Careful examination of the wound as well as the object is essential. Following careful inspection and irrigation, larger wounds should be closed in layers; smaller wounds may not require closure. If doubt exists concerning foreign bodies and/or contamination, a drain should be left in situ and proper antibiotics prescribed. The possibility of damage to large vessels should be recognized, especially when the perforation involves the posterolateral palate or a tonsillar pillar (see Chapter 22, Otolaryngology).

AVULSIONS (DEGLOVING INJURIES)
Avulsions of oral soft tissues are uncommon injuries, yet when they do occur they may involve deep as well as superficial tissues (Fig. 20.52A,B). Small avulsions can be treated by undermining and suturing surrounding tissues. Larger avulsions can be treated either by reattaching the avulsed tissues or by use of a graft.

LACERATIONS
Lacerations of facial and oral tissues are common in children. Small intraoral lacerations with well-approximated margins do not require suturing. Bleeding usually subsides spontaneously, and healing proceeds satisfactorily. Large lacerations,

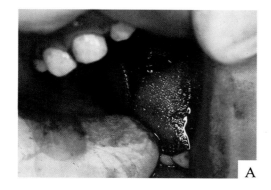

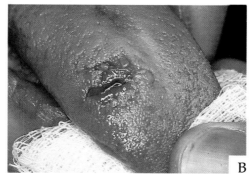

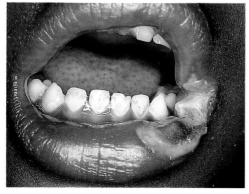

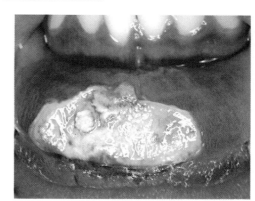

FIG. 20.55 Tongue lacerations. **A,** relatively large tongue laceration in a toddler produced by the upper front teeth being forced through the tissue by a fall with the tongue protruded. This type of injury usually requires suturing. **B,** this smaller laceration does not need surgical closure.

Fig. 20.56 This electrical burn was the result of chewing an extension cord. In this site, delayed hemorrage following separation of the eschar and deformity with scarring are particular problems.

FIG. 20.57 Traumatic lip ulceration caused by lip-biting following administration of local anesthesia.

through-and-through lacerations, and those associated with extensive, recurrent, or uncontrolled bleeding require careful assessment and surgical closure (Fig. 20.53).

Lip lacerations are often due to penetration of teeth through the labial soft tissues. Hence, the adjacent dentition must be carefully inspected for evidence of chipping as well as for signs of loosening or displacement. If chipping is found, imbedded tooth particles should be suspected. These may be difficult to palpate, but are easily detected radiographically. If present, they must be removed to prevent infection.

Because the trauma that results in chin lacerations commonly involves forced occlusion of the dentition, with transfer of impact forces to the underlying bone and condyles, these cases warrant assessment of underlying dental and bony structures (Fig. 20.54 and see Figs. 20.64 and 20.65). Forced occlusion injuries can also produce tongue lacerations. Closure is required for large, gaping wounds with persistent bleeding (Fig. 20.55A), but conservative management is best for smaller lesions (Fig. 20.55B).

Soft-palate lacerations require a thorough pharyngeal inspection. The possibility of foreign body entrapment, immediate or delayed vascular injury (particularly when the laceration involves posterolateral structures), or formation of pharyngeal abscesses should be seriously considered. Lacerations involving the labial frenulum of infants are common and usually require only restriction of lip manipulation and a soft diet.

BURNS

Burns involving the oral cavity usually heal rapidly, but with contracture and scarring. Burns at the angle of the mouth incurred by chewing on an electrical cord are particularly problematic. Following the injury an eschar forms over the necrotic tissue. This tends to separate approximately 10 days later, at which time profuse bleeding from the labial artery may occur (Fig. 20.56. Splints fabricated from dental materials are important in long-term management to prevent or minimize contracture by maintaining proper anatomic relationships during healing.

TRAUMATIC ULCERS

These painful ulcerations result from mechanical, chemical, or thermal trauma. Injury may be secondary to irritation by objects, trauma during mastication, toothbrush trauma, or abnormal habits. Large ulcerations involving the buccal mucosa or lower lip may be associated with cheek or lip biting following inferior alveolar nerve block (Fig. 20.57). Topical peroxide application (Gly-Oxide®) is useful in cleansing the area. Lesions usually heal without scarring, but secondarily infected lesions may require antibiotic therapy. Identification and elimination of the habit is necessary for resolution of habit-related lesions.

Trauma to the Dentition

As noted earler, facial injuries in childhood frequently involve the dentition and supporting bones. One prospective study showed that 50 percent of children had suffered at least one dental injury by age 14. While falls are the major source in early childhood, bicycle and skateboard accidents, contact sports, fights, and motor vehicle accidents become more important with advancing age. The risk of such injuries is relatively high in (1) children with neurologic disorders that impair coordination; (2) children with protruding maxillary anterior teeth; and (3) children with a deviant anatomic relationship, such as an anterior open bite or a hypoplastic upper lip. Preventive measures, such as use of helmets, mouthguards and seat belts, significantly reduce the incidence and severity of such injuries.

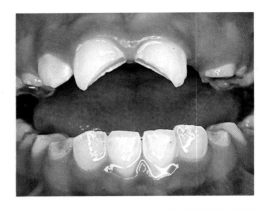

FIG. 20.58 These crown fractures demonstrate involvement of enamel and dentin, without exposure of the pulp. Immediate dental referral is necessary to prevent contamination of the pulp through the dentinal tubules.

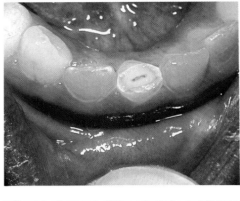

FIG. 20.59 This crown fracture involves not only enamel and dentin but the soft tissue of the pulp as well. Immediate dental referral is mandatory if the tooth is to be saved.

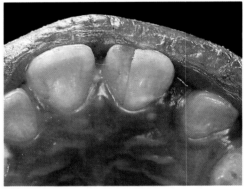

FIG. 20.60 A vertical fracture of the upper central incisor extending below the gum line resulted in pulp exposure.

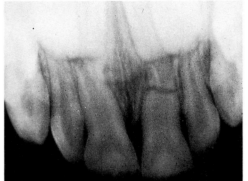

FIG. 20.61 This radiograph reveals a root fracture in the apical third of an upper primary incisor. This was suspected clinically because of tenderness and increased mobility.

Several extensive classifications of tooth injuries have been suggested, but for the purpose of this text a more simplified descriptive classification will now be presented.

CROWN CRAZE OR CRACK
A significant number of children are discovered during routine physical examination to have "cracks" in the enamel of their teeth. Such cracks are presumably caused by relatively minor trauma or temperature changes. The overwhelming majority of such teeth are asymptomatic and require no treatment.

CROWN FRACTURES WITHOUT PULPAL EXPOSURE
Fractures that traverse only the enamel layer often require no treatment other than smoothing down rough edges and ensuring close followup (see Fig. 20.46A). However, any fracture of the crown that results in exposure of the dentin requires urgent treatment to prevent infection and subsequent pulp necrosis (Fig. 20.58). The treatment of choice is to seal the exposed dentin with calcium hydroxide and to protect it with an acid-etched resin bandage for a minimum of 2 to 3 months to enhance pulpal healing. This procedure should be performed as soon as possible following the injury. As noted earlier, dental fragments are occasionally embedded in the soft tissues of the lip or tongue; therefore, appropriate examination and palpation of these areas is indicated. The presence of such fragments may be confirmed by radiographic examination.

CROWN FRACTURES WITH PULPAL EXPOSURE
Fractures that traverse all three tooth layers to expose the pulp usually involve a significant loss of tooth structure. On physical examination, the fracture surface reveals the pink central pulp surrounded by the brown or beige dentinal layer (Fig. 20.59). Severe vertical or diagonal fractures may also result in pulp exposure and can at times extend to involve the root (Fig. 20.60). Such teeth must be treated urgently with pulp capping, pulpotomy, or root canal therapy, depending on severity.

ROOT FRACTURES
Root fractures are less common in the primary dentition, and when they do occur they usually require no therapy. Root fractures of permanent teeth may occur with or without loss of crown structure, and may be asymptomatic (Fig. 20.61). If a seemingly normal tooth becomes tender or exhibits increased mobility following trauma, root fracture should be suspected and radiographs obtained. Generally the prognosis is good, and treatment may include splinting the involved segment for 6 to 10 weeks, with or without root canal therapy.

DISPLACEMENT INJURIES
These injuries result in extrusion, intrusion, or lateral displacement (labially or lingually), and are most commonly seen in the primary dentition where the combination of a short root length and a very "pliable" bony structure seem to permit displacement to occur (Fig. 20.62A,B). Displacement injuries are

ORAL DISORDERS

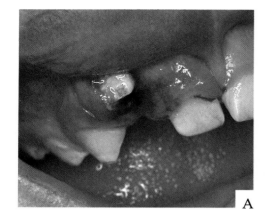

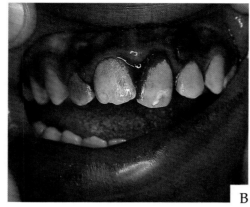

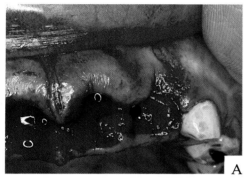

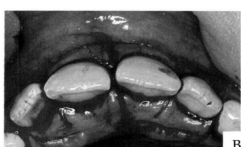

FIG. 20.62 Displacement injuries. **A,** *this primary lateral incisor was traumatically intruded. Such intrusions will usually spontaneously reerupt.* **B,** *lateral displacement. The left upper central incisor is lingually displaced and its crown appears elongated as a result of partial extrusion. This would require repositioning and splinting.*

FIG. 20.63 **A,** *four permanent incisors have been avulsed.* **B,** *the teeth have been reimplanted successfully.*

often the cause of significant discomfort, bleeding, and possible interference with mastication, and occlusion. All result in some degree of disruption of the periodontal ligament. Further, being the result of moderate to severe mechanisms of injury, fractures of underlying bony structures are common associated findings. Because the primary teeth are most vulnerable to these types of injury, there is always a risk of damage to and interference with normal development of permanent tooth buds. Therefore, immediate care is advised. Treatment may include observation with or without prophylactic antibiotic coverage, immediate correction in cases of lingual displacement due to interference with mastication, or extraction of the displaced tooth in cases of severe labial or vertical displacement. Most intruded primary teeth will reerupt within 6 to 8 weeks with antibiotic coverage, sensible oral hygiene, and an appropriate diet. In general, displaced permanent teeth should be surgically repositioned and splinted, with close followup. It is not uncommon for these teeth to require root canal therapy.

AVULSION AND REIMPLANTATION

Avulsion is the complete displacement of a tooth from its socket, and is seen mostly in preschool and early school-age children. Reimplantation of primary teeth is still experimental and should only be done under selective conditions. However, the prognosis is usually poor, and splinting is not easily carried out.

On the other hand, reimplantation of permanent teeth is an acceptable technique with a relatively good prognosis (Fig. 20.63A,B). The major factors in improving prognosis are:

1. A short period between avulsion and reimplantation, preferably less than half an hour.
2. Appropriate storage of the avulsed tooth (the most desirable "media" would be the socket itself, followed by saliva and milk).
3. Appropriate irrigation of the surgical site, replacing the tooth into the socket *without* pressure, and stabilizing it with the use of a resin-bonded splint.
4. Appropriate removal of the pulp within 2 weeks as a first step in completing root canal treatment, unless the tooth was immature with incomplete root formation.
5. Removal of the splint within 2 weeks.

It is generally accepted that scraping of the root or the socket is contraindicated, as preservation of adherent shreds of periodontal membrane appears to improve prognosis.

Trauma to Supporting Structures

In the young child the developing facial bones are small relative to the calvarium and thus somewhat protected by it. They are compact, spongy and have greater elasticity, which tends to reduce the risk of fractures. However, the relatively thin

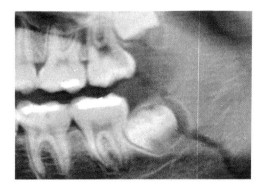

FIG. 20.64 A panoramic radiograph reveals a nondisplaced mandibular fracture originating in the third molar tooth bud.

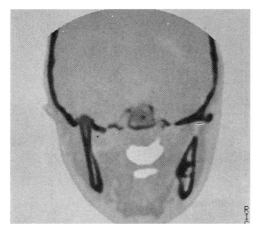

FIG. 20.65 CT scan reveals the intrusion of the mandibular condyle into the middle cranial fossa as a result of an extremely severe forced occlusion injury. Careful "pull back" and splinting is a common treatment for this type of injury.

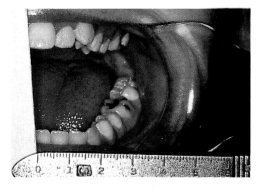

FIG. 20.66 A method of measuring deviation of the mandible on opening is illustrated in this picture showing a shift to the fracture side the width of one lower central incisor.

outer cortices make alveolar process fractures somewhat more likely with dental displacement injuries; and their growth centers and developing tooth buds serve as weak points and thus are major sites of fractures when they do occur (Fig. 20.64 and see Fig. 20.54). Finally, their thick periosteum has remarkable osteogenic potential, which speeds healing remarkably. Injuries to these bony supporting structures of the dentition may result from birth trauma, bicycle accidents, car accidents, various physical and sporting activities, child abuse, and animal bites. Because major forces are required to produce jaw fractures in children, one must carefully search for evidence of associated head and neck injuries (Fig. 20.65) and be vigilant in observing for evidence of expanding hematomas that may later compromise the airway.

In evaluating patients, first, a concise history must be obtained, including information concerning the circumstances of the accident. Then a careful clinical examination is necessary to determine the extent and nature of injury, which will help the physician select the needed diagnostic tools and take the appropriate course of action. The examination should include:

1. The overlying skin and soft tissues.
2. The dentition.
3. The gingiva and oral mucosa.
4. The facial and jaw bones.
5. Dental occlusion.

Tenderness on palpation, trismus, hemorrhage from the nose or the ear, deviation on opening or closing the mouth, periorbital ecchymosis or edema, subconjunctival hemorrhage or edema, diplopia, or the presence of sinus clouding on radiographs should call for a detailed evaluation of the suspected area.

FRACTURES OF THE MANDIBLE

Excluding nasal fractures, the most common facial fractures in children involve the mandible. The two major mechanisms are forced occlusion and lateral or frontolateral impact.

Forced occlusion can produce hemarthrosis of the temperomandibular joint, a compression fracture of the condylar process (see Fig. 20.54), or a greenstick condylar fracture. These injuries are often associated with fractures of the molar crowns. Lateral and frontolateral blows tend to produce fractures of the mandibular body, usually through the wall of a developing tooth bud (see Fig. 20.64). They also may be associated with a contralateral condylar fracture. Important diagnostic clues may include ecchymosis (see Fig. 20.68), facial swelling, deviation on opening or closing (Fig. 20.66), trismus, and malocclusion that may be apparent visibly or only subjectively evident to the patient. Palpation may reveal localized tenderness and hematoma formation, a step-off, or abnormal mobility with or without gingival tears. Examination of the child with a temperomandibular joint injury may reveal tenderness and decreased motion, or a snap when the examiner's fingers are pressed just anterior to the external auditory canal as the child opens and closes the mouth. A panoramic radiograph and a mandibular series should be ordered if there is clinical suspicion of a fracture. If routine views are unrevealing, tomography may be called for in certain unusual, difficult or complex cases.

Management requires careful assessment of the stability and type of erupted dentition as well as the location of the tooth buds. Nondisplaced fractures with no occlusal abnormalities may require no treatment other than a soft diet. Most displaced fractures can be treated conservatively: first, by appropriate reduction, followed by either simple intermaxillary fixation or by intraoral splints and circumferential wiring (closed reduction). Seldom is open reduction indicated; however, if this technique is used, careful placement of intraosseous holes is essential to avoid damage to the developing tooth buds.

FRACTURES OF THE MAXILLA AND THE MIDFACE

Fractures of the midface are especially uncommon in younger children and infants because of their relatively large cranial vault and the elasticity of their bones. When such fractures do occur, they are often associated with injuries to

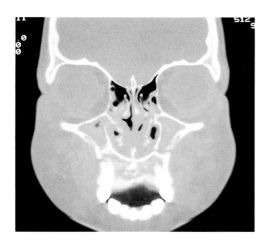

FIG. 20.67 CT scan shows a LeFort I fracture. The maxilla is separated from the midface. The degree is greater on the right.

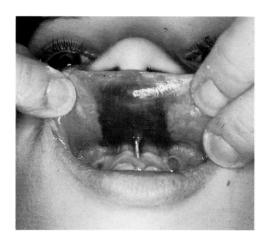

FIG. 20.68 Delineated ecchymosis with hematoma formation on the mucosa of the upper lip is a common sign associated with underlying fractures, in this case a fracture of the anterior nasal spine of the maxilla.

the frontal region, the orbits and overlying soft tissues, and the nose.

In 1901, LeFort divided midfacial fractures into three groups:

1. LeFort I, which primarily involves the maxilla (Fig. 20.67).
2. LeFort II, which primarily involves the maxilla and the nasal complex.
3. LeFort III, which involves separation of the midface from the cranium.

These fractures require a thorough and detailed examination to ensure proper care. Symptoms and signs are similar to those of mandibular fractures (Fig. 20.68). Exact diagnosis of the location and extent of maxillary fractures can be challenging and frequently requires specialized tomography since routine radiographic views such as anteroposterior, lateral, and Towne's are often inadequate.

Early treatment of facial injuries requires careful monitoring of vital signs, maintenance of an adequate airway, observation for progression of edema, and a careful neurologic evaluation. The need for intubation or even tracheotomy must be considered if airway difficulties arise. The next most important factor to consider is hemorrhage, which may become a critical problem in younger children. In such cases, total blood loss should be monitored, the patient typed and cross-matched, and replacement therapy initiated if necessary. Further definitive treatment can be completed following stabilization and appropriate radiographic evaluation.

TEMPOROMANDIBULAR JOINT DISORDERS (TMJD)

TMJ disorders are a heterogenous group of problems with only one common denominator—pain. Their incidence is not specifically known and the reported signs and symptoms vary considerably, probably due to lack of a scientifically acceptable definition of TMJD.

Origin of symptoms of TMJD can be traced to joint dysfunction or inflammation, muscle strain or spasm, trauma, significant malocclusion, and/or stress. In healthy adults, most recent evidence points to stress as a major contributor. As existing therapeutic modalities seem to have similar results, and as biofeedback has longer lasting effects when compared to

splints, it is recommended that the most noninvasive and the least expensive modality of treatment be used, with emphasis on stress control.

Specific signs and symptoms, such as clicking or popping of the TMJ, have never in controlled studies been proven reliable indicators of pathology. However, bruxism, clenching of the jaws or grinding of the teeth should be identified and their diagnostic relevance evaluated.

Examination of the TMJ should include palpation of the immediate area, including the surrounding muscles of mastication, and of movement of the condylar heads; assessment of maximum opening; and visual inspection for deviations of the mandible while opening and closing.

Required diagnostic data may include a thorough history, including behavioral assessment and clinical evaluation. Other diagnostic data such as tomography, transcranial radiography, and CT scanning have not been proven reliable under controled conditions.

In pediatric patients, no good data are yet available, but muscle fatigue and spasm must be first ruled out. History of repetitive habits or activities must be evaluated. Examples include prolonged violin playing, computer games, clenching, grinding and bruxism. As a general rule, the younger the child, the more likely it is that the pain is muscular in origin. Behavior modifications, rest, and changing or modifying repetitive habits, usually yield excellent results.

BIBLIOGRAPHY

Bhaskar SN: Oral lesions of infants and newborns. *Dent Clin North Am* 1966; July: 421–435.

Christensen RE Jr: Soft tissue lesions of the head and neck, in Sanders B (ed): *Pediatric Oral and Maxillofacial Surgery*. St. Louis, CV Mosby, 1979, 221–272.

Nazif MM, Ruffalo RC: The interaction between dentistry and otolaryngology. *Pediatr Clin North Am* 1981;28(4): 977–1010.

Rapp R: Dental and gingival disorders, in Bluestone CD, Stool SE (eds): *Pediatric Otolaryngology, ed 2*. Philadelphia, WB Saunders, 1990, 867–888.

Sanders B, et al: Injuries, in Sanders B (ed): *Pediatric Oral and Maxillofacial Surgery*. St. Louis, CV Mosby, 1979, 330–399.

Schuit KE, Johnson JT: Infections of the head and neck. *Pediatr Clin North Am* 1981;28 (4):965–971.

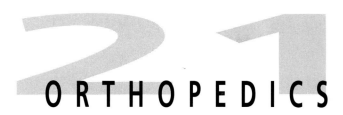

ORTHOPEDICS

W. Timothy Ward, M.D. ◆ Holly W. Davis, M.D. ◆ Edward N. Hanley Jr., M.D.

Children with musculoskeletal injuries and afflictions seek help because of pain, deformity, or loss of function. Often the clinical challenge lies not so much in recognizing the impaired or injured part, which in most cases is readily accessible to inspection and examination, but in making an accurate diagnosis in order to plan and initiate appropriate treatment. Because of their rapid physical growth and the special properties of their developing bones, children often pose special problems for the clinician.

Discussion is divided into six sections: (1) development of the skeletal system; (2) musculoskeletal trauma; (3) disorders of the spine; (4) disorders of the upper extremity; (5) disorders of the lower extremity; (6) generalized musculoskeletal disorders.

A number of other disorders generally classified under other subspecialties, but involving the musculoskeletal system, are covered in other chapters. Bone and joint infections are discussed in Chapter 12, collagen vascular diseases in Chapter 7, nutritional deficiencies and renal disorders affecting the skeletal system in Chapter 10, and neuromuscular disorders and spinal dysraphism in Chapters 15 and 13. Additional examples of trauma are present in Chapter 6.

DEVELOPMENT OF THE SKELETAL SYSTEM

The assessment, diagnosis, and management of pediatric orthopedic problems necessitate a clear understanding of the physiology of the growing musculoskeletal system and of the unique properties of growing bone especially. The process of growth begins in utero and continues until the end of puberty. Linear growth occurs as the result of multiplication of chondrocytes in the epiphyses, which align themselves vertically, forming a transitional zone of endochondral ossification in the metaphyses. The shafts of long bones widen and flat bones enlarge via deposition and mineralization of osteoid by the periosteum. Hence, genetic and congenital disorders that affect connective tissue (and thus the skeleton) tend to cause abnormal growth. Most commonly this results in dwarfism with varying degrees of deformity. However, in some conditions such as Marfan syndrome, excessive linear growth occurs, resulting in abnormally tall stature and unusually long fingers and toes.

The terminal arterial loops and sinusoidal veins that form the vascular bed of growing metaphyses have sluggish blood flow, which increases the risk of thrombosis and of deposition of bacteria during periods of bacteremia. As a result, pediatric patients are at greater risk of developing hematogenous osteomyelitis. Furthermore, the epiphyseal plates being incompletely formed in infancy are a less effective barrier to extension of infection into adjacent joints, and the relatively thin diaphyseal cortices tend to permit rupture outward under the overlying periosteum. Similarly, penetration of vascular channels through the vertebral end plates into the intervertebral discs makes discitis more likely than vertebral osteomyelitis in early childhood (see Chapter 12, Infectious Diseases).

A thorough understanding of musculoskeletal development and of radiographic findings at differing stages is particularly important in the diagnosis and management of orthopedic injuries. At birth only a few epiphyses have begun to ossify; the remainder are cartilaginous and, thus, are invisible radiographically. With development, other epiphyses begin to ossify, enlarge and mature in such an orderly fashion that one can estimate a child's age from the number and configuration of ossification centers (Figs. 21.1, 21.2). The epiphyseal plates (physes), being sites of cartilaginous proliferation and growth, do not begin to ossify until puberty (Fig. 21.3). When skeletal injuries involve sites where ossification has not begun or is incomplete, radiographs may appear normal or may not reflect the full extent of the injury. This necessitates greater reliance on clinical findings.

Prior to closure of the physis during puberty, the growth plate is actually weaker than nearby ligaments. As a result, injuries that occur near joints are more likely to result in physeal disruption than in ligamentous tearing (i.e., sprains and dislocations are seen less commonly in prepubertal children than in adolescents). When there is displacement of an epiphyseal fracture and the fragments are not anatomically reduced, growth disturbances may occur. Because the epiphysis may not be ossified, radiographs often may fail to reveal the injury, and for this reason children with injuries at or near joints must be examined with meticulous care in order not to miss epiphyseal fractures.

The periosteum of a child is much thicker than that of an adult, strips more easily from the bone, and rarely is disrupted

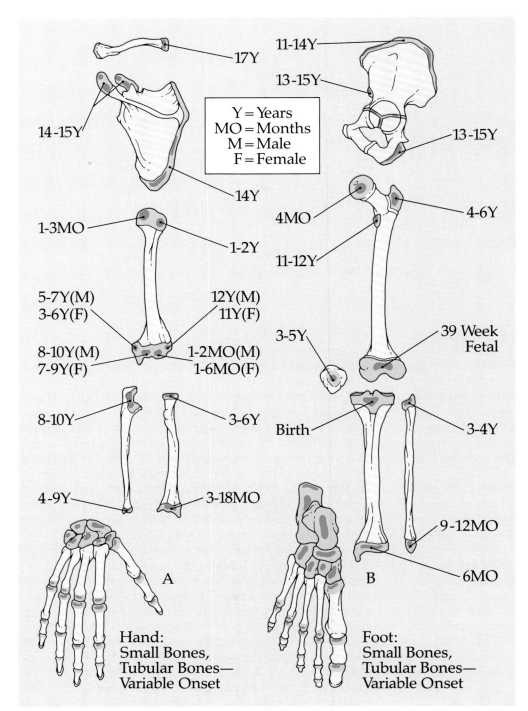

Y = Years
MO = Months
M = Male
F = Female

17Y

14-15Y

1-3MO

1-2Y

5-7Y(M)
3-6Y(F)

12Y(M)
11Y(F)

8-10Y(M)
7-9Y(F)

1-2MO(M)
1-6MO(F)

8-10Y

3-6Y

4-9Y

3-18MO

A

Hand:
Small Bones,
Tubular Bones—
Variable Onset

11-14Y

13-15Y

13-15Y

4MO

4-6Y

11-12Y

3-5Y

39 Week
Fetal

Birth

3-4Y

9-12MO

B

6MO

Foot:
Small Bones,
Tubular Bones—
Variable Onset

Fig. 21.1 Ages of onset of ossification. At birth only a few epiphyses have begun to ossify. The remainder are cartilaginous and therefore invisible radiographically. With development other epiphyses begin to ossify, enlarge, and mature in an orderly fashion, making it possible to estimate a child's age from the number and configuration of ossification centers. This forms the basis for the use of bone age as part of the evaluation of children with growth disorders. It is of crucial importance to bear in mind when evaluating the radiographs of injured children that fractures involving nonossified epiphyses are radiographically invisible until healing begins (see Figure 21.44).

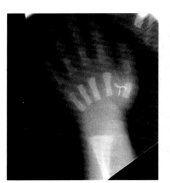 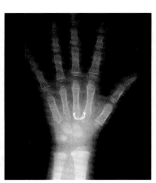 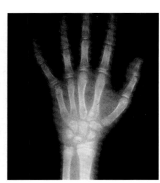

Fig. 21.2 Increasing numbers of ossification centers become radiographically visible with age. The hands shown are those of a toddler, a young school-age child, and a young adolescent. Injuries affecting unossified bones or growth centers are radiographically invisible.

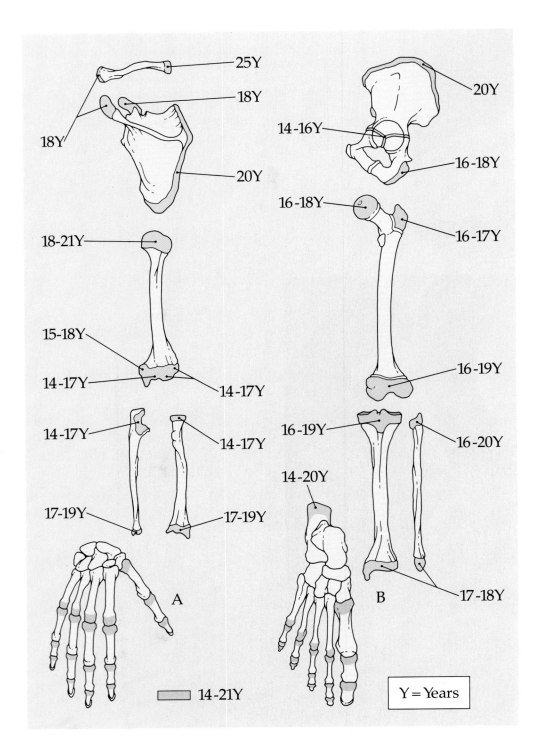

Fig. 21.3 Ages of physeal closure.

25Y
18Y
18Y
20Y
18-21Y
15-18Y
14-17Y
14-17Y
14-17Y
14-17Y
17-19Y
17-19Y
A
14-21Y

20Y
14-16Y
16-18Y
16-18Y
16-17Y
16-19Y
16-19Y
16-20Y
14-20Y
17-18Y
B
Y = Years

completely when the underlying bone is fractured. The immature, rapidly growing bone of the child is more porous than that of the adult and has a greater capacity for plastic deformation but less ability to withstand compressive or tensile forces. Consequently, a given compressive force that would produce a comminuted fracture in an adult tends to be dissipated in part by the bending that occurs in the more flexible bone of the child. Such a force is thus more likely to result in plastic deformation or to produce an incomplete fracture, such as a torus fracture or a greenstick fracture, in a child.

Thus, fracture patterns in children often differ from those in adults. Their fractures can be considerably harder to detect clinically and radiographically, and can potentially result in long-term growth abnormalities. Children do have advantages,

however, in that their activity growing bones heal with greater rapidity and have a remarkable capacity for remodeling.

Finally, numerous genetic, metabolic, endocrine, renal, and inflammatory processes can have impact not only on growth and ultimate height, but also on skeletal maturation—in some cases delaying it and in others accelerating it. Comparison of the patient's actual bone age, as determined by the number of radiographically visible ossification centers, with his chronologic age can help diagnose these underlying disorders.

MUSCULOSKELETAL TRAUMA

The normal impulsiveness and inquisitiveness of children combined with their lack of caution and love of energetic

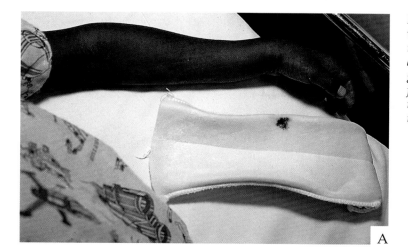

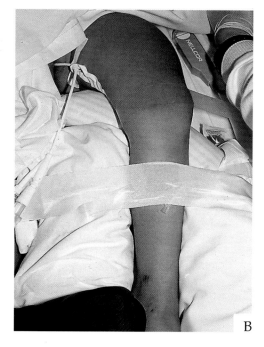

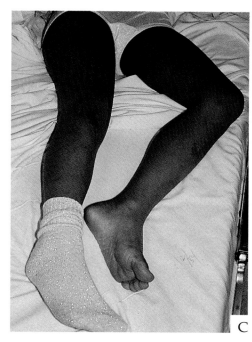

Fig. 21.4 Visible abnormalities seen on inspection in children with fractures. **A,** distortion and angulation of the distal forearm in a child with fractures of the radius and ulna. **B,** swelling and angulation of the proximal thigh due to a femur fracture. **C,** longitudinal shortening of the thigh in a child with a proximal femur fracture. Note the characteristic, externally rotated position of the injured leg. The child was struck by a car, sustaining a fracture of the femoral neck.

activities place them at a relatively high risk for accidental injury. The incidence of trauma is further elevated by the prevalence of child abuse (see Chapter 6). In fact, beyond infancy, trauma is the leading cause of death in children and adolescents, and is the source of significant morbidity. Musculoskeletal injuries are very common whether seen in isolation or as part of multisystem trauma. While management of life-threatening injuries to the airway, circulation, and CNS must take precedence over accompanying musculoskeletal injuries in cases of multiple trauma, it must be kept in mind that fractures can result in significant blood loss. This is particularly true of pelvic and femoral fractures. Furthermore, prompt attention must be given to assessment of the status of neurovascular structures distal to obvious fractures; failure to recognize compromise may result in permanent loss of func-

tion. Finally, traumatic hip dislocations must be reduced within 12 hours if the risk of aseptic necrosis and long-term morbidity are to be minimized.

Fractures

DIAGNOSIS

One of the many variables that complicate the diagnosis of the skeletally injured child is that the child, already in pain, is frightened by his recent experience and by the strangeness of the hospital or emergency room setting. Many children are too young to give a firsthand history, and the cooperation of toddlers is often limited. The parents are likely to be anxious as well. A calm, empathetic manner is needed to allay their fears. Taking a thorough history prior to any attempt at physical

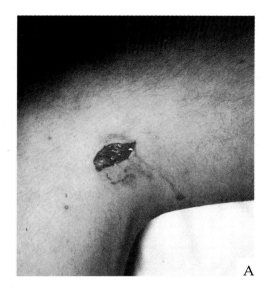

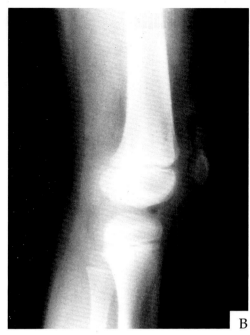

A

B

assessment will help establish rapport with the patient and the family. This should include questions concerning the type and direction of the injuring force, the position of the involved extremity at the time of the accident, as well as the events immediately following the injury, such as measures taken at the scene of the accident. The presence of underlying disorders and the possibility of contamination of an open wound should be determined as well. Physicians also should be alert to signs suggestive of inflicted injury or child abuse.

In cases of suspected fracture, splinting, elevation, and topical application of ice may help reduce discomfort and local swelling. Splinting is particularly important for displaced and unstable fractures as it prevents further soft tissue injuries and reduces the risk of fat embolization. When pain is severe and there are no cardiovascular or CNS contraindications, analgesia should be administered promptly. Contrary to the opinion of many physicians, this does not obscure physical findings. Tenderness will not be reduced significantly, swelling will remain, and patient cooperation for the examination may be considerably greater.

Before beginning the physical examination, it is wise to talk with the child to further gain his trust. Older infants and toddlers are often more comfortable when allowed to sit on a parent's lap, and use of puppets or toys can reduce fear and help engage their cooperation. As comparison of paired extremities is an integral part of orthopedic assessment, it is best to begin examining the uninjured side, and it is wise to defer palpation of the most likely site of the injury on the affected side until last. When young children are highly anxious, it can be useful to instruct the parent to perform a passive range of motion and palpation.

The first step in a physical examination is visual inspection of the injured area. The gross position of the extremity should be noted, and attention given to the presence or absence of deformity, distortion or abnormal angulation, and longitudinal shortening (Fig. 21.4). The overlying skin and soft tissues are examined for evidence of swelling, ecchymoses, abrasions, punctures or lacerations. Comparison with the opposite extremity and measurement of circumference can be very helpful when findings are subtle.

The location of open wounds is important in ascertaining whether an underlying fracture is open or closed and in assessing risk of joint penetration. Small puncture wounds or lacerations overlying bony structures that appear to be oozing a bloody, fatty exudate usually reflect communication with the medullary cavity of a fractured bone. Similarly, punctures or tears over joints that weep serous or serosanguinous fluid, especially when drainage is increased on moving the joint, must be assumed to communicate with the joint capsule (Fig. 21.5A). In patients with penetrating joint injuries, radiographs may demonstrate air in the joint, but absence of this does not rule out capsular penetration (Fig. 21.5B). Probing of open wounds that have a high likelihood of communication with a fracture or a joint is contraindicated. The wound should be cleaned and covered with a sterile dressing until its extent can be determined under sterile conditions in the operating room.

Following inspection of the most obviously injured area, palpation and assessment of active and passive motion can be performed. It is crucial to remember that in examining an injured limb the entire extremity must be evaluated in order to detect less obvious associated injuries. Localized swelling and tenderness on palpation are significant findings and should alert the examiner that there is a high likelihood of an underlying fracture. Pain on motion and limitation of motion signal the need for careful scrutiny as well. Assessment of motion involves observation of spontaneous movement, attempts to get the patient to voluntarily move the involved part through its expected range, and passive movement. Particular attention should be paid to the adjacent joints both proximal and distal to avoid missing associated injuries. It can be difficult, however, to determine whether motion is limited because of pain, an associated injury, or fear and lack of cooperation.

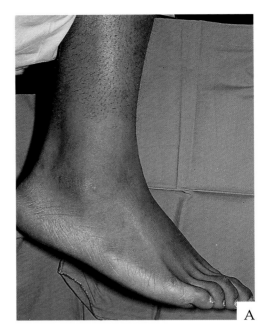
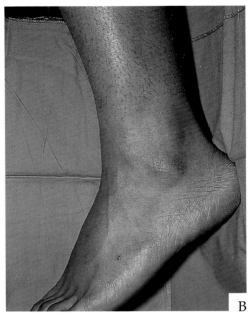

Fig. 21.6 Salter I fracture of the distal fibula. A, slight swelling is present over the lateral malleolus. The degree can only be truly appreciated by comparing the injured ankle to its normal counterpart shown in B. The patient had point tenderness over the affected malleolus. The findings differ from those of an ankle sprain in which tenderness and swelling are greatest over the ligaments inferior to the malleolus (see Fig. 21.53).

A

B

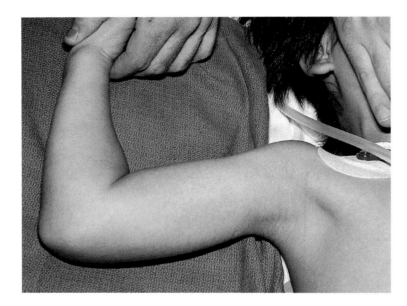

Fig. 21.7 Fracture with overlying soft tissue swelling. This child has a dislocated supracondylar fracture of the distal humerus with moderate soft tissue swelling. The degree becomes evident when the size of the elbow area is compared with the size of the patient's wrist.

Clinical findings vary depending on the nature of the fracture. Undisplaced growth plate fractures typically present with mild localized swelling and point tenderness at the level of the epiphysis (Fig. 21.6A,B). Since ligamentous injury is relatively uncommon in a child, the finding of such point tenderness should be sufficient evidence to treat the injury as a fracture until proven otherwise. Often initial radiographs appear normal and the fracture is confirmed only on followup when repeat radiographs disclose evidence of healing. Swelling is typically mild and occasionally imperceptible in cases of torus or buckle fractures and of undisplaced transverse and spiral fractures. Careful palpation should disclose focal tenderness, however. Usually, the patient will also experience some degree of discomfort on motion in some planes or on weight bearing, but it must be remembered that limitation of movement or

function can be minimal with such incomplete fractures. In contrast, fractures that completely disrupt the bone and displaced fractures are accompanied by more prominent swelling, more diffuse tenderness, and severe pain which is markedly increased on motion (Fig. 21.7). Crepitance may be evident also on gentle palpation. In examining children with these findings manipulation must be kept to a minimum to prevent further injury.

Assessment of neurovascular function distal to the injury is essential in evaluating any child with a potential fracture. This includes checking the integrity of pulses and speed of capillary refill as well as testing sensory and motor function. Strength and sensation should be compared to the contralateral extremity. Assessment of two point discrimination is probably the best test of sensory function. Evidence of neurovascular compromise necessitates urgent, often operative, orthopedic treatment. In addition, this assessment is crucial prior to and following reduction of displaced fractures in order to determine if the procedure itself has impaired function in any way. Supracondylar fractures of the humerus, fractures of the distal femoral shaft and proximal tibia, fracture/dislocations of the elbow and knee, and severely displaced ankle fractures have a particularly high risk of associated neurovascular injury. It is also important to be aware of the fact that vascular compromise can be present in a patient who has normal distal pulses and good peripheral perfusion. This should be suspected in patients who complain of intense muscle pain that is aggravated by stretching the muscle in an area distal to a displaced fracture. Persistence of intense pain following fracture reduction should also provoke suspicion of ischemia.

In all cases of suspected extremity fractures the injured part should be properly splinted and elevated, and an ice pack should be applied while awaiting transport to the radiography suite. However, in order to obtain high-quality radiographs, obstructing splints must be removed temporarily. This presents no major problem with partial or nondisplaced fractures, but can create difficulties in patients with severe displaced fractures. To insure that manipulation is minimal in these cases, splint removal, positioning for radiographs and splint reapplication should be supervised by a physician and not done merely at the discretion of the x-ray technician.

Fig. 21.8

PATTERNS OF FRACTURES

Fracture Pattern	Major Feature	Radiographic Appearance
Longitudinal	Fracture line is parallel to the axis of a long bone	Fig. 21.9
Transverse	Fracture line is perpendicular to the axis of a long bone	Fig. 21.10
Oblique	Fracture line is at an angle relative to the axis of a bone	Fig. 21.11
Spiral	Fracture line takes a curvilinear course around the axis of a bone	Fig. 21.12
Impacted	Bone ends are crushed together producing an indistinct fracture line	Fig. 21.13
Comminuted	Fracturing forces produce more than two separate fragments	Fig. 21.14
Bowing	Bone bends to the point of plastic deformation without fracturing	Fig. 21.15
Greenstick	Fracture is complete except for a portion of the cortex on the compression side of the fracture which is only plastically deformed	Fig. 21.16
Torus	Bone buckles and bends rather than breaking	Fig. 21.17

At a minimum, two radiographs taken at 90° angles are obtained, anteroposterior and lateral views being the most common. Oblique views are helpful in fully disclosing the nature and extent of many fracture patterns, especially when the injury involves the ankle, elbow, hand, or foot. They can also prove useful in detecting subtle spiral fractures, and in cases in which AP and lateral views are negative, yet a fracture is strongly suspected. Radiographs should include the joints immediately proximal and distal to a fractured long bone as there may be associated bony and/or soft-tissue injuries in these areas, as well. Such associated injuries easily can be missed on clinical examination when assessment of motion is limited by pain or when patient cooperation is limited. It is necessary to obtain comparison views of the opposite side, especially when evaluating patients with suspected physeal injuries who may have very subtle radiographic abnormalities. These views can also prove invaluable in detecting curtical disruptions. In some cases of displaced and/ or angulated fractures, tomograms and CT scans can be useful. Particular care should be taken in interpreting pediatric radiographs because of the high incidence of subtle or even negative findings in patients with fractures. When the clinical picture strongly suggests a fracture, appropriate treatment should be initiated even if the radiograph appears normal. Reassessment in 1 to 2 weeks can then clarify the exact nature of the injury.

FRACTURE PATTERNS

Fractures should be described in terms of anatomic location, direction of the fracture line, type of fracture, and degree of displacement. When the growth plate is involved, use of the Salter-Harris classification system is recommended.

Any specific mechanism of injury results in a readily definable pattern of force application, which tends to produce a typical fracture pattern. Because of this, it is often possible to infer the likely mechanism of injury once the fracture pattern is documented radiographically. If the vector of the direct force is perpendicular to the bone, a transverse fracture is most likely to result, whereas direct force applied at any angle to the bone produces an oblique fracture pattern. Examples of situations resulting in transverse and short oblique fractures include falls in which an extremity strikes the edge of a table, counter or chair, direct blows with an object such as a stick, and karate chops. These fractures are commonly seen as a result of accidents, fights, and in the battered child syndrome. Comminuted fractures generally are the result of high velocity direct forces such as those characteristic of vehicular accidents, falls from heights, or gunshot wounds. Impacted fractures are produced by forces oriented in a direction parallel to the long axis of the bone. Application of indirect force commonly results in spiral, greenstick, or torus fractures in children.

A common example of a nondisplaced spiral fracture is the *toddler's fracture* which results from a fall with a twist. Typically, the child either was running, turned, and then fell, or had gotten his foot caught and fell while twisting to extricate himself. When a child's arm or leg is forcibly pulled and twisted a similar fracture pattern may be seen. Greenstick and torus fractures of the radius and/or ulna are incurred usually by falling on an outstretched arm with the wrist in a dorsiflexed position. Vigorous repetitive shaking while holding a child by the hands, feet, or chest results in small metaphyseal chip or bucket handle fractures, a major feature of the shaken baby syndrome (see Chapter 6). Figure 21.8 describes the major features of these various fracture patterns, which are illustrated in Figures 21.9 through 21.17.

The anatomic location of the fracture line simply refers to that portion of the bone to which the injury force was applied. Figure 21.18 presents types of fractures classified by anatomic location. These fractures are illustrated in Figures 21.19 through 21.27. It should be noted that there is some degree of overlap in this method of categorization.

PHYSEAL FRACTURES

An estimated 15 percent of all fractures in children involve the physis. Because the adjacent epiphyseal plate is not ossified in the young child and therefore is invisible on a radiograph, the

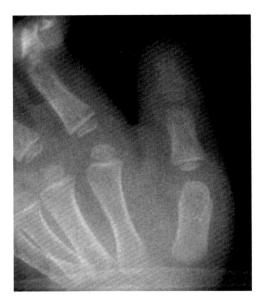

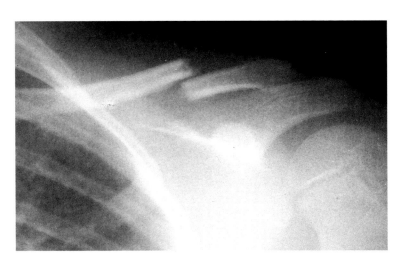

Fig. 21.9
Longitudinal fracture. A direct blow from above to the thumb produced this longitudinal fracture of the distal phalanx.

Fig. 21.10 Transverse fracture of the midportion of the clavicle. Fracture line is perpendicular to the long axis of the bone.

Fig. 21.11 Oblique fracture of the midportion of the femur. Fracture line is angled relative to the axis of the bone.

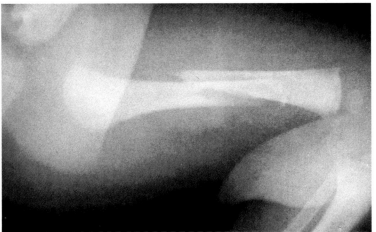

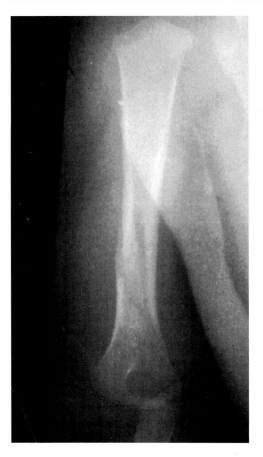

Fig. 21.12 Spiral fracture of the humerus. Fracture line takes curvilinear course around the axis of the bone.

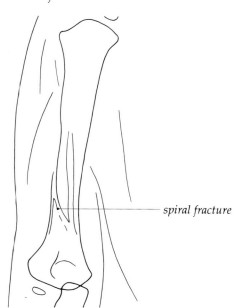

spiral fracture

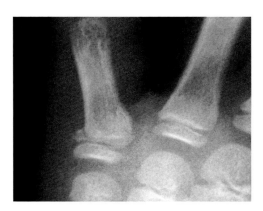

Fig. 21.13 Impacted fracture of the base of the proximal phalanx due to axial loading. The fracture line is indistinct and the fragments appear crushed together. The fracture does not actually involve the growth plate but is located just distal to it in the proximal metaphysis.

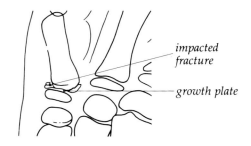

impacted fracture

growth plate

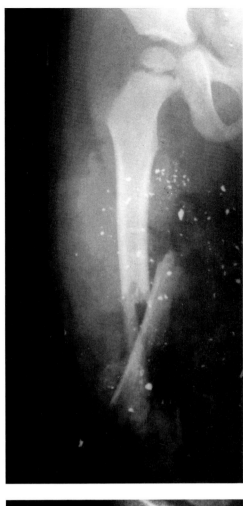

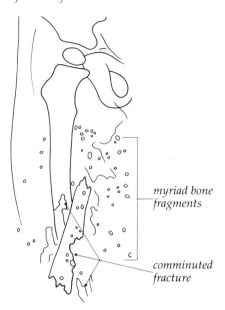

Fig. 21.14 Comminuted fracture of the femur secondary to gunshot wound. Notice the multiple small fragments of bone present in the adjacent soft tissues.

myriad bone fragments

comminuted fracture

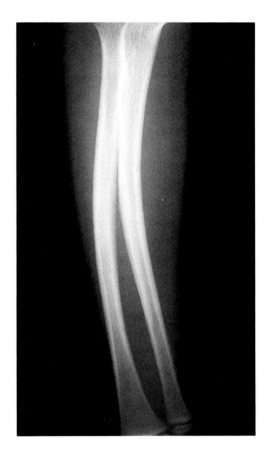

Fig. 21.15 Bowing of the forearm bones in an 8-year-old. This type of plastic deformation can be expected to remodel with time.

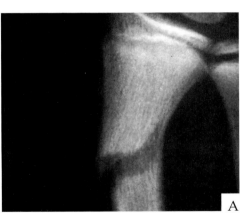

A

B

Fig. 21.16 Greenstick fracture of the distal radius. **A,** in the AP view of the distal radius a fracture line is seen that is complete except for a portion of the cortex on the compression side of the fracture. **B,** the lateral radiograph demonstrates more clearly the disrupted and compressed cortices. This resulted from a fall on the outstretched arm with the wrist in dorsiflexion.

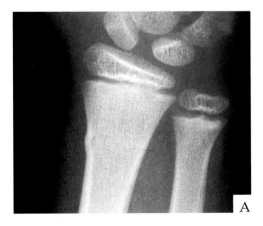

A

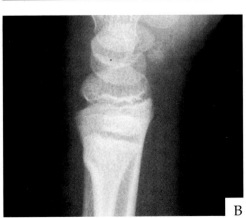

B

Fig. 21.17 Torus fracture of the distal radius due to a fall on an outstretched arm. **A,** an AP radiograph of the wrist demonstrates a minor torus or buckle fracture of the radius. **B,** the lateral radiograph shows the dorsal location of the deformity. This injury can be expected to completely remodel.

Fig. 21.18

CLASSIFICATION OF FRACTURES BY ANATOMIC LOCATION

Type	Site	Radiographic Appearance
Diaphyseal	Fracture involves the central shaft of a long bone	Fig. 21.19
Metaphyseal	Fracture involves the widened end of a long bone	Fig. 21.20
Epiphyseal	Fracture involves the chondro-osseous end of a long bone. Such fractures can also be classified as Salter-Harris fractures.	Fig. 21.21
Articular	Fracture involves the cartilaginous joint surface	Fig. 21.22 (see Figs. 21.31 and 21.32)
Intercondylar	Fracture is located between the condyles of a joint. This is one variant of articular fracture and could also be subclassified as a Salter-Harris fracture.	Fig. 21.22
Physeal	Fracture involves the growth center of long bone. These are subclassified according to the Salter-Harris system.	Fig. 21.23
Transcondylar	Fracture traverses the condyles of a joint	Fig. 21.24
Supracondylar	Fracture line is located just proximal to the condyles of a joint	Fig. 21.25
Epicondylar	Fracture involves an area juxtaposed to the condylar surface of a joint	Fig. 21.26
Subcapital	Fracture is located just below the epiphyseal head of certain bones	Fig. 21.27

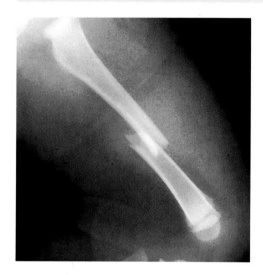

Fig. 21.19 Diaphyseal fracture. A transverse fracture line crosses the diaphyseal region of the femur. There is a moderate amount of overlap at the fracture site.

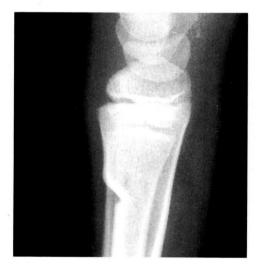

Fig. 21.20 Metaphyseal fracture. This lateral radiograph of the wrist shows a dorsal buckle fracture of the distal radial metaphysis. This fracture resulted from a fall on the outstretched arm with the wrist dorsiflexed and is a common injury in children.

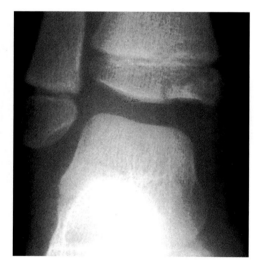

Fig. 21.21 Epiphyseal fracture. A fracture involving the medial aspect of the epiphysis of the distal tibia is seen in this AP radiograph of the ankle in a 4-year-old girl. A slight stepoff is present at the articular surface. This could also be classified as a Salter-Harris type III fracture.

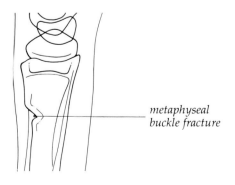

metaphyseal buckle fracture

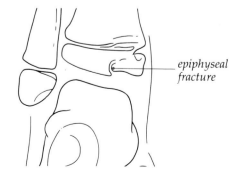

epiphyseal fracture

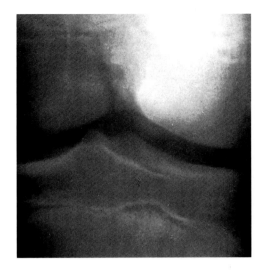

Fig. 21.22 Articular fracture. This AP view of the knee demonstrates intra-articular extension of a fracture line exiting at the junction of the medial and lateral femoral condyles. The condyles are separated by only a few millimeters. This can also be termed an intercondylar fracture.

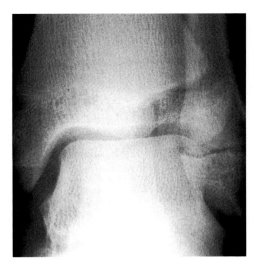

Fig. 21.23 Physeal fracture. A fracture of the lateral aspect of the epiphysis through the lateral aspect of the physeal plate is seen in this AP view of the ankle of a 13-year-old boy. Also called a "Tillaux" fracture, this pattern is seen in adolescents in whom the medial aspect of the distal tibial physis has closed but not the lateral aspect. Also termed a Salter-Harris type III fracture.

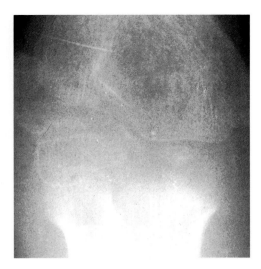

Fig. 21.24 Transcondylar fracture. This AP radiograph of the elbow reveals a fracture of the lateral condyle of the distal humerus. The condyle is displaced proximally and radially. The fragment is always larger than it appears on radiograph because of the large amount of unossified cartilage present in the distal humerus.

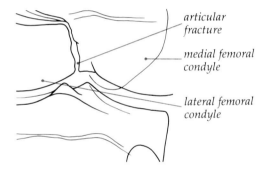

articular fracture

medial femoral condyle

lateral femoral condyle

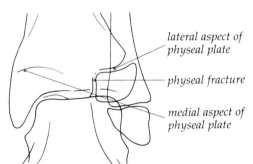

lateral aspect of physeal plate

physeal fracture

medial aspect of physeal plate

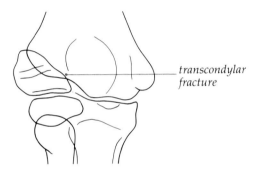

transcondylar fracture

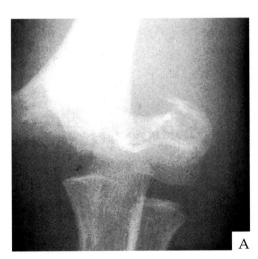

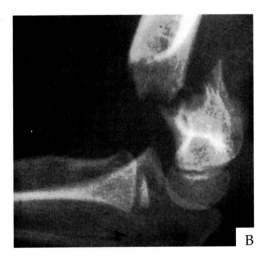

Fig. 21.25 Supracondylar fracture. These radiographs show the most common pattern of supracondylar humerus fracture seen in children. This injury resulted from a fall backwards on the outstretched arm with the elbow in hyperextension. This transmitted the force of the impact to the distal humerus driving the distal fragment posteriorly. **A,** the AP radiograph shows the distal fragment displaced radially. **B,** in the lateral view, posterior displacement is evident as well.

fracture may be mistaken for a minor sprain or missed altogether, only to manifest itself at a later date in slowed or failed longitudinal limb growth or in the development of an angular deformity. Even if diagnosed and properly treated, physeal injuries may still result in longitudinal or angular abnormalities. Most physeal disruptions occur through the zone of cartilage cell hypertrophy within the physeal plate and thus do not result in permanent damage to the plate. However, a small proportion of disruptions involve the resting or germinal layer of the physis and may disrupt the cells permanently, resulting in eventual deformity despite adequate reduction of the fracture fragments.

Because of their potential for long-term morbidity, great attention has been focused on the classification, diagnosis,

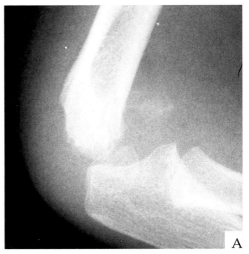
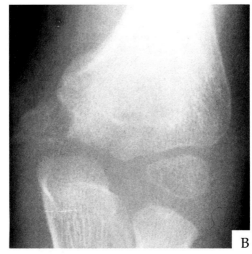

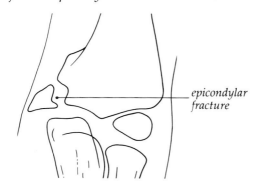

Fig. 21.26 Epicondylar fracture. **A,** lateral radiograph reveals significant proximal migration of medial epicondyle of distal humerus. **B,** the AP view shows slight medial displacement of medial epicondyle.

epicondylar fracture

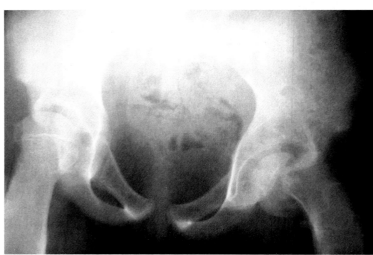

Fig. 21.27 Subcapital fracture. This AP radiograph of the pelvis shows a displaced subcapital fracture of the right femur. This particular injury may be seen acutely due to significant trauma, or may develop slowly as a result of gradual slipping at the physeal level.

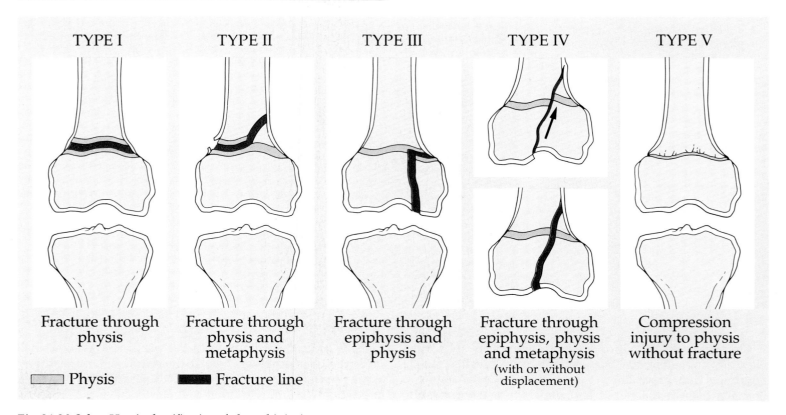

TYPE I	TYPE II	TYPE III	TYPE IV	TYPE V
Fracture through physis	Fracture through physis and metaphysis	Fracture through epiphysis and physis	Fracture through epiphysis, physis and metaphysis (with or without displacement)	Compression injury to physis without fracture

■ Physis   ■ Fracture line

Fig. 21.28 Salter-Harris classification of physeal injuries.

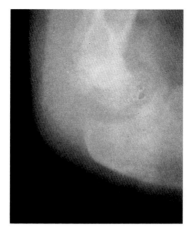
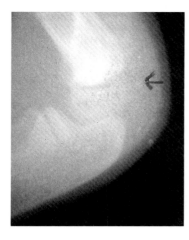

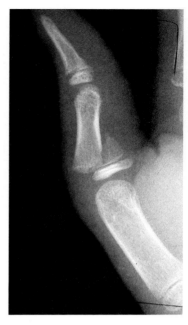

Fig. 21.30 Salter-Harris type II injury. On this lateral radiograph of the thumb the fracture is seen to involve the proximal phalanx. The fracture line runs through the physis and exits through the metaphysis on the side opposite the site of fracture initiation. A fragment consisting of the entire epiphysis with the attached metaphyseal fragment is produced.

Fig. 21.29 Salter-Harris type I injury. Close inspection shows slight widening of the distal humeral epiphysis. Clinically, the patient had pain, tenderness, and decreased range of motion of the elbow. (Courtesy of Dr. Jocelyn Ledisma Medina, Children's Hospital of Pittsburgh)

Fig. 21.31 Salter-Harris type III injury. Comparison view of both ankles reveals a fracture involving the lateral aspect of the right distal tibial epiphysis. This configuration creates a separate fragment without any connection to the metaphysis.

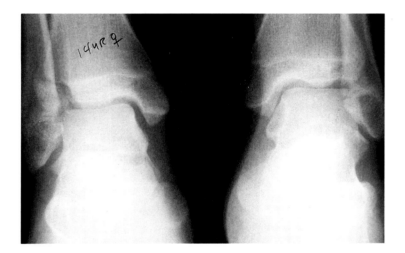

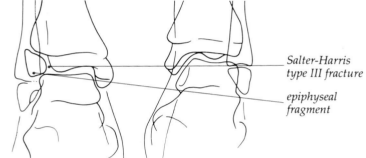

Salter-Harris
type III fracture

epiphyseal
fragment

treatment, and prognosis of physeal fractures. The Salter-Harris classification scheme is the system most commonly used in North America to classify physeal injuries (Fig. 21.28).

Salter-Harris Type I

This injury consists of a fracture running horizontally through the physis itself resulting in a variable degree of separation of the epiphysis from the metaphysis. The amount of separation depends on the degree of periosteal disruption. Radiographs are often normal, hence, the diagnosis frequently must be made clinically on the basis of point tenderness and mild soft tissue swelling over the site of an epiphysis (Fig. 21.29). This injury usually results from a shearing force. Prognosis is usually favorable.

Salter-Harris Type II

Also produced by shearing forces, this injury consists of a fracture line running a variable distance through the physis and exiting through the metaphysis on the side opposite the site of fracture initiation. A fragment consisting of the entire epiphysis with an attached metaphyseal fragment is thus produced (Fig. 21.30). Prognosis is generally favorable with adequate reduction.

Salter-Harris Type III

Intra-articular shearing forces can produce a fracture line running from the articular surface through the epiphysis then exiting through a portion of the physis. This creates a separate epiphyseal fragment with no connection to the metaphysis (Fig. 21.31). Prognosis may be quite poor. Accurate anatomic reduction is required to achieve the best possible outcome.

Salter-Harris Type IV

In this type the fracture line starts at the articular surface, runs through the physis across the epiphysis, and exists out the metaphysis. A single fragment consisting of both epiphysis

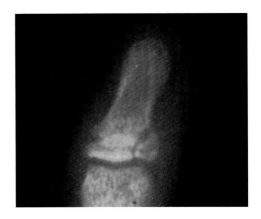

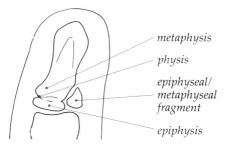

Fig. 21.32 Salter-Harris type IV injury. This patient incurred a fracture of the distal phalanx of the index finger. The fracture line starts at the articular surface, runs through the epiphysis across the physis, and exits through the metaphysis. A single fragment consisting of both epiphysis and attached metaphysis is thus created.

metaphysis

physis

epiphyseal/
metaphyseal
fragment

epiphysis

and attached metaphysis is thus created (Fig. 21.32). Like Salter-Harris Type III, the injury results from the application of a shearing force. Prognosis may be poor despite seemingly good anatomic restoration of the fracture fragments. Open reduction and internal fixation is virtually always necessary. Both Salter-Harris III and IV fractures also can be classified as intra-articular fractures.

Salter-Harris Type V

This type is the product of a crushing injury to the physis without physeal fracture or displacement. Radiographic diagnosis is virtually impossible to make at the time of injury, hence, this fracture must be diagnosed on clinical grounds. Distinction between a Salter-Harris I and a Salter-Harris V fracture is often possible only when a subsequent growth abnormality has been appreciated. Prognosis is quite poor for normal growth (Fig. 21.33).

FRACTURE TREATMENT PRINCIPLES

The healing and remodeling capacity of the growing bones of a child is considerably greater than that of an adult; the younger the child the greater is this capacity for regeneration. As a result, healing is rapid, necessitating a shorter period of immobilization; nonunion is rare. Furthermore, in planning fracture reductions, remodeling capability and the likely addition to bone length as a result of overgrowth must be considered. For example, in managing a toddler with a femur fracture that is displaced in the plane of motion of the adjacent joint, the bone ends must overlap to account for overgrowth, and a degree of angulation can be accepted, because this will ultimately be corrected by remodeling. The amount of angulation and the degree of overlap of fracture fragments that can be accepted is difficult to state in numeric terms. Acceptable position is determined in part by the child's age, the nature and position of the fracture, the bone involved, the appearance and condition of the adjacent soft tissues, and the presence or absence of other systemic injuries. Remodeling has its limitations, however. Rotational deformities and angular deformities which are not in the axis of adjacent joint motion are not effectively remodeled. Thus, these must be corrected at the time of initial fracture reduction.

Nondisplaced fractures are simply casted or splinted. Because of the relative rarity of ligamentous injuries prior to epiphyseal closure, patients with an appropriate clinical history and point tenderness over an epiphysis are presumed to have a fracture and should be treated accordingly even when radiographs are negative. Most displaced fractures not involv-

ing the physis can be treated by closed reduction and casting. As a general rule, open reduction and internal fixation is usually reserved for Salter-Harris Type III and Type IV fractures which have any degree of displacement, for certain open fractures, and for fractures associated with continued neurovascular compromise. Depending on the time of presentation, degree of displacement, and severity of soft tissue swelling, reduction and/or casting may have to be deferred pending application of traction and subsidence of edema.

The importance of adequate analgesia and sedation prior to closed reduction procedures warrants emphasis. Too often reduction is performed without the benefit of analgesia and justified by the rationale that "it will only hurt for a minute." This reasoning is callous and that excruciating "minute" may seem an eternity to the child. Following reduction and/or immobilization in a cast, pain should be markedly alleviated. Persistence or recurrence of significant discomfort suggests a complication and warrants prompt reevaluation.

Care must be taken in describing the nature of the injury and its prognosis, and in explaining the rationale for proposed treatment measures to the parents. A simpler explanation in terms geared to his developmental level should be given to the child. Use of written instructions regarding home care measures, necessary parent observations, and worrisome signs that signal need for prompt reevaluation is invaluable.

Special Cases

CLAVICULAR FRACTURES

Fractures of the clavicle are very common. They are caused by lateral compression forces (as can occur in the process of delivery of the newborn or in falls onto the shoulder), transmission of forces through the glenohumeral joint in a fall to the side on an outstretched arm, or occasionally by a direct blow or impact on the clavicle itself. Most involve the midshaft or distal clavicle. Greenstick fractures are more common in infants and toddlers, whereas through-and-through fractures are more typical of older children and adolescents (see Fig. 21.10). Clinically, the child is noted to avoid moving the arm on the involved side and often splints it by holding the arm close against the chest. Tenderness and mild swelling are evident on palpation of the fracture site. Complications are rare and treatment consists of application of a padded figure-of-eight splint for 2 to 3 weeks.

Rare medial clavicular fractures are due to high impact forces and may be accompanied by injuries of mediastinal structures.

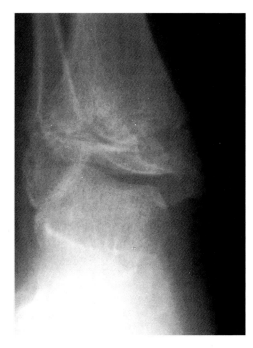

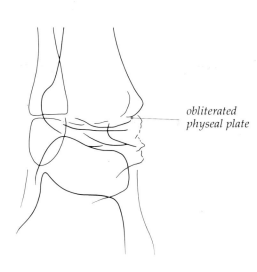

obliterated
physeal plate

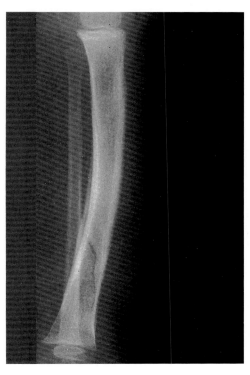

Fig. 21.33 Salter-Harris type V injury. This AP radiograph of the ankle taken several weeks after a crush injury sustained in an automobile accident reveals obliteration of the distal tibial physeal plate. As is often the case, original radiographs taken at the time of injury looked normal. This fracture must be suspected on clinical grounds and the patient treated and followed accordingly.

Fig. 21.34 Toddler's fracture. This spiral fracture of the distal tibia was the result of a fall with a twist.

TODDLER'S FRACTURE

One of the most common orthopedic injuries seen between the ages of 1 and 5 years is the toddler's fracture. The child usually has a sudden onset of refusal to bear weight on one leg or of an antalgic limp. Typically this develops following a fall with a twist, to which the unsteady toddler is unusually prone. The child may have gotten his foot caught and fallen trying to extricate himself, may have fallen while running and making a sudden change of direction, or fallen with a twist upon jumping. Not uncommonly the actual fall is unwitnessed, and the parents are unsure as to what happened. The injury results in a spiral or short oblique fracture of the distal tibia or the junction of the mid and distal tibia (Fig. 21.34). Because the thick periosteum tends to be only partially disrupted, soft tissue swelling is often minimal and tenderness may be subtle. Furthermore, many of these fractures are radiographically invisible or so subtle as to be difficult to detect, although some degree of soft tissue swelling may be evident on the film. Without radiographic evidence of a fracture, the physician must rely on the examination to make a clinical diagnosis.

It is generally best to allow the child to remain seated in the parent's lap during the examination. This will help calm the child and provide a more subdued response to palpation of the uninvolved areas. Attention should first be turned to the normal extremity. The ankle, knee, and hip should be placed through their range of motion. Next, the entire foot, tibia, fibula and femur should be palpated. If upset, the child will cry, but nothing about the examination will exacerbate the child's baseline irritability. Attention is then directed to the involved extremity, where a similar examination is performed. Palpation over the fracture site will be appreciated by either a withdrawal reaction or, more commonly, by an increase from baseline irritability, which can usually be seen in a change in the child's facial expression and appreciated in the pattern of crying. Localized bone tenderness in this setting is clinical proof of a fracture, even if radiographs are normal. In attempting to assess very frightened and highly uncooperative toddlers, it is best to give them time to calm down and then either to have the parents perform palpation or to introduce puppets and palpate using the puppet's hands.

Treatment consists of either long or short leg casting for approximately 4 weeks. Infection must be included in the differential diagnosis of the limping child in this 1- to 5-year age group, but usually can be ruled out by lack of fever, absence of local erythema, and normal blood work. When there is no clear history of a fall, only a mild limp, no evidence of localized tenderness, and radiographs are normal, it may be best to defer treatment and follow the child closely.

HAND AND FINGER FRACTURES

While a complete discussion of the examination of the hand and hand injuries is beyond the scope of this chapter, several key points bear emphasis, as appropriate assessment and management are essential if long-term dysfunction is to be prevented (see Figs. 21.74 and 21.75).

Phalangeal Fractures

The most common mechanism of injury producing phalangeal fractures in young children is a crush injury do to getting their fingers caught in a door or from the weight of a falling object. Crush injuries continue to be common in older children and adolescents, but contact sports and fist fights assume an increasing causative role.

Meticulous attention must be paid to the assessment of neurovascular and tendon function to detect subtle abnormalities that may reflect significant injury with the potential for long-term complications. This can be difficult in young children. However, much information can be gained from observing the position of the hands at rest, during spontaneous movement,

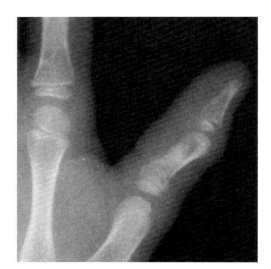

Fig. 21.35 Angulated phalanx fracture. Significant angular deformity is seen with this fracture of the proximal phalanx of the thumb. Such fractures require careful reduction to prevent permanent disability.

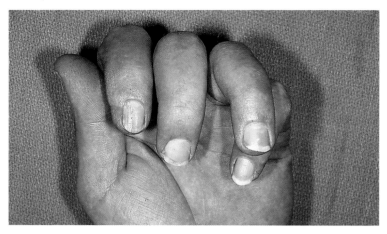

Fig. 21.36 Rotational deformity due to hand injury. With rotational deformity, the plane of the nail of the involved finger is seen to deviate from its normal plane of orientation. (Courtesy of Dr. Neil Jones, University Health Center of Pittsburgh)

and watching the motion as the parents give objects to the child. Any fracture associated with shortening, significant angulation (Fig. 21.35), or rotational deformity, and any intra-articular fracture must be appropriately reduced. Shortening and rotation are best detected by comparison of the injured hand with its normal opposite. Comparison of the plane of the fingernails of both hands with the forearms supinated and the fingers partially flexed is particularly useful in detecting rotational abnormalities (Fig. 21.36).

Determination of degree of angulation and identification of intra-articular fractures is best done radiographically. X-ray findings can be subtle, necessitating careful comparison with radiographs of the normal hand. It is also important to obtain oblique as well as AP and lateral views.

Chip fractures at the base of the middle or distal phalanges may be associated with avulsion of the flexor or extensor tendons, which may necessitate operative repair (Fig. 21.37). Clinically, an extensor tendon injury may be manifest by flexor tendon overpull when the fingers are flexed, and conversely, flexor tendon injuries may result in extensor overpull when the fingers are extended.

Crush injuries of the distal phalanges associated with partial or complete nail avulsions often result in open fractures with laceration of the nail bed (Fig. 21.38). These require careful cleansing, debridement, and nail bed repair.

The volar plate is a cartilaginous plate located at the base of the middle phalanx of each finger. Intra-articular fractures involving the proximal interphalangeal (PIP) joint may fracture or tear this structure as well. The typical mechanism of injury is usually a blow to the end of the finger in hyperextension. Often a chip of bone avulsed from the middle phalanx is seen radiographically. Clinically, pain and swelling are especially marked over the volar aspect of the PIP joint. A hyperextension deformity of the involved PIP joint may be seen when the fingers are extended, or pain or locking may be noted on attempted flexion. Pain is exacerbated on passive hyperextension and reduced on passive flexion. Volar plate injuries may also accompany dislocation of the PIP joint (see section on Ligamentous Injuries).

Metacarpal Fractures

The boxer's fracture, an impacted fracture of the neck of the fifth and often the fourth metacarpal, is among the most com-

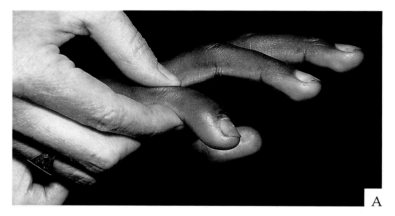

A

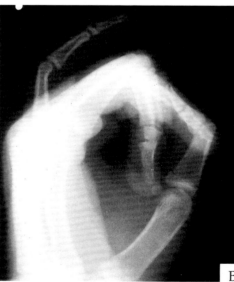

B

Fig. 21.37 Distal phalanx fracture with extensor tendon injury. **A,** another player's shoulder landed on this boy's finger. The finger was swollen and painful, maximally tender at the base of the distal phalanx, and the patient was unable to extend the distalinterphalangeal joint. **B,** radiographs revealed separation of the epiphysis at the base of the distal phalanx.

mon of these injuries (Fig. 21.39). It occurs as a result of direct impact with a partially clenched fist (typically due to punching another person or a wall), and is most commonly seen in aggressive adolescents. It can also follow a fall onto a clenched fist. Clinically, depression of the involved knuckle or knuckles may be noted along with more proximal swelling and discoloration. The involved metacarpals may also appear shortened. Associated rotational deformity when present is manifest by rotation of the nails of the corresponding fingers

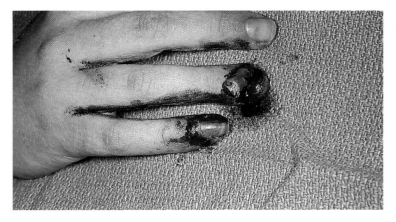

Fig. 21.38 Crush injury of distal phalanx. This child's finger was slammed in a car door. He incurred a crush fracture of the distal phalanx, partial avulsion of the nail, and a nail bed laceration. By definition, this is an open fracture. (Courtesy of Dr. Neil Jones, University Health Center of Pittsburgh)

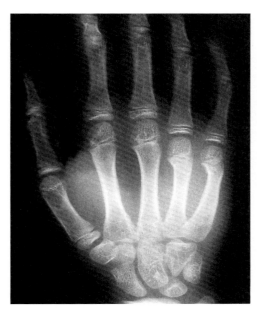

Fig. 21.39 Boxer's fracture. This adolescent presented with pain and swelling of the lateral aspect of his right hand after punching a wall in a fit of temper. Radiographically, he has a typical boxer's fracture of the neck of the fifth metacarpal with volar displacement of the distal fragment.

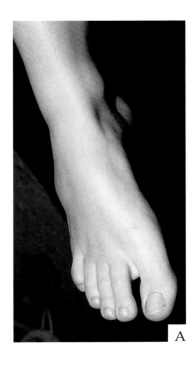

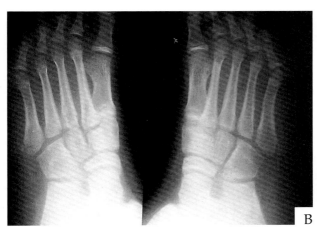

Fig. 21.40 Transverse metatarsal fracture. This adolescent fell forward with her forefoot twisted under her. A, swelling over the proximal portion of the fifth metatarsal was prominent. B, the transverse fracture is evident radiographically.

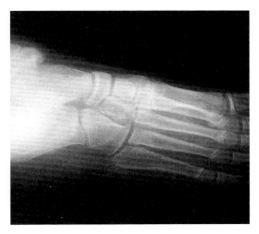

Fig. 21.41 Os vesaleanum. Many children have a secondary ossification center at the base of the fifth metatarsal. This can be distinguished from a fracture by the fact that its edges are smooth, rounded, and sclerotic. (Courtesy of Dr. Jocelyn Ledisma Medina, Children's Hospital of Pittsburgh)

(see Fig. 21.36). When the injury stems from punching another person in the mouth, care must be taken to check for overlying breaks in the skin caused by the opponent's teeth. These are infection-prone wounds and may communicate with metacarpophalangeal joints. Radiographically, volar angulation of the distal segment is typically found. If this exceeds 15 to 20 degrees or rotational deformity is present, referral to an orthopedist or hand surgeon for reduction is necessary. Nondis-placed, minimally angulated fractures can be treated with an ulnar gutter splint.

METATARSAL FRACTURES

Most metatarsal fractures are the result of dropping a heavy object on the foot and thus are crush injuries. Falls in which the patient twists the forefoot can produce transverse fractures at the base of the fifth metatarsal (Fig. 21.40), and injuries of the foot with the ankle inverted and the foot in plantar flexion can avulse the tuberosity from the base of the fifth metatarsal. This must be distinguished from the normal finding of a sec-

ondary ossification center, termed the os vesaleanum, at the base of the fifth metatarsal. The edges of the latter are smooth, rounded and sclerotic (Fig. 21.41). Mild, localized swelling, and point tenderness are noted over the site of a metatarsal fracture; weight-bearing is painful, if not impossible. Application of a short leg cast provides maximal relief.

Adolescents involved in long-distance running or walking may incur stress fractures on the shafts of the second and third metatarsals, which are the site of maximal stress and weight application during the push-off phase of walking and running. Pain often increases insidiously and tends to be poorly localized. Swelling may be imperceptible. These are often microfractures and may be radiographically invisible until healing becomes detectable 3 to 4 weeks after onset.

SEAT BELT FRACTURES

Increased awareness of the importance of using seat belts to prevent serious multiple trauma in auto accidents, and adherence to recommendations to place children in the back seat of

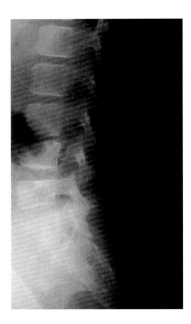

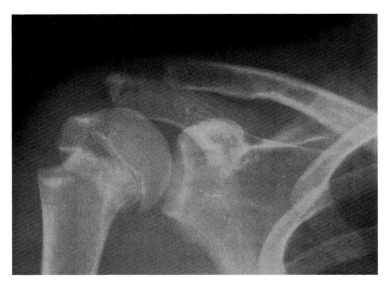

Fig. 21.42 Lap belt fracture. This compression fracture of the L-4 vertebral body was due to hyperflexion against the fulcrum of a back seat lap belt.

Fig. 21.43 Epiphyseal separation. Because of the elasticity and relatively greater strength of the ligaments, forces that would have resulted in dislocation in an older adolescent have instead caused epiphyseal separation and displacement of the proximal humeral epiphysis in this prepubertal child. (Courtesy of Dept. of Pediatric Radiology, Children's Hospital of Pittsburgh)

the car have resulted in an increase in the incidence of lap belt fractures in children, because most cars do not have three-point belts in the back seat. In a head-on collision, the child's head and torso are thrown forward, resulting in hyperflexion of the lumbar spine and often causing a compression fracture of the L-4 or L-5 vertebral body, or disruption of the posterior elements of one of these vertebrae. Pain from associated abdominal injuries may overshadow the pain of the vertebral injury; however, localized tenderness and/or spasm are present on examination of the back. Radiographic findings may include evidence of vertebral body compression, best seen on the lateral view (Fig. 21.42) or displacement of the shadow of the spinous process on the AP view in cases of disruption of the posterior elements. Identification of these fractures and determination of whether they are stable or unstable is essential before any undue movement is allowed.

PATHOLOGIC FRACTURES

Children with severe osteopenia or osteoporosis, whether due to an inherited disorder or disuse secondary to neurologic or neuromuscular disease, are at considerably increased risk of incurring fractures as the result of minor falls or even during routine physical therapy exercises. Localized bone lesions, including those due to osteomyelitis, tumors, or cysts can cause localized cortical thinning as they expand. Impact on the involved bone can then also result in pathologic fracture. Examples of these conditions and representative fractures are presented in Chapter 6.

Compartment Syndromes

A compartment syndrome arises in any situation in which interstitial tissue fluid pressure rises above that of capillary perfusion pressure. In clinical practice, this interstitial pressure elevation must reach approximately 35 to 45 mm Hg. Because the enclosed fascial boundary of the involved muscle compartment is unyielding, hemorrhage or edema within it can cause interstitial pressure to rise to such levels. Compartment syndromes are not rare in childhood and can be seen following open or closed fractures, crush injuries, or the prolonged pressure on an extremity that can occur in a comatose child who has been lying on an extremity for several hours. A displaced fracture of the proximal tibial metaphysis is the fracture most likely to be complicated by a compartment syndrome. Other fractures that are well documented as potentially predisposed to development of a compartment syndrome include supracondylar humerus fractures and displaced forearm fractures.

Prompt and accurate diagnosis is essential, as failure to implement definitive treatment within 4 to 6 hours of onset results in permanent neuromuscular damage. The clinical findings of compartment syndrome are quite classic. The involved extremity is swollen and tense to palpation. The patient complains of severe pain which is unrelieved by elevation, immobilization, and routine doses of narcotics. Passive movement of the terminal digits (fingers or toes) exacerbates the pain and active motion is avoided. In view of the fact that diminished or absent pulses may never develop despite a full-blown, florid compartment syndrome, the diagnosis and/or decision to treat should never be based on the presence or absence of the peripheral pulses. Because the clinical diagnosis of compartment syndrome can be difficult in the uncooperative or comatose child, intracompartmental needle pressure readings are recommended. Such readings are not necessary in awake and cooperative children, although they may be used to confirm the diagnosis.

Treatment necessitates emergent surgical decompression of the fascial covering of all involved compartments to prevent irreversible muscle and nerve damage. Following fascial decompression, relief of pressure, pain reduction, and return of active muscle power are immediate.

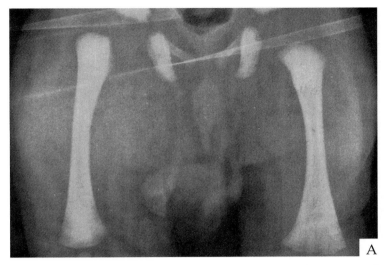

A

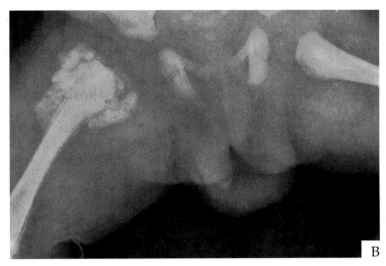

B

Fig. 21.44 Fracture dislocation, right hip. This young infant presented with what appeared to be a traumatic hip dislocation without an associated fracture. **A,** the right femoral head is displaced laterally and superiorly. **B,** the follow-up film taken 2 weeks later revealed vigorous callus formation around the proximal femur and periosteal new bone formation both proximally and distally, thus confirming associated fractures. (Courtesy of Dept. of Pediatric Radiology, Children's Hospital of Pittsburgh)

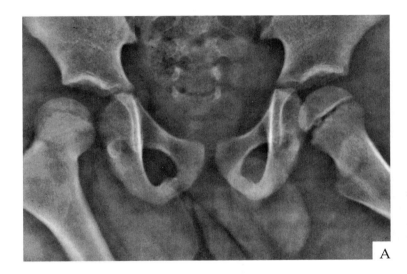

A

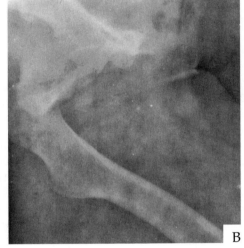

B

Fig. 21.45 Traumatic posterior hip dislocation. This child suffered an impaction injury in an automobile accident. **A,** in the AP view the femoral head appears to be displaced laterally and superiorly. The femur is also adducted and internally rotated. **B,** the frogleg view discloses the severity of displacement posteriorly.

Ligamentous Injuries

DISLOCATIONS

The ligaments of a child have great elasticity and are relatively strong as compared to bony structures, especially the physis (Fig. 21.43). Consequently joint dislocations and ligamentous disruptions are rather unusual in childhood; when seen, they are usually the result of severe trauma, and are commonly associated with fractures. In some instances the dislocation is obvious and the fracture subtle or even invisible radiographically (Fig. 21.44), but often the fracture is the prominent clinical finding and the dislocation less apparent. Hence, the emphasis in pediatric orthopedics is on examining the entire extremity, and including the joints proximal and distal to a suspected fracture site in radiographic examination. Failure to diagnose the full extent of injury can result in permanent morbidity. It must also be remembered that in infancy epiphyseal separations prior to ossification can simulate dislocations. For example, separation of the distal humeral epiphysis presents a radiographic picture suggesting posterior displacement of the olecranon. The most frequent sites of dislocation in childhood are the hip, the patellofemoral joint, and the interphalangeal joints.

Hip dislocations in the young are usually the result of falls. In a child under 5 years of age the softness of the acetabulum and relative ligamentous laxity enable dislocation without application of extreme force and thus there may be no associated fractures. In the older child violent force is required and dislocation is commonly accompanied by fractures of the femur and acetabulum. In most instances the femoral head dislocates posteriorly. The child presents in severe pain with the involved leg held in adduction, internally rotated and flexed (Fig. 21.45). Extension, external rotation, and abduction is the position adopted with the less common anterior dislocation. When the child also has an impressive femoral fracture, his pain may be interpreted as due to that and the positional findings missed unless the clinician specifically looks for them. Even in cases without an obvious associated fracture, epiphyseal separation or avulsion of an acetabular fragment may have occurred. Prompt reduction is important both for relief of pain and to reduce the risk of secondary avascular necrosis. Post-reduction films are important as these are more likely to disclose the fact that epiphyseal separation has occurred, and will tend to show incomplete reduction if a radiolucent intra-articular fragment is present.

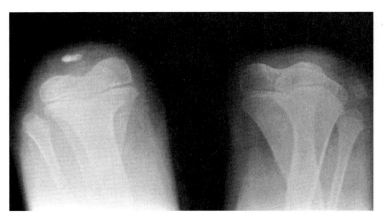

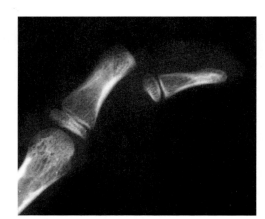

Fig. 21.46 Patellar dislocation. In this flexion view taken prior to relocation the left patella is displaced laterally and there is a marked degree of swelling. (Courtesy of Dept. of Pediatric Radiology, Children's Hospital of Pittsburgh)

Fig. 21.47 Interphalangeal joint dislocation. The distal phalanx of the thumb is dislocated dorsally. (Courtesy of Dept. of Pediatric Radiology, Children's Hospital of Pittsburgh)

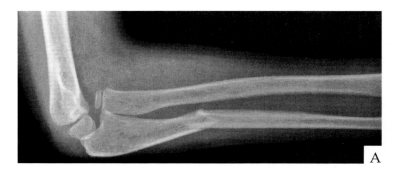

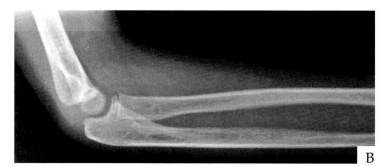

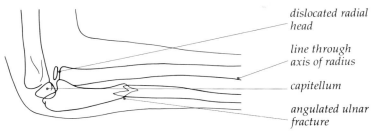

dislocated radial head

line through axis of radius

capitellum

angulated ulnar fracture

Fig. 21.48 Monteggia fracture. **A,** the displaced fracture of the proximal ulna is accompanied by dislocation of the radial head. A line drawn through the long axis of the radius would intersect the distal humerus above the level of the capitellum. **B,** the comparison view of the normal arm shows the normal position of the radial head. (Courtesy of Dept. of Pediatric Radiology, Children's Hospital of Pittsburgh)

In patellofemoral dislocations the patella usually dislocates laterally (Fig. 21.46). This may occur as the result of shearing forces or of a hyperextension injury. Patients with ligamentous laxity appear particularly susceptible. In most instances the patella has relocated by the time the patient is seen. If not, the leg should be extended immediately and the patella pushed back into place to alleviate pain. Findings on examination include prominent swelling and hemarthrosis, tenderness along the medial patellar border and increased lateral mobility of the patella. Avulsion fractures of the lateral femoral condyle and/or medial patella are common associated injuries. Application of ice, rest, and use of a knee immobilizer for 3 weeks is recommended. Currently there is disagreement on whether operative intervention should be considered following the first episode, or deferred until a recurrence.

Dislocation of an interphalangeal joint results in an obvious deformity and is an intensely painful injury (Fig. 21.47). Avulsion fractures, volar plate fractures, and tendinous or capsular injury may be associated and difficult to detect radiographically. These must be suspected if range of motion is incomplete following relocation. In some cases the associated injury makes closed reduction impossible.

Elbow dislocations are rare in the absence of an associated fracture. The fracture may be as subtle as a nonossified fragment avulsed from the medial epicondyle or the ulna, or as prominent as a displaced fracture of the ulna or radius. An example of the latter is the Monteggia fracture. Here a displaced fracture of the proximal ulna is accompanied by dislocation of the radial head. A radial dislocation should be suspected if a line drawn through the long axis of the radius fails to pass through the capitellum on any view (Fig. 21.48). Less frequently, fractures of the radius are associated with dislocation of the radioulnar joint, and fractures of the olecranon may be accompanied by dislocation of the radius.

True shoulder dislocations are seen only in adolescents after epiphyseal fusion (Fig. 21.49). Separation of the proximal humeral epiphysis or major fracture dislocations are seen in younger children subjected to forces that would cause dislocation after puberty (see Fig. 21.43).

SPRAINS

A sprain is a ligamentous injury in which some degree of tearing occurs, often as a result of excessive stretching or twisting. As noted in the section on fractures, sprains are less

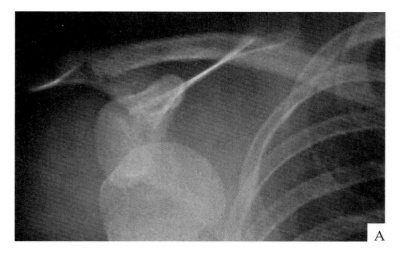

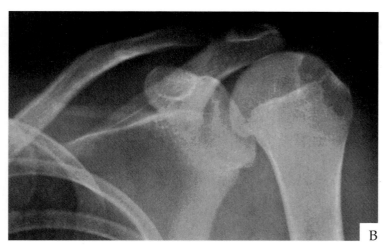

Fig. 21.49 **A,** anterior dislocation of the right shoulder. The humeral head is not in the glenoid fossa, but is displaced anteriorly. **B,** the normal relationship is seen in the left shoulder. The injury occurred when the patient was taking a back swing for a hockey shot. The patient felt a

pop and immediate onset of severe pain. Note that his epiphyses have fused. (Courtesy of Dept. of Pediatric Radiology, Children's Hospital of Pittsburgh)

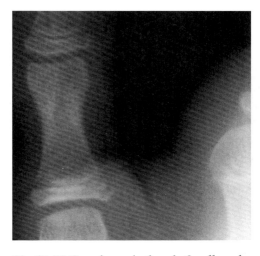

Fig. 21.50 Gamekeeper's thumb. Small avulsion fracture of the epiphysis at the base of the proximal phalanx associated with rupture of the ulnar collateral ligament. The injury occurred when the patient fell while skiing and the strap of his ski pole forcefully abducted his thumb on impact.

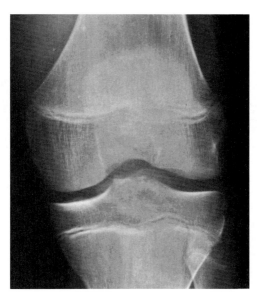

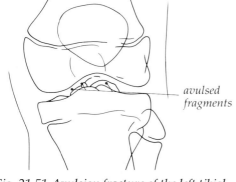

avulsed fragments

Fig. 21.51 Avulsion fracture of the left tibial spine due to soccer injury (AP view). Also present were a tear in the cruciate ligament and a lipohemarthrosis. (Courtesy of Dept. of Pediatric Radiology, Children's Hospital of Pittsburgh)

common in children with open epiphyses than they are in older adolescents who have fused their epiphyses. When sprains do occur, they tend to be milder and may be associated with Salter fractures. This stems from the fact that the growth plate, being weaker than the ligaments, tends to give before significant ligamentous tearing can develop. Thus, in children physeal fractures tend to result from forces that would produce a sprain in an older adolescent or adult. In many other instances, what appears to be a sprain is actually a small avulsion fracture. If the portion avulsed is ossified a small fragment may be detectable radiographically, but if the fragment is cartilaginous, it will be radiographically invisible. A particular example of this is the *gamekeeper's thumb,* often associated with a small avulsion fracture of the proximal phalanx (Fig. 21.50), in which an injury causing forceful abduction of the thumb results in rupture of the ulnar collateral lig-

ament at the base of the thumb. Adequate examination necessitates stress testing of the radial and ulnar collateral ligaments with the thumb in extension. This is often impossible until pain has been reduced by way of a digital nerve block. If greater than twenty degrees of instability is found on stressing the ulnar collaterals, the patient should be referred to an orthopedist or hand surgeon for possible operative repair. Failure to correct the problem results in a loss of resistance to abduction and a weak pinch.

Prior to epiphyseal closure, Salter-Harris fractures and avulsion fractures of the distal fibula or tibia should be strongly suspected in "sprain-like" injuries of the ankle. Similarly, injuries that rupture the cruciate ligaments of the knee in adults usually avulse the tibial spine in the child (Fig. 21.51). Following physeal closure in adolescence, sprains are seen with some frequency.

Fig. 21.52

CLASSIFICATION OF SPRAINS

Grade of Sprain	Degree of Tearing	Clinical Findings
I	A small fragment of ligamentous fibers is disrupted	Pain on motion Local tenderness Mild swelling
II	A moderate percentage of fibers is torn	Pain on motion More diffuse tenderness Moderate swelling, may have joint effusion Mild instability
III	The ligament is completely disrupted	Severe pain on motion Marked swelling usually with joint effusion Marked tenderness Joint instability

Sprains are classified in three grades according to severity (Fig. 21.52). In contrast to physeal fractures, swelling and tenderness are more likely to be prominent and to occur early and over the involved ligament or ligaments, not over the epiphysis (Fig. 21.53). Pain on motion is often more marked in patients with sprains than in patients with physeal fractures.

In evaluating patients with possible sprains, careful attention must be given not only to assessment of swelling, tenderness, and joint stability, but also to evaluation of adjacent bony structures and to musculotendonous function. Complete evaluation may be impossible if initial presentation has been delayed for several hours and secondary effusion, soft tissue swelling, and muscle spasm are pronounced. In such instances, it may be necessary to immobilize the affected joint with a splint and have the patient return for reevaluation in 24 to 72 hours when the swelling has abated.

Rest, application of ice, use of analgesic anti-inflammatory agents such as ibuprofen or aspirin, and perhaps use of an Ace® wrap or taping suffice for Grade I sprains. Subjective improvement occurs in a few days. Grade II and III sprains require a longer period of immobilization. Splinting or casting for a few to several weeks is generally necessary. Grade III sprains may necessitate operative intervention.

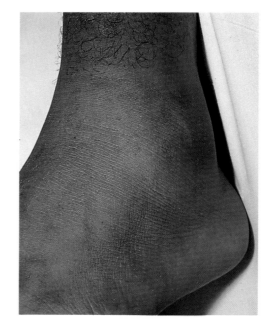

Fig. 21.53 Ankle sprain. Marked tenderness and swelling were maximal inferior to the malleolus of this 17-year-old youth. The anterior talofibular, calcaneofibular, and posterior talofibular ligaments were all tender. This is in contrast to the findings seen with a Salter I fracture of the distal tibia (see Fig. 21.6)

SUBLUXATION OF THE RADIAL HEAD (NURSEMAID'S ELBOW)

Subluxation of the radial head is the most common elbow injury in childhood and one of the most common ligamentous injuries. The mechanism is one of sudden traction applied to the extended arm. The injury is seen predominantly in children between the ages of 1 and 4 years. The typical history is one of a parent suddenly pulling the child by the arm to prevent a fall, of the child, in a fit of temper attempting to pull away from the parent, or of a child being swung by the arms. After a brief initial period of crying, the child calms down, but is unable to use the affected arm, which is held close to the body with elbow flexed and forearm pronated (Fig, 21.54A). Physical examination reveals no bony tenderness and no evidence of swelling, but on assessment of passive motion, the child resists any attempt at supination. Mild limitation of elbow flexion and extension may also be noted.

Pathologically, when the radial head is subluxed by the sudden pull on the arm, the annular ligament is torn at the site of its attachment to the radius and the radial head slips through the tear. When the traction is released and the radial head recoils, the proximal portion of the annular ligament becomes trapped between the radial head and the capitellum (Fig. 21.55). This limits motion and produces the child's pain.

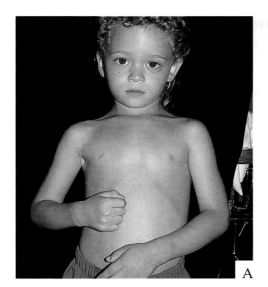

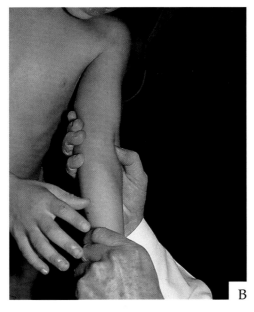

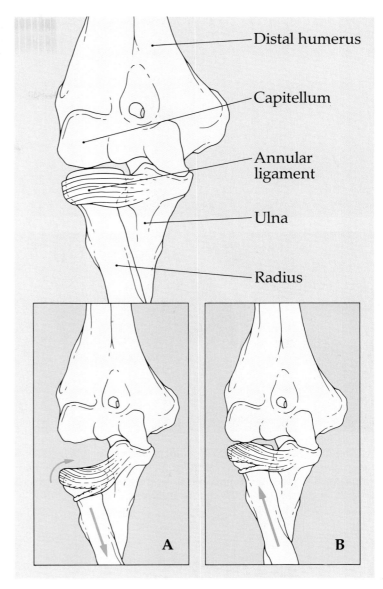

Fig. 21.54
Nursemaid's elbow.
A, note that the affected arm is held close to the body with the elbow flexed and the forearm pronated. B, reduction maneuver produces pain, as do attempts at supination during the examination.

Distal humerus

Capitellum

Annular ligament

Ulna

Radius

A B

Fig. 21.55 Nursemaid's elbow. **A,** *sudden traction on the outstretched arm pulls the radius distally causing it to slip partially through the annular ligament, and tearing it in the process.* **B,** *when traction is released, the radial head recoils trapping the proximal portion of the ligament between it and the capitellum.*

Radiographs are normal because the radial head is not truly subluxed.

Treatment consists of supinating the child's forearm with the elbow in a flexed position while applying pressure over the radial head (see Fig. 21.54B). A click can be perceived as the annular ligament is freed from the joint. Occasionally this maneuver fails, in which case the forearm should be supinated and extended with traction applied distally while pressing down on the radial head. Pain relief is immediate, return of function is evident within 10 to 15 minutes, and no cast is required. It is often recommended that the child wear a sling for 10 days to reduce use, and to allow the annular ligament to heal; compliance is difficult to assure, however.

When presentation has been delayed for several hours, it may be necessary to prescribe acetaminophen for 12 to 14 hours to relieve residual aching. Parents should be cautioned to avoid maneuvers that cause excessive traction on the arm, as there is a significant risk of recurrence.

EXTREMITY PAIN WITH LIGAMENTOUS LAXITY

Children with significant and generalized ligamentous laxity have hypermobile joints and are vulnerable to excessive stretching or stress on ligamentous and musculotendinous structures. They are also somewhat more susceptible to joint dislocations. The phenomenon is seen in up to 18 percent of girls and 6 percent of boys. Following periods of vigorous physical activity these children often complain of arthralgias and/or muscular pain, and occasionally have evidence of joint swelling. Episodes tend to occur in the evening or at night, are self-limited, lasting one to several hours, and respond to rest and aspirin, acetaminophen or ibuprofen. Many of these children have been accused of attention-getting behavior and hypochondriasis. Others have been dismissed as having "growing pains," and some have undergone extensive testing for rheumatic disorders. A history of greater than average activity on the preceding day and of recurrent short-lived pain usually without objective swelling, combined with findings of

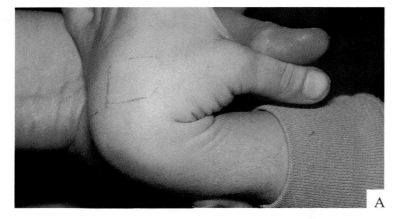

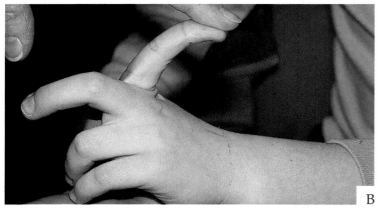

Fig. 21.56 Ligamentous laxity. This child demonstrates typical findings of joint hypermobility seen with ligamentous laxity. *A,* he is able to hyperflex the wrist on the forearm. *B,* he also is able to hyperextend the distal interphalangeal joint and the metacarpophalangeal joint.

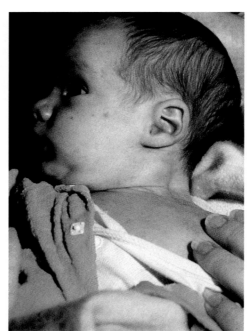

Fig. 21.57 Congenital torticollis. The "tumor" of congenital torticollis is seen as a swelling in the midportion of the sternocleidomastoid muscle. It is firm on palpation, and the muscle itself is shortened. The head tilts toward the affected side and the chin rotates in the opposite direction. (Courtesy of Dr. James Reilly, Children's Hospital of Alabama)

ligamentous laxity on examination (Fig. 21.56) should suggest this diagnosis. The rarity of joint swelling and the absence of fever and other systemic symptoms help to rule out rheumatic and collagen vascular disorders.

Once the problem is correctly diagnosed, patients can minimize discomfort by avoiding sudden increases in level of activity and by taking a mild analgesic prophylactically after a period of unusually vigorous activity. Graduated strengthening exercises may also be helpful. This is particularly true when children wish to participate in gymnastics or competitive sports.

DISORDERS OF THE SPINE

Children with disorders of the axial skeleton most commonly present with some type of deformity. Pain or dysfunction of the associated spinal cord and nerve roots may also prompt evaluation. As these conditions often progress with growth, awareness and early recognition are important to facilitate early institution of appropriate treatment measures, and to minimize resultant morbidity.

Congenital Torticollis

Congenital torticollis or "wry neck" is a positional abnormality of the neck produced by fibrosis and shortening of the sternocleidomastoid muscle. It is thought to be secondary to abnormal intrauterine positioning or birth trauma resulting in

formation of a hematoma within the muscle belly. Usually the condition is recognized at or shortly after birth. A palpable swelling or "tumor" is often noted within the muscle. With subsequent fibrosis, the characteristic deformity of torticollis develops, consisting of head tilt toward the affected side with rotation of the chin to the opposite side (Fig. 21.57). Passive rotation is diminished toward the side of the torticollis, while lateral side bending is limited toward the side away from the torticollis. While the mass usually disappears in the first several weeks of life, contracture of the muscle persists and, if untreated, may result in craniofacial disfigurement with flattening of the face on the affected side. Gentle passive stretching exercises and positioning the child's crib so that external stimuli will cause him to turn the head and neck away from the side of deformity may be beneficial. If these measures fail, surgical release of the contracted muscle may be indicated.

The differential diagnoses include Klippel-Feil syndrome, inflammatory or infectious conditions of the head, neck or nasopharynx, posterior fossa or brain stem neoplasm, traumatic cervical spine injury, or atlantoaxial rotary subluxation. However, with the exception of the Klippel-Feil anomaly, the other sources tend to occur considerably later in childhood. In addition, a hip examination and an AP pelvis x-ray should be taken in every child with torticollis, as hip instability or dysplasia is present in approximately 20 percent of these children.

Klippel-Feil Syndrome

This congenital malformation of the neck is the result of a failure of segmentation in the developing cervical spine. The condition varies greatly in severity depending on the number of vertebrae that are fused (Fig. 21.58A,B). More severely affected individuals exhibit a short broad neck with the appearance of "webbing," a low hairline, and gross restriction of motion (Fig. 21.58C,D). The condition may be associated with other congenital malformations, such as Sprengel's deformity, rib deformities, scoliosis, CNS defects, and cardiac, pulmonary, and renal anomalies. Secondary neurological problems are rare, but accelerated degenerative changes may occur at mobile spinal segments adjacent to the involved vertebrae.

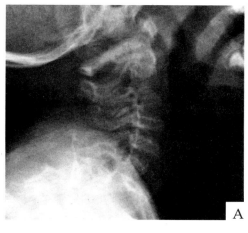

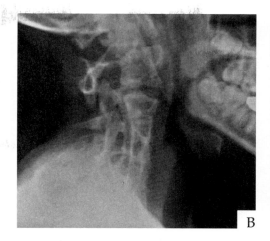

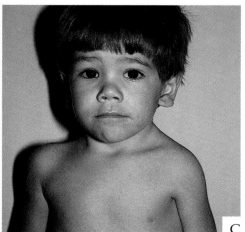

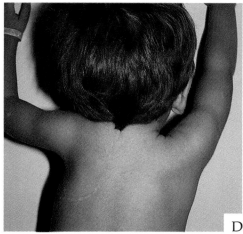

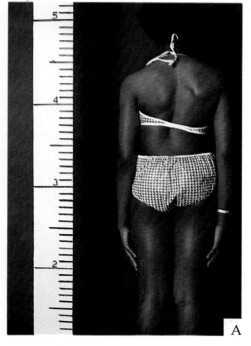

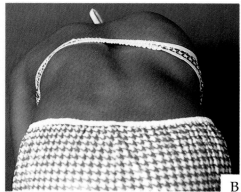

Fig. 19.58 Klippel-Feil syndrome. **A,** mild osseous involvement is seen in this radiograph in which there is fusion of the upper cervical segments. **B,** severe osseous involvement is demonstrated in this radiograph in which C-3 to C-7 are fused and hypoplastic. **C,** the neck appears short and broad in the anterior view of this young child. **D,** in the posterior view, the hairline is low and an associated Sprengel's deformity is present, the left scapula being hypoplastic and high-riding. As a result, the patient is unable to fully raise his left arm. Typical webbing is not appreciable in this child.

Fig. 21.59 Moderate thoracic idiopathic adolescent scoliosis. **A,** in the upright position, scapular asymmetry is easily discernible. This results from rotation of the spine and attached ribcage. **B,** forward flexion reveals a mild rib hump deformity.

On occasion, range of motion exercises or bracing may be tried to improve mobility or correct deformity. Surgery, except for cosmesis or neurological dysfunction, is rarely indicated. Individuals with mild forms of the malformation may be diagnosed only as a result of radiographs taken for other reasons.

Scoliosis

Scoliosis refers to curvature of the spine in the lateral plane. It occurs in structural forms characterized by a fixed curve and "functional" forms with a flexible or correctable curve. By anatomic necessity, this lateral deviation is associated with vertebral rotation such that when this deformity occurs in the thoracic spine, a chest wall deformity or "rib hump" develops (Fig. 21.59). When it occurs in the lumbar spine, a prominence of the flank may be noted (Fig. 21.60). Often there is a primary structural curve with an adjacent secondary compensatory curve. The majority of cases of structural scoliosis are idiopathic and have their onset in early adolescence. A familial predis-

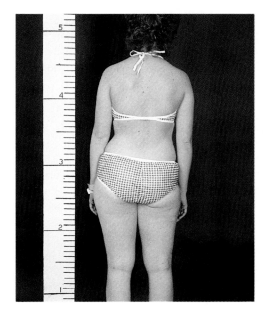

Fig. 21.60 Lumbar scoliosis. Pelvic obliquity is present, with prominence of the flank.

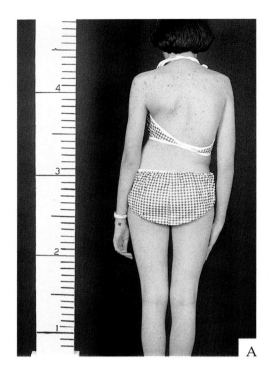

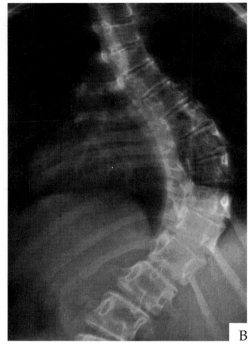

A

B

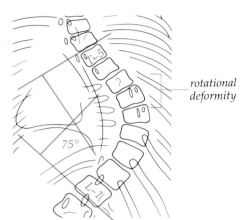

*Fig. 21.61 Severe thoracic scoliosis secondary to neurofibromatosis. **A,** note chest wall deformity and that patient's head is not centered over pelvis. **B,** the severe curvature is more apparent on this radiograph. The angle of measurement (here 75°) is determined by intersection of lines drawn perpendicular to end vertebrae of curve (Cobb method).*

rotational deformity

position has been documented, but inheritance of this appears to be multifactorial. Females are affected more often than males and are more likely to have progression of their curvature. Infantile (0 to 3 years) and juvenile (3 to 10 years) forms of idiopathic scoliosis are seen, though much less commonly. Affected infants rapidly develop plagiocephaly with flattening of the head on the concave side of the curve and a corresponding prominence on the opposite side of the head. They also have an increased incidence of associated hip dysplasia, congenital heart disease, inguinal hernias, and mental retardation. Structural scoliosis can also occur in conjunction with neuromuscular conditions (cerebral palsy, myelomeningocele, spinocerebellar degeneration, polio, spinal cord tumors, etc.); myopathic disorders (arthrogryposis or muscular dystrophy); congenital spinal anomalies (hemivertebrae, trapezoidal vertebrae, unsegmented vertebrae); neurofibromatosis and mesenchymal disorders (Fig. 21.61); and a variety of other conditions (Fig. 21.62). These neuromuscular and congenital forms tend to have more rapid progression of curvature than is true of idiopathic scoliosis, and infants with congenital spinal anomalies have a high incidence of associated genitourinary anomalies.

Apparent, nonstructural, flexible or "functional" scoliosis may be seen in association with poor posture, limb length inequality, or flexion contracture of a hip or knee, in which case the curve disappears when the child is seated. It can also be seen with paraspinous muscle spasm following back injury, due to splinting because of pain in cases of pyelonephritis, appendicitis, or pneumonia, or in patients with a herniated intervertebral disc and secondary nerve root pain (see Figs. 21.62 and 21.67A). These forms resolve with treatment of the primary disorder.

Except in curvatures resulting from inflammatory or neoplastic processes, pain is rarely a complaint in children and adolescents with scoliosis. In fact, patients with pain, signs of nerve root compression, or evidence of new onset peripheral

CAUSES OF SCOLIOSIS

Structural Scoliosis

Idiopathic
Congenital
Neuromuscular
Other conditions that may result in scioliosis:
   Myopathic disorders
   Neurofibromatosis
   Mesenchymal disorders
   Osteochondrodystrophies
   Metabolic disorders
   Posttrauma, surgery, irradiation, burns

Functional Scoliosis

Herniated lumbar discs
Postural derangements
Limb length inequality
Irritative or inflammatory disorders
Hysteria

Fig. 21.62

neurologic deficits should undergo thorough evaluation for a treatable underlying cause.

The clinical signs found on the scoliosis exam can be separated into true pathognomonic findings and associated stig-

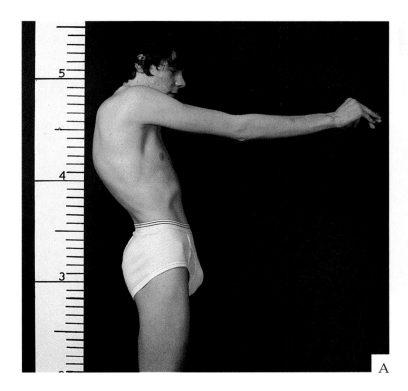

Fig. 21.63 *Moderate thoracic kyphosis secondary to Scheuermann's disease.* **A,** *the patient is attempting to correct the deformity, but due to its fixed nature, he cannot and must compensate for this with an increased lumbar lordosis.* **B,** *this tomographic cut demonstrates the anterior wedging of three consecutive vertebral bodies and clearly shows the associated erosion of the vertebral end plates and Schmorl's nodules.*

A

B

mata which may also occur in otherwise normal, nonscoliotic children. The only true pathognomonic sign of scoliosis is the presence of a curve noted on forward bending, termed a positive Adam's forward bending test. An associated convex posterior chest wall prominence (termed rib hump) or paralumbar prominence may also be noted on forward bending (see Fig. 21.59). The rib hump and paralumbar prominence are manifestations of the vertebral rotational deformity seen in scoliosis.

Frequently, a diagnosis of scoliosis is not based on a positive forward bending test, but rather on the presence of so-called stigmata signs. These signs include shoulder asymmetry, unilateral scapular prominence, waist asymmetry, and small chest or paralumbar humps. Any or all of these stigmata signs may be present in a child with true scoliosis, but the mere presence of these stigmata does not always imply scoliosis. Body assymetry is a frequent occurrence in the normal nonscoliotic child. A carefully performed Adam's forward bending test will always determine whether the stigmata signs are associated with true scoliosis, or simply provide evidence of body asymmetry—which does not warrant referral to an orthopedic specialist.

Because screening studies have found that up to 5 percent of school-age children and adolescents have lateral curvatures, routine screening by primary care physicians is important. Hence, the forward bending test should be part of all examinations from age 6 to 7 years until the end of puberty. When true clinical scoliosis is found, the patient should be referred for orthopedic evaluation no matter how small the curve is felt to be. It is probably safer and more cost-effective for the primary care physician to make the referral without

obtaining prior radiographs, because typical office radiographs done for scoliosis screening are usually not of high quality. Standing full torso, x-rays taken on 36-inch long cassette films with special grids are much more helpful and more readily available in the orthopedic clinic or office. Once a diagnosis of scoliosis has been made, followup x-rays are routinely obtained no more frequently than at 6- to 9-month intervals. The goal of close followup is to detect progression of curvature early and implement treatment to prevent or reduce it when needed. Idiopathic curves of 20° or more, or lesser curves with rapid progressions are treated with spinal bracing and an exercise program. Children with curves exceeding 40° or those that progress rapidly despite bracing require operative intervention.

Patients with untreated curvatures exceeding 60° inevitably develop significant secondary cardiopulmonary problems including decreased vital capacity, shunting, decreased oxygen saturation, and cor pulmonale.

Newborns and infants should be screened for scoliosis to detect congenital and infantile forms. This is often best done by holding the infant prone on the examiner's hand.

Kyphosis

Kyphosis refers to curvature of the spine in the sagittal plane. As opposed to scoliosis, this condition is generally not associated with a rotational spinal deformity. It may be purely postural in nature or associated with a number of pathologic conditions. The latter include congenital vertebral anomalies, spinal growth disturbance (Scheuermann's disease) (Fig. 21.63), neuromuscular afflictions, skeletal dysplasias, and

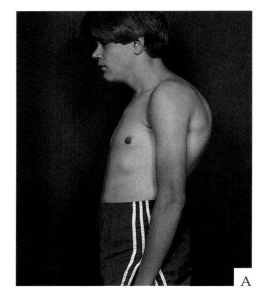

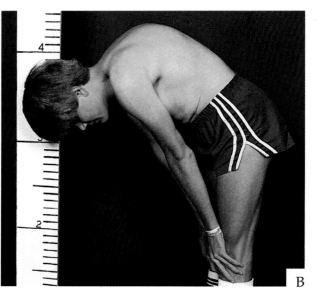

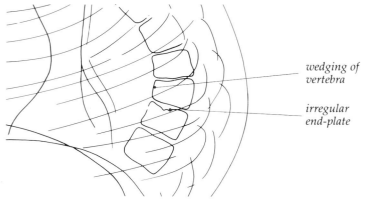

Fig. 21.64 *A, severe kyphosis of the thoracic spine secondary to vertebral wedging in glycogen storage disease. In order to stand upright, the patient must increase his lumbar lordosis and thrust his head forward to center it above the pelvis. **B,** the kyphotic deformity is accentuated on forward bending. **C,** radiographically the vertebral wedging which underlies the kyphotic deformity is evident.*

wedging of vertebra

irregular end-plate

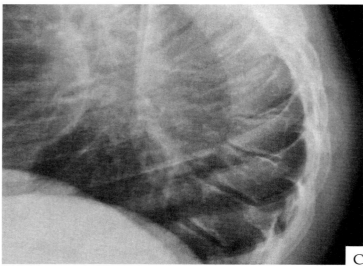

metabolic diseases (Fig. 21.64A–C). Kyphosis can also develop following spinal trauma or surgery. Patients with a structural deformity may complain of backache aggravated by motion. The deformity is best viewed from the lateral position on forward bending. Evaluation of the effects of posture and of application of pressure over the apex facilitates diagnosis and therapeutic decisions.

Postural kyphosis is usually seen in preadolescents and consists of a flexible thoracic kyphosis that is correctable on hyperextension. Most affected children have a compensatory increase in lumber lordosis. Radiographs are normal. Treatment consists of an exercise program designed to strengthen trunk and abdominal muscles, which are usually weak in these patients.

Scheuermann's disease, a disorder of unknown etiology, is the most common cause of fixed kyphotic deformity. It can be distinguished clinically from postural kyphosis by its inherent stiffness and greater magnitude. The deformity fails to correct, or is only partially correctable on hyperextension or upon application of pressure over the apex of the curve. Lateral radiographs reveal anterior wedging of three or more consecutive vertebral bodies which are located at the apex of the curve. There is often radiographic evidence of end-plate erosion of the involved vertebrae, and Schmorl's nodules are a common associated finding (see Fig. 21.63A,B).

Exercises and bracing are quite effective in treating mild structural kyphosis in the growing spine. However, when the deformity is severe and fixed, surgical correction and stabilization may be indicated.

Spondylolisthesis

Spondylolisthesis is a condition characterized by the translation or forward displacement of one vertebral body over another, and is seen most commonly at the lumbosacral articulation. The problem may develop as a result of insufficiency or fatigue fractures of the pars interarticularis (isthmic), congenital dysplasia of the posterior spinal elements (dysplastic), degenerative changes of the disc and facets (degenerative), or secondary to pathologic lesions within the vertebra and its elements (pathologic). Isthmic spondylolisthesis (spondylolysis) is by far the most common type (Fig. 21.65). Patients with a congenital predisposition may show alarming degrees of slippage. The condition is often associated with pain that increases with strenuous activities and improves with rest. Some patients have symptoms of nerve root irritation. This necessitates differentiation from inflammatory and neoplastic processes, and disc herniation.

Examination often reveals loss of normal lumbar lordosis, tenderness of the involved posterior elements, paravertebral

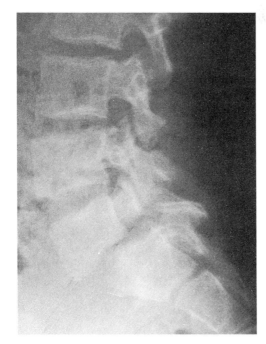

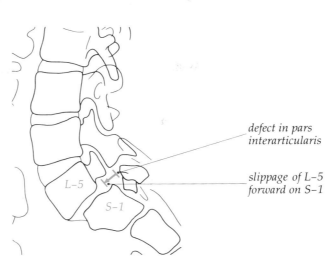

Fig. 21.65 Radiograph of moderate isthmic spondylolisthesis in a 14-year-old male. The forward slippage of L-5 on the sacrum is the result of a fatigue fracture of the pars interarticularis.

defect in pars interarticularis

slippage of L-5 forward on S-1

L-5

S-1

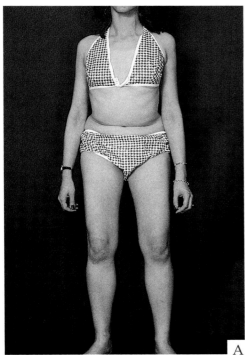

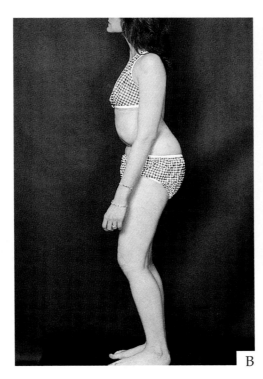

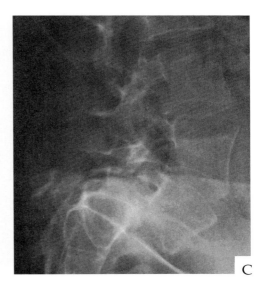

C

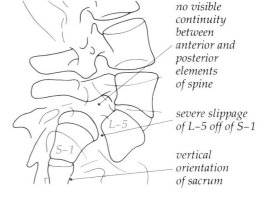

no visible continuity between anterior and posterior elements of spine

severe slippage of L-5 off of S-1

L-5

S-1

vertical orientation of sacrum

Fig. 21.66 Spondyloptosis in a 16-year-old female. **A,** a cosmetic deformity is common with this magnitude of spondylolisthesis. The torso is foreshortened and a transverse abdominal crease is present. **B,** in the lateral view, the torso is thrust forward, the buttocks are flattened, and there are flexion deformities of the hips and knees. **C,** the L-5 vertebra has completely translocated off the sacrum due to a congenital insufficiency of the posterior elements. The lumbar spine has essentially migrated anteriorly and into the pelvis.

muscle spasm and secondary tightness of the hamstring muscles. A step-off deformity may be evident on palpating the spinous processes. Range of motion is often limited in extension with complaints of pain. Nerve root signs may be present. In its most severe form, spondyloptosis, the L-5 vertebral body may completely translate off of the sacrum. These patients characteristically exhibit a waddling gait, a transverse abdominal crease, flattened buttocks and flexion deformities of the hips and knees. The torso may appear foreshortened (Fig. 21.66A,B). Characterization and grading of the process is made with radiographs. The oblique view may reveal a spondylolysis and the lateral view the degree of spondylolisthesis (Fig. 21.66C).

Treatment consists of appropriate exercises and bracing in mild to moderate cases. Patients with progressive slippage need surgical fusion, and those with neural involvement may

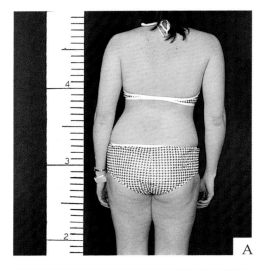

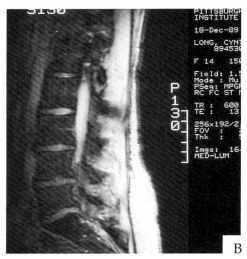

Fig. 21.67 Herniated intervertebral disc. **A,** discogenic scoliosis in a 16-year-old female with a herniated disc at L-4-5. The trunk is shifted away from the affected side. The normal lumbar lordosis is absent and spinal motion is severely limited. **B,** on this saggital MRI view, the L-4-5 disc bulges posteriorly compressing the cauda equina. (**B,** courtesy of the Department of Pediatric Radiology, Children's Hospital of Pittsburgh)

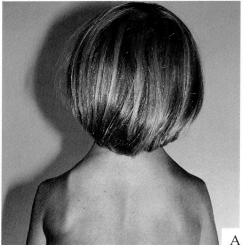

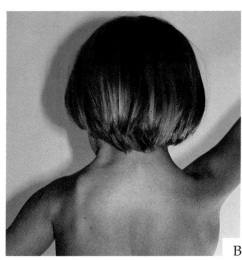

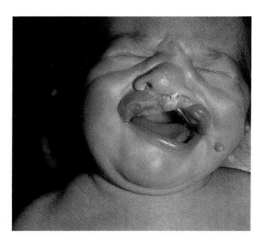

*Fig. 21.68 Sprengel's deformity. **A,** the left scapula is high-riding and hypoplastic, and its vertebral border is prominent **B,** shoulder motion is severely limited, particularly in abduction. (Courtesy of Dr. Dana Mears, Shadyside Hospital, Pittsburg)*

Fig. 21.69 Congenital pseudarthrosis of the clavicle. There is a bulbous, nontender swelling in the region of the midclavicle. The medial aspect of the clavicle is prominent. This patient has associated anomalies.

also require nerve root decompression. In severe spondylolisthesis with cosmetic deformity, functional impairment, and neurological dysfunction, surgical reduction of the deformity may be attempted, but this is not easy, nor is it without risk to the adjacent neural structures.

Herniated Intervertebral Disc

Although relatively common in adults, herniated discs occur rarely in children and are almost always limited to the lower two segments of the lumbar spine in adolescents. A history of trauma is not uncommon. Lower extremity radicular symptoms predominate. Patients often describe a peculiar "pulling" sensation in the lower extremity or liken their pain to a "toothache" in the distribution of the L-5 or S-1 nerve roots. They may complain of numbness or weakness in the involved limb. Forward flexion, sitting, coughing, or straining aggravate neural symptoms.

On examination, an antalgic scoliosis of the lumbar spine may be apparent which the patient is unable to reduce (Fig. 21.67A). Inability to reverse the normal lumbar lordosis is present and symptoms may be aggravated by attempts at flexion. The straight leg raising test is often positive (radicular symptoms are reproduced when the limb is raised by the examiner)

and neurological abnormalities on sensory, motor, and reflex testing may be found. Plain radiographs usually show no abnormality, other than a possible discogenic scoliosis, but the diagnosis may be verified by a myelogram, CT or MRI scan (Fig. 21.67B). The differential diagnosis may include hematogenous disc space infection or vertebral osteomyelitis, spinal cord or neural element tumor, and spondylolisthesis with nerve root irritation.

Nonoperative treatment consisting of rest and anti-inflammatory agents may be successful, but if profound neurologic deficit is present or incapacitating symptoms persist, surgical disc excision may be indicated. Intradiscal chemonucleolysis, as employed for adults, is contraindicated for children. Conservative treatment of radiographically proven disc herniation is not as effective in adolescents as it is in adults.

DISORDERS OF THE UPPER EXTREMITY

Because of the importance of prehensile function, disorders in any area of the upper limb can result in significant impairment of motor development during childhood. Knowledge of the normal anatomy and actions of the shoulder, arm, elbow, forearm, wrist, and hand is vital for assessment of abnormalities and institution of treatment.

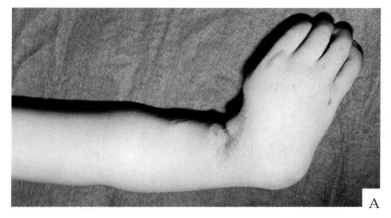

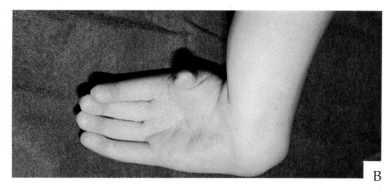

Fig. 21.70 Radial club hand deformity. **A,** the forearm is shortened with radial deviation of the hand and wrist on the ulna. **B,** there is a flexion deformity of the hand and wrist on the forearm and a hypoplastic thumb. **C,** this radiograph demonstrates absence of the radius, dislocation of the carpus, and a rudimentary thumb, all characteristic of radial club hand. (Clinical photographs courtesy of Dr. Joseph Imbriglia, Allegheny General Hospital, Pittsbiurg)

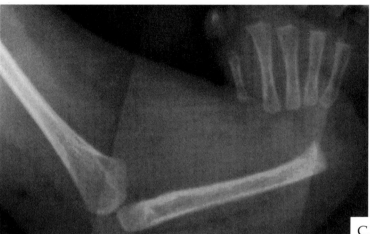

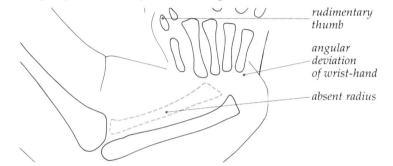

Sprengel's Deformity

Sprengel's deformity is a congenital malformation characterized by an abnormally small, high-riding scapula. In the majority of cases it is unilateral. The etiology is unknown, but there appears to be a familial predisposition, and the condition may be associated with a variety of other congenital anomalies, including Klippel-Feil syndrome, and rib and vertebral malformations. The small undescended scapula may be attached to the cervical spine by a band of fibrous tissue or bone (omovertebral bone). Scoliosis and torticollis may be associated. Complaints are usually those of cosmetic deformity and limited shoulder motion on the affected side.

On examination, the scapula is noted to be hypoplastic and high-riding in association with asymmetry of the base of the neck and shoulder. Shoulder motion is usually severely limited, particularly in abduction (Fig. 21.68). Radiography confirms the abnormal size and position of the scapula.

Nonoperative treatment measures consisting of stretching and range-of-motion exercises may be instituted, but are rarely successful. Surgery is usually undertaken for cosmetic and functional reasons and may consist of excision of the prominent superior aspect of the scapula, or release and reduction of the scapula by placing it inferiorly on the chest wall. The latter procedure is not without complication, as brachial plexus palsy may result from the maneuver.

Congenital Pseudarthrosis of the Clavicle

Congenital pseudarthrosis of the clavicle is a rare congenital disorder usually manifested by a painless, nontender bulbous deformity in the region of the midclavicle. It is thought to result from a failure of maturation of the ossification center of the clavicle. It generally involves the right side and, on occasion, may be associated with other congenital anomalies. In cleidocranial dysostosis the entire clavicle may be absent or may have an appearance similar to that of congenital pseudarthrosis.

On examination, the clavicle appears foreshortened with a prominence evident in its midportion (Fig. 21.69). Palpation reveals hypermobility of the two ends of the clavicle and crepitation. Range of motion of the shoulder is generally normal. This condition characteristically presents no functional impairment and requires no treatment. While clavicular fracture as a result of birth trauma may present a similar appearance, it is easily distinguished because of tenderness over the region of deformity.

Radial Club Hand

This condition is the result of congenital absence or hypoplasia of the radial structures of the forearm and hand. Associated muscular structures and the radial nerve are hypoplastic or absent. The anomaly is rare and affects males more frequently than females. Its characteristic clinical presentation is a small, short, bowed forearm and aplasia or hypoplasia of the thumb. The residual hand is deviated radially. Radiographs show absence of bones in the affected area (Fig. 21.70).

Treatment is best instituted early with passive stretching exercises and corrective casting. Surgical treatment consists of centralization of the hand on the "one bone forearm" to maximize function.

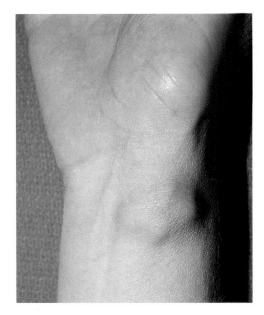 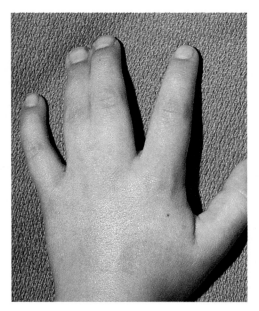 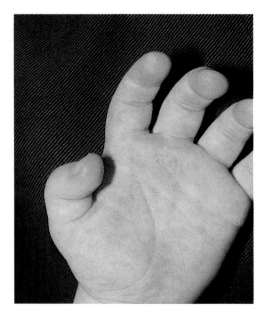

Fig. 21.71 Ganglion of the wrist. This cystic mass overlying the wrist joint and flexor tendons was asymptomatic and nontender.

Fig. 21.72 Mild syndactyly involving soft tissues of the middle and ring fingers without bony involvement. (Courtesy of Dr. Joseph Imbriglia, Allegheny General Hospital, Pittsbiurg)

Fig. 21.73 Congenital trigger thumb. There is a fixed flexion deformity at the interphalangeal joint of the thumb due to tightness of the tendon sheath of the flexor pollicus longus. The remainder of the hand appears normal.

Ganglion of the Wrist

A ganglion is a benign cystic mass consisting of an accumulation of synovial fluid or gelatin in an outpouching of a tendon sheath or joint capsule. The exact etiology is unknown, but it is thought to be related to a herniation of synovial tissue with a ball valve effect. Antecedent trauma may be reported. These masses may be present over the dorsal or volar aspects of the wrist and are generally located toward the radial side (Fig. 21.71). They are occasionally seen on the dorsum of the foot or adjacent to one of the malleoli of the ankle. Their size may fluctuate with time and activity. On examination, they may be either firm or fluctuant. Transillumination is positive. While most are asymptomatic, an occasional patient may have pain and tenderness.

Treatment is generally unnecessary for patients who are asymptomatic. Occasionally, patients desire removal for cosmetic or psychological reasons. Surgery is not routinely advised for asymptomatic cysts as recurrence may be as high as 20 percent. Aspiration, injection, or rupture of these cysts do not result in their elimination. Surgical excision with obliteration of the base of the ganglion is the most successful treatment for the occasional case in which treatment is indicated.

Syndactyly

Syndactyly is a relatively common congenital affliction involving failure of the digits of the hands or feet to separate. It is more common and disabling in the upper extremity. Bilateral involvement is usual and a positive family history is not uncommon. It may be associated with other congenital anomalies, particularly Apert's syndrome and Streeter's dysplasia. There is great variation in the degree of fusion. In mild cases, only the skin is joined, making reconstructive surgery simple (Fig. 21.72). In more severe cases, the nails, deeper structures and bones may be conjoined, contributing to deformity and growth abnormalities, and making reconstructive treatment more difficult.

Congenital Trigger Thumb

A congenital trigger thumb is characterized by a fixed or intermittent flexion deformity of the interphalangeal joint of the thumb that may be present at birth or may develop shortly thereafter (Fig. 21.73). The problem is thought to result from tightness of the tendon sheath of the flexor pollicus longus in the region of the metacarpophalangeal joint. The flexion deformity generally cannot be reduced, although in milder cases it may be passively correctable with a snapping sensation felt as the tendon passes through the stenosed pulley mechanism. If passively correctable, splinting in extension occasionally will result in correction; otherwise, surgery is required.

Boutonnière (Buttonhole) Deformity

A boutonnière deformity of the finger is the end result of a traumatic avulsion of the central portion of the extensor tendon at its insertion on the middle phalanx of the finger that went unrecognized at the time of initial injury. The mechanism of injury is usually a blow to the tip of the finger driving it into forced flexion against resistance. A laceration over the dorsum of the finger involving the extensor tendon may produce a similar deformity if tendon involvement is not recognized and

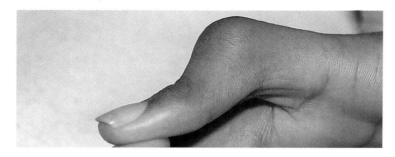

Fig. 21.74 Boutonnière deformity of the finger. There is a fixed flexion contracture of the proximal interphalangeal joint and hyperextension of the distal joint, secondary to volar migration of the lateral bands of the extensor mechanism. This is the result of unrecognized or inadequately treated injury to the extensor tendon at its insertion on the middle phalanx.

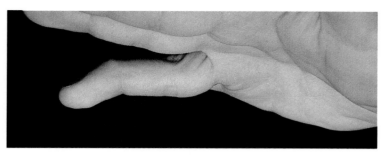

Fig. 21.75 Mallet finger with secondary "swan neck" deformity. This is the result of avulsion of the extensor tendon from its insertion at the base of the distal phalanx, which was not recognized at the time of injury. The patient demonstrates flexion deformity of the DIP joint and secondary hyperextension of the PIP joint.

repaired at the time. Initially, there may be local tenderness over the dorsal aspect of the proximal interphalangeal (PIP) joint without deformity. With time, however, the lateral bands of the extensor mechanism migrate volarly, producing a flexion deformity of the PIP joint with a secondary extension deformity of the distal joint (Fig. 21.74). When recognized early, healing may occur with splinting of the PIP joint in extension. Later, open surgical repair may be necessary to improve function.

Mallet Finger/Swan Neck Deformity

A mallet finger is the result of avulsion of the extensor tendon from its insertion at the base of the distal phalanx of a finger. It occurs as a result of a blow to the extended finger against resistance. The tendon alone, or a portion of the distal phalanx into which it inserts, may be involved. The clinical appearance is that of a "dropped finger" or flexion deformity of the distal interphalangeal (DIP) joint with inability to actively extend the joint. If not recognized and treated at the time of the initial injury the condition becomes chronic and contracture of the extensor mechanism may occur, with a secondary hyperextension deformity of the proximal interphalangeal joint producing a "swan neck deformity" (Fig. 21.75). Treatment consists of splinting the distal joint in an extended position, open reduction if a large fragment of bone is involved, or surgical repair in chronic cases.

DISORDERS OF THE LOWER EXTREMITY

Normally developed and functional lower extremities permit locomotion with ease and a minimal amount of energy expenditure. Disability from a deformed, shortened, or painful lower limb can be considerable.

Many problems of the lower extremities in childhood are congenital and, if they remain unrecognized or are unsuccessfully treated, can result in life-long disability. Knowledge of the normal anatomy and function of the hip, knee, ankle, and foot is necessary to accurately recognize and treat abnormalities in this region.

Congenital Dislocation of the Hip

Congenital dislocation of the hip, or displacement of the femoral head from its normal relationship with the acetabulum, is a relatively frequent problem with an incidence of 1 to 2 per 1,000 births. It is generally detectable at birth or shortly thereafter. Females are affected significantly more frequently than males and unilateral dislocation is twice as frequent as bilateral. Congenital dislocation may be divided into idiopathic and teratogenic types. Idiopathic congenital dislocation is more frequent and patients often have a positive family history. Its severity varies from subluxed, to dislocated and reducible, to dislocated and unreducible. This type of congenital dislocation may be related to abnormal intrauterine positioning, and/or restriction of fetal movement in utero, which impedes adequate development and stability of the hip joint complex. The relaxing effect of hormones acting on soft tissue during pregnancy may also contribute, with affected infants perhaps being more sensitive to the pelvic relaxation effects of maternal estrogen. A history of breech presentation is not uncommon and these patients often exhibit generalized ligamentous laxity. Teratogenic dislocations of the hip represent a more severe form of the disorder and are probably the result of a germ plasm defect. They occur early in fetal development and result in malformation of both the femoral head and the acetabular socket. Associated congenital anomalies are common in infants whose dislocations are teratogenic. There is a significant association with clubfoot deformity, congenital torticollis, metatarsus adductus, and infantile scoliosis.

The importance of careful hip evaluation in the newborn and at early infant visits cannot be overemphasized. Early diagnosis enables prompt institution of treatment measures and results in a better outcome. An understanding of clinical signs and skill in techniques of examination are necessary.

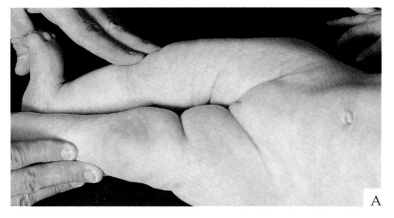
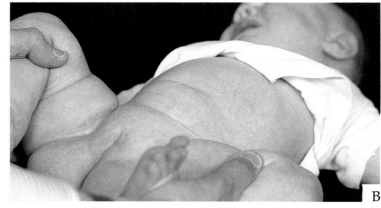

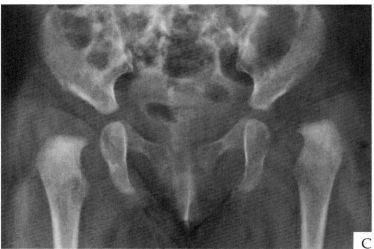
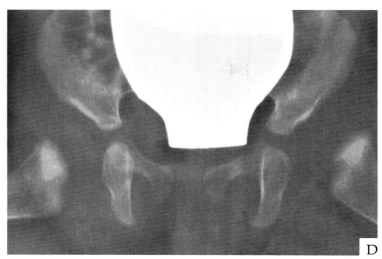

Fig. 21.76 Congenital dislocation of the hip. **A,** in cases of unilateral dislocation, the involved extremity is foreshortened and the thigh and groin creases are asymmetric. **B,** limited abduction of the involved hip is demonstrated. This is a consistent finding in infants with a dislocated and unreducible hip. **C,** in this AP radiograph of a 3-month-old child, the proximal femur is displaced upward and laterally and the

acetabulum is shallow. The femoral head is not visible on the radiograph because of the delayed ossification associated with congenital hip dislocation. **D,** in the "frogleg view" the long axis of the affected left femur is directed toward a point superior and lateral to the triradiate cartilage, in contrast to that of the right, which points directly at this structure.

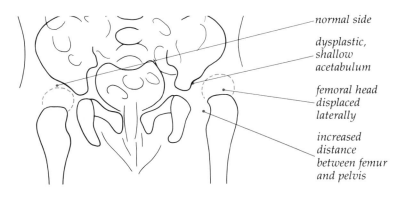

normal side

dysplastic, shallow acetabulum

femoral head displaced laterally

increased distance between femur and pelvis

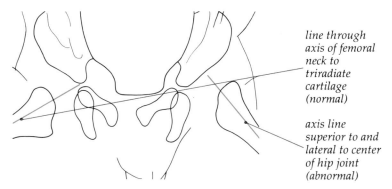

line through axis of femoral neck to triradiate cartilage (normal)

axis line superior to and lateral to center of hip joint (abnormal)

Typically, the infant with a dislocated hip holds the leg in a position of adduction and external rotation. When unilateral, the skin folds of the thighs and buttocks are often asymmetrical and the involved lower extremity appears shorter than the opposite side (Fig. 21.76A). This foreshortening is accentuated by holding the hips and knees in 90° flexion (Galeazzi's sign). In patients with bilateral dislocations, these asymmetric findings are not present. In a truly dislocated hip, the most consistent physical finding is that of limited abduction (Fig. 21.76C). Additional diagnostic maneuvers may assist in establishing and confirming the diagnosis. In patients with reducible dislocations, Ortolani's sign is positive when a palpable clunk is felt

upon abduction (relocation) of the hip. Barlow's test is positive when, with knees flexed and hips flexed to 90°, the hips are gently adducted with pressure applied on the lesser trochanter by the thumb. A palpable clunk indicating posterior dislocation is appreciated if the hip is unstable or dislocated. When the hip is dislocated and unreducible, only limitation of abduction will be apparent.

The radiographic findings of a congenital hip dislocation are characteristic. The femoral head is generally located lateral and superior to its normal position and the acetabulum may be shallow, with lateral deficiency and a characteristic high acetabular index or slope (Fig. 21.76C). Reduction of the dislo-

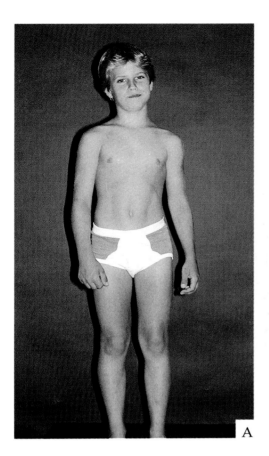

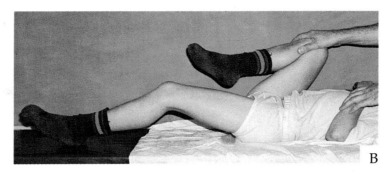

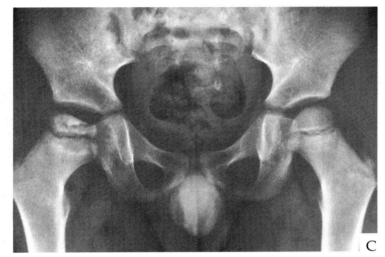

Fig. 21.77 Legg-Calvé-Perthes disease. **A,** this 7-year-old male is small for his chronologic age. He is bearing less weight on the involved right leg, and on examination a hip flexion contracture and abductor lurch gait were present. **B,** full flexion of the opposite hip eliminates lumbar lordosis and accentuates the contracture. This is an indication of irritation of the hip joint from the disease and associated synovitis. **C,** in this AP radiograph, the right femoral epiphysis is flattened and fragmented. The proximal femur is also displaced inferiorly and laterally.

cated hip is apparent when, upon abduction of the hip to 45°, a line drawn through the axis of the metaphysis of the neck crosses the triradiate cartilage (Fig. 21.76D). In idiopathic dislocation, ossification of the femoral epiphysis is delayed. Ossification is normally evident radiographically at 3 to 6 months of age, but is delayed in congenital dislocation because normal articulation forces are absent. In teratogenic hip dislocation, there may be hypoplasia of both the acetabular and femoral sides with noncongruent development of one or both of these structures. The radiographic findings early on, however, are similar to those mentioned above.

Successful correction depends on early diagnosis and institution of appropriate treatment measures. In the first 6 months of life, use of a Pavlik harness, which permits gentle motion of the hip in a flexed and abducted position, may achieve and maintain a satisfactory reduction. Between 6 and 18 months of age, gentle closed reduction and immobilization in a spica cast with or without surgical release of the contracted iliopsoas and adductor muscles is indicated. After the age of 18 months, reduction by manipulative measures is difficult owing to contractures of the associated soft tissues. In such instances, open reduction is usually indicated. In cases of teratogenic dislocation, underlying maldevelopment makes outcome less satisfactory even with optimal management.

With early recognition and appropriate treatment, a relatively normal hip with satisfactory function can be anticipated. Failure of concentric reduction or complications such as avascular necrosis of the femoral head, due to overzealous attempts at closed reduction in long-standing cases, may result in a life-long disability characterized by pain and stiffness in the hip, an antalgic lurching gait, and shortening of the involved limb.

Legg-Calvé-Perthes Disease

In Legg-Calvé-Perthes disease (coxa plana) impairment of the blood supply to the developing femoral head results in avascular necrosis. Etiology is unknown. Current theories implicate traumatic disruption of the blood supply and recurrent episodes of synovitis during which increased intra-articular pressure compromises blood flow to the developing ossific nucleus. The disorder generally becomes manifest between the ages of 4 and 11 years with a higher incidence in males. Affected children often exhibit delayed skeletal maturation and are small for their age. Unilateral involvement is the rule and, if a bilateral case is suspected, some form of epiphyseal dysplasia must be ruled out. The severity of the disease varies greatly, depending on how much of the femoral head is affected. Younger children generally have milder involvement, as a larger portion of the femoral head is still cartilaginous and less dependent on vascular supply.

Onset is often insidious. The child may present with symptoms characteristic of toxic synovitis without radiographic findings. Generally, there is a flexion contracture of the involved hip with the lower extremity positioned in a slightly externally rotated position. Pain and limitation of motion are encountered on attempts at internal rotation and abduction (Fig. 21.77A,B). Trendelenburg's sign (failure to maintain a level pelvis when standing on the involved limb) is positive. Many children present with a painless limp while others complain of thigh or knee pain, fatigue on walking, or hip stiffness. Early radiographic findings may include failure of progressive development of the femoral ossific nucleus, a subchondral radiolucent fracture line (Caffey's sign), or evidence of slight subluxation. However, in very early cases, radiographs may be

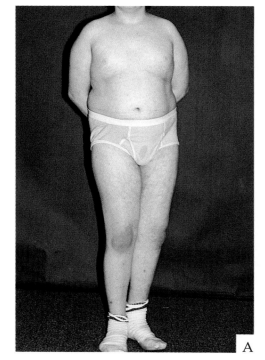

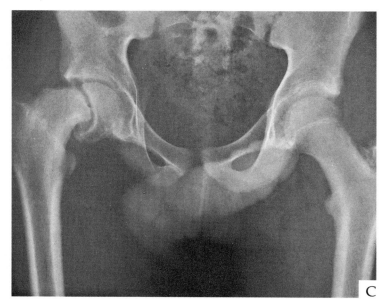

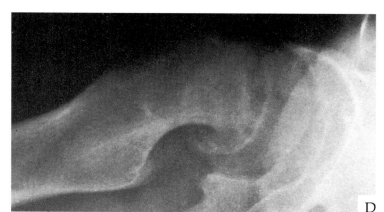

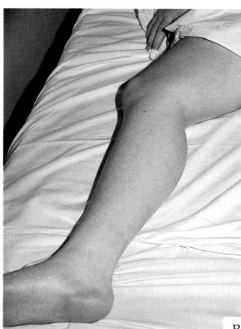

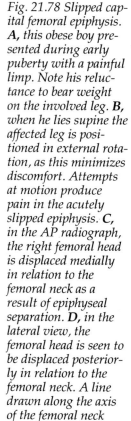

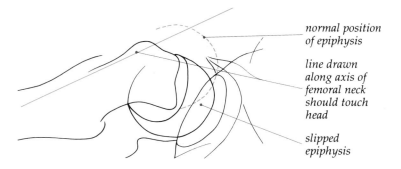

Fig. 21.78 Slipped capital femoral epiphysis. **A,** this obese boy presented during early puberty with a painful limp. Note his reluctance to bear weight on the involved leg. **B,** when he lies supine the affected leg is positioned in external rotation, as this minimizes discomfort. Attempts at motion produce pain in the acutely slipped epiphysis. **C,** in the AP radiograph, the right femoral head is displaced medially in relation to the femoral neck as a result of epiphyseal separation. **D,** in the lateral view, the femoral head is seen to be displaced posteriorly in relation to the femoral neck. A line drawn along the axis of the femoral neck should normally touch the head.

normal position of epiphysis

line drawn along axis of femoral neck should touch head

slipped epiphysis

completely normal and a nuclear bone scan may be useful in verification of impairment of the blood supply to this region. Later on, fragmentation of the femoral ossification center may be evident with flattening of the femoral head, extrusion, and frank subluxation (Fig. 21.77C).

The disease is self-limited, typically spanning a period of 1 to 2 years. While revascularization and reconstitution of the femoral head always occurs, loss of mechanical integrity of the head with flattening and fragmentation of its surface may result in irreversible predisposition to degenerative change. Most treatment methods are based on the principle of "containment" and the maintenance of a normal relationship of the femoral head within the acetabulum so as to minimize permanent joint incongruity. In young children with minimal symptoms and radiographic findings, decreased activity and close observation may be all that is necessary. Anti-inflammatory

agents and traction are used during episodes of synovitis. In more severe cases, abduction casting, bracing, or operative treatment with femoral or acetabular osteotomy to reposition the femoral head deeper within the acetabulum may be employed. In cases that are recognized late or those that fail to respond to appropriate measures, permanent degenerative change is common and salvage type surgery may be necessary.

Slipped Capital Femoral Epiphysis (SCFE)

Slipped capital femoral epiphysis (SCFE), a disorder seen early in puberty, involves displacement of the femoral head from the femoral neck through the epiphyseal plate. It is seen more frequently in males, and occurs bilaterally in approximately 25 percent of cases. Most commonly, it occurs at the onset of puberty in obese individuals with delayed sexual maturation.

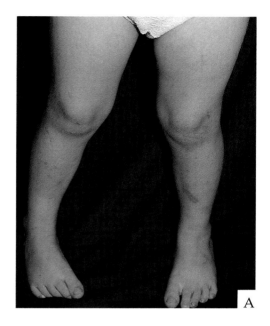

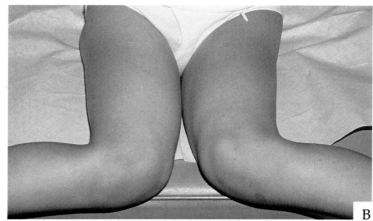

Fig. 21.79 Femoral anteversion. **A**, the condition is bilateral and in the standing view, both legs appear to turn inward from the hip down. **B**, on assessment of range of motion, the degree of internal rotation of the hips is found to be greater than normal. (Courtesy of Dr. M. Sherlock)

While etiology is unclear, it is generally thought that hormonal changes at the time of puberty may result in loss of mechanical integrity of the growth plate, and that if the epiphysis is then subjected to excessive shear stress, slippage through this area may occur. This condition differs from traumatic epiphyseal fractures because the translational displacement occurs through a different area of the growth plate. In some cases an underlying connective tissue disorder, such as Marfan's syndrome, or an endocrinologic problem, such as hypothyroidism, can be identified.

Clinical presentation is quite characteristic, although duration of symptoms varies. The patient presents with a painful limp and may or may not have a history of recent trauma, which is usually minor, or may have developed pain after jumping. This injury may have precipitated a slip in the previously weakened epiphysis, or may have increased the degree of displacement if a slip was already in progress. The pain may be perceived as being in the hip or in the thigh or knee. The lower extremity is held in an externally rotated position secondary to deformity at the site of physeal displacement. An antalgic and abductor lurch gait is usually apparent. A flexion contracture may be noted, and range of motion tends to be diminished in all planes, particularly internal rotation (Fig. 21.78A,B). Slight shortening of the involved lower extremity is observed in some cases.

Radiographic findings vary in severity from a widened and radiolucent physis (preslip) to frank deformity with displacement of the femoral head on the proximal femur posteriorly and inferiorly in relation to its normal counterpart (Fig. 21.78C,D). The degree of slippage and deformity correlates with the extent of incongruity of the hip joint and later development of degenerative change and painful symptoms. Prompt intervention to prevent further displacement is an important factor in preventing life-long problems, and awareness, a high index of suspicion, and early recognition are key factors in improving the prognosis.

In undisplaced or mildly displaced slips, cast immobilization or stabilization of the slip with in situ pin fixation is indicated. In acute slipped epiphyses of moderate or severe grade, an attempt at closed reduction followed by surgical pin fixation may be indicated. When the disease is recognized late and deformity is severe, proximal femoral osteotomy may be necessary. Children with unilateral slipped epiphyses must be monitored closely for signs of involvement of the opposite limb.

Femoral Anteversion

Femoral anteversion may be viewed as a normal variation of lower extremity positioning in the developing child. In utero and at birth, the femoral neck sits in an anteverted position relative to that of the adult. During childhood it will remodel to a position of slight anteversion and normal alignment of the lower extremities. In certain children, however, delayed rotational correction may result in persistent intoeing. An unsightly gait, kicking of the heels, or tripping on walking or running are frequently related complaints. There may be a history of sitting on the floor with the legs out in a "reversed Tailor position". Generally the condition is bilateral, and is not associated with other musculoskeletal problems.

On examination, the child is noted to stand with the entire lower extremities, including the knees and feet, turned inwards. An increase in internal rotation over external rotation is apparent on assessment of range of motion (Fig. 21.79). Radiographic examination is normal. No treatment is indicated other than reassurance that the condition will correct with growth and instructions to avoid sitting in the predisposing position.

Genu Varum (Physiologic Bowlegs)

Genu varum or bowlegs is a normal variation of lower extremity configuration, seen in the 1- to 3-year-old age group. It is generally recognized shortly after ambulation begins and may be associated with laxity of other joints and internal tibial torsion. Examination reveals diffuse bowing of the lower extremities with an increased distance between the knees that is accentuated on standing (Fig. 21.80). Varus positioning of the heel with pronation of the feet may be noted on weight-bearing. The child may walk with a waddling gait and kick the heels on running to clear the feet from the ground and avoid hitting the contralateral limb. Laxity of joint capsular structures may be noted with application of a reduction force.

Radiographs show normal osseous and physeal development and may reveal a gentle symmetrical bowing of the

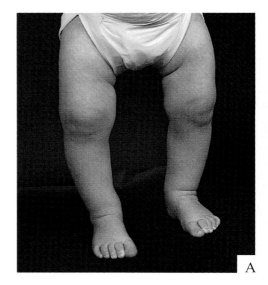
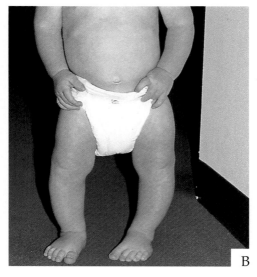
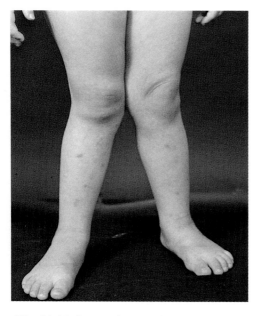

Fig. 21.80 Genu varum. **A,** the mild symmetric bowing seen in this 1-year-old male represents a normal variation of lower extremity configuration in toddlers; correction occurs with growth and remodeling. The bowing is diffuse and involves the upper and lower portions of the legs. **B,** this child has more severe physiologic bowing which resulted in frequent tripping and waddling gait. He also had associated ligamentous laxity and intoeing.

Fig. 21.81 Genu valgum. This 3½-year-old female exhibits a moderate knock-knee deformity. Ligamentous laxity and mild pes planus are associated.

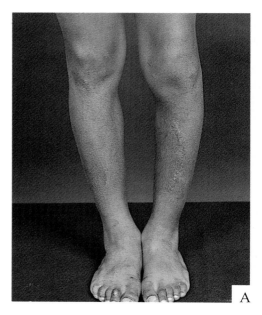
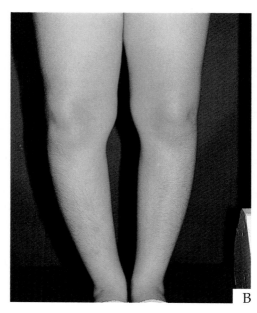
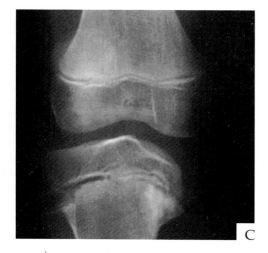
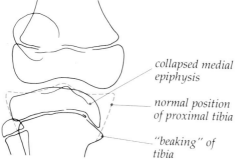

collapsed medial epiphysis

normal position of proximal tibia

"beaking" of tibia

Fig. 21.82 Blount's disease. **A,** the patient has a unilateral angular deformity of the proximal left tibia that gives the appearance of genu varum. **B,** both proximal tibiae are bowed in another patient as a result of fragmentation and loss of height of the medial epiphyses. In contrast to physiologic bowing, the thighs are straight. **C,** the radiograph demonstrates the typical fragmentation, loss of height, and angular deformity or beaking of the medial portion of the proximal tibia.

femur and tibia. While there may be slight beaking of the medial metaphysis of the femur and tibia adjacent to the knee joint, there is no fragmentation of the epiphysis or irregularity of the growth plate as is seen in Blount's disease. Conditions such as rickets or other metabolic abnormalities, epiphyseal dysplasia, various forms of dwarfism, or pathologic growth disturbances such as Blount's disease also can usually be ruled out by radiographs.

Treatment is rarely indicated, as this condition corrects with growth and, in fact, a valgus deformity of the knees may be noted later, at approximately 4 to 5 years of age. Casting, bracing, and corrective shoes are unnecessary and there is no indication for surgery.

Genu Valgum (Physiologic Knock-Knees)

Genu valgum or knock-knees is a normal variation of lower extremity configuration, generally noted in children between the ages of 3 and 5 years. The phenomenon is part of the normal process of remodeling of the lower extremities during

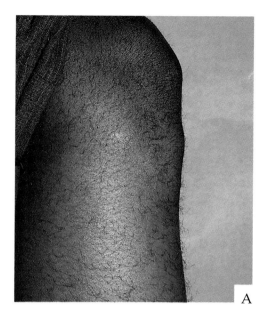 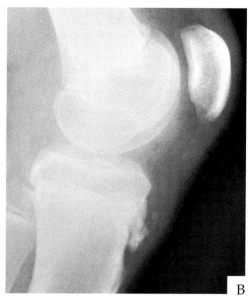

growth and development. It is more frequently seen in females and may be associated with ligamentous laxity. While standing the child is noted to have an increased distance between the feet when the medial aspects of the knees touch one another (Fig. 21.81). Not uncommonly, the child will place one knee behind the other in an attempt to get the feet together. In some cases valgus alignment of the feet and a pes planus deformity may be noted. Radiographs reveal no osseous or physeal abnormalities, but accentuation of the angular deformity of the knee is seen on weight-bearing views secondary to ligamentous laxity. One must rule out the possibility of an underlying metabolic condition such as rickets or renal disease. Treatment is generally not indicated as the condition gradually corrects with time.

Blount's Disease

Blount's disease is an isolated growth disturbance of the medial tibial epiphysis manifested as an angular varus deformity of the proximal tibia with apparent progressive genu varum. Unilateral and bilateral presentation are seen with nearly equal frequency. The etiology of this condition is unknown, although it appears to be more common in blacks. It may represent a compression injury to the medial growth plate of the proximal tibia.

On careful examination, a localized angular deformity of the proximal tibia is apparent, in contrast to the diffuse bowing of the lower extremities seen in patients with physiologic bowlegs (Fig. 21.82A,B). Generally there is no evidence of the ligamentous laxity commonly associated with physiologic bowing. Radiographs reveal fragmentation of the medial epiphysis of the tibia associated with beaking and loss of height in this region, and the characteristic angular deformity (Fig. 21.82C). Satisfactory treatment is dependent on accurate diagnosis and early recognition, as bracing or surgical osteotomy with realignment of the leg may prevent further progression.

Osgood-Schlatter Disease

Osgood-Schlatter disease is a traction apophysitis of the tibial tubercle which tends to develop during the adolescent growth spurt. It occurs somewhat more frequently in males than

females. It is thought that rapid differential growth between the osseous and soft tissue structures and stress on the apophysis produced by vigorous physical activity are contributing factors. Bilateral involvement is usual. Patients present with a history of gradually increasing pain and swelling in the region of the tibial tubercle. Discomfort is accentuated by vigorous physical activity, kneeling or crawling, and is relieved by rest.

On examination, a localized tender swelling is noted in the region of the tibial tubercle and patellar tendon. The knee joint is otherwise normal on examination, with the exception that some patients have findings of limitation of knee flexion with reproduction of their pain. Radiographs may reveal only soft tissue swelling in the region of the proximal tibial apophysis or irregularity of ossification of this structure (Fig. 21.83). In long-standing cases, frank fragmentation of the apophysis may be seen.

The problem, though self-limited, persists over a period of 6 to 24 months. If the condition is only occasionally bothersome and does not limit activities, treatment is unnecessary. If severe pain and a limp are present, a short period of immobilization in a splint or cast may be beneficial. Use of ibuprofen or aspirin as needed for pain and curtailing activities that produce pain is sufficient treatment for most patients. Steroid injection is contraindicated, as this may cause deterioration of the tendon and provides little in the way of long-term relief.

Popliteal (Baker's) Cyst

Popliteal cysts in childhood are encountered most commonly in children between 5 and 10 years of age and occur significantly more frequently in males than females. They are located in the posteromedial aspect of the knee joint in the region of the semimembranosus tendon and medial gastrocnemius muscle belly. The pathology is that of a fibrous tissue or synovial cyst filled with synovial-like fluid. In contrast to those seen in adults, popliteal cysts in childhood generally do not communicate with the joint capsule, but originate instead beneath the semimembranosus tendon, presumably as a result of chronic irritation. Occasionally vague pain is noted, but evaluation is usually sought because of a recently noted painless mass.

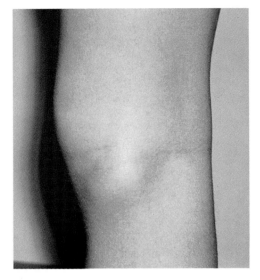 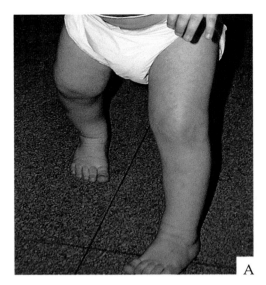 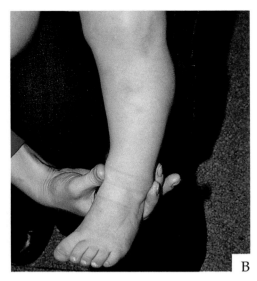

Fig. 21.84 Popliteal (Baker's) cyst. A local-ized swelling appears in the region of the semimembranosus tendon. This may arise from the synovial lining of the semimembra-nosus bursa.

Fig. 21.85 Internal tibial torsion. **A,** the hip, thigh, and knee are normally oriented and the patella faces anteriorly, but the lower leg and foot turn inward. The deformity results in prominent intoeing on walking, and may

cause the child to trip frequently. **B,** the later-al malleolus is positioned anterior to the medial malleolus, thus shifting the ankle mortise and foot to a medially oriented posi-tion. (Courtesy of Dr. M. Sherlock)

On examination, a soft, nontender, cystic mass is found in the described location (Fig. 21.84). Range of motion of the joint is normal unless the cyst is particularly large, limiting flexion. The knee is otherwise normal. Radiographs show no osseous abnormality. Popliteal cysts are benign and may resolve over time although their surgical excision is reasonable if desired.

Chondromalacia Patella

Chondromalacia patella is a disorder of as yet unclear etiology, although abnormal tracking of the patella is suspected to be causative in part. Patello-femoral incongruity due to develop-mental variations in the shape of the distal femur and patella, malalignment of the quadriceps and patellar tendons, abnor-mal positioning of the patella in the quadriceps tendon, and weakness of the quadriceps muscle have all been associated with the condition.

Onset of symptoms may be insidious or may abruptly follow trauma. The patient complains of diffuse aching behind the patella that is exacerbated by climbing stairs, pedaling a bicy-cle, or prolonged sitting. On examination, the patella is found to be tender along its medial border, and application of pres-sure over the patella with the knee slightly flexed elicits pain. When the examiner holds a hand over the patella as the patient flexes and extends the knee, a grating sensation may be felt.

Pathologically, softening and blistering of the articular carti-lage is found early on. With progression, the articular cartilage becomes fissured and ultimately eroded.

Treatment consists of quadriceps-strengthening exercises and use of oral anti-inflammatory agents such as ibuprofen or aspirin, along with avoidance of activities such as deep knee bends and weight lifting.

Internal Tibial Torsion

Internal tibial torsion is a nonpathologic variation in normal development of the lower leg in children under the age of 5. It consists of a rotational deformity thought to be the result of internal molding of the foot and leg in utero. The child is usu-ally brought for evaluation because of concern about promi-nent intoeing on walking and frequent tripping.

On examination, the hips and knees are normally aligned with the patellae facing anteriorly, the lower legs and feet are rotated inwardly. The lateral malleolus, which is normally positioned slightly posterior to the medial malleolus, may be in alignment with it or even anteriorly displaced, thus causing the ankle mortise to shift to a medially directed orientation, resulting in intoeing (Fig. 21.85A,B). The rotational deformity can also be detected by having the patient lie prone on the examining table with the knees flexed. In this position the feet turn toward the midline in children with tibial torsion. Radiographs reveal no osseous abnormalities. Treatment is sel-dom indicated; remodeling gradually corrects the condition as the child grows and develops. Children who have a habit of sitting on their feet on the floor may inhibit the normal remod-eling process and should be instructed not to do this. Bracing and special shoes have little effect, and are not recommended.

Congenital Clubfoot

Congenital clubfoot (talipes equinovarus) is a teratogenic deformity of the foot that is readily apparent at birth. It is seen more frequently in males than females and has an incidence of 1 in 1,000 live births. Etiology is probably multifactorial. Familial incidence studies suggest an underlying genetic pre-disposition. Abnormal intrauterine positioning and pressure at a critical point in development may contribute as well. Neural, muscular, and osseous abnormalities are other proposed pre-disposing conditions. There is a near equal frequency of unilat-eral and bilateral involvement. The deformity is characterized by three primary components: (1) the entire foot is positioned in plantar flexion (equinus); (2) the hindfoot is maintained in a position of fixed inversion (varus); and (3) the forefoot exhibits an adductus deformity often combined with supination (Fig. 21.86A–C). In the newborn period the deformity may be pas-sively correctable to some extent. With time, however, defor-

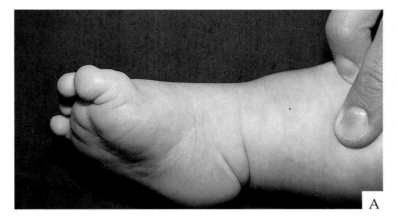

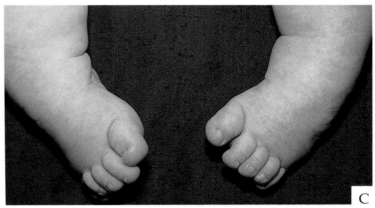

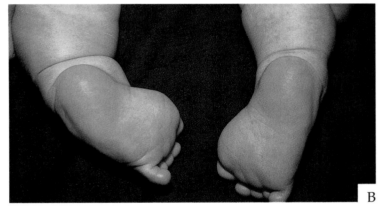

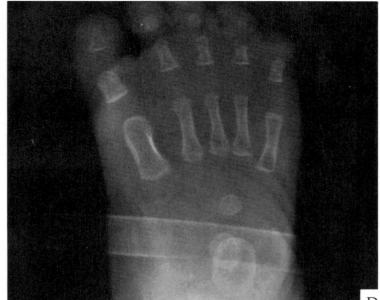

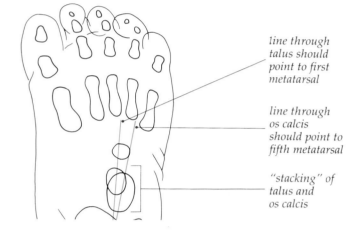

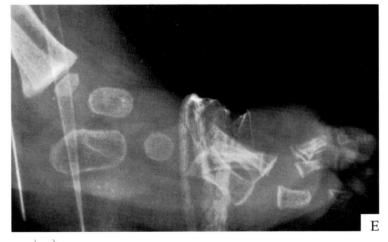

Fig. 21.86 Clubfoot. This deformity has three primary components. **A,** the foot is positioned in plantar flexion (equinus). Note the pathologic skin creases over the heel and arch. **B,** the heels or hindfeet are fixed in inversion (varus). **C,** the forefeet are fixed in an adducted and supinated position. **D,** in the AP radiographic view, the talus overlies the os calcis (stacking) and the forefoot is adducted. A line drawn through the longitudinal axis of the talus normally is in alignment with the first metatarsal, and one drawn through the axis of the os calcis normally aligns with the fifth metatarsal. **E,** the lateral radiograph shows the foot is in equinus and the axes of the talus and os calcis are nearly parallel. They normally intersect at an angle of approximately 45° (see Fig. 21.87 for comparison).

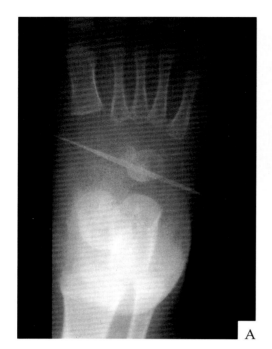

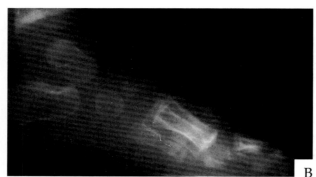

Fig. 21.87 Normal foot. **A,** *AP and* **B,** *lateral views of the foot of a slightly older child demonstrate the normal orientation of the tarsal bones in comparison with the findings in congenital clubfoot (shown in Fig. 21.86D and E).*

mities become more fixed due to contracture of soft tissue structures.

The primary pathologic finding is that of a rotational deformity of the subtalor joint with the os calcis internally rotated beneath the talus, producing the characteristic varus deformity of the heel and mechanically creating a block to dorsiflexion of the foot. The navicular is situated in a medially displaced position on the head or neck of the talus, producing the characteristic adductus deformity of the forefoot (Fig. 21.86D,E). Contractures of the Achilles and posterior tibial tendons, and the medial ankle and subtalor joint capsules appear to be secondary factors that contribute to the difficulty of obtaining anatomic reduction. Congenital absence of certain tendinous structures may be found in rare instances. A small atrophic-appearing calf is frequently noted without pathologic change in its osseous or soft tissue structures. The typical congenital clubfoot deformity must be differentiated from similar deformities present in the foot secondary to neurologic imbalance from myelodysplasia, spinal cord tethering, or degenerative neurological conditions. Occasionally, tibial hemimelia with deficiency of this bone may present a similar clinical picture. The condition should not be confused with the nonteratogenic occurrence of isolated metatarsus adductus. Its association with arthrogryposis and congenital dislocation of the hips should be kept in mind.

The roentgenographic difference between a clubfoot and a normal foot is established by comparing Figure 21.86D,E with Figure 21.87.

Early treatment consists of attempts at manipulation and serial casting or cast wedging with progressive correction. When the child presents late, and/or closed treatment is unsuccessful, open reduction and surgical release of the contracted soft tissues is indicated. Generally, these measures should be undertaken before the age at which walking is expected in order to prevent the deformity from impeding the child's motor and social development.

METATARSUS ADDUCTUS

Metatarsus adductus (metatarsus varus) is a deformity of the forefoot in which the metatarsals are deviated medially. The condition is probably the result of intrauterine molding and is usually bilateral. Other than the deviation, there are no pathologic changes in the structures of the foot. There is a wide spectrum of severity and resultant intoeing, but otherwise, patients are asymptomatic. Clinically, it should be distinguished from the more severe and complex deformity of congenital clubfoot, as it carries a more benign prognosis.

Examination is best performed with the foot braced against a flat surface or with the patient standing. With the hindfoot and midfoot positioned straight, the forefoot assumes a medially deviated or varus position (Fig. 21.88A,B). A skin crease may be located over the medial aspect of the longitudinal arch. When mild, the deviation may be passively correctable by the physician or actively correctable by the patient. Active correction may be demonstrated by gentle stroking of the foot, stimulating the peroneal muscles to contract. In more severe cases, the deviation may be only partially correctable by these maneuvers. Some patients have an associated internal tibial torsion deformity, but the calf muscle is normal in size. Radiographs demonstrate the abnormal deviation of the metatarsals medially without other osseous abnormalities (Fig. 21.88C).

Treatment depends on the severity of the condition. In very mild cases, passive manipulation of the deformity by the mother several times a day may suffice. In moderate cases, a combination of manipulative stretching and reverse or straight-last shoes may be indicated. More severe cases, which are not passively correctable and which exhibit a prominent deformity and skin crease, necessitate serial manipulation and casting over a period of 6 to 8 weeks. If the deformity persists despite these measures, surgical intervention may be required. Treatment should be undertaken prior to anticipated ambula-

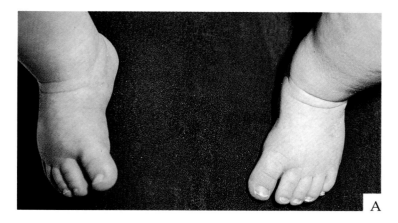

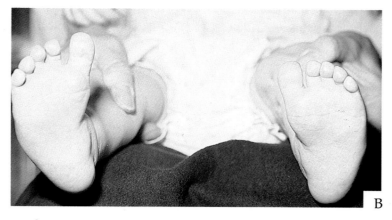

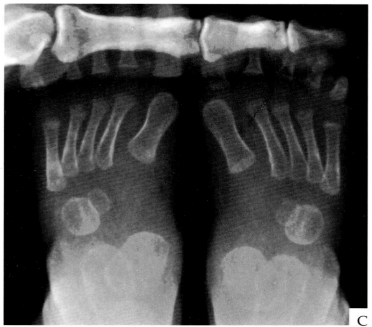

Fig. 21.88 Bilateral metatarsus adductus. *A,* in this view from above, the forefeet are seen to be deviated medially, but otherwise, the feet are normal. *B,* when viewed from the plantar aspect, rounding of the lateral border of the feet can be appreciated. *C,* in the AP radiograph note that all five metatarsals are deviated medially with respect to the remainder of the foot; otherwise, the bony structures are normal. In contrast to clubfoot deformity, the relationship of the talus and os calcis is normal.

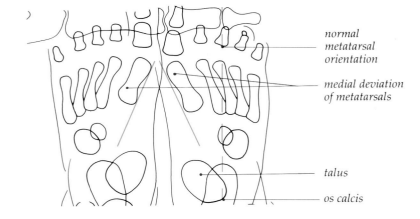

normal
metatarsal
orientation

medial deviation
of metatarsals

talus

os calcis

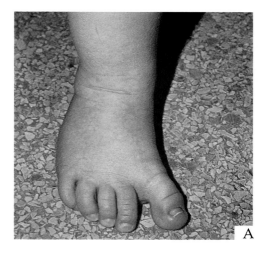

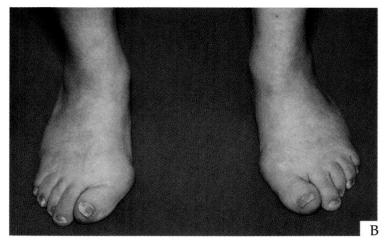

Fig. 21.89
*Metatarsus primus
varus. A,* the first
metatarsal and great
toe are deviated medi-
ally; the forefoot is
broad. The other
metatarsals are nor-
mal. *B,* bilateral
metatarsus primus
varus with hallux
valgus. The forefeet
are broad and the
great toes deviate
laterally. (*A,* courtesy
of Dr. Michael
Sherlock)

tion so as to avoid impairment of the patient's motor and social development.

Metatarsus Primus Varus (Adductus)

Metatarsus primus varus is a congenital and often hereditary foot deformity characterized by a broad forefoot with medial deviation of the first metatarsal. It is significantly more frequent in females than males.

Examination reveals a wide forefoot with medial deviation of the first metatarsal and normal orientation of the second through fifth metatarsals. There is often an associated varus deviation of the great toe (Fig. 21.89A). Over time, a secondary hallux valgus deformity and bunion may develop from the abnormal forces exerted on the great toe with weight-bearing and ambulation (Fig. 21.89B). The heel may seem narrow, but this is more apparent than real. Pronation of the forefoot may be present as well. Radiographs confirm the diagnosis by

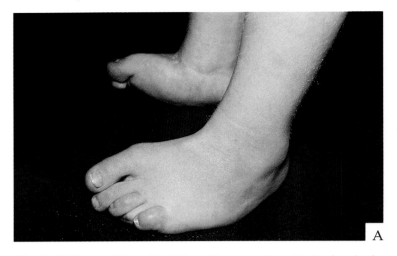

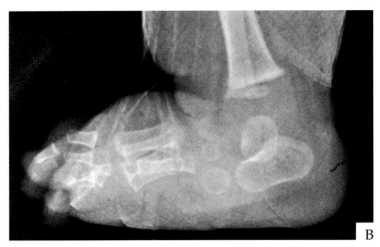

Fig. 21.90 Congenital vertical talus. The normal longitudinal arch of the foot is absent and a "rocker-bottom" type deformity is present. **A,**

the forefoot is fixed in dorsiflexion. **B,** note the vertical orientation of the talus in the radiograph (see Fig. 21.87 for comparison).

revealing an increased space between the first and second metatarsals and a large first intermetatarsal angle. The first ray through the tarsometatarsal joint may be medially oriented forming the basis for the deformity.

In mild cases, no treatment may be necessary. In moderate or severe cases, foot strain symptoms, bunion pain, and shoe-fitting problems may necessitate treatment. Surgical osteotomy of the medial cuneiform or first metatarsal in conjunction with bunion correction may satisfactorily correct the deformity.

Congenital Vertical Talus

Congenital vertical talus is a teratogenic anomaly of the foot noted at birth and characterized by a severe flatfoot deformity. The underlying pathology is a malorientation of the talus which assumes a more vertical position than normal. The adjacent navicular is dorsally displaced, articulating with the superior aspect of the neck of the talus and causing the forefoot to assume a dorsiflexed and valgus orientation. In effect, these deformities are the opposite of those seen in congenital clubfoot. The etiology of this condition is unknown, although it may be associated with other musculoskeletal or organ system anomalies. Pathologic analysis reveals normal development of the bones, but an abnormal relationship. As in clubfoot, associated soft tissue contractures may occur, particularly of the Achilles tendon, toe extensors, and anterior tibial tendon.

Clinically, the deformity is recognizable as a calcaneovalgus foot with loss of the arch, or on some occasions, a rocker-bottom type foot with a prominent heel (Fig. 21.90A). The head of the talus is often palpable on the medial plantar aspect of the midfoot. The deformity is usually fixed, but passive correction may be obtainable in some instances, particularly when the talus is oriented in a less severe oblique position. Radiographs mirror the clinical appearance with a vertical orientation of the talus, calcaneus deformity of the os calcis, and valgus orientation of the forefoot (Fig. 21.90B).

Initially, attempts at manipulation and serial casting are indicated. However, if this is unsuccessful, as is often the case, surgery may be necessary.

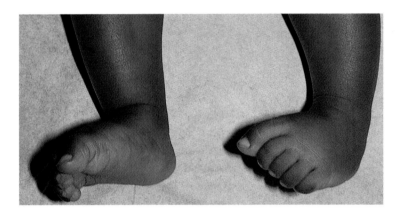

Fig. 21.91 Calcaneovalgus foot deformity. The right foot is held in a position of eversion and dorsiflexion. This deformity is supple, and thus is passively correctable. The contralateral foot exhibits a metatarsus adductus deformity, giving the feet a "windswept" appearance.

Calcaneovalgus Foot Deformity

Physiologic calcaneovalgus is another deformity of the foot thought to result from intrauterine molding. It is normally a supple deformity that is passively correctable in contrast to the rigid foot of congenital vertical talus. The condition is evident at birth and at times is associated with a contralateral metatarsus adductus deformity. There are no underlying pathologic changes in the foot and no osseous deformities other than the positional one. On examination, the foot is noted to be held in a dorsiflexed and everted position with some loss of the normal longitudinal arch (Fig. 21.91). Appreciable tightness of the anterior tibial tendon and laxity of the Achilles tendon may be noted in association with the positional deformity. Radiographs reveal no pathologic bony changes. Nonoperative treatment is usually successful and consists of serial casting to correct the deformity. Later, wearing shoes with inner heel wedges and longitudinal arch supports may help prevent recurrence and improve ambulation.

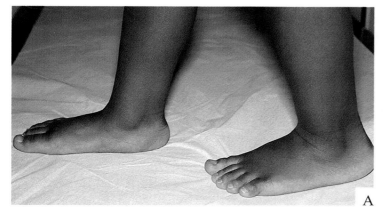

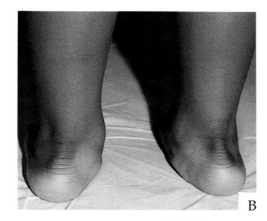

Fig. 21.92 Pes planus. **A,** laxity of the soft tissue structures of the foot results in a loss of the normal longitudinal arch and pronation or eversion of the forefoot. **B,** viewed from behind, the characteristic eversion of the heels is appreciated more readily.

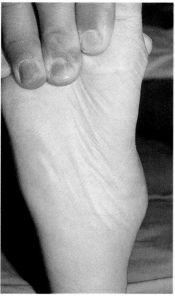

Fig. 21.93 Accessory tarsal navicular. A bony prominence produced by formation of a separate ossification center of the tarsal navicular is present over the medial aspect of the midfoot. It is covered by a painful bursa produced by chronic rubbing against the medial side of the patient's shoes Patients with this problem usually have a pes planus deformity as well..

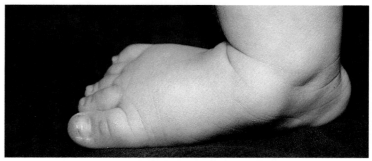

Fig. 21.94 Ganglion of the foot. A prominent soft tissue mass is present over the medial aspect of the midfoot. This represents a ganglion of the posterior tibial tendon sheath.

Pes Planus (Flatfeet)

Pes planus, or physiologic flatfeet, is an extremely common condition for which there is a familial predisposition. It is characterized by laxity of the soft tissues of the foot resulting in loss of the normal longitudinal arch, with pronation or eversion of the forefoot and valgus or lateral orientation of the heel (Fig. 21.92). There may be secondary tightness of the Achilles tendon. The condition is generally asymptomatic in children and evaluation is sought primarily because of parental concern with the appearance of the foot and the possibility of future problems. Occasionally, affected patients report discomfort after long walks or running.

On examination, the characteristic appearance is easy to recognize and laxity of other joints, particularly the thumb, elbow, and knee may be noted. Weight-bearing radiographs reveal loss of the normal longitudinal arch without osseous abnormality. Treatment is unnecessary when the condition is asymptomatic. Corrective shoes with arch supports are of no use unless symptoms of foot strain are present.

Accessory Tarsal Navicular

An accessory tarsal navicular results from formation of a separate ossification center on the medial aspect of the developing tarsal navicular at the insertion site of the posterior tibial tendon. The condition is not uncommon and is usually associated with a pes planus deformity. Clinically, patients exhibit a bony prominence on the medial aspect of the foot that tends to rub on the shoe, thus producing a painful bursa (Fig. 21.93). Radiographs reveal either a separate ossification center or bone medial to the parent navicular, or a medial projection of the navicular when fusion has occurred. Cast immobilization may be helpful in acutely painful cases. Long-term improvement can be obtained by wearing soft supportive shoes with longitudinal arches and a medial heel wedge. Recalcitrant symptoms warrant surgical intervention.

Ganglion of the Foot

A ganglion, or synovial cyst, may occur on the foot. These benign masses are similar to those commonly seen on the wrist. They originate from outpouchings of a joint capsule or tendon sheath. Trauma may be a predisposing factor in their growth. They are most commonly seen on the dorsal or medial aspect of the foot. The mass is soft, nontender, and transilluminates. It does not produce symptoms other than difficulty in fitting shoes (Fig. 21.94). If this occurs, surgical excision may be indicated.

Cavus Foot Deformity and Claw Toes

Cavus feet and claw toes are deformities produced by muscular imbalance within the foot. Although they may occur for unknown reasons, often they are manifestations of an underlying neurological disorder such as Charcot-Marie-Tooth dis-

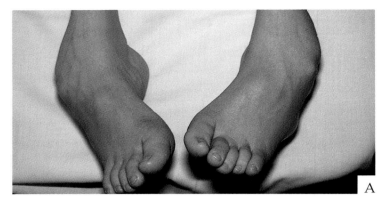

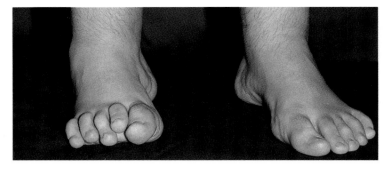

Fig. 21.96 Unilateral claw toes. This child with a tethered spinal cord has unilateral claw toe deformities. The MP joints are held in extension while the PIP joints are fixed in flexion.

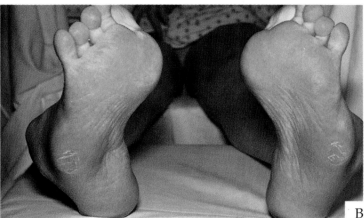

Fig. 21.95 Bilateral cavus feet. **A,** the feet are inverted and have high arches. The deformity is often a feature of neuromuscular disorders; this case is the result of Charcot-Marie-Tooth disease. **B,** in addition to the high arches and varus (inverted) heels seen in the view of the plantar surface, the prominence of the metatarsal head region is apparent. Callosities have developed over the lateral borders of the feet as a result of abnormal weight-bearing in this region.

GENERALIZED MUSCULOSKELETAL DISORDERS

A number of systemic disorders have significant musculoskeletal manifestations. Those relating to genetic, endocrine, collagen-vascular, neurologic and hematologic problems are discussed in their respective chapters. Three conditions with major musculoskeletal manifestations—cerebral palsy, osteogenesis imperfecta, and arthrogryposis—are discussed in this section.

Cerebral Palsy

The term cerebral palsy refers to a group of fixed, nonprogressive neurological syndromes resulting from static lesions of the developing central nervous system. Depending on the timing of injury, signs may be present at birth, or may become evident in infancy or early childhood. The primary cerebral insult may be intrauterine or perinatal infection; a pre- or perinatal vascular accident; anoxia due to placental insufficiency, difficult delivery, or neonatal pulmonary disease; hyperbilirubinemia resulting in kernicterus; or neonatal hypoglycemia. Following the newborn period, central nervous system infections, trauma, and vascular accidents may, when severe, produce the disorder. Abnormal motor function is the most obvious result, and may take the form of a spastic neuromuscular disorder (65 percent), athetosis (25 percent), or rigidity and/or ataxic neuromuscular dysfunction (10 percent). Sensory deficits and intellectual impairment are common, and there is a significant incidence of associated seizure disorders.

Because of the number and variety of possible insulting factors, each of which has its own spectrum of severity, there is a broad range in location and extent of neural damage, and thus in degree of functional impairment. Patients with severe afflictions generally have early evidence of gross neuromuscular dysfunction. Those with milder involvement may have subtler abnormalities and may be diagnosed only after failure to achieve normal developmental and motor milestones. Patterns of involvement include affliction of one or two limbs (monoplegia or hemiplegia), of both lower extremities (diplegia), of all four extremities (quadriplegia) (Fig. 21.97), or of all limbs with poor trunk and head control (pentaplegia). Those patients with a spastic disorder exhibit flexion contractures of the involved limbs, hyperreflexia, and spasticity, while those with athetosis exhibit the characteristic movement disorder. Mixed involvement is apparent in some individuals. Neurological examination often reveals persistence of primitive

ease, Friedreich's ataxia, or spinal cord tethering. These conditions should be considered in each patient presenting with these deformities, particularly when the problem is unilateral. Cavus feet exhibit a high arch with a varus or inversion deformity of the heel (Fig. 21.95). Usually the metatarsal heads appear prominent on the plantar aspect of the foot. This phenomenon is accentuated by overlying callosities that develop as a result of abnormal weight-bearing. With claw toes, the metatarsophalangeal joints are held in extension with the proximal interphalangeal joints in flexion, and the distal joint in the neutral or slightly flexed position (Fig. 21.96). Callouses tend to develop over the proximal interphalangeal joints from rubbing against shoes. Neurologic examination may reveal motor weakness, most often involving the anterior tibial, toe extensor, and peroneal muscles.

Logical treatment necessitates identifying and treating the underlying pathologic condition when possible. Nonoperative measures for control of the deformities and amelioration of symptoms consist of customized shoes and use of a metatarsal bar to relieve pressure on the metatarsal heads and to correct the extension deformities at the base of the toes. However, surgical correction is often necessary.

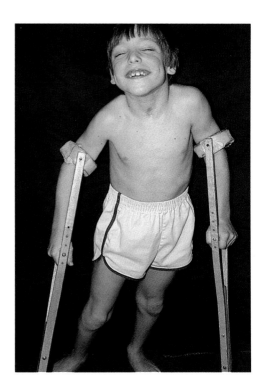

Fig. 21.97 Cerebral palsy. Typical patient with spastic quadriplegia. Note the secondary muscle atrophy especially evident in the lower extremities. He requires crutches to ambulate, seizure medication, and a specialized educational program. His neuromuscular abnormalities are the result of a one-time central nervous system insult and are not progressive.

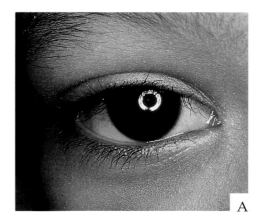

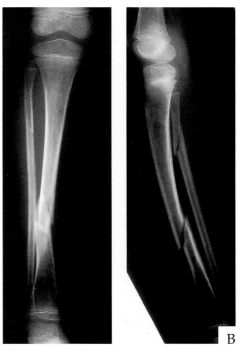

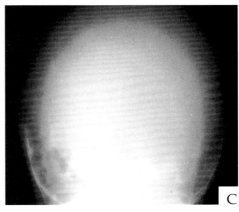

Fig. 21.98 Osteogenesis imperfecta Type I. **A,** blue sclera. **B,** cortical thinning is evident, especially distal to the spiral fracture of the tibia in this child with OI Type I. **C,** wormian bones. Multiple wormy irregular lucencies are seen over the occipitoparietal area. This finding is characteristic of all children with OI Types I, II, and II, and is seen in over 50 percent of patients with OI Type IV.

reflexes. Patients with severe involvement that inhibits sitting and ambulation develop disuse atrophy of involved muscles, and skeletal demineralization that increases their risk of fractures (see Chapter 6).

In evaluating such patients, one must be careful to rule out a progressive neurological disorder, such as intracranial or spinal cord neoplasms, degenerative neurological conditions, or tethering of the spinal cord.

Optimal treatment necessitates a team approach. In addition to general pediatric, neurologic, and orthopedic care, these patients often need the services of a urologist, physical and speech therapists, and individualized educational programs. Family counseling is a necessity. From an orthopedic standpoint, emphasis is placed on optimizing neuromuscular function by attempting to facilitate the achievement of progressive motor milestones, including the ability to sit, stand, walk, and perform activities of daily living. Exercises, bracing and surgical procedures all have a role, and institution of specific measures must be timed to fit the pace of growth and development of the individual child. Encouragement and cautious optimism are important. Surgical treatment usually takes the form of soft tissue release for flexion deformities, tendon transfer to optimize functional use of the extremities, osteotomy to correct deformities, and occasionally selective neurectomy to inhibit overactive muscle units.

Osteogenesis Imperfecta

Osteogenesis imperfecta (OI) is a family of inherited disorders in which Type I collagen formation is immature and characterized by abnormal cross-linking. While these disorders affect all connective tissue in the body, their primary clinical manifestations involve the skeleton because of the structural demands placed on the bones. Microscopically, osteoblasts are reduced in number, osteoid is disorganized and nonossified, and bony trabeculae are sparse. The end result is osteoporosis with increased susceptibility to fractures.

Formerly divided into two types (congenita and tarda), recent research using fibroblast culture techniques has now defined four major types and a number of subtypes. Overall, incidence is thought to be between 1 in 15,000 and 1 in 60,000 births.

OSTEOGENESIS IMPERFECTA TYPE I

This form accounts for 60 to 80 percent of cases and is transmitted as an autosomal dominant. In subtype A teeth are normal, and in subtype B dentinogenesis imperfecta is present (see Chapter 20, Oral Disorders). All affected patients have blue sclerae (Fig. 21.98A), although the degree of blueness

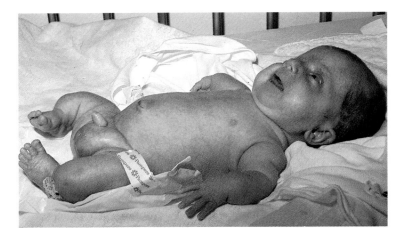

Fig. 21.99 Osteogenesis imperfecta Type II. This infant was born with multiple fractures and limb deformities. The thighs are fixed in abduction and external rotation. His sclerae are a dark blue-gray. His small thorax resulted in death due to respiratory insufficiency in the first month of life.

varies. Mild to moderate bony fragility is seen in 90 percent of affected individuals and is not present in the remaining 10 percent. Radiographs reveal mild to moderate generalized osteoporosis with cortical thinning (Fig. 21.98B). All affected children have significant wormian bones on skull radiographs (Fig. 21.98C). While the first fracture usually occurs during the preschool period, 8 to 10 percent of patients with Type IA and 25 percent of those with Type IB have one to a few fractures at birth. Fractures heal normally with normal callus formation and their frequency decreases after puberty.

Children with Type I OI tend to have generalized ligamentous laxity and joint hypermobility. Anterior and lateral bowing of the femurs and tibias is common as are valgus knees and pes planus. Ultimate stature is normal or mildly short. Three quarters of these children have easy bruisability, and approximately 35 to 55 percent develop conductive hearing loss in early adulthood.

OSTEOGENESIS IMPERFECTA TYPE II

This extremely severe form is lethal in the pre- or perinatal period. It is usually due to a new autosomal-dominant mutation, but rarely may be autosomal-recessive and accounts for less than 10 percent of all cases of OI. Intrauterine growth is severely retarded, and affected infants are born with multiple fractures and severe deformities due to extreme osteoporosis (Fig. 21.99). The extremities are short, bowed, and bent and the thighs are fixed in abduction and external rotation. The calvarium is large and soft with palpable bony islands, and poor mineralization and wormian bones are evident radiographically (see Fig. 21.98C). The face is triangular with a beaked nose and the sclerae are blue-black. The chest is so small that those who are liveborn die of respiratory insufficiency in the first few weeks. Three subtypes based on radiographic appearance of the ribs and long bones have been identified.

OSTEOGENESIS IMPERFECTA TYPE III

OI Type III, the severe progressive form accounting for approximately 15 percent of cases of OI, also is usually the result of a new autosomal-dominant mutation, although on rare occasion it is transmitted as an autosomal-recessive. Osteoporosis is severe, resulting in moderately severe to severe fragility. Most affected individuals are born with multiple fractures and deformities. Those who were not have multiple fractures by 1 to 2 years of age. The osteopenia and fractures produce progressive shortening, bowing, and angulation of the long bones (Fig. 21.100A,B) and severe progressive kyphoscoliosis, which results in marked dwarfism and ultimately causes cardiopulmonary compromise. The calvarium is large, thin, and radiographically is poorly ossified with multiple wormian bones (see Fig. 21.98C). Frontal and temporal bossing are common, and the facies are triangular (Fig. 21.100C). The sclerae can be normal or light blue or gray, changing to white by puberty. Approximately half of these patients have associated ligamentous laxity and half have dentinogenesis imperfecta. Easy bruising is seen in about 25 percent of cases.

OSTEOGENESIS IMPERFECTA TYPE IV

This mild form is rare, accounting for less than 5 percent of all cases of OI, with an estimated incidence of 1 in 1 to 3 million live births. It is inherited as an autosomal-dominant. There are two subtypes: IVA with normal teeth and IVB with dentinogenesis imperfecta. Bony fragility varies from mild to moderately severe, and osteoporosis is gradually progressive, although it may be minimal or absent at the time of the first fracture. About one-third have one to a few fractures at birth and the majority experience their first fracture by age 5. Over 50 percent have wormian bones on skull radiography (see Fig. 21.98C). Bowing of the lower extremities is common with or without fractures, and most affected individuals have short stature. The sclerae may be normal in color or light blue at birth, gradually changing to white later in childhood. Easy bruisability is unusual in this group.

TREATMENT

Patients with osteogenesis Types I and IV may require only routine orthopedic care for their fractures and counseling regarding accident prevention and safety. Palliative supportive care and minimum handling are the only measures available for infants with OI Type II. Treatment of infants and children with OI Type III is geared towards minimizing the frequency of fractures and preventing deformities. In infancy this may mean limited handling of the child, and use of a padded carrying device. Later, bracing and surgical treatment in the form of osteotomy and internal stabilization of long bones with intermedullary rod fixation may be necessary. Maintenance of activity and the avoidance of repeated prolonged periods of immobilization aid in the prevention of disuse atrophy.

Arthrogryposis

Arthrogryposis is a nonprogressive muscular disorder of unknown etiology, which appears to be related either to failure of development in or degeneration of muscular structures. Neural factors have been implicated in its origin, because in some instances the spinal cord has been found to be reduced in size, with a decreased number of anterior horn cells. Generally all limbs are involved. On occasion the disease may be confined to one or a few limbs only. Primary manifestations consist of joint contractures with secondary deformities and limited motion. Deformities include clubfeet, dislocated hips, and contractures of the knees, elbows, wrists and hands (Fig.

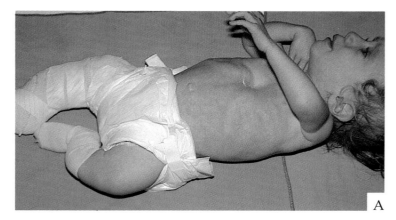

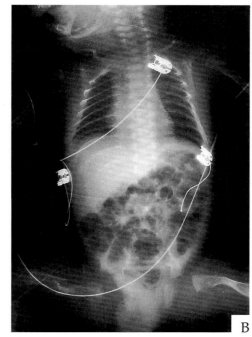

Fig. 21.100 Osteogenesis imperfecta Type III. **A,** note the extremely small stature of this 5-year-old child and the deformities of the rib cage. A recent fracture has been splinted. **B,** radiograph of an affected infant shows dwarfed, deformed femurs with a new fracture in the mid shaft of the right femur. Note also the thin, peculiarly shaped ribs.
C, in this close-up, the characteristic craniofacial features are seen, consisting of a triangular facies, a broad nose, and frontal and temporal bossing. The sclerae may be normal in color, as in this child, or light blue or gray.

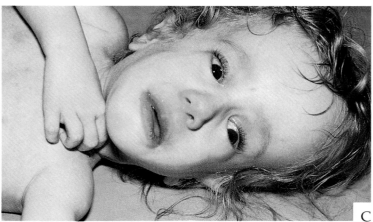

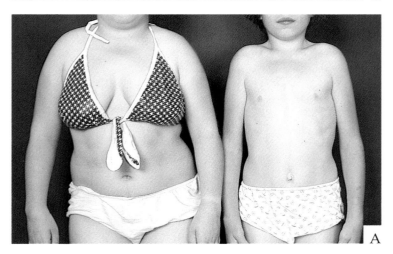

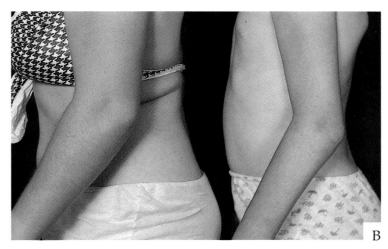

*Fig. 21.101 Arthrogryposis. **A,** two sisters with the generalized form of the disorder are shown. Note the stiff posture and tubular appearance of the limbs. Motion of all joints is limited either due to failure in development or degeneration of muscular structures. Their stature is short. **B,** the lateral view highlights flexion contractures of the elbows.*

21.101). Motion of involved joints is severely limited, but patients generally are able to compensate for this functional limitation. Radiographs show relatively normal appearing bones and joints, but fat density is noted in the areas where muscles are normally seen. On pathologic analysis, there is a striking absence of muscle tissue with strands of fat permeating the area.

Orthopedic treatment is aimed at providing optimal motor function. Range of motion exercises may maintain what motion is present, but rarely result in an increase. Surgery rarely results in improved range of motion, but is indicated to restore functional position when clubfeet and hip dislocation are part of the condition. Gradual recurrence of deformity after surgery is not uncommon, however.

BIBLIOGRAPHY

Ablin DS, Greenspan A, Reinhart M, Grix A: Differentiation of child abuse from osteogenesis imperfecta. *Am J Radiol* 1990;154:1035–1046.

Aegerter E, Kirkpatrick JA Jr: *Orthopedic Diseases, Physiology, Pathology, Radiology,* ed 4. Philadelphia, WB Saunders, 1975.

American Society for Surgery of the Hand: *The Hand: Examination and Diagnosis.* Edinburgh, Churchill Livingstone, 1983.

American Society for Surgery of the Hand: *The Hand: Primary Care of Common Problems.* Aurora, CO, 1985.

Edmonson AS, Crenshaw AH: *Campbell's Operative Orthopedics,* ed 6. St. Louis, CV Mosby, 1980.

Ferguson AB Jr: *Orthopedic Surgery in Infancy and Childhood,* ed 5. Baltimore, Williams & Wilkins, 1981.

Hoppenfeld S: *Physical Examination of the Spine and Extremities.* New York, Appleton-Century-Crofts, 1976.

Lovell WW, Winter RB: *Pediatric Orthopedics.* Philadelphia, JB Lippincott, 1978.

Moe JH, Winter RB, Bradford DS, Lonstein JE: *Scoliosis and Other Spinal Deformities.* Philadelphia, WB Saunders, 1978.

Ogden JA: *Skeletal Injury in the Child.* Philadelphia, Lea & Febiger, 1982.

Rang M: *Children's Fractures,* ed 2. Philadelphia, JB Lippincott, 1983.

Rockwood CA Jr, Wilkins KE, King RE: *Fractures in Children,* vol. 3. Philadelphia, JB Lippincott, 1984.

Salter RB: *Textbook of Disorders and Injuries of the Musculoskeletal System,* ed 2. Baltimore, Williams & Wilkins, 1983.

Scoles PV: *Pediatric Orthopedics.* Chicago, Year Book Medical Publishers, 1982.

Simon RR, Koenigsknecht SJ: *Orthopedics in Emergency Medicine: The Extremities.* New York, Appleton, 1982.

Tachidjian MO: *Pediatric Orthopedics,* ed 2. Philadelphia, WB Saunders, 1990.

PEDIATRIC OTOLARYNGOLOGY

Timothy P. McBride, M.D. ◆ Holly W. Davis, M.D. ◆ James S. Reilly, M.D.

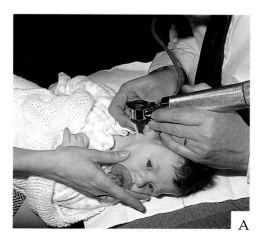
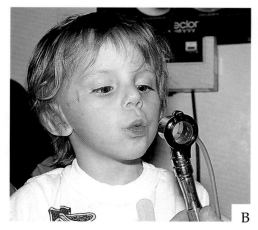
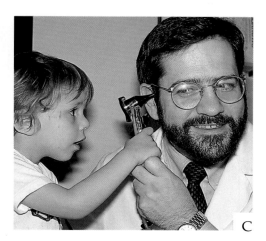

FIG. 22.1 *Techniques to facilitate examination of a child's ears, nose, and oropharynx.* **A,** *young infants often can be examined on their mother's lap, with gentle immobilization provided by the parent and* *the examiner's hand.* **B,** *and* **C,** *making a game of blowing out the otoscope light and allowing the patient to check the examiner first convey that otoscopy doesn't have to hurt.*

The importance for pediatricians and family physicians to have an understanding of and experience with otolaryngologic problems, and to be skilled in techniques of examination of the head and neck region, cannot be overemphasized. A recent study revealed that over one-third of all visits to pediatricians' offices were prompted by ear symptoms. When nasal and oral symptoms are included, ear, nose, and throat pathology accounts for over 50 percent of all visits. With patience and proper equipment, a thorough examination can be accomplished on almost all children. Then, if a disorder fails to respond to therapy, becomes chronic or recurrent, or if an unusual problem is encountered, consultation with a pediatric otolaryngologist should be sought.

Successful examination of the ears, nose, and oropharynx of a young child can present some challenges, especially with older infants and toddlers who fail to appreciate the need for (and thus often vigorously resist) examination. This can be a particular problem in children who have had previous bad experiences. Patience, warmth, and careful explanation on the part of the examiner are of great help in reducing fear and enhancing cooperation.

Whenever possible, the child should be allowed to sit on the parent's lap. Puppets, rubber gloves blown up into balloons, and tongue blades with faces drawn on them can all serve to reduce anxiety, enlist the child's trust, and distract attention. Gradual introduction of the equipment can also be most helpful, especially when done in a playful way. The child can be asked to blow out the otoscope light while the examiner turns it off, urged to catch the light spot as the examiner moves it around, and even allowed to look in the parent's or examiner's ears (Fig. 22.1A–C). Parents can also help demonstrate maneuvers for opening the mouth, panting to depress the tongue, and holding the head back. While this may take a little additional time at the outset, it often saves considerable time in the long run, and makes future followup exams far easier.

EAR DISORDERS

Ear pain (otalgia), discharge from the ear (otorrhea), and suspected hearing loss are three of the more common and specific otic symptons for which parents seek medical attention for their children. Less specific symptoms such as pulling or tugging at the ears, fussiness, and fever are also frequently encountered, particularly in children less than 2 years of age.

History should center on the nature and duration of symptoms, character of the clinical course, and possible antecedent treatment. Since many infections of the ear are recurrent and/or chronic, the parent should be asked about previous

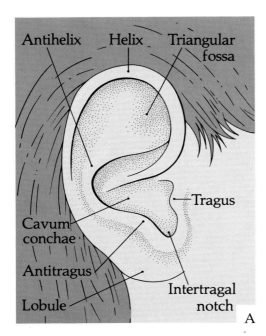

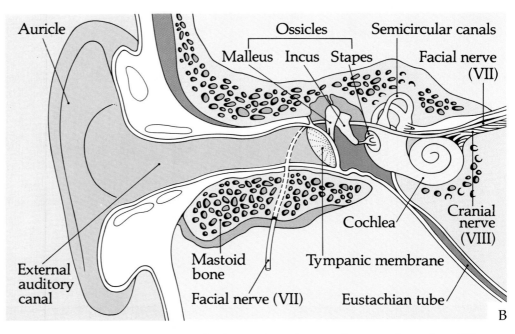

FIG. 22.2 Anatomy of the ear. **A,** a normal external ear (auricle or pinna) is shown, with its various landmarks labeled. It is helpful to refer to such a diagram in assessing congenital anomalies. **B,** this coronal section shows the various structures of the hearing and vestibular apparatus. The three main regions are the external ear, the middle ear, and the inner ear. The eustachian tube connects the middle ear and the pharynx, and serves to vent the middle ear.

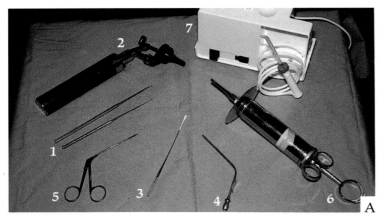

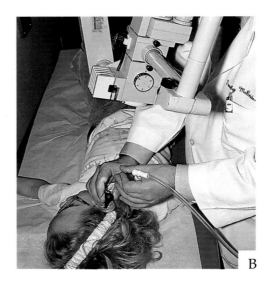

FIG. 22.3 **A,** equipment for cleaning the external auditory canal. The curette **(1)** is the implement most commonly used to remove cerumen. Use of a surgical otoscope head **(2)** makes the process considerably easier. Additional implements include cotton wicks **(3)** and a suction tip **(4)** for removal of discharge or moist wax; alligator forceps **(5)** for foreign bodies; an ear syringe **(6)** and motorized irrigation apparatus **(7)**, for removing firm objects or impacted cerumen. Lavage is contraindicated when there is a possible perforation of the tympanic membrane. If the motorized apparatus is used for irrigation, it must be kept on the lowest power setting to avoid traumatizing the eardrum. **B,** use of suction often is necessary when there is copious exudate.

medical or surgical therapy (e.g., antibiotics, myringotomy, and tubes).

A brief review of the anatomy of the ear is helpful in developing a logical approach to any encountered clinical abnormalities. The ear is conveniently divided into three regions (Fig. 22.2):

1. The *external ear* includes the pinna or auricle and the external auditory canal, up to and including the tympanic membrane.
2. The *middle ear* is made up of the middle-ear space, the inner surface of the eardrum, the ossicles, and the mastoid.
3. The *inner ear* comprises the cochlea (hearing), the semicircular canals (balance), and the main nerve trunks of the seventh and eighth cranial nerves.

The examination should include inspection of the auricle, periauricular tissues, and external auditory canal, as well as visualization of the entire tympanic membrane, including assessment of its mobility in response to positive and negative pressure. This often necessitates clearing the canal of cerumen or discharge by using a curette, cotton wick, lavage, or suction (Fig. 22.3A,B). These procedures should be performed carefully

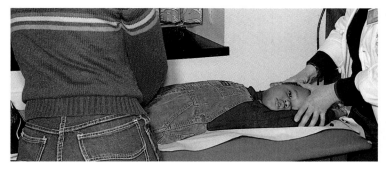

FIG. 22.4 Method of immobilization for cleaning. An assistant holds the arms and simultaneously immobilizes the child's head with the thumbs. The parent firmly holds the hips and thighs. This prevents motion by the child during cleaning of the ear canal and is also useful for otoscopy in young children.

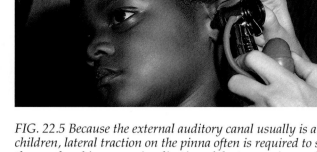

FIG. 22.5 Because the external auditory canal usually is angulated in children, lateral traction on the pinna often is required to straighten the canal and improve visualization of the tympanic membrane.

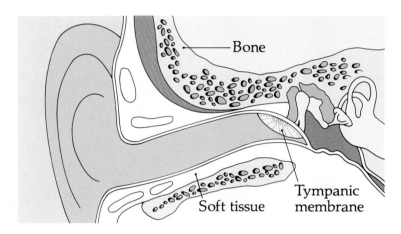

Bone

Soft tissue

Tympanic membrane

FIG. 22.6 Angulation of the tympanic membrane in infancy. The relationship between the ear canal and eardrum is different in the infant, with the drum being tilted at an angle of 130°. Greater care is required in examining an infant's eardrum because of this angulation and because the landmarks are less prominent.

and gently, and attempted only after the child has been carefully immobilized to avoid trauma (Fig. 22.4). It is extraordinarily easy to injure the canal during the process of cleaning the external ear. Hence, great care must be taken, otherwise bleeding from the ensuing trauma will obscure the examination and upset the patient and parent. Both the patient and parent should be given a clear explanation of the procedure beforehand.

Since the external auditory canal is often slightly angulated in infants and young children, gentle lateral traction on the pinna is frequently necessary to facilitate visualization of the eardrum itself (Fig. 22.5). In infancy, the tympanic membrane also tends to be oriented at an angle (Fig. 22.6), the landmarks are less prominent, and the canal mucosa, being loosely attached, moves readily on insufflation of air, simulating a normally mobile eardrum. To avoid confusion, it is important to inspect the canal as the speculum is inserted to ensure that the transition between canal wall and tympanic membrane is visualized.

The pneumatic otoscope is the most valuable diagnostic tool when signs or symptoms of otitis media are present. Pediatricians, family practitioners, and otolaryngologists who treat children should be skilled in its use. Practical advice on the use of this instrument is summarized by Schwartz as follows:

1. Use adequate light. A bright halogen lamp is better than an ordinary light bulb. Be sure to replace bulbs routinely every 4 to 6 months, and to provide for routine battery charging.
2. Choose a speculum the size of which allows adequate penetration (10 to 15 mm) into the external canal for good eardrum visualization.
3. Restrain the patient, either on the parent's lap or on the examining table.

When otoscopic findings are unclear or it is difficult to obtain a good air seal for pneumatic otoscopy, tympanometry can be highly useful in evaluating patients over 6 months of age (Fig. 22.7). The procedure is not of value in young infants, because the abundance of loose connective tissue lining the ear canal and the laxity of the cartilage at the entrance increases canal wall compliance and invalidates the results.

Recognition that otitis media is a reflection of both immunologic and anatomic abnormalities should lead the practitioner to be suspicious of possible underlying immune or temporal bone defects when seeing patients with chronic or frequently recurrent otitis media. The temporal bone is the bony housing for both the auditory and vestibular systems. In addition, it provides bony protection for the facial nerve as it crosses from the brainstem to the facial muscles. The growth and development of this bone is affected in syndromes such as Treacher-

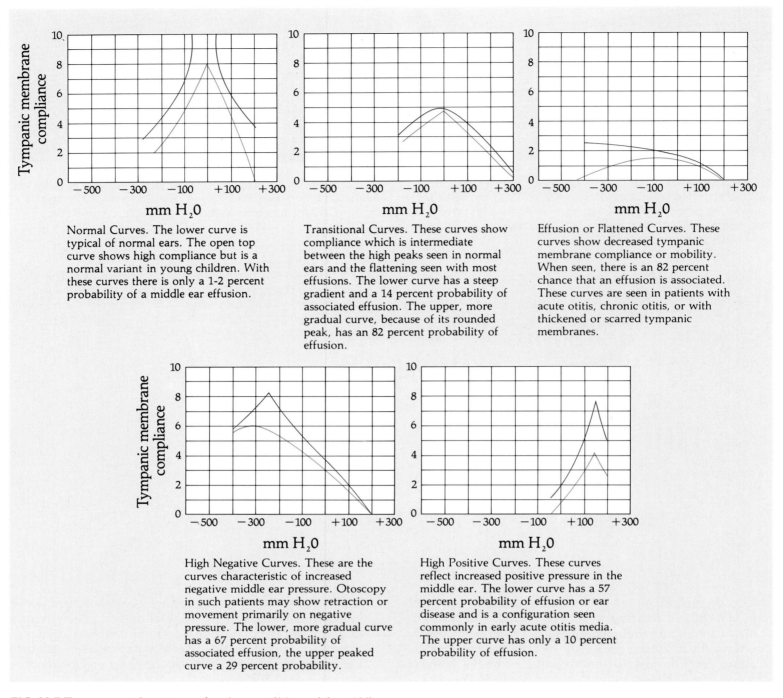

FIG. 22.7 Tympanometric patterns of various conditions of the middle ear.
(Courtesy of Mrs. Ruth Bachman, PNP, Children's Hospital of Pittsburgh)

Collins syndrome and others that involve altered mid-face growth (Fig. 22.8). The soft tissues attached to the temporal bone such as the muscles controlling eustachian tube function can be abnormal in children with cleft palates (see section on Palatal Disorders). As a result, children with these disorders tend to have an increased incidence of otitis media, and also may be vulnerable to recurrent sinus infections.

Children with chronic effusions who complain of hearing loss or whose parents complain that they do not listen, or those with suspected congenital malformations must have their hearing evaluated—either by audiometry or brainstem-evoked potentials. Patients with vertigo and/or problems of balance, and those with facial weakness or asymmetry, warrant testing of hearing *and* vestibular function. These children,

and those suffering from malformations, may require radiographic imaging in selected cases to clarify the nature of the problem.

Disorders of the External Ear

THE FOUR "D"S

Examination of every child's ear begins with inspection of the auricle and periauricular tissues for four very important signs: *discharge, displacement, discoloration,* and *deformity* (the four "D"s). The canal is normally smooth, and slightly angulated anteriorly. Cerumen is often present; it varies in color from yellowish-white to tan to dark brown. It is secreted from glands interspersed among the hair follicles at the entrance to the ear

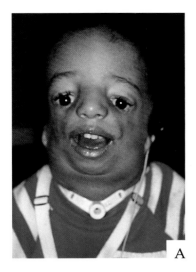 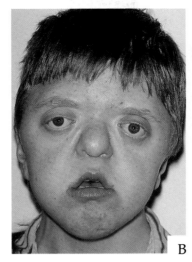 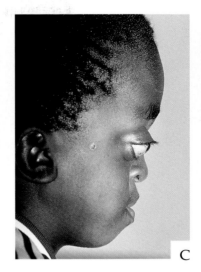 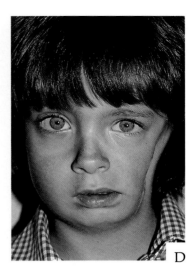

FIG. 22.8 Syndromes affecting growth of the temporal bone and mid-face that predispose patients to recurrent or chronic otitis media and chronic recurrent sinus infections. **A,** Treacher-Collins syndrome. **B,** Apert's syndrome. **C,** Crouzon's syndrome. **D,** hemifacial microsomia. (**B–D,** courtesy of Dr. Wolfgang Loskin, Children's Hospital of Pittsburgh)

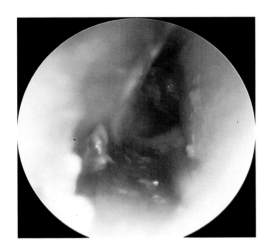

FIG. 22.9 External otitis. Acute bacterial external otitis is characterized by intense pain which is worsened by traction on the ear lobe, purulent exudate, and intense canal wall inflammation.

canal, and it may have some bacteriostatic activity. When cerumen obstructs the view, it must be removed to the extent that adequate visualization of the canal and tympanic membrane is achieved. When soft and moist, this is easily accomplished with a curette. It may be more difficult if the cerumen is dry and flaky, and at times may require instillation of drops. In some children, cerumen solidifies, forming a firm plug which impedes sound conduction and necessitates softening and irrigation for removal.

Discharge

Discharge is a common complaint with a number of possible causes. When there is thick white discharge and erythema of the canal wall, the physician should gently pull on the pinna. If this maneuver elicits pain and the canal wall is edematous, *primary otitis externa* is the likely diagnosis (Fig. 22.9), although prolonged drainage from untreated *otitis media with perforation* may present a similar picture (see section on Disorders of the Middle Ear). When the middle ear is the source of otic discharge, the tympanic membrane will be abnormal and should show evidence of perforation (see Fig. 22.27). The major predisposing condition to primary otitis externa is prolonged presence of excessive moisture in the ear canal which promotes bacterial or fungal overgrowth. Thus, this is a common problem in swimmers. Another major source is the presence of a *foreign body* in the ear canal (see Fig. 22.19) which stimulates an intense inflammatory response and production of a foul-smelling purulent discharge. Thus, when otic drainage is encountered, the discharge must be gently removed under appropriate magnification, in order to assess the condition of the tympanic membrane and rule out the presence of foreign objects. This can be accomplished either by gentle siphoning and wiping with cotton wicks or by careful suctioning (see Fig. 22.3).

If history indicates that the drainage is persistent or recurrent despite therapy, a culture should be obtained to determine both the causative organism and its sensitivity to antimicrobial agents. Treatment consists primarily of topical otic antibi-

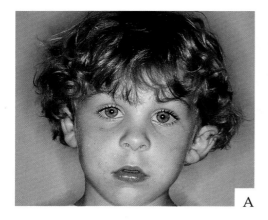
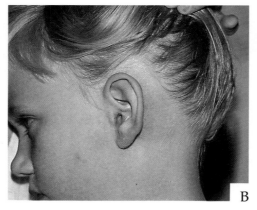
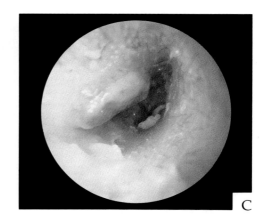

*Figure 22.10 Mastoiditis. **A,** this frontal photo clearly shows the left auricle displaced anteriorly and inferiorly. **B,** in another patient, seen from the side, one can appreciate erythema over the mastoid process.*

*C, on otoscopy, erythema and edema of the canal wall are evident, and the posterosuperior portion of the canal wall sags inferiorly. (**C,** courtesy of Dr. Michael Hawke)*

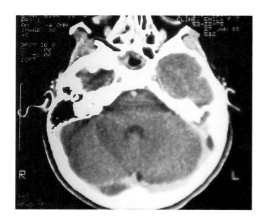

FIG. 22.11 *This CT image shows acute left-sided mastoiditis with the complication of an associated epidural abscess.*

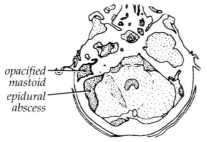

opacified mastoid
epidural abscess

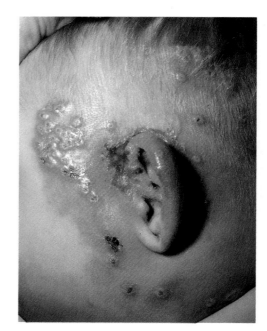

FIG. 22.12 *Periauricular and auricular cellulitis. This infant had mild postauricular seborrhea and developed varicella. This secondary infection progressed rapidly, producing intense erythema, edema, and tenderness of the auricle and periauricular tissues. In this case, the external canal was normal. (Courtesy of Dr. Ronald Chludzinski, Monroeville, PA)*

otic/steroid preparations. Systemic antibiotics should be given when pain is severe, when there is evidence of otitis media, or when, despite attempts at cleaning, there is still uncertainty about an infection of the middle ear. Parenteral antibiotics may be required when the process has extended to the point at which cellulitis occurs in the periauricular soft tissues.

Displacement

Displacement of the pinna away from the skull is a worrisome sign. The most severe condition causing displacement is *mastoiditis*, resulting from extension of a middle ear infection through the mastoid air cells and out to the periosteum of the skull. In addition to displacement, important clinical signs of mastoiditis include erythema and edema of the pinna and the skin overlying the mastoid, exquisite tenderness on palpation of the mastoid process, a sagging ear canal, purulent otorrhea, fever and, usually, toxicity (Fig. 22.10). This condition is now considered unusual, and is seen mainly in patients with long-standing, untreated, or inadequately treated otitis media. Recognition and prompt

institution of parenteral antibiotic therapy are crucial, as there is significant risk of central nervous system extension. Radiographs show haziness of the mastoid air cells; CT scanning helps delineate extent of involvement, and facilitates surgical approach (Fig. 22.11). Mastoidectomy is indicated in cases complicated by CNS extention and those in which IV antibiotics and myringotomy fail to produce complete resolution.

Other conditions characterized by displacement of the pinna away from the head include parotitis, primary cellulitis of periauricular tissues, and edema secondary to insect bites or contact dermatitis. *Parotitis* is differentiated by finding prominent induration and enlargement of the parotid gland anterior and inferior to the external ear, together with blunting of the angle of the mandible on palpation (see Chapter 12). *Primary cellulitis* is characterized by erythema and tenderness, but can often be distinguished clinically from mastoiditis by the presence of associated skin lesions which antecede the inflammation (Fig. 22.12). In cases secondary to untreated external otitis or otitis media with perforation, the picture may be clinically

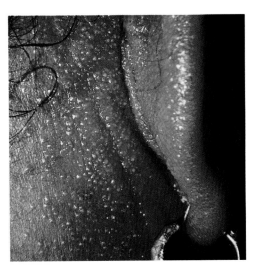

FIG. 22.13 This young girl became sensitive to the nickel posts of her earrings and developed periauricular contact dermatitis. The auricle and periauricular skin are erythematous and covered by a weeping, pruritic microvesicular eruption. (Courtesy of Dr. Michael Sherlock)

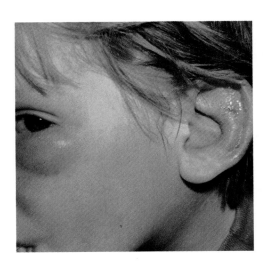

FIG. 22.14 Angioedema. This youngster presented with pruritic, nonpainful, nontender swelling of his ear and infraorbital region. Close examination of the latter revealed the punctum of an insect bite. This was obscured by the crusting on his ear which he had scratched. (Courtesy of Dr. Michael Sherlock)

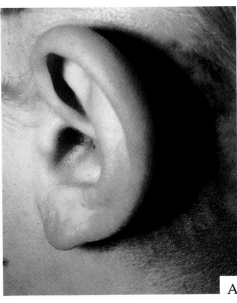

A

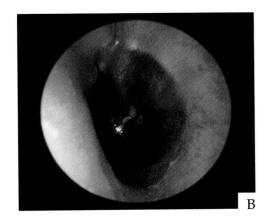

B

FIG. 22.15 Basilar skull fracture. **A,** the presence of a basilar skull fracture involving the temporal bone is often signaled by postauricular ecchymotic discoloration, termed Battle's sign. **B,** the force of the blow may also cause tearing of the ear canal or, as shown here, middle ear hemorrhage with hemotympanum. Depending on time of examination this may appear red or blue. (**B,** courtesy of Dr. Michael Hawke)

similar, but mastoid x-rays will be normal. Localized *contact dermatitis* and *angioedema* may be erythematous, but they will also be pruritic and nontender. The former condition is characterized by microvesicular skin changes (Fig. 22.13), while in the latter condition, a precipitating insect bite can often be identified on inspection (Fig. 22.14).

Discoloration

Discoloration is another important sign and is commonly a feature of conditions producing displacement. Erythema of the pinna is common when there is inflammation with or without infection (see Figs. 22.12–22.14). Ecchymotic discoloration may be encountered with trauma. When this overlies the mastoid tip, the area immediately posterior to the pinna, it is termed *Battle's sign* (Fig. 22.15A), and usually reflects a basilar skull fracture. In such cases, the canal wall should be checked for tears, and the tympanic membrane for perforation or a *hemotympanum* (Fig. 22.15B). In fact, these findings are generally more helpful in making the diagnosis than routine skull x-rays which are often negative. Of course, computed tomography can usually confirm the diagnosis of a basilar skull fracture.

Deformity

When the external ear is grossly misshapen or atretic, anomalies of middle and inner ear structures are often associated, and hearing loss may be profound (Fig. 22.16). Severe deformi-

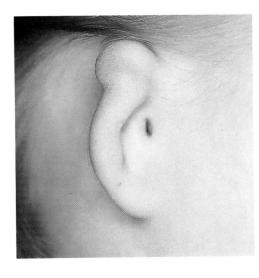

FIG. 22.16 Atresia of the right external ear. In this otherwise normal child, the pinna failed to develop properly, and the external canal was completely stenosed. Audiometric testing revealed a 60-dB hearing loss. Such isolated deformities stem from abnormal development of the first branchial arch.

ties stem from developmental anomalies of the branchial arches which contribute to both the external and middle ear structures. Such abnormalities warrant thorough evaluation in infancy in order to ensure early recognition and treatment of hearing loss. Deformity of the pinna can be the result of hereditary factors or exposure to teratogens but, at times, it is simply produced by unusual intrauterine positioning. Most deformi-

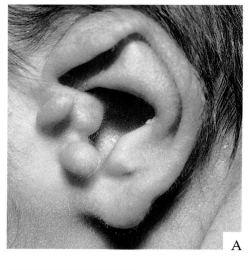

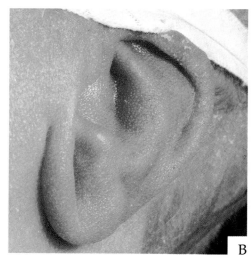

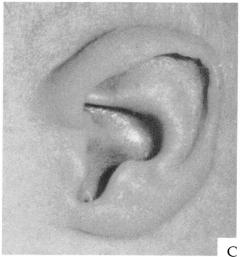

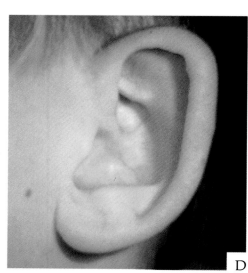

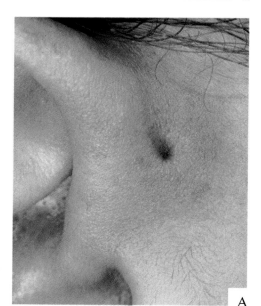

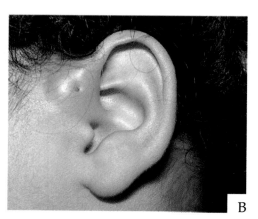

FIG. 22.17 Minor congenital auricular deformities. **A,** in this infant, the superior portion of the helix is folded over obscuring the triangular fossa, the antihelix is sharply angulated, and there are three preauricular skintags. **B,** this neonate with orofaciodigital and Turner syndromes has a simple helix and a redundant folded lobule. The ear is low set and posteriorly rotated, and the antitragus is anteriorly displaced. **C,** this infant with Rubinstein-Taybi syndrome has an exaggeratedly elongated intertragal notch. **D,** lop ear in an otherwise normal child. The auricular cartilage is abnormally contoured, making the ear protrude forward. (**C,** courtesy of Dr. Michael Sherlock)

FIG. 22.18 Preauricular sinuses. **A,** these branchial cleft remnants are located anterior to the pinna and have an overlying surface dimple. **B,** in this child, the sinus has become infected, forming an abscess. (**A,** courtesy of Dr. Michael Hawke)

ties are minor. In some instances, they may be part of a picture of multiple congenital anomalies (Fig. 22.17A–C; also see Fig. 22.8 and Chapter 1), but in most cases they represent isolated, minor malformations which are of little significance other than cosmetic (Fig. 22.17D).

Preauricular cysts constitute one of the more common congenital abnormalities. These are branchial cleft remnants located anterior to the pinna with an overlying surface dimple (Fig. 22.18A). These cysts are vulnerable to infection and abscess formation (Fig. 22.18B), which necessitates incision and drainage in conjunction with antistaphylococcal antibiotics. Once infected, recurrence will be common unless the entire cyst is completely excised. This procedure should be undertaken once inflammation has subsided.

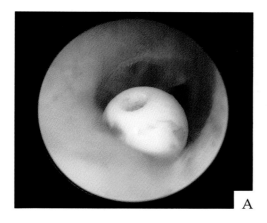

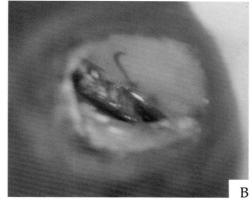

FIG. 22.19 Otic foreign bodies. **A,** this child had inserted a bead into her ear. The object must be removed carefully to prevent further trauma. **B,** this patient experienced a period of intense buzzing pain and itching in the ear which abated after a few hours. When the patient was taken to his physician, an insect was found to be the culprit. (**A,** courtesy of Dr. Michael Hawke. **B,** courtesy of Dr. Robert Gochman, Schneider Children's Hospital, Long Island Jewish Medical Center)

A   B

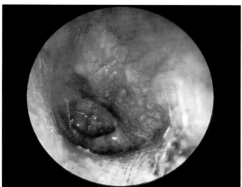

FIG. 22.20 Traumatic perforation of the tympanic membrane due to a blast injury such as one might see after close exposure to exploding fireworks.

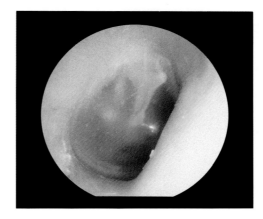

FIG. 22.21 Normal tympanic membrane. The drum is thin and translucent, and the ossicles are readily visualized. It is neutrally positioned with no evidence of either bulging or retraction. (Courtesy of Dr. Sylvan Stool, Children's Hospital of Pittsburgh)

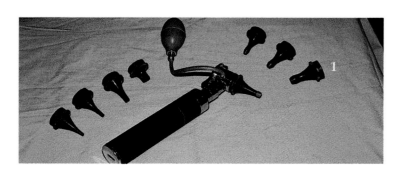

FIG. 22.22 Pneumatic otoscopy. This procedure requires proper equipment including a pneumatic otoscope head and an appropriately sized speculum to achieve a good air seal. When a seal is difficult to obtain despite proper speculum size, the head and tubing should be checked for air leaks. If none is found, application of a piece of rubber tubing to the end of the speculum (shown attached to the otoscope) or use of a soft speculum **(1)** may solve the problem.

FOREIGN OBJECTS AND SECONDARY TRAUMA

It is not unusual for children to put paper, beads, and other foreign objects into the ear canals (Fig. 22.19A). Small flying insects may also, on occasion, become trapped in the external ear (Fig. 22.19B). In some cases, small objects may be embedded in cerumen and missed on inspection. As noted earlier, if present for more than a few days, the foreign material stimulates an inflammatory response and production of a purulent discharge which is often foul-smelling and which may obscure the presence of the inciting foreign body. Removal of some objects can be accomplished by use of alligator forceps or by irrigation of the ear canal, while others—particularly spherical objects—require use of a Day hook or suction (see Fig. 22.3). Foreign objects may also be the source of painful abrasions or lacerations of the external auditory canal, or even perforation of the tympanic membrane. Insertion of pencils or sticks into the ear canal by the child, and parental attempts to clean the canal with a cotton swab are the most common modes of such injury. Exposure to concussive forces such as a direct blow or an explosion can also result in perforation (Fig. 22.20). Patients with traumatic perforations must be carefully assessed for signs of injury to deeper structures. If tympanic membrane perforation occurs either as a result of penetration by a foreign object or of concussive forces, one must be particularly aware of the possibility of middle or inner ear damage. Evidence of hearing loss, vertigo, or nystagmus should prompt urgent otolaryngologic consultation since an emergent surgical exploration may be indicated.

Disorders of the Middle Ear

The normal tympanic membrane is thin, translucent, neutrally positioned, and mobile. The ossicles, particularly the malleus, are generally visible through it (Fig. 22.21). Adequate assessment of the tympanic membrane requires that the examiner note four major characteristics: (1) thickness; (2) degree of translucence; (3) position relative to neutral; and (4) mobility. Application of gentle positive and negative pressure using the pneumatic otoscope (Fig. 22.22), produces brisk movement of the eardrum when the ear is free of disease, and abnormal movement when fluid is present, when the drum is thickened or scarred, or when there is an increase in either

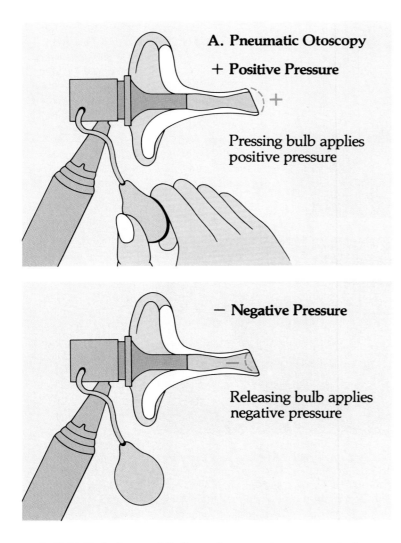

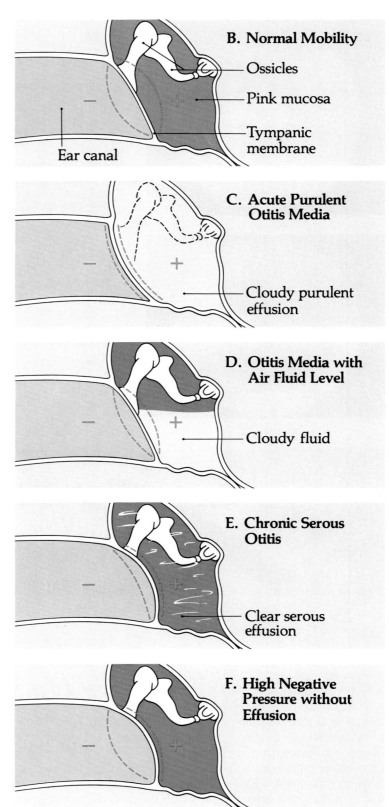

FIG. 22.23 Technique and findings of pneumatic otoscopy. **A,** the speculum is inserted into the ear canal to form a tight seal. The bulb is then gently and slowly pressed and released while the mobility of the drum is assessed. Pressing on the bulb applies positive pressure; letting up applies negative pressure. **B,** a normal drum moves inward and then back. **C,** in cases of acute otitis media in which the middle ear is filled with purulent material, the drum bulges toward the examiner and moves minimally. **D,** in cases of acute otitis media with an air-fluid level, mobility may be nearly normal. In some patients, however, the drum may be retracted, indicating increased negative pressure. If this is the case, mobility on positive pressure may be reduced while movement on negative pressure is nearly normal or only mildly decreased. This is the same pattern as that seen commonly in children with chronic serous otitis (**E**). In cases of high negative pressure and no effusion, application of positive pressure produces little or no movement, but on negative pressure the drum billows back toward the examiner (**F**).

positive or negative pressure (Fig. 22.23). An abnormality in *any one* of the four major characteristics is suggestive of middle ear pathology.

ACUTE OTITIS MEDIA

Acute otitis media is the term used to describe acute infection and inflammation of the middle ear. Associated inflammation and edema of the eustachian tube mucosa appear to play key roles in the pathogenesis by impeding drainage of the middle ear fluid. In some children, anatomic or chronic physiologic abnormalities of the eustachian tube predispose them to infection. The problem is commonly seen in conjunction with an acute upper respiratory infection, and its onset is often heralded by a secondary temperature spike one to several days after the onset of URI symptoms. The major offending organisms are bacterial respiratory pathogens. The most commonly iso-

DISTRIBUTION OF PATHOGENS CULTURED IN ACUTE OTITIS MEDIA (716 ISOLATES)

Streptococcus pneumoniae	44.5% (319)	
Haemophillus influenzae	31.4% (225)	Beta lactamase + 28%
Moraxella catarrhalis	16.9% (121)	Beta lactamase + 88%
Streptococcus pyogenes	4.9% (35)	
Staphylococcus aureus	1.7% (12)	
Pseudomonas aeruginosa	0.7% (5)	

FIG. 22.24 Distribtuion of pathogens cultured in acute otitis media (716 isolates).

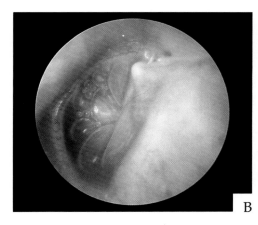 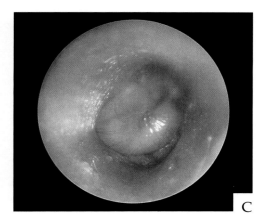

FIG. 22.25 Acute otitis media. **A,** this is the textbook picture: an erythematous, opaque, bulging tympanic membrane. The light reflex is reduced, and the landmarks are partially obscured. Mobility is markedly reduced **B,** in this acutely febrile child who complained of otalgia, the presence of both air and fluid formed bubbles separated by grayish-yellow menisci. Even though the drum was not injected, this finding, combined with fever and otalgia, is consistent with acute infection. **C,** in this child, the tympanic membrane was markedly injected superiorly, and a yellow purulent effusion caused the inferior portion to bulge outward. Mobility was markedly reduced. (**A,** courtesy of Dr. Michael Hawke)

lated organisms and their relative frequency are listed in Figure 22.24. A small portion of cases constitute an exception to these percentages, i.e., those in which otitis is accompanied by conjunctivitis. Here, nontypable *H. influenzae* have been found causative in 70 to 75 percent of cases. Increasing rates of beta-lactamase positivity in these organisms in certain regions of the country have led to use of beta-lactamase-resistant antibiotics by many practitioners whenever this syndrome is seen.

In acute otitis media, the classic findings on inspection of the tympanic membrane are erythema and injection; bulging which obscures the malleus; thickening, often with a grayish-white or yellow hue reflecting a purulent effusion; and reduced mobility (Fig. 22.25A,B). It must be remembered, however, that crying rapidly produces erythema of the eardrum, and thus, erythema in a crying child is of little diagnostic value. The patient is usually febrile and, if old enough, typically complains of otalgia. However, in many cases this "textbook picture" is not seen. This is probably due in part to time of presentation, the virulence of the particular pathogen, and host factors.

Accuracy in diagnosis necessitates meticulous care on otoscopy and knowledge of the various modes of presentation. Children may present with fever of a few hours duration and otalgia (or if very young with fever and irritability), yet have no abnormality on otoscopy. If reexamined the following day, many of these patients have clear evidence of acute otitis media. Some have erythema and bubbles or air-fluid or air-pus levels (due to venting by the eustachian tube) without bulging, and with nearly normal mobility (Fig. 22.25C). In still other cases, the drum may be full and poorly mobile with cloudy fluid behind it, but minimally erythematous. In some patients the drum is retracted, moves primarily or only in response to negative pressure, and shows signs of inflammation and/or a cloudy effusion.

Occasionally the signs and symptoms of otitis media may be accompanied by formation of a bullous lesion on the surface of the tympanic membrane, a condition termed *bullous myringitis* (Fig. 22.26). These children usually complain of intense pain. While this phenomenon is most commonly associated with *Mycoplasma* in adults, any of the usual pediatric pathogens (see Fig. 22.24) can be causative in children. Finally, acute otitis

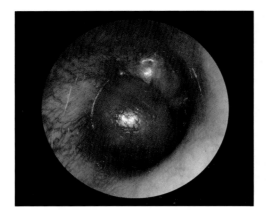

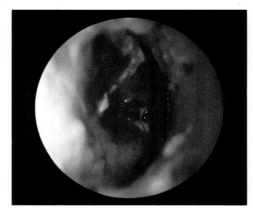

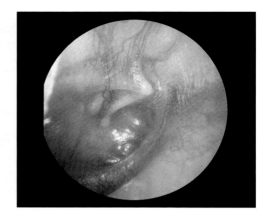

FIG. 22.26 Acute otitis media with bullous myringitis. This patient was febrile and extremely uncomfortable. On otoscopy, an erythematous bullous lesion is seen obscuring much of the tympanic membrane. This phenomenon, called bullous myringitis, is caused by the usual pathogens of childhood. The bullous lesion commonly ruptures spontaneously, providing immediate relief of pain.

FIG. 22.27 Acute otitis media with perforation. In this child, increased middle ear pressure with acute otitis resulted in perforation of the tympanic membrane. The drum is thickened, and the perforation is seen at 3 o'clock.

FIG. 22.28 Serous otitis media. This patient has a chronic serous middle ear effusion. The tympanic membrane is retracted, thickened, and shiny. Behind it is a clear yellow effusion. Mobility was decreased and primarily evident on negative pressure. The child was not acutely ill but did have decreased hearing. (Courtesy of Dr. Sylvan Stool, Children's Hospital of Pittsburg)

media may, by virtue of increasing middle ear pressure, result in acute perforation of the tympanic membrane. On presentation, the canal may be filled with purulent material; however, tugging on the pinna usually does not elicit pain, and erythema and edema of the canal wall are minimal or absent. Cleansing with a cotton wick will usually reveal an inflamed drum with a barely visible perforation (Fig. 22.27). Just as clinical findings vary, so do symptoms. While some patients present with severe otalgia, others may complain of sore throat, mild ear discomfort only, ear popping, or decreased hearing, yet have floridly inflamed eardrums. Fever may be absent.

Radiographic studies generally are of little value in the diagnosis of acute otitis media. When a temporal bone CT scan is obtained during acute otitis media in which fluid is present in the middle ear, fluid also will be present in the mastoid cavity. This will be read by a radiologist as clouding of the mastoid, as it may be difficult to distinguish between acute otitis media and acute mastoiditis. In such instances, it is important that the physician look at the patient's clinical signs rather than relying on radiographic findings to make the diagnosis.

In addition to treating patients with an appropriate antimicrobial agent and analgesics when needed, followup examination is important. This is best done 2 to 3 weeks after diagnosis, when complete resolution can be expected in over 50 percent of children. The purpose of reevaluation is to identify those patients who have persistent serous effusions and who require ongoing surveillance.

OTITIS MEDIA WITH EFFUSION ("SEROUS OTITIS MEDIA")

"Serous" effusion in the middle ear may result from an upper respiratory infection or it may be the residual of a treated acute otitis. In many instances, this effusion is not spontaneously cleared, but instead remains in the middle ear for weeks or months, resulting in a persistent clear gray or yellow effusion behind the eardrum (Fig. 22.28). Persistence

appears due in part to eustachian tube dysfunction. Pneumatic otoscopy often reveals poor mobility of the tympanic membrane, and then primarily on negative pressure. The latter is thought to develop as a result of consumption of middle ear oxygen by mucosal cells, creating a vacuum which persists with the fluid because of failure of ventilation by the eustachian tube. Such long-standing effusions impair hearing and are subject to bacterial invasion, and thus recurrent middle ear infection. Persistence of a serous effusion for more than 3-4 months is an indication for myringotomy and insertion of tubes (see Fig. 22.30) to facilitate hearing and reduce risk of recurrent infection.

CHRONIC/RECURRENT OTITIS MEDIA

Chronic or chronic/recurrent otitis media with effusion (COME) is not an uncommon finding in young children. Patients subject to this condition appear to have significant and prolonged eustachian tube dysfunction. This "otitis-prone" state may be a seemingly isolated phenomenon or it can be a feature of a number of syndromes characterized by palatal dysfunction or malformation, or by facial hypoplasia or deformity. These conditions include cleft palate, Crouzon syndrome, Down syndrome, the mucopolysaccharidoses, and mucolipidoses (see Figs. 22.8, 22.62 and 22.63). Chronic obstructive tonsillar and adenoidal hypertrophy may also be a predisposing condition. Less commonly, immunodeficiency and the immotile cilia syndrome are identified as underlying etiologic conditions.

Chronic otitis media is associated with significant morbidity in terms of intermittent or chronic hearing impairment, intermittent discomfort, and the ill effects of recurrent infection. Over months or years, the process produces permanent myringosclerotic changes in which the tympanic membrane becomes whitened, thickened, and scarred (Fig. 22.29A). Chronic perforations are not uncommon (Fig. 22.29B). Patients with persistent middle ear infections despite medical therapy, and those with frequent recurrences appear to benefit from

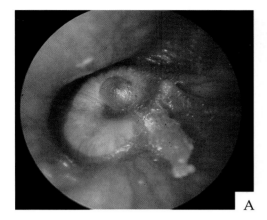
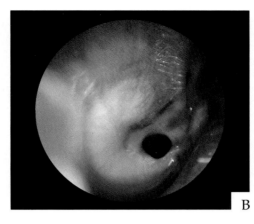
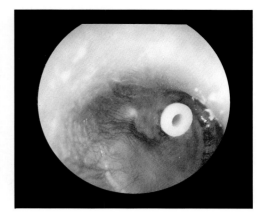

FIG. 22.29 Sequelae of chronic otitis media. **A,** much of this child's tympanic membrane is scarred and thickened, and a thinned dimeric area balloons out of the anterosuperior portion. **B,** the eardrum is markedly thick-

ened, scarred in an arc from 12 to 5 o'clock, and has a large chronic perforation. (Courtesy of Dr. Sylvan Stool, Children's Hospital of Pittsburg)

FIG. 22.30 Tympanic membrane of patient with chronic otitis media, with tympanostmy tube in place. The tubes serve to vent the middle ear, improve hearing, and reduce the frequency of infection. (Courtesy of Dr. Sylvan Stool, Children's Hospital of Pittsburg)

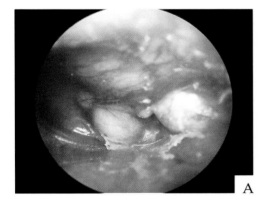
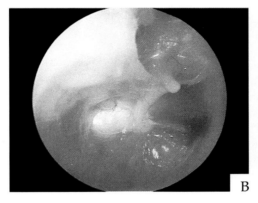
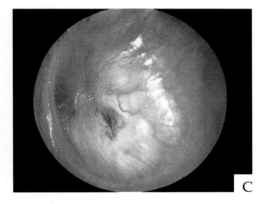

FIG. 22.31 Cholesteatomas. **A,** congenital cholesteatoma noted in a young child who presented with spontaneous ear drainage. There had been no previous history of ear infections. **B** and **C,** acquired cholesteatoma, which generally presents after a long history of chronic ear disease.

surgical drainage and insertion of tympanostomy tubes which vent the middle ear (Fig. 22.30). Persistence of a serous effusion for longer than 3 to 4 months is also an indication for myringotomy and insertion of tubes. Once placed, these should be checked at intervals for presence and patency. Spontaneous extrusion generally occurs 6 to 12 months after insertion. Children with chronic perforations or tubes must protect the ear from moisture to reduce risk of contamination of the middle ear and reinfection.

PROTECTION OF THE EXPOSED MIDDLE EAR BY EARPLUGS OR EAR DEFENDERS

Earplugs, or ear defenders, come in all shapes and sizes. They can vary in cost from inexpensive, premolded earplugs to expensive, custom-molded devices. The general purpose of an earplug is to prevent water from entering the external ear canal and contaminating the middle ear space. There are "wax" earplugs that act like a putty which can be molded into the particular shape that would seem to comfortably block the individual's ear canals. There is also a preformed ear defender which is held in place by the conchal bowl and provides quite reasonable protection for children. The ear defenders vary in shape, and a child needs to be fitted for an age-appropriate size. Custom-made earplugs are generally not neces-

sary except in the unusual case in which the child has a deformed ear and will not be able to utilize standard ones. Custom-made ear molds are obtained through audiological services. One should note that children have a propensity to lose or misplace these devices, and it is best to focus on obtaining functional earplugs that are easily replaceable at minimal cost to the family.

OTHER MIDDLE EAR DISORDERS

A number of other disorders involving the tympanic membrane, though considerably less common than otitis media and serous otitis media, are important because of potential seriousness.

Mass Lesions Involving the Tympanic Membrane

The most common and one of the most serious mass lesions of the eardrum is a *cholesteatoma.* It can present as a defect in the tympanic membrane through which persistent drainage occurs, or it can appear as a white cystic mass behind or involving the eardrum. It consists of trapped epithelial tissue which grows beneath the surface of the membrane (Fig. 22.31). While many are congenital, some are sequelae of untreated or chronic/recurrent otitis media. If a cholesteatoma is not removed surgically, it continues to enlarge, becomes locally

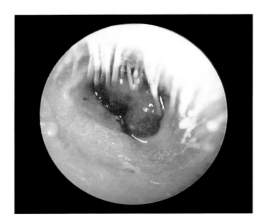

FIG. 22.32 Polyps of the tympanic membrane. These polyps, which protrude through a tympanic membrane perforation, have enlarged to entirely fill the external ear canal. Because of the possible attachment of the polyp to the ossicles of the middle ear, removal of polyps requires extreme caution.

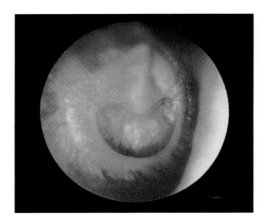

FIG. 22.33 Dimerism of the tympanic membrane. Otoscopy demonstrates a severely retracted atrophic segment of the eardrum which also has multiple white scars. The thinned portions are the result of abnormal healing of perforations, and tend to be hypermobile on otoscopy. (Courtesy of Dr. Sylvan Stool)

destructive, and can erode the mastoid bone, destroy the ossicles, and even invade the inner ear structures or cranium. A progressive hearing impairment usually occurs.

Granulomas or *polyps* of the tympanic membrane (Fig. 22.32) can also develop in children with chronic middle ear infections. These tissues often bleed easily and can be frightening to the patient, the parent, and the physician. Left untreated, polyps can enlarge to fill the canal and, by expansion, can progressively damage both the drum and the ossicles. Therefore, prompt surgical removal is indicated.

Distortions of the Tympanic Membrane

Thin, dimeric portions of the eardrum also may be observed in patients with chronic middle ear disease, or they may develop following extrusion of a tympanostomy tube (Fig. 22.33; see also Fig. 22.29A). These thinned areas are the result of abnormal healing of perforations, and are hypermobile on pneumatic otoscopy. The important points to note on examination are whether the pocket is fully visible or partly hidden, its location with respect to the ossicles, and whether or not it is dry. If the ear canal and drum are not dry, then an active infection and/or cholesteatoma will be present. In cases of severe deformity, aggressive therapy, including ventilation of the middle ear and excision of the pocket, may be necessary.

NASAL DISORDERS

A child's nose is most commonly examined for disturbances in external appearance, excessive drainage, or blockage of airflow and interference with breathing. Epistaxis is also frequently encountered.

Nasal Obstruction

UPPER RESPIRATORY INFECTIONS IN EARLY INFANCY

In infancy and early childhood, the nasal passages are small and easily obstructed by processes which produce mucosal edema and coryza, whether infectious, "allergic," or traumatic.

In the first 1 to 3 months, infants are obligate nose breathers, and therefore can have significant respiratory distress from nasal congestion alone. Young infants with upper respiratory infections may, in addition to nasal discharge, have tachypnea and mild retractions, and often have to interrupt feeding to breathe. This often results in the swallowing of significant amounts of air which leads to a secondary increase in spitting up after feeding, unless parents are instructed to hold these infants up on their shoulders and burp them a few extra times after completion of feedings. Instillation of saline nose drops to loosen secretions, followed by nasal suctioning prior to meals and naps, can provide a measure of relief. Oral decongestants are ineffective, and often produce marked irritability when given to infants in the first year of life. Fortunately, these upper respiratory infections are generally brief, and clear within a few days.

On occasion, infants with upper respiratory infection go on to have persistent, purulent, or serosanguineous nasal discharge. Culture of discharges persisting longer than 10 to 14 days may disclose heavy growth of a single pathogen. Preliminary studies of empiric antimicrobial therapy in such infants suggest that this produces rapid and effective resolution of symptoms when compared with placebo. Thus this picture of prolonged nasal discharge probably represents a bacterial ethmoiditis, the infant equivalent of sinusitis.

CONGENITAL CAUSES OF NASAL OBSTRUCTION

Congenital causes of nasal obstruction include choanal atresia, choanal stenosis, and mass lesions such as tumors, cysts, and polyps.

Choanal Atresia and Stenosis

Choanal atresia may be either bony (90 percent) or membranous (10 percent), bilateral or unilateral. Newborns with bilateral choanal atresia manifest severe respiratory distress at delivery, with cyanosis which is relieved by crying and returns with rest (paradoxical cyanosis). The true nature of the problem can elude detection if the physician relies solely on passing soft feeding catheters through the nose to determine paten-

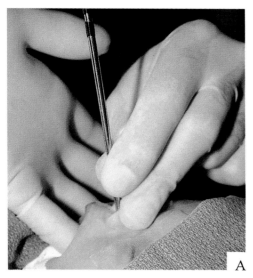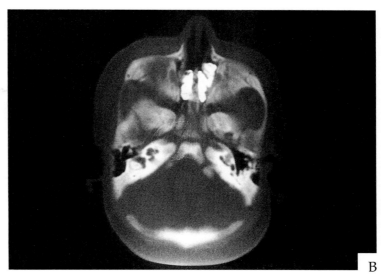

FIG. 22.34 Choanal atresia. **A,** this infant manifested severe respiratory distress at delivery, with paradoxical cyanosis. Attempts to pass a urethral sound revealed bony obstruction of the choanae bilaterally. **B,** a CT scan done following instillation of radiopaque dye reveals pooling of the dye within the nose anterior to the choane, confirming complete obstruction

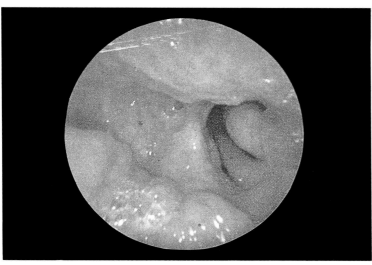

FIG. 22.35 Unilateral choanal atresia. Viewed through the nasopharyngoscope, the left choana is clearly patent while the right is atretic.

cy, as these can buckle or curl within the nose. The correct diagnosis is best made by using a Van Buren urethral sound or a firm plastic suction catheter (both #8 French). This is passed gently along the floor of the nose, close to the septum. If bony resistance is encountered, then the diagnosis of choanal atresia is suspected (Fig. 22.34A) and can be confirmed by placing barium into the nose and viewing lateral and basilar x-rays.

Immediate relief of respiratory distress may be accomplished by insertion of an oral airway (or a nipple from which the tip has been cut away) into the mouth. Definitive studies including computerized tomography can then be performed to aid in planning surgical correction (Fig. 22.34B). Infants with *unilateral choanal atresia* (Fig. 22.35) are usually asymptomatic at birth; however, with time, they develop a persistent unilateral nasal discharge.

Choanal stenosis also is generally asymptomatic in the newborn period, but acquisition of an upper respiratory infection can result in significant respiratory compromise. When suspected, probing with a urethral sound is indicated. If this meets resistance, further evaluation is required. In most cases,

symptomatic therapy using saline nose drops and nasal suctioning is sufficient to help the infants through their upper respiratory infections. With growth, the problem abates.

Congenital Mass Lesions

Congenital mass lesions are another source of nasal obstruction. These are particularly likely to become apparent during the first 2 years of life. The modes of presentation vary, some lesions manifesting primarily by symptoms of obstruction and detected via diagnostic radiography, others becoming visually evident either within a nostril or as a subcutaneous mass located near the root of the nose. Occasionally, these patients present with recurrent nasal infections and/or epistaxis. All such masses merit thorough clinical and radiographic evaluation, since many have intracranial connections.

An *encephalocele* is an outpouching of brain tissue through a congenital bony defect in the midline of the skull. Some patients present with craniofacial deformities and a rounded swelling between the eyes. In other instances, the neural tissue prolapses into the nasopharynx, resulting in signs and symp-

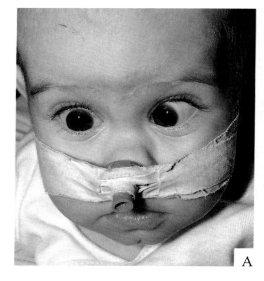
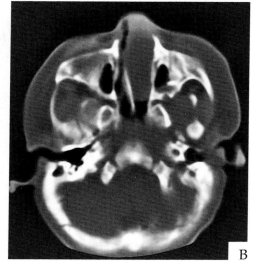
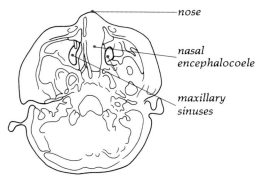

nose
nasal
encephalocoele
maxillary
sinuses

A

B

FIG. 22.36 Nasal encephalocele. **A,** this normal-appearing infant presented with signs of severe nasal obstruction, necessitating insertion of a nasopharyngeal airway to relieve distress. **B,** a CT scan shows a large nasal mass lesion which fills one nostril and pushes the nasal septum into the other. This lesion proved to be an encephalocele extruding through a bony defect in the skull (extrusion seen on another cut).

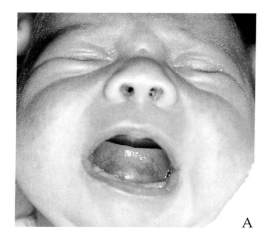
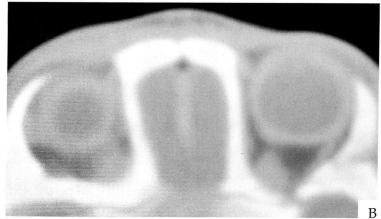

A

B

FIG. 22.37 Nasal dermoids. **A,** a firm round mass with a central dimple is seen over the bridge of this infant's nose. **B,** CT scan demonstrates a bony dehiscence of the nasal bridge with a nasal dermoid extending into the anterior cranial vault in the area of the foramen caecum.

toms of nasal obstruction without obvious external anomalies (Fig. 22.36A). Occasionally, a grapelike mass may be seen within the nares or (via direct nasopharynoscopy) protruding into the pharynx. The mass is usually identified by diagnostic radiography. Computerized tomography (Fig. 22.36B) is particularly helpful in delineating the extent of the mass and the underlying bony defect. Repair requires a collaborative effort by specialists in otolaryngology, neurosurgery, and in some cases, plastic surgery.

Nasal dermoids are embryonic cysts containing ectodermal and mesodermal tissue. They present as round, firm subcutaneous masses which are located on the dorsum of the nose, close to the midline (Fig. 22.37A). Examination of the overlying skin frequently reveals a small dimple, at times with extruding hair. Some of these cysts have deep extensions down to the nasal septum or through the cribriform plate into the cranium. Thorough evaluation using axial and coronal CT scans and MRI is necessary to determine extent and plan repair (Fig 22.37B). If not removed, secondary infection is common and often results in fistula formation.

Small skintags are frequently seen around the nasal vestibule, and should be removed to improve appearance. *Papillomas* (Fig. 22.38) are similar growths that occur on the distal nasal mucosa near the mucocutaneous junction. These

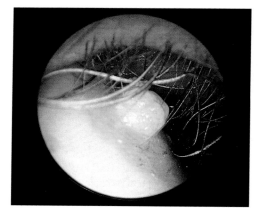

FIG. 22.38 Nasal papillomas present as warty growths at the mucocutaneous junction of the nares. (Courtesy of Dr. Michael Hawke)

should be excised both to improve appearance and confirm diagnosis; they do not cause obstruction.

ACQUIRED FORMS OF NASAL OBSTRUCTION
Adenoidal and Tonsillar Hypertrophy

The lymphoid tissue that constitutes the tonsils and adenoids is relatively small in infancy, gradually enlarges until 8 to 10 years of age, and then begins to shrink in size. In most instances, this normal process of hypertrophy results in mild to

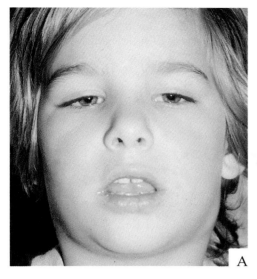

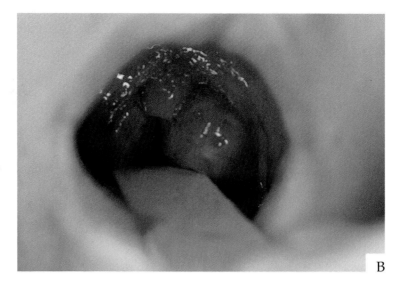

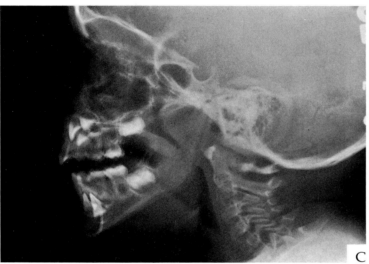

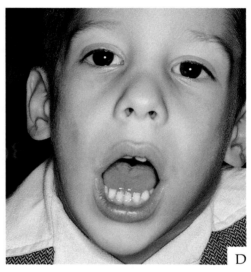

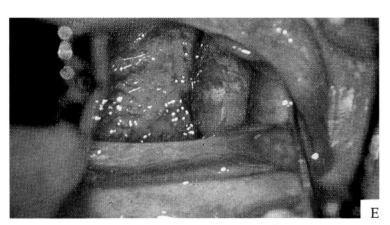

FIG. 22.39 Adenoidal and tonsillar hypertrophy. **A,** external appearance of a child with marked enlargement of tonsils and adenoids. He must keep his mouth open to breathe, and shows signs of fatigue as a result of sleep disturbance caused by his upper airway obstruction. **B,** on examination of the pharynx, his tonsils are seen meeting at the midline. **C,** a lateral neck radiograph shows a large adenoid shadow impinging on the nasal airway. **D,** if obstruction is prolonged, cor pulmonale, abnormal facial elongation, and widening of the nasal root may result. **E,** when the palate is retracted prior to adenoidectomy, the extent of overgrowth of adenoidal tissue is readily appreciated.

moderate enlargement of these structures and does not constitute a problem. A small percentage of children, however, develop marked adenoidal and tonsillar hypertrophy, with attendant symptoms of nasal obstruction and rhinorrhea. A few even have difficulty swallowing solid foods. Recurrent infection appears to be the most common inciting factor, although atopy may play a role in some cases. Occasionally, mononucleosis is the initiating event, resulting in rapid enlargement of adenoidal and tonsillar tissues which is then slow to resolve (see section on Tonsillopharyngitis and see also Chapter 12, Infectious Diseases). In most children, progressive adenoidal enlargement appears to be the cumulative result of

a series of upper respiratory infections. The consequent obstruction to normal flow of secretions then starts a vicious cycle, making the child even more vulnerable to recurrent infections of the ears, sinuses, and nasopharynx which, in turn, further exacerbate the adenoidal and tonsillar hypertrophy.

Regardless of mode of origin, when adenoidal hypertrophy is marked, blockage of the nasal airway becomes severe and results in mouth breathing, chronic rhinorrhea, inability to blow the nose, and snoring during sleep (Fig. 22.39A). Speech becomes hyponasal and muffled. The child holds his mouth open, has little or no airflow through the nares, and his tonsils may meet in the midline (Fig. 22.39B). A cephalometric lateral

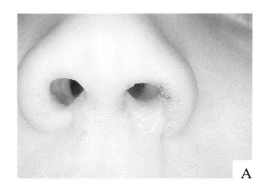 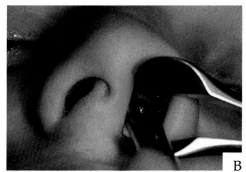

FIG. 22.40 Nasal foreign body. **A,** this child presented with a unilateral, foul-smelling nasal discharge. **B,** aspiration of the discharge in this patient revealed a red bead. (**A,** courtesy of Dr. Michael Hawke)

neck x-ray reveals a large adenoidal shadow impinging on the nasal airway (Fig. 22.39C). For many patients, these features are seen primarily in the course of acute illness; however, a number of children have symptoms even when free of acute infection. In a minority, obstruction is so severe as to produce sleep disturbance. This is characterized by restlessness and retractions when recumbent, stertorous snoring, and sleep apnea with frequent waking. Some patients actually begin to sleep sitting up, and many manifest daytime fatigue. Symptoms are worse during sleep because relaxation of the pharyngeal muscles further increases the degree of upper airway obstruction. In severe cases, this results in periods of hypoxia and hypercarbia, leading to intermittent apnea and waking. Because a patient may look relatively good when awake (with the exception of having to breathe through the mouth), it is important to study retractions and pattern of breathing after the child has been recumbent for a period of time or better still, during a nap. Use of continuous pulse oximetry during this period of observation enables documentation of presence or absence of oxygen desaturation. If an obstruction is prolonged, cor pulmonale (with signs of right ventricular hypertrophy on ECG and chest x-ray) and abnormal facial growth may result (Fig. 22.39D).

Management of patients with adenoidal hypertrophy is dependent in part upon the severity and the duration of the obstruction. In milder cases of short duration, or in patients with intermittent symptoms, careful monitoring, prompt institution of antimicrobial therapy for bacterial infections, and treatment of atopy, when present, may bring the problem under control. Children with persistent symptoms despite therapy, and those with sleep disturbance or cor pulmonale warrant adenoidectomy, during which the extent of adenoidal overgrowth can be fully appreciated (Fig. 22.39E). Children with major orthodontic abnormalities and nasal obstruction should also be considered for adenoidectomy prior to orthodontic correction.

Nasal Foreign Bodies

As is true of the external ear, it is not unusual for small children to put beads, paper, pieces of sponge, plastic toys, or other foreign material into their noses. Such foreign objects are irritating to the nasal mucosa and soon incite an intense inflammatory reaction with production of a thick, purulent, foul-smelling discharge that helps to hide their presence. Intermittent epistaxis may accompany the discharge. Since most children below 5 years of age are unable to blow their noses, and are afraid or unable to tell their parents what they've done, the object is not expelled and the problem often goes unrecognized until symptoms develop and medical attention is sought. A unilateral nasal discharge, a foul smell, or both are the typical chief complaints, and should lead the clinician to suspect a foreign body immediately.

Speculum examination may readily disclose the object (Fig. 22.40), but often, the purulent discharge obscures the view. Even when visualization is accomplished, removal can be difficult, as children are easily frightened at the prospect of instrumentation, and their struggling can result in mucosal injury during attempts at removal. To minimize problems, topical anesthetic spray and a topical vasoconstrictor can be applied, and the child restrained with a papoose board. Older patients or calm young children may do well sitting in a parent's lap, if the examiner is patient, reassuring, and willing to explain each step carefully. The discharge may then be removed by swab or suction. If the object is anterior to the turbinates, removal can be attempted using suction, a right angled Day hook for spherical objects, or alligator forceps for material that can be grasped. Consultation from an otolaryngologist should be sought for removal of objects located more posteriorly or those not readily removed on initial attempts. A major concern is that in the attempted removal, a deeply situated foreign body may be dislodged into the nasopharynx, leading to aspiration or worse, laryngeal obstruction. In such cases, the best course of action is to remove the object after the airway has been secured with an endotracheal tube, in the operating room, under a general anesthetic.

Nasal Polyps

Polyps are thought to be the end result of recurrent infection and/or inflammation, although in a proportion of cases, atopy may play a contributing role. Polyps originate in the ethmoid or less commonly, the maxillary sinuses and protrude through the sinus ostia into the nasal cavity. The phenomenon is unusual in children under 10 years of age, with the exception of patients with cystic fibrosis, 25 percent of

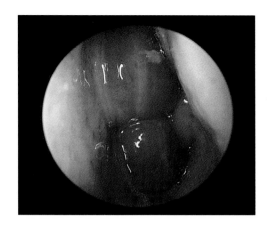

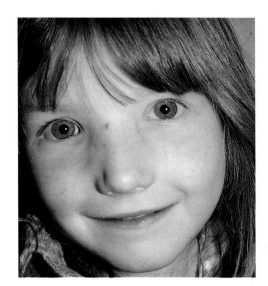

FIG. 22.41 Nasal polyp. This 2-year-old girl with cystic fibrosis was referred because of nasal obstruction and nocturnal snoring of a few months duration. A large grayish polyp was found in the left nostril.

FIG. 22.42 Sequela of chronic nasal polyps. This 7-year-old girl with cystic fibrosis and recurrent nasal polyps shows secondary alteration in facial growth consisting of a broadened nasal dorsum and prominence of the malar areas. This occurred despite several resections.

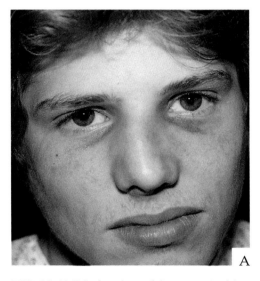

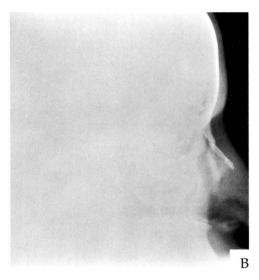

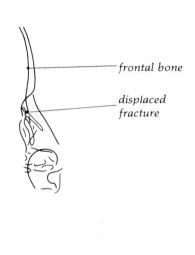

frontal bone

displaced fracture

A

B

FIG. 22.43 Displaced nasal fracture. **A,** this teenager was hit on the nose while playing football. On external inspection there is obvious deformity and there are ecchymoses under both eyes. Crepitance was evident on palpation. **B,** a lateral radiograph of another patient shows a displaced fracture of the proximal portion of the nasal bone.

whom develop polyps, some as early as infancy. Symptoms consist of progressive nasal obstruction, frequently with associated discharge. Recurrent sinusitis is a common complication as a result of impaired sinus drainage. In some cases, chronic sinusitis may be the cause of polyp formation. Affected patients with acute infections may also have intermittent epistaxis. Involvement may be unilateral or bilateral. On examination, moist, glistening pedunculated growths are seen that may have a smooth or a grapelike appearance (Fig. 22.41). Bilateral opacification of the ethmoid and maxillary sinuses is commonly found on radiography. Polyps must be distinguished from a nasal glioma or encephalocele which may have a similar appearance and can produce identical symptoms. These neural mass lesions are more common in infancy, but can present in older children. Therefore, computerized tomography of the nasopharynx should be considered for children under age 10 with polypoid nasal lesions without documented cystic fibrosis.

Surgical removal of the polyp is indicated to relieve nasal obstruction, reduce the risk of secondary sinusitis, and diminish the possibility of altered facial growth. The latter problem is seen in children with chronic polyps (most frequently those with cystic fibrosis) and consists of widening of the nasal dorsum and prominence of the malar areas of the face (Fig. 22.42).

Nasal Trauma

Blunt nasal trauma is frequently encountered in pediatrics. In the majority of instances it results only in minor swelling and mild epistaxis, which is readily controlled by application of pressure over the nares (see Chapter 2, Neonatology, for nasal trauma incurred during delivery). However, more severe injuries are not uncommon, and have a significant potential for long-term morbidity and deformity if not identified and treated appropriately. These include displaced nasal fractures (Fig. 22.43), which, if not reduced, result in permanent defor-

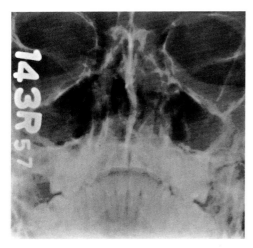

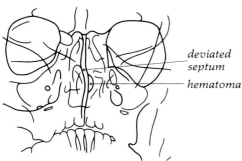

deviated
septum

hematoma

FIG. 22.44 Deviated nasal septum. This patient was punched in the nose, resulting in a leftward deviation of the cartilaginous portion of the nasal septum, which is clearly visible in this radiograph. The small arc of mucosal swelling along the septum proved to be a small septal hematoma. There is no visible fracture. Septal deviation requires correction to prevent deformity and relieve secondary nasal obstruction.

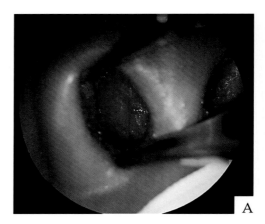

A

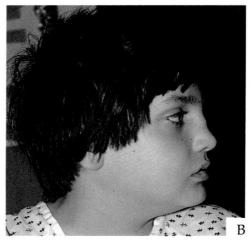

B

FIG. 22.45 Septal hematoma. A, this patient incurred facial trauma resulting in multiple fractures of the nasal and orbital bones and submucosal bleeding along the nasal septum. Such septal hematomas must be drained promptly to reduce the risk of abscess formation, and to prevent cartilage necrosis which ultimately results in B, a saddle nose deformity.

mity; septal deviation or dislocation, with or without an associated fracture (Fig. 22.44), which produces unilateral impairment of airflow; and septal hematomas (Fig. 22.45A), which, if not drained promptly, cause destruction of nasal cartilage resulting in a saddle nose deformity (Fig. 22.45B). Finally, profuse bleeding which is difficult to stop or recurs readily suggests trauma to deeper structures of the face or frontal bones, and warrants prompt stabilization and meticulous clinical and radiographic assessment.

In evaluating patients with nasal trauma, the nasal bridge should be inspected for swelling or deformity (the latter may not be apparent if swelling is marked), and the septum palpated for tenderness, crepitus, or excessive mobility. The nares should be cleared of clots and the septum assessed for position and presence of swelling, which would be suggestive of a hematoma. Examination of the oropharynx is also helpful in determining if blood is flowing posteriorly. When marked swelling, severe tenderness, deformity, crepitus, or septal deviation is found, radiography is indicated. However, radiographs should be interpreted with caution, since a large portion of the nasal skeleton in children is composed of cartilage rather than bone, and serious nasal injuries can be present despite a seemingly normal x-ray. Septal hematomas, displaced fractures, and bleeding which fails to cease readily with direct pressure necessitate prompt consultation with an otolaryngologist.

Epistaxis

Nasal bleeding in childhood has a number of causes including trauma, infection, mucosal irritation, bleeding disorders, vascular anomalies, and hypertension. Patients with these conditions may have apparently spontaneous bleeding, or may have epistaxis triggered by minor external trauma, forceful sneezing, and blowing. Profuse bleeding which is difficult to stop is most characteristic of acute thrombocytopenia, vascular anomalies, and hypertension. Mild bleeding which is readily controlled by application of pressure is more suggestive of mucosal infection or irritation which promote bleeding from small submucosal veins located on the anterior nasal septum (Fig. 22.46). In all cases, the problem should be taken seriously and investigated carefully in order to correctly diagnose and appropriately treat the primary source of the problem.

In approaching patients with epistaxis, the following historical points should be addressed:

1. Is the problem acute or recurrent?
2. Was external trauma, sneezing, or blowing a triggering event?
3. What is the duration of the current bleed and the approximate volume of blood loss (handkerchiefs soaked, hemodynamic status, etc.)?
4. Is the bleeding unilateral or bilateral?
5. Has the patient been having symptoms suggestive of an upper respiratory infection or nasal allergy?
6. Has the child manifested other signs and symptoms of an underlying coagulopathy or of hypertension?
7. Has the patient been taking medication, especially aspirin?

Physical assessment must address the patient's general well-being in addition to careful examination of the nose. Hemodynamic status is of particular import when hemorrhage has been profuse.

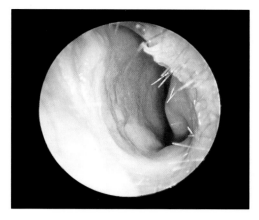

FIG. 22.46 Dilated septal vessels of Kesselbach's plexus which tend to bleed in response to mucosal infection or irritation.

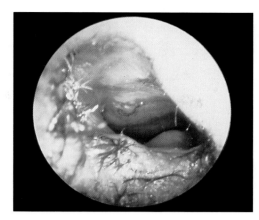

FIG. 22.47 Excoriated nasal septum. This child presented with URI and a history of intermittent epistaxis with nasal blowing and during the night. He had a purulent nasal discharge (on the lower right), and a diffusely excoriated erythematous septum. Cultures of his nose and throat grew group A beta-streptococci.

After observation of the external appearance of the nares, the nose should be cleared of clots and discharge, if present. Then, the septum and mucosa are inspected for possible points of hemorrhage, signs of obstruction, mass lesions, and foreign objects. The oropharynx should also be examined for posterior flow of blood, especially in cases in which no point of bleeding is evident on inspection of the nasal mucosa. Otolaryngologic consultation should be sought in cases involving profuse bleeding which does not readily cease upon application of pressure, and which may require nasal packing or other surgical treatment.

EPISTAXIS DUE TO INFECTION AND MUCOSAL IRRITATION

In many patients with nontraumatic epistaxis, examination reveals unilateral or bilateral septal erythema and friability or excoriation (Fig. 22.47). The history given is one of intermittent bleeding, especially with sneezing or blowing the nose, or during sleep (the child's pillow is found spotted with blood). The phenomenon is commonly attributed to picking the nose in response to itching. However, in view of the sensitivity of the mucosa to painful stimuli, picking to the point of excoriation is rather unlikely. In many instances, these lesions either are impetiginous or represent the combined effects of inflammation (due to nasopharyngitis, sinusitis, or allergic rhinitis) and trauma due to forceful sneezing and blowing. When infection is suspected, culturing of the friable area for a predominant bacterial pathogen (especially group A beta-streptococcus or coagulase-positive staphylococcus) may prove rewarding. In patients with no history of or findings consistent with upper respiratory infection, mucosal drying may be responsible. This is seen most commonly in winter, as a result of drying of the air by central heating systems. While application of topical antibiotic ointment, humidification, and antihistamines (for atopic patients) may provide some relief, oral antimicrobial therapy for bacterial pathogens, when found, is more likely to be successful.

Patients with nasal polyps who have an intercurrent infection, and children with nasal foreign bodies with secondary infection and inflammation are also highly prone to intermittent epistaxis and/or blood tinging of their nasal discharge.

EPISTAXIS DUE TO BLEEDING DISORDERS

Despite application of pressure, epistaxis in patients with coagulopathies is more likely to be prolonged, and carries a greater risk of significant blood loss. While many such patients have known bleeding disorders, a few may present with prolonged or recurrent nosebleeds as one of the initial manifestations of their problem. This is most typical of idiopathic thrombocytopenia, aplastic anemia, and acute leukemia. When epistaxis arises in the context of a bleeding disorder, the personal history, family history, and/or other physical findings should point to the diagnosis (see Chapter 11, Hematology and Oncology), which can then be confirmed by hematologic studies (CBC and differential, platelet count, PT and PTT, and coagulation profile).

Acute management is dependent in part on the source of the coagulopathy (e.g., factor replacement or platelet transfusion), and in part on severity of bleeding. Topical application of a vasoconstrictor such as epinephrine and insertion of absorbable synthetic material that aids coagulation (Gelfoam® or Surgicel®) can be very helpful in patients with thrombocytopenia and an anterior point of bleeding. The risks of secondary infection with packing must be given careful consideration when treating patients undergoing immunosuppressive therapy.

EPISTAXIS DUE TO VASCULAR ABNORMALITIES

In a minority of children with recurrent epistaxis, the history reveals significant bleeding which typically drains from one side of the nose. This suggests a localized vascular abnormality. The most commonly encountered problem is that of a *dilated septal vessel* or plexus, which may be a sequela of prior inflammation (see Fig. 22.46). This may be visible anteriorly, but can also be located high on the septum, requiring nasopharyngoscopy for identification. Cauterization is generally curative. In children over 7 years of age, anterior septal lesions can be cauterized in the office with silver nitrate after application of a topical anesthetic. Younger children, and many patients with posterior lesions, may need general anesthesia for cauterization.

Two relatively rare vascular anomalies may also be the source of recurrent nasal bleeding: telangiectasias and angiofi-

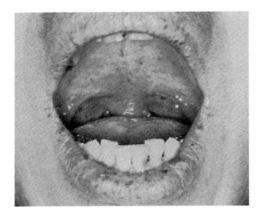

FIG. 22.48 Hereditary hemorrhagic telangiectasia. Numerous telangiectasias dot the lips and palatal mucosa of this boy who had problems with recurrent epistaxis. (Courtesy of Dr. Bernard Cohen, Children's Hospital of Pittsburgh)

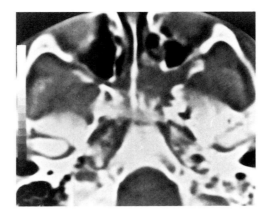

FIG. 22.49 Juvenile nasopharyngeal angiofibroma. CT scan is helpful in assessing the extent of this locally invasive vascular tumor. In this cut, an enhanced mass is seen occupying the posterior portion of the nostril, deviating the septum and compressing the ipsilateral maxillary sinus.

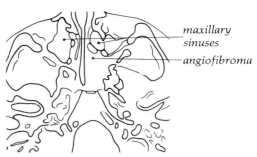

broma. Patients with *hereditary hemorrhagic telangiectasias* (Osler-Weber-Rendu disease) have an autosomal-dominant disorder characterized by formation of cutaneous and mucosal telangiectatic lesions which begin to develop in childhood and gradually increase in number with age. These lesions appear as bright red, slightly raised, star-shaped plexuses of dilated small vessels which blanch on pressure (Fig. 22.48). Mucosal telangiectasias may bleed spontaneously or in response to minor trauma. Recurrent epistaxis is a common mode of presentation in childhood. Multiple telangiectasias are evident on close examination. Hematuria and/or gastrointestinal bleeding may be seen separately or in combination with epistaxis.

Juvenile nasopharyngeal angiofibroma is a rare vascular tumor seen predominantly in adolescent males. While benign, it is locally invasive and destructive, and may involve the maxillary sinuses, palate, sphenoid sinus, and anterior portions of the skull. Its most common mode of presentation is profuse, often recurrent epistaxis. Some patients also have symptoms of nasal obstruction with secondary rhinorrhea, and a small percentage may have visual or auditory disturbances. On examination, a purplish soft-tissue mass may be seen through the nares or on nasopharyngoscopy. General radiographs, computerized tomography, and angiography may be needed to assess the extent of the tumor (Fig. 22.49). Carefully planned excision is then the treatment of choice.

EPISTAXIS DUE TO HYPERTENSION

In contrast to the adult population, hypertension is an unusual source of epistaxis in childhood. However, it should be considered, especially in patients with antecedent headache and spontaneous, profuse bleeding which is difficult to stop. It must be remembered that following significant blood loss, blood pressure may drop to normal limits. Patients with such a history may have previously undiagnosed coarctation of the aorta or chronic renal disease, and they should be examined with these possibilities in mind.

DISORDERS OF THE PARANASAL SINUSES AND ADJACENT STRUCTURES

The paranasal sinuses are air-filled, bony cavities that lie within the facial bones of the skull, adjacent to the nasal passage. They develop through a gradual enlargement of pneumatized cells that evaginate from the nasal cavity. This process occurs over the course of childhood and adolescence; there is a wide normal range in the duration of this process and in the ultimate size of the sinuses and their ostia (Fig. 22.50). In infancy, the ethmoid and maxillary sinuses are partially pneumatized, but they are small, and not readily demonstrable on x-rays (although they can be readily seen on CT scan). Therefore, radiographs are of little diagnostic value until after the first year of life. The sphenoid sinus is not evident until about 5 to 6 years, and the frontal sinuses are not well developed until after 7 to 8 years of age (Fig. 22.51).

The sinuses are lined by ciliated respiratory epithelium which both produces and transports mucous secretions. They drain through various small openings into the nasal cavity which are mainly under the middle and superior turbinates. Several points of clinical importance warrant emphasis. First, the ostia of the sinuses are small and thus, easily obstructed by mucosal edema. Further, there are many important structures adjacent to the sinuses that are vulnerable to involvement

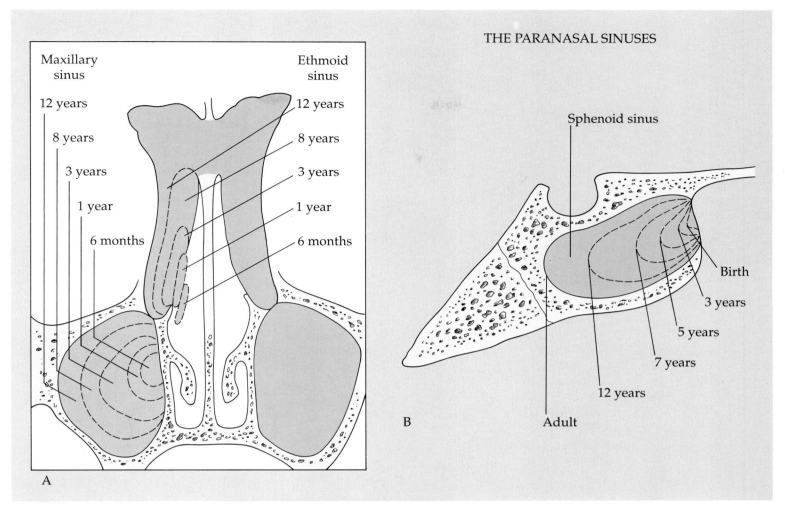

FIG. 22.50 Development of the paranasal sinuses. **A,** this schematic diagram shows the development of the maxillary, the ethmoid, and the frontal sinuses. Note that development occurs throughout childhood and may not be complete until 12 years of age. **B,** the sphenoid sinus, which sits under the pituitary fossa, develops very slowly, and may not even be present for the first 5 to 6 years of life.

should a disease process spread beyond a sinus. These include the orbit, the brain, and the cavernous sinus. The roots of the maxillary teeth lie in the floor of the maxillary sinuses. Therefore, dental infections may drain into the maxillary sinuses, resulting in recurrent or chronic sinusitis. Hence, the dentition should be thoroughly inspected in evaluating any child with suspected sinus infection (see Chapter 20, Oral Disorders).

Sinusitis

During the first several years of life, infection of the maxillary and/or ethmoid sinuses is more common than is generally appreciated. Frontal sinusitis assumes importance after about 10 years of age. The probable pathogenesis is mucosal swelling (whether due to upper respiratory infection, allergic rhinitis, or chemical irritation), resulting in obstruction of the sinus ostia. This impedes drainage of secretions, promotes mucous plugging, and if prolonged, sets the stage for proliferation of

bacterial pathogens with resultant infection. Both bacterial and viral pathogens have been isolated from pediatric patients. The most commonly identified bacteria are *Streptococcus pneumoniae*, nontypable *Haemophilus influenzae*, and *Moraxella catarrhalis*. The viral agents include adenoviruses and parainfluenza viruses. As in adults, there is no good correlation between results of nasopharyngeal and sinus aspirate cultures.

As is true of otitis media, a number of conditions have been identified as predisposing children to sinus infections by virtue of alterations in anatomy, physiology, or both. These include midfacial anomalies or deformities, particularly when maxillary hypoplasia is part of the picture (see Fig. 22.8); cleft palate (see section on Palatal Disorders); nasal deformity and/or septal deviation, whether congenital or acquired; mass lesions including hypertrophied adenoids, nasal foreign bodies, polyps, or tumors; abnormalities of mucus production and/or ciliary action such as cystic fibrosis and the immotile cilia syndrome; immunodeficiency; atopy; dental infection; and barotrauma.

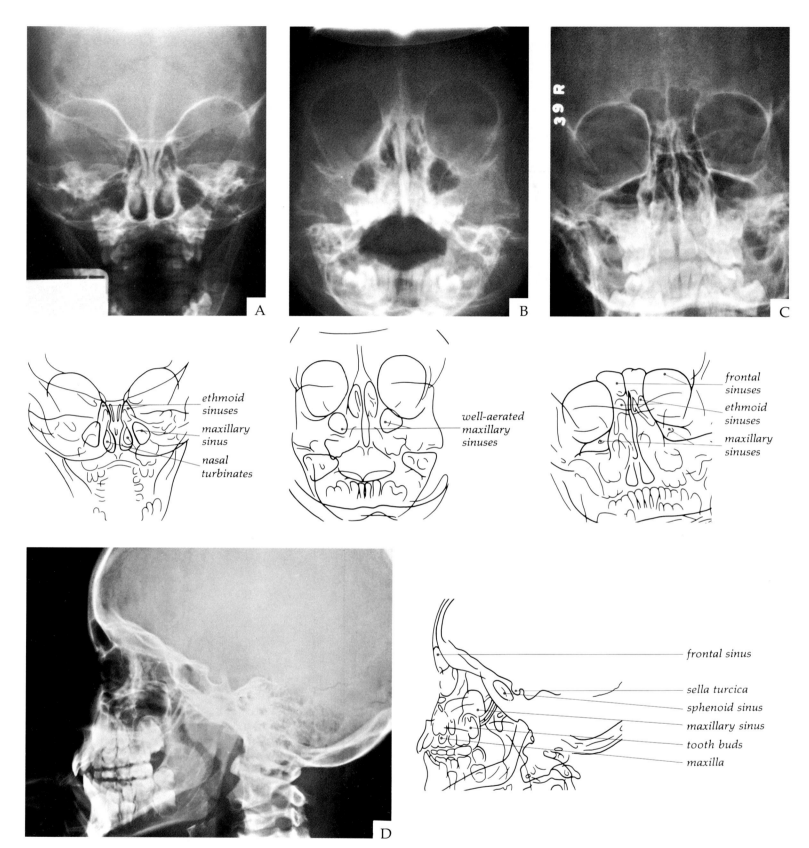

FIG. 22.51 Normal radiography of the sinuses. Radiography is currently the most helpful noninvasive tool for evaluating the paranasal sinuses. Interpretation requires appreciation of the normal pattern of development and the findings seen in health and with disease. **A**, AP or Caldwell view shows clear ethmoid sinuses in an 18-month-old child. The bony margins are sharp and the sinus cavities are dark. **B**, Waters view of the same child shows normal maxillary sinuses with sharply defined bony margins. The cavities appear black. **C**, after age 6 or 7, the Caldwell view is taken PA. In this 8-year-old boy, the bony margins of both the ethmoid and frontal sinuses are sharply defined.

Because the calvarium is superimposed, it can be difficult to distinguish frontal sinus clouding on this view alone, particularly with bilateral disease. Therefore, evaluation of the frontal sinuses requires close scrutiny of both Caldwell and lateral views. **D**, lateral view of an 8- year-old child shows pneumatization of the frontal and sphenoid sinuses. Bony margins are sharply defined. The frontal sinuses appear black, but the sphenoid is somewhat gray because there are more overlying structures. Note how the roots of the maxillary teeth are embedded in the floor of the maxillary sinus.

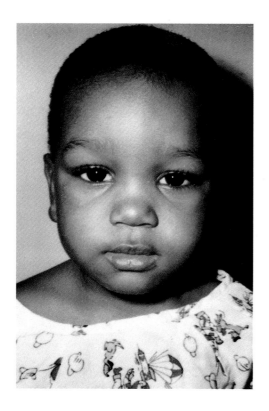

FIG. 22.52
Sympathetic perior-
bital swelling with
sinusitis. This 2-year-
old boy was seen late
in the afternoon with
high fever, wet cough,
decreased activity,
and mild infraorbital
puffiness. The latter
was neither red,
indurated, nor ten-
der, and reportedly
had been more
marked upon awak-
ening in the morning.
He also had a scant
cloudy nasal dis-
charge. His chest x-
ray was normal, but
sinus films showed
opacification of the
maxillary sinuses.

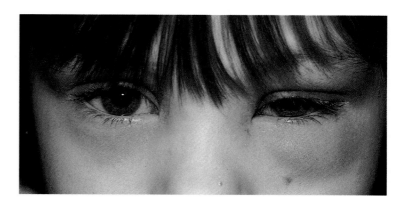

FIG. 22.53 This child with sinusitis presented with prominent erythematous periorbital edema and signs of purulent conjunctivitis. The
redness raised concerns of periorbital cellulitis, but the area was nontender and not indurated. Presence of periorbital swelling is a helpful
clue in diagnosing sinusitis in children with other suggestive signs
and symptoms. (Courtesy of Dr. Ellen Wald, Children's Hospital of
Pittsburgh)

CLINICAL PRESENTATIONS OF SINUSITIS

In young children, sinusitis is primarily a disorder of the ethmoid and maxillary sinuses, and the clinical picture differs
considerably from that of adolescents and adults. The most
common picture is one of a prolonged upper respiratory infection which has shown no sign of amelioration after 7 to 10
days. Cough and/or persistent nasal discharge (which may be
of any character—thin, thick; clear, cloudy; white, yellow, or
green) are the major complaints. The cough is usually loose or
wet; it is prominent during the day, but may be worse on waking in the morning and/or on first going to bed at night.
Patients tend to clear their throats and sniff or snort frequently.
Halitosis or "fetor oris" is commonly noted by parents. In a
minority of children, periorbital swelling, most noticeable on
awaking, may be reported (Fig. 22.52). A small percentage of
patients have low-grade fever, and a few may complain of
headache, facial discomfort, sore throat, or abdominal pain
(thought to be due to gastric irritation from swallowing the
purulent discharge).

Often, physical examination alone is of little help in distinguishing sinusitis from a URI. Findings may include purulent
nasal and postnasal discharge with erythema of the nasal
mucosa and pharynx; but, as noted above, this is not uniformly seen. Halitosis may be pronounced, and is strongly suggestive of sinusitis in the absence of evidence of dental infection,
severe pharyngitis, or nasal foreign body. Sinusitis is also probable when features of the above picture are accompanied by
signs of a maxillary dental abscess (see Chapter 20, Oral
Disorders). Tenderness to percussion over the sinuses is very
suggestive of—but not seen in the majority of patients with—
the "prolonged URI" picture. It is important to recognize that
the clinical spectrum is wide, that any combination of the
above symptoms and signs may be seen, and that sinusitis
should be suspected, even if the course is relatively brief,
whenever clinical findings are strongly suggestive.

A less frequent mode of presentation in young children is
that of an acute upper respiratory infection that is unusually
severe, characterized by high fever and copious purulent nasal
discharge. Facial discomfort and periorbital swelling (nontender, nonindurated, and most marked on waking) are not
uncommon with this picture. The edematous area may be normal in color or mildly erythematous (Fig. 22.53), and is
thought to result from impairment of venous blood flow
caused by increased pressure within the infected sinuses. If
erythema is intense, or the area is indurated or tender, periorbital cellulitis should be suspected. Some of these patients will
also have conjunctival erythema and discharge. Occasionally, a
child with sinusitis will present with the typical findings of
sympathetic edema, but without high fever or the prolonged
URI picture.

Older children and adolescents with acute maxillary
and/or ethmoid sinusitis may present with either of the
above symptom pictures, but are more likely to complain
specifically of headache and/or facial pain. The headache
may be perceived as frontal, temporal, or even retroauricular.
Facial discomfort can be described as malar pain, or a sense of
pressure or fullness. Occasionally, patients may complain that
their teeth hurt (in the absence of dental pathology). When the
frontal sinuses are involved, frontal or supraorbital headache
is prominent, often perceived as dull or pulsating. The sphenoid sinus is rarely a site of isolated sinus infection, but it is
often involved in pansinusitis, in which case occipital and
postauricular pain may be reported in addition to other sites
of discomfort. Not infrequently the headache is intermittent.
When constant, it varies in severity. This variability appears
related to degree of drainage. Patients reporting copious
"postnasal drip" tend to have less pain. Discomfort and congestion are often most marked on waking, probably as a
result of recumbency and lack of gravity-promoted drainage.
Some patients also report aggravation of pain with head

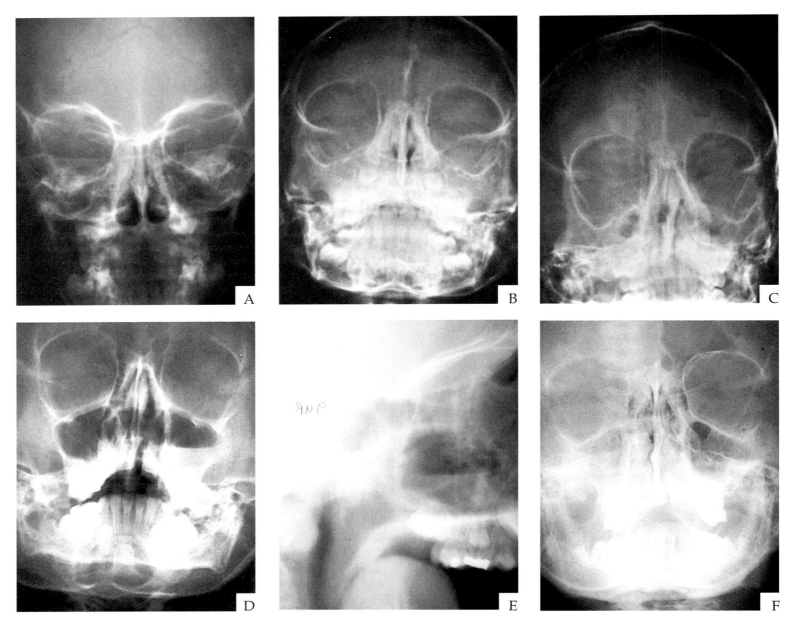

FIG. 22.54 Radiographic findings of sinusitis. *A,* in this Caldwell view, the right ethmoid is clouded, and the bony margins are less distinct than on the left. *B,* in this Waters view, complete opacification of both maxillary sinuses is evident. The bony margins are visible but faint. *C,* this child has significant mucosal thickening of the maxillary sinuses. Thickening of greater than 4 mm has *a strong association* with positive culture on sinus aspirate. An air-fluid level can be seen in the left maxillary sinus on both Waters (*D*) and lateral (*E*) views. *F,* differential opacification of the right frontal sinus is evident in this child who presented with fever and headache. (*D* and *E,* courtesy of Dr. J. Ledesma-Medina, Children's Hospital of Pittsburgh. *F,* courtesy of Dr. C. D. Bluestone, Children's Hospital of Pittsburgh)

movement, particularly with bending down and then straightening up. Swallowed discharge often produces significant abdominal discomfort as well. Cough is often a feature, but tends to be less prominent than in younger children. Physical findings may include purulent (often blood-streaked) nasal and postnasal discharge, erythema of the nasal mucosa, and halitosis. Tenderness on sinus percussion is more common. As with younger children, the clinical spectrum is wide and highly variable.

ANCILLARY DIAGNOSTIC METHODS

When patients have most of the signs and symptoms of sinusitis, the diagnosis can be made on clinical grounds. In less clear-cut cases, ancillary tools and tests are often needed. The usefulness of the various diagnostic methods in evaluating suspected sinusitis is still under study. Radiography does appear to be the most helpful noninvasive tool in children over 1 year of age. Findings of complete opacification, mucosal thickening greater than 4 mm, or an air-fluid level on standard radiography (Fig. 22.54) have a strong association with positive findings on sinus aspiration. However, the wide range of variability in development and configuration of the sinuses can make interpretation difficult. The CT scan is the most sensitive and useful modality for diagnosis, but it does require sedation of the younger patient for an adequate exam. Needle aspiration of the sinuses is conclusive but invasive, and not without risk. It is, however, justified in patients with very severe symptoms, patients with CNS or orbital extension,

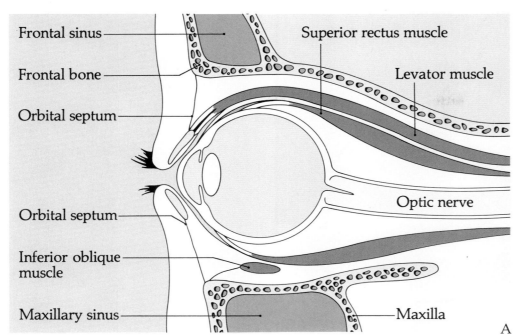

Frontal sinus

Frontal bone

Orbital septum

Superior rectus muscle

Levator muscle

Orbital septum

Inferior oblique muscle

Optic nerve

Maxillary sinus

Maxilla

A

FIG. 22.55 The anatomy of the orbit. **A,** sagittal section shows the relationship of the orbit to the maxillary and frontal sinuses, and the position of the orbital septum within the eyelid. The latter structure appears to serve as an anatomic barrier, helping to prevent the spread of infection from periorbital tissues into the orbit. **B,** in this horizontal section, the close relationship of the orbit to the ethmoid sinuses is apparent.

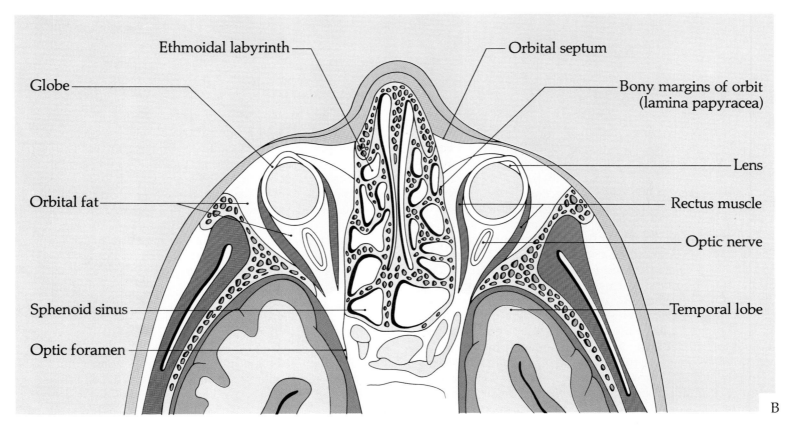

Ethmoidal labyrinth

Orbital septum

Globe

Bony margins of orbit (lamina papyracea)

Lens

Orbital fat

Rectus muscle

Optic nerve

Sphenoid sinus

Temporal lobe

Optic foramen

B

those not responding to treatment, and those who are immunocompromised or immunosuppressed.

At minimum, therapy consists of a 10- to 14-day course (perhaps longer, if duration of symptoms exceeds 3 to 4 weeks) of an antimicrobial agent suitable to the likely spectrum of organisms, analgesia as needed for discomfort, and perhaps, an oral antihistamine in patients known to have allergic rhinitis. Some children with intense headaches or facial pain may experience symptomatic relief from topical nasal vasoconstrictors and warm compresses during the first one or two days of therapy. Patients with sinusitis should be instructed to avoid swimming underwater or diving until completion of therapy, as the resultant barotrauma will aggravate symptoms, and may promote intracranial spread of infection.

COMPLICATIONS OF SINUSITIS

Infectious sinusitis is important not only because of the discomfort it causes, but also because there is a significant risk of extension of infection and secondary complications. This risk stems from several anatomic factors. First, the sinuses surround the orbits superiorly, medially, and inferiorly. The bony plates that make up their walls are very thin and porous, and their suture lines are open in childhood. This is especially true of the lamina papyracea which separate the ethmoid air cells from the orbits (Fig. 22.55). Increased sinus pressure as a result of ostial blockage and fluid collection can cause a separation of portions of these bony septa and can compromise their blood supply. The resultant necrosis thus promotes extension of infection. Facial vascular anatomy also contributes to the

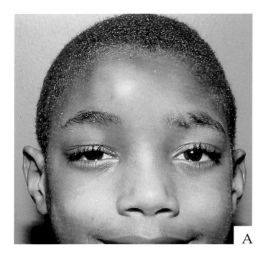
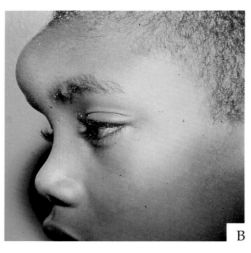
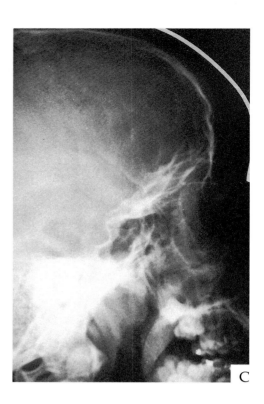

FIG. 22.56 Pott's puffy tumor. *A and B,* this patient presented with fever, headache, and an erythematous swelling over the forehead which was exquisitely tender and had a doughy consistency. *C,* a lateral radiograph shows frontal sinus clouding, irregularity of the frontal bone, and marked soft-tissue swelling which is highlighted by a wire placed over the forehead and scalp. *(C,* courtesy of Dr. Kenneth Grandfast, National Children's Medical Center)

spread of infection. The veins of the face, nose, and sinuses drain, in part, into the orbit, then into the ophthalmic venous system which is in direct continuity with the cavernous sinus. The ophthalmic veins are valveless and, thus, may present less of a defense against spread of infection. The orbit is also devoid of lymphatics, a fact that helps explain the ease of periorbital edema formation when there is increased sinus pressure. The relative looseness of the subcutaneous tissues of the face augments this, and may also aid in spread of infection. As a result of these factors, direct extension of infection can occur (1) into the periorbital soft tissues, producing periorbital cellulitis; (2) through the bony walls into the orbits, resulting in orbital cellulitis; (3) via erosion outward through the frontal bone, producing Pott's puffy tumor; or (4) via erosion inward through the frontal bone, resulting in an epidural abscess. On rare occasions, hematogenous seeding of bacteria may occur.

Fortunately, improved recognition of sinus infection and early use of antimicrobial therapy, whether before or early in the course of recognized extension, have reduced the frequency and severity of these disorders.

Pott's Puffy Tumor

Frontal sinusitis assumes importance after 8 to 10 years of age (once the frontal sinuses have begun to form), and has the potential for serious complications, particularly when neglected or inadequately treated. Erosion anteriorly through the frontal bone results in formation of a subperiosteal abscess classically known as Pott's puffy tumor. This is seen as an erythematous frontal swelling which has a doughy consistency and is exquisitely tender (Fig. 22.56). Affected patients are toxic, febrile, and extremely uncomfortable. Prompt surgical drainage is of utmost importance. A CT scan should be obtained prior to surgical drainage to evaluate the extent of the abscess, and to identify other sites of spread.

Epidural Abscess

Another potential complication of frontal sinusitis is the formation of an epidural abscess as the result of erosion through the posterior wall of the frontal bone. This should be suspected in patients with frontal sinusitis who have unusually high fever, unusually severe headache, signs of toxicity, or altered sensorium. Diagnosis is best confirmed by CT scan (Fig. 22.57). While intravenous antimicrobial therapy and careful monitoring may suffice in management of small lesions, larger abscesses necessitate surgical intervention.

Periorbital and Orbital Infections

PERIORBITAL CELLULITIS DUE TO SPREAD FROM ADJACENT SINUSITIS

This condition is the mildest of the complications of infectious sinusitis. The cellulitis is confined to tissues outside the orbit, with spread blocked in part by the orbital septum (see Fig. 22.55A). When sinusitis is the underlying condition, the ethmoid and/or maxillary sinuses are the structures primarily affected. Typically, patients are under 4 or 5 years of age, and have an antecedent history of upper respiratory infection (with or without conjunctivitis), otitis, or sinusitis. This is superseded by the sudden appearance of lid and periorbital swelling. In contrast to the uncomplicated sympathetic edema seen in some patients with sinusitis, the swelling in these children is usually unilateral, definitely erythematous, indurated, and tender (Fig. 22.58). Conjunctival infection and discharge may also be seen. In many patients, a secondary increase in temperature accompanies the onset of swelling, but while most appear uncomfortable, toxicity is unusual. The course of periorbital cellulitis resulting from extension of sinus infection is milder, and is characterized by much slower progression than is true of cases believed due to hematogenous spread.

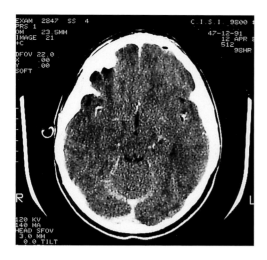 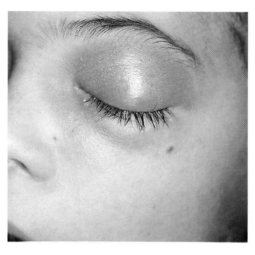 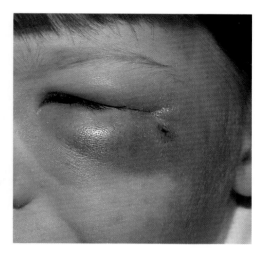

FIG. 22.57 Epidural abscess. This patient presented with lethargy, high fever, left eye pain, and periorbital swelling following 1 week of severe nasal congestion. A CT scan, obtained to rule out orbital involvement, revealed a small epidural abscess behind the left frontal sinus.

FIG. 22.58 Periorbital cellulitis. Intense erythema and edema of the lids are evident. The swollen tissues were indurated and very tender on palpation. Ocular motion was normal. Underlying ethmoid sinusitis was confirmed by CT scan.

FIG. 22.59 Periorbital cellulitis due to spread of an adjacent facial infection. This child developed fever and erythematous, tender periorbital swelling a few days after incurring an abrasion as a result of a fall.

Periorbital Cellulitis Due to Hematogenous Spread

When periorbital cellulitis is the result of hematogenous seeding, the organisms tend to be more virulent, the onset more explosive, and the course more fulminant. Typically, the patient experiences sudden onset of high fever (often following a mild URI) accompanied by the appearance of erythematous, indurated, and tender periorbital swelling. The infection progresses rapidly, and is accompanied by signs of systemic toxicity. The majority of these patients are under 1 year of age or only slightly older, and bacteremia with *H. Influenzae* type B or *S. pneumoniae* is usual.

PERIORBITAL CELLULITIS DUE TO SPREAD FROM ADJACENT FACIAL INFECTION

About 50 percent of periorbital cellulitis cases have neither sinusitis nor bacteremia as a predisposing condition. Rather, the patients appear to suffer from extension of facial infections to periorbital tissues. They tend to have a history of either antecedent trauma to the orbit or nearby facial structures (often with a break in the skin) (Fig. 22.59), or nearby skin infection (impetigo, a pustule, a chalazion, or an infected dermatitis or insect bite). They subsequently experience a temperature spike and evolution of periorbital and eyelid edema, but this is often less abrupt than in patients with underlying sinusitis. This group tends to be somewhat older, generally over 5 years of age. *S. aureus* and group A beta-hemolytic streptococci are the predominant offending organisms.

DIAGNOSTIC STUDIES

A number of cultures are often done in an attempt to isolate the causative pathogen in cases of periorbital cellulitis. Needle aspiration of the leading edge of the cellulitis has perhaps the highest yield, but requires caution. It is, perhaps, best avoided when the inflamed area does not extend beyond the orbital rim. Cultures of adjacent skin wounds, when present, are also commonly positive. Nasopharyngeal and conjunctival drainage reveals the offending organism in about one-half to two-thirds of cases, respectively. Blood cultures are positive in about one-third of patients overall, with the highest incidence found in cases due to hematogenous spread. Sinus x-rays show opacification in over two-thirds of patients without antecedent trauma or skin lesions, and in about 40 to 50 percent of patients with such a history. Ethmoid opacification is the predominant finding. Radiographic interpretation can be difficult, however, as overlying edema may give a false impression of clouding. In addition, x-rays are relatively useless in most cases of hematogenous origin, as the patients are typically under 1 year of age. Computed tomography is, however, an excellent tool for assessing the extent of infection, the presence or absence of sinus opacification, and for detecting evidence of early orbital involvement.

Because of the severity and potential for further extension and hematogenous spread, aggressive intravenous antimicrobial therapy is urgently required. This necessitates empiric selection of agents to cover likely pathogens, pending culture results. Patients also require close monitoring for signs of complications.

ORBITAL CELLULITIS

In this condition, infection extends into the orbit itself. It may take the form of undifferentiated cellulitis or it may evolve into a subperiosteal or orbital abscess. Patients tend to have a history similar to those with periorbital cellulitis, but are generally more ill, toxic, and lethargic. The most common source of spread is an adjacent, infected ethmoid sinus, although extension from a nearby facial infection is seen occasionally. Causative organisms are the same as in periorbital cellulitis. Patients old enough to be articulate describe intense, deep retro-orbital pain aggravated by ocular movement. Edema and erythema of the lid and periorbital tissues are so marked that

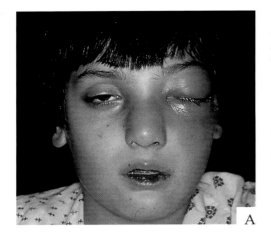 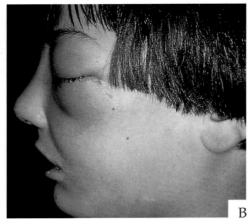 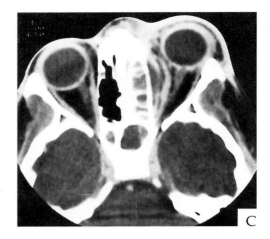

FIG. 22.60 Orbital cellulitis. **A** and **B**, this child presented with fever, severe toxicity, and marked lethargy. He experienced intense pain, and showed a limited range of ocular motion. **C**, this CT scan shows pre- septal swelling, protopsis, and lateral displacement of the globe and orbital contents by a subperiosteal abscess.

it is often impossible to open the eye without use of lid retractors (Fig. 22.60A,B). Tenderness is exquisite. If the lid can be retracted, one may find proptosis, conjunctival inflammation with chemosis and purulent discharge, decreased extraocular motion, and loss of visual acuity.

Aggressive intravenous antimicrobial therapy and close monitoring for evolution and central nervous system complications are vital in management of orbital cellulitis. Computed tomography is proving exceptionally useful for determining the presence or absence of abscesses (Fig. 22.60C). When a subperiosteal abscess is present, or the clinical ocular exam shows deterioration, then surgical drainage combined with an ethmoidectomy is indicated. Optimal management necessitates a team approach involving pediatrics, otolaryngology, ophthalmology, and at times, neurosurgery.

Local complications of orbital cellulitis include abscess formation, optic neuritis, retinal vein thrombosis, and panophthalmitis. Central nervous system complications may result from direct extension or spread of septic thrombophlebitis. Meningitis, epidural and subdural abscesses, and cavernous sinus thrombosis have been described. All are characterized by marked toxicity and alteration in level of consciousness. Cavernous sinus thrombosis is heralded by sudden, bilateral, pulsating proptosis in association with increased toxicity and obtundation.

Atopic Sinus Disorders

ALLERGIC SINUSITIS WITH POSTNASAL DISCHARGE

Patients with allergic rhinitis appear to be more susceptible to infectious sinusitis than nonatopic individuals, probably as a result of mucosal swelling in response to exposure to allergens, and perhaps as a result of alterations in ciliary action. They can also present with symptoms mimicking sinusitis in the absence of infection, and this can be a source of confusion. Two major clinical pictures are seen. In the first, nasal congestion, nighttime cough, and morning throat clearing are prominent. Some patients may complain of morning nausea, and a few may have morning emesis containing large amounts of clear mucus. Fever is absent, and in contrast to infectious sinusitis, nasal discharge is never purulent, there is no halitosis, and daytime cough is not prominent. Patients may complain of itching of the nose and eyes, and some have frequent sneezing.

On examination, the nasal mucosa is edematous, but does not appear inflamed. Discharge, if present, is clear. Patients also tend to have the typical allergic facies (see Chapter 4, Allergy and Immunology) with Dennie's lines, allergic shiners, and cobblestoning of the conjunctivae. Environmental control and antihistamines provide symptomatic relief for most of these children.

VACUUM HEADACHE

The second potentially confusing clinical picture is that of the allergic sinus headache or vacuum headache. In this condition, older atopic individuals complain of intense facial or frontal headache, without fever or other evidence of infection. This is seen during periods in which they are having exacerbation of allergic symptoms or following swimming in chlorinated pools. The phenomenon appears to be due to acute blockage of sinus ostia by mucosal edema, with subsequent creation of a vacuum within the sinus as a result of consumption of oxygen by mucosal cells. The resultant negative pressure pulls the mucosa away from the walls of the sinus, producing the pain. In these patients, the nasal mucosa will tend to be pale and swollen, but without discharge. Sinuses may be tender to percussion, but will be clear radiographically. Symptoms respond promptly to application of a topical vasoconstrictor and warm compresses over the face. Improvement is maintained by antihistamines.

OROPHARYNGEAL DISORDERS

Adequate examination of the pharynx is highly important in pediatrics because of the frequency of pharyngeal infections. However, the procedure can, at times, be challenging. The small size of the mouth and difficulty of depressing the tongue in infancy, lack of cooperativeness in toddlers, and fear of gagging with use of tongue blades in older children can impede efforts. These problems can be minimized by a few simple techniques. Infants and young children, when placed supine with the head hyperextended on the neck, tend to open their mouths spontaneously, enabling visualization of the anterior oral cavity, and facilitating insertion of a tongue blade to depress the tongue and inspect the posterior palate and pharynx. When examining older children, asking them to open their mouths as wide as possible and pant "like a

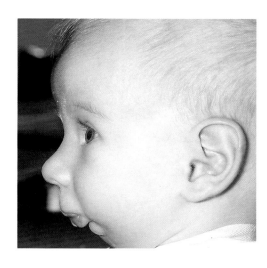

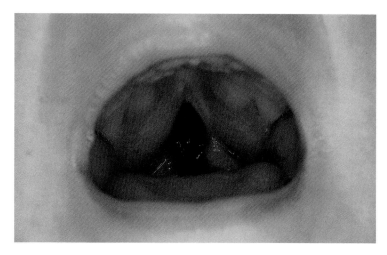

FIG. 22.61 Pierre-Robin syndrome, characterized by severe micrognathia and cleft palate. In this infant, the micrognathia produced posterior displacement of the tongue resulting in airway obstruction which necessitated a tracheostomy. (Courtesy of Dr. Wolfgang Loskin, Children's Hospital of Pittsburgh)

FIG. 22.62 Cleft palate. This child has a midline cleft of the soft palate. The hard palate, alveolar ridge, and lip are spared. (Courtesy of Barbara Elster, RN, PNP, Cleft Palate Center, Pittsburgh)

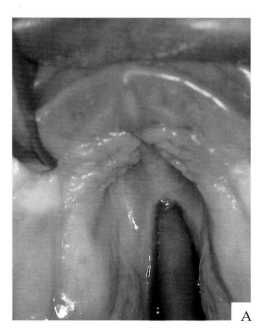

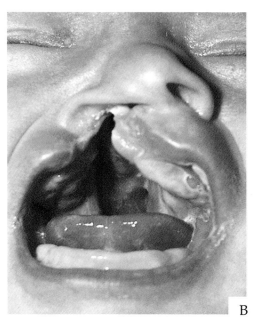

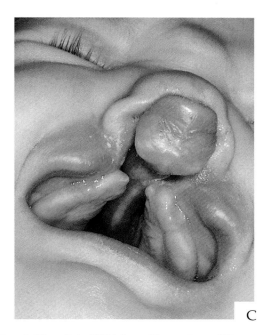

A   B   C

FIG. 22.63 Cleft palate. **A**, cleft of the hard and soft palate, sparing the alveolar ridge. Complete clefts of the palate, alveolar ridge, and lip may be unilateral (**B**) or bilateral (**C**). (**A** and **C**, courtesy of Dr. William Garrett, Children's Hospital of Pittsburg **B**, courtesy of Dr. Michael Sherlock)

puppy dog" or say "ha ha" usually results in lowering of the posterior portion of the tongue, revealing posterior palatal and pharyngeal structures. Because conditions involving the lips, mucosa, and dentition have been presented in Chapter 20, this section will concentrate on palatal and pharyngeal problems.

Palatal Disorders

Palatal malformations range widely in severity, and can have significant impact on feeding, swallowing, and speech. In addition, by altering normal nasal and oropharyngeal physiology, they place affected patients at increased risk for chronic recurrent ear and sinus infections.

CLEFT PALATE

Palatal clefts are among the most severe abnormalities encountered. They stem from a failure of fusion during the second month of gestation, and have an incidence of about 1 in every 2,000 to 2,500 births. They are usually but not always associated with a cleft lip. The defect is often isolated in an otherwise normal child. In many cases, there is a positive family history for the anomaly. A number of teratogens have also been linked to the malformation. In a small percentage of cases, the cleft palate is one of multiple congenital anomalies in the context of a major genetic syndrome such as the Pierre-Robin anomaly (Fig. 22.61) and trisomy 13 and 18.

The extent of the cleft varies: some involve only the soft palate (Fig. 22.62), others extend through the hard palate but spare the alveolar ridge. Still others are complete (Fig. 22.63). The defect may be unilateral or bilateral. The four major types of congenital cleft palate are:

Type I: Soft palate only (Fig. 22.62).

Type II: Unilateral cleft of soft and hard palate (Fig.22.63A).

Type III: Unilateral cleft of soft and hard palate extending through the alveolar ridge (Fig. 22.63B).

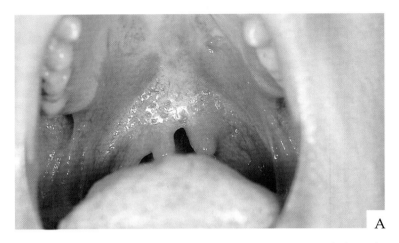 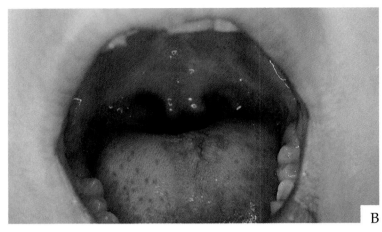

FIG. 22.64 Submucous cleft of the palate. **A,** this girl shows failure of normal midline fusion of the palatal muscles, resulting in midline thinning of the soft palate. Palpation confirms the area of weakness. A U-shaped notch can also be felt in the midline at the junction of the hard and soft palate. She also has a markedly bifid uvula. **B,** this child was found to have a notched uvula on pharyngeal examination. This may serve as a clue to the presence of a submucous palatal cleft, or it may be an isolated anomaly.

Type IV: Bilateral cleft of soft and hard palate extending through the alveolar ridge (Fig. 22.63C).

These anomalies create a number of problems beyond the obvious cosmetic deformity. In infancy, a cleft palate prevents the child from creating an effective seal when nursing and hampers feeding. In addition, formula tends to reflux into the nasopharynx with resultant choking. This necessitates patience in feeding and careful training of parents in feeding techniques to facilitate nursing and prevent failure to thrive. Eustachian tube function is uniformly abnormal and, prior to repair, all patients have chronic middle ear effusions which are frequently infected. Even following repair, recurrent middle ear disease (characterized by negative pressure and effusions) remains a problem. Hearing loss, with its potential for hampering language acquisition, ultimately occurs in over 50 percent of patients. Despite corrective surgery, palatal function is never totally normal, and many patients continue to have hypernasal speech and difficulties in articulation, necessitating long-term speech therapy. Secondary dental and orthodontic problems are routine as well.

The multitude of problems and the need for frequent medical visits and multiple operations, in combination with the oft-associated cosmetic deformity, can have significant psychological impact on both child and family. Optimal management necessitates a multidisciplinary team, preferably coordinated by a primary care physician who is aware of the patient's individual needs and those of his or her family. Timing of corrective surgery remains somewhat controversial. Cleft lips are repaired at about 3 months, but scheduling of palatal repair must be individualized depending on the size and extent of the cleft. Defects of the soft palate are generally repaired at about 8 months, and the hard palate is either closed surgically or by use of a prosthetic plate. Most patients also require early myringotomy with insertion of tubes to help in managing the chronic middle ear disease. Tonsillectomy and adenoidectomy are contraindicated because of adverse effects on palatal function.

Another disorder of clinical importance, *submucous cleft of the palate,* is often missed in infancy. The condition is characterized by a U-shaped notch, palpable in the midline, at the juncture of the hard and soft portions of the palate (Fig. 22.64A).

There may also be palpable midline thinning of the soft palate. The anomaly results from a failure of the tensor veli palatini muscle to insert properly in the midline. Some children have an associated double or notched uvula which, when present, serves as a clue to the existence of the palatal abnormality (Fig. 22.64B). The latter may be an isolated anomaly, however. While not subject to the feeding difficulties seen in children with overt clefts, children with submucous clefts do have similar problems with eustachian tube dysfunction and recurrent middle ear disease. Speech is often mildly hypernasal. Recognition is particularly important when considering tonsillectomy and adenoidectomy for recurrent tonsillitis and otitis, as surgical removal of the adenoids in these children can result. In severe speech and swallowing dysfunction; these procedures may be contraindicated.

HIGH-ARCHED PALATE

This minor anomaly is a common clinical finding (Fig. 22.65). While usually an isolated variant of palatal configuration, it is occasionally seen in association with congenital syndromes. Long-term orotracheal intubation of premature infants is now creating an iatrogenic form of the problem. While generally insignificant clinically, the high arch can be associated with increased frequency of ear and sinus infections, and with hyponasal speech when it is severe.

Tonsillar and Peritonsillar Disorders

PHARYNGITIS/TONSILLITIS

As noted earlier in the section, Acquired Forms of Nasal Obstruction, the tonsils and adenoids are quite small in infancy, gradually enlarge over the first 8 to 10 years of life, then start to regress in size. In evaluating the tonsils, particularly during the course of an acute infection, but also when following patients for chronic enlargement, it is helpful to use a standardized size-grading system, as shown in Figure 22.66. Inspection of the palate is also important in assessing patients with tonsillopharyngitis, as lesions characteristic of particular pathogens are often present on the soft palate and tonsillar pillars (see Chapter 12, Infectious Diseases).

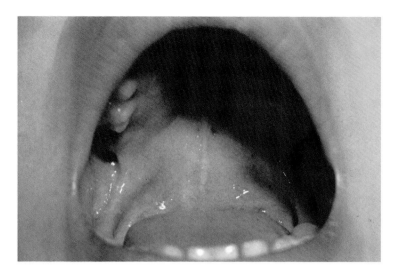

FIG. 22.65 High-arched palate. This is a common minor anomaly, usually isolated, but occasionally associated with genetic syndromes.

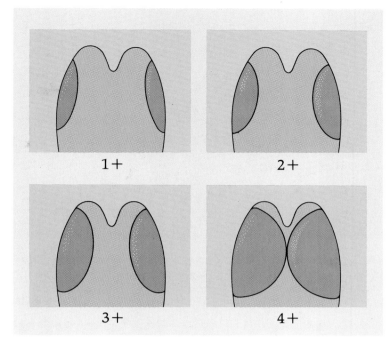

FIG. 22.66 Grading of tonsillar size for children with acute tonsillopharyngitis and those with chronic tonsillar enlargement. This grading system is particularly useful in the serial examinations of a given patient. (Adapted from Feinstein AR, Levitt M: Role of tonsils. N Engl J Med 1970;282:285–291)

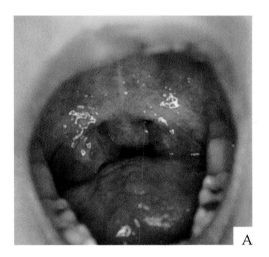

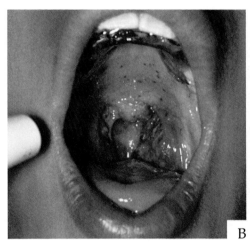

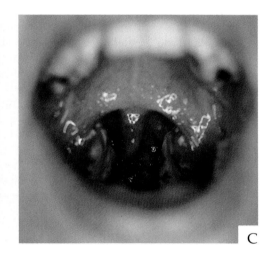

FIG. 22.67 Tonsillopharyngitis. This common syndrome has a number of causative pathogens and a wide spectrum of severity. **A,** the diffuse tonsillar and pharyngeal erythema seen here is a nonspecific finding that can be produced by a variety of pathogens. **B,** this intense erythema, seen in association with acute tonsillar enlargement and palatal petechiae, is highly suggestive of group A beta-streptococcal infection, though other pathogens can produce these findings. **C,** this picture of exudative tonsillitis is most commonly seen with either group A streptococcal or EB virus infection. (**B,** courtesy of Dr. Michael Sherlock)

The tonsils appear to serve as a first line of immunologic defense against respiratory pathogens, and are frequently infected by both viral and bacterial agents. The most commonly identified organisms are group A beta-hemolytic streptococci, adenoviruses, coxsackieviruses, and Epstein-Barr (EB) virus. There is a wide range of severity in symptoms and signs, regardless of the pathogenic organism. Sore throat is the major symptom, and it may be mild, moderate, or severe. When severe, it is typically associated with dysphagia. Erythema is the most common physical finding, and varies from slightly to intensely red (Fig. 22.67). Additional findings may include acute tonsillar enlargement, formation of exudates over the tonsillar surfaces, and cervical adenopathy. In a small percentage of cases, the findings are highly suggestive of a given pathogen. Patients with fever, headache, bright red, enlarged tonsils (with or without exudate), palatal petechiae (Fig. 22.67B), tender and enlarged anterior cervical nodes and, perhaps, abdominal pain are highly likely to have streptococcal infection. Patients with marked malaise, fever, exudative tonsillitis, generalized adenopathy, and splenomegaly are probably suffering from EB virus mononucleosis (Fig. 22.67C; see Chapter 12). Those with conjunctivitis, nonexudative ton-

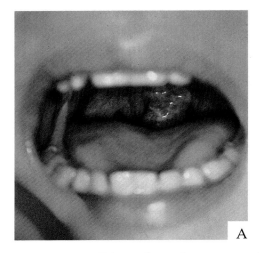 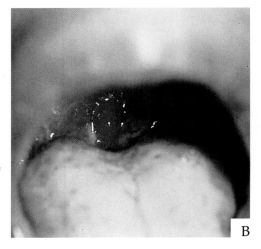 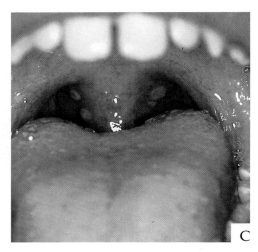

FIG. 22.68 Uvulitis. **A,** the uvula appears markedly erythematous and edematous, with pinpoint hemorrhages, in this case, due to beta-streptococci. **B,** in this child with mononucleosis, not only are the tonsils enlarged and covered with a gray membrane, but the uvula is edematous and erythematous. The patient had respiratory compromise due to the severity of his tonsillar and adenoidal hypertrophy. **C,** the vesicular lesions on the swollen, painful uvula of this patient suggest a viral etiology, probably an enterovirus.

sillar inflammation, and cervical adenopathy may have adenovirus. Presence of yellow ulcerations with red halos on the tonsillar pillars is highly suggestive of coxsackievirus infection whether or not other oral, palmar, or plantar lesions are present (see Chapter 12, Infectious Diseases). Unfortunately, the majority of patients with tonsillopharyngitis do not present with such clear-cut clinical syndromes. Patients with streptococcal infection may have only minimal erythema; in its early stages, mononucleosis may consist of fever, malaise, and nonexudative pharyngitis without other signs; and while streptococci and EB virus are the most common sources of exudative tonsillitis and palatal petechiae, other pathogens can produce these findings as well.

Because of the variability in the clinical picture and the importance of identifying and treating group A beta-streptococcal infection to prevent both pyogenic (such as cervical adenitis, peritonsillar and retropharyngeal abscesses) and nonpyogenic (rheumatic fever) complications, a screening throat culture is advisable for patients presenting with even mild signs and/or symptoms of tonsillopharyngitis. In obtaining this culture, both tonsils and the posterior pharyngeal wall should be swabbed to maximize the chance of obtaining the organism. In the first 3 years of life, when streptococcal infection is suspected (because of history of exposure, signs of pharyngitis, or scarlatiniform rash), it is helpful to obtain a nasopharyngeal (NP) culture as well. For reasons as yet unclear, the NP culture will often be positive while the throat culture is negative in this age group.

Treatment is symptomatic for all forms of tonsillopharyngitis except that due to group A beta-streptococci, which requires a 10-day course of penicillin or erythromycin. Followup is also important. As noted earlier, the tonsillitis of mononucleosis may appear mild early in the course of the illness, yet tonsillar inflammation and enlargement may progress over a few to several days to produce severe dysphagia

and even airway obstruction. Thus, parents should be instructed to notify the physician if such signs develop. Followup is also important in monitoring for other complications and for frequent recurrences.

RECURRENT TONSILLITIS

Frequent recurrences of tonsillitis, despite antibiotic therapy when indicated, must be handled on an individual basis. In some cases, frequent recurrences of streptococcal infection can be traced to another family member or members. When they are treated along with the patient, the cycle of recurrences often ends. In other instances, frequent recurrent tonsillar infections have no traceable source within the family, and they are significantly debilitating. In children with six or more episodes in any one year, or three episodes per year for three consecutive years, tonsillectomy does have a favorable outcome in reducing both frequency and severity of sore throats.

UVULITIS

Uvulitis is characterized by inflammation and edema of the uvula. In addition to throat pain and dysphagia, affected patients commonly complain of a sense of "something in their throat," or a gagging sensation. The phenomenon has been reported in association with pharyngitis due to the group A beta-hemolytic streptococcus, in which cases the uvula was bright red and often hemorrhagic (Fig. 22.68A). We have also noted the condition in association with mononucleosis, both in the presence of and in the absence of exudative tonsillitis (Fig. 22.68B), and we have seen it in association with other viral agents as well (Fig. 22.68C). Uvulitis has also been reported in a patient with concurrent epiglottitis. In this case, the child was anxious, toxic, had high fever, and was drooling, a more severe clinical picture than that seen with streptococcal or EB virus infection. Culture of the uvular surface grew *Haemophilus influenzae*, type B.

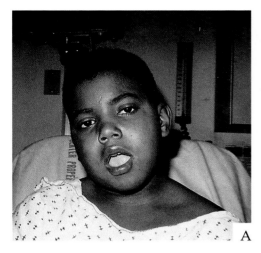
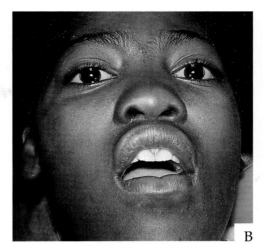
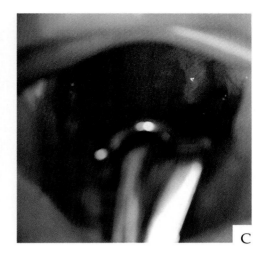

FIG. 22.69 Peritonsillar abscess. **A,** this patient demonstrates the torticollis often seen with a peritonsillar abscess in an effort to minimize pressure on the adjacent, inflamed tonsillar node. **B,** sympathetic inflammation of the pterygoid muscles causes trismus, limiting the patient's ability to open the mouth. **C,** this photograph, taken in the operating room, shows an intensely inflamed soft palatal mass that obscures the tonsil and bulges forward and toward the midline, deviating the uvula.

PERITONSILLAR ABSCESS/CELLULITIS

A peritonsillar abscess is actually an abscess which not only surrounds the tonsil but also extends onto the soft palate. Patients are usually school age or older, and typically have a history of an antecedent sore throat a week or two earlier. This either was not cultured or treated, or the patient took an incomplete course of antimicrobial therapy. The patient may experience initial improvement, but then has a sudden onset of high fever and severe throat pain, worse on one side. The pain usually radiates to the ipsilateral ear, and is associated with marked dysphagia, such that the patient spits out his saliva to avoid swallowing. On examination, the child often appears toxic, and has obvious enlargement of the ipsilateral tonsillar node, which is exquisitely tender. Many patients present with torticollis, tilting the head toward the involved side to minimize pressure of the sternocleidomastoid muscle on the adjacent tonsillar lymph node (Fig. 22.69A). Speech is thick and muffled due to splinting of the tongue and pharyngeal muscles. Trismus, or limitation of mouth opening, is often noted as a result of sympathetic inflammation of the adjacent pterygoid muscles (Fig. 22.69B). If visualization of the pharynx is possible (despite the trismus), a bright red, smooth mass is seen in the supratonsillar area projecting forward and medially, obscuring the tonsil, and deviating the uvula to the opposite side (Fig. 22.69C). Group A beta-streptococci and *Staphylococcus aureus* are the most common pathogens. Patients with mononucleosis, concurrently infected with group A strep and treated with steroids, have been reported to be at risk for a rapidly evolving peritonsillar abscess as well.

If the fluctuant abscess is evident on palpation, operative drainage is needed in addition to parenteral antibiotic therapy to prevent spontaneous rupture and secondary aspiration. When fluctuance is not present, the patient is in a cellulitic stage, and management consists of intravenous antimicrobial therapy and serial reexamination. Because of the risks of rupture, prompt otolaryngologic consultation is suggested from the outset.

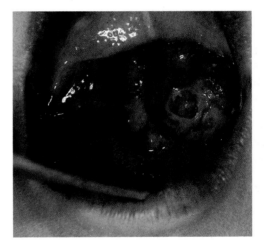

FIG. 22.70 Tonsillar lymphoma. This adolescent presented with painless dysphagia. Examination revealed marked unilateral tonsillar enlargement. The asymmetry and degree of enlargement prompted tonsillectomy. Pathologic examination confirmed a tonsillar lymphoma.

TONSILLAR LYMPHOMA

The vast majority of children, whether well or acutely ill with tonsillitis, have tonsils that are symmetrical in size. When a child is found to have an asymmetrically enlarged tonsil without evidence of infection, the possibility of a lymphoma should be considered (Fig. 22.70). Thorough history of recent health, and meticulous regional and general examination are in order. Particular attention should be paid to cervical and other nodes, and to the size and consistency of abdominal viscera. Hematologic studies may be helpful as well. In the absence of other evidence, a brief period of observation may be justified. If other findings are suggestive, or enlargement continues during observation, excisional biopsy is indicated.

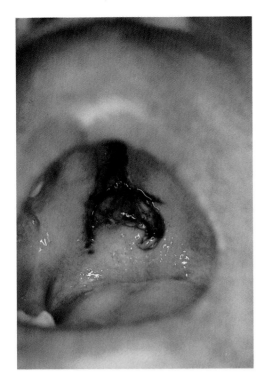

FIG. 22.71 Palatal laceration. This large, complex laceration occurred when this boy fell with a piece of metal tubing in his mouth. A flap of palatal tissue has retracted away from the tears, warranting surgical approximation.

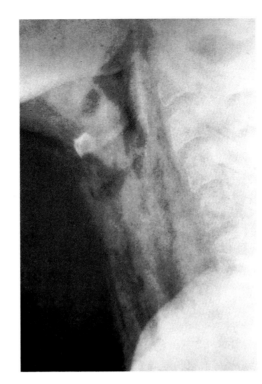

FIG. 22.72 Retropharyngeal air dissection. This lateral neck radiograph of a child with a puncture wound of the posterior pharyngeal wall reveals extensive air dissection through the retropharyngeal soft tissues. Subcutaneous air has tracked anteriorly as well.

Penetrating Oropharyngeal Trauma

Penetrating oral injuries are fairly frequent in childhood and are usually the result of falling with a stick, pencil, or lollipop in the mouth. Gunshot wounds and external stab wounds are unusual occurrences in the pediatric population, but begin to increase in incidence in adolescents.

The majority of intraoral injuries involve the palate and consist of simple lacerations. Many of these heal spontaneously and require no repair. Large lacerations producing mucosal flaps must be sutured (Fig. 22.71). Prophylactic penicillin is also indicated, because of the high risk of secondary infection.

Penetration of the posterior pharyngeal wall may result in a number of complications. Therefore, these patients merit careful clinical evaluation of the oropharynx and neck; neck radiographs should also be obtained. Whenever an object penetrates the pharyngeal wall, it introduces oral flora into the retropharyngeal soft tissues, setting the stage for development of infection and abscess formation (see section on Retropharyngeal Abscess). This complication is seen predominantly in patients who failed to seek care immediately following the injury. However, it can develop even in treated patients. Symptoms generally begin a few to several days following the initial trauma. Fever, pain, dysphagia, and signs of airway compromise predominate.

In a number of patients with posterior pharyngeal tears, penetration results in dissection of air through the retropharyngeal soft tissues (Fig. 22.72). Such children may complain of throat and neck pain. Subcutaneous emphysema may be noted clinically. Occasionally, signs of airway compromise develop with this complication. Therefore, hospitalization for observation is advisable when this sequela is encountered.

When penetration involves posterolateral structures (e.g., the tear is located near the tonsil or tonsillar pillar), the possibility of vascular injury must be considered. Deep penetration in this area can puncture or nick the internal carotid artery or nearby vessels, resulting in hemorrhage or, more commonly, in

CLINICAL FEATURES OF ACUTE UPPER AIRWAY DISORDERS

	Supraglottic Disorders	Subglottic Disorders
Stridor	Quiet and wet	Loud
Voice alteration	Muffled	Hoarse
Dysphagia	+	−
Postural preference*	+	−
Barky cough	−	+ especially with croup
Fever	+	+ usually in croup
Toxicity	+	−
Trismus	+ usually in peritonsillar abscess	−
Facial edema	−	+ usually with angioedema

* Epiglottitis—patient characteristically sits bolt upright, with neck extended and head held forward; retropharyngeal abscess—child often adopts opisthotonic posture; peritonsillar abscess—patient may tilt head toward affected side.

FIG. 22.73 (From Davis HW, et al: Acute upper airway obstruction: croup and epiglottitis. Pediatr Clin North Am 1981; 28:859-880)

ESTIMATION OF SEVERITY OF RESPIRATORY DISTRESS

	Mild	Moderate	Severe
Color	Normal	Normal	Pale, dusky or cyanotic
Retractions	Absent to mild	Moderate	Severe and generalized with use of accessory muscles
Air entry	Mild ↓	Moderate ↓	Severe ↓
State of consciousness	Normal or restless when disturbed	Anxious, restless when undisturbed	Lethargic, depressed

FIG. 22.74 (From Davis HW, et al: Acute upper airway obstruction: croup and epiglottitis. Pediatr Clin North Am 1981; 28:859-880)

gradual hematoma formation. Clues to vascular injury are lateral pharyngeal or peritonsillar swelling, and fullness and/or tenderness on palpation of the neck on the side of the wound. X-rays should confirm soft-tissue swelling. Patients with peritonsillar tears should be admitted for observation even in the absence of these signs. Those with findings suggestive of vascular involvement warrant angiography.

UPPER AIRWAY OBSTRUCTION
Acute Upper Airway Obstruction

Few conditions in pediatrics are as emergent and potentially life-threatening as those causing acute upper airway obstruction. In these conditions, expeditious assessment and appropriate stabilization are often lifesaving. In contrast, underestimation of severity of distress, overzealous attempts at examination or invasive procedures, and efforts by the unskilled to intervene may have catastrophic results.

The major causes are severe tonsillitis with adenoidal enlargement (see section on Tonsillar Disorders and Fig. 22.68B), retropharyngeal abscess, epiglottitis, croup or laryngotracheobronchitis, foreign body aspiration, and angioedema (see Chapter 4, Allergy and Immunology). All are characterized by stridor and retractions that are primarily suprasternal and subcostal (unless distress becomes severe and retractions generalize), and mild to moderate increases in heart rate and respiratory rate. For purposes of assessment, we have found it helpful to classify the disorders into two categories—supraglottic and subglottic—based on major signs and symptoms listed in Figure 22.73.

The key to appropriate management is a brief history detailing the course and associated symptoms, followed by rapid assessment of clinical signs to determine the approximate level of airway involvement and degree of respiratory distress (Fig. 22.74). This can be done for the most part by visual inspection, without ever touching the patient. It is particularly important to avoid upsetting a child with upper airway obstruction who shows signs of fatigue, cyanosis, or meets any of the other criteria for severe distress. Such disturbances can only serve to worsen distress and may precipitate complete obstruction. Therefore, when a child has signs of moderately severe or severe obstruction, his parents should be allowed to remain with him, any positional preference (if manifested) should be honored, and oral examination, venipuncture, IVs, and x-rays should be deferred until the airway is secure. Once the initial assessment is done, the most skilled personnel available are assembled to stabilize the airway. This procedure is best accomplished under controlled conditions in the operating room.

RETROPHARYNGEAL ABSCESS

A retropharyngeal abscess usually involves one of the retropharyngeal lymph nodes which run in chains through the retropharyngeal tissues on either side of the midline. Since these nodes tend to atrophy after 4 years of age, the disorder is seen primarily in children under 3 or 4 years. The major causative organisms are group A beta-streptococci, although Staphylococcus aureus is found in some cases.

The child with a retropharyngeal abscess generally has a history of an acute febrile upper respiratory infection or pharyngitis beginning several days earlier, which may have improved transiently. Suddenly, his condition worsens with development of high spiking fever, toxicity, anorexia, drooling, and dyspnea. On examination, the patient is restless and irritable, and tends to lie with his head hyperextended, simulating opisthotonus. Quiet gurgling stridor is heard. If respiratory distress is not severe, the pharynx can be examined, and a fiery red asymmetrical swelling of the posterior pharyngeal wall may be observed pushing the uvula and ipsilateral tonsil

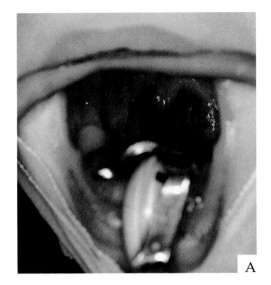
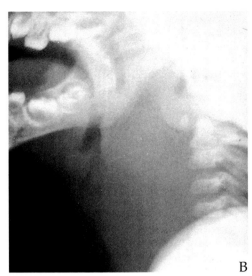
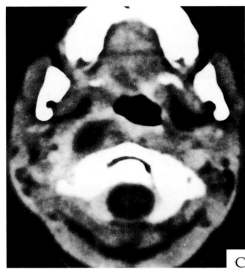

A   B   C

*FIG. 22.75 Retropharyngeal abscess. A young child presented with high fever, drooling, quiet stridor, and an opisthotonic postural preference. **A,** pharyngeal examination in the operating room revealed an intensely erythematous, unilateral swelling of the posterior pharyngeal wall. **B,** a lateral neck radiograph shows prominent prevertebral swelling which displaces the trachea forward. **C,** on CT scan, a thick-walled abscess cavity is evident in the retropharyngeal space. The highly vascular wall enhanced with contrast injection.*

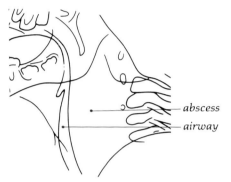

abscess

airway

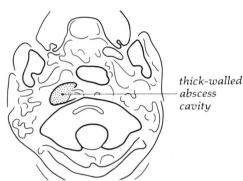

thick-walled abscess cavity

forward (Fig. 22.75A). Even with direct examination, this can be difficult to appreciate at times. A portable lateral neck x-ray (with a physician in attendance) taken on inspiration will show marked widening of the prevertebral tissues (Fig. 22.75B), which are normally no wider than the width of a vertebral body. When diagnosed, prompt otolaryngologic consultation should be sought to determine if the mass is fluctuant, necessitating surgical drainage, or if is in an early cellulitic phase requiring serial reexamination. A CT scan can be helpful in this regard (Fig. 22.75C). High-dose intravenous antimicrobial therapy is needed whether or not drainage is required.

As noted earlier, a retropharyngeal abscess may occasionally form in an older child following a puncture wound of the posterior pharyngeal wall (Fig. 22.76). Signs of infection develop acutely a few days later. In these cases, oral flora are found on culture.

PARAPHARYNGEAL ABSCESS

Lateral neck space abscesses can also occur in infants and young children. Most are toxic with high spiking fevers. The history and clinical picture are nearly identical to that of children with retropharyngeal abscess. However, these patients will have torticollis, bending toward the affected side, and examination of the neck reveals diffuse anterolateral swelling which is exquisitely tender (Fig. 22.77A). Oral inspection may show medial displacement of the tonsil or lateral pharyngeal wall. A CT scan is essential to confirm the diagnosis (Fig. 22.77B). Prompt drainage is important to prevent extension into the mediastinum.

EPIGLOTTITIS

Epiglottitis is an infection caused by *Haemophilus influenzae* type B. It is characterized by marked inflammation and edema of the pharynx, epiglottis, aryepiglottic folds, and ventricular bands. The peak age range is 1 to 7 years, but infants and older children may be affected. Onset is sudden and progression rapid, most patients being brought to medical attention within 12 hours of the first appearance of symptoms. Generally, the child is entirely well until several hours prior to presentation, when he abruptly spikes a high fever. This is rapidly followed by severe throat pain with dysphagia and drooling, and soon thereafter by dyspnea and anxiety.

On examination, the child is usually toxic, anxious, and remarkably still, sitting bolt upright with neck extended and head held forward (unless obstruction is very mild or fatigue has supervened) (Fig. 22.78A–C). Quiet gurgling, stridor, and drooling are evident, along with dyspnea and retractions. If the child will talk, which is unusual, the voice is muffled. This clinical picture is so typical that when seen, the best course of action following initial assessment is prompt airway stabilization, usually intubation under controlled conditions by experienced personnel in the operating room. At this time, the epiglottis will be found to be markedly swollen and erythematous (Fig. 22.78D). Following airway stabilization, cultures can be obtained and intravenous antimicrobial therapy initiated.

On occasion, children present with a similar history but milder symptoms and signs. In these cases, presentation is either very early, or the child is older than average. Respiratory distress is minimal, and visualization of the phar-

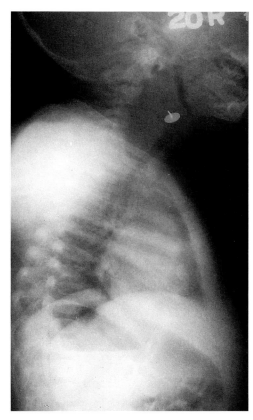

FIG. 22.76 Retropharyngeal abscess following a puncture wound. This child tried to swallow a tack which punctured and became lodged in the posterior pharyngeal wall. The incident was unwitnessed, and he came to medical attention only when he developed fever and began drooling.(Courtesy of Dr. Robert Gochman, Schneider Children's Hospital, Long Island Jewish Medical Center)

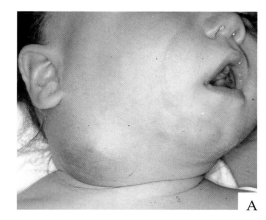

A

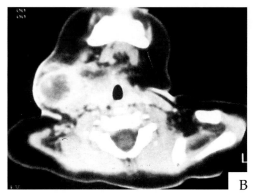

B

FIG. 22.77 Parapharyngeal abscess. **A,** this child presented with high fever, toxicity, and marked, exquisitely tender anterolateral neck swelling with overlying erythema. These manifestations followed a week of URI symptoms and decreased feeding. **B,** his CT scan reveals an encapsulated abscess in the right parapharyngeal area.

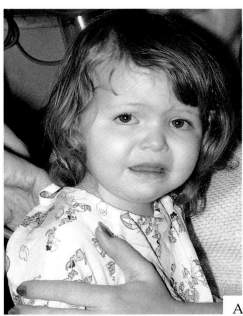

A

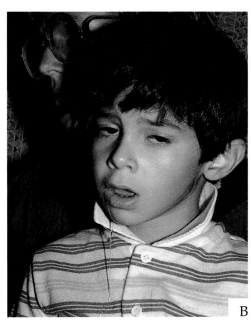

B

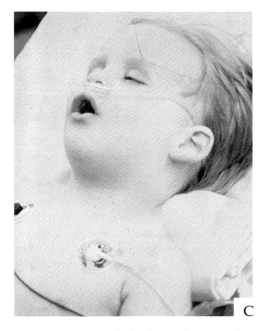

C

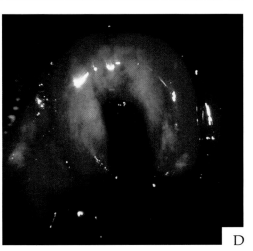

D

FIG. 22.78 Epiglottitis. **A–C,** these three patients with acute epiglottitis demonstrate the varying degrees of distress that may be seen, depending on age and time of presentation. **A,** this 3-year-old seen a few hours after onset of symptoms was anxious and still, but had no positional preference or drooling. **B,** this 5-year-old, who had been symptomatic for several hours, holds his neck extended with head held forward, is mouth breathing and drooling and shows signs of tiring. **C,** this 2-year-old was in severe distress, and was too exhausted to hold his head up. **D,** in the operating room the epiglottis can be visualized and appears intensely swollen.

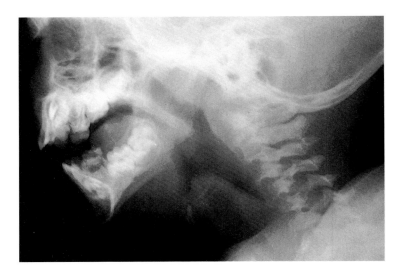

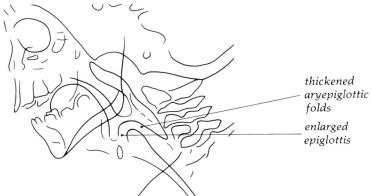

FIG. 22.79 Mild epiglottitis/supraglottitis. The lateral neck radiograph demonstrates mild epiglottic swelling and thickening of the aryepiglottic folds.

thickened
aryepiglottic
folds

enlarged
epiglottis

ynx can be attempted (without use of a tongue blade) if the child will voluntarily open his mouth. In some instances, a swollen epiglottis is seen projecting above the tongue. Where the history suggests epiglottitis, but clinical findings are mild, and the diagnosis is not confirmed by attempted noninvasive visualization, a portable lateral neck x-ray (done in the emergency room with physician in attendance) can be useful. It may reveal mild epiglottic enlargement (Fig. 22.79) or merely swelling of the aryepiglottic folds and ventricular bands: a condition called *supraglottitis*. If either is found, the diagnosis is confirmed. Intubation is generally advisable in the former instance despite mild symptoms, but close observation on intravenous antibiotic therapy (covering for *H. influenzae* type B) may suffice when supraglottitis is the only finding.

CROUP OR LARYNGOTRACHEOBRONCHITIS

This acute respiratory illness is characterized by inflammation and edema of the pharynx and upper airways, with maximal narrowing in the immediate subglottic region. There is probably a component of laryngospasm as well. The vast majority of cases are caused by viral pathogens, with parainfluenza, respiratory syncitial virus, adenoviruses, influenza viruses, and echoviruses being the agents most commonly identified. The peak season is between October and April in the Northern Hemisphere. The disorder primarily affects children between the ages of 3 months and 3 years. This is probably because their airways are narrower, and the mucosa is both more vascular and more loosely attached than in older children, enabling greater ease of edema. Older children can be affected, however.

Typically, the child has had symptoms of a mild upper respiratory infection with rhinorrhea, cough, low-grade fever, and perhaps a sore throat for 1 to 5 days prior to developing symptoms of croup. The change is generally sudden, and usually occurs at night or during a nap. The child awakens with fever, loud inspiratory and expiratory stridor, a loud "barky" or "seal-like" cough, and hoarseness. The severity of symptoms and the course vary widely, and are highly unpredictable. Duration averages 3 days, but can be as brief as 1 day or as long as a week. Most patients have a waxing and waning course, with symptoms more severe at night, but it is impossible to predict which night will be the worst. Some patients remain relatively mild throughout their course, while others

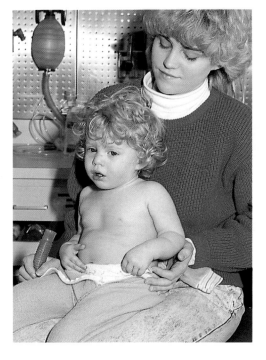

FIG. 22.80 Croup. This toddler with moderate upper airway obstruction due to croup had suprasternal and subcostal retractions. Her anxious expression was due to mild hypoxia confirmed by pulse oximetry.

progress either slowly or rapidly to severe distress. Airway drying, probably in part as a result of mouth breathing necessitated by nasal congestion, appears to aggravate the cough and possibly the element of laryngospasm.

Physical findings are highly variable depending on degree of distress at the time of presentation. Most affected children are moderately febrile but not toxic, and have a loud barky cough and loud inspiratory stridor, with suprasternal and subcostal retractions (Fig. 22.80), and a mild decrease in air entry. A small percentage of patients with more extensive airway inflammation may have wheezing on auscultation. Many improve substantially as a result of exposure to cool night air during the trip to the ER. Some have restlessness or agitation reflecting hypoxia, and a few have severe distress. In these more severely affected patients, stridor may be both inspiratory and expiratory, with generalized retractions. If impairment of air flow is extreme, fatigue supervenes, stridor abates, and retractions diminish. *This must not be mistaken for clinical*

CROUP SCORING SYSTEM

	0	1	2	3
Stridor	None	Mild	Moderate at rest	Severe, on inspiration and expiration, or none with markedly decreased air entry
Retraction	None	Mild	Moderate	Severe, marked use of accessory muscles
Air entry	Normal	Mild decrease	Moderate decrease	Marked decrease
Color	Normal	Normal (0 score)	Normal (0 score)	Dusky or cyanotic
Level of consciousness	Normal	Restless when disturbed	Anxious, agitated; undisturbed	Lethargic, depressed

FIG. 22.81 (Modified from Taussig et al: Treatment of laryngotracheobronchitis (croup): use of intermittent positive pressure breathing and racemic epinephrine. Am J Dis Child 1975; 129:790-793)

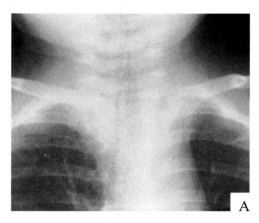

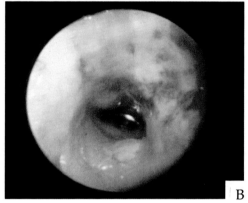

FIG. 22.82 Croup. **A,** this radiograph reveals a long area of narrowing extending well below the normally narrowed area at the level of the vocal cords. The finding is often termed the "steeple sign." **B,** in this patient, direct visualization revealed subglottic narrowing that was so severe, only tracheostomy would enable establishment of an adequate airway.

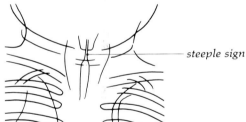

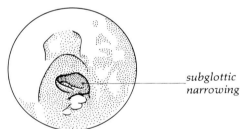

improvement. A clinical scoring system which helps in grading severity of distress is presented in Figure 22.81. In mild to moderate cases, the pharynx can be visualized and reveals only mild erythema. Oral examination should be deferred in severe cases until the airway is secure. Radiography can be helpful in demonstrating subglottic narrowing—the "steeple sign" (Fig. 22.82A). However, this is not necessary for patients with mild disease, and it is contraindicated for those with severe distress.

Management is dependent largely on severity of distress when seen, and on clinical response to mist therapy. Most patients have mild disease. They improve considerably on mist alone, and can be managed at home with humidification. Parents must, however, be instructed to watch for signs of increasing distress which would warrant return to the hospital. Aerosolized racemic epinephrine has been proven to be effective in reducing airway obstruction due to croup. It is particularly useful for children with moderate obstruction who do not show marked improvement on mist alone, and can provide significant relief for children with severe distress. This agent, though effective, is short-acting and rebound tends to occur. Thus, patients requiring racemic epinephrine should generally be admitted for further observation. The effectiveness of steroids is as yet unproved.

Patients in severe distress who do not improve dramatically following treatment with racemic epinephrine, and those who steadily worsen in the hospital despite mist and aerosol treatments warrant airway stabilization, either via intubation or tracheostomy under controlled conditions in the operating room. The choice of procedure remains controversial and is perhaps best made in accordance with the skills of the personnel and facilities available at the individual institution. In some instances, subglottic narrowing is so severe as to necessitate tracheostomy (Fig. 22.82B). Attempts at emergency tracheostomy are fraught with hazard and should be avoided at all costs.

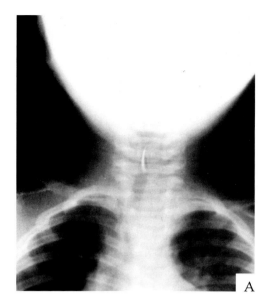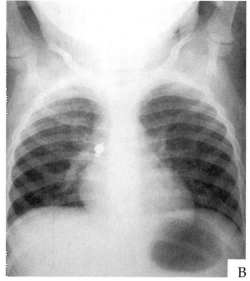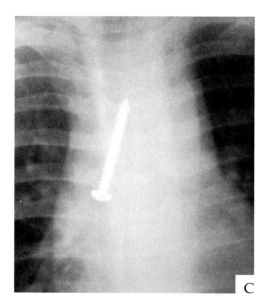

FIG. 22.83 Foreign body aspiration. Radiopaque objects and those well outlined by air are readily visualized on x-ray. **A,** a piece of eggshell is seen in the subglottic portion of the trachea, clearly outlined by the air column. **B,** an earring lies in the entrance of the right mainstem bronchus. **C,** a screw is seen lodged in the right mainstem bronchus and projecting into the trachea. (**A,** courtesy of Dr. Mananda Bhende, Children's Hospital of Pittsburgh. **B** and **C,** courtesy of Dr. Robert Gochman, Schneider Children's Hospital, Long Island Jewish Medical Center)

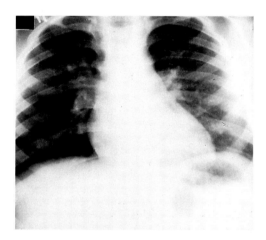

FIG. 22.84 Foreign body aspiration with ipsilateral hyperinflation. This 18-month-old child was eating popcorn when he suddenly began choking. Within a few hours, he developed significant respiratory distress and his chest x-ray revealed massive hyperinflation of the right lung due to the ball-valve effect of the popcorn lodged in the right mainstem bronchus. (Courtesy of Department of Radiology, Uniontown Hospital,Uniontown, PA)

BACTERIAL TRACHEITIS

In a small percentage of cases, children presenting with a croup-like picture are atypically toxic, markedly febrile, and have rapidly progressive airway obstruction necessitating urgent intubation. Bronchoscopy prior to airway stabilization reveals severe inflammation and edema, and a copious, purulent subglottic exudate which contains large numbers of bacteria. Most of these patients appear to have a history of viral croup with sudden worsening. It is thus thought that the disorder may represent secondary bacterial infection. However, there is still some question that this disorder may represent an unusually virulent form of viral laryngotracheobronchitis.

FOREIGN BODY ASPIRATION

This problem is seen for the most part in older infants and toddlers. The story is usually one of a sudden choking episode while the child was eating material that the immature dentition is ill equipped to chew. Such foods include nuts, seeds, popcorn, raw vegetables such as carrots and celery, and hot dogs. Occasionally, the episode occurs when the child is chewing on a small object, a toy, or a detachable portion of a toy. If the object lodges in the larynx, asphyxiation results unless the Heimlich maneuver or backslaps are performed promptly. In the majority of cases, the foreign material clears the larynx and lodges in the trachea or a bronchus (more commonly, the right mainstem). Following the choking spell, there is a silent period usually lasting a few to several hours (occasionally days or weeks), after which the child develops cough and either stridor (lodged in trachea) or wheezing (lodged in a bronchus), and respiratory distress. In this acute phase, when the object is situated in a bronchus, wheezing may be unilateral and associated with decreased breath sounds. Later, diffuse wheezing may be heard simulating asthma or bronchiolitis. Lateral neck and chest radiography will reveal aspirated objects that are radiopaque or outlined by the air column (Fig. 22.83A–C), enabling localization prior to endoscopy. However, most cases involve materials not visible on x-ray, although other radiographic clues may be present. Partial obstruction of a bronchus creates a ball-valve effect, allowing air in during inspiration but preventing its egress on expiration. This pro-

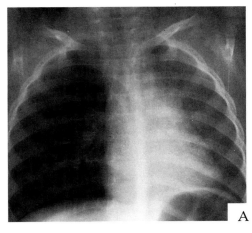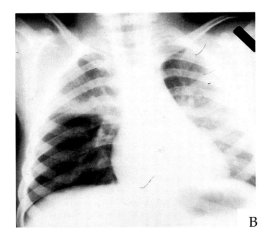

FIG. 22.85 *Foreign body aspiration, inspiratory and expiratory radiographs. A, this inspiratory film taken during fluoroscopy suggests hyperinflation of the right lower and middle lobes. B, this becomes much more evident on expiration when the hyperinflation persists, and the mediastinum shifts to the opposite side. (Courtesy of Dr. Robert Gochman, Schneider Children's Hospital, Long Island Jewish Medical Center)*

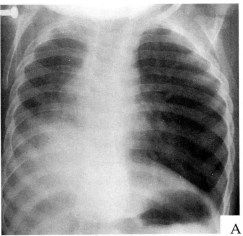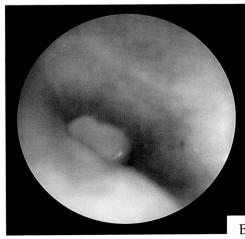

FIG. 22.86 *Foreign body aspiration—delayed presentaton. A, with delay in presentation of partial obstruction or with complete obstruction of a bronchus, radiographic findings consist of atelectasis and a mediastinal shift toward the side of the foreign body. B, in this case, a peanut was found completely obstructing the bronchus. (Courtesy of Dr. Robert Gochman, Schneider Children's Hospital, Long Island Jewish Medical Center)*

duces hyperinflation of one or more lobes of the lung on the same side as the foreign body (Fig. 22.84) which may be evident on the plain chest film. In subtler cases, chest fluoroscopy may highlight the differential inflation and deflation, showing mediastinal shift away from the side of the foreign body (Fig. 22.85). These findings are particularly likely if the patient is seen fairly soon after the aspiration episode. When there is a delay in seeking medical attention (usually because the aspiration episode was unwitnessed and onset of symptoms is insidious), the patient may present with cough and fever. In these instances, atelectasis and a mediastinal shift toward the side of the foreign body may be found on chest x-ray (Fig. 22.86). This finding may be seen acutely when the bronchus is totally obstructed. It is essential to recognize that many patients will have no detectable radiographic abnormality following foreign body aspiration. Hence, when clinical suspicion is high, given the history and physical findings, endoscopic examination is indicated despite normal plain films. Conversely, when physical findings and x-rays are normal, and the history is questionable, a period of close observation may be indicated.

Unfortunately, in up to 50 percent of cases, the aspiration episode is not reported, either because the parent does not relate it to the child's symptoms or did not witness the choking spell. For this reason, this diagnosis should be considered and specific questions asked regarding possible aspiration whenever a young child presents with acute onset of cough and stridor or experiences a first episode of wheezing.

Chronic Upper Airway Obstruction

SUBGLOTTIC STENOSIS

This is a disorder in which the subglottic region of the trachea is unusually narrow in the absence of infection. In some instances, the stenosis is the result of abnormal cricoid development and is, therefore, congenital. In other cases, narrowing is the long-term result of injury and scarring from prior intubation. Regardless of source, these children tend to develop stridor and respiratory distress with every upper respiratory infection. A few are identified by virtue of having an atypically prolonged episode of croup. Some also have stridor with crying, even when well. Neck x-rays may present a similar appearance to that seen with croup. The problem generally improves with growth, but up to 40 percent of these children develop such severe distress with colds that tracheostomy is required.

LARYNGOMALACIA

This congenital condition accounts for 60 percent of cases of persistent stridor in infants. The problem is the result of unusual flaccidity of the laryngeal structures, especially the epiglottis and the arytenoid cartilages. The etiology is uncer-

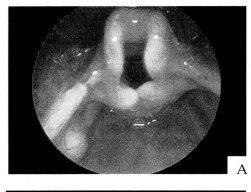

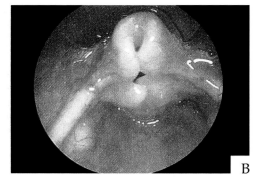

FIG. 22.87 Laryngomalacia. **A,** note the omegoid shape of the epiglottis, and the elongation of the arytenoid cartilages. **B,** this is the larynx during inspiration. Note that the forces of the inspired air lead to collapse of the laryngeal inlet. Infolding of the epiglottic surfaces and the arytenoid cartilages causes partial airway obstruction.

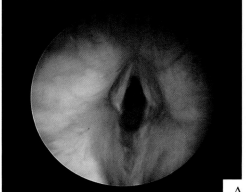

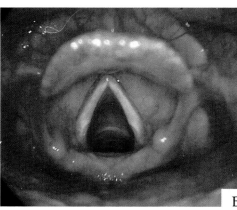

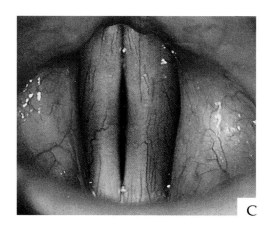

FIG. 22.88 Bilateral vocal cord paralysis. **A,** the marked narrowing of the aperture between the cords stems from loss of ability to abduct on inspiration. This is in contrast to normal opening and closing on inspiration and expiration as seen in **B** and **C.**

tain, but it is thought to be due to lack of neural coordination of the laryngeal muscles, with the result that supraglottic structures hang over the airway entrance like a set of loose sails over a sailboat (Fig. 22.87).

Clinically, these infants tend to have mild inspiratory stridor which is worse when lying supine, and which tends to improve when they are placed in the prone position or when their necks are slightly hyperextended. The condition is usually benign, and rarely interferes with feeding or respiration. The diagnosis can be confirmed only by direct visualization of the larynx during active respiration. This is important in that it is necessary to document that the stridor is not due to a more dangerous condition. Once the examination has been completed, one can reassure the parents that the condition is benign and that with growth, the stridor will usually abate by the end of the first year and a half of life. Management consists of observation, with particularly close monitoring during upper respiratory infections.

VOCAL CORD PARALYSIS

Paralysis of the vocal cords may be present at birth, or it may develop in the first 2 months of life. It may be bilateral or unilateral. The underlying problem generally is located somewhere along the vagus nerve, and may be found either in the central nervous system or in the periphery. Even though many paralyses are idiopathic, a thorough evaluation must be done to locate the lesion and identify its source. Ten percent of stridor in neonates is thought to be due to this condition.

Infants with unilateral cord paralysis present with stridor, hoarseness, and a weakened voice. The airway diameter is generally adequate for respiration, and unless a secondary lesion is present, it is rarely necessary to perform a tracheotomy. This lesion is most often due to a cardiac abnormality, because the recurrent laryngeal nerve is looped around these structures as it passes through the chest.

In contrast, bilateral vocal cord paralysis is a life-threatening condition, as the vocal cords are unable to abduct on inspiration and there is concomitant stridor and cyanosis due to severe narrowing of the aperture between the cords (Fig. 22.88). This condition usually is associated with a depressed laryngeal cough reflex, and therefore aspiration is common. A tracheotomy is essential to secure the airway. Hydrocephalus and Arnold-Chiari malformations often are the underlying problem, as they cause compression of the vagus nerve as it leaves the brainstem. Neurosurgical intervention may correct the problem and allow eventual decanulation.

JUVENILE LARYNGEAL PAPILLOMATOSIS

This is a condition in which multiple benign papillomas develop and grow on the vocal cords. In a few patients, they may extend to involve the pharyngeal walls or tracheal mucosa. They are apparently of viral origin, and there is some evidence of transmission during delivery to children born to mothers with condyloma accuminata. The main symptom is hoarseness, but stridor may develop in children with large lesions or tracheal extension. Radiographs are usually normal. The diagnosis should be considered in patients with chronic hoarseness and in those with atypically prolonged croup. On laryngoscopy, irregular warty masses are seen (Fig. 22.89). Biopsy is required to confirm the diagnosis. Excision can be attempted using forceps or a laser, but it is often followed by regrowth. Tracheostomy should be avoided if at all possible,

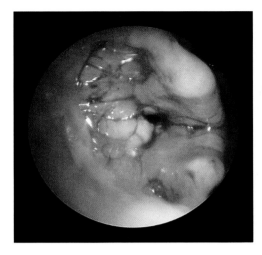

FIG. 22.89 Laryngeal papillomas. Multiple smooth, warty growths are seen nearly occluding the larynx in this child who had a history of chronic hoarseness.

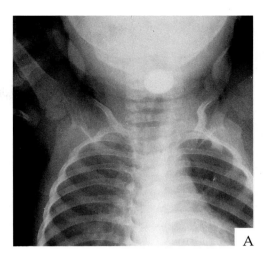

A

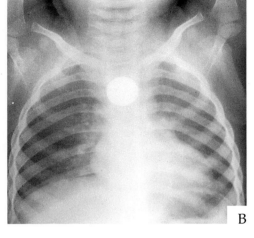

B

FIG. 22.90 Esophageal foreign bodies. **A,** this youngster accidentally swallowed a coin. He complained of throat pain and refused oral intake. When initially seen, the coin was lodged high in the esophagus. **B,** following observation overnight, repeat radiography revealed that the coin had moved but was still lodged in the esophagus. The patient under-

went endoscopic removal. Note that asymmetric objects in the esophagus are oriented in the coronal plane, whereas in the trachea they lie in the saggital plane (see Fig. 20.83A). (Courtesy of Dr. Robert Gochman, Schneider Children's Hospital, Long Island Jewish Medical Center)

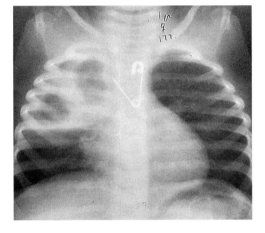

FIG. 22.91 Esophageal foreign body. An unwitnessed ingestion of this safety pin led to a period of anorexia followed by fever and respiratory distress. The point of the pin had perforated the esophageal wall and pleura, causing a secondary right upper lobe pneumonia. (Courtesy of Dr. Robert Gochman, Schneider Children's Hospital, Long Island Jewish Medical Center)

as this often promotes seeding further down the tracheobronchial tree.

ESOPHAGEAL FOREIGN BODIES

Ingestion of foreign objects is relatively common in older infants and toddlers, who are prone to putting almost anything they can pick up into their mouths. Coins, small toys, and pieces of toys are the objects most frequently found. Most traverse the esophagus, stomach, and intestines without incident and are of little concern. A small percentage of swallowed foreign bodies, being too large to pass through to the stomach, become lodged in the esophagus (usually at the level of the cricopharyngeus [C6] and, less commonly, at the level of the aorta [T4], or the diaphragmatic inlet [T11–12]). With mild obstruction the child may refuse solid foods (although 17 percent of patients are asymptomatic); with moderate obstruction liquids will often be refused as well, or the child may appear to choke with drinking. When obstruction is nearly complete, the child may begin drooling. If the object is particularly large, it may compress the trachea as well, producing signs of upper airway obstruction. Older patients may complain of neck or substernal pain or discomfort, especially with swallowing.

Patients who have significant symptoms of esophageal and/or respiratory obstruction, and those who have ingested sharp, potentially toxic, or caustic objects should undergo prompt endoscopic removal. Those who have ingested smooth objects and have mild symptoms can be observed for 12 hours and then have a repeat x-ray. If the object has passed into the stomach, then endoscopy can be avoided. Otherwise, such intervention is indicated.

While in many cases there is a clear history of ingestion, in a significant percentage, the ingestion was not witnessed. A high level of suspicion is often required to make the diagnosis, and the possibility of an esophageal foreign body should be considered in evaluating any young child for a sudden change in eating pattern. Plain radiographs will detect metallic and other radiopaque objects (Fig. 22.90). Most objects are plastic, however, and require barium swallow or, in some cases, endoscopy for detection. Delays in diagnosis can result in stricture formation or, more rarely, in esophageal perforation with secondary pneumomediastinum, mediastinitis, pneumonia (Fig. 22.91) and/or large vessel hemorrhage.

Note

Neck disorders, including adenitis, congenital cysts, vascular and lymphatic masses and tumors are commonly managed by otolaryngologists. Limitations of space have required us to be selective in presenting disorders in this chapter. The reader is referred to Chapter 12 for a discussion of cervical adenitis, and to Chapter 17 for a description of mass lesions.

Acknowledgments

The authors would like to acknowledge and thank Children's Hospital of Pittsburgh, Department of Radiology, and University Health Center of Pittsburgh, Department of Neuroradiology, for providing many of the radiographs and CT scans seen in this chapter.

BIBLIOGRAPHY

Bluestone CD, Stool SE (eds): *Pediatric Otolaryngology, ed 2.* Philadelphia, WB Saunders, 1990.

Bluestone CD: Recent advances in the pathogenesis, diagnosis, and management of otitis media. *Pediatr Clin North Am* 1981;28:727–755.

Bluestone CD, Wald ER, Shapiro GC: The diagnosis and management of sinusitis in children. Proceedings of a closed conference. *Pediatr Infect Dis J* 1985;4:549.

Bowen A'D, Ledesma-Medina J, Fujioka M, et al: Radiologic imaging in otorhinolaryngology. *Pediatr Clin North Am* 1981;28:905–939.

Davis HW, Gartner JC, Galvis AG, et al: Acute upper airway obstruction: croup and epiglottitis. *Pediatr Clin North Am* 1981;28:859–880.

Gellady AM, Shulman ST, Ayoub EM: Periorbital and orbital cellulitis in children. *Pediatrics* 1978;61:272–277.

Lim DJ, Bluestone CD, Klein JO, Nelson JD (eds): *Recent Advances in Otitis Media with Effusion.* Toronto, BC Decker, 1988.

McGuirt WF (ed): *Pediatric Otolaryngology Case Studies.* Garden City, NY, Medical Examination Publishing Company, 1980.

Wald ER: Acute sinusitis in children. *Pediatr Infect Dis J* 1983;2:61–68.

Wald ER, Milmoe GI, Bowen A'D, et al: Acute maxillary sinusitis in children. *N Engl J Med* 1981;304:749–754.

INDEX

Note: The numbers in bold refer to
Figure numbers.

Abdomen
    injuries, 6.11–6.12, **6.24**
    pain, 10.10–10.11, **10.27–10.29**
    signs and symptoms of cancer, 11.32,
        11.90–11.92
Abdominal masses, 17.20–17.25, **17.62,
    17.63**
    genitourinary obstructions,
        17.21–17.22, **17.64–17.69**
    inflammatory masses, 17.24–17.25,
        17.78
    neoplasms, 17.22–17.24, **17.70–17.77**
Abdominal pain, 17.18–17.20,
    17.55–17.61
Abdominal wall, 17.30–17.35
    gastroschisis and omphalocele,
        17.30–17.32, **17.104–17.108**
    inguinal hernia and hydrocele,
        17.32–17.35, **17.112–17.120**
    umbilicus, 17.32, **17.109–17.111**
Abrasions, 20.16
Abscesses
    dental, 20.14–20.15, **20.46–20.48**
    of the skin and soft tissues,
        12.20–12.22, **12.30–12.33**
Accessory tarsal navicular, 21.45, **21.93**
Accommodative esotropia, 19.7–19.8,
    19.15, 19.16
Acne, 8.27–8.28, **8.64**
Acquired immunodeficiency syndrome
    (AIDS), 4.26–4.30, **4.54–4.63**. *See also*
    Human immunodeficiency virus
    and nephrotic syndrome, 13.3
Acute necrotizing ulcerative gingivitis,
    20.15, **20.50**
Adenovirus, 12.4, **12.5**
Alagille syndrome, 10.14, **10.39,**
    13.17–13.18, **13.44**
Albinism, 8.42, **8.106,** 19.29, **19.88, 19.89**
Alder–Reilly bodies, 11.21, **11.55, 11.56**
Allergic rhinitis, 4.3–4.5, **4.4–4.11**
Allergies. *See* Hypersensitivity disor-
    ders
Alopecias, 8.43–8.45, **8.107–8.111**
Alport syndrome, 13.15, **13.36–13.18**
Amblyopia, 19.13–19.14, **19.29**
Anaphylactic laryngeal edema, 4.6
Amelogenesis imperfecta, 20.10, **20.32,
    20.33**
Anemia, 11.3–11.4
    and developmental delay, **3.27**
    chronic, renal failure of, 13.19–13.20,
        13.51

hemolytic, 11.10–11.14, **11.18–11.28**
hypochromic/microcytic, 11.3–11.6,
    11.6–11.17
macrocytic, 11.7–11.8
normocytic, normochromic,
    11.8–11.14
Aneurysm, coronary artery, **7.31**
Angelman syndrome, 1.16–1.18,
    1.28–1.30
Angioedema, 4.16–4.18, **4.33–4.37**
    hereditary, 4.31–4.32
Aniridia, 19.24, **19.68**
Anisocoria, 19.35
Ankyloblepharon, 19.17
Ankylosing spondylitis, **7.10**
Anthropometric measurements and lab-
    oratory tests, in nutrition, 10.3–10.4,
    10.10–10.13
Anus, 17.35–17.37, **17.121–17.128**
    imperforate, 3.10, **13.23**
Aphthous ulcers, 20.13–20.14, **20.45**
Apnea and sudden infant death syn-
    drome (SIDS), 16.15, **16.36**
Arthritis, septic,12.41–12.43, **12.57–12.59**
Arthrogryposis, 21.48–21.49, **21.101**
Ash leaf spots, 8.41–8.42, 15.4, **15.9**
Asthma, 4.6–4.14, **4.13–4.26**
    differentiating features and bronchi-
        olitis, **4.23**
    scoring system, **4.18**
Asymmetric tonic neck reflex (ATNR),
    3.2
Ataxia, and developmental delay, **3.27**
Ataxia telangiectasia, 4.25, 15.6, **15.18**
Audiogram, **3.45**
Autosome abnormalities, 1.7–1.11
Avulsions, 20.16, 20.19, **20.52, 20.62**

Band keratopathy, **7.9**
Bayley Scales of Infant Development,
    3.28
Bee sting, **4.27**
Behavior, developmental, 3.1–3.29
    assessment, 3.1
    cognitive development, 3.10–3.13
    assessment, 3.12–3.13, **3.27, 3.28**
    early sensory processing, 3.10
    logical thinking development,
        3.11–3.12, **3.26**
    sensorimotor intelligence develop-
        ment, 3.10–3.11, **3.23, 3.25**
    symbolic capability development,
        3.11
    and visual impairment, 3.28–3.29
    fine motor development, 3.7–3.10
    of complex skills, 3.8, **3.19**

evaluation and testing, 3.8–3.10, **3.21,
    3.22**
involuntary grasp, 3.7, **3.14**
and visual impairment, 3.28
voluntary grasp, 3.7–3.8, **3.15–3.18**
gross motor development, 3.1–3.7
antigravity muscular control, 3.3–3.5,
    3.5–3.10
assessment during health mainte-
    nance visits, 3.5–3.7
complex pattern development, 3.5
early reflex patterns, 3.1–3.3
locomotion development, 3.5, **3.11,
    3.12**
potential causes of delayed, **3.13**
and visual impairment, 3.28
language development, 3.13–3.16
assessment, 3.15–3.16
early skills in speech perception and
    production, 3.13
later development, 3.15, **3.30**
mastering intelligibility and fluency,
    3.15, **3.31**
and visual impairment, 3.29
principles of normal development,
    3.1
social development, 3.16–3.18
attachment development, 3.16–3.17
early capabilities, 3.16, **3.32, 3.33**
evaluation, 3.18
play development, 3.17
responsivity, 3.16, **3.32, 3.33**
self–development, 3.17–3.18, **3.34,
    3.35**
and visual impairment, 3.29
variations in developmental patterns,
    3.18–3.29
Biotin, as nutritional deficiency, **10.15**
Birth injury, 3.13
Bites. *See* Human bites; Insect bites
Bleeding disorders, 11.22–11.25, **11.59**
    coagulopathies, 11.24–11.25,
        11.64–11.67
    platelet disorders, 11.22–11.24,
        11.60–11.63
Blepharoptosis, 19.14, **19.33**
Blood pressure and pulse, 5.2
Blount's disease, 21.39, **21.82**
Bone cysts, 6.16, **6.37**
Bottle and pacifier habits, 20.5, **20.10**
Boutonnière deformity, 21.32–21.33,
    21.74
Brachial plexus injury, 3.13
Brain
    morphologic abnormalities, 3.13
Breast, abscess, 12.21–12.22, **12.32**

Breast feeding
    advantages, **10.2**
    comparison of milks, **10.3**
Bronchiolitis, differentiating features
    and asthma, **4.23**
Bronchopulmonary aspergillosis, aller-
    gic, 4.19, **4.38–4.40**
Brown's syndrome, 19.11, **19.25**
Bruises, 6.3–6.4, **6.1, 6.2, 6.13, 6.25, 6.26**
Bubonic plague, 12.34
Burns, 6.5–6.6, **6.7–6.11, 6.14, 6.15, 6.30,
    6.32**, 20.17

Caffey's disease, 6.17, **6.40**
Calcaneovalgus foot deformity, 21.44,
    21.91
Calcium, as nutritional deficiency, **10.15**
Cancer
    evaluation of bone pain, 11.35–11.36,
        11.103–11.106
    mediastinal masses, 11.35,
        11.100–11.102
    signs and symptoms of
        abdominal, 11.32, **11.90–11.92**
        chest, 11.31, **11.89**
        head, 11.28–11.31, **11.78, 11.79**
        musculoskeletal, 11.33–11.34, **11.97,
            11.98**
        nervous system, 11.34, **11.78**
        ophthalmologic, 11.29–11.30,
            11.80–11.82
        skin, 11.27–11.28, **11.71–11.77**
        urogenital, 11.32–11.33, **11.93–11.96**
Candida, 18.21–18.22, **18.35**
Candidiasis, 20.15–20.16, **20.51**
Canker sores. See Aphthous ulcers
Caput succedaneum, 2.10, **2.27**
Cardiology, 5.1–5.17
    congenital heart disease, physical
        diagnosis, 5.1–5.7, **5.1–5.4**
    bacterial endocarditis, 5.7, **5.15–5.17**
    blood pressure and pulse, 5.2
    cyanosis and clubbing, 5.1–5.2
    heart murmur, evaluation, 5.2–5.3,
        5.5
    rheumatic fever, 5.6, **5.13, 5.14**
    syndrome–associated physical find-
        ings, 5.3–6.5, **5.6–5.12**
    congenital heart disease, laboratory
        diagnosis, 5.7–5.17
    echocardiography, 5.14–5.17,
        5.39–5.46
    electrocardiography, 5.13–5.14, **5.37,
        5.38**
    roentgenogram, chest, 5.7–5.13,
        5.18–5.36
Cardiomyopathy, 4.29, **4.62**
Caries, 20.12, **20.41, 20.42**
Cataracts, 19.25–19.27, **19.72–19.80**
Cat scratch disease, 12.33–12.34, **12.50**
Cavus foot deformity, 21.45–21.46,
    21.95, 21.96
Celiac disease, 10.9, **10.21**
Cellulitis, 12.24–12.25, **12.36–12.39**
Central nervous system
    and motor dysfunction, **3.13**

Cephalohematoma, 2.10–2.11, **2.28**
Cerebral palsy, 3.19–3.22, 21.46–21.47,
    21.97
    associated findings, 3.21–3.22
    definition, 3.19
    physical examination, 3.19–3.20, **3.36**
    abnormalities in development of
        primitive reflexes and equilibrium
        responses, 3.20
    abnormalities of tone, 3.19–3.20,
        3.37–3.39
    prognosis, 3.22
    sub-types, 3.20–3.21
    dystonic–athetoid, 3.21
    hemiparesis, 3.20–3.21, **3.40, 3.41**
    hypotonic, 3.21
    quadriplegia, 3.21
    spastic diplegia, 3.21, **3.38, 3.42**
CHARGE association, 1.19–1.20, **1.32**
Chest
    signs and symptoms of cancer, 11.31,
        11.89
Chickenpox. See Varicella
Child abuse, 6.1–6.30
    and developmental delay, **3.27**
    emotional abuse, 6.28
    epidemiology, 6.1–6.2
    child risk factors, 6.1–6.2
    parental risk factors, 6.1
    neglect, 6.27–6.28, **6.52, 6.53**
    passive abuse, 6.27–6.28
    physical abuse, 6.2–6.18
    behavioral factors, 6.2–6.3
    differential diagnosis of inflicted
        injuries vs findings due to accident
        or illness, 6.12–6.18, 6.26–6.27
    historical factors, 6.2
    physical findings and patterns of
        injury, 6.3–6.12
    sexual abuse, 6.18–6.27
    differential diagnosis, 6.26–6.27,
        6.51
    examination techniques, 6.19–6.22,
        6.42–6.44
    physical findings, 6.22–6.24, **6.45–6.48**
    presentation modes, 6.19, **6.41**
    specimen collection, 6.24–6.26, **6.49,
        6.50**
Chalazion, 19.17, **19.42, 19.43**
Charcot-Marie-Tooth disease,
    15.20–15.21, **15.57, 15.58**
Chest wall, 17.29–17.30, **17.101–17.103**
Chlamydia, 18.28, **18.41**
Chondromalacia patella, 21.40
Chorioamnionitis, 2.8–2.9, **2.23**
Chronic granulomatous disease,
    4.30–4.31
Chronic inflammatory states, 11.7
Chronic mucocutaneous candidiasis,
    4.30
Chromosomal disorders, 1.1–1.23
    Angelman syndrome, 1.16–1.18,
        1.28–1.30
    autosome abnormalities, 1.7–1.11
    Down syndrome, 1.7–1.9, **1.14–1.18**
    Trisomy 13 and 18, 1.9–1.11, **1.19–1.21**

chromosomal–like syndromes,
    1.18–1.22
CHARGE association, 1.19–1.20, **1.32**
De Lange's syndrome, 1.20–1.21, **1.34**
fetal alcohol syndrome, 1.21–1.22,
    1.35
Noonan syndrome, 1.21
Smith-Lemli-Opitz syndrome, 1.19,
    1.31
VATER association, 1.20, **1.33**
general principles, 1.1–1.7
abnormality suspicions, 1.4–1.7,
    1.11–1.13
incidence of abnormalities, 1.4, **1.10**
nature of chromosomes, 1.1–1.4,
    1.1–1.9
molecular cytogenetic syndromes,
    1.13–1.16
fragile X syndrome, 1.13–1.16,
    1.24–1.27
Prader-Willi syndrome, 1.16–1.18,
    1.28–1.30
prenatal diagnosis, 1.22–1.23
sex chromosome disorders, 1.11–1.13
Klinefelter syndrome, 1.12–1.13, **1.23**
Turner syndrome, 1.11–1.12, **1.22**
XXX and XYY syndromes, 1.13
Claw toes, 21.45–21.46, **21.95, 21.96**
Clotting factor deficiencies, 6.13–6.14
Coats' disease, 19.29, **19.90**
Collodion baby, 8.34, **8.83**
Coloboma, 19.24, 19.28–19.29, **19.67,
    19.84**
Congenital cervical spinal atrophy,
    15.22, **15.59, 15.60**
Congenital clubfoot, 21.40–21.43, **21.86,
    21.88**
Congenital epulis in the newborn, 20.6,
    20.15
Congenital heart disease. See
    Cardiology
Congenital hip dislocation, 21.33–21.35,
    21.76
Congenital pseudarthrosis of the clavi-
    cle, 21.31, **21.69**
Congenital torticollis, 21.24, **21.57**
Congenital trigger thumb, 21.32, **21.73**
Conjunctivitis, 4.14, **4.28–4.32**,
    19.19–19.20, **19.51–19.57**
    atopic, 4.15, **4.29**
    bulbar, **7.22**
    vernal, 4.15–4.16, **4.30–4.32**
Constipation, 10.10, **10.26**
Contusions, 20.16
Convergency insufficiency, 19.10
Copper, as nutritional deficiency,
    6.16–6.17, **10.15**
Corticotropin-related peptide hor-
    mones, 9.1
Cough, 16.1–16.9, **16.3**
    age and cause of chronic, 16.2–16.7,
        16.4–16.16
    diagnostic approach, 16.8–16.9, **16.18**
    evaluation of, 16.7, **16.17**
Coxsackie hand-foot-and-mouth dis-
    ease, 12.4–12.5, **12.6**

CREST syndromes, 7.13–7.14, **7.34, 7.39**
Crohn's disease, 10.13, **10.31–10.33**
Crossed adductor reflex, **3.2**
Crossed renal ectopia, 13.11, **13.25**
Croup. *See* Laryngotracheobronchitis
Crown craze, 20.18
Crown fractures, 20.18, **20.57–20.59**
Cryptorchidism, neonatal, 14.2, **14.3**
Cushing syndrome, 9.10–9.13, **9.19–9.21**
Cutis marmorata, 8.33, **8.82**
Cyanosis and clubbing, 5.1–5.2
Cystic fibrosis (CF), 10.13, **10.37,** 16.12–16.15
    complications, 16.14, **16.34, 16.35**
    diagnosis, 16.14–16.15
    presentation, 16.12–16.13, **16.29–16.33**
    radiographic findings, 16.14, **16.35**
Cystinosis, 13.16, **13.40**
Cystitis, bacterial, 13.9, **13.19**
Cytomegalovirus (CMV), 19.31, **19.96**

Dandy-Walker malformation, 15.10–15.11, **15.25, 15.26**
DAP-Goodenough-Harris Drawing Test, **3.28**
Dehydration, 10.2, **10.4, 10.5**
De Lange's syndrome, 1.20–1.21, **1.34**
Dentinogenesis imperfecta, 20.10, **20.34**
Denver Developmental Screening Test (DDST), **3.28**
Dermatitides, 8.5–8.12, **8.10–8.30**
Dermatology, 8.1–8.48
    acne, 8.27–8.28, **8.64**
    bites, stings, and infestations, 8.23–8.27, **8.54**
    hymenoptera stings, 8.24, **8.57**
    infestations, 8.25–8.27, **8.59–8.63**
    insect bites, 8.23–8.24, **8.55**
    papular urticaria, 8.24–8.25, **8.58**
    spider bites, 8.24, **8.56**
    complications of topical skin therapy, 8.47–8.48, **8.121–8.123**
    examination and assessment of skin, 8.2–8.3
    hair and nail disorders, 8.43–8.47, **8.115–8.120**
    alopecias, 8.43–8.45, **8.107–8.111**
    congenital and genetic disorders, 8.46, **8.114**
    tinea capitis infections, 8.45–8.46, **8.112, 8.113**
    hemangiomas, 8.35–8.38
    flat, 8.36–8.37, **8.92, 8.93**
    pyogenic, 8.37–8.38, **8.94**
    raised, capillary and cavernous, 8.36, **8.88–8.91**
    neonatal, 8.32–8.35
    collodion baby, 8.34, **8.83**
    cutis marmorata, 8.33, **8.82**
    epidermolysis bullosa (EB), 8.34, **8.84–8.86**
    erythema toxicum neonatorum, 8.32, **8.78**
    incontinentia pigmenti (IP), 8.34–8.35, **8.87**
    mongolian spots, 8.32, **8.77**

sebaceous gland hyperplasia and acne, 8.33, **8.80, 8.81**
transient pustular melanosis (TNPM), 8.32–8.33, **8.79**
nevi and melanomas, 8.38–8.41
hamartomatous nevi, 8.40–8.41, **8.101, 8.102**
nevomelanocytic nevi, 8.38–8.40, **8.95–8.100**
papulosquamous disorders, 8.3–8.17
dermatitides, 8.5–8.12, **8.10–8.30**
diaper dermatitis, 8.15–8.17, **8.37–8.41**
fungal infections, 8.12–8.15, **8.31–8.36**
ichthyoses, 8.4, **8.6–8.9, 8.83**
psoriasis, 8.3–8.4, **8.2–8.5, 8.120, 8.141**
pigmentation disorders, 8.41–8.43
albinism, 8.42, **8.106**
ash leaf spots, 8.41–8.42
post-inflammatory pigmentary changes, 8.41, **8.103, 8.104**
vitiligo, 8.41, **8.105**
reactive erythemas, 8.19–8.23
drug eruptions, 8.22, **8.51, 8.52**
erythema multiforme (EM), 8.19–8.20, **8.46, 8.47**
erythema nodosum, 8.20, **8.48**
Henoch-Schönlein purpura (HSP), 8.22–8.23, **8.53**
urticaria, 8.20–8.22, **8.49, 8.50**
skin anatomy, **8.1**
signs and symptoms of cancer, 11.27–11.28, **11.71–11.77**
tumors and infiltrations, 8.28–8.32
granuloma annulare, 8.31–8.32, **8.76**
histiocytoses, 8.31, **8.75**
juvenile xanthogranuloma, 8.31, **8.74**
keloids, 8.29, **8.70**
mastocytosis, 8.30–8.31, **8.72, 8.73**
milia, 8.29, **8.69**
neurofibromas, 8.30, **8.71**
warts, 8.28–8.29, **8.65–8.68**
vesiculopustular disorders, 8.17–8.18
bacterial infections, 8.17
miliaria, 8.18, **8.43, 8.44**
toxic epidermal necrolysis (TEN), 8.17–8.18
vesiculation, 8.18, **8.45**
viral infections, 8.17, **8.42**
Dermatomyositis (DM), 7.5–7.7, **7.13–7.17**
Diabetes mellitus, 9.20, **9.30, 9.31,** 19.32
Diarrhea, 10.11–10.13
DiGeorge syndrome, 4.24, **4.47**
Dislocations, 21.19–21.20, **21.43–21.49**
Displacement injuries, 20.18–20.19, **20.61**
Districhiasis, 19.16, **19.35**
Down syndrome, 1.7–1.9, **1.14–1.18,** 3.22, **3.43, 3.44,** 5.3–5.4
Drash syndrome, 13.17, **13.43**
Draw-a-Person Test, **3.28**
Duane's syndrome, 19.8–19.9, **19.18**
Duchenne muscular dystrophy, 15.18–15.20, **15.50–15.56**
Dwarfism, short–limbed, 4.26, **4.53**
Dyshidrosis, **8.17**

Eagle–Barrett syndrome. *See* Prune–Belly syndrome
Ear, anatomy, **22.2**
Ear disorders, 22.1–22.14, **22.2–22.8**
    external ear disorders, 22.4–22.9
    deformity, 22.7–22.8, **22.16–22.18**
    discharge, 22.5–22.6, **22.9**
    discoloration, 22.7, **22.12–22.15**
    displacement, 22.6, **22.10–22.14**
    distortions of the tympanic membrane, 22.14, **22.33**
    foreign objects and secondary trauma, 22.9, **22.19, 22.20**
    middle ear disorders, 22.9–22.14
    acute otitis media, 22.10–22.12, **22.24–22.27**
    chronic/recurrent otitis media (COME), 22.12–22.13, **22.29, 22.30**
    mass lesions involving the tympanic membrane, 22.13–22.14, **22.31, 22.32**
    otitis media with effusion, 22.12, **22.28**
    protection of and prevention of otitis media, 22.13
Echocardiography, 5.14–5.17, **5.39–5.46**
Ecthyma, 12.19–12.20, **12.28, 12.29**
Ectropion, 19.16, **19.36**
Eczema, 8.5–8.9, **8.10–8.21**
Electrocardiography, 5.13–5.14, **5.37, 5.38**
ELISA (enzyme–linked immonosorbent assay) test, 4.30
Elliptocytosis, 11.12, **11.24**
Ellis-van Creveld syndrome, 5.4, **5.7**
Endocarditis, bacterial, 5.7, **5.15–5.17,** 19.32, **19.98, 19.99**
Endocrinology, 9.1–9.21
    endocrine deficiencies, **3.13**
    hormones, imbalance of, 9.6–9.13
    adrenal gland dysfunction, 9.10–9.13, **9.19–9.21**
    growth hormone deficiency, 9.6, **9.7–9.9**
    parathyroid gland dysfunction, 9.9–9.10, **9.18**
    thyroid gland disorders, 9.6–9.8, **9.10–9.14**
    Turner syndrome, 9.8–9.9, **9.15–9.17**
    insulin-dependent diseases, 9.20–9.21
    diabetes mellitus, 9.20, **9.30, 9.31**
    hypoglycemia, 9.21, **9.32–9.35**
    normal growth, 9.3–9.6, **9.5, 9.6**
    pituitary gland, anterior, 9.1–9.3, **9.1–9.4**
    sexual maturation, 9.14–9.19
    early sexual development, 9.14–9.16, **9.22–9.24**
    puberty, 9.16–9.19, **9.25–9.29**
Entropion, 19.16, **19.37**
Epiblepharon, 19.16–19.17, **19.38**
Epidermolysis bullosa (EB), 8.34, **8.84–8.86**
Epiglottitis, 22.38–22.40, **22.78, 22.79**
Epispadias, 14.7–14.8, **14.19**
Eruption cysts, 20.8, **20.22**
Erysipelas, 12.23, **12.35**

Erythemas, 8.19–8.23
  drug eruptions, 8.22, **8.51, 8.52**
  erythema infectiosum (fifth disease), 12.5–12.6, **12.7**
  erythema multiforme (EM), 8.19–8.20, **8.46, 8.47**
  erythema nodosum, 8.20, **8.48**
  erythema toxicum neonatorum, 8.32, **8.78**
  Henoch-Schönlein purpura (HSP), 8.22–8.23, **8.53**
  urticaria, 8.20–8.22, **8.49, 8.50**
Erythroblastosis fetalis, 20.11
Esophageal foreign bodies, 22.45, **22.90, 22.91**
Essential fatty acids, as nutritional deficiency, **10.15**
Exanthems, 12.1–12.16
Exstrophy
  classic, 14.6–14.7, **14.17**
  cloacal, 14.7, **14.18**
Extremity pain, in ligamentous laxity, 21.23–21.24, **21.56**
Eyelid colobomas, 19.17, **19.39**

Fabry's disease, 13.17, **13.41**
Facial weakness, 15.17–15.18, **15.47**
  central, 15.18, **15.49**
  peripheral, 15.17–15.18, **15.48**
Female genitalia, lesions, 14.15–14.17, **14.40**
  cysts, paraurethral, 14.16, **14.44**
  ureterocele, prolapsed, 14.16, **14.43**
  urethral polyps, 14.16, **14.42**
  urethral prolapse, 14.16, **14.41**
  vagina, congenital obstruction, 14.16–14.17
Femoral anteversion, 21.37, **21.79**
Fetal alcohol syndrome, 1.21–1.22, **1.35**
Fine pincer grasp, **3.18**
Fitz-Hugh-Curtis syndrome. *See* Perihepatitis
Folate, as nutritional deficiency, **10.15**
Folliculitis, 12.18, **12.25**
Fractures, 21.4–21.14, **21.4–21.33**
  and child abuse, 6.15–6.17, **6.36, 6.37**
  clavicular, 21.14, **21.10**
  diagnosis, 21.4–21.7, **21.4–21.7**
  hand and finger, 21.15–21.17, **21.35–21.39**
  of the mandible, 20.20, **20.65**
  of the maxilla, 20.21, **20.66, 20.67**
  metatarsal, 21.17, **21.40, 21.41**
  pathologic, 21.18
  patterns, 21.7, **21.8–21.27**
  physeal, 21.7–21.14, **21.28–21.33**
  seat belt, 21.17–21.18, **21.42**
  toddler's, 21.15, **21.34**
  treatment principles, 21.14
Fragile X syndrome, 1.13–1.16, **1.24–1.27**
Frenulae, abnormalities, 20.6, **20.18–20.20**
Fungal infections, 8.12–8.15, **8.31–8.36**
Furuncle, 12.21, **12.31**

Gallbladder, **7.30**
Galactosemia, and developmental delay, **3.27**
Ganglion of the foot, 21.45, **21.94**
Gastroenterology, 10.8–10.13
  abdominal pain, 10.10–10.11, **10.27–10.29**
  bleeding, 17.14–17.18, **17.42**
  in infants, 17.14–17.15, 17.43–17.47
  in older children, 17.17–17.18, **17.50–17.54**
  in toddlers, 17.16–17.17, **17.48, 17.49**
  chronic liver disease, 10.14–10.16
  during childhood, 10.14–10.16, **10.45–10.49**
  during infancy, 10.14, **10.38–10.44**
  constipation, 10.10, **10.26**
  cystic fibrosis, 10.13, **10.37**
  diarrhea, 10.11–10.13
  hemorrhage, 10.11, **10.30**
  inflammatory bowel disease, 10.13, **10.31–10.36**
  malabsorption, 10.9, **10.21**
  vomiting, 10.9–10.10
  reflux, 10.9–10.10, **10.24**
  pyloric stenosis, 10.9, **10.22, 10.23**
  trauma, 10.10, **10.25**
Genetic syndromes and chromosomal abnormalities, **3.13**
Genital trauma, 14.18, **14.47**
Genu valgum, 21.39, **21.81**
Genu varum, 21.37–21.39, **21.80**
Gesell Developmental Schedules, **3.28**
Gingival cysts in the newborn, 20.5–20.6, **20.12–20.14**
Gingival hyperplasia, 20.7–20.8, **20.21**
Glaucoma, 19.22–19.23, **19.63–19.66**
Glomerular disorders, 13.1–13.6
Glycoprotein hormones, **9.1**
Gonorrhea, 18.27–18.28, **18.41, 18.42**
Graves' disease, **12.45**
Growth curves, 10.3, **10.9**
Growth hormone (GH), 9.2–9.3, **9.4**
Gynecology, 18.1–18.33
  evaluation, 18.3–18.9
  examination of the adolescent or pubertal patient, 18.6–18.9, **18.8–18.11**
  examination of the prepubertal patient, 18.3–18.6, **18.5, 18.6**
  genitalia, normal female, 18.1–18.3
  newborn and prepubertal periods, 18.1–18.3, **18.1–18.3**
  peripubertal period, 18.3, **18.4**
  genital tract obstruction, 18.9–18.11
  imperforate hymen, 18.10–18.11, **18.13–18.15**
  labial adhesions, 18.9, **18.12**
  genital trauma, 18.11–18.13
  moderate, 18.12–18.13, **18.18–18.20**
  severe, 18.13, **18.21**
  superficial perineal injuries, 18.11–18.12, **18.16, 18.17**
  pregnancy, 18.30–18.32
  vulvovaginal disorders, nontraumatic, 18.13–18.30

adolescent complaints, 18.14–18.16, **18.24, 18.25**
  infectious, 18.18–18.30, **18.32–18.44**
  noninfectious, 18.16–18.18, **18.26–18.31**
  prepubertal "vulvovaginitis," 18.13–18.14, **18.22, 18.23**
Gynecomastia, 9.19, **9.29**

Hand grasp reflex, **3.2, 3.14**
Hashimoto's carcinoma, **12.45**
Head and neck, 17.25–17.29, **17.79, 17.80**
  control, **3.5**
  face, 17.25–17.26, **17.84**
  mouth, 17.26, **17.85**
  neck—lateral masses, 17.27–17.29, **17.90–17.100**
  neck—midline, 17.26–17.27, **17.86–17.89**
  scalp, 17.25, **17.81–17.83**
  signs and symptoms of cancer, 11.28–11.31, **11.78, 11.79**
Head grasp reflex, **3.2**
Head injuries, 6.10–6.11, **6.21–6.23**
Hearing
  and developmental delay, **3.27, 3.45–3.47**
Heart murmur. *See* Cardiology
Hemangiomas, 8.35–8.38
  differential diagnosis, **12.45**
  flat, 8.36–8.37, **8.92, 8.93**
  pyogenic, 8.37–8.38, **8.94**
  raised, capillary and cavernous, 8.36, **8.88–8.91**
Hematology, 11.1–11.36
  anemia, 11.3–11.14
  hemolytic, 11.10–11.14, **11.18–11.28**
  hypochromic/microcytic, 11.3–11.6, **11.6–11.17**
  macrocytic, 11.7–11.8
  normocytic, normochromic, 11.8–11.14
  bleeding disorders, 11.22–11.25, **11.59**
  coagulopathies, 11.24–11.25, **11.64–11.67**
  platelet disorders, 11.22–11.24, **11.60–11.63**
  hemolysis caused by extra red blood cell factors, 11.17–11.18
  intracellular red cell defects, 11.14–11.15, **11.29–11.32**
  oncology, 11.26–11.36
  laboratory aids to diagnosis, 11.34–11.36, **11.99–11.106**
  signs and symptoms, 11.26–11.34, **11.71–11.98**
  pancytopenia, 11.25–11.26, **11.68–11.70**
  peripheral blood smear, 11.1–11.2, **11.1, 11.2**
  red blood cell, 11.2,
  red blood cell enzyme abnormalities, 11.16–11.18, **11.33–11.37**
  red cell production, 11.2, **11.3–11.5**
  white blood cells, 11.18–11.22, **11.38–11.58**

Hematuria, 13.3–13.7, **13.7**
Hemoglobin C disease, 11.15, **11.28**
Hemoglobinopathies, 11.14–11.15, **11.27, 11.28**
Hemolysis, caused by extra red blood cell factors, 11.17–11.18
Hemophilia A and B, 11.25, **11.65–11.67**
Hemorrhage, 10.11, **10.30**
Henoch-Schönlein purpura (HSP), 7.7–7.9, **7.18–7.20**, 8.22–8.23, **8.53**, 13.3, **13.13, 13.14**
Hereditary sphenocytosis, 11.10–11.12, **11.20–11.23**
Hepatic discoloration, 20.11, **20.36**
Hepatomegaly, and developmental delay, **3.27**
Herniated intervertebral disc, 21.30, **21.67**
Herpes
    genital, 18.24–18.25, **18.38**
    simplex, 12.8–12.10, **12.41**, 19.31
    eczema herpeticum, 12.9, **12.13**
    primary, 12.8–12.9, **12.10–12.12**, 19.18, **19.44**
    recurrent, 12.9, **12.14**
    zoster, 12.10, **12.15**, 20.13, **20.44**
Herpetic gingivostomatitis, 20.12–20.13, **20.43**
Heterochromia iridis, 19.24–19.25, **19.70**
Hirsutism, 13.19, **13.48**
Hodgkin's disease, differential diagnosis, **12.45**
Holt-Oram syndrome, 5.4–5.5, **5.8**
Hordeolum, 19.17, **19.41**
Hormones, imbalance of, 9.6–9.13
    adrenal gland dysfunction, 9.10–9.13, **9.19–9.21**
    growth hormone deficiency, 9.6, **9.7–9.9**
    parathyroid gland dysfunction, 9.9–9.10, **9.18**
    thyroid gland disorders, 9.6–9.8, **9.10–9.14**
    Turner syndrome, 9.8–9.9, **9.15–9.17**
Horseshoe kidney, 13.11, **13.26**
Human bites, 6.5, **6.6**
Human immunodeficiency virus (HIV), 4.26–4.30. *See also* Acquired immunodeficiency syndrome
Human papilloma virus (HPV), 18.23
Hydranencephaly, 15.11, **15.27–15.29**
Hydrocele, 14.15, **14.39**
Hydrocephalus, 15.9–15.10, **15.23, 15.24**
Hydronephrosis, 14.3–14.4
    megaureter, 14.4, **14.7**
    ureteropelvic junction obstruction, 14.3–14.4, **14.6**
Hyperdontia, 20.9, **20.26–20.28**
Hyper-IgE syndrome, 4.26, **4.51, 4.52**
Hyperpigmented spots, 6.14, **6.29**, 8.32, **8.77**
Hypersensitivity disorders, 4.1–4.33
    cellular immunodeficient (T-lymphocyte), 4.23–4.24, **4.46**
    classification, **4.1**
    combined T- and B-lymphocyte, 4.25–4.30, **4.48, 4.49**

complement system, 4.31–4.32
    diagnostic techniques, 4.32–4.33
    nasal smear, 4.33
    skin testing, 4.32–4.33
    humoral immunodeficient (B-lymphocyte), 4.21–4.22
    immunological deficient, 4.19–4.32
    immune system
        normal development, 4.19–4.20, **4.41**
        abnormal function of, 4.20–4.21
    immunological hypersensitive, 4.1–4.18, **4.1**
    type I, 4.2–4.18, **4.2, 4.3**
    type III, 4.18–4.19
    mucosal barrier, 4.32
    phagocytic, 4.30–4.31
Hypersensitivity pneumonitis, 4.18–4.19, **4.38**
Hypervitaminosis A, 6.17
Hypogammaglobulinemia, congenital, 4.21, **4.42, 4.43**
Hypogammaglobulinemia, transient, of infancy, 4.22, **4.44**
Hypoglycemia, **3.13, 3.27**, 9.21, **9.32–9.35**
Hypotonic infant, 15.22–15.23, **15.63**
Hypocalcification, 20.10, **20.31**
Hypodontia, 20.9, **20.26–20.28**
Hypoplasia, 20.10, **20.32**
Hypothyroidism, **3.13, 3.27**
Hypotonia, **3.13**

Ichthyoses, 8.4, **8.6–8.9, 8.83**
"Id" reaction, 8.12
IgA defiency, 4.22
IgG defiency, 4.22, **4.45**
Immotile cilia syndrome, 4.32, **4.67, 4.68**
Impetigo, 6.15, **6.33**, 12.18–12.19, **12.26, 12.27**
Incontinentia pigmenti (IP), 8.34–8.35, **8.87**
Infancy, findings in failure to survive, 6.28, **6.53**
Infantile esotrophia, 19.7, **19.12–19.14**
Infectious disease, 12.1–12.46
    abscesses of the skin and soft tissues, 12.20–12.22, **12.30–12.33**
    acute suppurative lymphadenitis, 12.29–12.32, **12.47, 12.48**
    bacterial bone and joint infections, 12.35–12.43
    osteomyelitis, 12.35–12.41, **12.51–12.56**
    septic arthritis, 12.41–12.43, **12.57–12.59**
    bacterial skin and soft-tissue, 12.18–12.26, **12.25–12.29**
    cellulitis, 12.24–12.25, **12.36–12.39**
    congenital and perinatal, 12.43–12.45
    neonatal herpes simplex, 12.45, **12.62**
    rubella, 12.44–12.45, **12.61**
    toxoplasmosis, 12.43–12.44, **12.41, 12.60**
    erysipelas, 12.23, **12.35**
    exanthems, 12.1–12.16

bacterial, 12.10–12.16, **12.16–12.21**
    Rocky Mountain spotted fever, 12.16, **12.22**
    viral, 12.1–12.10, **12.1–12.15**
    lymphadenitis, 12.26–12.28
    diagnosis, 12.35
    lymphangitis, 12.22–12.23, **12.34**
    and motor dysfunction, **3.13**
    mumps, 12.16–12.18, **12.23, 12.24**
    mycobacterial lymphadenitis, 12.32–12.33, **12.49**
    necrotizing fasciitis, 12.26, **12.40, 12.41**
    oral, 20.12–20.16
    bacterial, 20.14–20.15, **20.46–20.50**
    fungal, 20.15–20.16, **20.51**
    viral, 20.12–20.14, **20.43–20.45**
    superficial regional lymph nodes, 12.28–12.29, **12.42–12.46**
Inflammatory bowel disease, 10.13, **10.31–10.36**
Insect bites, 6.14–6.15, **6.31, 6.34**, 8.23–8.27, **8.54, 8.55**
    hymenoptera stings, 8.24, **8.57**
    infestations, 8.25–8.27, **8.59–8.63**
    papular urticaria, 8.24–8.25, **8.58**
    spider bites, 8.24, **8.56**
Intelligence
    and visual impairment, 3.29
Intercellular adhesion molecule (ICAM) deficiency, 4.31, **4.65**
Iridocyclitis, **7.8**
Iron, as nutritional deficiency, **10.15**
Iron deficiency anemia, 11.4–11.5, **11.6, 11.7**

Jaundice, 10.14, **10.38**
Jeune's syndrome, 13.17, **13.42**
Juvenile laryngeal papillomatosis, 22.44–22.45, **22.89**
Juvenile xanthogranuloma (JXG), 19.25, **19.71**

Kaiser-Fleischer ring, 10.16, **10.47**
Kaposi's sarcoma, 4.29, **4.61**
Kawasaki syndrome, 7.9–7.13, **7.21–7.31**
Keloids, 8.29, **8.70**
Keratosis pilaris, **8.15**
Kernicterus, **3.13**
Klinefelter syndrome, 1.12–1.13, **1.23**
Klippel-Feil syndrome, 21.24–21.25, **21.58**
Koebner phenomenon, **8.4**
Kwashiorkor, 10.3, **10.7, 10.8**
Kyphosis, 21.27–21.28, **21.63, 21.64**

Lacerations, 20.17, **20.53–20.55**
Language and reading disorders, 3.24–3.27
    definition, 3.24
    physical examination, 3.24–3.27
    prognosis, 3.27
Lanugo hair, 2.4, **2.6**
Laryngomalacia, 22.43–22.44, **22.87**
Laryngotracheobronchitis, 22.40–22.41, **22.80–22.82**

Lead poisoning, 11.5–11.6, **11.8, 11.9**
Legg-Calvé-Perthes disease,
  21.35–21.36, **21.77**
Leiner syndrome, 4.31, **4.66**
Leiter International Performance Scale,
  3.28
Leukemia, 6.17, **6.39**, 11.19–11.20,
  11.43–11.49
  differential diagnosis, **12.45**
  ophthamologic evaluation, 19.32
Lethargy, and developmental delay,
  3.27
Leukorrhea, physiologic, 18.15–18.16,
  18.25
Lice, 8.26–8.27, **8.62, 8.63**
Lichenification, **8.14**
Ligamentous injuries, 21.19–21.24,
  21.43–21.56
Linear sebaceous nervus, 15.6–15.7,
  15.19
Liver disease, chronic, 10.14–10.16
  during childhood, 10.14–10.16,
    10.45–10.49
  during infancy, 10.14, **10.38–10.44**
Logic, preoperational, **3.26**
Lyme arthritis, **7.12**
Lymphadenitis
  acute suppurative, 12.25–12.32, **12.47,**
    12.48
  diagnosis, 12.35
Lymphangioma, differential diagnosis,
  12.45
Lymphangitis, 12.22–12.23, **12.34**
Lymphoid interstitial pneumonitis
  (LIP), 4.29, **4.59, 4.60**
Lymphoma, 22.35, **22.70**

Macrocephaly, 15.7–15.11, **15.20–15.26**
Malabsorption, 10.9, **10.21**
Malaria, 11.17–11.18, **11.37**
Male genitalia, anomalies, 14.9–14.15
  acute scrotum, 14.12–14.13
  buried penis, 14.10–14.11, **14.27**
  chordee, 14.10, **14.24**
  diphallus, 14.12, **14.32**
  epididymitis, 14.14, **14.36**
  hypospadias, 14.9–14.10, **14.23**
  microphallus, 14.12, **14.31**
  penile torsion, 14.10, **14.25**
  postcircumcision lesions, 14.11–14.12,
    14.28–14.30
  priapism, 14.12, **14.33**
  scrotal contents, lesions, 14.12
  scrotal swelling, chronic, 14.14–14.15,
    14.37–14.39
  spermatic cord torsion, 14.13–14.14,
    14.34
  testicular appendage torsion, 14.14,
    14.35
  webbed penis, 14.10, **14.26**
Mallet finger, 21.33, **21.75**
Malnutrition
  developmental delay, **3.27**
  clinical observations of, 10.1–10.3,
    10.4–10.9
Mandible, fractures, 20.20, **20.65**

Marasmus, 10.3, **10.6**
Marcus Gunn jaw winking phe-
  nomenon, 19.14–19.16, **19.34**
Marfan syndrome, 5.5, **5.9**
Marie-Foix maneuver, **3.39**
Mastocytosis, 8.30–8.31, **8.72, 8.73**
Maxfield-Buchalty Social Maturity for
  Blind Preschool Children, **3.28**
Maxilla, fractures of, 20.21,
  20.66, 20.67
Meningococcemia
  acute, 12.14–12.15, **12.20, 12.21**
  chronic, 12.15–12.16
Menkes' kinky hair syndrome, 6.17
Mental retardation, 3.22–3.23
  definition, 3.22
  physical examination, 3.22–3.23
  cranial abnormalities, 3.23
  facial abnormalities, 3.23
  growth pattern and vital signs, 3.22
  skin findings, 3.23
  prognosis, 3.23
Metabolism
  and motor dysfunction, **3.13**
Metatarsus primus, 21.43–21.44, **21.89**
Microcephaly, 15.11–15.12, **15.30**
Miliaria, 8.18, **8.43, 8.44**
"Mongolian spots." *See*
  Hyperpigmented spots
Mononucleosis, 12.6–12.8, **12.41**
  clinical features, 12.6–12.7, **12.9**
  diagnostic methods, 12.7
  differential diagnosis, 12.7–12.8
Morphea, 7.13, **7.32**
Moro response, **3.2, 3.40**
Motor automatism, **3.27**
Motor end-plate dysfunction, **3.13**
Mucocele, 20.8, **20.23**
Mucopolysaccharidoses (MPS), 19.33,
  19.101
Mumps, 12.16–12.18, **12.23, 12.24**
Muscular disorders, **3.13**
Musculoskeletal disorders, 21.46–21.49
  arthrogryposis, 21.48–21.49, **21.101**
  cerebral palsy, 21.46–21.47, **21.97**
  osteogenesis imperfecta (OI),
    21.47–21.48, **21.98–21.100**
Musculoskeletal system
  signs and symptoms of cancer,
    11.33–11.34, **11.97, 11.98**
Musculoskeletal trauma, 21.3–21.24
  compartment syndromes, 21.18
  fractures, 21.4–21.14, **21.4–21.33**
  ligamentous injuries, 21.19–21.24,
    21.43–21.56
  special cases, 21.14–21.18, **21.34–21.42**
Myasthenia gravis, **3.13**
Mycobacterial lymphadenitis,
  12.32–12.33, **12.49**
Myelinated nerve fibers, 19.29, **19.85**
Myelomeningocele, **3.13**
Myotonia congenita, 15.22, **15.61, 15.62**
Myxedema, **3.27**

Nasal disorders, 22.14–22.22
  epistaxis, 22.20–22.22, **22.46–22.49**

nasal obstruction, 22.14–22.19
  acquired forms of, 22.16–22.19,
    22.39–22.42
  congenital causes, 22.14–22.16,
    22.34–22.38
  upper respiratory infections in early
    infancy, 22.14
  nasal trauma, 22.19–22.20,
    22.43–22.45
Nasal smear, 4.33, **4.69**
Necrotizing fasciitis, 12.26, **12.40, 12.41**
Neonatal herpes simplex, 12.45, **12.62**
Neonatal stroke, **3.13**
Neonatology, 2.1–2.19
  birth trauma, 2.9–2.12
  bruises and petechiae, 2.11, **2.30**
  caput succedaneum, 2.10, **2.27**
  cephalohematoma, 2.10–2.11, **2.28**
  meconium staining, 2.11, **2.29**
  nasal deformities, 2.11, **2.32**
  peripheral nerve damage, 2.11–2.12,
    2.33, 2.34
  congenital anomalies, 2.12–2.14
  amniotic bands, 2.13, **2.42**
  digits, 2.12–2.13, **2.35–2.37**
  external ear, 2.13, **2.38, 2.39**
  midline defects, 2.13, **2.40, 2.41**
  oral clefts, 2.14, **2.45**
  scrotal swelling, 2.14, **2.44**
  umbilical hernia, 2.14, **2.43**
  examination techniques, 2.1–2.6, **2.1,**
    2.2
  abnormalities of growth, 2.6–2.7,
    2.15–2.18
  assessment of gestational age, 2.2–2.6,
    2.3–2.14
  newborn stools, 2.18–2.19, **2.60–2.63**
  placenta, 2.7–2.9, **2.19–2.26**
  primitive reflexes, 2.15, **2.46–2.50**
  respiratory distress, 2.15–2.18,
    2.51–2.59
Nephritis and nephrosis, 13.1–13.3,
  13.1–13.6
Nephrolithiasis, 13.5–13.6, **13.8–13.10**
Nephrology, 13.1–13.20
  bacterial cystitis, 13.9, **13.19**
  chronic renal failure, 13.19–13.20
  anemia of, 13.20, **13.51**
  renal osteodystrophy, 13.19–13.20,
    13.49, 13.50
  developmental/hereditary disorders,
    13.9–13.18
  abnormalities, 13.9–13.12, **13.20–13.27**
  hereditary and metabolic,
    13.12–13.18, **13.28–13.44**
  glomerular disorders, 13.1–13.6
  hematuria, 13.3–13.7, **13.7**
  nephrolithiasis, 13.5–13.6, **13.8–13.10**
  renal venous thrombosis, 13.6–13.7,
    13.11, 13.12
  nephritis and nephrosis, 13.1–13.3,
    13.1–13.6
  renovascular hypertension,
    13.18–13.19
  growth failure, 13.20
  hirsutism, 13.19, **13.48**

renal artery stenosis, 13.18–13.19, **13.45–13.47**
vesicoureteral reflux, 13.7–13.9, **13.13–13.18**
Nephrotic syndrome, 13.3, **13.5, 13.6**
Nervous system
  signs and symptoms of cancer, 11.34, **11.78**
Neurofibromas, 8.30, **8.71**
Neurofibromatosis 1, 15.1–15.2, **15.1–15.6**
Neurofibromatosis 2, 15.3–15.4
Neurology, 15.1–15.23
  central nervous system malformations, 15.7–15.13
  hydranencephaly, 15.11, **15.27–15.29**
  macrocephaly, 15.7–15.11, **15.20–15.26**
  microcephaly, 15.11–15.12, **15.30**
  spinal dysraphism, occult, 15.12–15.13, **15.31–15.33**
  facial weakness, 15.17–15.18, **15.47**
  central, 15.18, **15.49**
  peripheral, 15.17–15.18, **15.48**
  hypotonic infant, 15.22–15.23, **15.63**
  increased intracranial pressure, 15.13–15.17
  causes, 15.14–15.17, **15.37–15.46**
  primary signs and symptoms, 15.13–15.14, **15.34–15.36**
  neurocutaneous syndromes, 15.1–15.7
  ataxia telangiectasia, 15.6, **15.18**
  linear sebaceous nevus, 15.6–15.7, **15.19**
  neurofibromatosis 1, 15.1–15.2, **15.1–15.6**
  neurofibromatosis 2, 15.3–15.4
  Sturge-Weber syndrome, 15.5–15.6, **15.14–15.17**
  tuberous sclerosis, 15.4–15.5, **15.7–15.13**
  neuromuscular disorders, 15.18–15.22
  Charcot-Marie-Tooth disease, 15.20–15.21, **15.57, 15.58**
  congenital cervical spinal atrophy, 15.22, **15.59, 15.60**
  Duchenne muscular dystrophy, 15.18–15.20, **15.50–15.56**
  myotonia congenita, 15.22, **15.61, 15.62**
Neuropathy, heritable, **3.13**
Nevi and melanomas, 8.38–8.41
  hamartomatous nevi, 8.40–8.41, **8.101, 8.102**
  nevomelanocytic nevi, 8.38–8.40, **8.95–8.100**
Niacin, as nutritional deficiency, **10.15**
Nonaccommodative esotropia, 19.8, **19.17**
Noonan syndrome, 1.21, 5.5, **5.10**
Nursemaid's elbow, 21.22–21.23, **21.54, 21.55**
Nutrition, 10.1–10.8
  anthropometric measurements and

laboratory tests, 10.3–10.4, **10.10–10.13**
  clinical observations of malnutrition, 10.1–10.3, **10.4–10.9**
  feeding, **3.19**
  normal, 10.1, **10.1–10.3**
  therapy, 10.4–10.8, **10.14–10.20**

Object permanence, **3.24**
Ocular allergies, 4.14–4.16, **4.27–4.32**
Oncology, 11.26–11.36
  laboratory aids to diagnosis, 11.34–11.36, **11.99–11.106**
  signs and symptoms, 11.26–11.34, **11.71–11.98**
Ophthalmology, 19.1–19.39
  amblyopia, 19.13–19.14, **19.29**
  anatomy of the visual system, 19.1–19.2, **19.1–19.3**
  diseases of the eyes and surrounding structures, 19.14–19.37
  anterior chamber, 19.22–19.23, **19.63–19.66**
  conjunctiva, 19.19–19.20, **19.51–19.57**
  cornea, 19.20–19.22, **19.58–19.62**
  eyelid, anatomy, 19.14–19.18, **19.30–19.45**
  iris, 19.24–19.25, **19.67–19.71**
  lacrimal gland and nasolacrimal drainage system, 19.18–19.19, **19.46–19.50**
  lens, 19.25–19.27, **19.72–19.80**
  optic nerve, 19.34–19.36, **19.104–19.106**
  orbit, 19.36–19.37, **19.107–19.111**
  retina, 19.28–19.34, **19.84–19.103**
  uvea, 19.27–19.28, **19.81, 19.82**
  vitreous, 19.28, **19.83**
  ocular trauma, 19.37–19.39, **19.112–19.120**
  refractive errors, 19.4–19.6, **19.7–19.10**
  signs and symptoms of cancer, 11.29–11.30, **11.80–11.82**
  strabismus, 19.6–19.13, **19.11**
  esodeviation, 19.7–19.9, **19.12–19.19**
  exodeviations, 19.9–19.11, **19.20–19.23**
  tests for, 19.11–19.13, **19.26–19.28**
  vertical deviations, 19.11, **19.24, 19.25**
  vision, evaluation of, 19.3–19.4, **19.4–19.6**
Optic disc atrophy, 19.36, **19.105**
Optic neuritis, 19.35
Oral disorders, 20.1–20.21
  caries, 20.12, **20.41, 20.42**
  developmental abnormalities, 20.6–20.10
  hard-tissue abnormalities, 20.9–20.10, **20.26–20.34**
  soft-tissue abnormalities, 20.6–20.8, **20.17–20.25**
  discoloration, 20.10–20.12
  extrinsic, 20.11, **20.35**
  intrinsic, 20.11–20.12, **20.36–20.40**
  infections, 20.12–20.16
  bacterial, 20.14–20.15, **20.46–20.50**
  fungal, 20.15–20.16, **20.51**

viral, 20.12–20.14, **20.43–20.45**
  injuries, 6.7, **6.12**
  mixed dentition, 20.3–20.5, **20.4, 20.5**
  early permanent, 20.3–20.4, **20.6–20.8**
  harmful oral habits, 20.4–20.5, **20.9, 20.10**
  natal and neonatal abnormalities, 20.5–20.6,
  congenital epulis in the newborn, 20.6, **20.15**
  gingival cysts in the newborn, 20.5–20.6, **20.12–20.14**
  melanotic neuroectodermal tumor of infancy, 20.6, **20.16**
  teeth, 20.5, **20.11**
  normal structures, 20.1–20.3, **20.1**
  in the newborn, 20.2
  primary dentition, 20.2–20.3, **20.2, 20.3**
  trauma, 20.16–20.21
  dentition, 20.17–20.19, **20.57–20.62**
  soft-tissue, 20.16–20.17, **20.52–20.56**
  supporting structures, 20.19–20.21, **20.63–20.67**
Oropharyngeal disorders, 22.30–22.37
  palatal disorders, 22.31–22.32, **22.61–22.65**
  penetrating oropharyngeal trauma, 22.35–22.37, **22.71, 22.72**
  tonsillar and peritonsillar disorders, 22.32–22.35, **22.66–22.70**
Orthopedics, 21.1–21.50
  lower extremity disorders, 21.33–21.46
  accessory tarsal navicular, 21.45, **21.93**
  Blount's disease, 21.39, **21.82**
  calcaneovalgus foot deformity, 21.44, **21.91**
  cavus foot deformity, 21.45–21.46, **21.95, 21.96**
  chondromalacia patella, 21.40
  claw toes, 21.45–21.46, **21.95, 21.96**
  congenital clubfoot, 21.40–21.43, **21.86, 21.88**
  congenital hip dislocation, 21.33–21.35, **21.76**
  congenital vertical talus, 21.44, **21.90**
  femoral anteversion, 21.37, **21.79**
  ganglion of the foot, 21.45, **21.94**
  genu valgum, 21.39, **21.81**
  genu varum, 21.37–21.39, **21.80**
  internal tibial torsion, 21.40, **21.85**
  Legg-Calvé-Perthes disease, 21.35–21.36, **21.77**
  metatarsus primus, 21.43–21.44, **21.89**
Osgood-Schlatter disease, 21.39, **21.83**
pes planus, 21.45, **21.92**
popliteal cyst, 21.39–21.40, **21.84**
slipped capital femoral epiphysis (SCFE), 21.36–21.37, **21.78**
musculoskeletal disorders, 21.46–21.49
arthrogryposis, 21.48–21.49, **21.101**
cerebral palsy, 21.46–21.47, **21.97**

osteogenesis imperfecta (OI),
21.47–21.48, **21.98–21.100**
musculoskeletal trauma, 21.3–21.24
compartment syndromes, 21.18
fractures, 21.4–21.14, **21.4–21.33**
ligamentous injuries, 21.19–21.24,
21.43–21.56
special cases, 21.14–21.18, **21.34–21.42**
skeletal system, development,
21.1–21.3, **21.1–21.3**
spine, disorders of, 21.24–21.30
congenital torticollis, 21.24, **21.57**
herniated intervertebral disc, 21.30,
21.67
Klippel-Feil syndrome, 21.24–21.25,
21.58
kyphosis, 21.27–21.28, **21.63, 21.64**
scoliosis, 21.25–21.27, **21.59–21.62**
spondylolisthesis, 21.28–21.30, **21.65,
21.66**
upper extremity disorders,
21.30–21.33
boutonnière deformity, 21.32–21.33,
21.74
congenital pseudarthrosis of the clavicle, 21.31, **21.69**
congenital trigger thumb, 21.32,
21.73
mallet finger, 21.33, **21.75**
radial club hand, 21.31, **21.70**
Sprengel's deformity, 21.31, **21.68**
swan neck deformity, 21.33, **21.75**
syndactyly, 21.32, **21.72**
wrist ganglion, 21.32, **21.71**
Osgood-Schlatter disease, 21.39, **21.83**
Osler-Weber-Rendu disease, 7.15, **7.34**
Osteodystrophy, renal, 13.19–13.20,
13.49, 13.50
Osteogenesis imperfecta (OI), 6.16,
21.47–21.48, **21.98–21.100**
Osteomyelitis, 12.35–12.41, **12.51–12.56**
Otolaryngology, 22.1–22.46, **22.1**
ear disorders, 22.1–22.14, **22.2–22.8**
external ear disorders, 22.4–22.9,
22.9–22.20
middle ear disorders, 22.9–22.14,
22.21–22.33
esophageal foreign bodies, 22.45,
22.90, 22.91
nasal disorders, 22.14–22.22
epistaxis, 22.20–22.22, **22.46–22.49**
nasal obstruction, 22.14–22.19,
22.34–22.42
nasal trauma, 22.19–22.20,
22.43–22.45
oropharyngeal disorders, 22.30–22.37
palatal disorders, 22.31–22.32,
22.61–22.65
penetrating oropharyngeal trauma,
22.35–22.37, **22.71, 22.72**
tonsillar and peritonsillar disorders,
22.32–22.35, **22.66–22.70**
paranasal sinus disorders,
22.22–22.30, **22.50, 22.51**
atopic, 22.30
sinusitis, 22.23–22.30, **22.52–22.60**

upper airway obstruction,
22.37–22.45
acute, 22.37–22.43, **22.73–22.86**
chronic, 22.43–22.45, **22.87–22.89**

Palatal disorders, 22.31–22.32
cleft palate, 22.31–22.32, **22.61–22.64**
high-arched palate, 22.32, **22.65**
Pancytopenia, 11.25–11.26, **11.68–11.70**
Papilledema, 19.35, **19.104**
Papulosquamous disorders, 8.3–8.17
dermatitides, 8.5–8.12, **8.10–8.30**
diaper dermatitis, 8.15–8.17, **8.37–8.41**
fungal infections, 8.12–8.15, **8.31–8.36**
ichthyoses, 8.4, **8.6–8.9, 8.83**
psoriasis, 8.3–8.4, **8.2–8.5, 8.120, 8.141**
Parachute reflex, **3.2, 3.10**
Paranasal sinus disorders, 22.22–22.30,
22.50, 22.51
atopic, 22.30
sinusitis, 22.23–22.30, **22.52–22.60**
Parapharyngeal abscess, 22.38, **22.77**
Parinaud's syndrome, 15.15, **15.23**
Parasitic infestations, 18.23
Paronychia, 12.20–12.21, **12.30**
Partial combined immunodefiency dis-
orders, 4.25–4.30
acquired, 4.26–4.30
congenital, 4.25–4.26
Pelvic inflammatory disease,
18.29–18.30
Perforations, 20.16
Pericoronitis, 20.15, **20.49**
Perihepatitis, 18.29–18.30
Peripheral nerve dysfunction, **3.13**
Persistent hyperplastic primary vitreous
(PHPV), 19.29, **19.86, 19.87**
Pes planus, 21.45, **21.92**
Phenylketonuria, and developmental
delay, **3.27**
Phosphorus, as nutritional deficiency,
10.15
Phthiriasis, 19.18, **19.45**
Piebaldism, 8.42, **8.106**
Pigmentation disorders, 8.41–8.43
albinism, 8.42, **8.106**
ash leaf spots, 8.41–8.42, 15.4, **15.9**
post-inflammatory pigmentary
changes, 8.41, **8.103, 8.104**
vitiligo, 8.41, **8.105**
Pinworms, 18.21, **18.34**
Pityriasis alba, **8.16**
Pityriasis rosa, 8.10, **8.24**
Poison ivy, 8.11–8.12, **8.25, 8.26**
Polio, **3.13**
Polycystic kidney disorders (PKD),
13.12–13.14
autosomal dominant (adult-type)
PKD, 13.13, **13.31**
autosomal recessive (infantile) PKD,
13.12–13.13, **13.28–13.30**
cystic renal dysplasia, 13.13–13.14,
13.32–13.34
Porphyria, 20.12, **20.38**
Posterior urethral valves, 13.10, **13.24**
Posture, development, **3.6, 3.37**

sitting, **3.7**
standing, **3.8**
Potter's sequence, 13.14–13.15, **13.35**
Prader-Willi syndrome, 1.16–1.18,
1.28–1.30
Pregnancy, 18.30–18.32
Prehension, development, **3.17**
Prolactin (PRL), 9.2
Protective equilibrium reflex, **3.2, 3.9**
Prune-Belly syndrome, 13.9, **13.20**, 14.2,
14.4
Pseudopapilledema, 19.35–19.36
Pseudostrabismus, 19.9, **19.19**
Psoriasis, 8.3–8.4, **8.2–8.5, 8.120, 8.141**
Pulmonary disorders, 16.1–16.19, **16.1,
16.2**
apnea and sudden infant death syndrome (SIDS), 16.15, **16.36**
cough, 16.1–16.9, **16.3**
age and cause of chronic, 16.2–16.7,
16.4–16.16
diagnostic approach, 16.8–16.9, **16.18**
evaluation of, 16.7, **16.17**
cystic fibrosis (CF), 16.12–16.15
complications, 16.14, **16.34, 16.35**
diagnosis, 16.14–16.15
presentation, 16.12–16.13, **16.29–16.33**
radiographic findings, 16.14, **16.35**
diagnostic techniques, 16.16–16.19,
16.37–16.44
stridor, 16.9–16.11, **16.19–16.24**
wheezing, 16.11–16.12, **16.25–16.28**
Pulmonary lymphoid hyperplasia
(PLH), 4.29
Pulsus paradoxus, **4.17**
Pyloric stenosis, 10.9, **10.22, 10.23**

Radial club hand, 21.31, **21.70**
Ranula, 20.8, **20.24**
Rash
and malnutrition, **10.8**
and rheumatology, **7.14, 7.15, 7.18,
7.19, 7.24, 7.25, 7.40, 7.41, 7.47**
Raynaud's syndrome, **7.34**
Reflexes, primitive, **3.2**
Reflux, 10.9–10.10, **10.24**
Renal cysts, 14.5, **14.9**
Renal dysplasia, multicystic, 14.4, **14.8**
Renal venous thrombosis, 13.6–13.7,
13.11, 13.12
Renovascular hypertension, 13.18–13.19
growth failure, 13.20
hirsutism, 13.19, **13.48**
renal artery stenosis, 13.18–13.19,
13.45–13.47
Respiratory distress, 4.5–4.6, **4.12**,
17.1–17.7, **17.1**
extrathoracic causes, 17.7
thoracic, 17.2–17.7, **17.4–17.21**
upper airway, 17.1–17.2, **17.2, 17.3**
Retinal detachment, 19.30, **19.92**
Retinitis pigmentosa (RP), 19.29–19.30,
19.91
Retinoblastoma, 19.33–19.34, **19.102,
19.103**
Retinochoroiditis, 19.30

Retinopathy of prematurity (ROP), 19.30, **19.93**
Retropharyngeal abscess, 22.37–22.38, **22.75, 22.76**
Reynell-Zinkin Scales, **3.28**
Rhabdomyosarcoma, differential diagnosis, **12.45**
Rheumatic fever, 5.6, **5.13, 5.14**
Rheumatoid arthritis, juvenile (JRA), 7.1–7.5, **7.1–7.4**
    classification, **7.4**
    differential diagnosis, 7.5, **7.12**
    extra-articular manifestations, 7.4–7.5, **7.11**
    pauciarticular onset, 7.3–7.4, **7.8–7.10**
    polyarticular onset, 7.3, **7.6, 7.7**
    systemic onset, 7.3, **7.5**
Rheumatology, 7.1–7.19
    dermatomyositis (DM), 7.5–7.7, **7.13–7.17**
    juvenile rheumatoid arthritis (JRA), 7.1–7.5, **7.1–7.4**
    classification, **7.4**
    differential diagnosis, 7.5, **7.12**
    extra-articular manifestations, 7.4–7.5, **7.11**
    pauciarticular onset, 7.3–7.4, **7.8–7.10**
    polyarticular onset, 7.3, **7.6, 7.7**
    systemic onset, 7.3, **7.5**
    scleroderma, 7.13–7.15, **7.32–7.39**
    systemic lupus erythematosus (SLE), 7.16–7.19, **7.40–7.48**
    systemic vasculitis, 7.7–7.13
    Henoch-Schönlein purpura (HSP), 7.7–7.9, **7.18–7.20**
    Kawasaki syndrome, 7.9–7.13, **7.21–7.31**
Riboflavin B$_2$, as nutritional deficiency, **10.15**
Rickets, 6.16, 10.7, **10.16, 10.17**
    hypophosphatemic, 13.15–13.16, **13.39**
Rocky Mountain spotted fever, 12.16, **12.22**
Roentgenogram, chest, 5.7–5.13, **5.18–5.36**
Root fractures, 20.18, **20.60**
Roseola infantum, 12.6, **12.8**
Rubella, 12.1–12.2, 12.44–12.45, **12.2, 12.41, 12.61**, 19.30–19.31, **19.95**
Rubeola, 12.1, **12.1**

Salivary calculus, 20.8, **20.25**
Scabies, 8.25–8.26, **8.59–8.61**
Scalp, abscess, 12.22, **12.33**
Scarlet fever, 12.10–12.12, **12.16–12.19**
Scissoring, **3.38**
Sinusitis, 22.23–22.30
    allergic, with postnasal discharge, 22.30
    ancillary diagnostic methods, 22.26–22.27, **22.54**
    clinical presentations, 22.25–22.26, **22.52, 22.53**
    complications of, 22.27–22.28, **22.55**
    epidural abscess, 22.28, **22.57**

Pott's puffy tumor, 22.28, **22.56**
    periorbital and orbital infections, 22.28–22.30
    orbital cellulitis, 22.29–22.30, **22.60**
    periorbital cellulitis due to hematogenous spread, 22.28–22.29
    periorbital cellulitis due to spread from adjacent facial infection, 22.29, **22.59**
    periorbital cellulitis due to spread from adjacent sinusitis, 22.28, **22.58**
    vacuum headache, 22.30
Scoliosis, 21.25–21.27, **21.59–21.62**
Scurvy, 6.17, **6.38**
Seizures, **3.13**
Selenium, as nutritional deficiency, **10.15**
Scleroderma, 7.13–7.15, **7.32–7.39**
Seborrhea, 8.9–8.10, **8.22, 8.23**
Severe combined immunodeficiency disease (SCID), 4.25, **4.48, 4.49**
Sexual maturation, 9.14–9.19
    early sexual development, 9.14–9.16, **9.22–9.24**
    puberty, 9.16–9.19, **9.25–9.29**
Shaken baby syndrome, 6.9–6.10, **6.17–6.20**
Sharing, **3.34**
Shigella, 18.20–18.21
Shingles. *See* Herpes
Sialadenitis, **12.45**
Sickle cell disease, 11.15, 11.27, **11.30–11.32**, 19.32–19.33, **19.100**
Skeletal injuries, 6.7, **6.13–6.16**. *See also* Fractures
Skeletal system, development, 21.1–21.3, **21.1–21.3**
Skin. *See* Dermatology
Slipped capital femoral epiphysis (SCFE), 21.36–21.37, **21.78**
Smiling, **3.33, 3.35**
Smith-Lemli-Opitz syndrome, 1.19, **1.31**
Spermatocele, 14.14–14.15, **14.38**
Spinal cord dysfunction, **3.13**
Spinal dysraphism, occult, 15.12–15.13, **15.31–15.33**
Spine, disorders of, 21.24–21.30
    congenital torticollis, 21.24, **21.57**
    herniated intervertebral disc, 21.30, **21.67**
    Klippel-Feil syndrome, 21.24–21.25, **21.58**
    kyphosis, 21.27–21.28, **21.63, 21.64**
    scoliosis, 21.25–21.27, **21.59–21.62**
    spondylolisthesis, 21.28–21.30, **21.65, 21.66**
Sprains, 21.20–21.22, **21.50–21.53**
Sprengel's deformity, 21.31, **21.68**
Staphylococcal scalded skin syndrome, 12.12, **12.17**
Staphylococcal scarlet fever, 12.12–12.13, **12.18**
Stenosis, renal artery, 13.18–13.19, **13.45–13.47**
Stevens-Johnson syndrome, 8.19–8.20, **8.47**

Strabismus, 19.6–19.13, **19.11**
    esodeviation, 19.7–19.9, **19.12–19.19**
    exodeviations, 19.9–19.11, **19.20–19.23**
    tests for, 19.11–19.13, **19.26–19.28**
    vertical deviations, 19.11, **19.24, 19.25**
Strangulation, **6.3**
Stridor, 16.9–16.11, **16.19–16.24**
Sturge-Weber syndrome, 15.5–15.6, **15.14–15.17**
Subglottic stenosis, 22.43
Sudden infant death syndrome (SIDS), 16.15, **16.36**
Surgical disorders, 17.1–17.37
    abdominal masses, 17.20–17.25, **17.62, 17.63**
    neoplasms, 17.22–17.24, **17.70–17.77**
    genitourinary obstructions, 17.21–17.22, **17.64–17.69**
    inflammatory masses, 17.24–17.25, **17.78**
    abdominal pain, 17.18–17.20, **17.55–17.61**
    abdominal wall, 17.30–17.35
    gastroschisis and omphalocele, 17.30–17.32, **17.104–17.108**
    inguinal hernia and hydrocele, 17.32–17.35, **17.112–17.120**
    umbilicus, 17.32, **17.109–17.111**
    anus, 17.35–17.37, **17.121–17.128**
    chest wall, 17.29–17.30, **17.101–17.103**
    gastrointestinal bleeding, 17.14–17.18, **17.42**
    in infants, 17.14–17.15, 17.43–17.47
    in older children, 17.17–17.18, **17.50–17.54**
    in toddlers, 17.16–17.17, **17.48, 17.49**
    head and neck, 17.25–17.29, **17.79, 17.80**
    face, 17.25–17.26, **17.84**
    mouth, 17.26, **17.85**
    neck—lateral masses, 17.27–17.29, **17.90–17.100**
    neck—midline, 17.26–17.27, **17.86–17.89**
    scalp, 17.25, **17.81–17.83**
    respiratory distress, 17.1–17.7, **17.1**
    extrathoracic causes, 17.7
    thoracic, 17.2–17.7, **17.4–17.21**
    upper airway, 17.1–17.2, **17.2, 17.3**
    vomiting, 17.7–17.13
    in newborn infants, 17.8–17.12, **17.22–17.35**
    in older infants and children, 17.12–17.14, **17.36–17.41**
Swan neck deformity, 21.33, **21.75**
Syndactyly, 21.32, **21.72**
Syphilis, 18.24, **18.37**, 19.31
Systemic lupus erythematosus (SLE), 7.16–7.19, **7.40–7.48**
Systemic vasculitis, 7.7–7.13
    Henoch-Schönlein purpura (HSP), 7.7–7.9, **7.18–7.20**
    Kawasaki syndrome, 7.9–7.13, **7.21–7.31**

Tanner stages, 9.16–9.17, **9.26**
Target cells, 11.13–11.14, **11.26–11.28**
Teeth, 20.5, **20.11**
Telangiectasia, **7.16**
Telecanthus, 19.14, **19.31, 19.32**
Temporomandibular joint disorders
  (TMJD), 20.21
Teratoma, **12.45**
Tetracycline discoloration, 20.11, **20.37**
Thalassemia, 11.6–11.7, **11.10, 11.11**
Thiamine B$_1$, as nutritional deficiency,
  10.15
Third (oculomotor) cranial nerve palsy,
  19.10–19.11, **19.22, 19.23**
Thyroid goiter, differential diagnosis,
  12.45
Thrombocytopenia, 6.13, **6.27, 6.28**
Tinea capitis infections, 8.45–8.46, **8.112,
  8.113**
Tinea pedis, 8.14, **8.34**
Tinea versicolor, 8.14–8.15, **8.35, 8.36**
Toe grasp reflex, **3.2**
Tongue, geographic, 20.6, **20.17**
Tonsillar and peritonsillar disorders,
  22.32–22.35
    lymphoma, 22.35, **22.70**
    peritonsillar abscess/cellulitis, 22.35,
      22.69
    pharyngitis/tonsillitis, 22.32–22.34,
      22.66, 22.67
    recurrent tonsillitis, 22.34
    uvulitis, 22.34, **22.68**
Torch infection. *See* Toxoplasmosis
Tourniquet injury, 6.15, **6.4, 6.35**
Toxic epidermal necrolysis (TEN),
  8.17–8.18
Toxic shock syndrome (TSS),
  12.13–12.14, **12.19**
Toxocariasis, 19.31–19.32, **19.97**
Toxoplasmosis, 12.43–12.44, **12.60**, 19.30,
  19.94
Tracheitis, bacterial, 22.42
Transient pustular melanosis (TNPM),
  8.32–8.33, **8.79**
Trauma, 3.13, 10.10, **10.25**
Treacher-Collins syndrome, 22.3–22.4,
  22.8
Trench mouth, 20.15, **20.50**
Trichiasis, 19.16
Trichomonas, 18.25–18.27, **18.39, 18.40**
Trisomy 13 and 18, 1.9–1.11, **1.19–1.21**
Tuberous sclerosis, 13.9–13.10, **13.21,
  13.22**, 15.4–15.5, **15.7–15.13**
Tularemia, 12.34
Tumors and infiltrations, 8.28–8.32
    granuloma annulare, 8.31–8.32, **8.76**
    histiocytoses, 8.31, **8.75**
    juvenile xanthogranuloma, 8.31,
      8.74
    keloids, 8.29, **8.70**
    mastocytosis, 8.30–8.31, **8.72, 8.73**
    melanotic neuroectodermal tumor of
      infancy, 20.6, **20.16**
    milia, 8.29, **8.69**
    neurofibromas, 8.30, **8.71**
    warts, 8.28–8.29, **8.65–8.68**

Turner syndrome, 1.11–1.12, **1.22**, 5.5,
  9.8–9.9, **9.15–9.17**
Tzanck preparation, **8.42**

Ulcers, traumatic, 20.17, **20.56**
Upper airway obstruction, 22.37–22.45
    acute, 22.37–22.43, **22.73–22.86**
    chronic, 22.43–22.45, **22.87–22.89**
Urachus, 14.2–14.3, **14.5**
Urogenital tract
    duplication of the urinary collecting
      system, 13.11–13.12, **13.27**
    signs and symptoms of cancer,
      11.32–11.33, **11.93–11.96**
Urologic disorders, 14.1–14.18
    ambiguous genitalia, 14.17, **14.45,
      14.46**
    cryptorchidism, neonatal, 14.2, **14.3**
    cutaneous urinary diversion,
      14.5–14.6, **14.10–14.16**
    exstrophic anomalies, 14.6–14.8
    epispadias, 14.7–14.8, **14.19**
    exstrophy, classic, 14.6–14.7, **14.17**
    exstrophy, cloacal, 14.7, **14.18**
    female genitalia, lesions, 14.15–14.17,
      14.40
    cysts, paraurethral, 14.16, **14.44**
    ureterocele, prolapsed, 14.16, **14.43**
    urethral polyps, 14.16, **14.42**
    urethral prolapse, 14.16, **14.41**
    vagina, congenital obstruction,
      14.16–14.17
    genital trauma, 14.18, **14.47**
    hydronephrosis, 14.3–14.4
    megaureter, 14.4, **14.7**
    ureteropelvic junction obstruction,
      14.3–14.4, **14.6**
    male genitalia, anomalies, 14.9–14.15
    acute scrotum, 14.12–14.13
    buried penis, 14.10–14.11, **14.27**
    chordee, 14.10, **14.24**
    diphallus, 14.12, **14.32**
    epididymitis, 14.14, **14.36**
    hypospadias, 14.9–14.10, **14.23**
    microphallus, 14.12, **14.31**
    penile torsion, 14.10, **14.25**
    postcircumcision lesions, 14.11–14.12,
      14.28–14.30
    priapism, 14.12, **14.33**
    scrotal contents, lesions, 14.12
    scrotal swelling, chronic, 14.14–14.15,
      14.37–14.39
    spermatic cord torsion, 14.13–14.14,
      14.34
    testicular appendage torsion, 14.14,
      14.35
    webbed penis, 14.10, **14.26**
    neurovesical dysfunction, 14.8–14.9,
      14.21
    non-neurogenic vesical dysfunction,
      14.9, **14.22**
    prenatal urinary tract dilation,
      14.1–14.2, **14.1, 14.2**
    prune-belly syndrome, 14.2, **14.4**
    renal cysts, 14.5, **14.9**
    renal dysplasia, multicystic, 14.4, **14.8**

urachus, 14.2–14.3, **14.5**
urinary retention, 14.8, **14.20**
Urticaria, 4.16–4.18, **4.33–4.37**, 8.20–8.22,
  8.49, 8.50
    papular, 8.24–8.25, **8.58**
Uvulitis, 22.34, **22.68**

Varicella, 12.2–12.4, **12.3, 12.4**
Varicocele, 14.14, **14.37**
Vasculitis, 6.14
VATER association, 1.20, **1.33**
Vesicoureteral reflux, 13.7–13.9,
  13.13–13.18
Vesiculopustular disorders, 8.17–8.18
    bacterial infections, 8.17
    miliaria, 8.18, **8.43, 8.44**
    toxic epidermal necrolysis (TEN),
      8.17–8.18
    vesiculation, 8.18, **8.45**
    viral infections, 8.17, **8.42**
Vincent's infection, 20.15, **20.50**
Visual impairment, **3.27**, 3.28–3.29, **3.48**
    and cognitive development, 3.28–3.29
    and gross and fine motor develop-
      ment, 3.28
    and language and intellectual devel-
      opment, 3.29
    and social development, 3.29
Vitamin A, as nutritional deficiency,
  10.15
Vitamin B$_6$, as nutritional deficiency,
  10.15
Vitamin B$_{12}$, as nutritional deficiency,
  10.15
Vitamin C, as nutritional deficiency,
  10.15
Vitamin D, as nutritional deficiency,
  10.15
Vitamin E, as nutritional deficiency,
  10.15
Vitamin K, as nutritional deficiency,
  10.15
Vitiligo, 8.41, **8.105**
Vocal cord paralysis, 22.44, **22.88**
Vomiting, 10.9–10.10, 17.7–17.13
    in newborn infants, 17.8–17.12,
      17.22–17.35
    in older infants and children,
      17.12–17.14, **17.36–17.41**
    reflux, 10.9–10.10, **10.24**
    pyloric stenosis, 10.9, **10.22, 10.23**
    trauma, 10.10, **10.25**

Warts, 8.28–8.29, **8.65–8.68**
Werdnig-Hoffmann disease, **3.13**
Wechsler Intelligence Scale for
  Children—Revised (WISC-R), **3.28**
Wheezing, **4.24**, 16.11–16.12, **16.25–16.28**
Williams syndrome, 5.5, **5.11**
Wiskott-Aldrich syndrome, 4.25, **4.50**
Wrist ganglion, 21.32, **21.71**

Xanthogranuloma, juvenile, 8.31, **8.74**
XXX and XYY syndromes, 1.13

Zinc, as nutritional deficiency, **10.15**